Turnbull's Obstetrics

Cover figure appears courtesy of
Dr Pamela Johnson, St George's Hospital, London, UK

For Churchill Livingstone

Publisher: Lucy Gardner
Project Editor: Tim Atkinson
Project Controller: Mark Sanderson
Copy Editor: Pat Croucher
Indexer: Michele Clarke

Turnbull's Obstetrics

Edited by

Geoffrey Chamberlain RD MD FRCS FRCOG FACOG (Hons) FSLCOG (Hon)

SECOND EDITION

CHURCHILL LIVINGSTONE
EDINBURGH HONG KONG LONDON MELBOURNE NEW YORK TOKYO 1995

CHURCHILL LIVINGSTONE
Medical Division of Pearson Professional Limited

Distributed in the United States of America by Churchill
Livingstone Inc., 650 Avenue of the Americas, New York,
N.Y. 10011, and by associated companies, branches and
representatives throughout the world.

First published 1995

ISBN 0 443 04998 X

British Library Cataloguing in Publication Data
A catalogue record for this book is available from the British Library.

Library of Congress Cataloging in Publication Data
A catalog record for this book is available from the Library of Congress.

The
publisher's
policy is to use
**paper manufactured
from sustainable forests**

Printed in Hong Kong
NPC/01

Contents

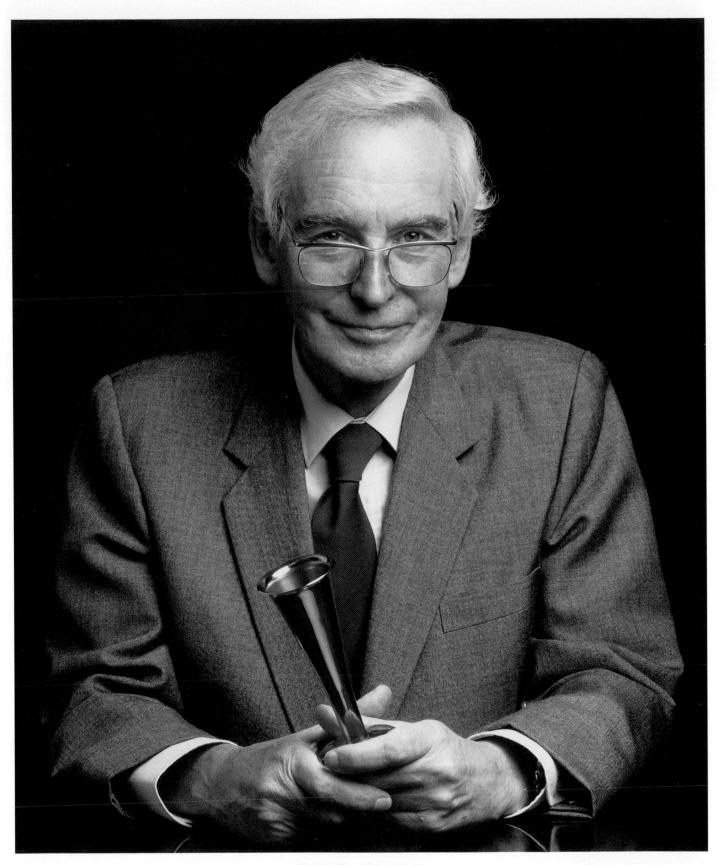

Sir Alec Turnbull 1925–86

Sir Alec Turnbull

The architects of the first edition of *Obstetrics*, Professors Turnbull and Chamberlain, laid their opening plans in the gardens of an hotel in Chandigar in the Punjab in 1984. They were lecturing at the Postgraduate Medical Centre as part of a British Council course and one evening were sitting and talking about the future of postgraduate medical education in the United Kingdom. They both realized that a big definitive postgraduate work, a compendium of the best in obstetrics, was required in Britain and agreed that evening to co-edit such a volume. In the foothills of the Himalayas, the first discussions took place and a provisional list of authors was considered. This was modified several times and, as soon as they returned to Britain, invitations went out.

At the time, the editors were both Vice-Presidents of the Royal College of Obstetricians and Gynaecologists. The book, therefore, had an emphasis from that educational establishment, and had a Commonwealth flavour. During the course of the next two or three years, unfortunately the senior editor developed a recurrence of his previous malignancy. He still, however, worked hard at the planning and editing of the first edition. The publication of *Obstetrics* in 1986 corresponded with one of the last appearances of Alec Turnbull on the international scene in London at the XXV British Congress of Obstetrics and Gynaecology.

Years have gone by and the science of obstetrics has advanced. A new edition of the 1986 volume was required and, with the permission of Lady Elsie Turnbull, we decided to turn the title into *Turnbull's Obstetrics*, thus creating a memorial for a man who was probably the greatest British obstetrician of his generation. The junior editor was happy to edit this new edition as a memorial to Alec Turnbull who did so much for his College, his

science and for womankind. Alec's influence is still with us in obstetrics; in all he touched, he left his mark for the betterment of women in childbirth.

Alec was born in Aberdeen in 1925. He went to school and medical school there, qualifying in 1947. With the exception of a period with Professor James Walker at Dundee, he stayed in the Aberdeen school until 1975. Whilst there, he met Elsie, a noted clinical scientist herself, and they married. She was his staunch companion for the rest of his life.

From Aberdeen, Alec Turnbull moved to Cardiff as Professor and then on to Oxford. In all these changes he was accompanied by his colleague, Anne Anderson, with whom he made a strong team examining much of the physiology of labour and control of uterine contractions. Anne unfortunately died in 1983 and Alec continued in his department at Oxford with other workers. As well as his grasp of science, Sir Alec Turnbull was a great humanitarian, looking at the woman as an individual and caring for all those who consulted him. Alec was the ideal obstetrician, and in 1984 *The Observer* honoured him with the title of The Obstetricians' Obstetrician. With Lady Turnbull's permission, we use the photograph of that occasion on the facing page.

Alec developed a secondary malignancy and became ill in 1985. In July of the following year, a great scientific meeting was held in Oxford at which all his friends gathered and he died in September of that year.

This book is a memorial to Alec Turnbull. It is hoped that it will go through many editions with many editors, but all of them will be remembering and paying respect to a great British obstetrician. We all owe Alec a debt.

London 1994   Geoffrey Chamberlain

Preface

After eight years, a new edition of this book was needed. In preparing this second edition, the editor approached the previous authors in many cases. In other chapters, to get a different slant, he has asked new authors to update material or has requested them to group together material from the previous chapters. In doing this, both Churchill Livingstone and Professor Chamberlain are grateful to the contributors of the first edition for the use of their work. The science of medicine is a continuum and as some authors become more senior, we must expect that others will take up the batton. The editor is grateful to all those authors who responded in reasonable time and only mildly chastises those who took a little longer to submit their material. Life now is extremely complex and revising or writing chapters for big volumes is a stint which goes with international fame and ability.

This volume has been thoroughly revised. New material to the winter of 1993 is included and future trends hinted at. We are happy to receive letters about the new edition and the Editor will try to answer any questions if you write to him.

Please note that there is no gender neutral pronoun in English, only he, she or it, and we are loath to refer to a baby as it. Hence the convention for using he for the baby is used. Readers, if they wish, may mentally add 'or she' each time but it would be repetitive to do that in the script.

London 1994   G. C.

Preface to First Edition

In obstetrics there have been great advances in knowledge over the past 30 years while more has changed in the last decade than in the whole of the history of the subject. Advance has been particularly rapid in the prenatal diagnosis of fetal anomaly, the assessment of intrauterine fetal growth retardation, the detection and effective augmentation of slow labour and the treatment of many neonatal disorders.

Although many books have been written about specialized aspects of obstetrics, there is a dearth of major books covering the whole modern field. *Obstetrics* provides a comprehensive account of current knowledge and practice in the specialty by choosing a full spectrum of experts. Authors have shown how their field has developed over the years, described the present scene and, by providing extensive references to the literature, given readers an opportunity to achieve deeper knowledge. We are proud to have such a distinguished team of authors.

Both the editors are consultants in active clinical practice, looking after patients while teaching undergraduate and postgraduate students. Not only are we kept aware of new developments in the clinical field by our junior staffs but we learn of topics about which there is controversy, argument and confusion. In planning this book, we have ensured that new developments and obstetric controversies are covered. We have also included chapters presenting the views of women themselves on their care in labour and on the role of the modern midwife for we consider these issues of importance to the contemporary obstetrician. We believe that *Obstetrics* will make a major contribution to the training of young specialists.

Advances in clinical practice should depend on new scientific knowledge which itself is based upon appropriate and valid measurements. A strong basic science foundation has been provided in the first quarter of the book. Subsequent chapters deal with normal pregnancy, labour and the puerperium, each section being followed by consideration of abnormal variations of these processes. There are two important groups of chapters on fetal assessment: the first deals with fetal monitoring up to 28 weeks, covering the new areas of prenatal diagnosis, including biophysical and biochemical methods as well as molecular biology and DNA technology; the second group is on fetal diagnosis in late pregnancy and draws attention to the recent trend away from biochemical assessment towards the modern biophysical methods which have revolutionized antenatal care of the fetus at higher risk of various unfavourable outcomes.

Obstetrics includes a large section on the care of the newborn, indicating our opinion that obstetricians need to have a good working knowledge of neonatal disorders and of advances in neonatal care. We also consider it important to include two chapters on assisted fertility, while three chapters on perinatal epidemiology emphasize how correct interpretation of vital statistics can help clinical practice. The book is completed by a major chapter on contraception in relation to the recently pregnant and by another on the vitally important topic of medicolegal problems in obstetrics.

We are grateful to all our authors for the work they have done in preparing the chapters. Our publishers have been particularly helpful and we are especially grateful to Mrs Elif Fincanci-Smith who has survived the brunt of being our real working editor. Mrs Anne Fraser at St George's Hospital has been the stage manager, expertly juggling the various drafts of 80 chapters. We are grateful to Jonathan Frappell and Richard de Chazal, also of St George's Hospital, for proofreading under pressure.

It is our hope that *Obstetrics* will provide a comprehensive account well into the 1990s of the knowledge and practice of the specialty for young obstetricians in training, for practising clinicians and for undergraduates who wish to take a special interest.

Oxford and London 1989   A. T.
G. C.

Contributors

S. Leonard Barron MB BS FRCS FRCOG
Emeritus Consultant Obstetrician and Gynaecologist,
Royal Victoria Infirmary, Newcastle upon Tyne, UK

Felix Beck MD DSc
Senior Principal Research Fellow, Howard Florey
Institute of Experimental Physiology and Medicine,
University of Melbourne, Australia

Phil R. Bennett BSc PhD MD MRCOG
Senior Lecturer, Honorary Consultant, Action Research
Laboratory for Molecular Biology, Queen Charlotte's
and Chelsea Hospital, London, UK

John Bonnar MA MD(Hons) FRCOG
Professor and Head, Trinity College Department of
Obstetrics and Gynaecology, University of Dublin;
Consultant Obstetrician and Gynaecologist, St James's
Hospital and Coombe Women's Hospital, Dublin,
Ireland

Andrew A. Calder MD FRCS(Ed) FRCP(Glas & Ed) FRCOG
Professor and Head of Obstetrics and Gynaecology,
University of Edinburgh, Centre for Reproductive
Biology, Edinburgh, UK

J. Brian Capstick MA
Solicitor, London, UK

Linda Cardozo MD FRCOG
Professor of Urogynaecology, King's College, University
of London; Consultant Gynaecologist, King's College
Hospital, London, UK

Geoffrey Chamberlain RD MD FRCS FRCOG
FACOG(Hon) FSLCOG(Hon)
Professor and Head of Department of Obstetrics and
Gynaecology, St George's Hospital Medical School,
University of London, London, UK

Michael G. Chapman MD MBBS FRCOG
Professor of Obstetrics and Gynaecology, University
of New South Wales, St George Hospital, Kogarah,
New South Wales; Consultant, Sydney IVF Ltd,
New South Wales, Australia; Consultant, Bridge Fertility
Centre, London, UK

Jean Chapple MBGB MCommH FFPHM
Consultant in Perinatal Epidemiology, North Thames
Region, London, UK

Rowena J. Davies RN RH MTD MSc
Assistant Director of Nursing Services (Womens
Health), St George's Health Care (NHS) Trust,
London, UK

John M. Davison BSc MD MSc FRCOG
Consultant Obstetrician and Gynaecologist, Professor of
Obstetric Medicine, University of Newcastle upon Tyne,
Royal Victoria Infirmary, Newcastle upon Tyne, UK

Noel Dilly GM MB BS BSc PhD DO FRCOphth
Professor and Chairman, Department of Anatomy, St
George's Hospital Medical School, London, UK

William Dunlop PhD MB ChB FRCOG FRCS(Ed)
Professor and Head, Department of Obstetrics and
Gynaecology, University of Newcastle upon Tyne, Royal
Victoria Infirmary, Newcastle upon Tyne, UK

Gillian C. Forrest MB BS FRCPsych MRCGP DCH
Consultant Child Psychiatrist, Park Hospital for
Children, Oxford, UK

H. Fox MD MRCPath FRCOG
Professor of Reproductive Pathology, Department of
Pathological Sciences, University of Manchester,
Manchester, UK

C. J. van Gelderen MB ChB FRCOG
Professor and Chief Specialist, Department of Obstetrics
and Gynaecology, Baragwanath Hospital and the
University of the Witwatersrand, Johannesburg,
South Africa

Ian A. Greer MD FRCP MRCOG MFFP
Muirhead Professor and Head of Department of
Obstetrics and Gynaecology, University of Glasgow;
Honorary Consultant Obstetrician and Gynaecologist,
Glasgow Royal Infirmary and Royal Maternity Hospital,
Glasgow, UK

J. G. Grudzinskas BSc(Hons) MB BS(Hons) MD FRACOG
FRCOG
Professor of Obstetrics and Gynaecology, London
Hospital Medical College; St Bartholomew's Hospital
Medical College, London, UK

Marion H. Hall MD(Aberd) FRCOG
Consultant Obstetrician and Gynaecologist, Aberdeen
Royal Hospitals Trust, Honorary Clinical Senior
Lecturer, University of Aberdeen, Aberdeen, UK

Michael Harmer MB BS FRCA
Consultant Anaesthetist, University Hospital of Wales,
Cardiff, UK

G. Justus Hofmeyr MBBCh MRCOG
Professor and Head, Department of Obstetrics and
Gynaecology, Coronation and Jgstrijdom Hospitals and
University of the Witwatersrand, Johannesburg,
South Africa

P. W. Howie MD FRCOG FRS FRCP(Glas)
Head of Department, Department of Obstetrics and
Gynaecology, University of Dundee Medical School,
Dundee, UK

Sir David Hull BSc MB FRCP DObst RCOG DCH
Professor of Child Health, Department of Child Health,
University Hospital, Queen's Medical Centre,
Nottingham, UK

Dame Rosalinde Hurley DBE LLB MD FRCPath FRCOG
Professor of Microbiology, Royal Postgraduate Medical
School's Institute of Obstetrics and Gynaecology, Queen
Charlotte's and Chelsea Hospital, London, UK

Mark R. Johnson MRCP
Senior Lecturer, Academic Department of Obstetrics
and Gynaecology, Charing Cross and Westminster
Medical School, Chelsea and Westminster Hospital,
London, UK

Pam Johnson MD MRCGP MRCOG
Lecturer/Senior Registrar, Department of Obstetrics and
Gynaecology, St George's Hospital Medical School,
London, UK

Peter M. Johnson DSc FRCPath
Professor of Immunology, University of Liverpool,
Liverpool, UK

I. Kola PhD
Reader, Institute of Reproduction and Development,

Monash University, Monash Medical Centre, Clayton,
Victoria, Australia

Elizabeth A. Letsky MB BS FRCPath
Consultant Perinatal Haematologist, Queen Charlotte's
and Chelsea Hospital, London; Honorary Senior
Lecturer, Royal Postgraduate Medical School, London,
UK

Frank Loeffler FRCS FRCOG
Consultant Obstetrician and Gynaecologist, St Mary's
Hospital, London; Consultant Obstetrician and
Gynaecologist, Queen Charlotte's and Chelsea Hospital,
London, UK

John Malvern BSc FRCSE FRCOG
Consultant, Queen Charlotte's and Chelsea Hospital,
London; Honorary Senior Lecturer, Institute of
Obstetrics and Gynaecology, Royal Postgraduate
Medical School, London, UK

Iain R. McFadyen MB ChB
Senior Lecturer and Honorary Consultant, Department
of Obstetrics and Gynaecology, Liverpool Women's
Hospital, Liverpool, UK

Ann Oakley MA PhD
Director, Social Science Research Unit, London, UK

Philip Owen MB BCh MRCOG
Lecturer and Honorary Senior Registrar, Department of
Obstetrics and Gynaecology, Ninewells Hospital and
Medical School, Dundee, UK

Naren B. Patel MB FRCOG
Consultant Obstetrician and Gynaecologist, Department
of Obstetrics and Gynaecology, Ninewells Hospital and
Medical School, Dundee, UK

J. Malcolm Pearce MD FRCS FRCOG
Consultant Obstetrician, St George's Hospital, London,
UK

Christopher Redman MB BChir FRCP FRCOG
Nuffield Department of Obstetrics and Gynaecology,
John Radcliffe Hospital, Oxford, UK

Gillian Robinson MD MRCOG
Consultant Obstetrician, Mayday University Hospital,
Thornton Heath, UK

Jeffrey S. Robinson BSc MB BCh BAO(Belf) FRACOG
FRCOG
Professor of Obstetrics and Gynaecology, University of
Adelaide, South Australia

C. H. Rodeck DSc FRCOG
Professor of Obstetrics and Gynaecology, Head of
Department, Department of Obstetrics and
Gynaecology, University College London Medical
School, London, UK

P. A. W. Rogers PhD
National Health and Medical Research Council Senior
Research Fellow, Senior Lecturer, Department of
Obstetrics and Gynaecology, Monash University,
Monash Medical Centre, Clayton, Victoria, Australia

A. H. Sathananthan PhD
Senior Lecturer, Faculty of Health Sciences, La Trobe
University, Bundoora, Victoria; Honorary Research
Fellow, Institute of Reproduction and Development,
Monash University, Monash Medical Centre, Clayton
Victoria, Australia

H. F. Seeley MA MSc FRCA
Dean of Postgraduate Medicine, (University of London),
South Thames (West), London, UK

Fiona J. Stanley MB BS MSc MD FFPHM FAFPHM MFCCH
FRACP
Director, Institute for Child Health Research and Variety
Club Professor of Paediatrics, University of Western
Australia

Philip J. Steer BSc MD FRCOG
Professor and Head of Department, Academic
Department of Obstetrics and Gynaecology, Charing
Cross and Westminster Medical School, Chelsea and
Westminster Hospital, London, UK

Terence Stephenson BSc BM BCh DM MRCP(UK)
Senior Lecturer, Department of Child Health,
Nottingham University; Honorary Consultant
Paediatrician, University and City Hospitals,
Nottingham, UK

Michael de Swiet MD FRCP
Consultant Physician, Queen Charlotte's and Chelsea
Hospital, London; Consultant Physician, University

College Hospital, London; Consultant Physician,
Northwick Park Hospital, London, UK

Alan O. Trounson PhD
Professor of Obstetrics and Gynaecology and Paediatrics
Director, Centre for Early Human Development,
Monash University; Deputy Director, Institute of
Reproduction and Development, Monash University,
Monash Medical Centre, Clayton, Victoria, Australia

Sir Alec Turnbull CBE MD ChB FRCOG
Formerly Professor and Head of Nuffield Department of
Obstetrics and Gynaecology, University of Oxford,
Oxford, UK

Nicholas J. Wald MBBS DSc FRCP FFPHM FRCOG
Professor and Head of Department of Environmental
and Preventive Medicine, St Bartholomew's Hospital
Medical College, London, UK

Stephen A. Walkinshaw BSc(Hons) MD MRCOG
Consultant in Maternal-Fetal Medicine, Fetal Centre,
Liverpool Women's Hospital, Liverpool, UK

William A. W. Walters MBBS(Adel) PhD(Lond) FRCOG
FRACOG
Professor of Reproductive Medicine, Faculty of Medicine
and Health Sciences, The University of Newcastle;
Chairman, Department of Obstetrics and Gynaecology,
John Hunter Hospital, Newcastle, New South Wales,
Australia

C. R. Whitfield MD FRCOG FRCP (Glas)
Emeritus Regius Professor of Midwifery, University of
Glasgow, Glasgow, UK

Martin J. Whittle MD FRCOG FRCP(Glas)
Professor of Fetal Medicine, Birmingham Maternity
Hospital, Birmingham, UK

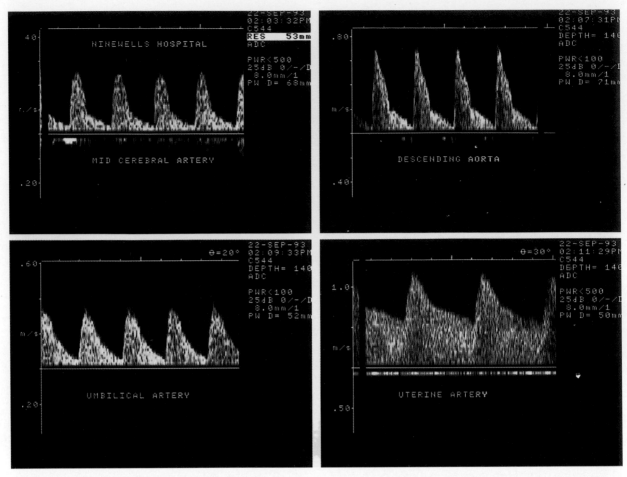

Plate 1. Flow velocity waveforms obtained from the umbilical, fetal aortic and middle cerebral arteries and maternal uterine artery at 19 weeks' gestation. Courtesy of Dr A.D. Christie, Dundee. (Also reproduced as Fig. 14.8, pp 239.)

Basic sciences

1. The continuum of obstetrics

Geoffrey Chamberlain

Obstetrics is the art and science of caring for women and their unborn progeny during pregnancy, labour and continuing into the immediate puerperium. In earlier times there was much craft and not much science. Now there is an increasing amount of well understood science but a lot of the craft is still required; the one has not given way to the other; rather, science has augmented craft.

THE PAST

Early times

Long before physicians took an interest in obstetrical matters, midwives or guid women were supervising labour. With no formal training but a variable heritage of experience, such women have been working since biblical times (Genesis 35.17 and Genesis 38.27) and were well known in the Egyptian and Greek civilizations. Training was usually obtained by learning from another more experienced guid woman—an apprentice system—and there was usually no checking of standards. The first formal training for midwives was laid down by Hippocrates in the fifth century BC, followed by intermittent efforts in Italy and Greece in the second and third century AD. In the UK, William Chamberlin, father of Chamberlin the forceps, started a midwifery school in Southampton; however, a uniform formalization of midwifery training was not undertaken until the Midwives Acts were passed in the early days of this century.

Doctors came into obstetrics comparatively late. At first they were resisted by midwives who saw them as competition, but gradually a team approach evolved so that both professionals worked together. One feature which may have catalysed this was the abundant extra-marital activity of the courts of France and England during the later 17th century. In both countries, monarchs and their imitators led a merry life of multiple coitus which, in the days before contraception, led to many pregnancies. In both countries, in consequence, obstetricians were used because of the confidentiality and secrecy required to handle the results of royal dalliance. From such unsalubrious beginnings rose to fame several of the great obstetricians of the 17th and 18th centuries.

The first aid service for delivery

Forceps came into use with Peter Chamberlin, although possibly as a re-invention of a much earlier instrument used for extracting dead babies. A century of manipulative skills then followed with increasingly complex instruments evolved to help deal with problems. A woman did not have access to powerful anesthesia at this time and so a vaginal delivery had to be successful, even at the expense of the baby's life. Nearly all manipulations were very intrusive, requiring long apprenticeship and practice for training. Hence obstetricians were great mechanists, inventing ingenious instruments to extract babies from awkward corners. Some appliances were modifications of existing tools and the destructive instruments of the previous generation. Most well known obstetricians had their trained mechanic (often the blacksmith) around the corner to make their own variation of the various vaginal instruments. With the aid of personalized tools, these obstetricians would go on using their own eponymous variant. If they were influential and had apprentices, the latter would be taught their skills on their master's instruments, thus perpetuating the innumerable ramifications of the obstetrical armamentorium which flourished into the 19th and early 20th centuries.

Safer Caesarean section came in the mid 1800s (inhalation anaesthesia was first used in 1851); the increase in the use of this route, bypassing the more difficult vaginal procedures, sounded the knell of mechanistic obstetrics. The attitude of vaginal delivery at all costs still persisted for a few decades since obstetricians were still concerned about infection. Puerperal sepsis (childbed fever) killed some women after vaginal delivery but peritoneal infection after abdominal operative delivery was a death sentence with no cure until chemotherapy and antibiotics were introduced in the 1930s. Maternal mortality was sharply reduced as a result and only then could obstetricians start to consider a Caesarean section as a comparatively safe substitute for a vaginal delivery.

The beginnings of science

All science depends upon measurement. Among the first steps in obstetrics was the measurement of various aspects of the pelvis by Levret in 1753. Like many enthusiasts, he over-elaborated the complexities of pelvic axes and planes, and Smellie, in the following year, first proposed a measurement which has been continued into current obstetrics, the diagonal conjugate anterioposterior diameter of the pelvis. All sorts of measuring instruments were used and external pelvimetry became fashionable, but was mostly dismissed after the analysis of Michaelis in 1851. In vivo measurements followed the invention of Roentgen when the first X-ray pelvimetries were performed by Albert in 1897.

The more recent surge in biophysical estimations in obstetrics may be considered to have started with fetal heart auscultation in the early 19th century but really came to prominence with the work of the Glaswegian obstetrician, Ian Donald. He, more than any other single person, led biophysics into obstetrics with the use of ultrasound and his work will always be acknowledged. He was a pioneer in all ultrasound measurement of the fetus. Dynamic measurements of blood flow in the placental bed and the fetal blood vessels followed the static ones which provided a system of measuring fetal growth from serial readings. These are entering practice and research now extends to magnetic resonance and infrared wave absorption for measuring the fetus.

Biochemistry in medicine owes much to another obstetrician, Robert Barnes of St George's Hospital, London. He was an obstetric physician and then consultant from 1875 to 1907. In this time he set up the first biochemical laboratory in the world for the measurement of levels of body constituents such as sodium, potassium, proteins and urea in human blood. Another great advance came after the Second World War when miniaturization of biochemical processes, automation and the use of radioactive labels allowed steroid biochemistry to forge ahead. While the value of the steroid markers as a measure of fetal well-being in late pregnancy has mostly been overshadowed by ultrasound, the assessing of pregnancy-associated placental proteins is helping in the management of first-trimester problems. Again, measurement is leading research.

Epidemiology, the measurement of numbers of people, has been a major part of modern obstetrics. The counting of heads started with epidemics of infectious diseases in the Victorian days and went on to quantify birth rates and death rates; from 1830 these measurements were under the control of the Registrar General's Office in England and equivalent bodies in other countries. The Office of Population Censuses and Surveys performs this task for England and Wales. This is an important area: epidemiology in this country has led obstetrics in the rest of the world. Measures of fetal and antenatal outcome can be firmly established, so providing a rapid medical audit of procedures or of doctor groups. Comparisons can be made from one centre to another or even from one country to another, provided the data compare like with like. The ready acceptance of randomized controlled trials and meta-analysis of results by obstetricians has allowed even more sophisticated analyses with more valid results; multicentre studies on cervical cerclage and the use of aspirin to prevent pre-eclampsia have provided results which have influenced management.

Clinical care

Epidemiology however has not always been used in the evaluation of systems of management; antenatal care, for example, evolved piecemeal. Starting in Edinburgh at the turn of the century, current practice owes much to Doreen Campbell in the mid 1920s; it was she who in London laid down the pattern of antenatal visits followed today in most of the western world.

The place of delivery has shifted from the home to the institution. This is partly following the trend of hospitalization of much western medicine, with primary care becoming a service dealing mostly with ambulatory care and a diagnosis only. Further, most obstetricians, concerned with the unexpected serious complications to mother and baby which arise suddenly in labour, wish to have close access to the full facilities which will be required if labour deviates from the normal. Institutional delivery in the UK has increased from 20% in the 1920s to 98% currently. A move by a few to return to home births is happening, for these women often feel they have more control over events when they are not in hospital.

Contemporary obstetrics

The years of the Second World War (1939–1945) provide a convenient division between the end of a long-standing period of conservative maternity care and the beginning of contemporary obstetrics. The older practice was dominated by fear of maternal death: rightly so—the maternal mortality rate in England and Wales remained between 4 and 5 per 1000 births until 1937. The introduction of sulphonamides in 1937 and subsequently newer antibiotics, safe blood transfusion and other advances led to the dramatic reduction in maternal mortality rates (see Ch. 50). As a result, obstetricians returning to practice after the end of the war in 1945 began to realize that the maternal mortality rate had fallen to such an extent that they could now concentrate more on improving perinatal mortality and morbidity.

ADVANCES IN PERINATAL CARE

Perinatal medicine

One of the earliest obstetricians who practised what developed into perinatal medicine was Dugald Baird in Aberdeen; he classified the clinical causes of perinatal death and demonstrated the importance of good maternal health as well as expert perinatal care in achieving a low perinatal mortality rate. By describing the circumstances of perinatal death, he drew attention to those obstetric conditions for which better management was needed to improve fetal outcome. The conditions initially stressed were labour disorders such as prolonged first stage, manipulative vaginal delivery, preterm labour and prolonged pregnancy. Disorders of pregnancy carrying special risks for the fetus included severe pre-eclampsia, antepartum haemorrhage, rhesus disease and maternal medical disorders such as diabetes. He naturally recognized fetal abnormality as a major cause of fetal death, but like others at the same time, considered that much of this was unavoidable.

Biochemical assessment of fetus and placenta

For many years it was considered that poor placental function was the probable explanation for complications such as intrauterine fetal death in pregnancy, intrauterine death of the fetus during labour or unexpected birth asphyxia. However it was not possible to make any measurements of placental function or fetal well-being until the mid 1950s, when reliable methods were developed by Arnold Klopper and Jim Brown in Edinburgh for measurement of pregnanediol and oestrogens in urine. At first, urinary pregnanediol was used to assess placental function, but this was soon superseded by urinary oestriol which gave an indication not only of placental function but also of fetal well-being. Scientists made great efforts to provide quicker and simpler methods to measure oestriol in urine and blood, and clinicians hastened to apply these methods widely in practice. Other hormones, such as human placental lactogen, were measured in the quest for the best biochemical method for assessing the con-

dition of the fetus and placenta. After about 20 years the popularity of this biochemical approach waned because of the increasing realization that the assessment provided was inconsistent: with urinary oestriol, for example, the daily background coefficient of variation was almost 40%.

Nevertheless, attempts to assess the condition of the fetus by biochemical means showed obstetricians how important it was to have reliable knowledge of the condition of the intrauterine fetus; better biophysical methods were becoming available and finally in 1984, one large unit took the plunge and formally reported that discontinuing oestriol assay in the third trimester in clinical practice had no effect on perinatal outcome.

Many biochemical measurements however are still of value, including serum alpha-fetoprotein assay in maternal blood and amniotic fluid. High levels in early second-trimester pregnancy indicate increased risks of fetal neural tube defect and of later fetal compromise. Unduly low levels of serum alpha-fetoprotein, serum oestriol and human chorionic gonadotrophin in early second-trimester pregnancy indicate increased risks of Down's syndrome in the fetus.

Biophysical assessment of fetus and placenta

Biophysical methods of making direct observation of intrauterine conditions have proved more valuable than biochemical methods, which tend to be indirect. Diagnostic ultrasound, pioneered by Ian Donald in Glasgow, has made possible accurate measurements of the parameters of normal and abnormal fetal growth with advancing pregnancy. Pathological growth retardation of the intrauterine fetus is readily detectable by measurements made by serial scans. The first scanners provided only a static picture but now most function in real time and can assess fetal function in dynamic fashion. Frank Manning and Larry Platt in the USA utilized real-time ultrasound to derive a fetal biophysical profile, which gives a dynamic assessment of the fetus. Doppler ultrasound techniques now enable the characteristics of blood flow in specific vessels of the fetal and placental circulation to be assessed with considerable accuracy and prognostic ability.

Another important biophysical measurement, first developed in Germany by Fred Hammacher, is fetal cardiotocography. Fetal heart rate is recorded continuously and the tracing is related to a recording of uterine contractions, originally measured by the changes in intrauterine pressure. Although this method was first developed for use in labour, the application of sophisticated ultrasound techniques has enabled it to be used during pregnancy. It is now a technique of major importance for assessment of the fetus during pregnancy.

Even more recent is the introduction of cordocentesis, by which samples of blood are taken from the umbilical artery or vein through a needle passed, under ultrasound control, through the maternal abdomen into the uterus and then into the cord. This was first developed in France by Daffos in the early 1980s and has since been used extensively in the UK, USA, Europe and Scandinavia in the intrauterine assessment of the potentially jeopardized fetus.

While it is now possible to assess the condition of the intrauterine fetus with some precision in most cases, it must be remembered that in a minority of cases, even the most careful and skilful assessment may be misleading, and that repeated assessment is especially important when there is any uncertainty.

Antenatal diagnosis

Interauterine diagnosis of the sex of the fetus was first reported by Fritz Fuchs in Copenhagen in the mid 1950s when he performed amniocentesis, enabling cells of fetal origin in the amniotic fluid to be cultured and the fetal karyotype determined. Progress was initially slow but improvements in amnion cell culture meant that by the mid 1960s the method was reliable enough for clinical application of amniocentesis. National studies on the safety of genetic amniocentesis in the USA, Canada and the UK indicated that the risks were low enough to be clinically acceptable. Since then, amniocentesis has become the standard technique for prenatal diagnosis. Initially used mainly for the diagnosis of chromosomally determined abnormalities such as Down's syndrome, this application has been rather patchy and, disappointingly, the incidence of Down's syndrome at birth has not been reduced over the past 20 years or so. Now amniocentesis can be done earlier in pregnancy (12–13 weeks), so allowing earlier chromosome analysis. It has been joined by chorionic villus sampling at 10–12 weeks with swift results following. Research proceeds rapidly in the isolation of fetal cells in the mother's circulation and the karyometric assay for these may warn of chromosomally flagged abnormalities even earlier in the first trimester.

Advances have been made in the application of DNA technology to clinical diagnosis so that disorders associated with gene abnormalities and deletions are now increasingly detectable. Fetal cells can be obtained at amniocentesis or chorionic villus sampling provides small samples of fetal tissue. From these samples results can be obtained rapidly and a reliable diagnosis can be made of fetal disorders such as thalassaemia major, Duchenne's muscular dystrophy, cystic fibrosis or Huntington's chorea.

By contrast, the first demonstration that serum and amniotic fluid alpha-fetoprotein levels were elevated in women carrying a baby with an open neural tube defect (NTD) led to the rapid application of maternal serum alpha-fetoprotein screening. This, coupled with ultrasonic confirmation of the diagnosis, made possible screening programmes which have been associated with a consider-

able reduction in the incidence of NTD. Although this reduction had started spontaneously, availability of NTD screening procedures has contributed to the reduced incidence of these disorders. Since ultrasound examination can detect NTD by itself, many units have given up the alpha-fetoprotein screening and depend entirely on routine fetal anomaly scanning at about 18 weeks to detect NTD and other fetal abnormalities. However, the association between elevated alpha-fetoprotein at 16 weeks and later pregnancy complications, such as fetal growth retardation and preterm labour, and between very low alpha-fetoprotein at 16 weeks and Down's syndrome represent additional reasons for considering alpha-fetoprotein screening at 16–18 weeks' gestation. Besides, in many parts of the world ultrasound services are not expert.

CONTROL OF FERTILITY

Scientific advances are making it increasingly possible for women to bear the number of children they wish, rather than being at the mercy of their own fertility. In the mid 1950s the first combined oral contraceptive preparations became available and were improved rapidly; as major side-effects were found to be dose-related, equally effective lower-dose preparations were introduced. Improved intrauterine devices also became available but medicolegal problems are now causing the manufacturers to reduce production. Hormone-impregnated intrauterine devices are now used as a source of continuous release, while subcutaneous and deep intramuscular depots of progesterone provide good contraception.

The technique of laparoscopic sterilization was pioneered in France by Raoul Palmer and popularized in the UK by Patrick Steptoe. This quickly replaced laparotomy for sterilization. Therapeutic abortion for a series of indications was legalized in England, Wales and Scotland in 1967.

The UK birth rate reached its peak in 1964 and then fell steadily to 1977 as a result of many factors, helped by the increased availability of contraception, sterilization and pregnancy termination. From 1980 the general fertility rate (see Ch. 48) has been maintained at around this levels with small fluctuations. There has been a slight shift to the older mother, particularly among first babies.

PERINATAL MORTALITY AND MORBIDITY

In the UK perinatal mortality has continued to fall steadily. Surveys performed in 1958 and 1970 clarified many aspects of causation and pointed to the directions in which further improvements could be achieved. Improved methods of fertility control helped women to avoid pregnancy at extremes of age and parity or if there was an unduly high risk of perinatal death. The perinatal mortality rate combines the stillbirth and first week neonatal death rates and is therefore expressed as the rate per 1000 live and stillbirths. In 1992 the rate in England and Wales was 7.4 per 1000 (see Ch. 49).

NEONATAL INTENSIVE CARE

Among the many specialties with which obstetricians and midwives collaborate in none do they work closer than with neonatology. Peter Dunn carried out much of the pioneering work in the UK, and the clinical use of new knowledge of neonatal cardiorespiratory and metabolic functions, combined with impressive technology, has made possible an increasing rate of high quality survival of extremely immature babies. Advances in neonatal surgery have corrected many congenital fetal disorders previously thought to be lethal.

OBSTETRIC ANAESTHESIA

Anaesthesia and analgesia are essential for good obstetric practice. Although the number of women having general anaesthesia for vaginal operative delivery has been reduced in recent years, there has been an increase in the use of regional methods, especially epidural anaesthesia: currently 17% of women in the UK use this form of analgesia. In the early 1960s the technique of paracervical block was popular but proved less effective for the mother and sometimes dangerous to the fetus and has largely been abandoned in this country. Apart from providing anaesthesia for operative delivery, anaesthetists are often involved with intensive care in obstetrics, for conditions such as severe pre-eclampsia or eclampsia, excessive bleeding with or without coagulation defect and many other conditions requiring intensive care.

CONTROL OF LABOUR

Although the use of a continuous intravenous oxytocin infusion was first reported in 1947 by Geoffrey Theobald in the UK, and in the same year by Louis Helman in the USA, it was not widely used at first because of the relative unreliability of the preparations of oxytocin available. With the synthesis of oxytocin in 1962, various investigators recognized that intravenous administration could be used more efficiently than was previously the case for the induction of labour and to augment uterine contractions in slowly progressing labour of spontaneous onset. Alec Turnbull published in 1967 and 1968 studies in Aberdeen which pioneered the use of oxytocin titration for induction and augmentation of labour. The philosophy of active management of labour, in which almost 50% of primigravidae may have their labour augmented by intravenous oxytocin to ensure normal progress, was pioneered at the National Maternity Hospital in Dublin by Kieran O'Driscoll. Oxytocin works best when the

membranes are ruptured. Amniotomy and intravenous oxytocin administration remained popular for over 10 years until the mid 1970s, when after work by Kavim at Queen Charlottes Hospital, local administration of prostaglandins proved able to initiate labour without amniotomy and more gradually and physiologically than amniotomy and oxytocin. Prostaglandin E_2 proved to have fewer side-effects than prostaglandin $F_{2\alpha}$. Given intravenously, prostaglandins have no advantages over oxytocin but administered extra-amniotically, intracervically or intravaginally in appropriate doses they are effective and more acceptable to women than the more invasive amniotomy and intravenous oxytocin administration.

WOMEN'S WISHES

Throughout the 1960s, advances in obstetric care involved the introduction of many technological innovations. The continuing fall in perinatal mortality reassured obstetricians that these innovations were beneficial. However, many women were frightened by what they regarded as unnecessary interference in the physiological process of birth and concerned by the potentially serious complications of some of the technology. They felt that women were no longer in control of their own labour. The Caesarean section rate rose steadily and although perinatal mortality fell, the two rates were not necessarily related to each other.

In the UK, obstetricians and women's organizations continued on a collision course until the mid 1970s when there was a major confrontation. Women's organizations vilified obstetric technology on the television, radio and in the newspapers, while obstetricians defended their record of improving results. It became clear that many innovations had not been subjected to trials to assess their efficacy. Subsequently there was a significant reduction in the use of interventions which could not be clearly justified. Obstetricians recognized that they had failed to convince women of the value of many useful advances in technique and so have now involved women increasingly in the decision-making processes of pregnancy management. They need to convince women of the necessity of relevant high technology methods when there is a high risk for the mothers or their infants.

Midwives are coming back into their rightful place. More women are being cared for throughout pregnancy and labour by the midwife, an independent practitioner in her own right. The emphasis on choice combined with midwife care has been made in the UK by the initiative 'Changing Childbirth' (1993), steered through the Department of Health by Baroness Cumberledge.

In many units there has been a considerable reduction in the use of interventions previously thought to be essential, including episiotomy, epidural anaesthesia, induction of labour and electronic fetal heart rate monitoring in labour. Women have encouraged their husband or partner to be present during labour and at the birth of the baby. Analgesic drug use in labour has been reduced, with many multiparous women requiring no analgesia at all. Ambulation in labour has been encouraged, as has delivery with the mother in any position she cares to adopt.

All these changes in practice seem to have lightened the atmosphere in UK maternity hospitals, with many now more orientated towards fulfilling the expectations of pregnant women and their families, even when this involves accepting requests for less usual forms of management. Pregnancy and labour are important days for women and must be seen to be so. It is important that the woman is centre-stage and all the attendants, their equipment and their science are supportive.

While most pregnancies end with mother and baby fit and well, the baby may be born dead or may die in the neonatal period. It was customary to try to protect such mothers from as much of the experience as possible by not letting her see the dead baby, discharging her from hospital as soon as possible. Although this was meant well, it is now recognized that this management caused untold misery to bereaved mothers. Grief is normally an intense process but once completed, normal life can start again. She should be properly counselled and given an opportunity to talk about her feelings of loss in the weeks or months after the baby's death.

THE FUTURE

Women in the developed world will be having fewer babies; obstetricians will continue to add the fine tuning of safety and comfort to the natural process. With fewer perinatal and maternal deaths, even more individual attention will be paid to those women at higher risk and perhaps fetal and maternal monitoring will be applied more rationally. Individual methods will be more carefully assessed so that we reject the less useful tests but apply more widely those investigations which can be shown to be powerful in their capacity to predict with reasonable precision. If obstetricians concentrate on detecting and protecting this smaller group of higher-risk pregnancies, the majority of healthy women will be cared for by other members of the obstetric team. In the British Commonwealth, these will be the midwives whose natural place in caring for the normal will be better fulfilled as they find their rightful place in obstetrics.

In providing better support for the woman who is having a baby, a new wave of education and understanding is starting in the developed world. This will spread so that women are more aware and in a better position to discuss with their doctor or midwife what is happening. The Victorian barriers between the professional and the woman will continue to break down and a wider and better understanding will take their place. In non-drug analgesic techniques, we will refine and use what can be more widely applied.

The most important problems facing obstetricians are the prevention of preterm delivery and of intrauterine growth retardation. These two overlapping but separate conditions need much more research into their causes before correct preventive measures can be applied; this will be much more effective than the current emphasis of treating the established conditions.

The precise tests which will be used by obstetricians in the next century have not yet been developed. They will probably involve non-invasive techniques with a biophysical basis. Functions of fetal heart and brain and of uterine muscle will be more precisely measured; so possibly a better understanding of fetal and maternal physiology in pregnancy will follow. The indirect assessment of the body state from blood gas levels and acidaemia will have to continue until better measures are perfected. Probably these too will be derived non-invasively by magnetic resonance imaging rather than blood samples taken from the body.

In the developing world, many of the obstetrical problems are political ones. The provision of health care for such large numbers so widely spread is the major hurdle. Those who come from countries that went through the Industrial Revolution almost two centuries ago must remember that improvements in health care have to take their place among other social priorities in building a country's economy. Politicians perceive different goals from those seen by the medical profession. They are looking at different priorities and if they are good politicians, they seek the good of the whole of society of which health is a part and obstetrics a subpart of that good. Health care professionals know that maternal and child health preventive measures will in the long run yield greater returns per unit of money spent than on virtually anything else. Some politicians grasp this principle, but forget that they must also provide some improvements in care for the present generation of women and their babies. They must build for the future but not turn their backs on the present.

2. Anatomy of the female pelvis

Noel Dilly

INTRODUCTION

This chapter contains a clinically oriented introduction to functional anatomy and histology of the female genital organs. The tract has been approached from the vulva upwards as it is seen in clinical medicine. Some areas such as lymphatic drainage and nerve supply will be discussed in two contexts, once as a general overview, then in a more specific context of individual regions.

THE VULVA

The vulva consists of the vaginal orifice, the urethral orifice and those structures associated with them which make up the floor of the anterior part of the pelvic outlet. It extends upwards to include the mons pubis (Fig. 2.1). It is supported by the largely transverse fibres of the inferior fascia of the urinogenital diaphragm, a part of the perineal membrane. This fascia has three holes, one just behind the pubic bone, one for the urethra and one for

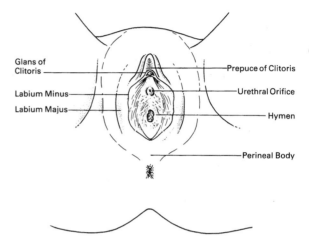

Fig. 2.1   The female external genitalia. This represents the classical portrait of the female external genitalia, but in life the labia majora are normally in contact with each other except during intercourse and labour.

the vagina. It is strengthened posteriorly by the perineal body, an aponeurosis for the fibres of the perineal, levator ani and external and internal anal sphincter muscles.

Above this membrane lies the deep perineal pouch and beneath it the superficial pouch that contains the terminal portions of the vagina and urethra as well as their associated structures, the clitoris, the bulb of the vestibule, the vestibular glands, the superficial perineal muscles and their nerves and vessels.

The perineum

The perineum is the pelvic outlet below the pelvic diaphragm. It is usually divided by a line joining the anterior end of the ischial tuberosities into an anterior urogenital area and a posterior anal triangle. The anal triangle contains the anal canal and the surrounding ischiorectal fossae. It is bound posterolaterally by the sacrotuberous ligaments. The fossa itself is filled with fat. Its lateral wall is the fascia over obturator internus and the edge of the sacrotuberous ligaments; medially the fossae are separated

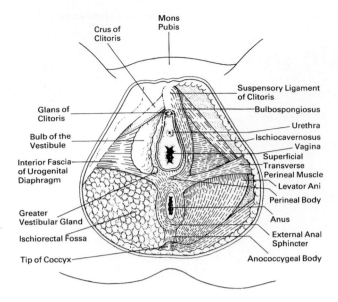

Fig. 2.2   The perineum. A view from below of the pelvic outlet showing its boundaries and triangles.

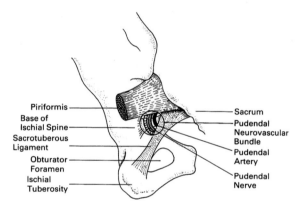

Fig. 2.3   Nerve supply of the perineum. The pudenal nerve usually leaves the pelvis via the greater sciatic foramen and enters the perineum via the lesser sciatic foramen, running forwards along its lateral wall in the pudendal canal.

by the perineal body, the anal canal and the anococcygeal body (Fig. 2.2).

The pudendal nerve and vessels leave the pelvis through the greater sciatic foramen then hook around the ischial spine. They enter the perineum through the lesser sciatic foramen into the pudendal canal where they run forwards to supply the perineum (Fig. 2.3). The pudendal canal runs on the lateral wall of the fossa from the lesser sciatic foramen to the perineal membrane.

The urogenital triangle

The perineal membrane is a narrow shelf of fibrous tissue attached along the pubic rami. Anteriorly the crurae of the clitoris are attached to it. Each crus is covered by the ischiocavernosus muscle. Medial to each crus is the

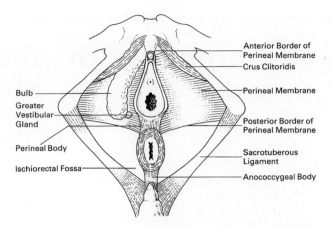

Fig. 2.4   Diagram of the superficial layers of the urogenital triangle. The bulbospongiosus and ischiocavernosus muscles have been removed to reveal the structure of the clitoris and the glands associated with it.

erectile tissue of the bulb of the vestibule and separating the bulbs on either side are the openings of the urethra and vagina. The bulbs fuse anteriorly in front of the urethral orifice and extend to the glans of the clitoris. The bulbospongiosus muscle lies superficial to the bulb, extending from the perineal body where it also covers the vestibular glands forwards around the vagina and urethra to the clitoris (Figs 2.2, 2.4).

The deep perineal pouch is also perforated by the vagina and urethra. The perineal body is the fibrous tissue aponeurosis of the fibres of the bulbospongiosus, the transverse perinei, the sphincter vaginae and the external anal sphincter. It is somewhat mobile but provides support for the levator ani above.

The nerve supply of the urogenital triangle is derived from the ilioinguinal nerve, the perineal branch of the posterior cutaneous nerve of the thigh, and the pudendal nerve. The ilioinguinal nerve supplies the anterior part of the labia majora, the posterior part being supplied by the posterior cutaneous nerve of the thigh laterally. Its remaining area together with the labia minora is supplied medially by branches of the pudendal nerve. The clitoris is supplied by one of the terminal branches of the pudendal nerve, the dorsal nerve of the clitoris. It runs forwards along the ischiopubic ramus above the inferior fascia of the urogenital diaphragm, and reaches the dorsum of the clitoris through the gap between the anterior end of the inferior fascia and the inferior pubic ligament. The major specialized receptors in the clitoris are Pacinian corpuscles.

The mons pubis

The mons pubis is an area over the pubic bone which develops at puberty as a secondary sexual characteristic. The pubic hair is usually distributed upon its surface in a characteristic triangular fashion but a significant proportion of normal woman have male-type distribution with the hair extending up the midline of the lower abdomen. The probable functions of the mons include acting as a buffer between the male and female pubic bones during intercourse and as a source of arousal responses when stimulated. It is also said to provide tissue for the increase in size of the labia minora as they expand during coitus.

The labia majora

The labia are a pair of fatty folds which are continuous anteriorly with the mons. Posteriorly they peter out but small continuations come together between the vagina and the anus. In the adult their outer surfaces are covered with pubic hair and their medial surfaces are usually in apposition, closing off a potential aperture called the pudendal cleft. They are sometimes separated by a piece of the labia minora. This surface contains many large sebaceous and sweat glands.

The labia consist of skin-covered loose fibrofatty tissue similar to that of the mons, but containing some muscle, as well as the termination of the round ligament of the uterus.

The labia minora

The labia minora are a pair of fleshy folds containing erectile tissue, usually contained within the folds of the labia majora and separated from them by a deep cleft. They surround the vestibule of the vagina. Posteriorly in the virgin the labia minora join each other with a delicate fold of skin called the fourchette just deep to the labia majora. Anteriorly they divide into a pair of folds that split to enclose the clitoris. The outer surface is hairy and contains many sweat and sebaceous glands but the inner hairless surface is covered by a poorly keratinized stratified squamous epithelium with sweat and sebaceous glands. The labia minora contain extensive vascular spaces surrounded by delicate connective tissue and a little smooth muscle. Their probable functions are to increase the depth of the vaginal canal during intercourse and afterwards probably to help in maintaining the vaginal continence to the ejaculate. They are a potent source of stimuli resulting in sexual arousal.

The vestibule

The vestibule is the space between the labia minora bounded anteriorly by the clitoris and posteriorly by the fold of skin joining the labia minora, the fourchette. Opening into the vestibule are the vagina, the urethra and the ducts of the great and lesser vestibular glands. The bulborectal glands with their alkaline mucous secretion also drain into the vestibule posteriorly. The vaginal orifice may contain a hymen or hymenal remnants. Its lining is similar to the vaginal epithelium and is stratified

squamous non-keratinized epithelium. Its glands are one of the two major natural sources of lubrication during coitus.

The clitoris

The clitoris is a small but variable-sized organ made mainly of erectile tissue situated at the anterior end of the vestibule. It is suspended from the lower border of the pubic arch by a small triangular ligament. It is made from two corpora cavernosa, the cavernous blood spaces of which are separated from each other by fibromuscular trabeculae. Each corpus cavernosum arises from a crus near the ischiopubic ramus and this crus is palpable. The free extremity of the clitoris is made up of a rounded mass of erectile tissue—the glans—which, when not aroused, is normally covered by the anterior folds of the labia minora to form a prepuce. This prepuce contains vast numbers of sebaceous and sweat glands. However the glans of the clitoris has neither sweat nor sebaceous glands.

The clitoris is an important source of stimuli and is responsible for sexual arousal and reflex lubrication; it contains a considerable number of mechanoreceptors.

Vestibular bulb

The vestibular bulb consists of two masses of erectile tissue, one on either side of the vaginal orifice. They are covered by the bulbospongiosus muscle and lie deep in the labia majora. They are joined by a commissure in front of the vagina, which is in contact with the lower surface of the urinogenital diaphragm.

Musculature of the vulva

Superficially these muscles are the transverse perinei, the bulbospongiosus and the ischiocavernosus muscles, and deeper, the parts of the urinogenital diaphragm surrounded by the superficial and deep layers of fascia. The deeper muscles are the deep transverse perinei and the sphincter urethrae. The superficial muscles are slender and delicate; the transverse perinei run horizontally from the inferior ramus of the ischium to the perineal body superficial to the posterior part of the inferior fascia of the urinogenital diaphragm. On each side, the bulbospongiosus comes from the perineal body and passes forwards encircling the external end of the vagina, superficial to the bulb and the greater vestibular glands. It ends in the dorsal aspect of the connective tissue capsule of the corpus cavernosus of the clitoris.

The deep transverse perinei also meet at the perineal body. The sphincter urethrae fibres not only encircle the anterior and lateral parts of the urethra but also the corresponding parts of the vagina.

Nerve supply

Nerves come from the anterior divisions of the anterior rami of the second, third and fourth sacral spinal nerves. The principal named nerve is the pudendal nerve but the labia and the adjacent skin of the perineum also have a sensory supply from the perineal branch of the posterior cutaneous nerve of the thigh.

The pudendal nerve is a mixed nerve and travels together with the internal pudendal artery in the fascial canal on the lateral wall of the ischiorectal fossa. In this region it usually branches away from the inferior rectal branch, that is crossing to provide the sensory supply to perianal skin and the lower part of the anal canal, and the vital motor supply to the external anal sphincter.

The pudendal nerve itself divides into two branches in the anterior part of the pudendal canal. The terminal branches are the dorsal nerve of the clitoris and the perineal nerve (Fig. 2.5). The dorsal nerve of the clitoris runs above the inferior fascia of the urinogenital diaphragm alongside the ischiopubic ramus. It then passes out between the anterior border of the urogenital diaphragm and the pubis to reach the clitoris and glans (Fig. 2.5).

The perineal nerve gives motor branches to the striated muscles of the vulva, some of the anterior fibres of the external anal sphincter and the levator ani. Its sensory terminations are a pair of posterior labial nerves.

The vulva contains large numbers of special nerve endings and a corresponding rich supply of sensory nerves. Many of these specialized endings are mechanoreceptors, but they are absent from the region of the vestibule surrounding the vagina where there is a dense arborization of free nerve endings.

Most of the sensory fibres are conveyed by the pudendal nerve, but those in the mons and the anterior parts of the labia major go to the lumbar plexus via the ilioinguinal and genitofemoral nerves. Some fibres from the posterior parts of the labia major are conveyed with the perineal branch of the posterior femoral cutaneous nerve to the sacral plexus.

There is also a dense autonomic nerve supply—the postganglionic sympathetic fibres arising from the hypogastric plexus, and the pelvis plexus; these are distributed to their endings via the pudendal nerve. The parasympathetic fibres come from S2, S3 and S4, as the nervae erigentes to join with the pelvic plexus; they are distributed with either the pelvic blood vessels or the pudendal nerves.

Blood supply

The arteries spring mainly from the internal iliac artery with a significant contribution from the femoral artery. The internal pudendal artery arises from the internal iliac artery and runs in the pudendal canal to the labia majora where it forms a very rich anastomosis with the deep external pudendal branches from the femoral artery. There are also communications between the vessels on either side (Fig. 2.5).

The pudendal artery gives off the inferior rectal artery which supplies the skin and musculature around the anal canal but provides blood for only a small area—the posterior aspect of the lower end of the vagina. Although the pudendal artery is near the ischiopubic ramus, it gives off branches that penetrate the inferior fascia of the urinogenital diaphragm to supply the labia, the erectile tissue of the bulb, the lower end of the vagina and associated muscles. Its final branches are the deep and dorsal arteries of the clitoris. It is the deep branch that is the main supply to the corpus cavernosus. The branches of the femoral artery, the superficial and deep external pudendal vessels, pass medially to reach the anterior portion of the labia majora.

The venous drainage of this area is basically a vast intercommunicating plexus that drains to the internal pudendal veins and hence to the internal iliac veins, with a small part of the anterior region of the labia majora draining to the greater saphenous vein.

Lymphatic drainage

The initial drainage from the vulva, the lower part of the urethra, the vagina and anal canal is mostly to the medial group of superficial inguinal lymph nodes. From here they drain into the deep inguinal lymph nodes in the femoral canal. The glans clitoridis drains directly into these nodes. There is considerable overlap in the drainage, which is bilateral. This overlap is of crucial importance during radical surgery for malignant disease.

THE VAGINA

The vagina is a distensible fibromuscular tube extending

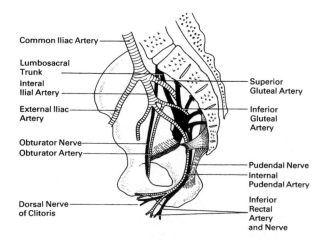

Fig. 2.5   Pelvic nerves and blood supply of the pudenda. The major nerve is the pudendal, but it is supplemented by the posterior cutaneous nerve of the thigh and the ilioinguinal and genitofemoral nerves.

from the vestibule to the cervix of the uterus. It runs backwards and upwards with the anterior and posterior walls in close contact reducing the lumen to a mere slit. The lining epithelium is thrown into transverse folds or rugae. It is probably the slack in these folds that accommodates the considerable distension of the vagina during intercourse and, later, parturition so that the vagina does not tear.

The vagina is related anteriorly to the base of the bladder and the urethra. It is separated from the bladder base by loose connective tissue, but the urethra is firmly bound to the adventitia of the anterior surface of the lower two-thirds of the vagina. Where the vagina is related to the bladder base it is separated from it in part by the two ureters, as their terminal portions pass in front of the anterior fornix.

Posteriorly the vagina is related to the rectum and the retrouterine pouch of Douglas. The lowermost part of the vagina is separated from the anal canal by the mass of dense connective tissue, the perineal body (Fig. 2.6).

Laterally the upper vagina is related to the pelvic fascia and the lower part is embraced by the anteromedial fibres of pubococcygeus and the urogenital diaphragm. Near its outermost extremity the bulb of the vestibule, the greater vestibular glands and the bulbospongiosus muscles are its lateral relations.

The epithelium lining the vagina lies upon a dense fibrous lamina propria. The epithelium is stratified, squamous and non-keratinized and does not contain mucous glands and so should never be referred to as vaginal mucosa. It is unusual in that even the most superficial shrunken cells retain their nuclei. The apparent emptiness of many of the cells in the epithelium results from the fact that they contain glycogen which does not show up on routine histological stains.

The submucosa consists of loosely arranged connective tissue with many elastic fibres and numerous large venous spaces together with occasional lymphoid patches. The muscularis is relatively thin, with both longitudinal and circular smooth muscle and is continuous above with the uterine muscle. The outer layer of the vagina, the adventitia, is a fibrous tissue coat that binds the vagina to the surrounding structures.

Blood supply

The vagina has a rich and variable blood supply. The major vessels are the uterine arteries and the vaginal branches of the internal iliac arteries. From the anastomosis of these vessels, azygos arteries extend on the anterior and posterior surfaces of the vagina. Other contributions, especially to the lower end of the vagina, are from the artery to the bulb, the pudendal arteries, and the middle and inferior rectal vessels. Because the vagina is distensible these vessels have a very tortuous course in its contracted state. The venous drainage, in common with the other pelvic viscera, starts as a series of plexuses associated with the vesicle, rectal and uterine plexuses and drains eventually by vaginal veins to the internal iliac veins (Fig. 2.7).

Lymphatic drainage

Drainage differs for the upper two-thirds compared with the lower third and for the anterior wall as opposed to the posterior wall. From the upper two-thirds the drainage is to the internal and external iliac lymph nodes. The difference between the anterior and posterior walls is that while drainage from the anterior wall is direct to the internal iliac nodes, that from the posterior wall relays first in a node lying in the connective tissue between the vagina and rectum. From the lower third of the vagina, lymph drains to the superficial inguinal nodes on both sides.

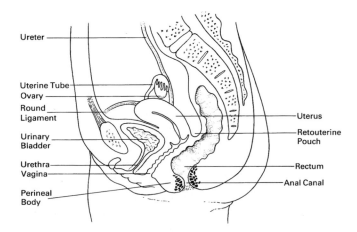

Fig. 2.6 Sagittal section of the female pelvis. The peritoneal covering of the pelvic organs is organized much as if a cover had been draped over them. Note the close relationship between the posterior fornix of the vagina and the rectouterine pouch.

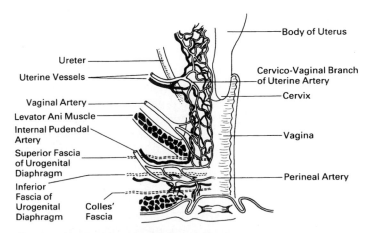

Fig. 2.7 Blood supply to the vagina. The deeper structures are supplied mainly from the uterine vessels, whereas the more superficial structures have a complex supply from the rectal and pudendal arteries.

Nerve supply

The major nerve supply to the vagina is autonomic arising from the pelvic plexuses, but the lower end has a sensory supply from the pudendal nerve.

The sympathetic fibres come from the lower lumbar sympathetic ganglia via the hypogastric plexus. The parasympathetic outflow is through the second, third and fourth sacral nerves. The fibres are distributed mainly in company with the arterial supply. The parasympathetic ganglia are found between the bladder and vagina and in association with the lateral walls of the vagina. The majority of nerve endings are undecorated, but Pacinian corpuscles are found within the vaginal adventitia.

THE UTERUS

The uterus is usually described in terms of cervix, body and fundus. In the nulliparous woman it is pear-shaped and measures about $7.5 \times 5 \times 2.5$ cm. There is a cavity which communicates with the peritoneal cavity via the Fallopian tubes and with the cavity of the vagina via the cervical canal. The fundus is that part of the uterus which lies above the openings of the tubes, while the tapering body lies below the fundus. It is somewhat flattened anteroposteriorly and is continuous with the cervix below. The cervix protrudes into the vault of the vagina. The gap between the cervix and the vaginal wall is called the fornix of the vagina; it is deepest posteriorly.

The uterus is described as having four layers—firstly, there is an outer peritoneal or serous coat below which is a subserous connective tissue layer that is densest where the various ligaments attach to the cervix. Third is the myometrium, the muscle layer of the uterus; it is the thickest layer, made up of interlacing bundles of smooth muscle fibres separated by connective tissue sheets containing blood vessels. This layer is about 15 mm thick in the nulliparous uterus of the adult. The fourth, innermost layer is the endometrium, surrounding the cavity of the uterus; the endometrium undergoes considerable changes during the menstrual cycle.

The cervix has a central canal that extends from the internal os, where it becomes continuous with the cavity of the uterus, to the external os, where it becomes continuous with the cavity of the vagina. It forms a narrow bottleneck between these two organs.

The cervix is divided from the corpus by a fibromuscular junction which acts as a sphincter; its competence is important, especially during the second trimester of pregnancy.

The cervix projects into the vagina, surrounded by a gutter-like fornix. The vaginal cervix has a short anterior lip and a longer posterior lip. It is penetrated by the endocervical canal which joins the uterine cavity to the vagina. The canal is fusiform in shape, flattened from front to back and measures 7 mm across at its widest part and about 3 cm long.

Anteriorly the supravaginal part is separated from the bladder by the connective tissue layer, the parametrium. The uterine arteries run in this tissue while the ureter runs downwards and forwards within the parametrium about 2 mm from the cervix.

Posteriorly the supravaginal cervix is covered with the peritoneum lining the rectouterine pouch of Douglas. The cervix is supported posteriorly by the uterosacral ligaments which extend from this part of the cervix to the second, third and fourth sacral vertebrae. The cardinal ligaments support the cervix laterally and are the major support of the cervix and uterus.

The cervix shares its blood supply with that of the body of the uterus. Coming from the uterine artery, the cervicovaginal branch runs down the lateral margins of the cervix where it anastomoses with branches of the vaginal artery, forming a rich plexus of vessels (Fig. 2.7). The venous drainage is lateral into a plexus on either side of the cervix and from there into veins that follow the arteries.

The nerve supply to the cervix is autonomic, with the densest innervation being at the level of the internal os and most of these fibres supplying the smooth muscle in this region. The fibres appear to follow the arterially derived vessels. In contrast with the body of uterus, many of these nerve fibres are cholinesterase-positive. There are both adrenergic and cholinergic fibres within the cervix: their distribution is very similar, but overall there are fewer cholinergic fibres. Most of these fibres disappear after the menopause. Sensory fibres travel with both divisions of the autonomic nervous system.

The cervix has a rich lymphatic drainage with a three-layered arrangement of beds of vessels: a subepithelial bed, a stromal bed and a serosal bed which gives rise to a series of larger vessels that drain along the base of the broad ligament. The most anterior are closely related to the uterine artery and eventually reach the external iliac nodes. Slightly posteriorly the vessels also follow the uterine artery to its origin where they join the internal iliac nodes. The most posterior group leave the cervix posterolaterally and pass along the uterosacral fold to reach the nodes situated over the sacrum.

The bulk of the cervix consists mainly of fibrous tissue containing varying proportions of smooth muscle—usually about 10%, but it can vary between 2 and 40%.

The vast amount of collagen is probably the reason for the rapid dilatation of the cervix during labour. It may be that during the later stages of pregnancy, the ratio of glycosaminoglycans to collagen exceeds some critical level when there is an influx of water into the tissues. There is also a reduction in the cohesive forces between cervical collagen filaments, so that the adhesion between the fibrils breaks down, producing a soft tissue which is dilated by the mechanical forces of uterine contraction during labour.

Blood supply

This is through the uterine arteries supported superiorly by the terminal branches of the ovarian arteries. The uterine artery arises from the internal iliac artery, passing medially across the pelvic floor and lying in the base of the broad ligament. As the artery reaches the uterus near the supravaginal part of the cervix, it passes above the ureter and turns upwards to pass close to the lateral side of the body of the uterus as far as the entrance of the Fallopian tube into the uterus. Here it anastomoses with the ovarian artery. Throughout its course it gives off many branches that penetrate the wall of the uterus (Fig. 2.8).

The venous drainage of the uterus consists of a plexus of veins that starts in the broad ligament, spreading out across the pelvic floor to communicate with the rectal and vesicle plexuses and draining into the internal iliac veins.

Lymphatic drainage

In general this follows the arteries.

Nerve supply

This system is poorly understood. The main sensory fibres from the cervix run in the nervi erigentes from the sacral segments 2 and 3, while those from the body of the uterus travel with the hypogastric plexus to the lower thoracic segments. Some sensory fibres from the fundus travel in the ovarian and renal plexuses to reach their dorsal nerve roots of T11 and T12.

Peritoneal relations

The uterus is draped in a fold of peritoneum which extends forwards to cover the bladder and backwards to the rectum. It spreads laterally as the broad ligament, and the peritoneum then spreads to cover the pelvic wall. It is as if these organs had been pushed up into the pelvic cavity from below, carrying the peritoneum to various degrees into the cavity of the pelvis.

Anteriorly the peritoneum extends downwards as far as the attachment of the base of the bladder at the level of the internal os, whereas posteriorly the bladder is completely covered by peritoneum.

Fascia and ligaments of the uterus

These ligaments contain a remarkably high proportion of smooth muscle besides the usual collection of collagen. The cardinal and uterosacral ligaments assist the fibrous tissue in fixing the anterior aspect of the uterus to the bladder base and in maintaining the stability of the bladder. This connective tissue extends inferiorly to bind the urethra to the anterior wall of the vagina. It is probable that the broad and round ligaments have little function in uterine stability.

The uterosacral ligaments, arising from the supravaginal part of the cervix, pass backwards, embracing the rectum, to be attached to the front of the lower part of the sacrum. Posteriorly the vagina and anal canals are separated but bound together by the fibromuscular mass of the perineal body. The lateral ligaments, the main ligaments of uterine stability, extend laterally from the cervix to the side wall of the pelvis (Fig. 2.9). The round and broad ligaments are associated with the body of the uterus. The round ligament arises from the junction between the body of the uterus and the uterine tube passes via the broad ligament

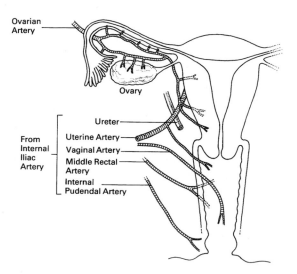

Fig. 2.8 Blood supply of the genitalia. The uterus has an anastomotic supply from both the ovarian and uterine arteries, both vessels running in the broad ligament.

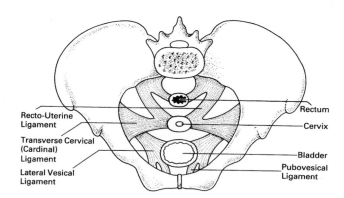

Fig. 2.9 Pelvic ligaments. The transverse or cardinal ligament is probably the major supporting structure of the cervix.

where it raises a ridge on the anterior surface. It eventually runs along the inguinal canal to the labium majus of the vulva. It is mostly made up of smooth muscle. It probably functions as an anchor for the uterus in the anteverted position during recumbent sleep and against the pressure of a full bladder.

The broad ligament is no ligament: it is little more than a fold of peritoneum extending between the lateral aspect of the body of the uterus and the lateral wall of the pelvis. Superiorly, there is a free border, while inferiorly it merges with the pelvic floor. It contains the ovarian artery and uterine tube, the round and ovarian ligaments superiorly, and the uterine artery medially. There are extensive lymphatics associated with the arteries. The ovary is attached to the posterior surface of the broad ligament by the mesovarium, a fold of peritoneum from the posterior side of the ligament (Fig. 2.10).

MENSTRUATION

In the prepubertal period the epithelium lining the uterine cavity is only a single layer of cuboidal cells and the mucosal glands are simple unbranched tubes. For two or three years before puberty there is considerable growth of the uterus in line with the increased ovarian activity. By menarche the uterus has almost reached its adult size.

The menstrual debris comes from the endometrium above the internal os. It is composed of blood and epithe-

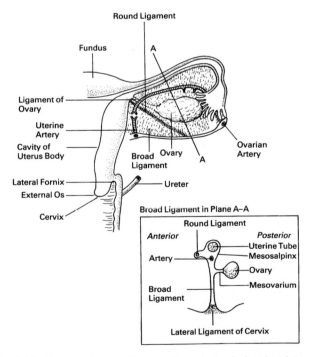

Fig. 2.10 Ovary and broad ligament from the back showing the relations of structures within the broad ligament. There are multiple small branches from the ovarian artery to the Fallopian tube.

lial detritus and averages between 50 and 60 ml in healthy adults. The cyclical changes of the endometrium are directly related to changes occurring in the ovary. It is easiest to consider the menstrual changes from the end of menstruation, that is about day 5 of a 28-day cycle. At this stage the endometrium consists of little else but the stumps of glands in a dense stroma. This part of the lining, the stratum basale, usually has variable amounts of stratum spongiosum on its surface. There is a very rapid spread of epithelial cells from the mouths of the gland remnants so that by the end of the first week of the cycle the surface has a complete epithelial cover (Fig. 2.11).

The second week of the cycle is a time of considerable growth and cell division. The glands increase in size, the blood vessels dilate and the stroma becomes oedematous as a result of the oestrogens secreted by the ovary.

During the third week of the cycle, after ovulation and under the influence of progesterone from the corpus luteum, the endometrium becomes even more oedematous, boggy and pale. The cells in the stroma enlarge and fill with glycogen, the glands become more coiled and swollen and some begin to release their contents into the lumen of the glands.

In the last week of the cycle the endometrium is at its thickest—some 10 times thicker than at the beginning—and is described as having three layers; a narrow stratum compactum below the surface of the epithelium, a thick stratum spongiosum occupying most of the endometrium, and the inactive stratum basale. At the end of this time the strata compactum and spongiosum are shed and the whole cycle begins again.

These cyclical changes, under the control of the ovarian hormones, are brought about by changes in the arterioles supplying the endometrium. There are two types of arterioles—the straight and the spiral. The straight arterioles only supply the basal layer, but the spiral ones supply the whole thickness of the endometrium. It is ischaemia of the spiral arteries which produces the necrosis that results in the menstrual discharge. By the second day of menstruation the endometrium has been lost down to the basal layer.

THE UTERINE TUBES

The uterine (Fallopian) tubes are between 10 and 14 cm long, lying for the middle three-quarters in the upper border of the broad ligament. The lateral extremity is free of the broad ligament and is in close association with the surface of the ovary. The end is open and expanded with a bunch of finger-like processes, the fimbriae (Fig. 2.12). There can be more than one ostium to a Fallopian tube. It is said that one of the fimbriae—the ovarian fimbria—is longer than the others and is attached by its tip to the ovary.

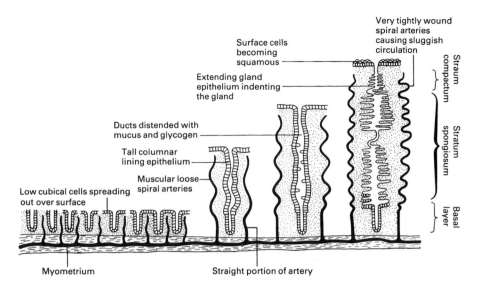

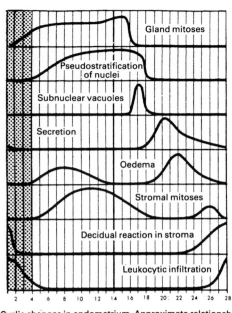

Cyclic changes in endometrium. Approximate relationship of useful microscopic changes

Fig. 2.11 Diagram of the menstrual cycle.

The uterine tube is usually considered to have four regions—the fimbriated infundibulum outside the broad ligament, a dilated ampulla, followed by a narrow isthmus with a lumen 1–2 mm in diameter within the broad ligament, and finally an intramural part of the tube which lies within the muscular wall of the uterus. Thus the cavity of the uterus is continuous with the peritoneal cavity. However the circular muscle at the uterine end of

the Fallopian tube is thickened and is regarded by some as a sphincter controlling the flow of fluids from the uterus into the tube. The tube is capable of producing secretions; the nature of these secretions is poorly known, but the amounts vary during the ovarian cycle, being greatest in the post-ovulation phase.

The tube consists of smooth muscle surrounding a mucous membrane which is ciliated and thrown into many complex longitudinal folds. The isthmus differs in that here the lumen is narrow, the folds disappear and there are only a few cilia.

The tube has a rich blood supply via many small branches from the ovarian artery and its inner end from the uterine artery. The veins of the tube drain to the pampiniform plexus, while the lymphatics follow the course of the ovarian arteries.

Fig. 2.12 Uterine (Fallopian) tubes. The functional anatomy of the tube is poorly understood. The variations in lumen size probably act as a baffle to stop too large objects passing and the highly convoluted wall with ciliated crests to the folds functions to allow sperm to move in one direction and the egg in the opposite way.

THE OVARIES

The ovaries lie free within the cavity of the pelvis; they are without a covering of peritoneum except along the equatorial attachment of the mesovarium. The ovary is attached to the uterus at its upper angle by the ligament of the ovary. This mass of fibrous tissue and smooth muscle lies between the two layers of the broad ligament.

The ovary lies obliquely, with its upper pole medial and its lower pole lateral. It touches the side wall of the pelvis between the internal and external iliac vessels and lies upon the obturator nerve. The peritoneum, against which the ovary lies, is supplied by the obturator nerve. The ovary receives its blood from the ovarian arteries—

direct branches of the abdominal aorta—while the ovarian veins form a plexus in the mesovarium that eventually drains into a pair of veins which run with the ovarian artery. Those from the left unite to form a single vein that drains into the left renal vein. Those on the right fuse and join the inferior vena cava.

The ovarian lymph drainage follows the course of the ovarian artery.

Structure

The ovary consists of a cuboidal epithelium surrounding a fibrous stroma. Initially each ovary contains about 3 million potential ova which have migrated along the dorsal mesentery during development.

In the newborn baby the ovaries are very large compared with the uterus. They increase in weight some 20 times before maturity, but the relative growth of the uterus is such that by puberty they are relatively much smaller than the uterus. There is practically no recognizable germinal tissue in the fully involuted ovary after the menopause.

THE BLADDER

The bladder is fixed at the trigone and has a mobile and distensible fundus above it. The trigone is generally immobile; it is attached by ligaments and tough fascia to the cervix and anterior fornix, as well as by the lateral ligaments which pass across the pelvic floor covering the vesicle veins, the inferior vesicle artery and its associated lymphatics, together with the nerves of the bladder.

There are three ligaments extending from the fundus of the bladder to the umbilicus—the median umbilical ligament, the remains of the urachus in the midline, and a pair of lateral umbilical ligaments (the remains of the umbilical arteries of the fetus) extending obliquely upwards to the umbilicus. Each of these ligaments is retroperitoneal and raises a ridge of peritoneum on the internal surface of the anterior abdominal wall. Only the superior surface of the bladder is firmly attached to peritoneum; elsewhere it is surrounded by loose areolar tissue. The potential space between the anterior aspect of the bladder and the pubic symphysis is the cave of Retzius. Posteriorly lies the uterus. Between the uterus and the trigone of the bladder the fascia is strong and it is this fascia that helps the ligaments to anchor the bladder (Fig. 2.13).

The triangular trigone lies between the openings of the ureters into the bladder and the midline internal urethral orifice. The openings of the two ureters are found at either end of a transverse ridge, the interureteric bar. The track of the ureters through the muscle of the bladder wall is oblique, and it is debated whether it is this oblique course or the flap of mucous membrane

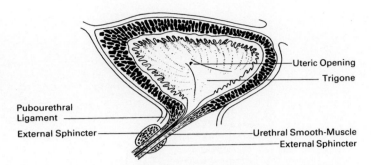

Fig. 2.13 Except where it is fixed at its base, the bladder is a highly distensible structure, and urinary continence probably depends upon the physical relations of the fixed/mobile junction.

associated with the opening that has the major role in preventing urinary reflux.

In life, the base of the bladder lies flat; this flat area is greater than the area of the trigone but is of prime importance in maintaining urinary continence. There are said to be three sphincters controlling micturition—an internal, urethral and external urinary sphincter. The internal sphincter is complex. It probably does not exist as such but its effect is produced by a series of muscle actions. It is really the tone of the detrusor loop from the outer longitudinal layer of bladder muscle that forces the urethra backwards and it is the tone of the base plate that forces the trigone forwards into the concavity formed by the circular fibres of the fundus. Thus the trigone comes to lie in front of the urethral orifice, so that as long as the base plate remains flat the bladder neck remains closed.

In order to convert the base plate into a funnel-like tube during voiding, considerable force is required. The human is probably alone amongst animals in being able to hold urine for a considerable time after bladder-filling has reached the point where the bladder would empty reflexly. This can even be achieved during sleep. At birth this bladder control is not possible because the base plate is rounded and does not fit into the concavity formed by the detrusor. In stress incontinence it is probably a sagging of the anterior vaginal wall that causes a descent of the bladder, distorting it in the base and so reducing its ability to resist increases in intra-abdominal pressure.

The bladder wall is made of smooth muscle fibres which run in spirals. The apparently randomly arranged muscle fibres produce a series of trabeculated ridges which at cystoscopy show through the mucous membrane. The muscle as a whole is called the detrusor. The mucous membrane of the bladder is thick and lax and lined with a transitional epithelium which is urine-proof because of the specialized junctions between the inner edges of the adjacent cells. There is said to be a ring of fibres around the internal urethral orifice. The membrane has neither glands nor muscularis mucosa.

The blood supply to the bladder is from the superior and inferior vesicle arteries, assisted by a few branches from the pubic branch of the inferior epigastric artery.

The veins of the bladder become a plexus at the base of the bladder. The vesicle plexus communicates with veins in the broad ligament, and drains to the internal iliac veins.

The lymph drainage follows the course of the arteries. Its nerve supply is autonomic from the pelvic plexus, the parasympathetic segments are S2, S3 and S4 and the fibres reach the plexus via the nervi erigentes. The sympathetic nerves are inhibitory to the detrusor muscle and motor nerves to the internal sphincter.

THE URETHRA

This tube extends from the bladder to the vestibule—a distance in the normal non-pregnant adult female of about 5 cm. It penetrates the urinogenital diaphragm. The vagina is closely related to it posteriorly and the urethra is closely bound to the vagina in its lower two-thirds; the upper part is loose and held only by loose connective tissue. The urethra is a very distensible organ which has muscular, submucous and mucous layers; the smooth muscle is made up of an outer circular and inner longitudinal layer. In its lower part there is a ring of striated muscle fibres, the sphincter urethrae. The submucosa is remarkable in that it contains numerous venous channels surrounded by loose elastic connective tissue. The mucous membrane itself is thrown into a series of longitudinal folds with an especially prominent one posteriorly.

The epithelium is stratified and columnar in the middle third of the urethra, merging with bladder epithelium upwards and with the stratified squamous non-kcratinized epithelium of the vestibule inferiorly. There are numerous small and a pair of large periurethral glands that drain via short ducts into its lumen.

The blood supply of the main part of the urethra is from branches of the vaginal vessels and the upper part is supplied by terminations of the vesicle arteries. The venous plexuses have a corresponding drainage, either to the vesicle veins or to the venous plexuses of the vulva.

The urethral sphincter has inner longitudinal and outer circular smooth muscle layers around the urethra and some striated paraurethral muscle. It is normally closed except during micturition when the inner longitudinal muscle contracts, shortening the urethra and therefore increasing the bore of its lumen.

The external urinary sphincter is located between the layers of the urinogenital diaphragm. It is made up of striated muscle innervated by the pudendal nerve. It can stop the voluntary urinary stream.

The lymph drainage is either to inguinal nodes or to the internal and external iliac nodes. The nerve supply is autonomic from the pelvic and hypogastric plexuses.

THE RECTUM

The rectum—despite its name—is anything but straight. It curves to follow the anterior curve of the sacrum and also deviates towards the left in its middle part, whereas the upper and lower thirds lie in the midline. The rectum begins at the level of the third segment of the sacrum and extends as far as the perineal body, where it becomes the anal canal. The rectum has no mesentery but its upper third has pelvic peritoneum on its anterior and lateral surfaces, the middle third only on its anterior surface and the lowest third has no contact with the peritoneum.

Unlike the large intestine, the external layer of longitudinal muscle is complete over the surface of the rectum. Internally the junctions between the curves of the rectum are marked by horizontal folds, the valves of Houston. These folds contain circular muscle of the gut.

Three arteries contribute to the blood supply of the rectum. The principal supply is from the inferior mesenteric artery via the superior rectal branch which supplies the mucous membrane of the organ as far as the rectoanal junction. At the beginning of the rectum the superior rectal arteries divide into a left and right branch. The right branch soon divides into anterior and posterior branches (Fig. 2.14). The venous return mimics the arterial supply but there are considerable anastomoses between the vessels. The submucous plexus of veins communicates with the venous plexus at the base of the broad ligament. This venous plexus is the site both of haemorrhoidal dilation and of portosystemic anastomosis.

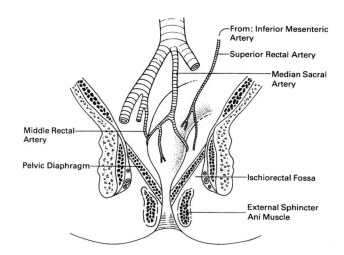

Fig. 2.14 The rectum has a rich anastomotic blood supply, from the median sacral, the internal iliac and the inferior mesenteric arteries and this arrangement is reflected in its venous drainage.

Anorectal lymphatic drainage

The rectosigmoid and upper rectum drain via the mesentery to the inferior mesenteric group of nodes. The middle and lower part of the rectum drains both to the mesenteric group and to the internal iliac nodes. The anal canal below the levator ani muscle drains across the thigh to the inguinal and gluteal nodes.

The rectum has an autonomic nerve supply which is sympathetic directly from the pelvic plexus and parasympathetic via S2 and S3 and the nervi erigentes.

BLOOD VESSELS OF THE PELVIS

The pelvic contents and walls are supplied by branches of the internal iliac artery and are drained to the internal iliac veins. The vessels lie with the parietal pelvic fascia and only those branches that leave the pelvis pierce this membranous structure. The obturator vessels leave the obturator foramen via the obturator canal, which is a hole in this fascia. The internal iliac artery divides into a large anterior branch and a smaller posterior branch, the anterior branch supplying the pelvic viscera (Fig. 2.15).

The venous drainage is via the internal iliac veins to the inferior vena cava, but there are anastomoses through the superior rectal and inferior mesenteric veins to the portal system. There is also a drainage passage of the internal vertebral plexus via the lateral sacral veins to the internal iliac veins, the flow in which can be reversed by raised intra-abdominal pressure. This is a potential route of spread of pelvic inflammatory and malignant disease.

THE NERVES OF THE PELVIS

Besides nerves of passage such as the obturator nerve, the nerves whose function lie with the pelvis are branches of the sacral plexus and the pelvic autonomic system. The sacral plexus is a broad structure formed by the fusion of nerves from L4 to S4 and lies lateral to the

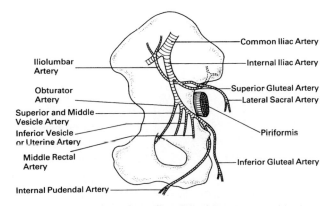

Fig. 2.15 The blood supply to the pelvic viscera is derived in the main from the internal iliac artery.

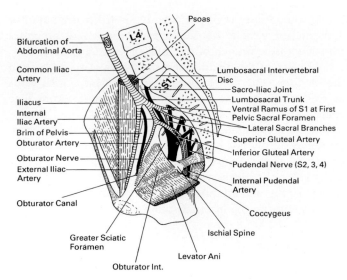

Fig. 2.16 Pelvic musculature. Muscles leave the pelvis either above the superior ramus of the pubis or through the greater or lesser sciatic foramina. Nerves and vessels also leave via the obturator foramen.

anterior sacral foramina. It lies upon the piriformis muscle and is covered anteriorly by the parietal pelvic fascia (Fig. 2.16).

The parasympathetic nerves travel with some branches of this plexus and arise by several rootlets from the anterior surfaces of S2, S3 and sometimes S4. They are called the nervi erigentes.

The pudendal nerve which is sensory to pudenda arises from S2, S3 and S4; it then passes backwards between the piriformis and coccygeus to round the sacrospinous ligament and enter the ischiorectal fossa. The perineal branch of S4 passes between the coccygeus and iliococcygeus to be distributed to the external anal sphincter and the perianal skin.

The pelvic autonomic plexus lies on the side wall of the pelvis lateral to the rectum. The sympathetic fibres are derived from the hypogastric plexus as well as a contribution from the upper sacral ganglia of the sympathetic trunk. The plexus is ganglionated. About half of the fibres in the hypogastric plexus are preganglionic and synapse in these ganglia; the rest are post-ganglionic and do not synapse. The parasympathetic fibres of the nervi erigentes do not synapse here but in the walls of the viscera.

The autonomic system is organized so that the sympathetic fibres are vasoconstrictor and the parasympathetic fibres are motor to the smooth muscle of the bladder and gut, and secretomotor to the gut glands. The sympathetic fibres are motor to the bladder and anal canal sphincters as well as to the smooth muscle of the seminal vesicles in the male. The course of pain and sensory fibres is complex and not fully understood. Most pain fibres travel with the sympathetic system, especially those from the gut and the gonads. However, pain fibres from the bladder and rectum as well as those conveying the sensation of distension probably travel in the nervi erigentes. Pain fibres from the cervix also follow this course, but those from the body of the uterus travel mainly in the hypogastric nerves, especially to thoracic dorsal roots 11 and 12.

THE PELVIC CAVITY

The pelvic cavity is a part of the abdominal cavity surrounded by the bony pelvis. It is bound inferiorly by the urogenital diaphragm separating the pelvis from the perineum. In the female the pelvis contains the organs of reproduction as well as the bladder and the terminal portion of the alimentary canal.

The urogenital diaphragm and perineum are penetrated in the midline by three tubes. From before backwards, they are the urethra, the vagina and the anal canal. The urethra and vagina are surrounded by a series of structures which together constitute the vulva (Fig. 2.17).

The bony pelvis surrounds a cavity shaped like a pudding basin lying on its side, such that the anterior superior iliac spine and the pubic symphysis are in the same vertical plane. The brim of the cavity is made from the promontory and alae of the sacrum, the arcuate line of the ilium, the pectineal line of the pubis; the pubic crest lies at about 30° to this plane. The upper border of the symphysis pubis, the spine of the ischium and the tip of the coccyx define a plane that can just be reached by the tip of a finger placed in the vagina (Fig. 2.18).

The pelvic cavity aspect of the bony pelvis is mostly covered by muscles—superiorly by the psoas and iliacus muscles, below the pelvic brim by the obturator internus muscle and posteriorly by pyriformis and coccygeus muscles arising from the anterior surface of the sacrum (see Fig. 2.16). The fascia covering these muscles is a tough membrane attached to the periosteum at the edges. The bare bone of the pelvic wall is not covered by fascia.

The pelvic floor is a V-shaped gutter of muscles which is higher posteriorly than anteriorly to produce the base

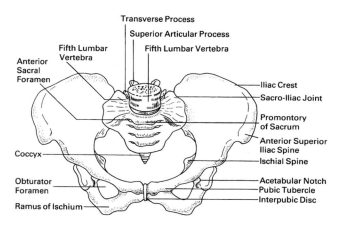

Fig. 2.18 The bony pelvis. The bones both enclose the birth canal and provide support for the body on the legs. There are notable sexual differences between the male and female bony pelvis.

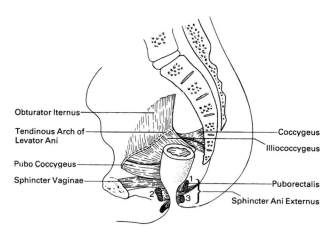

Fig. 2.19 Muscles of the pelvic floor. The slings of muscle that surround and separate the major body effluents have an important role as sphincters.

of the V, formed by the midline raphe of these muscles. The raphe and muscles are penetrated by the urethra, vagina and rectum. The direction of the muscle fibres forming the anterior part of this diaphragm of muscles is backwards and medially, such that they form a series of slings encircling the posterior aspects of the penetrating structures and thus have a potential sphincter-like action (Fig. 2.19). There is a hole anteriorly between the muscles arising from the posterior aspect of the pubis. This gap is closed by the pubovesical ligaments, between which passes the deep dorsal vein of the clitoris.

The muscles arise peripherally from a continuous line starting at the spine of ischium, which proceeds as the white line over the fascia covering the medial aspect of obturator internus, and from the body of the pubis. The midline raphe extends from the coccyx forwards.

The function of this gutter during labour is to deflect anteriorly the first part of the baby which comes into contact with it and later to rotate the head or buttocks so that the shortest diameter lies transversely at the brim

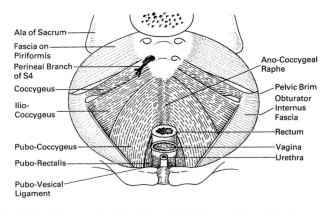

Fig. 2.17 The urogenital diaphragm. The floor of the pelvis slopes steeply forwards and plays an important role in continence and childbirth.

of the bony pelvis. The muscles of the pelvic diaphragm are supplied in the main by the perineal branch of S4, and anteriorly by branches from the inferior rectal and perineal nerves.

The function of these muscles is to respond to changes in intra-abdominal pressure, assisting in maintaining faecal and urinary continence. In micturition and defecation the relevant portion of the muscle is relaxed, but the remainder maintains its tone to prevent prolapse of the pelvic organs. Most of the weight of the gut is borne by the superior aspect of the pubic symphysis.

The fascia of the pelvic floor is little more than loose areolar tissue. Separating the pelvic floor from the pelvic peritoneum are the pelvic viscera. The space around these organs provides room for distension of the bladder and rectum.

THE LYMPHATIC DRAINAGE OF THE PELVIS

The lymphatics in the pelvis originate as tiny lymphocapillaries that form complex nets of interconnecting vessels. They are without valves and their walls consist solely of endothelial plates. These networks join to form lymphatic vessels with smooth muscle in their walls and have valves. Eventually lymph vessels lead to lymph nodes. The lymphatics of the perineum, together with those of the lower limb, go to a collection of lymph nodes below the inguinal ligament. Some of the deeper lymphatics of the buttock follow the superior and inferior gluteal arteries and penetrate into the pelvic cavity (Fig. 2.20). In general these lymphatics are found between the membranous layer of superficial fascia and the deep fascia. The nodes are classified into three major groups—superficial inguinal, deep inguinal and pelvic lymph nodes.

Superficial drainage

The superficial inguinal nodes radiate outwards from the saphenous opening, in the form of the letter T. The

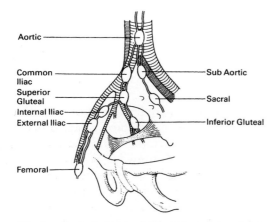

Fig. 2.20 The lymphatic drainage of the pelvis and associated structures.

Aortic

Common Iliac
Superior Gluteal
Internal Iliac
External Iliac

Femoral

Sub Aortic

Sacral

Inferior Gluteal

stem of the T is made by the group associated with the terminal part of the great saphenous vein, while the arms of the T follow the inguinal ligament. The vulva drains initially to the medial horizontal group. In most cases the vulval lymphatics do not cross the labia crural fold, but reach the nodes by traversing the mons pubis.

From the posterior part of the vulva and the perineum the lymphatics drain into the thigh and the lower lymph nodes, together with those from the lower limb. The deep inguinal nodes lie in relation to the junction between the femoral vein and the great saphenous vein after it has passed through the deep fascia at the saphenous opening. It is no longer believed that all efferents from the inguinal region pass through this group.

Internal iliac system

The pelvic lymph nodes are usually related to the major blood vessels and are named after them. The internal iliac vessels drain the pelvic contents. Unfortunately there are several common variations amongst the veins, and the distribution of the lymphatics may vary with the veins. Usually the internal iliac vein is formed from an anterior, a middle and a posterior branch. Variations include how the vessels join with each other and the territories they drain. There is frequently variation between the two sides of the pelvis. Usually nodes are named external iliac when related to the external iliac artery. All nodes inferior to the external iliac vein and anterior to the internal iliac artery are named interiliac. Lymph nodes behind the anterior division of the internal iliac artery are called the internal iliac group. Since there are three main arteries entering the pelvis—one paired, the common iliac arteries, and two single, the median sacral and the superior haemorrhoidal arteries—there are three possible routes for lymphatic drainage.

The external iliac nodes

This system is much confused, as several surgical and anatomical descriptions describe the same structures, giving them differing names. Basically there is a system of chains of nodes and vessels surrounding the external iliac artery and vein with a few related nodes associated with them. Although these lymph chains are interconnected it is usual to describe them as anterior–superior, intermediate and posteromedial (Fig. 2.21).

The associated glands are those within the inguinal canal, those associated with the inferior epigastric artery and those associated with the first part of the obturator artery. They are named after their associated vessels. It is the posteromedial group that is the important lymphatic relay for the genital tract and the cervix.

The internal iliac nodes, like the arterial supply, are in two main divisions: those from the pelvic viscera and

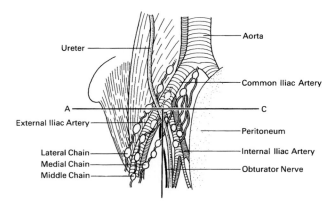

Fig. 2.21 The iliac group of lymph nodes and their related structures. The complex system of interconnections between individual nodes probably precludes any functional significance being correlated with concise anatomical localization. The horizontal line and the vertical line are superimposed to emphasize that the lateral group of lymph nodes associated with the external iliac artery is relatively superficial and is associated mainly with the lymphatic drainage of the limb, whereas the lymph nodes medial to the vertical line are deep within the pelvic basin and are closely associated with the pelvic organs. Those lymph nodes above the horizontal line drain lymph from both groups below the line.

those from the buttock and leg. Since the viscera within the pelvis are separated from the pelvic wall, the peripheral lymph nodes are associated with the walls of the organs rather than with the pelvic wall. Both the internal and external iliac system of lymphatics drain to the common iliac nodes. They are most easily visualized as a continuation of the three chains of nodes surrounding the external iliac vessels. These chains continue to the bifurcation of the aorta where they anastomose freely with each other and with those from the other side. The symmetry of the two sides is disturbed by the left common iliac vein.

Besides this system there are a few nodes associated with the median sacral artery, and with the superior haemorrhoidal artery. The median sacral vessels join the common iliac lymphatics at the bifurcation of the aorta.

It is important to realize that this classification in terms of adjacent vessels gives very little clue to the drainage of these nodes; structures like the urethra and vagina straddle the territories of several vessels. Even structures such as the bladder and uterus, which are supplied by the visceral division of the internal iliac artery, drain to nodes associated with other vessels. Indeed the ovary can drain almost anywhere—to the renal region via the gonadal vessels; to the iliac nodes via the uterine vessels; to the adjacent pelvic wall, and even to the inguinal nodes via the round ligament.

Nevertheless it is a reasonable generalization that the lymphatic drainage of the pelvic viscera follows the vessels that supply them. The posteromedial group of the external iliac lymph nodes is functionally more related to the visceral branches of the internal iliac artery than to external iliac artery territory.

THE BONY PELVIS

The pelvis is constructed from the two innominate bones and posteriorly, the sacrum, wedged like a keystone between them. Each innominate bone is divided into three parts—an ilium, an ischium and a pubis. The innominate bones come together anteriorly at the symphysis pubis.

The pelvic brim comprises the promontory of the sacrum, the alae of the sacrum, the arcuate line of the ilium, the iliopubic eminence, the pectineal line and the pubic crest, which, together with the upper surface of the symphysis pubis, separates the false pelvis above from the true pelvis below. The outlet of the pelvis is diamond-shaped, bound in front by the lower surface of the symphysis pubis and the ischiopubic ramus, laterally by the ischial tuberosities, posterolaterally by the sacrotuberous ligament and posteriorly by the tip of the coccyx (Fig. 2.22).

The planes of the anterior urogenital triangle and the posterior anal triangle lie at about 150° to each other.

The sacrum is formed by the fusion of the five sacral vertebrae. This classical condition is frequently changed, either by the fusion of the fifth lumbar vertebra to the sacrum, or when the fifth sacral is separated and fused with the coccyx. The sacral hiatus—the inferior opening of the sacral canal—is very variable in size but the two bony prominences on either side of the aperture are usually felt easily—a fact which is of importance when performing caudal anaesthesia. The sacrum joins the innominate bones at the sacroiliac joints.

The major obstetric interest in the bony pelvis is that it is not distensible; only minor degrees of movement are possible at the pubic and sacroiliac joints. Its dimensions are therefore critical during childbirth. Furthermore the diameters of the true pelvis vary in different parts of the

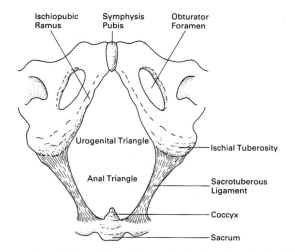

Fig. 2.22 Boundaries of the pelvic outlet. By the time the fetal head reaches this region it has usually been orientated by the pelvic diaphragm such that its long axis is antero-posterior and the face faces posteriorly.

Table 2.1 Comparison between the male and female pelvis

	Male	Female
Subpubic angle	45–55°	70–80°
Ratio of width of acetabulum to distance from anterior edge to the symphysis pubis	<1	1
Sciatic notch	75°	50°
Ischial spines point	Inwards	Downwards
Shape of obturator foramen	Triangular	Oval
Sacral index: $\dfrac{\text{width}}{\text{height}} \times 100$	115	105
Ratio of ala of sacrum to width of body of S1	1	<1
Cavity	Short segment of wide cone	Long segment of narrow cone

pelvis. The pelvic cavity is widest transversely at the inlet and anteroposteriorly at the outlet. Most attempts to classify the shape of the pelvis fail because there appears to be a continuous series of pelves extending from the classical gynaecoid, the anteroposteriorly flattened and platypelloid. Although it is possible to list the salient features of the classical female pelvis and contrast them with the male pelvis, in a large series the differences are by no means always apparent. The commonly quoted distinctive features of the female pelvis are given in Table 2.1.

The pelvic joints

The sacroiliac joint is a synovial joint between the articular surfaces of the ilium and the sacrum. The facets have interlocking facies and, at least posterosuperiorly, the two bones are united by fibrous tissue typical of a fibrous joint, especially in later life. Indeed, in old age bony fusion may take place. The joint has considerable support from its associated ligaments. The strong posterior superior interosseous ligaments and the posterior sacroiliac ligaments prevent the weight of the body pushing the sacrum

downwards and forwards. The sacrotuberous and sacrospinous ligaments also contribute to this stability.

The symphysis pubis is a secondary cartilaginous joint. The adjoining surfaces of the pubic bones are covered with hyaline cartilage, between which there is a disc of fibrocartilage joining the two bones. The joint is further strengthened by ligaments superiorly, and inferiorly by direct fibres, but anteriorly and obliquely by interdigitating fibres that interlace with fibres from the rectus abdominis and external oblique muscles.

There is an increase in movements of these joints, especially during the third trimester of pregnancy. The net result is to increase the sagittal diameter of the outlet and true conjugate. Studies of these movements suggest that as far as pelvic capacity is concerned, squatting during uterine contractions and lying recumbent between them may provide a helpful routine during labour.

CONCLUSIONS

The anatomy of the female urogenital tract is highly dynamic and undergoes vast changes at all stages of the reproductive cycle, from the vast increase in size of the labia minora during copulation to the recovery of the prepregnant uterine size after parturition. The tract is under the control of multiple influences—psychogenic, emotional, sensory, autonomic and hormonal—but seems capable of fulfilling its role in reproduction in the absence of many of them. Its design faults, if they may be considered as such, are the narrowness of the bony pelvic canal and the great vulnerability of the narrow lumen of the Fallopian tubes.

Acknowledgements

I have borrowed heavily from the standard anatomical textbooks and from the advice of my colleagues. The standard diagrams are in such a highly evolved state that it would be a research project in itself to trace them to their origins. I have done little except tinker with their details. To these unknown original artists and ancestors I offer my sincere thanks.

3. Fertilization, early development and implantation

Alan O. Trounson   Peter A. W. Rogers   Ismail Kola
A. Henry Sathananthan

INTRODUCTION

The events which mark the onset of embryonic development are exceedingly complex and finely balanced between continuation, abnormal change and cessation of development. Given the understanding that a major modification to one of the composite events could be an effective contraceptive it is slightly easier to comprehend the genesis of infertility. In this chapter we explore the events which determine normal fertilization and embryo development and try to illustrate how these events are controlled by many other interacting factors.

THE OVULATED OOCYTES

Oocyte maturation

Fertilization and normal embryonic development can only be achieved if the ovulated oocyte has progressed through complete maturation within the ovarian follicle or in culture in vitro (Cha et al 1991). It is not known whether immature oocytes may be ovulated in the spontaneous menstrual cycle but in the artificially manipulated and superovulated cycles of treatment for in vitro fertilization (IVF), incomplete oocyte maturation is frequently observed. Immature oocytes may be obtained even after administration of large doses (10 000 iu) of human chorionic gonadotrophic (hCG) (Veek et al 1983) which could be expected to saturate all luteinizing hormone (LH) receptor sites on growing ovarian follicles and thereby initiate the final phase of oocyte maturation. There are maturation inhibitors within follicular fluid which maintain even fully grown oocytes in meiotic arrest.

The induction of the normal process of oocyte maturation is mediated by the signals from granulosa cells (Moor et al 1981) and involves the action of follicle-stimulating hormone (FSH) as well as specific changes in ovarian steroids. Absence of the granulosa cells, inhibition of their normal function or alteration to the sequence of hormonal changes and cytological events may result in incomplete oocyte maturation, despite the completion of chromosomal changes which are frequently used as indicators of oocyte maturity (Moore et al 1981, Staigmiller & Moor 1984). The sequelae of incomplete or incorrect oocyte maturation are: failure of fertilization and pronuclear formation (Thibault 1977); polyspermic fertilization (Sathananthan & Trounson 1982); oocyte or embryo fragmentation; retardation of embryonic cleavage and inviability of early cleavage stage embryos (Moor & Trounson 1977, Moor et al 1980, Crosby et al 1981).

If, in spontaneous ovulation, oocytes which have not completely matured are produced at times, this will be a source of reproductive failure. In the case of superovulation and IVF, the wastage will be exaggerated by the lack of synchrony in the growth of multiple follicles and the aspiration of oocytes from follicles which would not normally be ovulated. Despite attempts to identify follicular components which completely identify mature oocytes (Carson et al 1982) there is no consensus on any single parameter which can completely identify viable oocytes (Hillier et al 1985). As a result of this difficulty all oocytes obtained for IVF are normally inseminated so that the regularly cleaving embryos can be selected for transfer to the uterus. Since there is no information on the incidence of abnormally matured oocytes and premature or postmature oocytes in natural ovulatory cycles, the contribution of this factor to human reproductive failure cannot be estimated.

Chromosomal abnormalities of human oocytes

Martin et al (1986) found that in 50 oocytes which were quinicrine-banded to determine structural normality of chromosomes, 16 (32%) had abnormal chromosome numbers or had chromosomal structural abnormalities. The data were obtained from karyotyping spare oocytes from an IVF programme in which the patients were super-ovulated with fertility drugs. The chromosomal abnormalities observed in this study may include a component due to superovulation. However, recent data (Gras et al 1992) have shown that the incidence of chromosomal eneuploidies are not significantly different in oocytes retrieved from patients stimulated with Clomid/HMG/HRG and buserulin-flare protocol compared with oocytes obtained from IVF patients in the natural cycle. The vast majority of studies on the rates of chromosomal aneuploidies in human oocytes preimplantation human embryos put the incidence at between 20% and 35% (Kola et al 1993). This figure is significantly higher than that found in animal studies. It is unknown whether the higher incidence in humans is due to a species difference or the fact that these studies have been carried out on oocytes or embryos derived from infertile patients.

Aneuploidy in human spermatozoa is more consistently estimated at about 9% (Martin 1984) which means that there is probably a higher incidence of chromosomal abnormalities in human oocytes than in sperm. The excessive loss of chromosomes in oogenesis could be due to anomalies in meiosis, such as anaphase lag, and excess hypoploidy has been observed in females of other species. There is a concern about the accumulation of chemicals collectively referred to as biozides in the follicular fluid of women (Trapp et al 1984), which may increase the possibility of chromosomal aberrations. This becomes more concerning if the higher estimates of oocyte abnormality of around 30% are correct because this is substantially higher than for other species. The human female is also unusual in that oocytes formed before birth are not used for reproduction on average for 20–25 years which represents a very long period for the accumulated effects of any biozides. It would certainly be of interest to know whether oocyte chromosomal abnormalities vary according to the type of environmental exposure or community in which women are living.

FERTILIZATION

Sperm capacitation

Human sperm, unlike those of many other species, develop the ability to fertilize the oocyte under relatively non-specific conditions. Removal of the seminal plasma component of the ejaculate will result in the progressive capacitation of human sperm and, at any time during incubation after separation of the sperm from seminal plasma, highly motile and acrosome-reacted sperm may be observed to be present. Capacitation includes specific morphological, biochemical and physiological changes in the membranes of the sperm head (Meizel 1978, Yanagimachi 1981).

During capacitation there are marked changes in sperm membrane binding of many substances, including immunoglobulins and lectins (Koehler 1978) and these changes involve glycosylation in order to transform surface glycoproteins into those which enable sperm to bind and fertilize oocytes (Ahuja 1985a). There is also increased sperm motility observed during capacitation and finally the acrosome reaction occurs (Figs 3.1, 3.2). The acrosome reaction involves the fusion and vesiculation of the plasma membrane with the outer acrosomal membrane (Soupart 1980, Sathananthan 1984). The acrosome consists of a cap and an equatorial segment and the acrosome reaction may occur in two stages, with the cap reacting first followed by the equatorial segment (Fig. 3.1).

Capacitation usually occurs within the female reproductive tract and is difficult to initiate in vitro in many species. Human sperm capacitate spontaneously in vitro in chemically very simple culture media. It is not necessary for human sperm to be exposed to follicle cells or to follicular fluid for fertilization to occur (Mahadevan & Trounson 1985) nor to supplement culture medium which contains oocytes surrounded by follicle cells with any other protein (Caro & Trounson 1986). A comprehensive review of conditions which enable human sperm

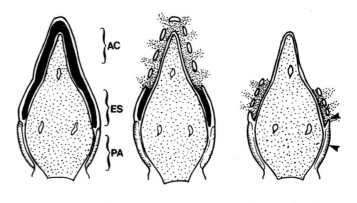

ACROSOME REACTION

NON-REACTED   REACTING   REACTED

Fig. 3.1 Human sperm acrosome reaction. The illustration of sperm heads shows progressive vesiculation of surface membranes caused by fusion of the plasma and outer acrosomal membranes. The acrosome is the dark structure and consists of a cap (AC) and and equatorial segment (ES). The anterior region of the postacrosomal region (PA) is the fusogenic midsegment of the spermhead (arrowheads). The acrosomal enzymes are shown diffusing out of the acrosome after vesiculation. The nucleus (stippled) occupies most of the head region of the sperm. Reproduced with permission from Sathananthan et al (1986b).

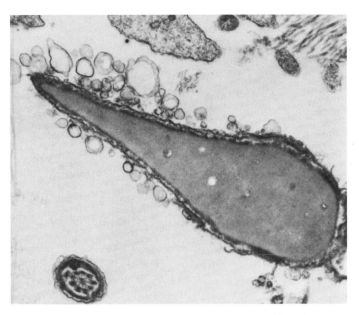

Fig. 3.2 Human sperm head, entering the zona pellucida and undergoing the acrosome reaction by vesiculation of surface membranes. Electron micrograph × 44 100.

to fertilize zona-free hamster oocytes has been published by Yanagimachi (1984). These conditions appear to be the same as those required for human sperm to fertilize human oocytes in vitro.

There are sufficient levels of the enzyme hyaluronidase in seminal plasma or released by the sperm themselves during the acrosome reaction to digest the cumulus oophorus, which is a complex of granulosa and corona radiata cells embedded in a matrix of hyaluronic acid. In fact, the acrosome releases two major enzymes, hyaluronidase and acrosin, a protein-digesting enzyme which is believed to be involved in sperm penetration of the zona pellucida. Both acrosome-reacted and unreacted sperm can be observed in the close vicinity of the zona pellucida but it is only the acrosome-reacted sperm that are capable of penetrating through the glycoprotein matrix of the zona. Sperm bind to the zona pellucida and capacitated sperm are acrosome reacted by a glycoprotein component of the zona (ZP3) which aggregates receptors on the sperm head, exposing proteolytic enzymes on the inner acrosomal membrane and secondary binding receptors, allowing sperm penetration of the zona. The attachment of sperm to the zona is species-specific, involving the binding of specific glycoprotein moieties of the zona and sperm surface membranes (Yanagimachi 1981, Ahuja 1985b).

Sperm transport can also be influenced by a number of conditions within the female reproductive tract. Sperm more readily capacitate under alkaline conditions than in acid conditions which prevail in the vagina. Sperm may be quickly immobilized by immunoglobulins in cervical mucus or by subtle changes in the physical and chemical nature of cervical mucus. It is considered that abnormalities of sperm transport are probably responsible for idiopathic (undiagnosed) infertility because both IVF and gamete intrafallopian tube transfer (GIFT), where sperm and oocytes are transferred together into the Fallopian tube (Asch et al 1984), are effective therapies for this type of infertility. Subtle changes in the chemical composition of cervical mucus and in uterine and tubal secretions may reduce the number of capacitated sperm in the tubal ampulla, reducing the chance of fertilization.

The process of fertilization

Fertilization normally occurs in the ampulla of the Fallopian tube. The actual fertilizable lifespan of the human oocyte after ovulation is not known precisely, but apparently mature oocytes obtained for IVF may be inseminated with sperm 19–25 hours after aspiration from the follicle. They can be fertilized and develop normally to term when transferred to the uterus (Fishel et al 1984). Fertilization may also occur outside the Fallopian tube, for example in the uterus (Craft et al 1982), and very rarely, intraovarian pregnancies may occur when the oocyte is retained in the ruptured follicle. Sperm can be found in the pouch of Douglas within a few hours of intercourse or artificial insemination (Templeton & Mortimer 1980). There are no accurate data on the fertilizable lifespan of human sperm in vivo, but they may retain their capacity to fertilize zona-denuded hamster oocytes for 6–14 days and human oocytes for 5 days when kept at room temperatures (Cohen et al 1985).

There are relatively few sperm at the site of fertilization in most species following natural intercourse, in contrast with the number of sperm (10 000–200 000/ml) used in IVF or transferred with oocytes to the ampulla in the GIFT technique. Reduction of sperm concentration below 10 000/ml in vitro may result in a lowering of fertilization rate (Wolf et al 1984) and the apparent difference in sperm concentrations required for fertilization in vivo and in vitro may be due to selection of sperm by the natural barriers in vivo and more effective capacitation of sperm which migrate to the ampulla in vivo. The presence of the large sticky cumulus at the time of ovulation is important for transport of the oocyte from the surface of the ovary into the ampulla. Cilia on the surface of the fimbria of the Fallopian tube sweep the oocyte cumulus mass into the ciliated ampulla and may assist in moving the oocyte towards the ampulla–isthmus junction. The oocyte is progressively denuded of follicle cells by tubal proteases and never remains stationary because of cilial agitation and ampullary contractions. These movements effectively increase the chance of the few sperm present making contact with the oocyte. Damage to the tubal transport mechanisms may reduce the chance of fertilization and may contribute to the incidence of infertility.

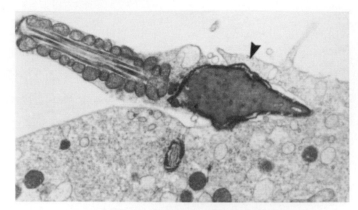

Fig. 3.3 Sperm–egg fusion in the human: the spermhead has been engulfed by a tongue-like process extended from the egg-surface (arrowhead) and the midsegment of the sperm plasma membrane has fused with the oolemma on either side. Electron micrograph × 27 300. Reproduced with permission from Sathananthan et al (1986a).

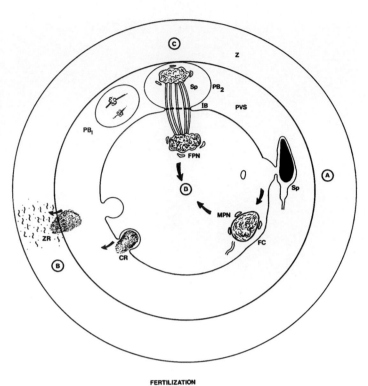

FERTILIZATION

Fig. 3.4 Illustration of the morphological events of fertilization: Ⓐ Sperm–egg fusion and sperm incorporation. Ⓑ Cortical and zona reactions. Ⓒ Completion of meiotic maturation by extrusion of the second polar body. Ⓓ Early formation and associated of pronuclei. CR = cortical reaction; FC = fertilization cone; FPN = female pronucleus; IB = interbody; MPN = male pronucleus; PB_1 = first polar body; PB_2, = second polar body; PVS = perivitelline space; Sp = maturation spindle; Z = zona pellucida; ZR = zona reaction. Reproduced with permission from Sathananthan et al (1986b).

The initial process of fertilization involves passage of the sperm through the cumulus and zona pellucida, entry of the sperm into the perivitelline space, fusion of the mid-segment of the sperm head to oocyte plasma membrane (oolemma; Fig. 3.3), release of cortical granules at the surface of the oolemma (Sathananthan & Trounson 1982), and the gradual incorporation of the whole sperm including the flagellum into the ooplasm. These events have been described at the ultrastructural level in an atlas of human IVF by Sathananthan et al (1986b) and are summarized in Figure 3.4.

During fertilization in vitro, sperm enter the zona pellucida obliquely or tangentially but may be observed entering at all angles in the absence of the cumulus. The acrosomal enzymes help to digest a furrow around the apical and lateral segments of the head in the direction of motion propagated by the vigorously moving flagellum. High sperm concentrations around the oocyte result in many sperm entering the zona and may increase the incidence of polyspermic fertilization (Wolf et al 1984). Incomplete zona formation or incomplete oocyte maturation, where cortical granules have not distributed under the surface of the oolemma, also results in polyspermy (Sathananthan & Trounson 1982).

The mature oocyte has many microvilli on the surface of the oolemma which make the initial contact with the sperm head. Sperm incorporation after the initial contact and fusion appears to be an active process because sperm are engulfed by extrusions of the oocyte (Fig. 3.3) and are taken into the ooplasm by the process of phagocytosis (Sathananthan & Chen 1986). Sperm which enter the perivitelline space through the zona are drawn close to the oolemma and held tangentially along one side of the head during the process of membrane fusion. Perpendicular entry of the apex of the sperm head is a feature of zona-denuded oocytes (Sathananthan et al 1986b) in which

the forward thrust of highly motile sperm results in entry with fusion still along the mid-segment of the sperm head. There appears to be no such forward progressive momentum in sperm which enter the perivitelline space through the zona in the human. Only acrosome-reacted or reacting sperm are observed to fuse with the oolemma. The fusion of human sperm with the oolemma may be also mediated by specific molecules but their exact nature is still to be elucidated. Immotile sperm from a patient with Kartagener's syndrome has also resulted in fertilization of zona-denuded human oocytes, showing that sperm motility may not be essential for sperm fusion and incorporation by the oolemma (Ng et al 1987).

The initial reaction of the oocyte to fusion with the sperm head is a rapid and progressive release of the cortical granule contents (Fig. 3.4) from under the oolemma (Sathananthan & Trounson 1982). This appears to progress from the site of sperm fusion and may be accelerated by the rapid efflux of calcium ions from the oocyte. Rapid movement of molecules between closely apposed membranes such as those surrounding the cortical granules and the plasma membrane result in their fusion, releasing cortical contents into the perivitelline space.

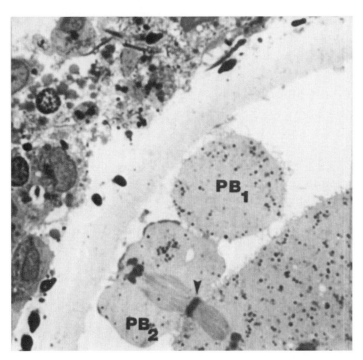

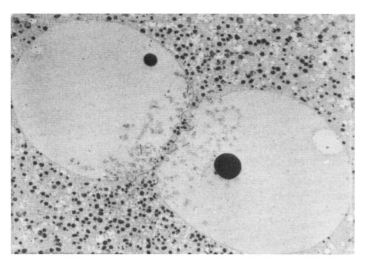

Fig. 3.6 Association of male and female pronuclei in the central ooplasm of a fertilized human ovum. Electron micrograph × 2940. Reproduced with permission from Sathananthan et al (1987).

Fig. 3.5 Extrusion of the second polar body into the perivitelline space at fertilization. Chromosomes are located at each pole of the telophase II spindle, associated with an interbody (arrowhead). Supplementary sperm are seen in the outer zona. PB_1 = first polar body; PB_2 = second polar body. Light micrograph × 1500. Reproduced with permission from Sathananthan (1984).

Cortical granules may fuse with one another at the same time. The cortical contents contain a zona hardening substance which diffuses into the inner zona causing the zona reaction. Alteration occurs to the chemical structure of the inner zona which becomes more electron-dense, traps any sperm in the vicinity and prevents them from penetrating though the zona pellucida. This is the mechanism which normally blocks polyspermy and any delay of the cortical reaction or breach in the zona will usually result in fertilization by more than one sperm.

Sperm fusion with the oolemma also initiates the completion of meiosis in the oocyte (Fig. 3.5). The daughter chromatids held in the second metaphase stage are separated by the microtubules of the anaphase spindle and one complete set of chromosomes is expelled from the oocyte in the extrusion of the second polar body (Sathananthan et al 1986b). Nuclear membranes begin to form around the set of chromosomes retained by the oocyte in close proximity to the second polar body. The sperm head decondenses in the ooplasm and detaches from the flagellum. Specific cytoplasmic factors (proteins) are required for this, and are generated during oocyte maturation (Thibault 1977). A nuclear membrane is also formed around the sperm chromosomes.

Decondensing sperm heads can be located in the ooplasm within 3 hours of inseminating oocytes in vitro (McMaster et al 1978, Sathananthan et al 1986a,b).

Pronuclei are visible by 6 hours and may move from peripheral locations to the centre of the oocyte by 12 hours after insemination. The male and female pronuclei in the human are of about equal size (Fig. 3.6) and remain separate but very close together until 20–24 hours after insemination, at which time the nuclear membranes are dismantled (Sathananthan & Trounson 1985). At the time the nuclear membrane disappears, a bipolar spindle forms with apices at opposite poles of the pronuclei. The condensing chromosomes are mixed on the metaphase plate of the first cleavage division in a stage termed syngamy. The pronuclei are no longer visible during syngamy and the time between disappearance of the pronuclei and the first cleavage division is 3–6 hours.

It is at syngamy that the maternal and paternal chromosomes are mixed for the first time, restoring the normal diploid constitution of the cell. DNA replication occurs during the pronuclear stage so that equal numbers of paternal and maternal chromosomes will be drawn into each daughter cell by the microtubules during anaphase of the first cleavage division. The cleavage furrow separates the identical components of the new embryonic genome at telophase into equal sized daughter cells or blastomeres. Cleavage is a rapid event, taking less than 10 minutes, and it is at this time that fragmentation may occur. The formation of small anucleate fragments does not normally effect embryonic viability (Killeen & Moore 1971) but severe fragmentation of many different sized anucleate bodies can be a lethal abnormality. Fragmentation occurs frequently in vitro under suboptimal culture conditions and may also be due to incomplete or abnormal oocyte maturation.

Syngamy, rapidly followed by the first cleavage division, marks the completion of fertilization. The pronuclear oocyte has been termed the zygote and initial cleavage stage have been also termed zygote or conceptus. The first cleavage stage until blastocyst stage is usually termed preimplantation embryo (pre-embryo), cleavage stage embryo or conceptus.

Recently we discovered sperm centrioles in human embryos at the pronuclear stage and at syngamy (Sathananthan et al 1991). The centriole is an enigma in cell biology and its role in cell division is little understood. Most cells have centrioles but oocytes do not. It is a minute object composed of microtubules organized in triplets resembling a pinwheel. There are usually two centrioles aligned perpendicular to one another and surrounded by dense material, the centrosomes nucleate spindle microtubules during mitosis.

The sperm cell has a single functional centriole in its neck region, which is thought to be the kinetic centre of sperm motility. At fertilization, the whole sperm including its tail is incorporated into the ooplasm and the centriolar complex, centriole and surrounding pericentriolar substance (centrosome), remains in close association with the developing male pronucleus and is finally located at one pole of the first mitotic spindle at syngamy (Fig. 3.7). The human embryo thereby inherits the paternal centriole from the fertilizing sperm. There is further evidence that this paternal centriole duplicates and continues to be involved during preimplantation embryonic cleavage (Sathananthan et al 1990). The inheritance of paternal centrioles in the human follows the sea urchin pattern of inheritance, a theory first postulated by Bovem

in 1900, and is common to most animals, except the mouse where the centrosome is maternally derived (Schatten et al 1991).

Fertilization rates

There are very few data on the failure of fertilization in vivo after natural intercourse. Factors contributing to fertilization failure may be both maternal and paternal in origin and will include reduced semen quality, intercourse at an inappropriate time relative to ovulation and factors within the female reproductive tract which reduce sperm transport and survival.

Both IVF and GIFT have been used as treatments for male factor infertility because pregnancy rates with these techniques are higher than those achieved by carefully timed intercourse and artificial insemination with the husband's semen. The probability of pregnancy in male factor infertility may be computed by life table analyses (Baker et al 1986) and compared with pregnancy success rate by IVF (Yates & de Kretser 1987). From data available in IVF, it is apparent that implantation and pregnancy rates for couples with male factor infertility are similar to those with tubal infertility if fertilization can be achieved.

Polyspermy

Multipronuclear oocytes are observed to occur in 2–10% of fertilized oocytes in IVF. The majority (>80%) are tripronuclear and are due primarily to dispermic fertilization (Sathananthan et al 1986b). This is considered the major cause of triploidy which may result in failure of preimplantation embryo development, spontaneous abortion, hydatiform moles and occasionally chorionic tumours or the birth of severely abnormal infants.

A study of tripronuclear oocytes (Kola et al 1987) has shown that the majority (62%) cleave directly to three cells rather than two cells at the first cleavage division. Indeed, recent data (Sathananthan et al 1991) has shown that three cornered spindles are found in dispermic human oocytes; thus providing a mechanism for the cleavage from one to three cells.

Chromosome numbers in the three individual cells are variable but are never exactly diploid. This may be a lethal condition of chromosome mosaicism with severe hypoploidy and hyperploidy and development is probably limited to preimplantation cleavage. The remainder (38%) of tripronuclear oocytes cleave either to two cells (24%) which are triploid or to two cells which are diploid and an extrusion (14%) which probably contains a haploid set of chromosomes. It is possible that the diploid embryos could contain either maternal and paternal chromosomes and develop normally or contain two sets of paternal chromosomes and be androgenones which

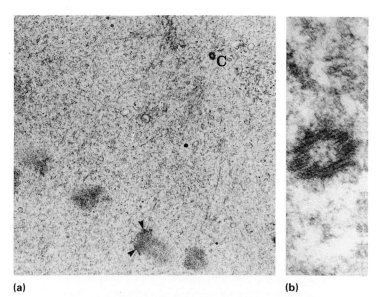

(a)   **(b)**

Fig. 3.7 Bipolar spindle of a human I-cell embryo in syngamy. (**a**) A centriole (C) is visible at one pole of half a spindle depicted in this electron micrograph. Spindle MT extend from the pole to chromosomes, connecting at kinetochores (arrows). The spindle zone is usually devoid of other organelles. × 13 200. (**b**) Centriole in oblique cross section at higher magnification. It presents the typical '9 + 0' structure consisting of nine triplets of MT arranged in a circle. × 35 750. Reproduced from Sathananthan et al 1991.

develop abnormally, including the possibility of tropho-blastic disease (hydatiform moles and chorionic cancer; Patillo & Hussa 1984).

Androgenones have been made in the mouse using nuclear transplantation techniques. The maternal pronucleus is removed and a second paternal pronucleus introduced by micromanipulation. The majority of these artificial androgenones do not implant and those that do, develop abundant trophoblast whilst the embryonic component fails to develop normally (Barton et al 1984). Gynogenones made by transferring a second maternal pronucleus to an oocyte after removal of the paternal pronucleus or by parthenogenetic activation (Barton et al 1984) develop to about the 25 somite stage of embryonic development with inadequate trophoblast and other extraembryonic tissue. These experiments amply demonstrate that both maternally and paternally derived chromosomes are essential for normal embryogenesis in mammalian species (McGrath & Solter 1984, Mann & Lovell-Badge 1984, Surani et al 1984, 1986) and provide evidence for genomic imprinting.

EMBRYONIC DEVELOPMENT

Preimplantation embryonic cleavage

The first cleavage stage occurs about 16–22 hours after penetration of the oocyte by the fertilizing sperm (Trounson et al 1982). The second and third cleavage stages (Fig. 3.8) occur at 12–20-hour intervals (Cummins et al 1986). In the mouse the first major product of the new embryonic genome appears at the mid 2-cell stage and has been identified as heat shock protein 70 (Bensaude et al 1983). It is interesting that the embryonic genome may be activated by production of a stress protein and that this occurs in the mouse at the time when many strains of mice have a block (2-cell block) of cleavage in vitro (Fig. 3.9). It is not certain when the human embryonic genome is activated but preliminary experiments suggest this may be between the 4- and 8-cell stage (Tesarik et al 1986, Braude et al 1988).

In the mouse at the late 8-cell stage a process of compaction occurs when the cells flatten against each other and become firmly adherent by specific glycoproteins and focal tight junctions (Kimber et al 1982, Pratt et al 1982). Blastomeres of the compacting 8-cell embryo become polarized (Ziomek & Johnson 1980) and give rise to a heterogeneous population of large polar cells or small non-polar cells when they divide to 16 cells (Johnson & Ziomek 1981). The small non-polar cells are completely internalized and the large polar cells form the outside cells of the morula. It can be shown that the inside or non-polar cells develop into inner cell mass cells and the outside or polar cells develop into the trophoblast lineage (Johnson 1986). Compaction occurs at the late 8-cell

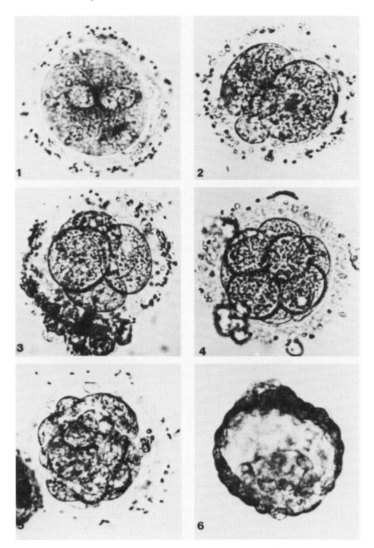

Fig. 3.8 Stages of human preimplanatation development. 1. Pronuclear oocyte 16 hours after insemination. 2. Two-cell embryo. 3. Four cell embryo. 4. Eight cell embryo. 5. Compacted morula (16 cells). 6. Hatched blastocyst. The inner cell mass is at the lower pole surrounded by trophoblast cells and blastocelic cavity above. Reproduced with permission from Trounson et al (1982).

stage or during the next cleavage division in human embryos cultured in vitro (Trounson et al 1982). Figure 3.10 shows the compaction of individual blastomeres in a late 8-cell stage human embryo. It is presumed that the blastomeres of the human embryo undergo the same polarization and positioning within the morula as mouse embryos.

Individual blastomeres of the 8-cell mouse embryos lose their totipotency or capacity to form a complete embryo by themselves (Tarkowski & Wroblewska 1976). This may be due to their inability to form sufficient daughter blastomeres before blastulation rather than any intrinsic differentiation. Single blastomeres of 8-cell embryos often cleave and one daughter cell completely internalizes the other in the attempt of compaction (Johnson 1986). Division then ceases. In other species such as the sheep,

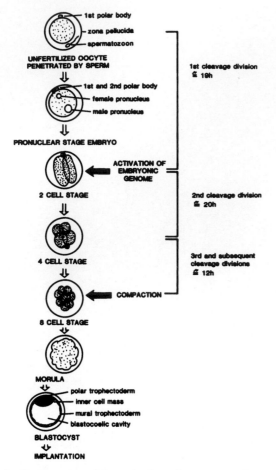

Fig. 3.9 Development of the preimplantation mouse embryo.

totipotency still exists at the 8-cell stage; live lambs have been obtained from single blastomeres of this cleavage stage (Willadsen 1981). Compaction occurs at the 16-cell stage and blastulation at the sixth cleavage division in sheep embryos. Interestingly, even single blastomeres of more than 50 cells and inner cell mass cells of the blastulating sheep and cow embryo, when fused into enucleated oocytes, can develop to term, indicating that the nuclei of these late preimplantation embryos have not differentiated and retain their totipotency if cycled through oocyte cytoplasm. In the mouse, blastulation occurs at the fifth cleavage division irrespective of the number of cells. In an intact embryo there are 32 cells with both inside (non-polar) and outside (polar) cells. Blastulation occurs by the pumping of extracellular fluid by outside cells into an intercellular space in the compacted embryo. This fluid-filled cavity, a blastocele, increases in size, flattening the outside cells against the zona pellucida. The inside cells remain closely attached together at one pole of the blastocyst, becoming the inner cell mass. The flattened outside cells are structurally differentiated into a single layer of flattened trophoblast cells connected by tight junctions and gap junctions. Blastulation in the human occurs at the sixth cleavage

division and the morphological structure of the blastocyst is similar to other species (Fig. 3.8; Mohr & Trounson 1982).

Inner cell mass cells are primarily undifferentiated cells which eventually develop into both embryonic and extra-embryonic lineages. The blastocyst emerges from the zona pellucida by the pressure of the expanding blastocele forcing a crack in the thinned zona. The trophoblast cells emerge through the crack, giving a dumb-bell appearance to the hatching blastocyst. Our observations of human embryos in vitro suggest that division of the inner cell mass during hatching through the crack made in the zona can form two inner cell masses, and may be a mechanism involved in the formation of identical twins. For the first time the cells of the embryo escaping from the zona are able to make direct contact with the endo-metrial cells and it is the trophoblast cells which initiate the maternal–embryonic association necessary for con-tinued embryonic development and the maintenance of pregnancy.

Preimplantation embryonic cleavage is relatively syn-chronous up to the third cleavage stage; thereafter the cell cycles are less and less synchronized and by the blas-tocyst stage usually only 10–20% of cells are in mitosis at the same time. From observations in IVF, embryos are 2-celled 24–36 hours after insemination, 4-celled 40–50 hours, 8-celled 52–70 hours, compact 70–86 hours and begin blastulation around 100–120 hours, hatching from the zona 110–140 hours (Trounson et al 1982, Cummins et al 1986). Implantation begins on the fifth or sixth day after fertilization.

DNA methylation in germ cells and embryos

Interest in DNA methylation in the developing embryo is generated by its relationship to gene expression. Current data suggest that a difference exists in the DNA methylation patterns of male and female germ cells. Sanford et al (1984) have shown that the DNA of oocytes is undermethylated for the repetitive sequences, both centromeric and dispersed; it seems probable that oocytes are globally undermethylated. In contrast, the DNA of male germ cells becomes remethylated during sperma-togenesis (perhaps at the stage of meiotic arrest) and remains methylated overall. It has been shown (Waalwijk & Flavell 1978) that certain structural genes in sperm are highly methylated. Centromeric sequences in sperm, however, have been shown to be undermethylated (Chapman et al 1984, Ponzetto-Zimmerman & Wolgemuth 1984). The significance of the differential pattern of DNA methylation of male and female germ cells remains to be elucidated.

In other cells a considerable body of evidence now exists which correlates the methylation status of cytosine moieties at certain sites within and near an autosomal

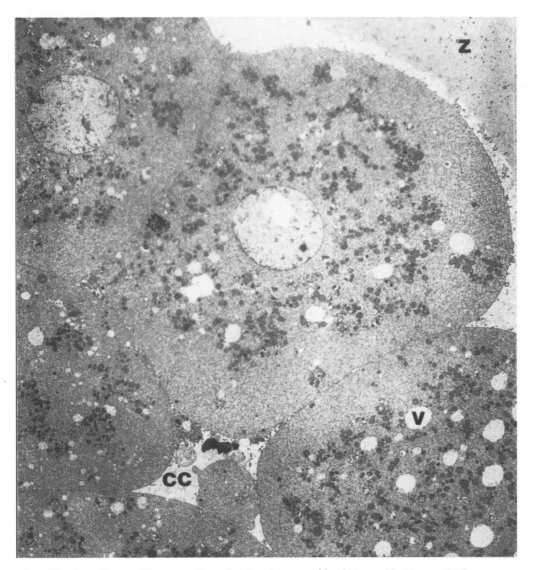

Fig. 3.10   Part of an 8-cell human embryo showing close apposition between blastomeres (early compaction). CC = cleavage cavity; V = vacuole; Z = zona pellucida. Electron micrograph × 2940. Reproduced with permission from Sathananthan et al (1982).

gene with its potential to be expressed (Razin & Riggs 1980, Doerfler 1983). Thus when a gene is expressed in a particular tissue, the tendency is for it to be under-methylated and to reside in regions of chromatin more accessible to digestion by the enzyme deoxyribonuclease (Groudine et al 1980, Doerfler 1983). Chapman et al (1984) have also shown that DNA from all derivatives of the two extraembryonic mouse embryo lineages, troph-ectoderm and primitive endoderm, was substantially undermethylated compared with primitive ectoderm de-rivatives and adult somatic tissues. These same sequences, however, appear to be fully methylated at 7.5 days of development in the primitive ectoderm cell lineage, which gives rise to the embryo. It has been suggested (Chapman et al 1984) that both specific demethylation of some cytosine CpG sites and failure of de novo methylation may be occurring in preimplantation embryos.

Data on the molecular basis of X chromosome inactiva-tion in mammals suggest that regulation is due to multiple events, one of which is DNA methylation. Holliday & Pugh (1975) proposed that methylation of the pyrimidine base cytosine in DNA might provide a molecular mecha-nism for X chromosome inactivation in female cells. Inactivation of the X chromosome during mouse embryonic development occurs sequentially; firstly as the extra-embryonic lineages differentiate, the paternally inherited X chromosome is inactivated preferentially (Monk 1981) and secondly, just prior to gastrulation the X chromo-some is randomly activated, i.e. either the maternal or paternal X chromosome is inactivated. Interestingly, when cells in which the X chromosome is inactive are treated with azacytidine (a chemical which demethylates DNA), the X chromosome is reactivated. Monk (1981) has pro-posed that X chromosome inactivation is coupled to cell differentiation. It has been shown that not all the genes on the inactive X chromosome are inactivated, e.g. the *Xist* gene on the inactive X chromosome is transcriptionally active. Curiously, however, it is not translated into a protein. Similarly, the H19 gene, which is also imprinted, is not translated into a functional protein. The relationship between genomic imprinting and DNA methylation could prove intriguing.

Teratogens and the preimplantation embryo

Most of the research on the effects of exposure of teratogenic stimuli has been directed at the postimplantation stages of pregnancy and more specifically during the period of organogenesis. It is generally agreed that the developing embryo is most susceptible to the induction of malformations during the period of organogenesis. The preimplantation mammalian embryo however, has been shown to be relatively refractory to teratogenesis (i.e. malformations) and this has led to the wide acceptance of the all-or-none phenomenon. This has been interpreted by some teratologists as meaning that the exposure of preimplantation mammalian embryos to noxious physical and chemical stimuli may result in the death of the embryo before implantation or the embryo will survive to term without being malformed (see Spielmann et al 1981).

The effects on preimplantation mouse embryos have been investigated using the immunosuppressive and alkylating agent cyclophosphamide (a potent teratogen in animals) as a model. Cyclophosphamide was shown to have a significant effect on preimplantation embryo viability (Kola & Folb 1986). Viable cyclophosphamide-treated blastocysts were shown to have fewer cells (Eibs & Spielmann 1977, Kola & Folb 1985) and the cells displayed a significant increase in chromosomal aberrations (Kola et al 1986) and sister chromatid exchanges. Preimplantation embryo differentiation was adversely affected and a significantly higher number of embryos were resorbed during organogenesis (Kola et al 1986). However, the number of malformed embryos retrieved at term was not significantly affected. The only detectable difference at term was that the cyclophosphamide-treated fetuses were lower in weight than corresponding controls.

These data demonstrate that teratogenic exposure of preimplantation mammalian embryos induces embryo and fetal loss and that the embryos appear to be refractory to the induction of morphologically detectable abnormalities. However, caution should be exercised in drawing firm conclusions about whether or not malformations can be induced by expressing preimplantation mammalian embryos to teratogens, as Takeuchi (1984) has reported that the exposure of preimplantation mouse embryos to methylnitrosurea induced malformations in embryos retrieved at term. Iannaccone (1984) has shown that methylnitrosurea-treated neonatal mice (exposed to the drug at the blastocyst stage and then transferred into pseudopregnant recipients) had a three-fold higher crude mortality rate than corresponding controls.

Nutrition and transport of the preimplantation embryo

Although preimplantation cleavage stage embryos can develop in vitro in the absence of any exogenous fixed nitrogen source (protein or amino acids) from the 1-cell to the blastocyst stages (Cholewa & Whitten 1965, Caro & Trounson 1984, 1986), development in culture (as determined by increases in blastocyst formation and cell number) is significantly increased by the inclusion of specific amino acids (Gardner & Lane 1993, Gardner et al 1993). In the mouse embryo, non-essential amino acids promote cleavage stage development (Gardner & Lane 1994) whilst essential amino acids are required for blastocyst hatching and outgrowth in vitro (Spindle & Pedersen 1973). The capacity to develop without exogenous amino acids or protein shows that the early cleavage stages are able to utilize endogenous fixed nitrogen sources for protein synthesis or they convert exogenous energy substrates (glucose, lactate and pyruvate) into amino acids (glutamate, aspartate and alanine; Wales 1975). The protein content of mouse embryos decreases by 26% during the first 3 days of embryonic development (Brinster 1967), as do some of the amino acid pools (Schultz et al 1981) and there is relatively little uptake of exogenous protein before the blastocyst stage (Pemble & Kaye 1986). These observations suggest a preferential utilization of endogenous fixed nitrogen during early cleavage and development. The oocyte and preimplantation embryo can synthesize protein from radiolabelled amino acids (Levinson et al 1978) and it is apparent that both endogenous and exogenous amino acids may by used for metabolism in vivo. There is a marked increase in the utilization of exogenous amino acids and protein at the blastocyst stage.

The preimplantation embryo requires exogenous energy sources, primarily lactate and glucose (Brinster 1963). However only pyruvate can act as a single energy source for the first cleavage division (Biggers et al 1967) and the combination of pyruvate and lactate as well as glucose in culture media enables cleavage readily to occur from the 1-cell to blastocyst stage in vitro (Biggers et al 1965). These studies provided the basis for all embryo culture media presently in use.

As distinct from many other species, the human preimplantation embryo can complete development and implant in either the Fallopian tube or the uterus. In the human, ectopic or tubal pregnancy occurs quite frequently but this is exceedingly rare in other species. Fertilization and complete preimplantation development in the uterus was demonstrated by Craft et al (1982), who reported pregnancies after the transfer of sperm and oocytes into the uterus. Others had demonstrated that pronuclear and 2-cell embryos transferred to the uterus result in pregnancy (Trounson et al 1982). These observations show that human tubal and uterine secretions or even peritoneal fluid are relatively non-specific for embryonic nutrition and that embryonic transport from the Fallopian tube to the uterus is not essential for preimplantation embryonic survival, growth and development. Embryos which implant in the tube are unable to proceed to term because of space limitations. The expanding embryo may often cause rupture of the tube, resulting in serious haemorrhage. Ectopic pregnancies which do grow outside the tube or rupture the tube without causing maternal death may develop to term.

The fimbria of the Fallopian tube is responsible for removal of the ovulated oocyte–cumulus mass from the surface of the ovary. Fimbriectomy has been used as a method of sterilization and in most species ovulated oocytes remain on the surface of the ovary if the fimbria is interfered with around the time of ovulation. The oocyte is moved in ampulla by the action of cilia and slow peristaltic contractions of the ampulla. These contractions run from the fimbrial end towards the isthmus, fading at the ampulla–isthmus junction. This is the primary mechanism of oocyte and embryo transport in the Fallopian tube (Thibault 1972) and is supported by reports of fertility in women with Kartagener's syndrome where cilia are immotile (Jean et al 1979). There are strong antiperistaltic contractions in the isthmus under the control of oestrogen and progesterone. These contractions maintain the early

cleavage stage embryo at the ampulla–isthmus junction for about 3 day (Croxatto et al 1978). With increasing dominance of progesterone to oestrogen, the antiperistaltic contractions weaken and the embryo passes rapidly into the uterus. It has been shown that surgical removal of the isthmus has no effect on fertility or on embryo survival and development in the pig (Paterson et al 1981).

It is also of interest to note that embryos of many species may develop for 3–4 days in the Fallopian tubes of another species. For example, cow embryos develop normally in the rabbit oviduct (Lawson et al 1972). This supports the notion that the nutritional requirements of the early cleavage stage embryo are relatively non-specific but the cleavage rate of embryos in vitro is usually retarded (Harlow & Quinn 1982) so that prolonged culture in vitro reduces embryo viability in all species studied to date.

Pre- and postimplantation embryonic normality and survival

Accurate figures for embryonic wastage during the first 2 weeks of development in the human are not readily available. Estimates by Leridon (1977; based on the work of Hertig et al 1956, French & Bierman 1962) calculate embryonic wastage in the first week (from fertilization to the commencement of implantation) at 18% with a further 39% of embryos failing in the second week of development (Table 3.1). Further support for this high early embryonic wastage rate in the human compared with most other mammalian species studied comes from the work of Buster et al (1985). Of 25 preimplantation

Table 3.1 Embryonic and fetal wastage in vivo and vitro*

Source of pregnancy, wastage and outcome	Natural conception		In vitro fertilization†	
	Wastage (%)	Cumulative survival (%)	Wastage (%)	Cumulative survival (%)
		100		100
Fertilization failure	16	84	14	86
Failure of preimplantation zygote development				
days 14–16 for IVF			2	84
days 14–21 for natural conception	18	69		
Implantation failure				
days 17–28 for IVF			82	15
days 22–28 for natural conception	39	42		
Pregnancy loss between weeks 5 and 40	26	31	34	9
Live births	—	31	—	9

*These estimates were of embryonic wastage following natural conception (based on Leridon 1977) and IVF (based on unpublished data from the Monash IVF programme, 1983–86). These calculations assume that the sperm and ova are brought into contact in all cases. (This is obviously not the case under natural circumstances where a number of problems, including anovulation, reduced semen quality and intercourse at the incorrect time can interfere. Estimates of maximum human fecundability calculated to include these additional factors range from 14.4% to 31.8% for various populations and age groups of women; Leridon 1977.)
†IVF figures for fertilization, embryo development and implantation are per patient, not per embryo. Following superovulation an average of five oocytes is normally collected. The respective failure rates per oocyte or embryo are: fertilization 30%, early development 10%; implantation 90%.

embryos flushed from the uterus between 93 and 130 hours after ovulation, only five (20%) were at the expected blastocyst stage of development. Studies on the chromosomal numbers of preimplantation embryos also reveal a high rate of abnormalities. In two studies on human embryos obtained either from volunteer egg donors or as spare or reject embryos from IVF, two out of three and eight out of 22 were chromosomally abnormal (Angell et al 1983, 1986). However, these studies may not reflect the normal in vivo situation for three reasons: the high age of the maternal donors (mean 34 years); the fact that all women had undergone superovulation, and the in vitro treatment of the gametes. Karyotyping studies do not identify those embryos with normal chromosome compliments but carrying other genetic abnormalities. Although only 0.56% of liveborn babies are chromosomally abnormal (Evans 1977), over 50% of spontaneous abortions carry a lethal chromosome anomaly (Hassold et al 1980). These figures demonstrate that although there is a high incidence of chromosomal and genetic abnormality in the human preimplantation embryo, such defective embryos are usually lost by pregnancy wastage well before birth.

IMPLANTATION

Embryo implantation encompasses a complex series of events that vary quite markedly between different mammalian species. Understanding of the processes involved in implantation is poor even in the frequently studied laboratory rodents. Needless to say, morphological and physiological information on human implantation is very scarce, with most descriptions relying on a few classical publications (Hertig et al 1956, Knoth & Larsen 1972, O'Rahilly 1973).

In its broadest sense, implantation is taken to include orientation of the blastocyst within the uterus, dissolution of the zona pellucida, attachment, migration through the epithelium, localized disruption of the endometrial capillaries and the formation of trophoblastic lacunae. In the human, these processes take place during the 6th to 12th days after ovulation (ovulation is day 0) although some uncertainty exists about the exact timing of individual events.

It has been estimated that the preimplantation embryo passes through the isthmus into the uterine cavity 68–80 hours after ovulation (Croxatto et al 1978). For the next 40–76 hours the embryo is free-floating within the uterus, which at this stage has a flattened or slit-like lumen. Animal studies have demonstrated precise uterine control over blastocyst orientation and positioning within the uterus during this period (Rogers et al 1983b), and since human implantation generally occurs on the median portion of the uterine wall (equivalent to antimesometrially in a bicornuate uterus) with the embryonic disc oriented towards the endometrium, it is probable that similar mechanisms exist in the human.

In rodent blastocysts, trophoblast cells at the abembryonic pole (opposite to the inner cell mass) become sticky and contain large vesicles of unknown substances. This transformation at the abembryonic pole occurs within a few hours of implantation and is probably the reason why rodent embryos adhere to the endometrium and implant with the embryonic disc orientated away from the endometrium (Lindenberg et al 1989). Secretory vesicles similar to those released from mouse blastocysts can be observed bulging from the surface of human trophoblast cells allowed to implant on endometrial cells in culture (Lindenberg et al 1986, Lindenberg & Hyttel 1988).

In the human, as in the guinea-pig, lemming and chimpanzee, the blastocyst attaches to the uterine wall after escape from the zona pellucida before migrating through the epithelium into the underlying endometrial stroma (Finn & Porter 1975). Since blastocysts can be flushed from the uterine cavity 5 days after ovulation (Buster et al 1985) no firm attachment to the uterine epithelium occurs until about the sixth day. In vitro studies by Lindenberg et al (1986) with implanting human blastocysts show that the polar trophoblast cells adjacent to the inner cell mass are involved in the primary adhesion to the endometrial cells (Fig. 3.11). These in vitro studies show that initial penetration of the epithelium by the polar trophoblast is via long slender ectoplasmic protrusions which insinuate themselves between the endometrial cells (Fig. 3.12). The trophoblast cells were not phagocytotic at this stage as no degenerating epithelial cells were observed. Endometrial cells respond to the initial penetration of the cytotrophoblast by increased membrane activity which may represent either endo- or exocytosis (Fig. 3.13). In most other species similar membrane activity is endocytotic (Parr & Parr 1977). This process may be responsible for the transfer of messengers, which probably include glycoproteins such as hCG necessary for maternal recognition and the maintenance of pregnancy.

Little is known about the local endocrine requirements for human implantation. Local effects of cAMP (Holmes & Bergstrom 1975, Webb 1975) and prostaglandins, particularly PGE_2 (Holmes & Gordashko 1980), have been shown to induce implantation in diapausing mouse blastocysts. Endometrial production of leukaemia inhibitory factor (LIF) is essential for successful implantation in the mouse, as was elegantly demonstrated using homologous recombination in embryonic stem cells containing a non-functional mutant LIF gene (Stewart et al 1992). Females lacking a functional LIF gene can produce normal viable blastocysts, however without LIF production the uterus will not support implantation. Prostaglandins also play a role in the vascular changes seen within the endometrium at the time of implantation (Kennedy &

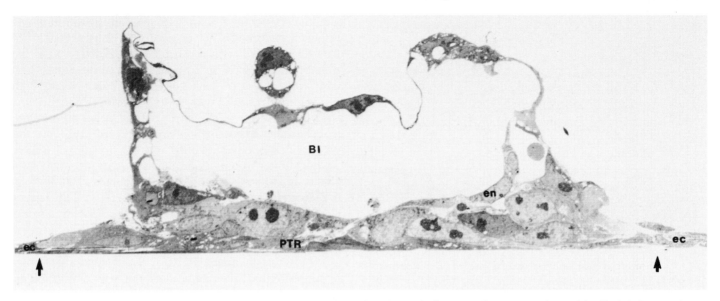

Fig. 3.11   Human blastocyst implanted in vitro with expanded blastocele (BI). Arrows indicate attachment to endometrial cells (ec). Inner cell mass cells, polar trophoblast cells (PTR) and endodermal cells (en) are at the pole of attachment to endometrial cells, and mural trophoblast cells are at the opposite pole. Reproduced by kind permission of Dr Svend Lindenberg.

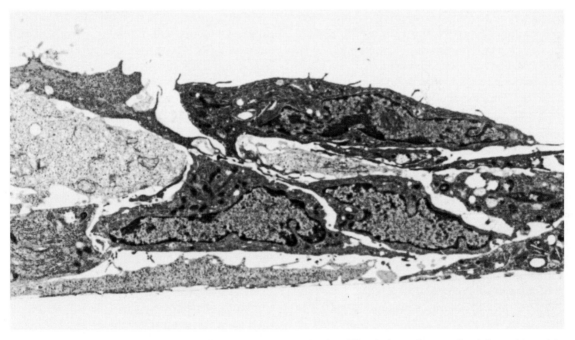

Fig. 3.12   Peripheral implantation zone of a human blastocyst in vitro. The darker cells are cells of the endometrial monolayer and the lighter cells are trophoblast cells with their long protrusions intruding between the endometrial cells. Reproduced by kind permission of Dr Svend Lindenberg.

Armstrong 1981). It is likely that these substances are also involved during human implantation. In addition the production of steroids, such as the sulphated oestrogens by the pig blastocysts may be required for implantation and the maintenance of pregnancy (Perry et al 1973). Reports of plasminogen activator secretion by early embryonic trophoblast and parietal endoderm cells are consistent with the highly invasive nature of the early embryo

and the major tissue reorganization that follows implantation (Strickland et al 1976). It is interesting that in the pig, where the implanting embryo does not breach the uterine epithelium, a uterine-derived progesterone-dependent inhibitor of plasminogen activator nullifies the embryonic secretion of this proteolytic activator (Mullins et al 1981). In comparison, the implantation stage pig embryo is highly invasive when placed in contact with

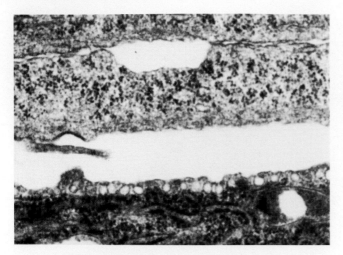

Fig. 3.13 A higher magnification electron micrograph of a trophoblastic ectoplasmic protrusion (see Fig. 3.12) between endometrial cells. Note the pinocytotic activity of closely associated endometrial cells. Reproduced by kind permission of Dr Svend Lindenberg.

non-uterine tissues. The role of plasminogen activator in human implantation is unknown at this time.

By 7–8 days after ovulation the embryo is fully embedded in the superficial layers of the endometrium, and the epithelium has started to migrate inwards to cover the exposed area. At this time the embryonic trophoblast begins to differentiate into syncytiotrophoblast and cytotrophoblast, with the syncytiotrophoblast forming the outermost layer between the endometrium and the invading embryo. The syncytial tissues project into the surrounding endometrium, in what appears to be an invasive growth phase. Intact maternal capillaries can be traced to and from the syncytiotrophoblast, although within these areas red blood cells occupy a series of irregularly shaped spaces (Harris & Ramsey 1966). Macroscopically no congestion or haemorrhage is visible in the endometrium at this time, although microscopic examination reveals dilated capillaries and sinusoids. The embryonic disc is composed of two layers, the epiblast and the primary endoderm. The first signs of an amniotic cavity also appear, probably arising from cells of the embryonic disc (Luckett 1973), although it has been postulated that cytotrophoblastic cells are also involved in its formation.

By the ninth day after ovulation the syncytial mass surrounding the embryo is some 500–600 μm in diameter, while the embryonic disc remains at approximately 100 μm. Maternal endometrial vessels form communications with the numerous lacunae that develop within the syncytiotrophoblast at this stage, as a prelude to the placental circulation. It is not until this stage (9 days after ovulation or 23 days of a standard 28-day menstrual cycle) that predecidual cells first appear in the endometrium surrounding the embryo. Animal studies have shown a major localized increase in uterine vascular permeability and capillary dilatation around the implantation site (Rogers et al 1983a, Tavis & Rogers 1992) leading to significant oedema. Oedema is also clearly seen surrounding the human implantation site at this time. It is probably this oedema, coupled with localized hyperaemia, that makes it possible to visualize human implantation sites from about this stage of development onwards using high-resolution ultrasound with a vaginal probe. The amniotic cavity has nearly developed to a fully enclosed structure by this stage, bordering on an embryonic disc that has not changed size significantly over the previous 3–4 days.

The human implantation site 11–12 days after ovulation is readily recognizable macroscopically as a 1 mm diameter red spot on the mucosal surface of the uterus. This appearance is due to maternal blood passing through the lacunar spaces within the syncytiotrophoblast. By this stage the syncytial mass surrounding the embryo is 750–1000 μm in diameter, with the syncytiotrophoblast forming about three-quarters of the whole trophoblast. Along with the developing lacunar circulation, large numbers of maternal red blood cells appear within the syncytiotrophoblast, apparently undergoing phagocytosis. Oedema around the implantation site is still present, while stromal cells show more signs of decidualization.

At this stage, cells forming the extraembryonic mesoderm, which is still lined by cytotrophoblast, begin to aggregate as precursors to chorionic villus formation. The combined syncytiotrophoblast, cytotrophoblast and extraembryonic mesoderm are collectively termed the chorion by this stage. Ultrastructural studies of an implantation site at this time (Knoth & Larsen 1972) show the syncytiotrophoblast invading maternal vessels, with the syncytium having many microvilli and pinocytotic vesicles at its surface.

Uterine factors in successful implantation

There are considerable data to support the view that the uterus, rather than the embryo, predominantly controls the success or failure of the implantation process. Among well-studied species such as laboratory rodents, it has been shown that the uterus becomes receptive to the implanting blastocyst for a short period of time a few days after the commencement of continuous progesterone administration (De Feo 1963). These and other studies have led to the concept of an implantation window, defined as the period of time when the uterus is receptive to the implanting blastocyst. In addition to the receptive state, it has also been postulated that the uterus goes through 'implantation neutral' and 'implantation hostile' states (Psychoyos & Casimiri 1980). During the neutral phase the embryo can survive in the uterus but will not implant, while during the hostile phase the embryo is actively destroyed. A number of mammalian species utilize embryonic diapause or delayed implantation to maximize reproductive efficiency (Sandell 1990). During diapause blastocyst development is arrested by the uterus until conditions are suitable for pregnancy to continue.

That control over diapause is entirely a uterine phenomenon can easily be shown by removing the blastocyst from the uterine environment, at which time normal development will recommence (Lundkvist & Nilsson 1982). Conversely, recent studies in cattle have shown that under certain conditions the uterus can induce the preimplantation embryo to accelerate its development in order to catch up to the uterus and implant at the optimal time in terms of uterine receptivity (Garrett et al 1988). How the uterus controls diapause, accelerates rates of embryo development, and produces receptive, neutral and hostile states remains largely unclear, although embryo-toxic compounds have been demonstrated in uterine flushings from rats and mice taken at times other than when implantation normally occurs (Weitlauf 1978, Psychoyos & Casimiri 1980) and there is a suggestion that similar embryo-toxic compounds occur in the human (Psychoyos et al 1989).

In a review of more than 120 published pregnancies established in patients receiving donated oocytes for premature ovarian failure (Rogers, 1993), it was estimated that successful implantation occurred when the embryo was anything from 39 hours in front to 48 hours behind the uterus. These calculations give an implantation window in the human of at least 3½ days, and are based on the assumption that the commencement of progesterone in the human initiates a 'clock' that results in the uterus passing through a receptive phase. In a study where human embryo-uterine synchrony was systematically varied to explore the length of the implantation window (Navot et al 1991a), pregnancies were achieved over a 6-day window equivalent to days 18–24 of the menstrual cycle. Numbers were not large enough in this study to determine whether differences in success rate existed within this time frame. It may also be possible to artificially widen the implantation window by manipulating the pre- and peri-implantation endocrine environment. It has been reported that ovarian stimulation with gonadotrophin releasing-hormone agonist and human menopausal gonadotrophin (hMG) compared with hMG alone appears to widen the implantation window (Tur-Kaspa et al 1990). Knowledge of the length of the human implantation window is of critical significance to all future studies aimed at identifying endometrial markers for uterine receptivity.

The large amount of human implantation data produced following superovulation and multiple embryo transfer by various IVF groups has provided a mathematical avenue for exploring the relative contributions of embryonic and uterine factors to implantation failure in stimulated cycles (Rogers et al 1986, Walters et al 1985). In summary, these data showed that for four IVF groups using the antioestrogen clomiphene citrate for superovulation, theoretical uterine receptivity values ranged from 0.31 to 0.42. By contrast, one IVF group not using clomiphene citrate as a superovulation drug had a theoretical

uterine receptivity of 0.64. In addition to indicating that some superovulatory drugs may act to reduce uterine receptivity, these data provide the first evidence that the human uterus has selective mechanisms by which the implanting embryo can be accepted or rejected. It is interesting to note that many IVF centres performing donor oocyte transfers report higher success rates for their oocyte recipients than for the donors undergoing ovarian stimulation for IVF (Rogers et al 1988, Paulson et al 1990, Navot et al 1991a). This observation, where oocytes and embryos of similar quality are placed in uteri that have seen different endocrine environments, provides strong evidence that either the superovulatory drugs or the elevated levels of circulating oestrogen and progesterone are acting to reduce uterine receptivity. The relative contributions of uterine receptivity and oocyte quality to successful implantation is an as yet unresolved issue. In a recent study involving oocyte donation to 35 infertile women over the age of 40, 15 ongoing pregnancies were achieved by using oocytes donated from younger women (Navot et al 1991b). One conclusion from this study was that the primary determinant of age-related decline in female fertility was poor oocyte quality, with endometrial receptivity having a secondary though important role. By contrast, a second study reporting 100 cycles of oocyte donation (Abdalla et al 1990) resulting in 27 clinical pregnancies, concluded that the age of the recipient (i.e. the uterus) significantly affects pregnancy rate, falling from 50% in the 25–29 year age group to 9.7% in the 45–49 year age group, while the age of the donor (i.e. the oocyte) does not.

An ability to identify receptive human endometrium would be of major clinical value in both infertility and contraceptive medicine. There have been numerous studies describing and quantifying morphological and histological changes in the endometrium during the menstrual cycle in an attempt to identify markers for uterine receptivity. It is well documented that the endometrium undergoes a cyclical series of changes in histological appearance under the influence of oestrogen and progesterone during the menstrual cycle (Noyes et al 1950). However, the functional importance of these morphological changes remains unclear (Rogers et al 1989a), as was highlighted in recent work where a single biopsy taken inadvertently from a conception cycle produced an endometrium that rated as non-receptive by morphometric analysis (Rogers et al 1989b). Tight junctions play an important role in joining adjacent cell walls closely together and thus maintaining the integrity of the epithelium. It has been suggested that endometrial epithelial integrity plays a major role in determining uterine receptivity for implantation, since removal of the epithelium from a non-progestational rat uterus will overcome the block to implantation that normally occurs (Cowell 1969). Recent studies (Murphy et al 1991) using freeze-fracture followed by morphometry have shown a significant decrease in human epithelial tight junction area between days 13 and 23 of the menstrual cycle, as well as a reduction in geometrical complexity. This data supports the hypothesis that sex steroid conditioning of the human uterus for implantation causes a reduction in epithelial integrity. In a related study (Rogers et al 1992) the surprising observation was made that in endometrial biopsies from Turner's syndrome patients there were minimal or no tight junctions, despite successful pregnancies occurring. This observation that a compromised epithelium does not appear to interfere with implantation is consistent with the hypothesis that the uterine epithelium normally acts as a barrier to the embryo, only becoming receptive for implantation when appropriately conditioned with oestrogen and progesterone.

CONCLUSIONS

The knowledge which is rapidly accumulating on fertilization, preimplantation embryo development and implantation in the human from a number of new research initiatives and medical applications is providing much-needed illumination into the problems of infertility, pregnancy failure, the reasons for birth defects and fetal abnormalities. Already this information has had a profound effect on the treatment of infertility, raising great ethical and social debates; these have resulted in legislative action to regulate and control many aspects of the new reproductive technologies. It is rare that developments in medicine have such deeply felt consequences for all of us. Modern day clinicians should be well informed of the recent expansion of knowledge in the area of conception and early embryonic development in order to comprehend the clinical significance of the new reproductive technologies for their patients. This is also necessary for any reasonable discussion of the medical, social, ethical and legal issues which are raised by these new technologies. The information provided in this chapter will be helpful in this.

REFERENCES

Abdalla H I, Baber R, Kirkland A, Leonard T, Power M Studd J W W 1990 A report on 100 cycles of oocyte donation, factors affecting the outcome. Human Reproduction 5: 1018–1022

Ahuja K K 1985a Inhibitors of glycoprotein biosynthesis block fertilization in the hamster. Gamete Research 11: 179–189

Ahuja K K 1985b Carbohydrate determinants involved in mammalian fertilization. American Journal of Anatomy 174: 207–223

Aitken R J, Maathuis J B 1978 Effect of human uterine flushings collected at various states of the menstrual cycle on mouse blastocysts in vitro. Journal of Reproduction and Fertility 53: 137–140

Anderson T L, Hoffmann L H 1984 Alterations in epithelial glycocalyx of rabbit uteri during early pseudopregnancy and pregnancy, and following ovariectomy. American Journal of Anatomy 171: 321–324

Angell R R, Aitken R J, van Look P F A, Lumsden M A, Templeton A A 1983 Chromosome abnormalities in human embryos after in vitro fertilization. Nature 303: 336–338

Angell R R, Templeton A A, Aitken R J 1986 Chromosome studies in human in vitro fertilization. Human Genetics 72: 333–2339

Asch R H, Ellsworth L R, Balmaceda J P, Wong P C 1984 Pregnancy after translaparoscopic gamete intrafallopian transfer. Lancet ii: 1034–1035

Baker H W G, Burger H G, de Kretser D M, Hudson B 1986 Relative incidence of etiological disorders in male infertility. In: Santen R J, Swerdloff R S (eds) Diagnosis and management of hypogonadism, infertility and impotence. Marcel Dekker, New York, pp 341–372

Barton S C, Surani M A H, Norris M L 1984 Role of paternal and maternal genomes in mouse development. Nature 311: 374–376

Bensaude O, Babinet C, Morange M, Jacob F 1983 Heat shock proteins, first major products of zygotic gene activity in mouse embryo. Nature 305: 331–333

Biggers J D, Moore B D, Whittingham D G 1965 Development of mouse embryos in vivo after cultivation from the two-cell ova to blastocysts in vitro. Nature 206: 734–735

Biggers J D, Whittingham D G, Donahue R P 1967 The pattern of energy metabolism in the mouse oocyte and zygote. Proceedings of the National Academy of Sciences (USA) 58: 560–567

Braude P, Bolton V, Moore S 1988 Human gene expression first occurs between the four- and eight-cell stages of preimplantation development. Nature 332: 459–461

Brinster R L 1963 A method for in vitro cultivation of mouse ova from two-cell to blastocyst. Experimental Cell Research 32: 205–208

Brinster R L 1967 Protein content of the mouse embryo during the first five days of development. Journal of Reproduction and Fertility 13: 413–420

Buster J E, Bustillo M, Rodi I A et al 1985 Biologic and morphologic development of donated human ova recovered by nonsurgical uterine lavage. American Journal of Obstetrics and Gynecology 153: 211–217

Caro C M, Trounson A 1984 The effect of protein on preimplantation mouse embryo development in vitro. Journal of In Vitro Fertilization and Embryo Transfer 1: 183–187

Caro C M, Trounson A 1986 Successful fertilization, embryo development, and pregnancy in human in vitro fertilization (IVF) using chemically defined culture medium containing no protein. Journal of In Vitro Fertilization and Embryo Transfer 3: 215–217

Cha K Y, Koo J J, Ko J J, Choi D H, Han S Y, Yoon T K 1991 Pregnancy after in vitro fertilization of human follicular oocytes collected from non-stimulated cycles, their culture in vitro and their transfer in a donor oocyte program. Fertility and Sterility 55: 109

Carson R S, Trounson A O, Findlay J K 1982 Successful fertilization of human oocytes in vitro: concentration of estradiol-17β, progesterone and androstenedione in the antral fluid of donor follicles. Journal of Clinical Endocrinology and Metabolism 55: 798–800

Chapman V, Forrester L, Sanford J, Hastie N, Rossant J 1984 Cell lineage specific undermethylation of mouse repetitive DNA. Nature 307: 284–286

Cholewa J A, Whitten W K 1965 Development of 2-cell mouse embryos in vitro. III. The effect of fixed nitrogen source. Journal of Experimental Zoology 158: 69–78

Cohen J, Fehilly C B, Walters D E 1985 Prolonged storage of human spermatozoa at room temperature or in a refrigerator. Fertility and Sterility 44: 254–262

Cowell T P 1969 Implantation and development of mouse eggs transferred to the uteri of non-progestational mice. Journal of Reproduction and Fertility 19: 239–245

Craft I L, Djahanbakheh O, McLeod F et al 1982 Human pregnancies following intrauterine transfer of preovulatory oocytes and sperm. Lancet ii: 1031–1033

Crosby I M, Osborn J C, Moor R M 1981 Follicle cell regulation of protein synthesis and developmental competance in sheep oocytes. Journal of Reproduction and Fertility 62: 575–582

Croxatto H B, Ortiz M E, Diaz S, Hess R, Balmaceda J, Croxatto H-D 1978 Studies on the duration of egg transport by the human oviduct

II. Ovum locations at various intervals following luteinizing hormone peak. American Journal of Obstetrics and Gynecology 132: 629–634

Cummins J M, Breen T M, Harrison K L, Shaw J M, Wilson L M, Hennessey J F 1986 A formula for scoring human embryo growth rate in in vitro fertilization: its value in predicting pregnancy and in comparison with visual estimates of embryo quality. Journal of In Vitro Fertilization and Embryo Transfer 3: 284–295

De Feo V J 1963 Determination of the sensitive period for the induction of deciduomata in the rat by different inducing procedures. Endocrinology 73: 488–497

Doerfler W 1983 DNA methylation and gene activity. Annual Review of Biochemistry 52: 93–124

Eibs H G, Spielmann H 1977 Inhibition of postimplantation development of mouse blastocysts in vitro after cyclophosphamide treatment in vivo. Nature 270: 54–56

Eppig J J, Downs S M, Schroeder A C 1985 Perspectives of mammalian oocyte maturation in vitro and practical applications. In: Testart J, Frydman R (eds) Human in vitro fertilization. Elsevier, Amsterdam, pp 33–43

Evans H J 1977 Chromosome anomalies among live births. Journal of Medical Genetics 14: 309–312

Fawcett D W, Wioslocki G B, Waldo C M 1947 The development of mouse ova in the anterior chamber of the eye and in the abdominal cavity. American Journal of Anatomy 81: 413–443

Finn C A, Porter D G 1975 Implantation of ova. In: Finn C A (ed) The uterus. Reproductive Biology Handbooks, Elek Science, London, pp 55–73

Fishel S B, Edwards R G, Purdy J M 1984 Births after a prolonged delay between oocyte recovery and fertilization in vitro. Gamete Research 9: 175–181

French F E, Bierman J E 1962 Probabilities of fetal mortality. Public Health Report 77: 835–847

Gardner D K, Lane M 1993 Amino acids and ammonium regulate the development of mouse embryo in culture. Biology of Reproduction 48: 377–385

Gardner D K, Lane M, Spitzer A, Batt P A 1994 Enhanced rates of cleavage and development for sheep zygotes cultured to the blastocyst stage in vitro in the absence of serum and somatic cells: amino acids, vitamins, and culturing embryos in groups stimulate development. Biology of Reproduction 50: 390–400

Garrett J E, Geisert R D, Zavy M T, Morgan G L 1988 Evidence for maternal regulation of early conceptus growth and development in beef cattle. Journal of Reproduction and Fertility 84: 437–446

Gianaroli L, Serracchioli R, Ferraretti A P, Trounson A, Flamigni C, Bovicelli L 1986 The successful use of human amniotic fluid for mouse embryo culture and human in vitro fertilization, embryo culture and transfer. Fertility and Sterility 46: 907–913

Gras L, McBain J, Trounson A, Kola I 1992 The incidence of chromosomal aneuploidy in stimulated and unstimulated (natural) uninseminated human oocytes. Human Reproduction 7: 1391–1401

Groudine M, Eisenmann R, Weintraub H 1980 Chromatin structure of endogenous retroviral genes and activation by an inhibitor of DNA methylation. Science 292: 311–317

Harlow G M, Quinn P 1982 Development of preimplantation mouse embryos in vivo and in vitro. Australian Journal of Biological Science 35: 187–193

Harris J W S, Ramsey E M 1966 The morphology of human uteroplacental vasculature. Carnegie Institute of Washington, Publication 625, Contributions to Embryology 33: 43–58

Hassold T, Chen N, Funkhouser J et al 1980 A cytogenetic study of 1000 spontaneous abortions. Annals of Human Genetics 44: 151–176

Hertig A T, Rock J, Adams E C 1956 A description of 34 human ova within the first 17 days of development. American Journal of Anatomy 98: 435–493

Hillier S G, Wickings E J, Afnan M, Margara R A, Harlow C R, Winston R M L 1985 Sex steroids and oocyte function. In: Rolland R, Heineman M J, Hillier S G, Vemer H (eds) Gamete quality and fertility regulation. Excerpta Medica, Amsterdam, pp 43–52

Holliday R, Pugh J E 1975 DNA modification mechanisms and gene activity during development. Science 187: 226–232

Holmes P V, Bergstrom S 1975 Induction of blastocyst implantation in mice by cyclic AMP. Journal of Reproduction and Fertility 43: 329–332

Holmes P V, Gordashko B J 1980 Evidence of prostaglandin involvement in blastocyst implantation. Journal of Embryology and Experimental Morphology 55: 109–122

Iannaccone p M 1984 Long-term effects of exposure to methylnitrosurea on blastocysts following transfer to surrogate female mice. Cancer Research 44: 2785–2789

Jean Y, Langlais J, Roberts K D, Chapdelaine A, Bleau G 1979 Fertility of a woman with nonfunctional ciliated cells in the fallopian tubes. Fertility and Sterility 31: 349–350

Johnson M H, Ziomek C A 1981 The foundation of two distinct cell lineages within the mouse morula. Cell 24: 71–80

Kennedy T G, Armstrong D T 1981 The role of prostaglandins in endometrial vascular changes at implantation In: Glasser S R, Bullock D W (eds) Cellular and molecular aspects of implantation. Plenum Press, New York, pp 349–364

Killeen I D, Moore N W 1971 The morphological appearance and development of sheep ova fertilized by surgical insemination. Journal of Reproduction and Fertility 24: 63–70

Kimber S J, Surani M A H, Barton S C 1982 Interactions of blastomeres suggest changes in cell surface adhesiveness during the formation of inner cell mass and trophectoderm in the preimplantation mouse embryo. Journal of Embryology and Experimental Morphology 70: 133–152

Kirby D R S 1963 The development of mouse blastocysts transplanted to the scrotal and cryptorchid testis. Journal of Anatomy 97: 119–130

Knoth M, Larsen J F 1972 Ultrastructure of a human implantation site. Acta Obstetricia et Gynecologica Scandinavica 51: 385–393

Koehler J K 1978 The mammalian sperm surface: studies with specific labelling techniques. International Reviews of Cytology 54: 73–105

Kola I, Folb P I 1985 The effects of cyclophosphamide on alkaline phosphatase activity and on in vitro postimplantation murine blastocyst development. Development Growth and Differentiation 27: 645–651

Kola I, Folb P I 1986 An assessment of the effects of cyclophosphamide and sodium valproate on the viability of preimplantation mouse embryos using the fluorescein diacetate test. Teratogenesis, Carcinogenesis and Mutagenesis 6: 23–31

Kola I, Folb P I, Parker M I 1986 Maternal administration of cyclophosphamide induces chromosomal aberrations and inhibits cell number, histone and DNA-synthesis in preimplantation mouse embryos. Teratogenesis, Carcinogenesis and Mutagenesis 6: 115–127

Kola I, Trounson A, Dawson G, Rogers P 1987 Tripronuclear human oocytes: altered cleavage patterns and subsequent karyotypic analysis of embryos. Biology of Reproduction 37: 395–401

Kola I, Sathananthan A H, Gras L 1993 Chromosomal analysis of preimplantation mammalian embryos. In: Trounson A, Gardner D (eds) Handbook of in vitro fertilization. CRC Press, Boca Raton, Florida, pp 173–193

Lawn A M 1973 The ultrastructure of the endometrium during the sexual cycle. In: Bishop M W H (ed) Advances in reproductive biology, vol 6. Elek, London, pp 61–95

Lawson R A S, Rowson L E A, Adams C E 1972 The development of cow eggs in the rabbit oviduct and their viability after retransfer to heifers. Journal of Reproduction and Fertility 28: 313–315

Leridon J 1977 Human fertility. University of Chicago Press, Chicago

Levinson J, Goodfellow P, Vadeboncoeur M, McDevitt H 1978 Identification of stage-specific polypeptide synthesis during murine preimplantation development. Proceedings of the National Academy of Sciences USA 75: 3332–3336

Lindenberg S, Hyttel P 1988 In vitro studies of the peri-implantation phase of human embryos. In: Van Blerkom J, Motta P (eds) Ultrastructure of human gametogenesis and early embryogenesis. Martinus Nijhof, Amsterdam, pp 201–211

Lindenberg S, Hyttel P, Lenz S, Holmes P V 1986 Ultrastructure of the early human implantation in vitro. Human Reproduction 1: 533–538

Lindenberg S, Hyttel P, Sjøgren A, Greve T 1989 A comparative study of attachment of human, bovine and mouse blastocysts to uterine epithelial monolayer. Human Reproduction 4: 446–456

Ljungkvist M D 1972 Attachment reaction of rat uterine luminal epithelium. IV. The cellular changes in the attachment reaction and its hormonal regulation. Fertility and Sterility 23: 847–865

Luckett W P 1973 Amniogenesis in the early human and rhesus monkey embryos. Anatomical Record 175: 375 (abstract)

Lundkvist Ö, Nilsson B O 1982 Endometrial ultrastructure in the early uterine response to blastocysts and artificial deciduogenic stimuli in rats. Cell and Tissue Research 225: 355–364

Lutjen P, Trounson A, Leeton J, Findlay J, Wood C, Renou P 1984 The establishment and maintenance of pregnancy using in vitro fertilization and embryo donation in a patient with primary ovarian failure. Nature 307: 174–175

Mahadevan M M, Trounson A 0 1985 Removal of the cumulus oophorus from the human oocyte for in vitro fertilization. Fertility and Sterility 43: 263–267

Mann J R, Lovell-Badge R H 1984 Inviability of parthenogenesis determined by pronuclei, not egg cytoplasm. Nature 310: 66–67

Martin R H 1984 A comparison of chromosomal abnormalities in hamster egg and human sperm pronuclei. Biology of Reproduction 31: 819–825

McGrath J, Softer D 1984 Mouse embryogenesis requires a maternal and paternal genome. Cell 37: 179–183

McMaster R, Yanagimachi R, Lopata A 1978 Pentration of human eggs by human spermatozoa in vitro. Biology of Reproduction 19: 212–216

Meizel S 1978 The mammalian sperm acrosome reaction, a biochemical approach. In: Johnson M H (ed) Development in mammals, vol 3. North Holland, Amsterdam, pp 1–64

Menezo Y, Testart J, Perrone D 1984 Serum is not necessary for human in vitro fertilization, early embryo culture and transfer. Fertility and Sterility 42: 750–755

Mohr L R, Trounson A O 1982 Comparative ultrastructure of the hatched human, mouse and bovine blastocysts. Journal of Reproduction and Fertility 66: 499–504

Monk M 1981 A stem-line model for cellular and chromosomal differentiation in early mouse development. Differentiation 19: 71–76

Moor R M, Trounson A O 1977 Hormonal and follicular factors affecting maturation of sheep oocytes in vitro and their subsequent developmental capacity. Journal of Reproduction and Fertility 49: 101–109

Moor R M, Polge C, Willadsen S M 1980 Effect of follicular steroids on the maturation and fertilization of mammalian oocytes. Journal of Embryology and Experimental Morphology 56: 319–335

Moor R M, Osborn J C, Cran D, Walters D E 1981 Selective effect of gonadotrophins on cell coupling, nuclear maturation and protein synthesis in mammalian oocytes. Journal of Embryology and Experimental Morphology 61: 347–365

Morton H, Rolfe B, Clunie G J A, Anderson M J, Morrison J 1977 An early pregnancy factor detected in human serum by the rosette inhibition test. Lancet i: 394–397

Mullins D E, Bazer F W, Roberts R M 1981 The pig uterus secretes a progesterone-induced inhibitor of plasminogen activator In: Glasser S R, Bullock D W (eds) Cellular and molecular aspects of implantation. Plenum Press, New York, pp 420–422

Murphy C R, Martin B 1985 Cholesterol in the plasma membrane of uterine epithelial cells: a freeze-fracture cytochemical study with digitonin. Journal of Cell Science 78: 163–172

Murphy C R, Swift J G, Mukherjee T M, Rogers A W 1982a Changes in the fine structure of the apical plasma membrane of endometrial epithelial cells during implantation in the rat. Journal of Cell Science 55: 1–12

Murphy C R, Swift J G, Need J A, Mukherjee T M, Rogers A W 1982b A freeze-fracture electron microscopic study of tight junctions of epithelial cells in the human uterus. Anatomy and Embryology 163: 367–370

Murphy C R, Rogers P A W, Leeton J, Hosie M, Beaton L, Macpherson A 1987 Surface ultrastructure of uterine epithelial cells in women with premature ovarian failure following steroid hormone replacement. Acta Anatomica 130: 348–350

Murphy C R, Rogers P A W, Leeton J, Hosie M, Beaton L 1991 Tight junctions of human uterine epithelial cells change during the menstrual cycle: a morphometric study. Acta Anatomica 144: 36–38

Navot D, Bergh P A, Williams M et al 1991a An insight into early reproductive processes through the in vivo model of ovum donation. Journal of Clinical Endocrinology and Metabolism 72: 408–414

Navot D, Bergh P A, Williams M A et al 1991b Poor oocyte quality rather than implantation failure as a cause of age-related decline in female fertility. Lancet 337: 1375–1377

Ng S C, Sathananthan A H, Edirisinghe W R et al 1987 Fertilization of a human egg with sperm from a patient with immotile cilia syndrome. Case report. In: Ratnam S S, Teoh E S, Anandakumar C (eds) Advances in fertility and sterility Parthenon Lancaster, pp 71–76

Noyes R W, Hertig A T, Rock J 1950 Dating the endometrial biopsy: Fertility and Sterility 1: 3–25

O'Neil C, Gidley-Baird A A, Pike I L, Porter R N, Sinosich M J, Saunders D M 1985 Maternal blood platelet physiology and luteal phase endocrinology as a means of monitoring pre and post implantation embryo viability following in vitro fertilization. Journal of In Vitro Fertilization and Embryo Transfer 2: 87–93

O'Rahilly R 1973 Developmental stages in human embryos. Part A: embryos of the first 3 weeks (stages 1 to 9). Carnegie Institution of Washington, Publication 631, Washington, DC

Parr M B, Parr E L 1977 Endocytosis in the uterine epithelium of the mouse. Journal of Reproduction and Fertility 50: 151–153

Paterson P, Downing B, Trounson A O, Cumming I A 1981 Fertility and tubal morphology after microsurgical removal of segments of the porcine fallopian tube. Fertility and Sterility 35: 209–213

Patillo R A, Hussa R 0 1984 Human trophoblastic neoplasms: advances in experimental medicine and biology, vol 176. Plenum Press, New York

Paulson R J, Sauer M V, Lobo R A 1990 Embryo implantation after human in vitro fertilization: importance of endometrial receptivity. Fertility and Sterility 53: 870–874

Pemble L B, Kaye P L 1986 Whole protein uptake and metabolism by mouse blastocysts. Journal of Reproduction and Fertility 78: 149–157

Perry F S, Heap R B, Amoroso E C 1973 Steroid hormone production by pig blastocysts. Nature 245: 45–47

Ponzetto-Zimmerman C, Wolgemuth D J 1984 Methylation of satellite sequences in mouse spermatogenic and somatic DNAs. Nucleic Acids Research 12: 2807–2822

Pratt H P M, Ziomek C A, Reeve W J D, Johnson M H 1982 Compaction of the mouse embryo: an analysis of its components. Journal of Embryology and Experimental Morphology 70: 113–132

Psychoyos A, Casimiri V 1980 Factors involved in uterine receptivity and refractoriness. Progress in Reproductive Biology 7: 143–157

Psychoyos A, Casimiri V 1981 Uterine blastotoxic factors. In: Glasser S R, Bullock D W (eds) Cellular and molecular aspects of implantation. Plenum Press, New York, pp 327–334

Psychoyos A, Roche D, Gravanis A 1989 Is cholic acid responsible for embryo-toxicity of the post-receptive uterine environment? Human Reproduction 4: 832–834

Quinn P, Kerin J F, Warnes G M 1985 Improved pregnancy rate in human in vitro fertilization with the use of a medium based on the composition of human tubal fluid. Fertility and Sterility 44: 493–498

Razin A, Riggs A D 1980 DNA methylation and gene function. Science 210: 604–610

Rogers P A W 1993 Uterine receptivity. In: Trounson A O, Gardner D K (eds) Handbook of in vitro fertilization. CRC Press, Boca Raton, Florida, pp 263–285

Rogers P A W, Murphy C R, Rogers A W, Gannon B J 1983a Capillary patency and permeability in the endometrium surrounding the implanting rat blastocyst. International Journal of Microcirculation: Clinical and Experimental 2: 241–249

Rogers P A W, Murphy C R, Squires K R, MacLennan A H 1983b Effects of relaxin on the intrauterine distribution and antimesometrial positioning and orientation of rat blastocysts before implantation. Journal of Reproduction and Fertility 68: 431–435

Rogers P A W, Milne B J, Trounson A O 1986 A model to show human uterine receptivity and embryo viability following ovarian stimulation for in vitro fertilization. Journal of In Vitro Fertilization and Embryo Transfer 3: 93–98

Rogers P, Leeton J, Cameron I T, Murphy C, Healy D, Lutjen P 1988 Oocyte donation. In: Wood C, Trounson A O (Ms) Clinical in vitro fertilization and embryo transfer, 2nd edition. Springer-Verlag, Berlin, pp 143–154

Rogers P, Murphy C, Cameron I, Leeton J, Hosie M, Beaton L, Macpherson A 1989a Uterine receptivity in women receiving steroid replacement therapy for premature ovarian failure: ultrastructural and endocrinological parameters. Human Reproduction 4: 349–354

Rogers P A W, Murphy C R, Leeton J, Hosie M, Beaton L, Macpherson A 1989b An ultrastructural study of human uterine epithelium from a patient with a confirmed pregnancy. Acta Anatomica 135: 176–179

Rogers P A W, Murphy C R, Leeton J, Hosie M J, Beaton L 1992 Turner's syndrome patients lack tight junctions between uterine epithelial cells. Human Reproduction 7: 883–885

Sandell M 1990 The evolution of seasonal delayed implantation. Quarterly Reviews of Biology 65: 23–42

Sanford J, Forrester L, Chapman V, Chandley A, Hostie N 1984 Methylation patterns of repetitive DNA sequences in germ cells of *Mus musculus*. Nucleic Acids Research 12: 2823–2836

Sathananthan A H 1984 Ultrastructural morphology of fertilization and early cleavage in the human. In: Trounson A, Wood C (eds) In vitro fertilization and embryo transfer. Churchill Livingstone, Edinburgh, pp 131–158

Sathananthan A H, Chen C 1986 Early penetration of human sperm through the vestments of human eggs in vitro. Archives of Andrology 16: 183–197

Sathananthan A H, Trounson A O 1982 Cortical granule release and zona interaction in monospermic and polyspermic human ova fertilized in vitro. Gamete Research 6: 225–234

Sathananthan A H, Trounson A 0 1985 Human pronuclear ovum: fine structure of monospermic and polyspermic fertilization in vitro. Gamete Research 12: 385–398

Sathananthan A H, Wood C, Leeton J 1982 Ultrastructural evaluation of 8–16 cell human embryos cultured in vitro. Micron 13: 193–203

Sathananthan A H, Ng S C, Edirisinghe R, Ratnam S S, Wong P C 1986a Sperm–oocyte interaction in the human during polyspermic fertilization in vitro. Gamete Research 15: 317–326

Sathananthan A H, Trounson A O, Wood C 1986b Atlas of fine structure of human sperm, eggs and embryos cultured in vitro. Praeger Scientific, Philadelphia

Sathananthan A H, Trounson A, Freemann L 1987 Morphology and fertilizability of frozen human oocytes. Gamete Research 16: 343–354

Sathananthan A H, Bongso A, Ng S C, Ho J, Mok H, Ratnam S 1990 Ultrastructural of preimplantation human embryos cocultured with human ampillary cells. Human Reproduction 5: 309–318

Sathananthan A H, Kola I, Osborn J et al 1991 Centrioles in the beginning of human development. Proceedings of the National Academy of Sciences USA 88: 4806–4810

Schatten G, Simerly C, Schatten H 1991 Maternal inheritance of centrosomes in mammals? Studies on parthenogenesis and polyspermy in mice. Proceedings of the National Academy of Sciences USA 88: 6785–6789

Schultz G A, Kaye P L, McKay D L, Johnson M H 1981 Endogenous amino acid pool sizes in mouse eggs and preimplantation embryos. Journal of Reproduction and Fertility 61: 387–393

Soupart P 1980 Fertilization. In: Hafez E S E (ed) Human reproduction: conception and contraception. Harper & Row, New York, pp 453–470

Spielmann H, Habernicht U, Eibs H G, Jacob-Muller U, Schimmell A 1981 Investigations on the mechanism of action and on the pharmacokinetics of cyclophosphamide treatment during the preimplantation period in the mouse. In: Neubert D, Merker J H (eds) Culture techniques: applicability for studies on differentiation and toxicity. Walter de Gruyter, Berlin, pp 436–445

Spindle A I, Pedersen R A 1973 Hatching, attachment and outgrowth of mouse blastocysts in vitro: fixed nitrogen requirement. Journal of Experimental Zoology 186: 305–318

Staigmiller R B, Moor R M 1984 Effect of follicle cells on the maturation and developmental competence of ovine oocytes matured outside the follicle. Gamete Research 9: 221–229

Stewart C L, Kaspar P, Brunet L J, Bhatt H, Gadi I, Köntgen F, Abbondanzo S J 1992 Blastocyst implantation depends on maternal expression of leukaemia inhibitory factor. Nature 359: 76–79

Strickland S, Reich E, Sherman M 1 1976 Plasminogen activator in early embryogenesis: enzyme production by trophoblast and parietal endoderm. Cell 9: 231–240

Surani M A H, Barton S C, Norris M L 1984 Development of reconstituted mouse eggs suggests imprinting of the genome during gametogenesis. Nature 308: 548–550

Surani M A H, Barton S C, Norris M L 1986 Nuclear transplantation in the mouse: heritable differences between parental genomes after activation of the embryonic genome. Cell 45: 127–136

Takeuchi I K 1984 Teratogenic effects of methylnitrosurea on pregnant mice before implantation. Experientia 40: 879–881

Tarkowski A K, Wroblewska J 1967 Development of blastomeres of mouse eggs isolated at the 4- and 8-cell stage. Journal of Embryology and Experimental Morphology 18: 155–180

Tawia S A, Rogers P A W 1992 In vivo microscopy of the subepithelial capillary plexus of the endometrium of rats during embryo implantation. Journal of Reproduction and Fertility 96: 673–680

Templeton A A, Mortimer D 1980 Laparoscopic sperm recovery in infertile women. British Journal of Obstetrics and Gynaecology 87: 1128–1131

Tervit H R, Whittingham D G, Rowson L E A 1972 Successful culture in vitro of sheep and cattle ova. Journal of Reproduction and Fertility 30: 493–497

Tesarik J, Kopecny V, Plachot M, Mandelbaum J 1987 Activation of nucleolar and extranucleolar RNA synthesis and changes in the ribosomal content of human embryos developing in vitro. Journal of Reproduction and Fertility 78: 463–470

Thibault C 1972 Physiology and physiopathology of the fallopian tube. International Journal of Fertility 17: 1–13

Thibault C 1977 Are follicular maturation and oocyte maturation independent processes? Journal of Reproduction and Fertility 51: 1–15

Trapp M, Baukloh V, Bohnet H-G, Heeschen W 1984 Pollutants in human follicular fluid. Fertility and Sterility 42: 146–148

Trounson A O, Mohr L R, Wood C, Leeton J F 1982 Effect of delayed insemination on in vitro fertilization, culture and transfer of human embryos. Journal of Reproduction and Fertility 64: 285–294

Tur-Kaspa I, Confino E, Dudkiewicz A B, Myers S A, Friberg J, Gleicher N 1990 Ovarian stimulation protocol for in vitro fertilization with gonadotropin-releasing hormone agonist widens the implantation window. Fertility and Sterility 53: 859–864

Veeck L L, Wortham J W E, Witmyer J et al 1983 Maturation and fertilization of morphologically immature human oocytes in a program of in vitro fertilization. Fertility and Sterility 39: 594–602

Waalwijk C, Flavell R A 1978 Mspl an isoschizomer of HPA2 which cleaves both unmethylated and methylated HPA2 sites. Nucleic Acids Research 5: 3231–3236

Wales R G 1975 Maturation of the mammalian embryo: biochemical aspects. Biology of Reproduction 20: 985–990

Walters D E, Edwards D G, Meistrich M L 1985 A statistical evaluation of implantation after replacing one or more human embryos. Journal of Reproduction and Fertility 74: 557–563

Webb F T G 1975 Implantation on ovariectomized mice treated with dibutyryl adenosine 3′,5′-monophosphate (dibutyryl cyclic AMP). Journal of Reproduction and Fertility 42: 511–517

Weitlauf H M 1978 Factors in mouse uterine fluid that inhibit the incorporation of ^{3}H-uridine by blastocysts in vitro. Journal of Reproduction and Fertility 52: 321–325

Willadsen S M 1981 The developmental capacity of blastomeres from 4- and 8-cell sheep embryos. Journal of Embryology and Experimental Morphology 65: 165–172

Wolf D P, Byrd W, Dandekar P, Quigley M M 1984 Sperm concentration and the fertilization of human eggs in vitro. Biology of Reproduction 31: 837–848

Yanagimachi R 1981 Mechanisms of fertilization in mammals. In: Mastorianni L, Biggers J D (eds) Fertilization and embryonic development in vitro. Plenum, New York, pp 81–182

Yanagimachi R 1984 Zona-free hamster eggs: their use in assessing fertilizing capacity and examining chromosomes of human spermatozoa. Gamete Research 10: 187–232

Yates C A, de Kretser D M 1987 Male-factor infertility and in vitro fertilization. Journal of In Vitro Fertilization and Embryo Transfer 4: 141–147

Ziomek C A, Johnson M H 1980 Cell surface interaction induces polarization of mouse 8-cell blastomeres at compaction. Cell 21: 935–942

4. The placenta, membranes and umbilical cord

Harold Fox

THE PLACENTA

The human placenta is a villous haemochorial structure which is of critical importance in materno–fetal transfer, has a complex synthetic capacity and plays a fundamental role in the immunological acceptance of the fetal allograft. The placenta is unique in its range of functional activities, its ability to flourish in an immunologically alien environment and, because it depends upon maternal blood for its oxygenation and nutrition, its vascular parasitism.

The placenta, as expelled from the uterus, appears to be a complete organ: this, the fetal placenta, is not the total structure, however, for there is also the maternal component of the placenta which comprises the placental bed and the uteroplacental vessels.

Development of the fetal placenta

The fertilized ovum enters the uterine cavity as a morula which rapidly converts into a blastocyst and loses its surrounding zona pellucida (Fig. 4.1). The outer cell layer of the blastocyst proliferates to form the primary trophoblastic cell mass from which cells infiltrate between those of the endometrial epithelium: the latter degenerate and the trophoblast thus comes into contact with the endometrial stroma; this process of implantation is complete by the 10th or 11th postovulatory day. In the 7-day ovum the trophoblast forms a peripheral circumferential plaque which rapidly differentiates into two layers, an inner layer of large, mononuclear cytotrophoblastic cells with well defined limiting membranes and an outer layer of multinucleated syncytiotrophoblast, this latter being a true syncytium (Fig. 4.2). That the syncytiotrophoblast is derived from the cytotrophoblast, not only at this early stage

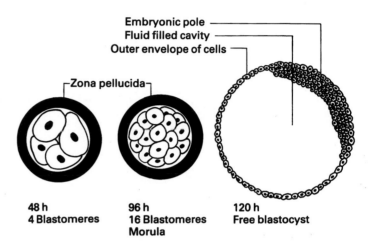

Fig. 4.1   Formation of the blastocyst. The morula sheds the zona pellucida and forms a blastocyst with an embryonic pole, or inner cell mass, and an outer envelope of cells from which the primary trophoblastic cell mass develops. Reproduced with permission from McLean (1987).

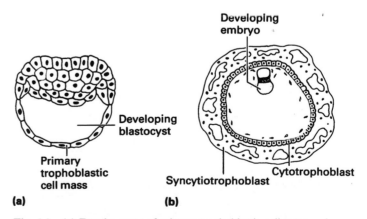

Fig. 4.2   (a) Development of primary trophoblastic cell mass and (b) its differentiation into cytotrophoblast and syncytiotrophoblast. Reproduced with permission from Fox (1986b).

but throughout gestation, is now well established for even when the trophoblast is growing rapidly DNA synthesis and mitotic activity occur only in the nuclei of the cytotrophoblastic cells (Richart 1961, Galton 1962), the

45

syncytiotrophoblast being a postmitotic, terminally differentiated tissue. The syncytiotrophoblast appears to be formed by a breaking down of the limiting membrane of the cytotrophoblastic cells for although no true intercellular membranes are present in the syncytial layer, remnants of such membranes can occasionally be found on electron microscopy (Enders 1965). Cells with a cytoplasmic complexity and nuclear structure intermediate between those of the trophoblastic layers can also be identified on electron microscopy and these intermediate-type cytotrophoblastic cells appear to be ones which are beginning to differentiate into syncytiotrophoblast but have not yet lost their limiting membranes. It is worth noting that the syncytiotrophoblast is the only true syncytial human tissue: this must have some currently unidentified biological advantage for the trophoblast and it has also been suggested that, in teleological terms, the lack of any necessity for the syncytiotrophoblast to synthesize DNA and undergo mitotic activity allows the full metabolic activity of the tissue to be directed towards its transfer and synthetic functions.

Between the 10th and 13th postovulatory days a series of intercommunicating clefts, or lacunae, appear in the rapidly enlarging trophoblastic cell mass (Fig. 4.3): these are probably formed as a result of engulfment of endometrial capillaries within the trophoblast. These lacunae soon become confluent to form the precursor of the intervillous space which, as maternal vessels are progressively eroded, become filled with maternal blood. At this stage the lacunae are incompletely separated from each other by trabecular columns of syncytiotrophoblast which, between the 14th and 21st postovulatory days, tend to become radially orientated (Fig. 4.4) and come to possess a central cellular core produced by proliferation of the cytotrophoblastic cells at the chorionic base. These trabeculae are not true villi but serve as the framework from which the villous tree will later develop, the placenta at this time being a labyrinthine rather than a villous structure and

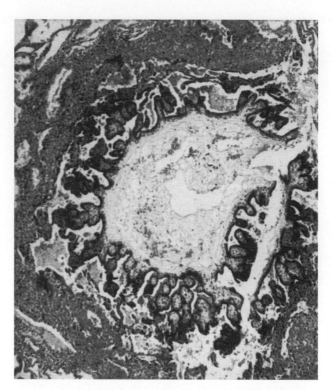

Fig. 4.4 A developing conceptus approximately 14 days after conception. Trabecular primary villous stems are arranged radially and divide the precursor of the intervillous space into a labyrinth. Haematoxylin and eosin. × 24. Reproduced with permission from Fox (1978).

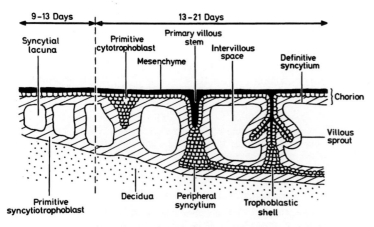

Fig. 4.3 Early development of the placenta. Reproduced with permission from Fox (1978).

the trabeculae being best known as primary villous stems (Boyd & Hamilton 1970). Continued growth of the cytotrophoblast leads to its distal extension into the region of decidual attachment (Fig. 4.5) whilst, at the same time, a mesenchymal core appears within the villous stems, formed by a distal extension of the extraembryonic mesenchyme. Later, the villous stems become vascularized; the vessels develop from mesenchyme within the core and establish, in due course, functional continuity with others differentiating in the body stalk and inner chorionic mesenchyme.

The distal part of the villous stems is now formed almost entirely by cytotrophoblastic cells which form columns anchored to the decidua of the basal plate. The cells in these cytotrophoblastic cell columns proliferate and spread laterally to form a continuous cytotrophoblastic shell which splits the syncytiotrophoblast into two layers; the definitive syncytium is on the fetal aspect of the shell and the peripheral syncytium is on the maternal side. The definitive syncytium persists as the lining of the intervillous space but the peripheral syncytium eventually degenerates and is replaced by fibrinoid material (Nitabuch's layer). The establishment of the cytotrophoblastic shell is a mechanism to allow for rapid circumferential growth of the developing placenta and this leads to an expansion of the intervillous space into which sprouts extend from

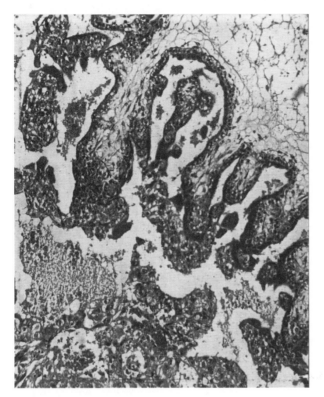

Fig. 4.5 Detail of primary villous stem in a 14-day-old conceptus. The stems have a mesenchymal core and the growing tip of each is formed by a mass of proliferating cytotrophoblastic cells. Haematoxylin and eosin. × 68. Reproduced with permission from Fox (1978).

the primary villous stems. These off-shoots consist initially only of syncytiotrophoblast but as they enlarge they pass through the stages previously seen during the development of the primary villous stems, i.e. intrusion of cytotrophoblast, formation of a mesenchymal core and eventual vascularization. These sprouts are the primary stem villi and, since they are true villous structures, the placenta is a vascularized villous organ by the 21st postovulatory day. The primary stem villi later grow and divide to form secondary and tertiary stem villi and these latter eventually break up into the terminal villous tree.

Between the 21st postovulatory day and the end of the fourth month of gestation there is not only continuing growth but also considerable remodelling of the placenta. The villi oriented towards the uterine cavity degenerate and form the chorion laeve whilst the thin rim of decidua covering this area gradually disappears to allow the chorion laeve to come into contact with the parietal decidua of the opposite wall of the uterus. The villi on the side of the chorion oriented towards the decidual plate proliferate and progressively arborize to form the chorion frondosum which develops into the definitive fetal placenta. During this period there is some regression of the cytotrophoblastic elements in the chorionic plate and in the trophoblastic shell, whilst the cytotrophoblastic cell columns largely degenerate and are replaced by

fibrinoid material (Rohr's layer): clumps of cells persist, however, as the cytotrophoblastic cell islands.

The placental septa appear during the third month of gestation: they protrude into the intervillous space from the basal plate and divide the maternal surface of the placenta into 15–20 lobes. These septa are simply folds of the basal plate, being formed partly as a result of regional variability in placental growth and partly by the pulling up of the basal plate by the anchoring columns which have a poor growth rate (Boyd & Hamilton 1970). As the basal plate is formed principally by the remnants of the trophoblastic shell embedded in fibrinoid material it follows that the septa are similarly constituted, though some decidual cells may also be carried up into the folds. The septa are simply an incidental byproduct of the architectural remodelling of the placenta and have no physiological or morphological role to play.

By the end of the fourth month of gestation the fetal placenta has achieved its definitive form and undergoes no further anatomical modification. Growth continues, however, until term and is due principally to continuing branching of the villous tree and formation of fresh villi.

Development of the maternal placenta

During the early weeks of gestation cytotrophoblastic cells stream out from the tips of the anchoring villi, penetrate the trophoblastic shell and extensively colonize the decidua and adjacent myometrium of the placental bed, these cells being known as the interstitial extravillous cytotrophoblast: in addition, trophoblastic cells stream into the lumina of the intradecidual portions of the spiral arteries of the placental bed where they form intraluminal plugs and constitute the intravascular extravillous cytotrophoblast. These endovascular trophoblastic cells destroy and replace the endothelium of the maternal vessels and then invade the media with resulting destruction of the medial elastic and muscular tissue (Brosens et al 1967): the arterial wall becomes replaced by fibrinoid material which appears to be derived partly from fibrin in the maternal blood and partly from proteins secreted by the invading trophoblastic cells (de Wolf et al 1973). This process is complete by the end of the first trimester, at which time these physiological changes within the spiral arteries of the placental bed extend to the myometriodecidual junction.

After this there is a rest phase in this process but between the 14th and 16th week of gestation there is a resurgence of endovascular trophoblastic migration with a second wave of cells moving down into the intramyometrial segments of the spiral arteries, these cells extending as far as the origin of these vessels from the radial arteries. Within the intramyometrial portion of the spiral arteries the same process as occurs in their intradecidual portion is repeated, i.e. replacement of the

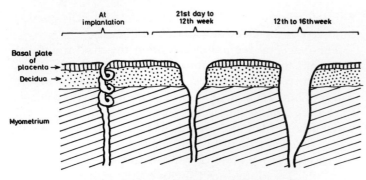

Fig. 4.6 Conversion of spiral arteries into uteroplacental vessels. Reproduced with permission from Fox (1986b).

endothelium, invasion and destruction of the medial musculoelastic tissue and fibrinoid change in the vessel wall. The end result of this trophoblastic invasion of, and attack on, the vessels is that the thick-walled muscular spiral arteries are converted into flaccid, sac-like uteroplacental vessels (Fig. 4.6) which can passively dilate in order to accommodate the greatly augmented blood flow through this vascular system required as pregnancy progresses.

The extravillous population of trophoblastic cells therefore plays a key role in placentation and through these cells the placenta establishes its own low-pressure, high-conductance, vascular system, simultaneously ensuring an adequate maternal blood flow to itself and an ample supply of oxygen and nutrients to the fetus. The factors which control and limit intravascular invasion by extravillous trophoblast are unknown but the crucial importance of this process is shown by the finding that in women destined to develop pre-eclampsia in the later stages of their pregnancy there is a partial failure of placentation which results in a markedly restricted blood flow to the placenta. This failure has two components: firstly, unlike a normal pregnancy in which all the spiral arteries in the placental bed are invaded by trophoblast, this process occurs in only a proportion of these vessels in women who later develop pre-eclampsia, with a significant fraction of the placental bed arteries in such cases showing a complete absence of physiological change (Khong et al 1986). Secondly, although the first stage of the arterial invasion process occurs quite normally, with trophoblast evoking physiological changes in their intradecidual segments, there is complete failure of the second stage, with endovascular trophoblast failing to advance into the intramyometrial portion of these vessels (Robertson et al 1967, 1975, Pijnenborg et al 1991). As a result, there is incomplete transformation of the spiral arteries to uteroplacental vessels and this abnormality, leading to restriction of maternal uteroplacental blood flow, accounts for all the placental abnormalities and fetal complications seen in pre-eclampsia. Pre-eclampsia is not the only serious consequence of inadequate placentation for

it is now becoming clear that defective invasion of the spiral arteries by extravillous trophoblast is also a feature of many cases of intrauterine fetal growth retardation in normotensive women, the deficit in fetal growth being due to the reduced maternal supply of oxygen and nutrients (Robertson et al 1981).

Whilst the function of intravascular extravillous trophoblastic cells appears clear, that of the interstitial trophoblastic cells is obscure. The number of these cells has, in the past, been seriously underestimated for it is now known that they are a major component of the placental bed (Pijnenborg et al 1981). Interstitial trophoblastic cells tend to aggregate around spiral arteries and may prime these vessels to allow them to react to their eventual invasion by endovascular trophoblast (Pijnenborg et al 1983): if this is indeed the function of these cells, their mode of action is unknown.

Extravillous trophoblastic cells differ from villous trophoblast in their ability to express an unusual type of class 1 major histocompatibility antigen (Redman et al 1984, Sargent et al 1993) and in that their principal synthetic product is human placental lactogen rather than human chorionic gonadotrophin (Gosseye & Fox 1984, Kurman et al 1984). Studies with monoclonal antibodies have, however, shown that the morphologically homogeneous extravillous trophoblastic cells actually comprise a number of antigenically heterogeneous populations (Bulmer & Johnson 1985).

Anatomy of the fetal placenta

The fetal placenta is made up of a number of subunits, generally known as lobules. The injection studies of Wilkin (1965) have shown that the primary stem villi break up just below the chorionic plate into a number of secondary stem villi which, after running for a short distance parallel to the chorionic plate, divide into a series of tertiary stem villi. The lobule are formed by these tertiary stem villi sweeping through the intervillous space to anchor on to the basal plate. As they traverse the intervillous space, they give off multiple branches which ramify into the terminal villous network. As the tertiary stem villi pass down towards the basal plate they are arranged in a circular fashion around the periphery of an empty cylindrical space; the lobule thus forms a hollow globule (Fig. 4.7) with the bulk of the terminal villi being mainly in the outer shell and the centre relatively empty and free of villi. The lobules are separated from each other by interlobular areas which are in continuity with the subchorial space.

There has been considerable confusion as to the meaning of the term cotyledon when applied to the human placenta. This name should not be used to describe the lobes seen on the maternal surface for these are merely the areas lying between the septa and lack any other morphological significance. A cotyledon is the functional unit of

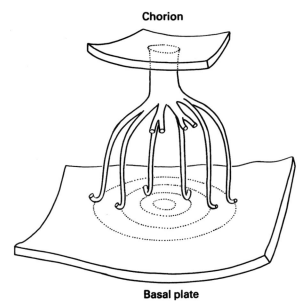

Fig. 4.7 Fetal lobule. The stem villi are arranged in a circular fashion around a central hollow core. Reproduced with permission from Fox (1978).

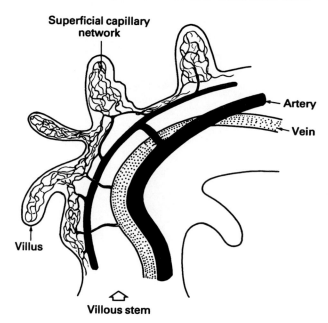

Fig. 4.8 The fetal circulation through the villi. Reproduced with permission from Fox (1978).

the placental villous tree, which is best defined as the part derived from a single primary stem villus (Ramsey 1959). Such a villus can, however, give rise to a varying number of secondary stem villi and thus to a differing number of lobules, for there is no fixed relationship between cotyledons and lobules. Thus centrally placed cotyledons may contain as many as five lobules whilst those situated laterally may have only one or two lobules. The nomenclature has, however, been complicated because some have used the word cotyledon to describe maternal surface lobes, while others have used it to describe the lobule. In fact, the human placenta is not really a cotyledonary structure and Ramsey (1975) has suggested that the word cotyledon should be abandoned when referring to human and primate placentas.

The fetal circulation through the placenta

Fetal blood passes to the placenta through the two umbilical arteries which spiral around the umbilical vein. Shortly before reaching the placenta the two arteries are connected by one or more anastomotic vessels and may even fuse into a single trunk which subsequently divides into two rami (Szpakowski 1974). On reaching the placenta the arteries run in the chorion, usually being of equal size and each supplying one-half of the organ. As the arteries run across the chorion they branch repeatedly, a proportion of the branches at each division entering the placental substance to run in the primary stem villi. The cotyledonary arteries soon divide into secondary stem arteries which in turn arborize into tertiary stem arteries running through the intervillous space within the tertiary stem villi giving

off, throughout their course, many villous branches which eventually break up into a villous capillary system.

The villous capillary system was studied by Boe (1953) using an Indian ink injection technique (Fig. 4.8). He showed that not only is there a terminal villous network but also a paravascular capillary network, formed by branches arising directly from the main artery. Boe thought that this plexus communicated directly with the main vein, was of arteriolar rather than truly capillary nature and could serve as a shunt to buffer against focal overloading of the terminal villous circulation. Penfold et al (1981) found no evidence, however, of large-diameter vascular shunts within the lobule and Habashi et al (1983), in a scanning electron microscopic study of corrosion casts (Fig. 4.9), demonstrated that the paravascular plexus is found predominantly in those areas of the villous tree which are bathed with relatively poorly oxygenated maternal blood, prompting their suggestion that this network could be responsible for the transport of oxygen and nutrients to the stroma of larger villi. Leiser et al (1985) believe that the paravascular network plays a role in materno-fetal transfer in the earlier stage of placental development but has no functional role in the mature placenta. The terminal villi are vascularized only by capillary vessels and these are arranged in such a way that 3–5 terminal villi are supplied by the same multiply-coiled capillary loop (Kaufmann et al 1985).

The fetal blood flow through the placenta is about 500 ml/min and, although the main propelling force is clearly the fetal heart, it is possible that there is also a peripheral villous pulse: smooth muscle fibres are present in the stem and anchoring villi (Krantz & Parker 1963)

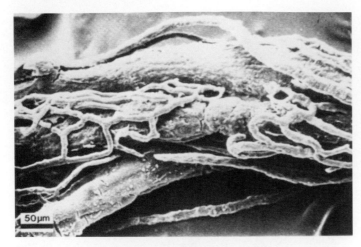

Fig. 4.9 Scanning electron micrograph of the cast of a paravascular network encircling a straight vessel of larger calibre. Reproduced with permission from Habashi et al (1983).

and it has been suggested that contraction of these fibres may help to pump blood from the placenta back to the fetus (Huszar & Bailey 1979). More recently it has been demonstrated that the fetal vessels in the placenta are ensheathed in myofibroblastic cells (Feller et al 1985), and contraction of these cells could be a more important factor in establishing the villous pulse than smooth muscle cells in stem villi.

The maternal uteroplacental circulatory system

Maternal blood enters the intervillous space via arterial inlets in the basal plate (Fig. 4.10) and is then driven by the head of maternal pressure towards the chorionic plate as a funnel-shaped stream (Ramsey & Donner 1980). The driving head of maternal pressure is gradually dissipated, a process aided by the baffling effect of the villi, and

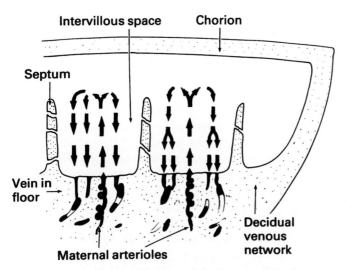

Fig. 4.10 Maternal circulation through the placenta. Reproduced with permission from Fox (1978).

lateral dispersion of the blood occurs. This forces the blood already present in the intervillous space out through basally sited wide venous outlets into the endometrial venous network. Indian ink injection studies originally suggested that the maternal blood entered the intervillous space as a jet or spurt but cineangiography has shown that these terms give an undue impression of both speed and intermittency, the maternal blood entering the space 'much as water from an actively flowing brook penetrates a reed filled marsh' (Ramsey 1965).

The physiological basis for this circulatory system is a series of pressure differentials, the pressure in the maternal arterioles being higher than the mean intervillous space pressure which in turn exceeds that in the maternal veins during a myometrial diastole. This entire system is, however, a low-pressure one for whereas in most organs there is a progressive decrease in the diameter of the arteries as they approach their target tissues, the reverse is true for the placenta; the uteroplacental vessels assume an increasing diameter as they approach their entry into the intervillous space. There is therefore a considerable drop in pressure from the proximal to the distal portion of these vessels and the full arterial pressure is not transmitted to the intervillous space. The placenta itself offers little flow resistance to maternal blood and has a high vascular conductance: there is thus very little fall in pressure across the intervillous space and the main factor governing the rate of maternal blood flow in a normal pregnancy is the vascular resistance within the radial branches of the uterine arteries as they run through the myometrium (Moll et al 1975, Moll 1981). Despite the fact that the pressure difference between arterial and venous sides of the intervillous space is small, it is apparently sufficient to drive arterial blood towards the chorionic plate, to stop short-cutting of the stream into adjacent venous outlets and to prevent mixing of neighbouring arterial inflows.

Cineangiography has shown that the individual uteroplacental arteries act independently of each other and are not all patent and discharging blood simultaneously into the intervillous space. Furthermore, during myometrial contractions, the afferent blood flow through the intervillous space may be markedly reduced or can even cease. This is probably due to compression and occlusion of the veins draining the intervillous space (Adamson & Myers 1975) but ultrasonic studies have shown that during a myometrial contraction the intervillous space distends (Bleker et al 1975) and thus the fetus is not severely deprived of oxygen supply during myometrial systole.

Relationship of maternal circulatory system to fetal lobule

The haemodynamic system originally proposed by Ramsey (1965) postulated that the maternal blood flow into the

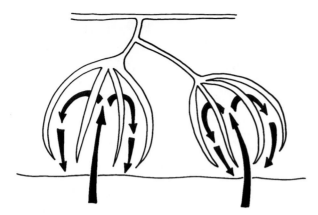

Fig. 4.11 Relationship between maternal uteroplacental blood flow and the fetal lobule, as envisaged by Freese (1966) and Wigglesworth (1967). Reproduced with permission from Fox (1986b).

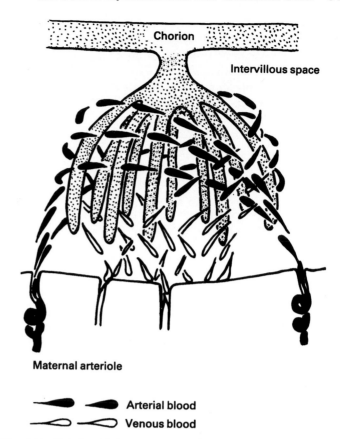

Fig. 4.12 Relationship between maternal uteroplacental blood flow and the fetal lobule, as envisaged by Lemtis (1970) and Gruenwald (1973). Reproduced with permission from Fox (1978).

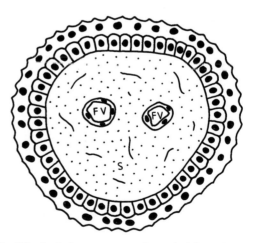

Fig. 4.13 Histological appearances of a typical first trimester villus. FV = fetal vessels; S = villous stroma. Reproduced with permission from Fox (1986b).

intervillous space was through randomly situated arterial inlets. However, it has since become clear that a definite relationship exists between the maternal vessels and the fetal lobules, probably because the lobules tend to develop preferentially around the flow from eroded maternal vessels (Reynolds 1966). The exact nature of this relationship is still not fully determined and two contrasting schemes have been proposed. Thus, Freese (1966) and Wigglesworth (1967) thought that arterial inlets into the intervillous space are situated such that the inflow from each uteroplacental vessel is into the central villus-free space of a fetal lobule and the maternal blood then flows laterally through the lobule into the interlobular area from which it is drained by basal venous outlets (Fig. 4.11). Others (Lemtis 1970, Gruenwald 1973, Schuhmann 1981) consider that the maternal vessels open, not into the central space of a lobule, but into the interlobular spaces and that the maternal blood then encircles the lobule in streams to form a shell around them, entering and leaving the lobule whilst doing this and before draining through the basal outlets (Fig. 4.12).

Whichever of these two concepts is correct it is clear that materno-fetal exchange takes place principally in those villi that form the shell of the lobule and that it is only here that a true functional intervillous space, which is probably only of capillary calibre, exists; elsewhere, in the subchorial lake, the interlobular spaces and the central intralobular spaces, villi are either sparse or absent and these areas are in functional terms physiological dead spaces.

Histology of the placental villi

In the first two months of pregnancy the villi are relatively few in number, have a homogeneous pattern and measure approximately 170 μm in diameter (Fig. 4.13). Their outer mantle is covered by a two-layered trophoblastic mantle, an outer layer of syncytiotrophoblast and an inner layer of cytotrophoblastic cells (Langhans' cells). The latter, which form a complete layer, are cuboid, polyhedral or ovoid and have well marked cell borders: their cytoplasm is clear or slightly granular whilst the nucleus is pale staining with finely dispersed chromatin. No cell boundaries are visible between the nuclei of the syncytiotrophoblast and, indeed, microinjection studies have shown that substances flow freely through this layer and can pass from one villus to another, indicating that there is a continuous common cytoplasm over the entire surface of the placental villi (Gaunt & Ockleford 1986). The syncytiotrophoblast is of uniform thickness, whilst the syncytial nuclei are regularly spaced, smaller and more densely staining than those of the cytotrophoblast.

The syncytial cytoplasm may be homogeneous, finely granular or vacuolated. A delicate brush border is often discernible on the outer surface of the syncytium and this corresponds with the microvilli seen on electron microscopy: these probably have no absorptive function but may play a role in pinocytotic vesicle formation and could also serve to increase the density of specific surface receptor sites (Dearden & Ockleford 1983). It is worth noting that the syncytiotrophoblast lines the intervillous space and thus acts in the manner of an endothelium; since the structure of syncytiotrophoblast is quite unlike that of an endothelial cell, its ability to function in this manner is somewhat of a mystery. It is possible, however, that some of the many placental proteins secreted by the syncytiotrophoblast act to prevent coagulation. Furthermore, studies with monoclonal antibodies have shown that, despite their structural dissimilarity, syncytiotrophoblast and endothelial cells share otherwise specific antigens (Voland et al 1986).

The villous stroma is at this stage formed by loose mesenchymal tissue. The exact stage of gestation at which fetal vessels appear within the stroma is variable but by the end of 8 weeks small centrally placed vessels, lined by large immature endothelial cells, are present (Demir et al 1989). Hofbauer cells are a prominent feature of the villous stroma: these cells may be round, ovoid or reniform, measure about 25 μm in diameter and have an eccentrically placed nucleus (Fig. 4.14). There is now overwhelming morphological, cytochemical and immunological evidence that the Hofbauer cells are fetal tissue macrophages (Fox & Kharkongor 1969, Moskalewski et al 1975, Castellucci et al 1980, Demir & Erbengi 1984, Castellucci & Kaufmann 1990). Their origin is obscure for they are present in the villi before they are vascularized by fetal vessels and before haematopoiesis begins in the fetus. It has recently been suggested that there are several populations of Hofbauer cells, those in early pregnancy developing from chorionic mesenchyme but later being supplemented by cells derived either from the fetal liver or bone marrow (Castellucci et al 1986). The number of Hofbauer cells has in the past been seriously underestimated (Wood 1980); they probably play a number of roles, some related to transport mechanisms and others to immunological protection of the fetus; in this latter respect their ability to trap maternal antibodies crossing over into the placental tissues is almost certainly of considerable importance.

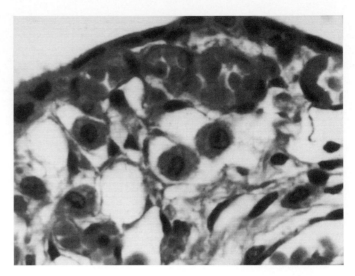

Fig. 4.14 Several typical Hofbauer cells in the stroma of a placental villus. Haematoxylin and eosin. × 840. Reproduced with permission from Fox (1967).

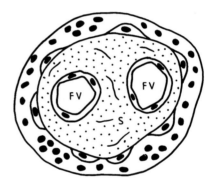

Fig. 4.15 Histological appearances of a typical second-trimester villus. FV = fetal vessels; S = villous stroma. Reproduced with permission from Fox (1986b).

Between the eighth and 30th weeks of gestation the villi become more numerous and the predominant form of villus has an average diameter of about 40 μm (Fig. 4.15). In these villi the cytotrophoblastic cells are less prominent whilst the syncytiotrophoblast is thinner and somewhat irregular: the syncytial nuclei are less evenly distributed than in the first trimester and often show a degree of clustering. A distinct, but thin, trophoblastic basement membrane is present, separating the trophoblast from the stroma. The stroma is more compact than is the case in the villi of early gestation and contains a variable number of fibroblasts, myofibroblasts and delicate collagen fibres. Hofbauer cells are seen in the stromal interfibrillary spaces but appear less numerous than in the villi of the early placenta. The villous fetal capillaries are quite prominent, tend to lie more towards the villous periphery and are lined by flattened, fully mature endothelial cells.

From about the 30th week of gestation small terminal villi, measuring about 40 μm in diameter, begin to appear

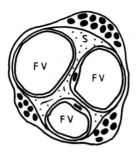

Fig. 4.16 Terminal villus—the predominant type of villus in the term placenta. FV = fetal vessels; S = villous stroma. Reproduced with permission from Fox (1986b).

and these are the predominant form of villi seen in the term placenta (Fig. 4.16). Their trophoblastic covering layer is irregularly thinned whilst cytotrophoblastic cells are few and inconspicuous. The cytotrophoblastic cells do however retain their proliferative capacity and represent a largely quiescent germinative zone in which a recrudescence of growth occurs, if the necessity arises, to replace damaged syncytiotrophoblast, e.g. in severe pre-eclampsia where ischaemically damaged syncytiotrophoblast is readily repaired by cytotrophoblastic proliferation; this phenomenon is easily recognized by the undue prominence and number of cells in which mitotic figures may be seen (Jones & Fox 1980).

In terminal villi the syncytial nuclei are irregularly distributed and are often aggregated to form multinucleated protrusions into the intervillous space (Fox 1978). It has been claimed that many—even most—of these knots (Fig. 4.17) are histological artefacts due to tangential sectioning of the villi (Cantle et al 1986) but the nuclei within these knots differ considerably from those in the

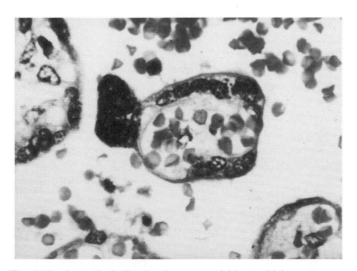

Fig. 4.17 A terminal villus bearing a syncytial knot which appears as a multinucleated protrusion from the free surface of the trophoblast. Haematoxylin and eosin. × 660. Reproduced with permission from Fox (1978).

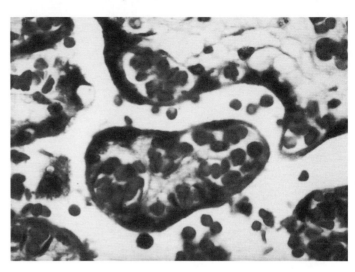

Fig. 4.18 A terminal villus with a vasculo-syncytial membrane (on the right). Haematoxylin and eosin. × 680. Reproduced with permission from Fox (1985b).

rest of the villous syncytiotrophoblast and show all the ultrastructural features of senescence. Syncytial knots are therefore seen to be formed of aged nuclei sequestrated from functional areas of the syncytium, their loss being compensated by the formation of fresh syncytial nuclei from the cytotrophoblast (Jones & Fox 1977).

In many terminal villi, the syncytiotrophoblast is focally attenuated and anuclear (Fig. 4.18): these thinned areas commonly overlie a dilated fetal capillary vessel and may, on light microscopy, appear to fuse with the vessel wall to form a vasculo-syncytial membrane (Getzowa & Sadowsky 1950). Electron microscopy shows that there is no real fusion between trophoblast and vessel wall but nevertheless these membranous areas of the syncytiotrophoblast differ markedly from the non thinned areas of the syncytium in their content of histochemically detectable enzymes (Amstutz 1960), in their ultrastructure (Burgos & Rodriguez 1966) and in their surface characteristics (Fox & Agrofojo-Blanco 1974); it is almost certain that they are specialized zones of the placenta for the facilitation of gas transfer across the placenta. The formation of vasculo-syncytial membranes is not due simply to stretching the trophoblast by dilated fetal vessels, for scanning electron microscopy shows that they are randomly situated and very localized, often occurring along the course of a vessel; this distribution is incompatible with a purely mechanical origin (Fox & Agrofojo-Blanco 1974). Thus the functional, regional differentiation which can be detected ultrastructurally in the villous syncytiotrophoblast of the immature placenta (Dempsey & Luse 1971, Kaufmann & Stegner 1972) is sufficiently overt in the terminal villi of the mature placenta to be easily discernible on light microscopy.

The trophoblastic basement membrane of the terminal villi is well defined while the villous stromal tissue is

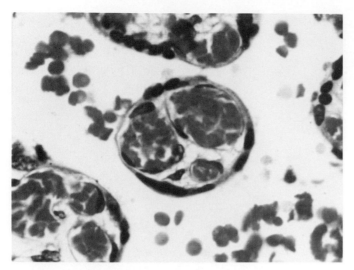

Fig. 4.19 A terminal villus with sinusoidally dilated fetal vessels. Haematoxylin and eosin. × 580. Reproduced with permission from Fox (1978).

reduced to a thin layer between the sinusoidally dilated villous capillaries. Hofbauer cells are present in the stroma but are difficult to recognize because of their compression by vessels and collagen fibres. A sprinkling of mast cells is also present in the villous stroma (Mahnke & Emmrich 1973, Durst-Zivkovic 1973); their function in this site is uncertain.

In the terminal villi there are usually 2–6 fetal capillary vessels characteristically situated towards the periphery of the villus in close approximation to the covering trophoblast. These vessels are commonly sinusoidally dilated and occupy most of the cross-sectional area of the villus (Fig. 4.19). Aherne (1975) thought that the dilatation of the fetal villous vessels was a mechanism for crowding flow lines, and hence increasing concentration gradients, for substances crossing from maternal to fetal blood and was thus a mechanism for augmenting the efficiency of placental transfer mechanisms. By contrast, Kaufmann et al (1985) considered that the sinusoidal dilatation of these vessels was a method of decreasing blood flow resistance, allowing an evenness of blood flow throughout the placenta and facilitating fetal placental perfusion.

Growth, maturation and ageing of placental villi

It will be clear from the description of villous histology that the villous morphology alters considerably during pregnancy. It should not be considered that these changes occur in individual villi i.e. a first-trimester villus does not gradually transform into a third-trimester villus. The observed changes reflect the progressive growth and evolution of the villous tree (Sen et al 1979, Kaufmann et al 1979, Kaufmann 1982, Castellucci et al 1990, Jauniaux et al 1992). The villi present in the first 2 months of pregnancy develop into stem villi, later giving off inter-

mediate villi which represent the growth zone of the placenta; as they mature they begin to give out small outgrowths which develop into terminal villi. Thus in the second trimester the villous population consists of an admixture of immature and mature intermediate villi whilst in the term placenta nearly 60% of the villi are of the terminal type. These latter villi with their high surface area : volume ratio, their laterally placed sinusoidal vessels and with a trophoblastic layer specifically differentiated in some areas for gas transport, represent the form of villous structure which provides optimal conditions for maternofetal transfer. The changes in villous morphology during gestation reflect a continuing process of maturation of the villous tree with a progressive increasing functional efficiency (Jackson et al 1992, Mayhew et al 1993).

This maturational process within the villous tree has been widely misinterpreted as ageing; there is a tenaciously held belief that during the course of normal pregnancy the placenta progressively ages and at term is on the verge of a decline into morphological and functional senescence. An extension of this attitude is the concept of premature or accelerated ageing that used to be thought a feature of the placenta in certain complications of pregnancy, such as pre-eclampsia. In purely morphological terms there are no histological or ultrastructural changes in the villi which can be considered as indicative of an ageing process (Fox 1979) whilst the claim by Parmley et al (1981) that lipofuscin pigment accumulates in the villous syncytiotrophoblast, a change generally accepted as being a feature of ageing cells, has been shown to be erroneous (Haigh et al 1984).

It has been suggested that a sign of placental ageing is the cessation of placental DNA synthesis and growth which occurs at the 36th week of gestation (Winick et al 1967). More recent studies have however shown that total placental DNA levels continue to rise in a linear fashion until and even beyond the 40th week of gestation (Sands & Dobbing 1985). This finding is in accord with histological evidence of fresh villous growth in the term placenta (Fox 1978) and with autoradiographic and cytophotometric studies which have shown continuing DNA synthesis in the villi of the placenta at term (Geier et al 1975, Hustin et al 1984, Iversen & Farsund 1985). The continuing growth of the placenta has also been confirmed by morphometric techniques showing a continuing expansion of the villous surface area and progressive branching of the villous tree up to and past term (Boyd 1984).

Placental growth certainly slows during the last few weeks of gestation, although this decline in growth rate is neither invariable nor irreversible, for the placenta can continue to increase in size when faced with an unfavourable maternal environment (e.g. pregnancy at high altitude or severe maternal anaemia), whilst the potential for a recrudescence of growth is shown by the proliferative response mounted to repair syncytial damage in conditions such as pre-eclampsia (Jones & Fox 1980, Hustin et al 1984, Redman 1993). Those arguing that decreased placental growth during late pregnancy is evidence of senescence often appear to be comparing the placenta to the gut; in such an organ continuing viability is dependent upon a constantly replicating stem cell layer producing short-lived postmitotic cells. A more apt comparison would be with an organ like the liver, formed principally of long-lived postmitotic cells and which, once an optimal size has been attained to meet metabolic demands, shows little evidence of cell proliferation whilst still retaining a latent capacity for growth activity. Certainly there seems to be no good reason why the placenta, having reached a size sufficient to meet its transfer function adequately, should continue to grow. The term placenta, with its considerable functional reserve capacity, more than meets this need.

Functional adequacy of the placenta

The placenta has many functions but its most important role is to transfer oxygen and nutrients from the maternal circulation to the fetal blood. Many have thought that the placenta frequently fails to meet the demands placed upon it and that this condition of placental insufficiency is responsible for many instances of fetal hypoxia, intra-uterine growth retardation or death. In reality the placenta rarely becomes insufficient, for it has a considerable functional reserve capacity. Histopathological studies clearly indicate that the placenta can withstand the functional loss of 30–40% of its villous population without any evidence of a decline in its physiological capacity (Fox 1985a, 1986a). Experimental studies, involving either surgical reduction of placental mass (Robinson et al 1979) or artificially increased fetal oxygen consumption (Lorijn & Longo 1980), have confirmed the striking functional reserve of the placenta. Very few pathological lesions of the placenta are sufficiently extensive to dissipate this physiological reserve and it is difficult to accept that intrinsic placental damage is an important factor in the aetiology of inadequate materno-fetal transfer. It has become increasingly clear that the common factor in most cases of presumed placental insufficiency is reduced maternal utero-placental blood flow which is, in turn, due to inadequate conversion of the spiral arteries into uteroplacental vessels by extravillous trophoblast during the early stages of pregnancy.

THE FETAL MEMBRANES—AMNION AND CHORION

Development of the fetal membranes

The conversion of the early morula to a blastocyst is facilitated by the formation of a central fluid-filled cavity.

This separates the primary trophoblastic cell mass, which develops into the placenta and extraplacental chorion, from those cells which give rise to the embryo and contribute to the formation of the yolk sac and the amnion. The latter cells form the eccentrically situated inner cell mass which remains in contact with the cytotrophoblast on the inner aspect of the blastocyst wall.

During the 8th and 9th days postovulation the inner cell mass arranges itself into a bilaminar disc, with the inner layer, i.e. that facing the blastocyst cavity forming the primitive embryonic endoderm while the outer, in contact with cytotrophoblast, forms the primitive embryonic ectoderm. The amniotic cavity first appears as a slit-like space between embryonic ectoderm and the adjacent cytotrophoblast. This enlarges by the 12th postovulatory day to form a small cavity, of which the base is formed by embryonic ectoderm and the walls and roof by cytotrophoblast. At the same time endodermal cells migrate out from the deeper layer of the embryonic disc to line the blastocyst cavity and thus form the primary yolk sac.

Extraembryonic mesenchyme subsequently appears (Fig. 4.20), possibly derived from the trophoblast, and separates the primary yolk sac from the blastocyst wall. Extraembryonic mesenchyme also intrudes between, and largely separates off, the roof of the amniotic sac and the trophoblast of the chorion. A connection between the two is, however, maintained for a time by the persistence of a column of cells, the amniotic duct, which provides a pathway for continuing migration of trophoblastic cells into the amniotic epithelium. Mitotic activity at the margin of the embryonic ectodermal disc suggests that the ectoderm is also a continuing source of amniotic epithelial cells.

The extraembryonic mesenchyme forms a loose reticulum in which small cystic spaces appear. The spaces

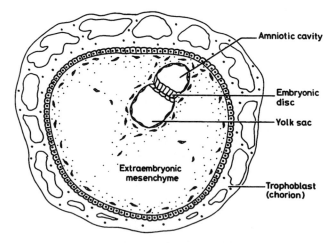

Fig. 4.20 Relationship between developing amniotic cavity and extraembryonic mesenchyme. Reproduced with permission from Fox (1986b).

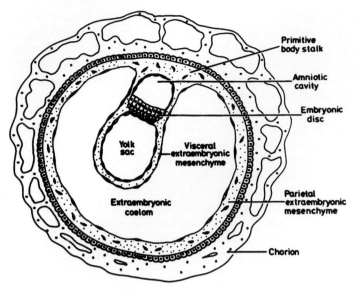

Fig. 4.21 Relationship between developing amniotic cavity, extraembryonic mesenchyme, extraembryonic coelom and primitive body stalk. Reproduced with permission from Fox (1986b).

gradually enlarge and fuse to form the extraembryonic coelom which splits the extraembryonic mesenchyme into two layers (Fig. 4.21), one apposed to the trophoblast covering the amnion (the parietal extraembryonic mesenchyme) and the other covering the yolk sac (the visceral extraembryonic mesenchyme). The progressively enlarging extraembryonic coelom also separates the amnion from the inner aspect of the chorion, except at the caudal end of the embryo where an attachment of extraembryonic mesenchyme persists, to form the body stalk from which the umbilical cord will eventually be derived. Subsequently the amniotic space enlarges at the expense of the extraembryonic coelom and the developing embryo bulges into the expanding amniotic cavity (Fig. 4.22). Meanwhile the yolk sac becomes partially incorporated into the embryo in which it gives rise to the gut. The part of the yolk sac remaining outside the embryo communicates with the primitive gut, but this communicating

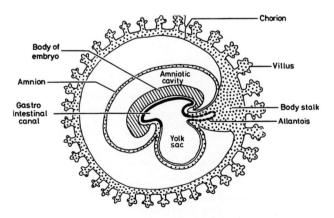

Fig. 4.22 Relationship between the expanding amniotic cavity and the developing embryo. Reproduced with permission from Fox (1986b).

channel gradually becomes elongated and attenuated to form the vitelline duct; the extraembryonic yolk sac becomes progressively removed away from the embryo, and eventually is incorporated into the lower end of the body stalk.

A further expansion of the amniotic cavity leads to more or less complete obliteration of the extraembryonic coelom with the eventual fusion of the extraembryonic mesenchyme covering the amnion with that lining the chorion. At the same time the extraplacental chorion (chorion laeve) ceases to produce syncytiotrophoblast and the cytotrophoblastic component undergoes a partial regression. The single, fused amniochorionic membrane is now fully formed.

Structure of the amnion and chorion

Bourne (1960), using a combination of light and electron microscopy, was able to define seven distinct layered components of the amniochorion but on routine histological examination of the membranes it is difficult to detect more than five histological strata (Kohler 1987). This is the number one would expect from a knowledge of the development of the amniochorion. These layers from fetal to maternal side would be:

1. Amniotic epithelium.
2. Amniotic connective tissue.
3. Spongy layer.
4. Chorionic connective tissue.
5. Trophoblast.

On embryological grounds it would be assumed that the amniotic connective tissue is derived from visceral extraembryonic mesenchyme, that the spongy layer is a vestige of the extraembryonic coelom and that the chorionic connective tissues originate from the parietal extraembryonic mesenchyme. This is probably not the entire story, however, for it is probable that the amniotic connective tissue is produced at least partly by the amniotic epithelial cells (Aplin et al 1985).

The amniotic epithelial cells are usually described as cuboidal, but there are also subpopulations of flat and columnar cells, the flattened cells being more common in the extraplacental amnion and umbilical cord and columnar cells in the placental amnion (Kohler 1987). The amniotic cells have prominent intercellular bridges near their free margins which increase the mechanical stability and coherence of the layer. It should not be thought that the amniotic cells serve only a mechanical function for they play an important role in water transport and appear to have a significant secretory capacity (Ho et al 1982). Amniotic epithelial cells do not manifest trophoblastic antigens but have a unique plasma membrane (amniotic) antigen specific to that epithelial tissue (Hsi et al 1982). The trophoblastic component of the amniochorion varies from 2 to 10 cell layers in thickness, expresses specific trophoblastic antigens and does not react with antisera to amniotic epithelium.

Macrophages, comparable in all ways with the Hofbauer cells of the chorionic villi, are present in the amnio-chorion: they are usually inconspicuous but can become prominent if they take up meconium. Myofibroblasts have also been described in the membranes (Wang & Schneider 1982).

UMBILICAL CORD

The umbilical cord links the fetus with the placenta. Although often regarded simply as a mechanical conduit, it also plays a role in the movement of water and other substances between the fetal circulation and the amniotic fluid.

Structure

The basic structure of the cord is simple: it consists of two arteries and a vein embedded in Wharton's jelly covered by one or more layers of amniotic epithelium. Vestigial structures are not uncommon. Remnants of the allantoic and vitelline ducts are usually lined by a simple flat or cuboidal epithelium which may differentiate into fully fledged gastrointestinal-type epithelium.

Wharton's jelly, a mucomyxoid tissue, consists of an abundant ground substance, rich in mucopolysaccharides, in which are embedded collagen fibres, mast cells and sparse large flat stellate cells arranged concentrically around the vessels. Clearly, Wharton's jelly has as its salient function a mechanical cushioning effect which protects the umbilical vessels from trauma. The tissue is metabolically very active, however (Zawisch 1955), and it would be unwise to allot to it only a mechanistic function.

The umbilical cord arteries are unusual in lacking an internal elastic lamina. They have a well formed media zone containing both myocytes and myofibroblasts arranged in a helical fashion (Gebrane-Younes et al 1986). The arteries lack an adventitia; Zawisch (1955) pointed out that Wharton's jelly appears to substitute for this layer. The umbilical vein differs from the arteries less than is the case elsewhere in the body but has a thinner media and a better developed mural elastic component. Both arteries and veins have endothelial cells which appear to be metabolically highly active. It has been suggested that these vessels may play a role in water transfer to the amniotic fluid (Gebrane-Younes et al 1986). The umbilical vessels lack vasa vasorum and the long-standing controversy over whether or not they are innervated has still not been resolved (Reilly & Russell 1977, Bettzieche 1978).

Length of the cord

The average length of the cord is between 54 and 61 cm (Fox 1978). There is a wide variability but the minimum length of the cord which allows a normal cephalic delivery at term is 32 cm, whilst an arbitrary length of 100 cm has been accepted as the maximum which does not predispose to complications such as knotting, torsion or prolapse. Although there is a wide scatter within these extremes, Mills et al (1983) have formulated standard tables for cord length based on measurements of over 18 000 cords from babies ranging in gestational age from 34 to 43 weeks. These tables show that the cord continues to grow in length up to and beyond term and that male babies tend to have longer cords than females. This may be related to greater intrauterine movement of male fetuses, for there is both clinical and experimental evidence that restriction of fetal activity results from a short cord. Fetal movement appears to have a stimulatory effect on the longitudinal growth of the cord (Miller et al 1981, Moessinger et al 1982).

Site of cord insertion

There is a widespread impression that the cord should insert into the central portion of the placental disc. The fallacy of this belief has been admirably summarized by Kohler (1987):

In discussing what is the normal site of insertion some authors appear to have been influenced by perfectionist idiosyncrasies: a central insertion is more gratifying, therefore it must be normal. On the other hand, the contention that eccentric insertion is more common than central and must therefore represent the norm, is also not free from fallacy. There are no natural categories of central, moderately eccentric, markedly eccentric and marginal insertions, but a continuous series and the frequency of insertion at various points within this series is, therefore, determined by the laws of probability.

This view is confirmed by the finding that the site of cord insertion into the placental disc is of no clinical significance (Fox 1978).

Velamentous insertion of the cord is not, however, a normal event. In this condition the cord does not insert into the placental surface but into the extraplacental membranes so that unprotected umbilical vessels, divested of Wharton's jelly, run for some distance between the amnion and chorion exposed to the risk of mechanical injury before reaching the placental margin. This risk is greatest when the vessels overlie the internal os (vasa praevia); as the presenting part of the fetus descends during labour it will inevitably lacerate and rupture the unprotected vessels. Bleeding from velamentously inserted vessels can occur even in sites well away from the internal os. Despite a plethora of theories, neither the aetiology nor the pathogenesis of velamentous insertion is understood (Fox 1978, Kohler 1987).

Acknowledgements

Figures 4.6, 4.13, 4.15, 4.16, 4.20, 4.21 and 4.22 were drawn by Dr Carolyn J. P. Jones. I am indebted to Dr P. Wilkin for supplying me with Figure 4.3 and to the late Dr F. Boe for Figure 4.8.

REFERENCES

Adamson K, Myers R E 1975 Circulation in the intervillous space: obstetrical considerations in fetal deprivation. In: Gruenwald P (ed) The placenta and its maternal supply line. Medical and Technical Publishing, Lancaster, pp 158–177

Aherne W 1975 Morphometry. In: Gruenwald P (ed) The placenta and its maternal supply line. Medical and Technical Publishing, Lancaster, pp 80–97

Amstutz E 1960 Beobachtungen über die Reiung der Chorionzotten in der menslichen Plazenta mit besonderer Berückichtigung der Epithelplatten. Acta Anatomica 42: 12–30

Aplin J D, Campbell S, Allen T D 1985 The extracellular matrix of human amniotic epithelium: ultrastructure, composition and deposition. Journal of Cell Science 79: 119–136

Bettzieche H 1978 Studien zur Frage der Innervation der Nabelschnur. Zentralblatt für Gynäkologie 100: 799–804

Bleker O P, Kloosterman G J, Mieras D J, Oosting J, Sallé H J A 1975 Intervillous space during uterine contractions in human subjects: an ultrasonic study. American Journal of Obstetrics and Gynecology 123: 697–699

Boe F 1953 Studies on the vascularization of the human placenta. Acta Obstetricia et Gynecologica Scandinavica 32 (suppl 5): 1–92

Bourne G L 1960 The microscopic anatomy of the human amnion and chorion. American Journal of Obstetrics and Gynecology 79: 1070–1073

Boyd J D, Hamilton W J 1970 The human placenta. Heffer, Cambridge

Boyd P A 1984 Quantitative studies of the normal human placenta from 10 weeks of gestation to term. Early Human Development 9: 297–307

Brosens I, Robertson W B, Dixon H G 1967 The physiological response of the vessels of the placental bed in normal pregnancy. Journal of Pathology and Bacteriology 93: 569–579

Bulmer J N, Johnson P M 1985 Antigen expression by trophoblast populations in the human placenta and their possible immunobiological relevance. Placenta 6: 127–140

Burgos M H, Rodriguez E M 1966 Specialized zones in the trophoblast of the human term placenta. American Journal of Obstetrics and Gynecology 96: 342–356

Cantle S J, Kaufmann P, Luckhardt M, Schweikhart G 1987 Interpretation of syncytial sprouts and bridges in the human placenta. Placenta 8: 221–234

Castellucci M, Kaufmann P 1990 Hofbauer cells. In: Benirschke K, Kaufmann P (eds) Pathology of the human placenta, 2nd edn. Springer, Berlin, pp 71–80

Castellucci M, Scheper M, Scheffen I, Celona A, Kaufmann P 1990 The development of the human placental villous tree. Anatomy and Embryology 181: 117–128

Castellucci M, Zaccheo D, Pescetto G 1980 A three-dimensional study of the normal human placental villous core. I. The Hofbauer cells. Cell and Tissue Research 210: 235–247

Castellucci M, Celona A, Bartels H, Steininger B, Benedetto V, Kaufman P 1987 Mitoses of the Hofbauer cell: possible implications for a fetal macrophage. Placenta 8: 65–75

Dearden I, Ockleford C D 1983 Structure of human trophoblast: correlation with function. In: Loke Y W, Whyte A (eds) Biology of trophoblast. Elsevier, Amsterdam, pp 69–110

Demir R, Erbengi T 1984 Some new findings about Hofbauer cells in the chorionic villi of the human placenta. Acta Anatomica 119: 18–26

Demir R, Kaufmann P, Castellucci M, Erbengi T, Kotowski A 1989 Fetal vasculogenesis and angiogenesis in human placental villi. Acta Anatomica 136: 117–128

Dempsey E W, Luse S A 1971 Regional specialisations in the syncytial trophoblast of early human placenta. Journal of Anatomy 108: 545–561

de Wolf F, de Wolf-Peeters C, Brosens I 1973 Ultrastructure of the spiral arteries in the human placental bed at the end of normal pregnancy. American Journal of Obstetrics and Gynecology 117: 833–848

Durst-Zivkovic B 1973 Das Vorkommen der Mastzellen in der Nachgeburt. Anatomischer Anzeiger 134: 225–229

Enders A C 1965 A comparative study of the fine structure of the trophoblast in several hemochorial placentae. American Journal of Anatomy 116: 29–67

Feller A C, Schneider H, Schmidt D, Parwaresch M R 1985 Myofibroblast as a major cellular constituent of villous stroma in human placenta. Placenta 6: 405–415

Fox H 1967 The incidence and significance of Hofbauer cells in the mature placenta. Journal of Pathology and Bacteriology 93: 710–717

Fox H 1978 Pathology of the placenta. Saunders, London

Fox H 1979 The placenta as a model of organ ageing. In: Beaconsfield P, Villee C (eds) Placenta—a neglected experimental animal. Pergamon, Oxford, pp 351–378

Fox H 1985a Placental pathology: a contemporary approach. Obstetrics and Gynecology Annual 14: 427–440

Fox H 1985b Placental structure. In: Macdonald R R (ed) Scientific basis of obstetrics and gynaecology, 3rd edn. Churchill Livingstone, Edinburgh, pp 1–38

Fox H 1986a Pathology of the placenta. Clinics in obstetrics and gynaecology, vol 13. Churchill Livingstone, Edinburgh, pp 1–28

Fox H 1986b Development of the placenta and membranes. In: Dewhurst J, De Swiet M, Chamberlain G (eds) Basic sciences in obstetrics and gynaecology. Churchill Livingstone, Edinburgh, pp 34–41

Fox H, Agrofojo-Blanco A 1974 Scanning electron microscopy of the human placenta in normal and abnormal pregnancies. European Journal of Obstetrics, Gynecology and Reproductive Biology 4: 45–50

Fox H, Kharkongor N F 1969 Enzyme histochemistry of the Hofbauer cells of the human placenta. Journal of Obstetrics and Gynaecology of the British Commonwealth 76: 918–921

Freese U E 1966 The fetal–maternal circulation of the placenta. I. Histomorphologic, placental injection and X-ray cinematographic studies on human placenta. American Journal of Obstetrics and Gynecology 94: 354–360

Galton M 1962 DNA content of placental nuclei. Journal of Cell Biology 13: 183–203

Gaunt M, Ockleford C D 1986 Microinjection of human placenta: 2. Biological application. Placenta 7: 325–331

Gebrane-Younes J, Minh H N, Orcel O 1986 Ultrastructure of human umbilical vessels: a possible role in amniotic fluid formation. Placenta 7: 173–183

Geier G, Schuhmann R, Kraus H 1975 Regional unterschiedliche Zellproliferation innerhalb der Plazenteone reifer menschlicher Plazenten: autoradiographische Untersuchungen. Archiv für Gynäkologie 218: 31–37

Getzowa S, Sadowsky A 1950 On the structure of the human placenta with full-term and immature foetus, living or dead. Journal of Obstetrics and Gynaecology of the British Empire 57: 388–396

Gosseye S, Fox H 1984 An immunohistological comparison of the secretory capacity of villous and extravillous trophoblast in the human placenta. Placenta 5: 329–348

Gruenwald P 1973 Lobular structure of hemochorial primate placentas, and its relation to maternal vessels. American Journal of Anatomy 136: 133–152

Habashi S, Burton G J, Steven D H 1983 Morphological study of the fetal vasculature of the human term placenta: scanning electron microscopy of corrosion casts. Placenta 4: 41–56

Haigh M, Chawner L E, Fox H 1984 The human placenta does not contain lipofuscin pigment. Placenta 5: 459–464

Ho P C, Haynes W D G, Ing R M Y, Jones W R 1982 Histological, ultrastructural and immunofluorescence studies of the amniochorionic membrane. Placenta 3: 109–126

Hsi B-L, Yeh C-J G, Faulk W P 1982 Human amniochorion: tissue-specific markers, transferrin receptors and histocompatibility antigens. Placenta 3: 1–12

Hustin J, Foedart J M, Lambotte R 1984 Cellular proliferation in villi of normal and pathological pregnancies. Gynecologic and Obstetric Investigation 17: 1–9

Huszar G, Bailey P 1979 Isolation and characterization of myosin in the human term placenta. American Journal of Obstetrics and Gynecology 135: 707–712

Iversen O E, Farsund T 1985 Flow cytometry in the assessment of human placental growth. Acta Obstetricia et Gynecologica Scandinavica 64: 605–707

Jackson M R, Mayhew T M, Boyd P A 1992 Quantitative description of the elaboration and maturation of villi from 10 weeks of gestation to term. Placenta 12: 357–370

Jauniaux E, Burton G J, Jones C J P 1992 Early human placental morphology. In: Barnea E R, Hustin J, Jauniaux E (eds) The first twelve weeks of gestation. Springer, Berlin, pp 45–64

Jones C J P, Fox H 1977 Syncytial knots and intervillous bridges in the human placenta: an ultrastructural study. Journal of Anatomy 124: 275–286

Jones C J P, Fox H 1980 An ultrastructural and ultrahistochemical study of the human placenta in maternal pre-eclampsia. Placenta 1: 61–76

Kaufmann P 1982 Development and differentiation of the human placental villous tree. Bibliotheca Anatomica 22: 29–39

Kaufmann P, Stegner H E 1972 Uber die funktionelle Differentzeitung des Zottensyncytium in der mesnchlichen Plazenta. Zeitschrift für Zellforschung und Mikroskopische Anatomie 135: 361–382

Kaufmann P, Sen D K, Schwikhart G 1979 Classification of human placental villi. I. Histology. Cell and Tissue Research 200: 409–423

Kaufmann P, Bruns U, Leiser R, Luckhardt M, Winterhager E 1985 The fetal vascularization of term human placental villi. II. Intermediate and terminal villi. Anatomy and Embryology 173: 203–214

Khong T Y, de Wolf F, Robertson W B, Brosens I 1986 Inadequate maternal vascular response to placentation in pregnancies complicated by preeclampsia and by small-for-gestational-age infants. British Journal of Obstetrics and Gynaecology 93: 1049–1059

Kohler H G 1987 Pathology of the umbilical cord and of the fetal membranes. In: Fox H (ed) Haines and Taylor's textbook of obstetrical and gynaecological pathology, 3rd edn. Churchill Livingstone, Edinburgh, pp 1079–1116

Krantz K E, Parker J G 1963 Contractile properties of the smooth muscle in the human placenta. Clinical Obstetrics and Gynecology 6: 26–38

Kurman R J, Main C S, Chen H-H 1984 Intermediate trophoblast: a distinctive form of trophoblast with specific morphological, biochemical and functional features. Placenta 5: 349–370

Küstermann W 1981 Uber 'Proliferationsknoten' und 'Syncytialknoten' der menschlichen Plazenta. Anatomischer Anzeiger 150: 144–157

Leiser R, Luckhardt M, Kaufmann P, Winterhager E, Bruns U 1985 The fetal vascularisation of term human placental villi. I. Peripheral stem villi. Anatomy and Embryology 173: 71–80

Lemtis H 1970 Physiologie der Plazenta. Fortschritte der Geburtshilfe und Gynäkologie 41: 1–52

Lorijn R H V, Longo L D 1980 Clinical and physiologic implications of increased fetal oxygen consumption. American Journal of Obstetrics and Gynecology 136: 451–457

Mahnke P F, Emmrich P 1973 Zur Mastzellhaufigkeit der menschlichen Plazentarzotte. Zentralblatt für Gynäkologie 95: 730–732

Mayhew T M, Jackson M R, Boyd P A 1993 Changes in oxygen diffusive conductances of human placentae during gestation (10–41 weeks) are commensurate with the gain in fetal weight. Placenta 14: 51–61

McLean J M 1987 Embryology and anatomy of the female genital tract and ovaries. In: Fox H (ed) Haines's & Taylor's textbook of gynaecological and obstetrical pathology. Churchill Livingstone, Edinburgh, pp 1–50

Miller M E, Higginbottom M, Smith D W 1981 Short umbilical cord: its origin and relevance. Pediatrics 67: 618–621

Mills J L, Harley E E, Moessinger A C 1983 Standards for measuring umbilical cord length. Placenta 4: 423–426

Moessinger A C, Blanc W A, Marone P A, Polsen D C 1982 Umbilical cord length as an index of fetal activity: experimental study and clinical implications. Pediatric Research 16: 109–112

Moll W 1981 Physiologie der maternen placentaren Durchblutung. In: Becker V, Schiebler Th H, Kubli F (eds) Die Plazenta des Menschen. Thieme, Stuttgart, pp 172–194

Moll W, Kunzell W, Herburger J 1975 Hemodynamic implications of hemochorial placentation. European Journal of Obstetrics,

Gynecology and Reproductive Biology 5: 67–74

Moskalewski S, Ptak W, Czernik Z 1975 Demonstration of cells with IgG receptor in human placenta. Biology of the Neonate 26: 268–273

Parmley T H, Gupta P K, Walker M A 1981 'Aging' pigments in term human placenta. American Journal of Obstetrics and Gynecology 139: 760–763

Penfold P, Wooten R, Hytten F E 1981 Studies of a single placental cotyledon in vitro III. The dimensions of the villous capillaries. Placenta 2: 161–168

Pijnenborg R, Bland J M, Robertson W B, Dixon G, Brosens I 1981 The pattern of interstitial trophoblastic invasion of the myometrium in early human pregnancy. Placenta 2: 303–315

Pijnenborg R, Bland J M, Robertson W B, Brosens I 1983 Uteroplacental arterial changes related to interstitial trophoblast migration in early human pregnancy. Placenta 4: 397–414

Pijnenborg R, Anthony J, Davey D A et al 1991 Placental bed spiral arteries in hypertensive disorders of pregnancy. British Journal of Obstetrics and Gynaecology 98: 648–655

Ramsey E M 1959 Circulation in the placenta. In: Villee C A (ed) Gestation: transactions of the fifth conference. Macy Foundation, New York

Ramsey E M 1965 Circulation in the placenta. Birth Defects, Original Articles Series 1: 5–12

Ramsey E M 1975 Discussion of Gruenwald P. European Journal of Obstetrics, Gynecology and Reproductive Biology 5: 31

Ramsey E M, Donner M W 1980 Placental vasculature and circulation. Thieme, Stuttgart

Redman C W G 1993 The placenta, pre-eclampsia and chronic villitis. In: Redman C W G, Sargent I L, Starkey P M (eds) The human placenta. Blackwell Science, Oxford, pp 414–467

Redman C W, McMichael A J, Stirrat G M, Sunderland C A, Ting A 1984 Class I major histocompatibility complex antigens on human extravillous trophoblast. Immunology 52: 457–468

Reilly F D, Russell P T 1977 Neurohistochemical evidence supporting an absence of adrenergic and cholinergic innervation in the human placenta and umbilical cord. Anatomical Record 188: 277–285

Reynolds S R M 1966 Formation of fetal cotyledons in the hemochorial placenta: a theoretical consideration of the functional implications of such an arrangement. American Journal of Obstetrics and Gynecology 94: 425–439

Richart R 1961 Studies of placental morphogenesis. I. Radiographic studies of human placenta utilizing tritiated thymidine. Proceedings of the Society for Experimental Biology and Medicine 106: 829–831

Robertson W B, Brosens I, Dixon H G 1967 The pathological response of the vessels of the placental bed in hypertensive pregnancy. Journal of Pathology and Bacteriology 93: 581–592

Robertson W B, Brosens I, Dixon H G 1975 Uteroplacental vascular pathology. European Journal of Obstetrics, Gynecology and Reproductive Biology 5: 47–65

Robertson W B, Brosens I A, Dixon H G 1981 Maternal blood supply in fetal growth retardation. In: Van Assche A, Robertson W B (eds) Fetal growth retardation. Churchill Livingstone, Edinburgh, pp 126–138

Robinson J S, Kingston E J, Jones C T, Thorburn G D 1979 Studies of experimental growth retardation in sheep: the effect of removal of endometrial caruncles on fetal size and metabolism. Journal of Developmental Physiology 1: 379–398

Sands J, Dobbing J 1985 Continuing growth and development of the third-trimester human placenta. Placenta 6: 13–22

Sargent I L, Redman C W G, Starkey P M 1993 The placenta as a graft. In: Redman C W G, Sargent I L, Starkey P M (eds) The human placenta. Blackwell Science, Oxford, pp 334–361

Schuhmann R 1981 Plazenten: Begriff, Entstehung, funktionelle Anatomie. In: Becker V, Schiebler Th H, Kubli F (eds) Die Plazenta des Menschen. Thieme, Stuttgart, pp 199–207

Sen D K, Kaufmann P, Schweikhart G 1979 Classification of human placental villi. II Morphometry. Cell and Tissue Research 200: 425–434

Szpakowski M 1974 Morphology of arterial anastomoses in the human placenta. Folio Morphologica 33: 53–60

Voland J R, Frisman D M, Baird S M 1986 Presence of an endothelial antigen on the syncytiotrophoblast of human chorionic villi:

detection by a monoclonal antibody. American Journal of
Reproductive Immunology and Microbiology 11: 24–30
Wang T, Schneider J 1982 Myofiblasten in Bindegewebe des
menschlichen Amnions. Zeitschrift für Geburtshilfe und
Perinatologie 186: 164–168
Wigglesworth J S 1967 Vascular organisation of the human placenta.
Nature 216: 1120–1121

Wilkin P 1965 Pathologie du placenta. Masson, Paris
Winick M, Coscia A, Noble A 1967 Cellular growth in human
placenta. I. Normal cellular growth. Pediatrics 39: 248–251
Wood G W 1980 Mononuclear phagocytes in the human placenta.
Placenta 1: 113–123
Zawisch C 1955 Die Whartonische Sulze und die Gefässe des
Nabelstranges. Zeitschrift für Zellforschung 42: 94–133

5. Structural development of the embryo and fetus

Felix Beck

INTRODUCTION

Human implantation takes place between the sixth and eighth day after fertilization. At this stage the conceptus is in the blastocyst stage, weighs less than 1 μg and contains a few hundred cells (Fig. 5.1).

The first morphological evidence of post-implantation differentiation is manifest in the deepest cells of the inner cell mass (i.e. those facing the blastocyst cavity). They become cuboidal and form a single layer of primary embryonic endoderm. The remainder of the inner cell mass then gradually forms a layer of columnar cells which are the precursors of the embryonic ectoderm and will also give rise to the embryonic mesoderm. The amniotic cavity appears between these cells and those overlying them, which form the amniotic ectoderm derived from the deep aspects of the polar trophoblast (Fig. 5.2). At

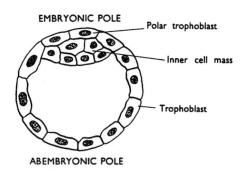

EMBRYONIC POLE

— Polar trophoblast

— Inner cell mass

— Trophoblast

ABEMBRYONIC POLE

Fig. 5.1 The human blastocyst. Reproduced with permission from Beck et al (1985).

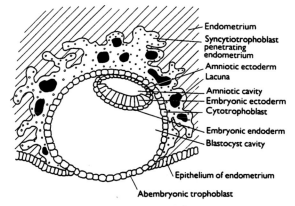

— Endometrium
— Syncytiotrophoblast penetrating endometrium
— Amniotic ectoderm
— Lacuna
— Amniotic cavity
— Embryonic ectoderm
— Cytotrophoblast
— Embryonic endoderm
— Blastocyst cavity
— Epithelium of endometrium
— Abembryonic trophoblast

Fig. 5.2 The implanted conceptus. The embryo forms a bilaminar disc, above which the amniotic cavity lies. Reproduced with permission from Beck et al (1985).

this stage (9–13 days postfertilization) the cells of the future embryo, having been derived from the inner cell mass, form a bilaminar embryonic disc and the whole of the remainder of the conceptus goes on to form the fetal membranes.

Soon the blastocyst cavity becomes lined by squamous extraembryonic endoderm separated from the thick outer trophoblast by a loose reticular layer of extraembryonic mesoderm. The extraembryonic endoderm, in continuity with the cuboidal embryonic endoderm, forms the yolk sac (Fig. 5.3). In the future cranial area of the embryo the cuboidal cells of the yolk sac roof become columnar and form the prochordal plate which, together with overlying ectoderm, forms the buccopharyngeal membrane. Meanwhile, the extraembryonic mesoderm develops fluid-filled spaces which, becoming confluent, form the extraembryonic coelom (Fig. 5.4). Extraembryonic splanchnopleure and extraembryonic somatopleure (amnion and chorion) are therefore delineated about 15 days after fertilization.

FORMATION OF THE TRILAMINAR DISC

Between 14 and 16 days after fertilization the trilaminar

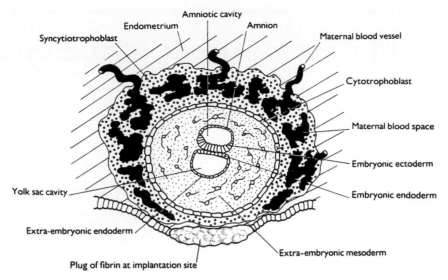

Fig. 5.3 The formation of the extraembryonic endoderm and mesoderm around the yolk sac. Reproduced with permission from Beck et al (1985).

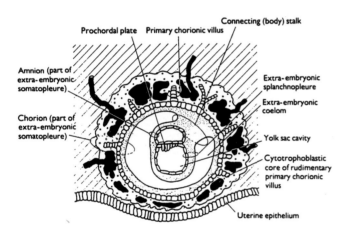

Fig. 5.4 Day 15: chorionic vesicle after the formation of the extraembryonic coelom. Reproduced with permission from Beck et al (1985).

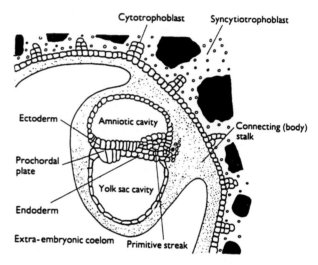

Fig. 5.5 Sagittal section of day 15 embryo within chorionic vesicle, showing formation of prochordal plate and primitive streak. Reproduced with permission from Beck et al (1985).

embryonic disc is formed by interposition of a notochord and mesoderm (the chordamesoderm) between embryonic ectoderm and endoderm. The cells of the upper layer of the bilaminar disc proliferate and migrate backwards and medially to amass at the posterior part of the embryonic midline forming the primitive streak (Fig. 5.5). Once within the streak the cells lose their columnar form, become rounded and spread laterally and forward between ectoderm and endoderm as intraembryonic mesoderm. At the lateral border of the embryonic disc the migrating cells become continuous with the extraembryonic mesoderm covering both yolk sac and amnion. Anteriorly the embryonic mesodermal cells of each side become continuous across the midline in front of the prochordal plate, although in the region of the plate itself ectoderm and

endoderm remain in contact forming the buccopharyngeal membrane. The primitive streak elongates by addition of cells to its posterior extremity (Fig. 5.6). The endoderm in the roof of the yolk sac behind the primitive streak remains (like that of the prochordal plate) adherent to the overlying ectoderm to form the cloacal membrane but some of the embryonic mesodermal cells migrate backwards from the streak, mingling with and contributing to the extraembryonic mesoderm of the connecting stalk (Fig. 5.5). At 16 days a further amassing of cells takes place at the anterior extremity of the primitive streak. This is the primitive knot which will form an elongated notochordal process running backwards from the posterior

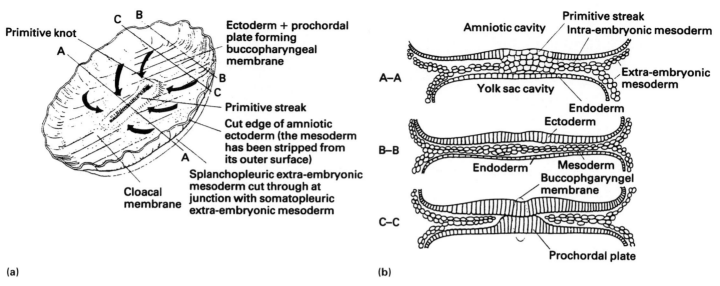

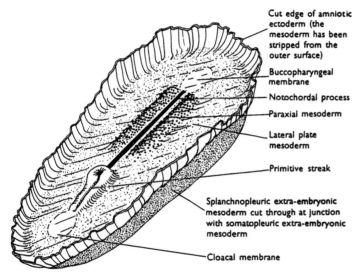

Fig. 5.6 (a) Diagram of the embryonic disc revealed by cutting away the overlying amnion. Intraembryonic ectoderm is represented as being transparent, showing the stippled intraembryonic mesoderm beneath. Note the absence of mesoderm from the region of the buccopharyngeal and cloacal membranes. Arrows indicate the direction of migration of cells towards the primitive streak. (b) Transverse sections through the embryo shown in Fig. 5.6(a) at A–A, B–B and C–C. Reproduced with permission from Beck et al (1985).

Fig. 5.7 A more advanced stage of development than that shown in Fig. 5.6(a). The notochord is elongated and the paraxial mesoderm is heaped up on either side of it as the somites begin to form. Reproduced with permission from Beck et al (1985).

edge of the prochordal plate (Figs 5.7, 5.8). The notochordal process undergoes a series of changes, including a stage of canalization and intercalation into the yolk sac roof (Fig. 5.7), which may be of clinical importance. At 17–18 days ectoderm overlying the notochordal process and the region immediately anterior to it forms a thickened neural plate from which the neural tube arises. Mesoderm on either side of the notochord forms thickened strips of paraxial mesoderm which become segmented to

form 44 somites. More anteriorly this area of thickened mesoderm remains unsegmented. Lateral to the paraxial mass the mesoderm forms lateral plate mesoderm but a longitudinal tract of intermediate mesoderm (the intermediate cell mass) remains interposed between the two. This will give rise to the nephrogenic chord (Fig. 5.9). While still in the trilaminar disc stage, a small diverticulum—the allantois—grows into the connecting stalk immediately behind the cloacal membrane (Fig. 5.8).

The genetic basis of regional specification in mammalian development is being elucidated gradually. For example, series of closely linked developmental control genes, the Hox genes, are expressed in the primitive streak and somite stages of development. These code for transcription factors that regulate the expression of further sets of genes and are fundamentally important in basic pattern formation. A large literature has been established (see for example Gehring 1987, Hunt et al 1991), discussion of which is beyond the scope of this chapter.

THE INTRAEMBRYONIC COELOM AND FORMATION OF THE BODY FOLDS

A horseshoe-shaped cavity, the intraembryonic coelom, appears in the lateral plate mesoderm at 19–20 days of development (Fig. 5.10). The lateral arms of the horseshoe are connected across the midline just anterior to the buccopharyngeal membrane and this is the site of the future pericardial cavity. Caudally the horseshoe communicates with the extraembryonic coelom on either side (Figs 5.9, 5.10) in the region of the future midgut.

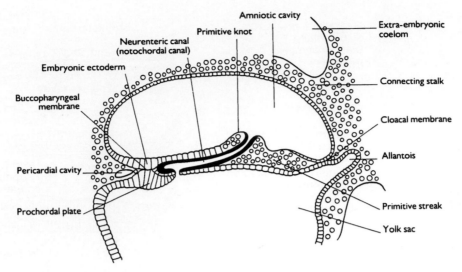

Fig. 5.8 A diagrammatic sagittal section through the embryonic disc at 16 days. Reproduced with permission from Beck et al (1985).

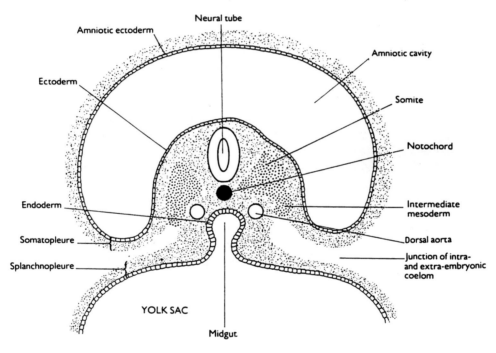

Fig. 5.9 The embryonic disc is beginning to bulge into the amniotic cavity forming lateral folds. The intraembryonic mesoderm has split to form the intraembryonic coelom which is continuous at the edges of the disc with the extraembryonic coelom (see Fig. 5.10, A–A). Reproduced with permission from Beck et al (1985).

The embryonic splanchnopleure and somatopleure are thus formed (Fig. 5.9).

During the fourth week after fertilization the trilaminar embryonic disc bulges into the amniotic cavity. A head and tail fold are formed by folding under of the cranial and caudal parts of the disc (Fig. 5.11). Concurrently, quite marked folding takes place along the lateral margins of the embryo (Fig. 5.12). As a consequence a primitive endodermally lined foregut is formed within the head fold

and a hindgut with an allantoic diverticulum is present in the tail fold. Between them the midgut is continuous inferiorly with the yolk sac (Fig. 5.11). Gradually, the lateral folds constrict the cavity of the midgut from the remainder of the yolk sac, producing an elongated vitello-intestinal duct (Fig. 5.12) which connects the midgut with a shrivelled yolk sac remnant until quite late in pregnancy.

When the head and tail folds have formed, the caudal wall of the pericardial cavity forms an important landmark

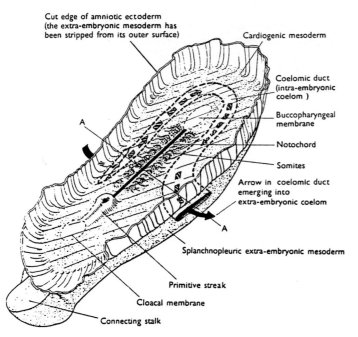

Fig. 5.10 19–20-day embryo showing the intraembryonic coelom. A section through A–A is shown in Fig. 5.9. Reproduced with permission from Beck et al (1985).

called the septum transversum (Fig. 5.13). The latter is, in fact, a broad ventral mesentery for the caudal portion of the foregut and also forms the anterior extremity of the midgut. It is also the anterior limit of the connection between the intra- and extraembryonic coelom, as can be seen in Figure 5.13, and is therefore a region in which vessels can pass from the somatopleure to the splanchnopleure.

The 26-day embryo shown in Figure 5.13 illustrates the relationship between the gut and the intraembryonic coelom. In the tail fold region the attachment of the connecting stalk can now be seen on the ventral aspect of the embryo. The main part of the allantois has been taken into the embryo but it still extends into the stalk for a short distance. Behind the connecting stalk the cloacal membrane (see above) separates the hindgut from the amniotic cavity. The hindgut itself forms a single chamber which gives rise to the greater part of the cloaca. This will become subdivided by a septum, thus forming the primitive urogenital sinus anteriorly and the rectum posteriorly. The primitive urogenital sinus eventually forms much of the bladder and urethra (see below).

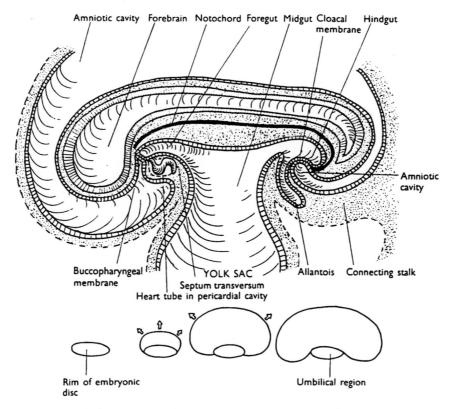

Fig. 5.11 Sagittal section through the embryo during the fourth week showing the formation of the head and tail folds. The four lower diagrams show how the head, tail and lateral folds result from the bulging upwards and outwards of the embryonic disc from its relatively fixed rim. Reproduced with permission from Beck et al (1985).

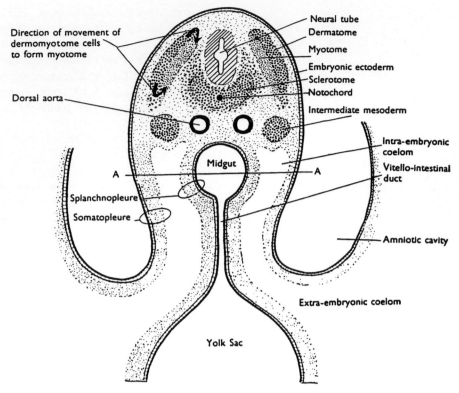

Fig. 5.12 Transverse section through the embryo after the formation of the lateral folds in the region of the midgut. Reproduced with permission from Beck et al (1985).

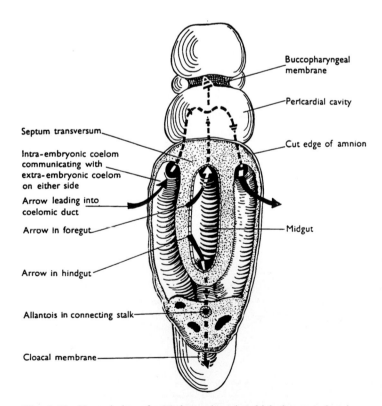

Fig. 5.13 Ventral view of a 26-day embryo in which the ventral region has been removed along the line A–A in Fig. 5.12. Reproduced with permission from Beck et al (1985).

DEVELOPMENT OF THE MAJOR ORGAN SYSTEMS

In this chapter it is clearly impossible to review human organogenesis comprehensively. The approach has been, therefore, to highlight the central issues in developmental anatomy using a visual approach based upon the copious use of diagrams. These are based upon, or reproduced from, *Human Embryology* by Beck et al (1985), where there is further detail and reference to clinical significance. In the present chapter particular attention is paid to the temporal sequence of events.

The mesodermal somites

The embryo illustrated in Figure 5.13 has about 20 somites, although these are not visible in ventral view. An embryo towards the end of the somite stage (approximately 33 somites) is illustrated in Figure 5.14. The somites have developed from the parachordal mesoderm (see above) and at this stage have the appearance of square opacities in the rather transparent tissues of the embryo. They form the basic segmental structure of the body and somite-derived tissue will spread medially to form vertebrae, dorsally to form the extensor musculature of the back and ventrally into the body wall to form ribs, intercostal muscles and abdominal muscles. The dermis

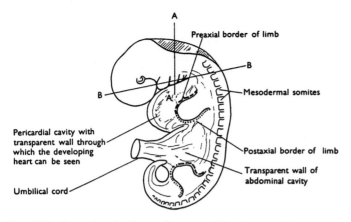

Fig. 5.14 An embryo in the somite stage of development (about 33 days) before invasion of the body wall by cells from the somites. The limb buds have just begun to develop. Reproduced with permission from Beck et al (1985).

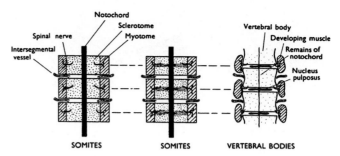

Fig. 5.15 Each vertebral body is formed from the adjacent halves of two somites. A segmental nerve supplies the myotome of each somite and an intersegmental artery passes between each somite pair. With the formation of the vertebral bodies the nerves become intervertebral in position and the arteries run in relation to the vertebral bodies. Reproduced with permission from Beck et al (1985).

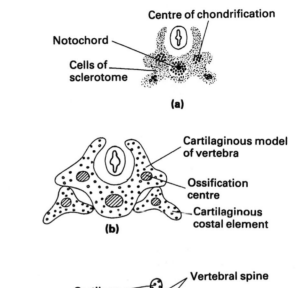

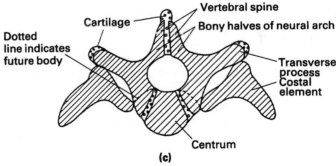

Fig. 5.16 (**a**) The cells of the sclerotome migrate towards the neural tube and form the rough shape of a vertebra. (**b**) Cartilaginous models of vertebrae and costal elements develop, with centres of ossification for the centrum, for each half of the neural arch and for each rib. (**c**) The vertebra and costal elements are almost completely ossified but some cartilage remains so that at birth each bony vertebra is in three pieces. Reproduced with permission from Beck et al (1985).

of the skin is also of somite origin; without it the skin would remain a thin and semi-transparent somatopleure and eventually would lose its viability. The somites form a craniocaudal gradient of maturity, the first appearing in the future occipital region at about 21 days after fertilization. Caudal somites remain visible until 40–45 days but after the first month (26 somites) it is usual to stage embryos by reference to the crown–rump length rather than by somite number.

In total, about 44 somites develop in the human although the most cranial ones begin to break up before the caudal ones are completed. There are 4 occipital, 8 cervical, 12 thoracic, 5 lumbar, 5 sacral and 8–10 coccygeal somites.

The ventro-medial part of each somite forms the sclerotome (Sensenig 1949) and its cells stream medially to surround the neural tube (Figs 5.9, 5.12). The largest accumulation of cells surrounds the notochord. At 4 weeks the caudal portion of each sclerotome begins to unite with the cranial portion of the next to form the vertebral body which is, therefore, an *intersegmental structure* so that the nerves which originally innervated each of the somites now lie between the vertebrae, while the arteries which originally passed between the somites now lie close to the vertebral bodies (Fig. 5.15). Each sclerotome, in addition to forming the vertebral centrum, also forms a neural arch and transverse processes and these elements begin to chondrify in the cervical region in the seventh week. Ossification begins between T5 and S2 in the eighth week, between C5 and T4 and L5 and S2 after 12 weeks, in C2 and C4 and S3 by about 16 weeks, at C1 and S4 after 20 weeks and at S5 at about 28 weeks. At birth the vertebrae have three ossific centres—one in the centrum and one on each side of the neural arch. Costal elements develop in close relation to the transverse processes and their ultimate fate varies in different regions of the spine (Figs 5.16, 5.17).

The tissue remaining after segregation of the sclerotome (Fig. 5.12) differentiates into an inner myotome and an outer dermatome. The spindle-shaped myoblasts of the myotome form the epaxial and hypaxial skeletal musculature, the former by moving into a position between the

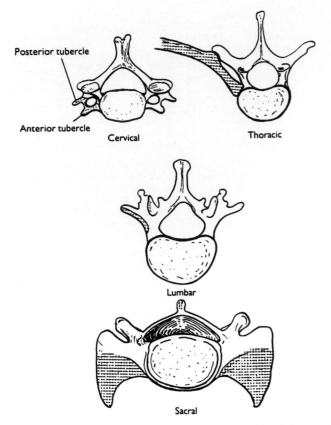

Fig. 5.17 Cervical, thoracic, lumbar and sacral vertebrae. The costal element is shaded. Reproduced with permission from Beck et al (1985).

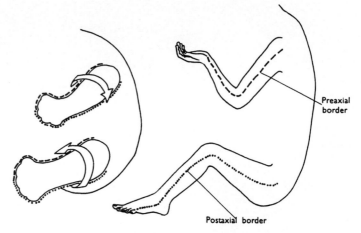

Fig. 5.18 Stages in the development of the limbs to show their changes in position. Reproduced with permission from Beck et al (1985).

transverse processes and the spines of the vertebrae, while the latter moves into the body wall which thus becomes thicker and less transparent. The myotomes of certain somites adopt an atypical location giving rise, for example, to tongue, diaphragmatic and pelvic floor musculature. In the whole of the trunk (including the pectoral and pelvic girdles) migrating myoblasts are followed by their nerves so that it becomes a simple matter to deduce the origin of any trunk muscle. Even though the subjective sensation of quickening is not appreciated until about 20 weeks, the first local reflexes, i.e. mouth-opening after stimulation of the facial skin, are present at 8 weeks and motor end-plates are well developed by the 12th week. Motor responses to cutaneous stimulation occur in the hands by 12 weeks and in the feet by 16 weeks. The definitive body wall is complete by 12 weeks.

Like the myotomes, the dermatomes take their nerve supply with them and the dermis is established by 12 weeks. By 10 weeks the nail anlagen appear, as do lanugo hairs. By 20 weeks the vernix caseosa is present and at around 28 weeks of gestation the scalp and eyebrow hairs develop. At birth the nails reach the end of the fingers and the nipples are everted.

As in birds, the limb musculature of mammals probably develops from the somites. Limb buds appear at the somite stage of development (Fig. 5.14) and at about 5 weeks the prominences of the future knee and elbow region can be recognized, projecting both laterally and backwards. Hand and foot plates appear as flattened expansions and between 36 and 38 days the digital rays become apparent. The limb bones differentiate from the mesenchyme of the limb bud. The limb buds grow in such a way that they appear to rotate in different directions (Fig. 5.18) so that the preaxial border of the hand is located laterally and that of the foot medially.

The nervous system

The development of the primitive neural tube from the neural groove overlying the notochord is illustrated in Figure 5.19. The afferent and efferent columns of grey matter which develop in the alar (sensory) and basal (motor) laminae of the spinal cord are illustrated in Figure 5.20. The visceral afferent and efferent columns are restricted to the thoracolumbar and sacral outflow regions. In the brain stem additional special visceral afferent (gustatory) and special visceral efferent (branchial) columns appear in connection with the special sense of taste and the voluntary muscles associated with the branchial arches. This is illustrated in a diagrammatic transverse section through the fourth ventricle (Fig. 5.21). Excellent reviews of the histogenesis and general development of the central nervous system are available (Langman 1968, O'Rahilly & Gardner 1971, S. Jacobson 1972, M. Jacobson 1978, Lemire et al 1975).

At 21 days the neural groove begins to form the neural tube at the level of somites 4–6; by 25 days the groove is closed except for its anterior and posterior ends (neuropores) and by day 30 closure is complete. By this time it is possible to recognize three well defined

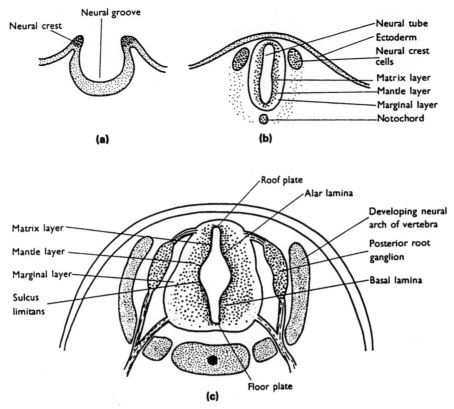

Fig. 5.19 (a) The neural groove and neural crest. (b) and (c) The neural crest cells form inter alia the posterior root ganglia. The three layers of the neural tube can be distinguished. Reproduced with permission from Beck et al (1985).

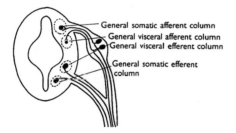

Fig. 5.20 Schematic section of the developing spinal cord to show the two types of efferent and afferent columns of grey matter. Reproduced with permission from Beck et al (1985).

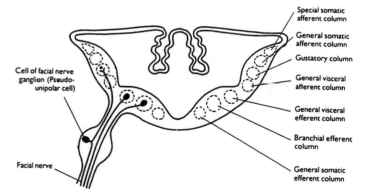

Fig. 5.21 Transverse section of hindbrain to show columns of grey matter. The constituents of the facial nerve are illustrated on the left as an example of the connections of a cranial nerve. Reproduced with permission from Beck et al (1985).

subdivisions of the brain—the forebrain (prosencephalon), midbrain (mesencephalon) and hindbrain (rhombencephalon; Fig. 5.22). The cervical and midbrain flexures have formed. By 35 days the pontine flexure forms as a corollary to a thinning of the roof of the hindbrain in the region of the fourth ventricle (Figs 5.23, 5.24). Within the fifth week the optic vesicles become invaginated and the lens of the eye is formed from an ectodermal placode. By this time the otic vesicles, which will develop into the inner ear, have formed from ectodermal placodes situated in the rhombencephalic region. Meanwhile the forebrain shows signs of increasing complexity with the

formation of the telencephalic vesicles (Fig. 5.25). The two vesicles and the intervening part of the forebrain together form the telencephalon while the posterior part of the forebrain forms the diencephalon (Fig. 5.26). The telencephalic vesicles increase rapidly in size and soon hide the diencephalon completely. Their walls remain relatively thin except in the floor and lateral walls where

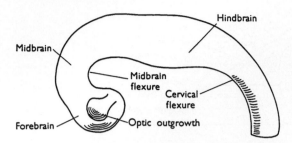

Fig. 5.22 The cranial end of the neural tube at 28 days showing the primitive forebrain, midbrain and hindbrain. Reproduced with permission from Beck et al (1985).

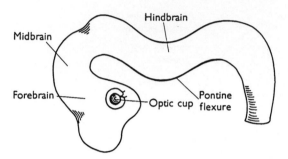

Fig. 5.23 The development of the pontine flexure at approximately 35 days. Reproduced with permission from Beck et al (1985).

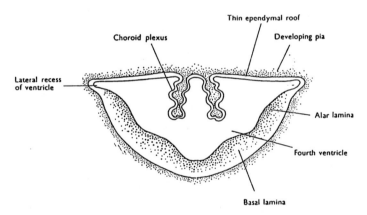

Fig. 5.24 The pontine flexure causes the lateral walls of the hindbrain to spread out so that the roof plate is thinned. Note its invagination by the choroid plexus. Reproduced with permission from Beck et al (1985).

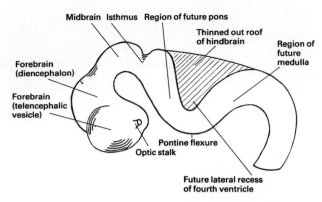

Fig. 5.25 The brain at 37 days. The pontine flexure is further developed and the telencephalic vesicles are forming. Reproduced with permission from Beck et al (1985).

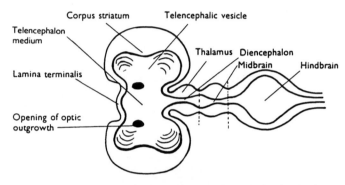

Fig. 5.26 Diagrammatic horizontal section through the developing brain. Reproduced with permission from Beck et al (1985).

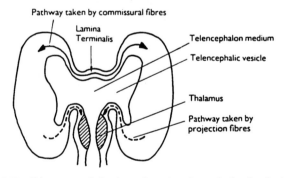

Fig. 5.27 Diagrammatic horizontal section through the developing forebrain to show how the commissural fibres use the lamina terminalis as a pathway while the projection fibres bend sharply round into the diencephalon. Reproduced with permission from Beck et al (1985).

the corpus striatum develops. A further thickening, the thalamus, appears in the lateral wall of the diencephalon. The original cranial end of the neural tube—the lamina terminalis—is a region in which commissural fibres develop and the corpus callosum begins to develop here (Fig. 5.27). Projection fibres develop and fill up the space between the telencephalon and diencephalon until eventually these two parts of the forebrain fuse so that the projection fibres and the developing corpus striatum lie immediately lateral to the thalamus (Fig. 5.28).

Around the developing brain a condensation of vascular mesenchyme, the meninx primitiva, gives rise to the membranous neurocranium and to the three layers of the meninges. The choroid plexuses are formed because the medial wall of the telencephalic vesicle remains very thin in one region and the vascular pia, together with the ependyma, becomes invaginated into the medial walls of the lateral ventricle and also forms the roof of the third ventricle (Fig. 5.28). A slight longitudinal swelling above

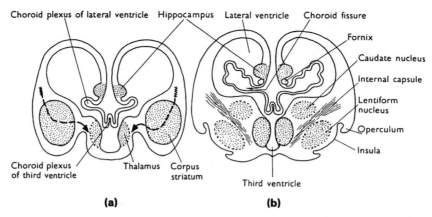

Fig. 5.28 Frontal section through the forebrain. (**a**) Arrows show the pathway taken by projection fibres through the corpus striatum and into the diencephalon. (**b**) Fusion has taken place between the lateral sides of the diencephalon and the medial side of the telencephalon lateral to the thalamus. The corpus striatum is divided into lentiform and caudate nuclei. The choroid fissure is developing in relation to the hippocampus and fornix. Reproduced with permission from Beck et al (1985).

the thin part of the medial wall of the telencephalon develops into the hippocampus. A bundle of nerve fibres of hippocampal origin decussate in the fornix, and the choroid fissure through which the choroid plexuses invaginate the ventricle lies immediately below this (Fig. 5.28). The cerebral hemispheres grow caudally and the caudal pole folds under to form the temporal lobe in which lies the inferior horn of the lateral ventricle. As a result the choroid fissure, fornix and hippocampus become reversed in position in the temporal lobe. This is illustrated in Figure 5.29, which also shows the development of the corpus callosum from the region of the lamina terminalis. The events described above happen early in gestation. At 7 weeks there is already a large corpus striatum and thalamus and at 8 weeks, the meninges have formed and the cerebral cortex is differentiating. At this stage the downgrowth of the forebrain, which will form the posterior lobe of the pituitary, fuses with an upgrowth from the primitive mouth (Rathke's pouch) to form the pituitary gland (Fig. 5.30). Gonadotrophs are immunocytochemically identifiable in the pars distalis at the beginning of the fourth month and gradually other cell types differentiate, ending with follicle-stimulating hormone-secreting cells at about 30 weeks.

By 12–16 weeks the brain begins to resemble that of the adult and the corpus callosum together with the other commissures are formed. From 16 weeks to full term, the cerebral gyri and sulci appear, the insula sinks below the surface and considerable myelinization takes place, though this is not complete until well after birth. By about 16 weeks the neuronal cell complement of the brain is almost complete. There follows a brain growth spurt beginning at 20 weeks of gestation, reaching a maximum at 40 weeks and completed by about the fifth year after conception. The growth spurt involves multiplication of glia and increasing myelinization. Figure 5.31 illustrates the formation of the cerebellum which first grows into the fourth ventricle (contained in the hindbrain) and then evaginates to its adult position. Its relationship to the choroid plexus of the fourth ventricle should be noted. The cerebellum begins to develop at 6 weeks and its main lobes are large and clearly delineated by the fourth month.

Detailed consideration of the special senses is beyond the scope of this review; Figures 5.32–5.35 illustrate the basic development of the eye. Optic pits appear in the floor of the neural plate as early as 4 weeks; the optic cup is formed in the fifth week, the lens vesicle in the sixth, the cornea and sclera in the seventh. By the eighth week the retina has eight layers and optic nerve fibres are well established. By 12 weeks the eyelids have fused and the ciliary muscles of the eye have developed, while by 24 weeks myelination is present in the optic tract and a few weeks later separation of the eyelids is complete. The maculae differentiate late by about 32 weeks and, at this stage, the pupillary light response appears. At full term myelination of the optic nerve—which is proceeding distally—reaches the lamina cribrosa sclerae.

The face, mouth, palate and branchial region

At about the 20-somite stage (Fig. 5.13) the stomatodaeum, or primitive mouth, has been delineated. The mesenchyme covering the forebrain is seen to form its cranial boundary, the mandibular arches are lateral and the pericardial cavity is placed inferiorly. These topographical relations can be seen in sagittal section in Figure 5.11. With the breakdown of the buccopharyngeal membrane

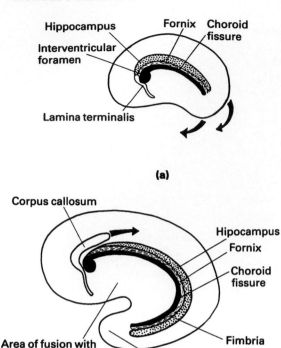

(a)

(b)

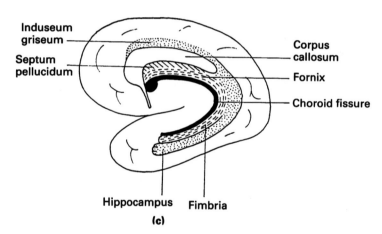

(c)

Fig. 5.29 Diagram of the medial side of the telencephalic vesicle detached from the mesencephalon. (**a**) Arrows show the main direction of growth. (**b**) Growth of the caudal part of the telencephalic vesicle has formed the temporal lobe. The fornix lies above the choroid fissure but its continuation, the fimbria, lies *below* the choroid fissure in the *temporal* lobe. (**c**) The corpus callosum has grown caudally and the upper part of the hippocampus is represented only by the indusium griseum. Reproduced with permission from Beck et al (1985).

the ectodermally derived stomatodacum becomes continuous with the endodermally lined foregut. The transition occurs at the level of Rathke's pouch but leaves no visible sign after the disappearance of the buccopharyngeal membrane.

Figure 5.36 illustrates the subsequent development of

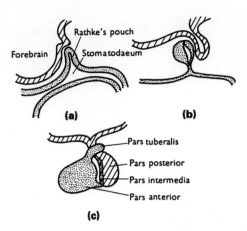

(a)   **(b)**

(c)

Fig. 5.30 The development of the pituitary gland. (**a**) An upgrowth (Rathke's pouch) from the stomatodaeum meets a downgrowth from the forebrain. (**b**) The walls of Rathke's pouch become thicker, particularly the anterior wall, and the pouch separates from the stomatodaeum. (**c**) The mature pituitary gland. Reproduced with permission from Beck et al (1985).

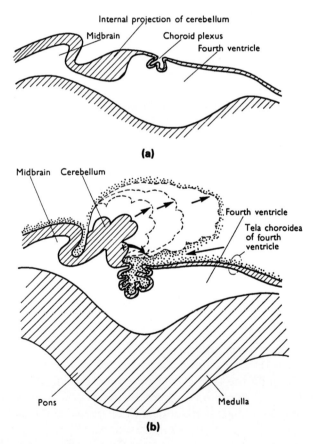

(a)

(b)

Fig. 5.31 (**a**) The cerebellum begins to grow into the fourth ventricle. (**b**) It then becomes everted to overhang the thin roof of the fourth ventricle. The small arrows indicate the backward growth of the neocerebellum. The long arrow indicates the cerebello-medullary subarachnoid cistern of the adult. Reproduced with permission from Beck et al (1985).

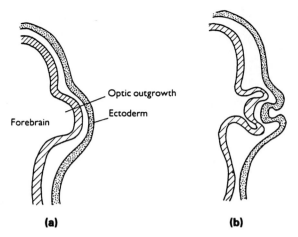

Fig. 5.32 (a) The optic outgrowth from the forebrain. (b) The formation of the lens vesicle and the optic cup. Reproduced with permission from Beck et al (1985).

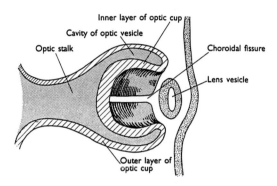

Fig. 5.33 Horizontal section through the optic cup viewed from above. The lens vesicle has detached itself from the surface ectoderm. Reproduced with permission from Beck et al (1985).

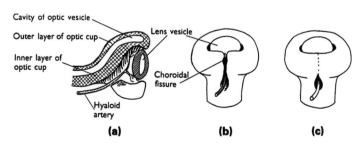

Fig. 5.34 (a) Midline section through the developing eye. The section passes through the choroidal fissure. (b) The optic vesicle seen from below. The hyaloid artery enters through the choroidal fissure. (c) Closure of the choroidal fissure. Reproduced with permission from Beck et al (1985).

the face (Slarkin 1979). The mandibular arches fuse below the stomatodeal opening and a dorsal wing from each mandibular arch gives rise to the maxillary process on that side. Bilateral thickenings in the ectoderm, the olfactory placodes, sink beneath the surface each to lie in the floor of a nasal sac. The external opening of the sac forms the external nares with mesodermal thickenings—

the medial and lateral nasal processes—on each side of it. The mesoderm of the lateral nasal process soon becomes continuous with the maxillary processes and the line of junction between them runs up to the eye. The two medial nasal processes together form the frontonasal process, and the maxillary processes growing further medially fuse with each other and with the frontonasal process in the midline. The embryological basis of hare lip and oblique facial cleft is therefore clear.

The nasal sac establishes continuity with the stomatodaeum posteriorly to form the primitive posterior nares (Fig. 5.37) and the mesoderm of the maxillary processes becomes continuous with that of the frontonasal process to form the upper lip. The primitive palate is thus established but the greater part of the definitive palate is formed behind this when the palatal processes on each side grow medially from the inner surface of the maxillary processes (Fig. 5.38). At first the palatal processes hang down on either side of the tongue but they eventually rise to meet and fuse with each other and with the edge of the nasal septum. The adoption of the horizontal attitude by the palatal processes is multifactorial, including an increased turgor due to water imbibition, extension of the embryonic head, movements of the tongue etc.

The maxillary processes appear and the buccopharyngeal membrane ruptures at about 4 weeks. The upper lip is completed in the seventh week though it does not separate from the gums until about 12 weeks. The face is recognizably human at 8 weeks and palatal fusion is complete at 11 weeks. This marks one of the final events of organogenesis of the human embryo.

Figure 5.14 is a lateral view of a somite stage (33 days) embryo. The developing face is seen to be pressed against the pericardium and a little more caudally the lateral surface of the embryo shows a series of elevations, the branchial (or pharyngeal) arches. The two most cranial are clearly marked but, behind these, the arches are progressively smaller and, at about 40 days, they are completely overgrown by the second arch so that the smooth surface of the neck is established (Fig. 5.39). The external groove between the first and second arches forms the external auditory meatus.

The relationship of the branchial arches and the brain is illustrated by Figure 5.40, which passes through the second arch. The arch consists of a thickening of the mesoderm on each side of the pharynx. This mesoderm blends with mesoderm in the roof and floor of the pharynx. In the floor lies the aortic sac which is the cranial end of the heart tube. From the sac an artery passes dorsally through the arch substance to join one of the paired dorsal aortae which further caudally fuse to form a midline vessel. From the brain one of the cranial nerves (in this case, the seventh) passes ventrally into the arch eventually to supply skeletal muscle of branchial arch

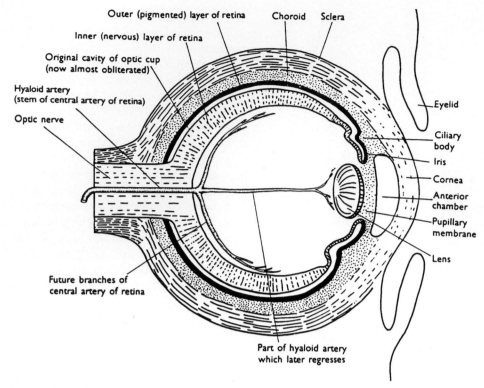

Outer (pigmented) layer of retina
Inner (nervous) layer of retina
Original cavity of optic cup (now almost obliterated)
Hyaloid artery (stem of central artery of retina)
Optic nerve
Choroid
Sclera
Eyelid
Ciliary body
Iris
Cornea
Anterior chamber
Pupillary membrane
Lens
Future branches of central artery of retina
Part of hyaloid artery which later regresses

Fig. 5.35 Vertical section through the developing eye. Reproduced with permission from Beck et al (1985).

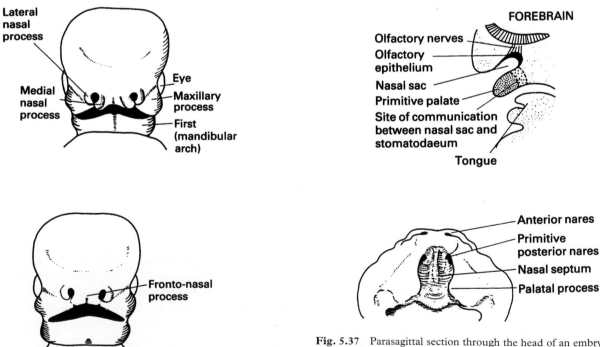

Lateral nasal process
Medial nasal process
Eye
Maxillary process
First (mandibular arch)

Fronto-nasal process

Fig. 5.36 The developing face. Reproduced with permission from Beck et al (1985).

FOREBRAIN
Olfactory nerves
Olfactory epithelium
Nasal sac
Primitive palate
Site of communication between nasal sac and stomatodaeum
Tongue

Anterior nares
Primitive posterior nares
Nasal septum
Palatal process

Fig. 5.37 Parasagittal section through the head of an embryo passing through the nasal sac. The sparsely dotted area will later break down to form a communication between nasal sac and stomatodaeum (the primitive posterior nares). Reproduced with permission from Beck et al (1985).

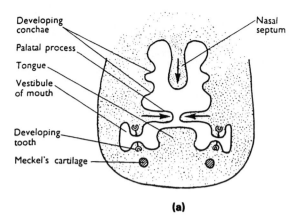

(a)

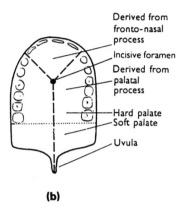

(b)

Fig. 5.38 (**a**) Coronal section through the head to show the formation of the palate and nasal septum. The diagram is simplified—in a real embryo the tongue at first lies between the palatal processes so that its dorsum is in contact with the free border of the nasal septum. (**b**) The origin of the constituents of the adult palate. Reproduced with permission from Beck et al (1985).

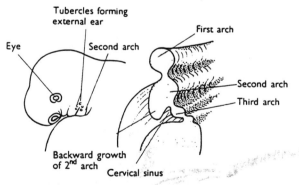

Fig. 5.39 Diagram to show how backward growth of the second arch forms the cervical sinus. Its obliteration will form the smooth line of the neck. Reproduced with permission from Beck et al (1985).

origin. Some of the arch mesoderm will also differentiate into skeletal tissue (cartilage, bone). The other branchial arches are very similar, each containing an aortic arch artery, a nerve, muscle and skeletal tissue. Altogether there are six branchial arches; the first gives rise to the

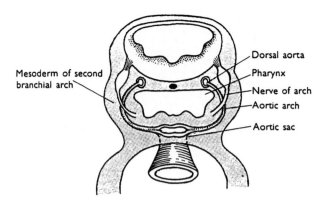

Fig. 5.40 A section through the pharynx at the level of the second branchial arch (A–A in Fig. 5.14), seen from the front. Each arch contains a nerve and an artery. Reproduced with permission from Beck et al (1985).

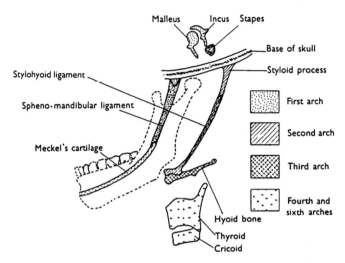

Fig. 5.41 The derivatives of the skeletal elements of the branchial arches. Reproduced with permission from Beck et al (1985).

muscles of mastication (V); the second the muscles of facial expression (VII); the third to the stylopharyngeus muscle (IX); and the fourth and sixth to the pharyngeal and laryngeal muscles (X). The fifth arch has never developed in mammals. Skeletal elements of branchial arch origin are depicted in Figure 5.41 and the arch arteries are discussed below in connection with the cardiovascular system.

Between the branchial arches lie the endodermally lined branchial pouches which at first are continuous with the cavity of the pharynx (Fig. 5.42). The endodermal lining of these pouches differentiates into various important structures situated chiefly in the neck and these are illustrated in Figure 5.43. Of particular note is the position of the inferior parathyroid gland which, although derived from a more anterior arch than the superior gland, is nevertheless dragged to its final position by the descent of the inferior part of the pouch (which gives rise to

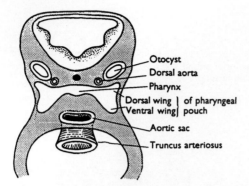

Fig. 5.42   Vertical section through the pharyngeal region (just posterior to Fig. 5.40) passing through the second pharyngeal pouch on each side. Reproduced with permission from Beck et al (1985).

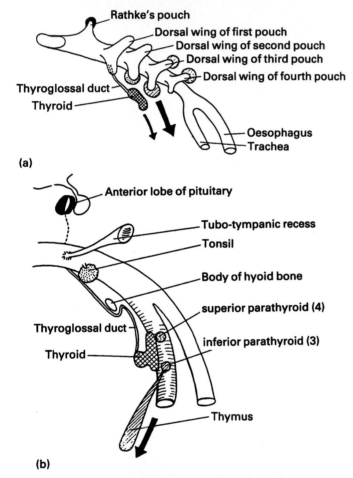

Fig. 5.43   Side view of the pharynx to show: (**a**) the origin of the endodermal proliferations giving rise to the pharyngeal pouch derivatives. Also shown is Rathke's pouch and the thyroid outgrowth. (**b**) The fate of the structures depicted in (a). Reproduced with permission from Beck et al (1985).

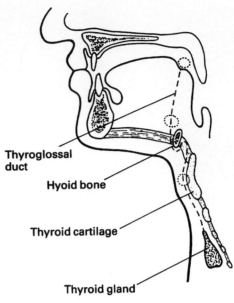

Fig. 5.44   The path of the thyroglossal duct, indicating the possible sites of aberrant thyroid tissue or thyroglossal cysts. Reproduced with permission from Beck et al (1985).

become functional at various stages of gestation, thus parathormone is demonstrable by 12 weeks and T3 by the 20th week of gestation. It will be seen that the thyroid anlage becomes attached to the ventral part of pouch 4. Here its cells are joined by cells which have migrated from the neural crest via the more caudal pouches (the ultimobranchial body). These will form the calcitonin-secreting C cells of the gland.

The floor of the pharynx at the end of the somite period is illustrated in Figure 5.45. From its lining the mucous membrane of the tongue will develop by overgrowth of the second arch mesoderm by that of the third (Fig. 5.46). The musculature of the tongue, however, is of occipital somite origin. Tongue development is reflected in its nerve supply both for taste and general sensation as well as for the musculature. The tongue primordia (Fig. 5.46) are first recognizable at 5 weeks of development.

The cardiovascular system

The blood vascular system, including the heart, is formed initially from endothelial tubes which develop in mesenchyme both within the embryo and in the extraembryonic tissues. Blood islets first appear in the yolk sac, although some authorities have recently suggested that haematopoietic stem cells originate in the embryo itself (Le Dourain 1982). The scattered endothelial tubes link up to form a primitive circulatory system in which the first peristalsis-like heart beats begin on day 21. At this stage a single heart tube which has formed by fusion of right and left tubes (Fig. 5.47) lies in the pericardium ventral

the thymus) into the thorax. Figure 5.43 also illustrates the development of the pituitary and thyroid glands (see also Fig. 5.44). The pharyngeal arches and hyoid rudiment are first recognizable at 4 weeks and their derivatives

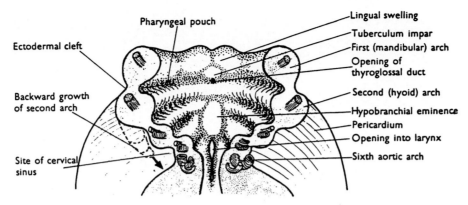

Fig. 5.45 Horizontal section through the pharyngeal region (B–B in Fig. 5.14) viewed from above. The first and second aortic arch arteries have already regressed. Reproduced with permission from Beck et al (1985).

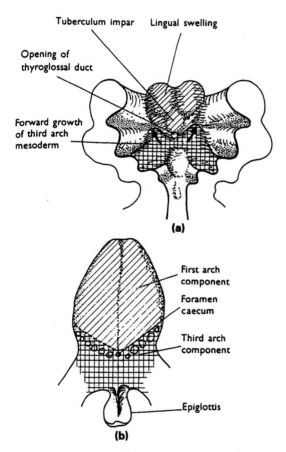

Fig. 5.46 (a) The tongue, with the exception of its muscles, develops from the first and third arches in the floor of the embryonic pharynx. (b) Adult tongue showing first and third arch components. Reproduced with permission from Beck et al (1985).

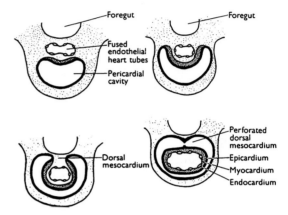

Fig. 5.47 The heart develops from a pair of endothelial tubes which fuse and invaginate the pericardial cavity. The dorsal mesocardium, which is thus formed, becomes perforated so that the heart tube runs freely through the pericardial cavity. Reproduced with permission from Beck et al (1985).

runs into an aortic sac. Two vessels pass dorsally from the sac on either side of the foregut in the mesenchyme of the first branchial arch. These are the first aortic arch arteries and they join the corresponding dorsal aortae in the roof of the pharynx (O'Rahilly 1971).

A cranial prolongation of each dorsal aorta (the future internal carotid artery) supplies the forebrain. Caudal to the branchial region the paired dorsal aortae eventually fuse to form a single midline vessel. At about 28–30 days the first aortic arch arteries are followed by second and third arch arteries which lie in the succeeding branchial arches. By the time the third arch has formed, the first aortic arch artery has begun to break up (about 30 days) and, a short time later, the fourth develops and the second disappears. Finally, at about 37–39 days, the sixth aortic arch artery forms (it will be remembered that there is no fifth arch in the human embryo); Figures 5.49a and 5.50a illustrate this stage. The further development of the aortic arch arteries is illustrated in Figures 5.49b

to the foregut and delineated posteriorly by the septum transversum (Fig. 5.48). The heart tube is divided into four primitive chambers of which the most caudal (the sinus venosus) is still embedded in the septum. The cranially situated bulbus cordis leads into a short wide segment, the truncus arteriosus, which, further forward,

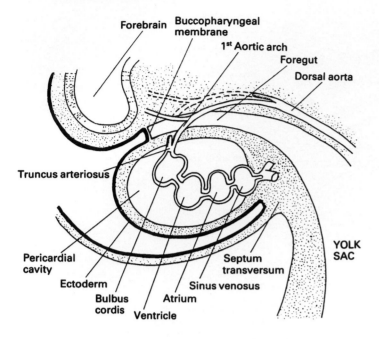

Fig. 5.48 The heart tube consists of four chambers. The first aortic arch arteries only have developed at this stage. Reproduced with permission from Beck et al (1985).

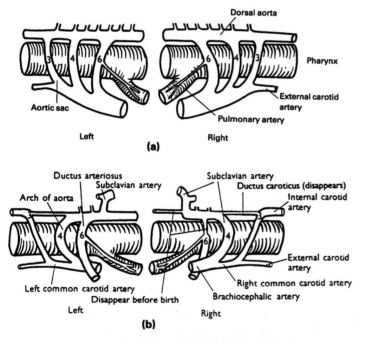

Fig. 5.49 The aortic arch arteries. (a) The right and left third, fourth and sixth aortic arch arteries when fully developed. (b) The subsequent fate of these arteries. Reproduced with permission from Beck et al (1985).

and 5.50b. From the ventral end of the third arch the external carotid artery grows forward to the face. From the middle of the sixth arch another vessel grows down to the developing lung. The dorsal aorta between the third and fourth arches (ductus caroticus) disappears

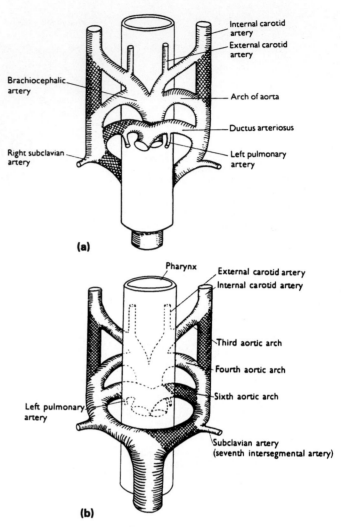

Fig. 5.50 The relation of the aortic arch arteries to the pharynx viewed from in front (a) and from behind (b). The cross-hatched vessels will later disappear. Reproduced with permission from Beck et al (1985).

and the third arch, together with the cranial part of the dorsal aorta, thus forms the internal carotid artery while the common carotid results from the elongation of the aortic sac proximal to the junction of the internal and external carotids.

On the left side the fourth arch artery forms the arch of the aorta from which the left common carotid may now be said to arise. The sixth arch artery, together with the vessel that passes down to the lung, forms the left pulmonary artery while the distal part of the sixth arch artery becomes the ductus arteriosus. The seventh intersegmental artery forms the subclavian artery and the subsequent relative descent of the heart causes it to adopt its adult position. On the right side the fourth arch artery, together with a part of the right dorsal aorta and the seventh intersegmental artery, forms the right subclavian artery. The proximal part of the right sixth aortic arch artery, together with its branch to the lung, forms the right pulmonary artery but the distal part of the sixth arch and the dorsal aorta caudal to the seventh intersegmental artery disappear at about 45 days of development.

From its inception the heart tube (Fig. 5.48) grows faster than the pericardium. Since it is fixed both cranially and caudally it becomes kinked and this occurs in both the anteroposterior and the transverse planes. These acute bends of the heart tube are shown in Figure 5.51. In a lateral view (Fig. 5.51a) at about 25–26 days it will be seen that the bulbus cordis and ventricle lie ventral to the atrium and sinus venosus. Endocardial cushions have begun to form in the atrioventricular canals. Figure 5.51b (at about 32 days) indicates how a further lateral twist of the tube brings the bulbus cordis to lie to the right of the ventricle so that the two form a common chamber in which a depression corresponding to the interventricular septum can already be seen. The thin-walled atrium is clearly bulging forward on either side of the truncus arteriosus.

At this stage the sinus venosus has become asymmetrical due to shunting of the venous return from the

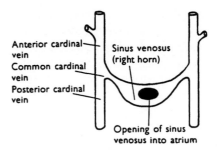

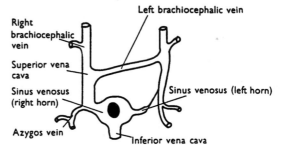

Fig. 5.52 The shunting of blood from left to right by the development of the brachiocephalic vein causes the right horn of the sinus venosus to enlarge at the expense of the left. Reproduced with permission from Beck et al (1985).

head and neck to the right by development of the brachiocephalic vein (Fig. 5.52). As a result of the relative decrease in size of the left horn it is now the right horn of the sinus venosus that opens into the posterior wall of the common atrial cavity, rather to the right side, by a slit which is guarded by two venous valves. This is shown at a slightly later stage of development in Figure 5.53

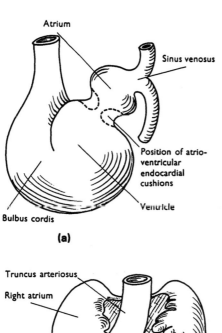

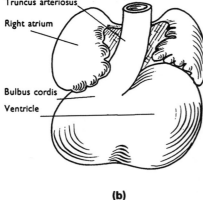

Fig. 5.51 Lateral (a) and anterior (b) views of the developing heart after the formation of the acute bends in the heart tube. (a) is at a slightly earlier stage of development than (b). Reproduced with permission from Beck et al (1985).

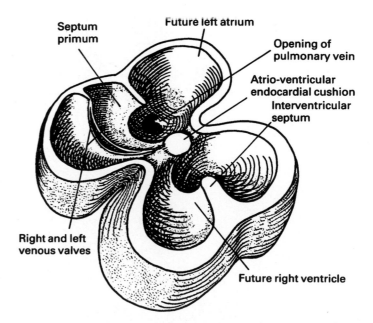

Fig. 5.53 Coronal section through the plane of the developing heart at about 37 days. Reproduced with permission from Beck et al (1985).

which also indicates that the atrioventricular cushions have fused across the atrioventricular canal which thus becomes divided into right and left canals.

At about 32 days or so the growth of the septum primum begins the formation of the interatrial septum, illustrated in Figure 5.54. The fully functional foramen ovale is present towards the end of the organogenetic period, though the septum secundum is quite well developed by about 46 days. Two other changes take place in the atria; on the left the walls of the pulmonary vein become incorporated into the atrial wall to form its smooth-walled part and on the right the sinus venosus is incorporated into the right atrium. The left venous valve disappears, the right horn of the sinus venosus forms the smooth posterior portion of the right atrium and into it opens the coronary sinus which is the original left horn of the sinus venosus. The embryology of the interior of the right atrium (Fig. 5.55) is thus clear.

Septation of the bulbo-ventricular cavity is illustrated in Figure 5.56. It will be seen that the common outflow tract (truncus arteriosus) becomes divided into two at about 42 days of development by a spiral aorticopulmonary septum formed by fusion of bulbar ridges developed in its walls. The lower ends of these bulbar ridges, together with a contribution from the atrioventricular cushion, fuse with the crescentric upper edge of the muscular interventricular septum. The result is the formation of the membranous part of the interventricular septum which causes blood from the left ventricle to empty exclusively into the aorta and from the right into the pulmonary trunk. Septation of the ventricles is complete at about 46 days of development. The fetal circulation is depicted in Figure 5.57 and the changes occurring at birth are discussed in Chapter 8.

The development of the aortic and pulmonary valves is shown in Figure 5.58, and a summary diagram of the development of the inferior vena cava is given in Figure 5.59.

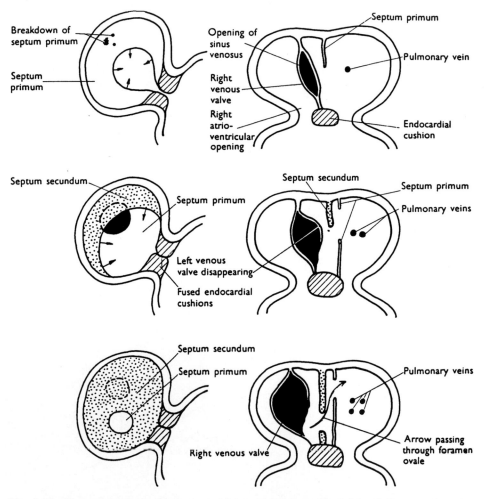

Fig. 5.54 Three stages in the development of the atrial septum. The left-hand diagrams show the right side of the developing septum and the right-hand diagrams show a coronal section in the plane of the atria. The septum secundum is stippled. Reproduced with permission from Beck et al (1985).

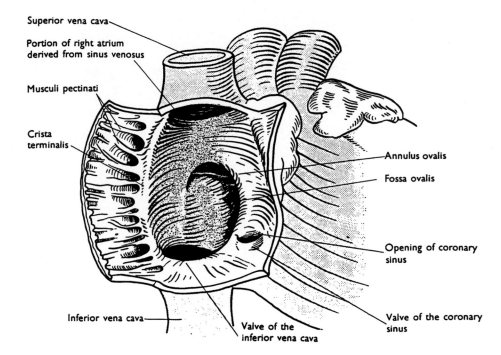

Fig. 5.55 The interior of the adult right atrium seen from in front. Reproduced with permission from Beck et al (1985).

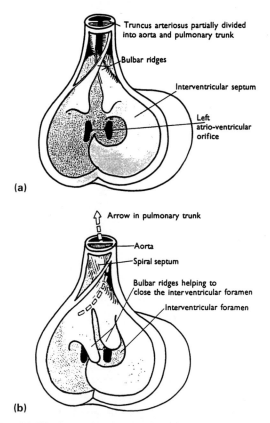

Fig. 5.56 (a) The heart viewed open from the front to show the spiral bulbar ridges. (b) Fusion of the right and left bulbar ridges has formed a separate aorta and pulmonary trunk. The interventricular foramen is partly closed and will later completely close by further development of the bulbar ridges and by proliferation of the tissues of the atrioventricular cushions. After closure of the interventricular septum the right atrioventricular orifice will open exclusively into the right ventricle and the left orifice into the left ventricle. Reproduced with permission from Beck et al (1985).

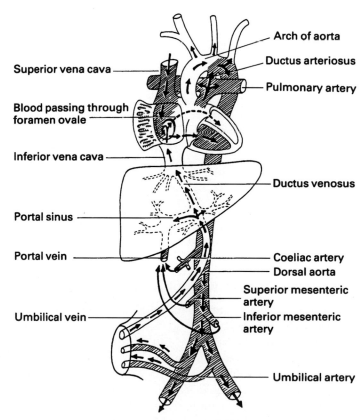

Fig. 5.57 Diagram of the fetal circulation. The cross-hatching represents deoxygenated or mixed blood. Reproduced with permission from Beck et al (1985).

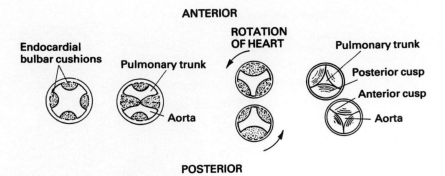

Fig. 5.58   The development of the aortic and pulmonary valves viewed from above. Reproduced with permission from Beck et al (1985).

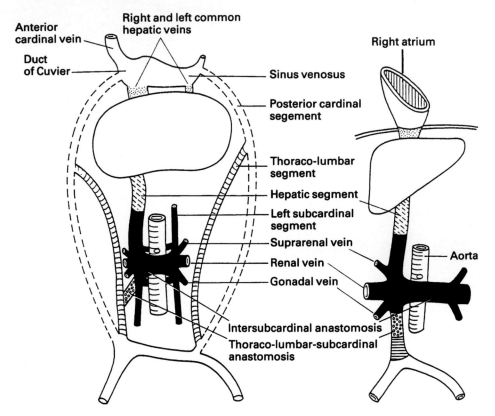

Fig. 5.59   Development of the inferior vena cava. The segments which make up the adult vessel are shown in the right-hand diagram. Reproduced with permission from Beck et al (1985).

The coelom, lungs and diaphragm

The early development of the coelom is illustrated by reference to Figures 5.10 and 5.11. Figures 5.60–5.63 illustrate the detailed relationship of the coelomic cavity to the foregut and midgut in the middle of the somite period of development. Figure 5.64 shows how the right lung bud (developed from a midline ventral foregut diverticulum at the caudal extremity of the pharynx) grows into the coelomic cavity. This section of the coelom now becomes the pleural cavity because, as the heart descends relatively, the common cardinal veins become

increasingly vertical and raise prominent ridges which eventually fuse with the mesoderm covering the front of the oesophagus. Figures 5.65a and b illustrate this process; Figure 5.65c shows the further growth of the lungs around the heart by burrowing into the body wall. The growing lungs raise a septum (the pleuroperitoneal membrane) situated on their caudal aspect and eventually the adult diaphragm is formed as shown in Figure 5.66.

The small remaining pleuroperitoneal opening is crowded out as a result of invasion of the diaphragm by myotomes from C3 to C5 and by growth of the subjacent liver

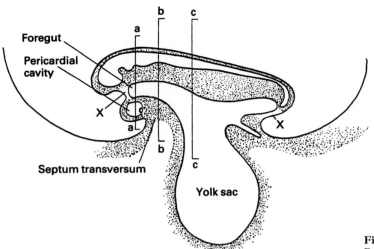

Fig. 5.60 Sagittal section through an embryo to show the planes of Figures 5.61, 5.62 and 5.63. Reproduced with permission from Beck et al (1985).

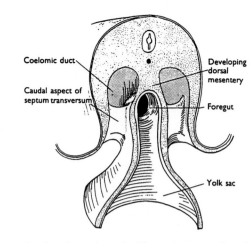

Fig. 5.63 Section through c–c in Figure 5.60 seen from behind. Reproduced with permission from Beck et al (1985).

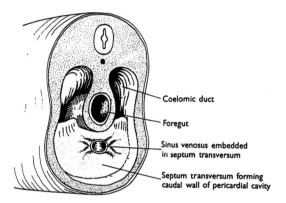

Fig. 5.61 Section through a–a in Figure 5.60 seen from in front. Reproduced with permission from Beck et al (1985).

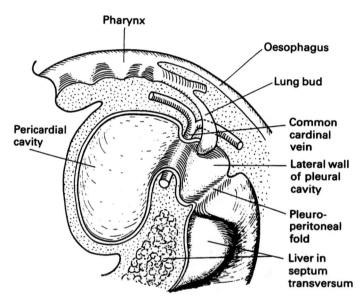

Fig. 5.64 Parasagittal section through the region of the septum transversum to show the right lateral wall of the pericardial cavity and the right coelomic duct (pleural cavity). Reproduced with permission from Beck et al (1985).

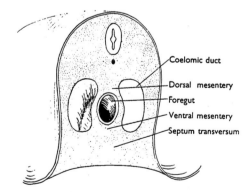

Fig. 5.62 Section through b–b in Figure 5.60 seen from in front. Reproduced with permission from Beck et al (1985).

At this stage the lobar bronchi are recognizable. At 5 weeks the pericardium and pleura separate and at 7 weeks pleura and peritoneum separate. The *glandular* stage of lung development is present at 4 months, giving rise to a *canalicular* stage at 4–6 months and an alveolar stage beginning at 6 months. New alveoli form as the lungs grow until the eighth year of life. The development and significance of surfactant is discussed in Chapter 47.

The urogenital system

Reference to Figures 5.10 and 5.11 will remind the reader of the cloacal membrane lying behind the remnants of the primitive streak. When the tail fold is formed the

and suprarenal glands. The derivation of the trachea is shown in Figures 5.45 and 5.67. The laryngotracheal groove (Fig. 5.45) appears at 22 days but the trachea does not fully separate from the oesophagus until 4–5 weeks.

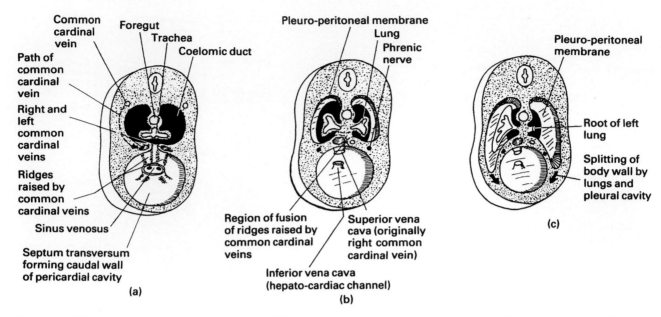

Fig. 5.65   Three sections showing the development of the lungs and the pleuroperitoneal membranes. The lungs grow ventrally in the direction of the arrows in (**c**). Reproduced with permission from Beck et al (1985).

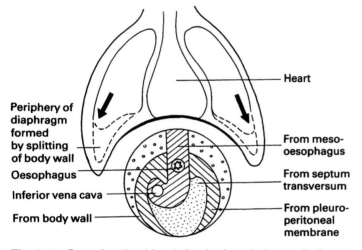

Fig. 5.66   Coronal section (above) showing how the lungs split the body wall to form the peripheral portion of the diaphragm. The arrows show the direction of lung growth in this plane. The lower diagram shows the embryonic constituents of the adult diaphragm viewed from above. Reproduced with permission from Beck et al (1985).

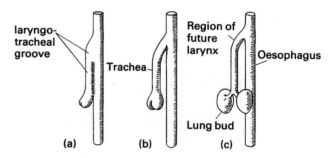

Fig. 5.67   Three stages in the development of the trachea. Reproduced with permission from Beck et al (1985).

cloacal membrane comes to lie on the ventral aspect of the embryo (Fig. 5.68). The proximal end of the allantois now opens into the cloaca just anterior to the cloacal membrane and takes part in the formation of the apex of the adult bladder. The cloaca is thus common to the hindgut and a portion of the allantois. Later in development the urinary system establishes an opening into the cloaca which becomes split into a urinary and rectal part by the development of the urorectal septum (Fig. 5.68).

At 23–24 days of development the intermediate cell mass (Figs 5.9, 5.12) proliferates to give rise to two long nephrogenic ridges lying one on either side of the midline from the cervical region to the caudal end of the coelomic cavity. From it will develop the mesonephros as well as the stroma of the gonads and their associated ducts (Fig. 5.69). On the ventrolateral aspect of the ridge the mesonephric (Wolffian) duct develops and grows caudally to open into the ventral (urinary) region of the cloaca (Fig. 5.68). The mesonephros consists of a series of glomeruli and tubules which are similar to, but less complicated than, those of the adult kidney and develop in a craniocaudal direction between days 24 and 28. It functions as an excretory organ during embryonic life. A second longitudinal duct (Fig. 5.69) develops at between 5 and 6 weeks lateral to the mesonephric duct. This is the paramesonephric (Müllerian) duct which will form much of the reproductive system in the female.

The urorectal septum divides the cloaca into a dorsal region, which forms part of the hindgut, and a ventral primitive urogenital sinus (Figs 5.68, 5.70). The primitive urogenital sinus then becomes further subdivided by the entrance of the mesonephric ducts at about 28 days

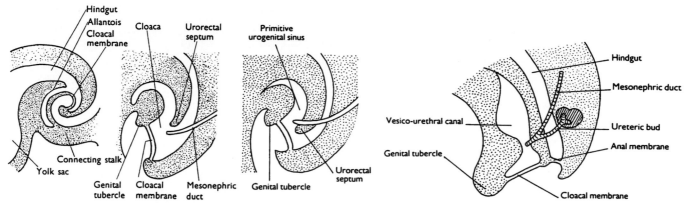

Fig. 5.68 The splitting of the cloaca by the urorectal septum to form the primitive urogenital sinus; also shown is the ureteric bud. Reproduced with permission from Beck et al (1985).

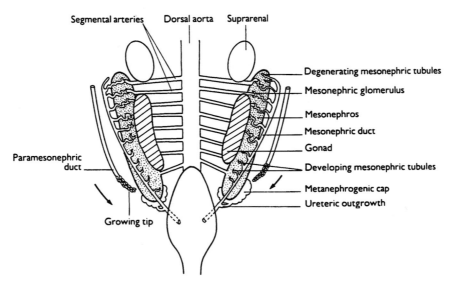

Fig. 5.69 The mesonephros and its relations. The glomeruli are functional at this stage but will disappear later. Reproduced with permission from Beck et al (1985).

into an upper portion (the vesico-urethral canal) from which the bladder and part of the urethra develop and a lower definitive urogenital sinus. The lower part has a short, narrow cylindrical pelvic portion lying above a laterally compressed phallic portion (Fig. 5.70). The phallic portion extends forwards on to the ventral surface of a midline mesodermal swelling covered by ectoderm called the genital tubercle which develops at about 5 weeks. At first this is similar in both males and females (Fig. 5.71). On either side of the urogenital membrane a ridge of ectoderm-covered mesoderm forms the urethral folds. Outside this lies a less well defined elevation, the genital swelling. Further growth in the region between the genital tubercle and the umbilicus leads to the development of the infraumbilical abdominal wall which will become invaded by tissues of dermatomyotome origin. From the lower end of the mesonephric duct at about 5 weeks of development a diverticulum grows dorsally and cranially

to meet the lower end of the nephrogenic ridge. This is the ureteric bud and a slightly dilated ampulla at its upper end becomes surrounded by a mass of cells from the ridge (Fig. 5.70). These cells form the greater part of the permanent kidney (the metanephros) which begins to function as an excretory organ at the end of embryonic and the beginning of fetal life (8 weeks). At this stage the cells form the metanephrogenic cap. A complex pattern of branching of the ureteric bud results in the establishment of the renal pelvis. Junction of the portion of the kidney derived from the metanephrogenic cap and that from the ureteric bud occurs just distal to the distal convoluted tubule of the nephrons. The kidneys undergo relative ascent during development and rotate so that the hilum faces medially instead of forwards. Figure 5.70 illustrates that the lower ends of the mesonephric ducts up to and beyond the ureteric buds become taken into the endo-dermal vesico-urethral canal so that part of the wall of

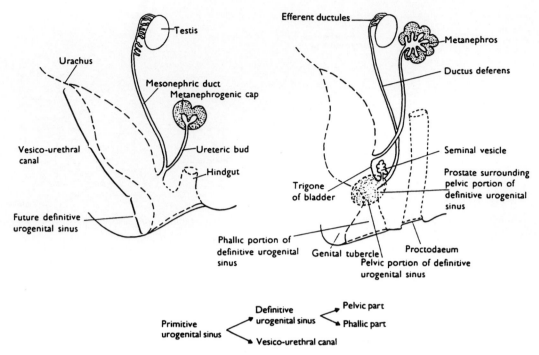

Fig. 5.70   The development of the bladder and internal genitalia. The endodermal derivatives are dotted. The flow chart shows how the primitive urogenital sinus becomes divided. Reproduced with permission from Beck et al (1985).

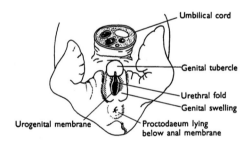

Fig. 5.71   The external genitalia at the end of the second month. There is little development of the infraumbilical abdominal wall at this stage; the genital tubercle reaches up as far as the umbilicus. Reproduced with permission from Beck et al (1985).

the canal becomes mesodermal. At the same time complicated growth changes occur so that the ureters finally open into the definitive bladder while the mesonephric ducts open lower down into the pelvic part of the definitive urogenital sinus. This results in the formation of the trigone of the bladder. The bladder is therefore derived mainly from the vesico-urethral canal and from the lower ends of the mesonephric ducts. The allantois makes a small contribution to its apex but largely regresses to form the urachus.

The gonads, which at first have a similar appearance in both sexes, are first seen as thickenings along the middle two quarters of the medial aspect of the nephrogenic ridge (Figs 5.69, 5.72). They first appear during the fifth week of development and become colonized by primordial

germ cells which originate in the yolk sac wall, having segregated there at an early stage of development. At 7–8 weeks (but not earlier) it becomes possible to determine sex by the histology of the gonad. Prior to this cytogenetic techniques are required to establish sex. The histological differentiation of the gonads has been well documented (Gillman 1948, Pinkerton et al 1961, Zuckerman & Weir 1977, Guraya 1980, Steinberger & Steinberger 1980) and good reviews concerning the genetic and endocrinological basis of sexual differentiation are available (Visser 1974, Short 1979). The precise location on the human Y chromosome of the SRY gene which determines that the indifferent gonad shall differentiate into testis, rather than enter a 'default' pathway leading to ovarian development, has now been demonstrated (Sinclair et al 1990).

In the male the mesonephric duct, after the mesonephros has ceased to function, becomes taken over by the genital system. Mesonephric tubules in the region of the testis link up with the rete testis to become the efferent ductules which constitute much of the caput epididymis and are continued into the mesonephric duct which becomes tightly coiled to form the body and tail of the epididymis followed by the ductus deferens (Fig. 5.73). Atavistic mesonephric tubules form various remnants around the testis and epididymis which can give rise to cysts in later life.

As the testis and epididymis form, a thick column of mesodermal tissue, called the gubernaculum, is separated

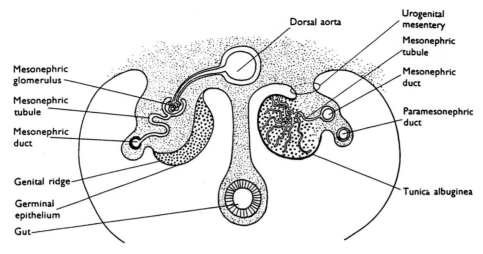

Fig. 5.72 Transverse section through the abdomen. The right side of the diagram shows a more advanced stage of development than the left. Reproduced with permission from Beck et al (1985).

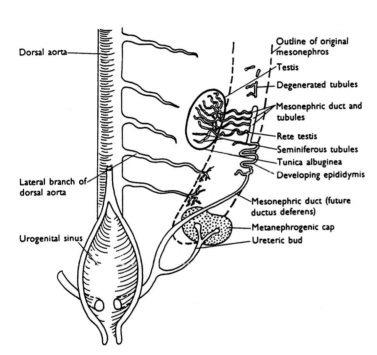

Fig. 5.73 Diagram to show the takeover of the mesonephric duct by the testis and the development of the metanephros. Reproduced with permission from Beck et al (1985).

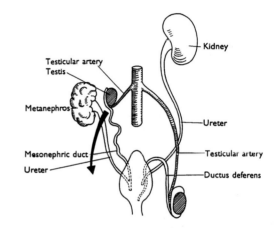

Fig. 5.74 Diagram to explain the adult relations of the testicular artery and ductus deferens to the ureter. The arrow shows the path of testicular descent. Reproduced with permission from Beck et al (1985).

from the dorsal body wall. This structure remains attached to the lower pole of the testis and, passing through the tissues around which the abdominal muscles will develop, ends in the genital swelling, which will eventually form the scrotum. By a complex series of morphological changes which are not completely understood in mechanical terms but are known to include differential growth and swelling of the gubernaculum to dilate the inguinal canal, the testis—together with its vessels, nerves and lymphatics as well as the tunica vaginalis—is guided into the scrotum.

An interesting, if controversial, contribution to the problem of testicular descent has been made by Hutson et al (1992). True testicular descent, i.e. from the region of the internal ring to the scrotum, usually takes place during the last weeks (32–36) of intrauterine life and the tunica vaginalis is separated from the general peritoneal cavity shortly after birth (Fig. 5.74). Prostatic buds begin to proliferate from the urethral epithelium at about 12 weeks and a diverticulum of the lower end of each ductus deferens grows out to form the seminal vesicles.

The ovary remains histologically undifferentiated until 16 weeks; like the testis, it undergoes a relative descent but remains in the pelvis. The paramesonephric ducts lie laterally at the cranial end of the nephrogenic ridge but caudally they meet in the midline. Their fused lower portions are closely related to the dorsal wall of the urogenital sinus (Fig. 5.75) where, by 15 weeks, they produce

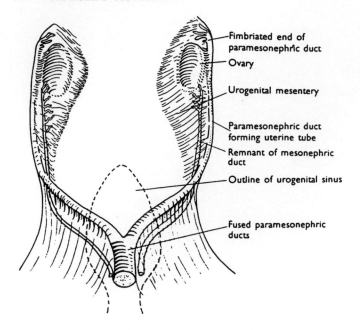

Fig. 5.75 Development of the urogenital mesentery into the broad ligament of the uterus. The mesonephros, together with its ducts and tubules, has almost completely disappeared. Reproduced with permission from Beck et al (1985).

an elevation, the Müllerian tubercle. The fused portions of the ducts, known as the uterovaginal canal, form the uterus and probably a part of the vagina. The original urogenital mesentery will form the broad ligament of the uterus and the gubernaculum develops in it. The latter gains a secondary attachment to the uterus and becomes converted into a fibrous cord. It thus becomes converted into two ligaments—the ligament of the ovary and the round ligament of the uterus (Fig. 5.76). The Müllerian

tubercles become pushed away from the urogenital sinus by a solid mass of cells growing posteriorly from the sinus, known as the sinus upgrowth. The sinus upgrowth and Müllerian tubercles together form the vagina, and much of the pars phallica of the definitive urogenital sinus forms the vestibule (Fig. 5.77). Reference to Figures 5.71 and 5.77 explains the development of the female external genitalia.

The male phallus is developed from the genital tubercle, which enlarges greatly. A proliferation of endodermal cells from the anterior extremity of the phallic part of the urogenital sinus extends forwards into it to form the urethral plate. From this the penile urethra will develop, as shown in Figure 5.78. After dissolution of the urogenital membrane, the urethral folds begin to fuse with each other from behind forwards (Fig. 5.79). This process involves the urethral plate and the development of the male external genitalia may therefore be understood by reference to Figures 5.71, 5.78 and 5.79. In Figure 5.79 the completion of the penile urethra by an ectodermal plate which canalizes the glans is shown.

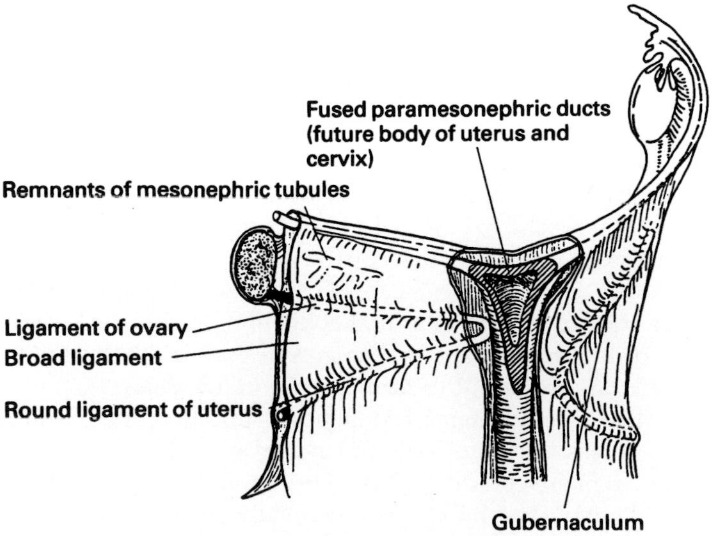

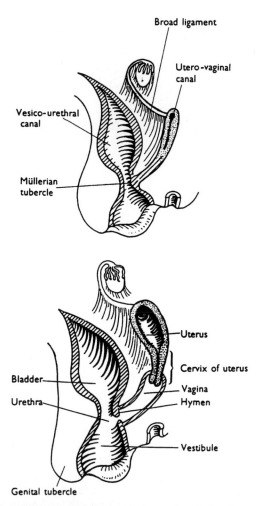

Fig. 5.76 Diagram to show how the gubernaculum becomes the round ligaments of the uterus and the ligament of the ovary. Reproduced with permission from Beck et al (1985).

Fig. 5.77 Development of the female internal genitalia. Reproduced with permission from Beck et al (1985).

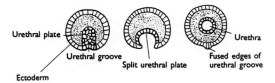

Fig. 5.78 Transverse sections through the phallus of a male embryo to show the development of the urethra from the urethral plate. Reproduced with permission from Beck et al (1985).

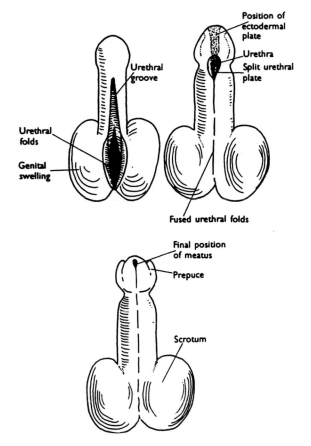

Fig. 5.79 Development of the male external genitalia. Reproduced with permission from Beck et al (1985).

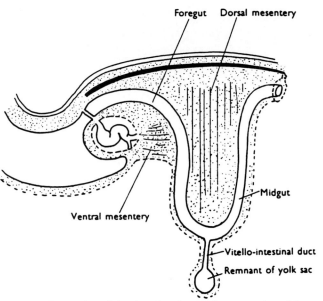

Fig. 5.80 Formation of the dorsal and ventral mesenteries of the gut. Reproduced with permission from Beck et al (1985).

It becomes possible to distinguish the sexes by examination of the external genitalia at 12–16 weeks of development.

The digestive system

The division of the primitive gut into foregut, midgut and hindgut, which begins to be apparent at 21–22 days of development, is shown in Figure 5.13. Histogenesis of the gut has been extensively reviewed (Tench 1936, Salenius 1962, Deren 1968, Severn 1971, 1972, Grand et al 1976, McLean 1979, Trier & Moxey 1979).

As development proceeds the gut pulls away from the dorsal body wall mesoderm to form a dorsal mesentery and from the septum transversum to form a ventral me-

sentery (Fig. 5.80). The liver bud grows into the ventral mesentery between 24 and 26 days at the junction of the foregut and midgut (Fig. 5.81) and a ventral division of this outgrowth forms the gallbladder. The liver is gradually everted from its intraseptal position and, in the adult, remains attached to the diaphragm only by its bare area (Fig. 5.82). The lesser sac is formed by an erosion of the right side of the dorsal mesentery (the bursa omentalis; Fig. 5.83), followed by rotation of the stomach so that its left surface comes to face anteriorly (Fig. 5.84). Finally, the portion of the mesentery lying between the aorta and left kidney fuses with the posterior abdominal wall; the spleen develops at about 6 weeks (Fig. 5.85) and the inferior wall of the sac is extended downwards to form the

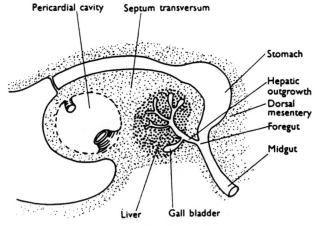

Fig. 5.81 The hepatic outgrowth grows into the ventral mesentery from the end of the foregut. Liver cells invade the septum transversum. Reproduced with permission from Beck et al (1985).

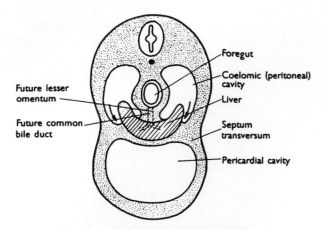

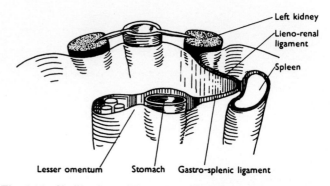

Fig. 5.82 Transverse section through the peritoneal and pericardial cavities to show the position of the liver within the septum transversum. To a large extent the liver becomes separated from the diaphragm except for the region lying between the arrows (the bare area). Reproduced with permission from Beck et al (1985).

Fig. 5.85 Similar view to Figure 5.84 after fusion of part of the dorsal mesentery to the dorsal body wall. Reproduced with permission from Beck et al (1985).

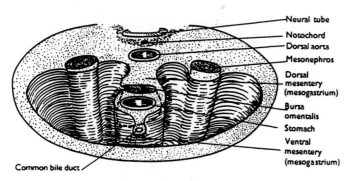

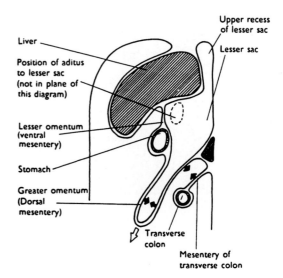

Fig. 5.83 The bursa omentalis grows into the mesentery from the (embryo's) right. Its lower part is indicated by a dashed line. Reproduced with permission from Beck et al (1985).

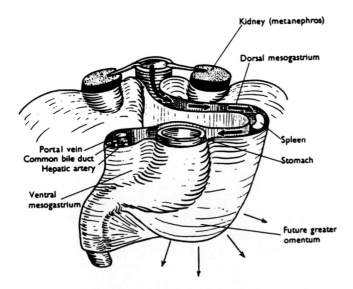

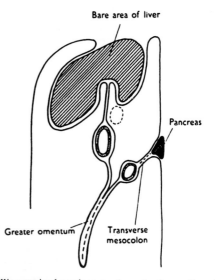

Fig. 5.84 Rotation of the stomach causes the dorsal mesentery to be diverted to the left. It also grows in the direction of the thin arrows. The darker arrows show the course of the arteries to the spleen and stomach. Reproduced with permission from Beck et al (1985).

Fig. 5.86 Midline sagittal sections to show the formation of the lesser sac. Reproduced with permission from Beck et al (1985).

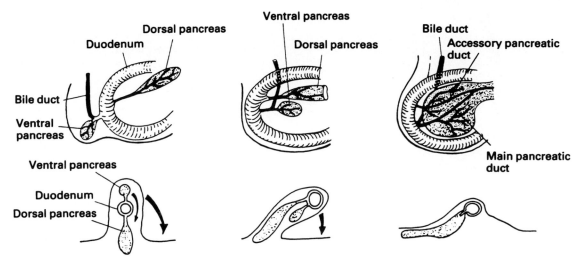

Fig. 5.87 The development of the pancreas. Upper diagrams show the pancreas and bile duct seen from in front; the lower row is a series of cross-sections seen from above. Reproduced with permission from Beck et al (1985).

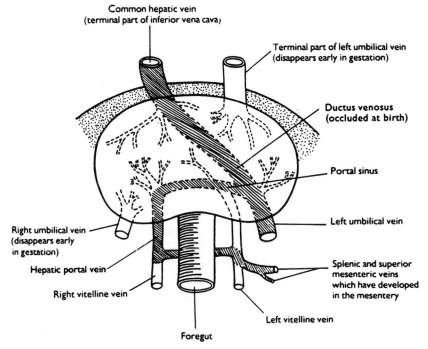

Fig. 5.88 The vessels in the region of the liver. The cross-hatched vessels persist at least until birth, while the others disappear. Reproduced with permission from Beck et al (1985).

greater omentum and to fuse with the transverse mesocolon (Fig. 5.86). The pancreas also develops (24–26 days) at the junction of the foregut and midgut (Fig. 5.87). This figure also explains the retroperitoneal position of both the duodenum and the pancreas. The development of the portal vein is shown in Figure 5.88. The ductus venosus is occluded at birth to form the ligamentum venosum and the position of the terminal part of the inferior vena cava is apparent from reference to Figure 5.59.

The large size of the liver at 5 weeks causes most of the midgut, which has an extensive dorsal mesentery (Fig. 5.80), to be forced into the extraembryonic coelom (Fig. 5.89). At 6 weeks external inspection of the embryo demonstrates that the liver is large enough to produce an external bulge above the midgut hernia. While in the extraembryonic situation the midgut loop forms a caecal swelling and undergoes rotation through 90° (Fig. 5.90). Between 8 and 9 weeks the relative size of the liver allows

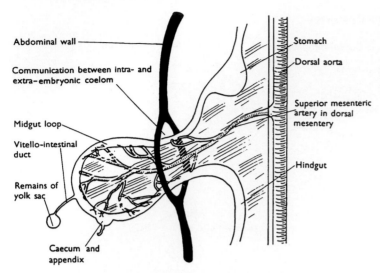

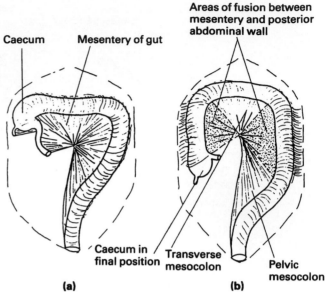

Fig. 5.89 Side view of the midgut loop herniated out into the extraembryonic coelom. Reproduced with permission from Beck et al (1985).

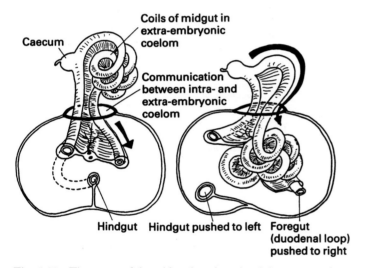

Fig. 5.90 The return of the midgut loop into the abdomen, seen from above. The right (proximal) limb returns first; the caecum is the last to return and comes to lie high in the abdomen on the right side. Reproduced with permission from Beck et al (1985).

Fig. 5.91 (a) The colon and its mesentery immediately after the return of the midgut loop. (b) The final stage of rotation of the gut. The caecum has attained its final position and the ascending and descending colon have become retroperitoneal. Reproduced with permission from Beck et al (1985).

EXTERNAL FEATURES DURING THE EMBRYONIC AND EARLY FETAL PERIOD
(Fig. 5.92)

The embryonic period of development extends from conception to 8 weeks and the post-implantation formation of the germ layers has been described in the introduction to this chapter. The crown–rump length (4 mm) can first be measured at 28 days when the embryo has between 28 and 30 somites. At this stage there is a large pericardial cavity which forms a bulge below the developing facial and pharyngeal regions, although the branchial arches are not yet all present. The neural tube is completely closed and the mesodermal somites are a prominent feature. Shortly thereafter the limb buds appear. The embryo is growing in length at about 1 mm per day and by the end of the embryonic period has reached a length of 30 mm. Thereafter, during the early fetal period, the rate of growth increases to 1.5 mm per day.

The early fetal period lasts from 8 to 28 weeks (Fig. 5.93). There is very rapid growth of the body, together with maturation of tissues and organs. The average crown–rump length at 8 weeks is 29 mm whilst, at 28 weeks, measurement of 28 cm and weight of 1000 g are recorded. Accompanying this growth there are profound changes in external form. At 12 weeks the embryo has a disproportionately large head and the physiological hernia has just re-entered the abdominal cavity. Sex is easily identified. At 16 weeks the human appearance is even clearer, with the eyes looking forward rather than laterally, the

the herniated gut to return to the abdominal cavity; the proximal part of the midgut loop returns first (because of the caecal swelling on the distal part of the loop) and this results in a further rotation of 90°. On return the gut lies in the position it will occupy in the adult. The remaining development concerns the formation of the ascending colon and the fixation of the descending colon (Fig. 5.91). Peristalsis begins at about the tenth week. It is interesting to note that, while the buccopharyngeal membrane disappears between 24 and 26 days, the cloacal membrane persists until 7–8 weeks.

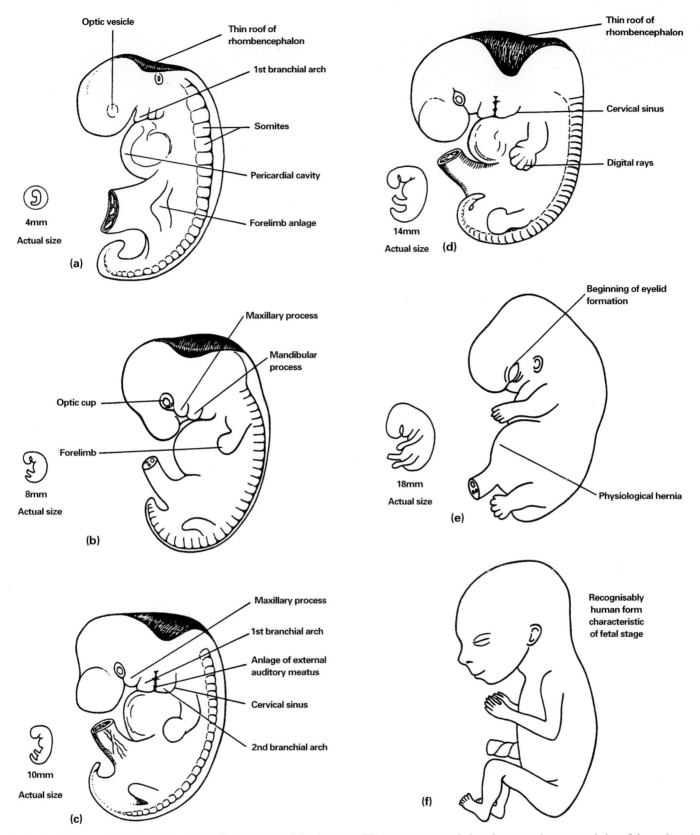

Fig. 5.92   Human embryos and fetuses at different stages of development. These are not to scale but the approximate actual size of the embryo is shown in the insets: (**a**) 28 days 4 mm O'Rahilly (1979) stage 13; (**b**) 35 days 8 mm O'Rahilly (1979) stage 15; (**c**) 37 days 10 mm O'Rahilly (1979) stage 16; (**d**) 40 days 13.5 mm O'Rahilly (1979) stage 16/17; (**e**) 47 days 18 mm O'Rahilly (1979) stage 19; (**f**) 100 days 100 mm. Reproduced with permission from Beck et al (1985).

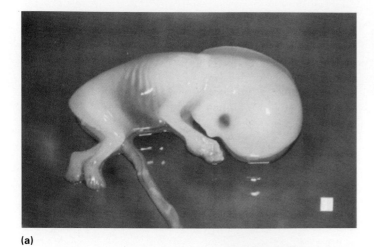

(a)

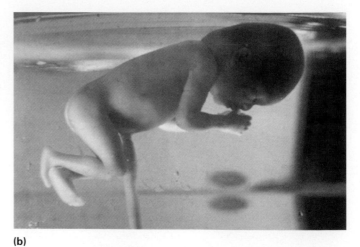

(b)

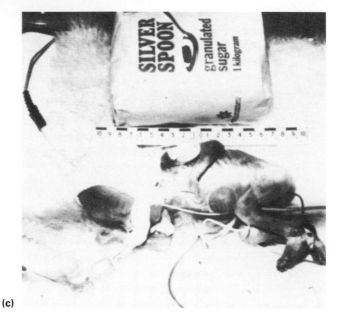

(c)

Fig. 5.93   The fetus at (**a**) 8 weeks; (**b**) 18 weeks; (**c**) 27 weeks.

ears much closer to their definitive positions and the infraumbilical region of the abdominal wall beginning to expand so that the umbilicus lies relatively higher in the abdomen. At 20 weeks lanugo hair covers the whole body, including the head. Between 24 and 28 weeks there is still almost complete absence of subcutaneous fat. Extensive documentation of timed stages in human development were first produced by Streeter (1942, 1945, 1948, 1951) and have been added to and improved by O'Rahilly & Müller (1987).

REFERENCES

Beck F, Moffat D B, Davies D P 1985 Human embryology, 2nd edn. Blackwell, Oxford

Deren J J 1968 Development of intestinal structure and function. In: Cook C F (ed) Handbook of physiology, vol 3. American Physiological Society, Bethesda, Maryland, p 1099

Gehring W 1987 Homeoboxes in the study of development. Science 236: 1245–1252

Gillman J 1948 The development of the gonads in man with a consideration of the role of fetal endocrines and histogenesis of ovarian tumours. Contributions to Embryology, Carnegie Institute 32: 81

Grand R J, Watkins J B, Troti F M 1976 Progress in gastroenterology. Development of the human gastrointestinal tract. A review. Gastroenterology 70: 790

Guraya S S 1980 Recent progress in morphology, histochemistry, biochemistry and physiology of developing and maturing human testes. International Review of Cytology 62: 187–309

Hunt P, Whiting J, Muchamore I, Marshall H, Krumlauf R 1991 Homeobox genes and models for patterning the hindbrain and branchial arches. Development (suppl 1): 187–197

Hutson J M, Baker M L, Griffiths A L et al 1992 Endocrine and morphological perspectives in testicular descent. Reproductive Medicine Review 1: 165

Jacobson M 1978 Developmental neurobiology. Plenum Press, New York

Jacobson S 1972 Neuroembryology. In: Curtis B H, Jacobson S (eds) An introduction to neurosciences. Saunders, Philadelphia

Langman J 1968 Histogenesis of the central nervous system. In: Bourne G H (ed) The structure and function of nervous tissues. Academic Press, New York

Le Dourain 1982 In: Cohen N, Segal M M (eds) The reticulo endothelial system 3. Phylogeny and ontogeny. Plenum Press, New York

Lemire R J, Loeser J D, Leech R W, Alvord E C 1975 Normal and abnormal development of the human nervous system. Harper & Row, Hagerstown

McLean J M 1979 Embryology of the pancreas. In: Howart H T, Sarles H (eds) The exocrine pancreas. Saunders, London, p 3

O'Rahilly R 1971 The timing and sequence of events in human cardiogenesis. Acta Anatomica 79: 70

O'Rahilly R 1979 Developmental stages in human embryos. European Journal of Obstetrics, Gynecology and Reproductive Biology 9: 273

O'Rahilly R, Gardner E 1971 The timing and sequence of events in the development of the human nervous system during the embryonic period proper. Zeitschrift vür Anatomie und Entwicklungsgeschichte 134: 1

O'Rahilly R, Müller K 1987 Developmental stages in human embryos. Carnegie Institute of Washington, Publication 637

Pinkerton J H M, McKay D G, Adams C, Hertig A T 1961 Development of the human ovary—a study using histochemical techniques. Obstetrics and Gynecology 18: 152

Salenius P 1962 On the ontogenesis of the human gastric epithelial cells. A histologic and histochemical study. Acta Anatomica 50 (suppl 46): 1

Sensenig E C 1949 The early development of the human vertebral column. Contributions to Embryology, Carnegie Institute 33: 23

Severn C B 1971 A morphological study of the development of the human liver. I. Development of the hepatic diverticulum. American Journal of Anatomy 131: 133

Severn C B 1972 A morphological study of the development of the human liver. II. Establishment of liver parenchyma, extrahepatic ducts and associated venous channels. American Journal of Anatomy 133: 85

Short R V 1979 Sex determination and differentiation. British Medical Bulletin 35: 121

Sinclair A H, Berta P, Palmer M S et al 1990 A gene from the human sex-determining region encodes a protein with homology to a conserved DNA-binding motif. Nature 346: 240–244

Slarkin H C 1979 Developmental craniofacial biology. Lea & Febiger, Philadelphia

Steinberger H, Steinberger E 1980 Testicular development structure and function. Raven Press, New York

Streeter G L 1942 Developmental horizons in human embryos, description of age group XI, 13–20 somites and age group XII 21–29 somites. Contributions of Embryology, Carnegie Institute 30: 211

Streeter G L 1945 Developmental horizons in human embryos, description of age group XIII embryo of about 4 or 5 mm long and age group XIV period of indentation of lens vesicle. Contributions to Embryology, Carnegie Institute 31: 27

Streeter G L 1948 Developmental horizons in human embryos, description of age groups XV. Being the 3rd issue of a survey of the Carnegie Collection XVI, XVII and XVIII. Contributions to Embryology, Carnegie Institute 32: 133

Streeter G L 1951 Developmental horizons in human embryos, description of age groups XIX, XX, XXI, XXII and XXIII. Being the 5th issue of a survey of the Carnegie Collection. Contributions to Embryology, Carnegie Institute 34: 165

Tench E M 1936 Development of the anus in the human embryo. American Journal of Anatomy 59: 333

Trier J S, Moxey P C 1979 Morphogenesis of the small intestine during fetal development. Ciba Foundation Symposium 70: 3

Visser H K A 1974 Sexual differentiation in the fetus and newborn. In: Davies J A, Dobbing J (eds) Scientific foundation of paediatrics. Saunders, Philadelphia, p 455

Zuckerman S, Weir B J 1977 The ovary, 2nd edn. Academic Press, New York

6. Fetal growth and development

Jeffrey S. Robinson

Material in this chapter contains contributions from the first edition and we are grateful to the previous author for the work done.

INTRODUCTION

Fetal growth is of most concern to the clinician when it deviates from normal. However, this can be difficult and sometimes impossible to detect in obstetric or midwifery practice. Two common forms of altered growth that place the fetus at increased risk are the large-for-dates and small-for-dates fetus. Although acceleration of fetal growth is commonly associated with maternal diabetes or abnormal glucose tolerance, the majority of macrosomic babies weighing more than 4000 g at birth are born at term to healthy mothers. In this chapter, large-for-dates and big babies (macrosomia) will be considered together. In the first edition, slow fetal growth was described as intrauterine growth retardation; however, in keeping with the view that this term raises unnecessary concern for the lay community (Bastian 1992) the term growth restriction will be used in preference.

It has been recognized for a long time that there are tiny puny infants with great vitality. Their movements are untiring and their cry lusty, for their organs are quite capable of performing their allotted functions. These infants will live although their weight is inferior . . . their sojourn in the womb was longer (Budin 1907).

Obstetric recognition of this problem of intrauterine growth restriction was delayed, in part because a weight of < 2500 g was defined as representing prematurity. In 1947, McBurney noted that slow growth caused some babies to be small at birth. The formal definition of preterm babies came in 1961 (World Health Organization 1961) and soon afterwards the morphological characteristics of the small-for-dates baby dying in the perinatal period were described (Gruendwald 1963, Naeye 1965). Perinatal mortality correlates closely with birthweight and is highest in small-for-dates or growth restricted fetuses and is also increased in the large-for-dates or macrosomic fetus.

The small-for-dates fetus is also likely to deliver or be delivered prematurely, and to suffer from fetal distress or perinatal asphyxia especially when it is born at term. The neonate who is growth restricted may also have significant morbidity due to hypoglycaemia, hyperbilirubinaemia or asphyxia which began before birth (Robinson 1979). Perhaps of greater concern in a developed society is the comparatively slow decline in the rate of unexplained stillbirth, many of whom are normally formed but small-for-dates (Northern Region 1984). Unexplained stillbirths now account for more than 25% of all perinatal deaths. These deaths are difficult for women and their families to accept as they do not have the reassurance of a diagnosis. The number of unexplained deaths has been related to the number of babies still undelivered at each week of gestation. This ratio of unexplained stillbirths to undelivered babies rises with increasing gestational age (Yudkin et al 1987b). However, this epidemiological finding makes counselling more difficult when women ask if induction would have prevented their tragedy. Unfortunately, the large-for-dates baby is also more likely to die late in gestation.

Long term follow-up studies have shown that growth-restricted babies, especially if born prematurely, are more frequently handicapped either physically or neurologically

(Comney & Fitzharding 1979, Ounsted et al 1982, 1984, Rantakallio 1985). The risk of poor developmental outcome relates to the time when failure of fetal growth was estimated to have begun by extrapolation from ultrasound scans (Harvey et al 1982). Not all authors agree that the risk of handicap is increased in growth-restricted babies born at term (Low et al 1982). However, when the prevalence of cerebral palsy in a community was determined, the relative risk of cerebral palsy was increased in growth-restricted babies born at term (Blair & Stanley 1990, 1992).

Perinatal morbidity in the large-for dates infant relates to its body proportions. The disproportionate baby has more complications in the neonatal period. Long-term follow-up has shown that larger babies are less likely to develop hypertension, coronary artery disease or diabetes in adult life (Barker 1992). The latter studies have important implications, particularly if it is established that these problems are preventable by interventions to improve the health or nutrition of the mother during pregnancy.

There have been a number of advances in the last decade which have made it possible to recognize deviations from normal fetal growth on most if not all occasions, enabling selective early delivery of compromised fetuses. New interventions, such as maternal hyperoxia (Nicolaides et al 1987, Battaglia et al 1992) or low-dose aspirin therapy (Wallenberg & Rotmans 1987, Trudinger et al 1988a) have been proposed, but await full evaluation in randomized trials. The CLASP study (CLASP 1994) has not provided support for use of aspirin. More than nine thousand women were recruited into this large multi-centre study. Aspirin was associated with a non-significant reduction in the incidence of proteinuric pre-eclampsia and there was no significant effect on the incidence of intrauterine growth restriction. Use of aspirin was associated with a slight increase in use of blood transfusions after delivery. The overview provided in the report on the CLASP study highlights another concern; the trend to a smaller benefit observed in the larger trials compared to the earlier small trials. The study design of at least one of the small trials was poor and led to unrealized expectations for aspirin. This reinforces the caution which should be exercised in the use of aspirin. Other large trials are in progress and the results of these should be interpreted together with the CLASP study before offering aspirin in clinical practice outside a clinical trial. It also provides greater urgency for well-designed randomized trials of use of aspirin in the lupus obstetric syndrome.

The purpose of this chapter is to provide an account of the factors associated with abnormal rates of fetal growth and their management when it is diagnosed. In addition the physiological changes which have been observed in experimental growth restriction or maternal undernutrition will be outlined. These provide the necessary scientific basis for new interventions which should or already are being subjected to clinical trial.

DEFINITIONS

A number of criteria have been used to define intrauterine growth restriction, small-for-dates, large-for-dates and big or macrosomic babies. Small-for-dates is easier to define than growth restriction. However, it should be remembered that there is only a partial overlap of the babies who are light-for-dates with those who are short-for-age. The most commonly used definition is a baby whose birthweight is below the 10th percentile allowing for both age and sex. Additional criteria such as maternal size (weight, height or weight-for-height) and parity may also be used to determine centiles for birthweight within subpopulations. Since these definitions include many healthy but genetically small fetuses, more extreme limits—less than the 3rd percentile or more than two standard deviations below the mean weight-for-age and sex—are also used. Large-for-dates is categorized in an analogous fashion as more than the 90th or 97th percentiles or more than two standard deviations above the mean. Macrosomia is commonly defined as a birthweight of more than 4000 g. Since small-for-dates presents the greater clinical problem, this will receive greater emphasis in this chapter.

Many charts of centiles for birthweight for gestational age have been produced (see Dunn 1981). In the USA, the chart prepared by Lubchenco et al (1963) was widely used before others charts became available but suffered the disadvantage of being derived from a population which lives at altitude and contains on unusual race distribution. Accurate assessment of gestational age remained a problem and was addressed statistically by Milner & Richards (1974). More recently it was proposed that an international reference chart should be made available (Dunn 1985). Factors adversely affecting fetal growth are more likely to be present when preterm delivery is undertaken electively for maternal or fetal reasons (Yudkin et al 1987a). These authors noticed that this can have a major effect on mean weight for gestation since as many as 28% were delivered before 34 weeks for fetal problems. The difference in mean birthweight for spontaneous compared with elective preterm birth ranged from 169 to 569 g and was significant at all weeks from 27 to 34 except for 28 weeks. Estimates of fetal weight obtained from ultrasound measurements of healthy fetuses who later deliver at term, provide a different picture of the growth of the human fetus (Persson 1989) more akin to that described for other species. These show a decline in the velocity of fetal growth with increasing gestational age. When preterm babies are compared to this chart a high proportion of them have grown slowly (Persson 1989). The national trends in birthweight need to be re-examined from time to time. Recently, it has been shown that the current birthweight norms are heavier for full-term infants than those described in the 1970s (Arbuckle et al 1993). Indeed the incidence of babies over 4000 g has risen dramatically in Scotland between 1975 and 1992 from 6.79% to 9.93%. There is a suggestion that the same trend occurred in England a little earlier (Power 1994).

Normal growth is the expression of the genetic potential to grow which is neither abnormally constrained nor promoted by internal or external factors. This is a nebulous concept for clinical purposes and it may be difficult to identify real or true variations from normal growth in a particular fetus. Intrauterine growth restriction is often loosely defined as being the same as small-for-dates but it should also include fetuses which remain within the normal limits but which fail to maintain growth. This is sometimes recognized by ultrasound with measurements showing that the fetus is crossing to lower centiles as pregnancy proceeds. Whenever possible, it is better to define the factors constraining or promoting growth and causing the fetus to be growth restricted or accelerated respectively. Thus, intrauterine growth restriction can be caused by fetal malnutrition and hypoxia, or by problems such as congenital viral infections or chromosomal anomalies. It is obvious that each of these has a different prognosis for the fetus during pregnancy and parturition and for its subsequent development. Furthermore, fetal malnutrition and hypoxia may result from many different aetiological factors, e.g. starvation or living at altitude. In affluent societies, pre-existing or pregnancy-induced disease may play a more significant role but socio-economic circumstances still remain very important and interact with lifestyle problems, e.g. maternal smoking. In many developing countries maternal protein-energy malnutrition has a major influence on growth of the fetus.

PREVENTION AND PREPREGNANCY COUNSELLING

Successful management of abnormal intrauterine growth has to begin with knowledge of the factors which may alter fetal growth. When these (Tables 6.1, 6.2) have been defined, education to avoid their consequences must begin in the community. For example, most of the community is aware of the adverse effects of alcohol and smoking on growth and development of the fetus. However, most strategies only have a small effect on long-standing habits and, therefore emphasis should be placed on programmes that alter community attitudes. Since reproduction can begin in the young teenager, school children need to be informed of some of the common factors adversely affecting prenatal growth.

Prepregnancy counselling may identify factors in previous pregnancies, family or medical history which may increase the risk of either a growth-restricted or large-for-dates fetus. However, it must be acknowledged that often the causes of growth acceleration or restriction remain obscure. Despite this, identification of putative factors before pregnancy enables counselling of the woman and her partner so that risks of factors constraining growth can be minimized.

FACTORS ASSOCIATED WITH GROWTH ACCELERATION AND RESTRICTION

Growth acceleration

Macrosomia has been defined earlier as a weight at birth of more than 4000 g. There is a matrilineal trend for macrosomia and the majority of these babies are born to healthy mothers who have uncomplicated pregnancies. Maternal diabetes mellitus and carbohydrate intolerance are both associated with macrosomia and large-for-dates babies, although they account for only a small proportion of these babies. However, it is important that the woman is aware of the need for control of blood sugars before and during pregnancy to reduce the risk of malformation associated with insulin dependent diabetes mellitus. The benefits of strict control of blood sugars by reducing the risk of large-for-dates infants may be more than balanced by an increase in the proportion of small-for-dates babies with a different set of problems. Other factors associated with macrosomia and large-for-dates babies include large

Table 6.1 Factors associated with intrauterine growth restriction

Medical complications	Maternal behavioural conditions	Fetal problems	Environmental problems	Abnormalities of the placenta
Pre-eclampsia	Malnutrition	Multiple births	High altitude	Reduced blood flow
Acute or chronic hypertension	Low pre-pregnancy weight for height	Malformation	Toxic substances	Reduced area for exchange
Severe chronic disease	Low maternal weight gain	Chromosomal anomalies		Focal lesions: infarcts
Severe chronic infections	Delivery < 16 years	Inborn errors of metabolism		Haematomas
Disseminated lupus erythematosus	Drug use: smoking alcohol hard drugs	Intrauterine infections		Placenta praevia
Lupus obstetric syndrome	Low socioeconomic status			Placenta membranacae
Anaemia				Extrachorial placenta
Malignancy				Circumvallate placenta
Abnormalities of the uterus				Chromosomal mosaicism
Uterine fibroids				

Table 6.2 Factors associated with intrauterine growth acceleration

Matrilineal tendency   DM
Maternal size
Weight gain > 20 kg
Previous big baby
Male fetus
Maternal diabetes
Glucose intolerance
Hydrops fetalis
Beckwith–Weidemann syndrome
Cerebral giantism

maternal size, birth of a previous large baby, hydrops fetalis, cerebral gigantism and the Beckwith–Weidemann syndrome, which provides clues to the paternal drive to growth of the fetus through imprinting of the gene for insulin-like growth factor II. These children are more likely to develop tumours in adult life (Henry et al 1991). Studies in mice provide evidence for a potential constraint to growth mediated by the maternally derived type-2 receptor for this growth factor (Barlow et al 1991, Stoger et al 1993).

Growth restriction

Low birthweight is the birth of a baby of less than 2500 g. The percentages of babies with low birthweight vary widely in different communities. In some, the incidence is more than 30% and even in affluent communities with well developed community services, including those for health and welfare, the rate is usually between 5% and 10% (Ebrahim 1984). Communities with a high proportion of low birthweight babies have a high percentage of these born at term, suggesting that growth restriction is common, although genetic effects on size could not be excluded by this analysis (Vilar & Belizan 1982). Later studies in India show a close relationship between birthweight and social class. However, nutritional problems, recognized by low fasting glucose (less than 50 mg per 100 ml) or low maternal weight-for-height, can identify a group of women across the social classes who are at risk of having a low birthweight baby (Raman 1987). In contrast, in a similar community, evidence of good nutrition determined by the increasing size of the mother's fat store over the thigh in mid-pregnancy predicts a well-grown baby (Vilar at al 1992).

Failure of normal fetal growth is common in preterm babies. This was recognized by examination of birthweight curves, where it was shown that the coefficient of birthweight around the mean weight-for-age increased with prematurity (Dunn 1985). Ultrasonic measurements indicated that growth may decelerate and remain within normal limits some weeks before women go into unexplained premature labour (Persson et al 1978). Others have indicated that elective preterm delivery for maternal

or fetal indications is associated with significantly lower mean birthweight than for babies born after spontaneous preterm labour (Yudkin et al 1987a). Overall, almost 30% of preterm babies are light compared with ultrasound estimates of weight for fetuses of the same gestational age who subsequently deliver at term (Persson 1989).

Surveys conducted in Britain at different times have highlighted a small number of factors which have strong associations with low birthweight (Peters et al 1983). Smoking, maternal size, low parity and pre-eclampsia were identified by both the 1958 (Butler & Bonham 1963, Butler & Alberman 1969) and 1970 (Chamberlain et al 1975, 1978) British Births Surveys despite substantial changes in the maternity services, promoting the comment: *plus ça change*. Unfortunately, maternal smoking continues to be a major factor and increases the odds ratio for a small-for-dates baby in older multiparous women (Cnattingus et al 1993) and is the single most important preventable cause of perinatal death (Cnattingus et al 1988). Many studies have shown that stopping smoking in the first half of pregnancy has a beneficial effect on birthweight.

Many years ago it was suggested that disorders of the placenta could account for a significant proportion of small-for-dates babies in a developed community. Recent studies have shown that fetal growth restriction can result when a trisomy is present in the placenta and not in the fetus who may have uniparental disomy (Kalousek et al 1993). This placental mosaicism is an uncommon cause of fetal growth restriction (Fryburg et al 1993). Many other factors have been identified as adversely affecting fetal growth and will be divided into behavioural, medical, fetal and environmental factors and abnormalities of the placenta (Table 6.1).

Maternal behavioural factors

Another facet of education of the school child is the benefit of delaying pregnancy until at least the later teens. Pregnancy in the under 16 year old is more often complicated by poor fetal growth, even after social circumstances have been taken into account (Russell 1982, Zhang & Chan 1992). It is more difficult to alleviate the effects of poor social circumstances, but in at least one affluent society (Australia) the differences in birthweight in different socioeconomic groups could be largely ascribed to the differences in smoking across the groups (Lumley et al 1985). Unfortunately a high incidence of teenage smoking is present in this society. In poorer communities other factors obviously play a more significant role, e.g. nutrition, poor housing and heavy manual work. Pressure to improve these must come from many parts of the community and will often be political in nature. Maternal nutritional supplements have little effect on birthweight (Rush 1989) but this may be the wrong end point—children of mothers receiving energy supplements in the last trimester were taller for the next 5 years than the unsupplemented group (Kusin et al 1992). Similarly providing advice to women to stop work outside the home may achieve an unexpected outcome as it can lead to an even heavier workload as they then have to assume responsibilities in the home instead, looking after other children, doing housework, shopping and other home duties. Others who may be better off financially often indulge in some strenuous leisure activities.

Maternal smoking remains a major factor constraining the growth of the fetus. On average, smoking reduces birthweight by 13 g per cigarette smoked daily (Anderson et al 1984). Numerous studies have shown a similar effect of smoking on growth of the fetus. Intervention studies have been successful in reducing or stopping smoking with improvements in birthweight even if cessation of smoking was delayed to the second trimester (MacArthur et al 1987). A beneficial effect may also accrue to the fetus since the risk of preterm delivery and the impact of severe pre-eclampsia may also be reduced. Cessation of smoking in pregnancy should be a major goal for all providers of antenatal care, however some staff have shown a reluctance to be proactive (MacArthur et al 1987), even though more women stop smoking if they are provided with self-help smoking-cessation manuals and support from those providing antenatal care (Lumley 1991). Interestingly, discussion about the effects of smoking on the fetus at the time of an ultrasound examination may be beneficial (Waldenstrom et al 1988). The infants of mothers who stop smoking in early pregnancy have similar outcomes to those of non-smokers, with increases in birthweight and lower perinatal morbidity relative to babies of smokers (Ahlsten et al 1993).

Other drugs affect the growth of the fetus. The fetal alcohol syndrome is found more often in women who are heavy drinkers (> 60 g/day). There is a concern that moderate amounts of alcohol adversely affect growth of the fetus. However, there is an interaction between cigarette smoking and alcohol especially in older women that accounts for poorer fetal growth. A recent analysis of babies born in New York City demonstrates a rise in the proportion of low birthweight babies that was greater in black-skinned than white-skinned women, and this has been attributed to the increase in substance abuse (Joyce 1990).

DETECTION OF LARGE- OR SMALL-FOR-DATES FETUS

Detection of the woman who is at risk for acceleration or restriction of growth of her fetus should begin at the first antenatal visit. Detailed history should be obtained about her family history. There is a matrilineal trend for both large and small babies. Alternatively a strong family history for pre-eclampsia may indicate that the woman may have a 25% or greater chance of this condition, especially if her mother had severe pre-eclampsia or eclampsia in the pregnancy leading to her birth (Chesley & Cooper 1986, Cooper et al 1988, Arngrimsson et al 1990). Previous history or a large- or small-for-dates fetus would be a strong indicator to seek recurrent causes of the altered growth to ensure that increased monitoring of fetal growth occurs in the current pregnancy. Previous studies from Aberdeen (Hall & Chng 1982) suggest that a history of growth restriction in previous pregnancies is often overlooked, although previous stillbirth is not. Problems in labour such as shoulder dystocia or fetal distress should also be recorded.

The traditional method of palpation of the maternal abdomen is not effective in detecting either the large- or small-for-dates fetus. The success rate is low and many fetuses are considered to be small but are subsequently shown to be normally grown. Several studies have suggested that serial measurement of symphysial–fundal height improves the detection of both the growth-restricted baby (Belizan et al 1978, Quaranta et al 1981, Calvert et al 1982, Taylor et al 1984) and the large baby which causes problems with delivery (Hughes et al 1987). The only randomized trial of symphysial–fundal height measurements showed that fewer small-for-dates fetuses were detected in the measurement group (28 vs 48%, Lindhard et al 1990). This result was supported by the earlier finding from Sweden that symphysial–fundal height and risk factor analysis after confirmation of dates using ultrasound only detected a minority of small-for-dates fetuses (Gemiser & Persson 1986). However, before abandoning symphysial–fundal height measurements, it is worth noting that the protagonists noted above were able to detect more small-for-dates babies with the addition of this measurement. Further studies of this simple measurement in randomized trials seem worthwhile.

Ultrasound scanning programmes which include a dating scan combined with an assessment of fetal morphology, followed later by a second scan in the third trimester, offer the highest detection rates for growth-restricted fetuses (Neilson et al 1980). Some 20% of small-for-dates fetuses were not detected. Almost all multiple pregnancies are detected in the first scan (Persson & Kullander 1983). An audit in the unit where a two-stage ultrasound screening programme was recommended found a disappointingly low detection rate for growth restriction (Hepburn & Rosenberg 1986). Mortality and morbidity of the growth-restricted baby remained higher in these babies. More disturbingly, the management of women with suspected fetal growth restriction bore no relationship to the test results and was not in keeping with agreed policies. More recently, a computer program has been devised that takes into account a number of variables to make antenatal assignment of a particular fetus to the category of small-for-dates easy in clinical practice (Gardosi et al 1992).

Detection of a growth-restricted fetus should prompt a repeat careful anatomical survey, particularly if polyhydramnios is present, since some problems only become apparent later than the normal time of a first dating and morphology ultrasound scan (about 18 weeks). These later manifestations of intrauterine problems include microcephaly, hydrocephaly and some cardiac lesions. Detailed descriptions of the growth of many organs with gestational age are available. For example the size of the ventricular walls of the heart has been measured using M-mode ultrasound and the heart is large in proportion to estimated body weight. In addition, it was found that the free ventricular walls are hypertrophied (Veille et al 1993) and it was suggested that this may be due to increased peripheral resistance (after load).

Recognition of malformation or very severe growth restriction presenting early in the second half of pregnancy is an indication for cordocentesis or a late chorion villous biopsy. Oligohydramnios often accompanies severe growth restriction and together they may be relative contraindications to cordocentesis. The former can be overcome by amnio-infusion to provide a better view of the fetus (Fisk et al 1991). Cordocentesis has allowed a dramatic picture of the metabolic and endocrine states of both the growth-restricted and macrosomic fetuses (see below).

Separation of the normally grown but premature fetus from the growth-retarded one continues to be a problem if the woman presents late in pregnancy with uncertain dates. If circumstances allow, assessment of the rate of growth of the abdominal circumference or length of the femur over a period of at least 14 days will identify most of the growth-restricted fetuses. Indeed wasting or reduction of the abdominal circumference has been observed in a few small fetuses (Divon et al 1986). Since the publication of this report, anecdotal comment suggests that this may not be too rare a finding on ultrasound examination of the growth-restricted fetus. Without an obvious cause (e.g. renal agenesis), oligohydramnios identified by the absence of a pocket of amniotic fluid of more than 2 cm adds further evidence supporting a diagnosis of a growth-retarded fetus (Divon et al 1986). Further, a high perinatal mortality was found in women whose pregnancies were complicated by oligohydramnios (Chamberlain et al 1984). Oligohydramnios should lead to a careful assessment of the fetal urinary tract and this should include determination of the rate of urine production (Wladimiroff & Campbell 1974). In the presence of obstruction, urine may have to be aspirated before this evaluation can be made. Determination of urinary electrolytes and protein in the urine sample allows further assessment of renal function (Crombleholme et al 1990).

Assessment of the appearance of the placenta on ultrasound is another means of identifying the growth-restricted fetus (Fisher et al 1975). A grading system for the maturation in the appearance of the placenta has been devised (Grannum et al 1979). Early placental maturation identifies a group of women with a high incidence of growth-restricted fetuses and, in contrast, a low incidence when this early maturation is absent (Patterson et al 1983). Unfortunately this assessment of the placenta is subject to observer error or bias and this led to the abandonment of a randomized trial of report and non-report groups when a new ultrasonographer was unable to grade placentas (Proud & Grant 1987). It will be interesting to re-examine the role of placental grading by ultrasound when objective measures exist.

PLACENTA AND FETAL GROWTH

Placental weight and fetal weight are closely correlated in most circumstances. The placenta increases in weight more slowly than the fetus in late pregnancy and the ratio of fetal weight : placental weight (FP) increases (Molteni et al 1978, Bonds et al 1984). High FP ratio is associated with fetal distress and meconium staining. Villous surface area of the placenta is also related to both gestational age and fetal weight (Boyd & Scott 1985). The expansion of the total volume and surface area of villi in normal pregnancies can be explained by a dramatic linear growth of the terminal villi which begins at about mid-pregnancy. At the same time there is an increase in the capillary volume in the villi and a decrease in the harmonic thickness of the villous membrane (Jackson et al 1992). This latter effect is exaggerated in placentas obtained from women giving birth at altitude (Jackson et al 1988) and the placentae are larger (Jackson et al 1987). Overall these changes lead to a reduction in oxygen diffusive conductance (Mayhew et al 1990). Morphological examination of the placenta has shown that the surface area for exchange is substantially reduced in pregnancies complicated by growth restriction (Aherne & Dunnill 1966, Teasdale 1984, Boyd & Scott 1985). In contrast, the morphological features of placentas from women with diabetes mellitus include increases in the parenchyma which includes villi, fetal vessels and the maternal intervillous spaces, and these placentas had greater surface areas (Boyd et al 1986).

It has been much harder to provide a quantitative description of the changes in the maternal component of the placenta with growth restriction or acceleration. However, biopsy of the placental bed has provided a qualitative description and on a few occasions hysterectomy specimens with the placenta in situ have provided quantitative data. Initially, the trophoblast occludes the lumen of the spiral arterioles and protects the conceptus from the high oxygen tensions (Rodesch et al 1992) and pressure of arterial blood. Brosens, Dixon and Robertson noted that invasion of the spiral arterioles by the trophoblast extends as far as its myometrial segment and converts the vessel into a wide bore conduit with low resistance to flow and presumably unresponsive to vasoactive substances. Normally about 120 spiral arterioles are recruited to form the placental bed (Brosens 1988). Late in pregnancy the trophoblast withdraws leaving a vessel wall composed of endothelium, fibrinoid and just a few scattered trophoblast cells. This change has been referred to as the physiological change (see Khong et al 1986, Robertson et al 1986, Khong 1991b). In pre-eclampsia and idiopathic growth restriction these physiological changes are reduced or absent in the spiral arterioles. However, a third wave of invading trophoblast that partially occludes the vessel may be found in the third trimester. In one specimen from a woman with severe intrauterine growth restriction only 72 spiral arterioles formed the maternal placental vascular supply (Brosens 1988). These placentas may also be further compromised by acute atherosis as indeed may the placenta from women with diabetes mellitus (Khong 1991a).

Attempts have been made to assess placental size from linear measurements made using ultrasound and an association of the small placenta with small-for-dates baby was found (Hoogland et al 1980). A compound B-scan has been used to obtain parallel transverse scans at intervals of 2 cm. When the placenta was oblique to the horizontal plane 1 cm intervals were used. Computer reconstructions were made and placental volume determined. There was a large difference between antepartum placental volume and postpartum placental weight with a volume : weight ratio of 1.6 : 1 (Wolf et al 1987). Serial measurements showed that the placenta stopped increasing in volume at least 3 weeks before a slowing of fetal growth or other sign of fetal compromise were apparent (Wolf et al 1989). More recently, measurements of placental volume were made to assess the effects of exercise on pregnancy outcome. Exercise in the first half of pregnancy is associated with a substantial increase in the volume of the placenta by as early as 16 weeks and this persisted to 24 weeks (Clapp & Rizk 1992). It may be suggested that this is an adaptation to sustain fetal growth when there is competition for nutrients or oxygen. This idea is not new since Godfrey et al (1991) noted a relatively heavy placenta in women with anaemia and suggested that a nutritional deficiency enhanced placental growth. Evidence for this enhancement of placental growth by moderate nutritional deficit has been found in sheep studies (Faichney & White 1987, McCrabb et al 1992). This is complicated by an interaction between maternal nutritional reserves in early pregnancy and diet in pregnancy (DeBarro et al 1992).

METABOLIC STATE OF THE FETUS

In 1987, Peter Soothill and his colleagues published their seminal paper on the metabolic state of the growth-restricted fetus. Since that time there has been an exponential growth in our knowledge of oxygenation, metabolism and the endocrine state of the growth-restricted fetus. By and large, these studies, using the technique of cordocentesis, have show that there is a remarkable similarity between these observations and earlier studies of experimental animals where fetal blood samples have been obtained from chronically indwelling catheters (Soothill et al 1987, Owens et al 1989a, Economides & Nicolaides 1990, Harding & Charlton 1990). Intrauterine growth restriction is characterized by fetal hypoxaemia and hypoglycaemia, at least in late gestation. In sheep, consumption of oxygen and glucose by the growth-restricted fetus is similar per unit weight to that of the normally growing fetus suggesting that fetal growth may by limited by the supply of these substrates (Owens et al 1987a,b). However, in sheep the fetal supply is maximized as far as possible in growth restriction by a large reduction in placental oxygen and glucose consumption. In order to maintain placental function despite this reduction, there are dramatic changes in amino acid metabolism within the uterus. Late in pregnancy, the fetus loses amino acids to its placenta. This loss of amino acids is selective, with alanine and the branched-chain amino acid making the greatest contribution (Owens 1991; Fig. 6.1). The growth-restricted human fetus has lowered concentrations of amino acids in its blood, and again alanine and the branched-chain amino acids show the greatest changes (Cetin et al 1988, 1989, 1990, Economides et al 1989). Cetin and her colleagues have used stable isotopes to show that the human fetus may also lose the amino acid, leucine, to the placenta. Triglyceride concentrations are higher in the growth restricted fetus and correlate with the degree of hypoxaemia (Economides et al 1990).

The changes in oxygenation and metabolite concentrations are probably responsible for many other changes within the fetus. Soothill et al (1987) showed that the number of erythroblasts in the fetal blood relative to white cells related to the severity of hypoxaemia. The endocrine changes in the growth-restricted fetus include lower concentrations of a range of anabolic or growth-promoting hormones including insulin, thyroxine and insulin-like growth factor-I (IGF-I). Stress and catabolic hormones such as beta-endorphin, adrenaline, nor-adrenaline, cortisol and glucagon are elevated. These endocrine changes may account for the slowing of growth and also for the

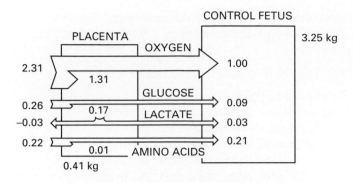

CONTROL FETUS

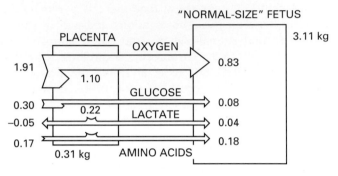

"NORMAL-SIZE" FETUS

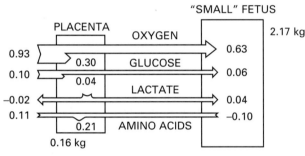

"SMALL" FETUS

Fig. 6.1 Partition of substrates between the fetus and its placenta in sheep when growth of the placenta is restricted. Rates of flux of substrates in mmol/min between mother, placenta and fetus in 30 control sheep, 13 sheep with restricted placental growth but normal fetal growth (normal-sized) and six sheep with restricted placental and fetal growth (small) in late gestation. Reproduced with permission from Owens et al (1989b).

different pattern of growth. In sheep there was an elevation in basal cortisol before the prepartum rise in its concentration. Furthermore, in this period there is a greater increase in the concentrations of catecholamines, ACTH and cortisol in response to acute hypoxia than in the normally grown fetus. These endocrine changes are likely to influence the timing of maturation of fetal organs.

MATURATION OF FETAL ORGANS

In all species studied, there are important maturational processes in fetal organs in preparation for independent life after birth. The timely and coordinated maturation of these organs is due to activation of the pituitary–adrenal axis combined with other endocrine signals such as pro-

lactin and tri-iodothyronine. The peripheral endocrine organs such as the adrenal and thyroid glands and the islet cells of the pancreas all have significant maturational changes prepartum. Growth restriction reduces the number of the beta cells in the pancreas (van Assche et al 1977). Epidemiological evidence suggests that there may be some catch-up in the first year of life. However, the pancreas may not recover fully and a permanent reduction in the number of beta-cells of the pancreas caused by intrauterine growth restriction makes the adult susceptible to type 2 diabetes (Hales et al 1991). Although cortisol is high in the growth-restricted fetus, thyroid hormone concentrations are low (Economides & Nicolaides 1990, Thorpe-Beeston et al 1991) and, in animals, hypoxia can delay the rise in tri-iodothyronine. Other hormones (e.g. prostaglandin E_2) that are elevated in blood of growth-restricted animals modify the activation of the pituitary–adrenal axis and the function of other endocrine glands.

Many organs and body systems are affected by these maturational changes. Emphasis will be placed on the lung, liver and gut here. In the liver, glycogen accumulation, gluconeogenesis, enzyme maturation, suppression of the IGF-II gene, and loss of erythropoiesis to the bone marrow are all part of preparation for independent life. In the haemopoietic system, there is also a switch from fetal to adult haemoglobin. In the growth-restricted sheep fetus this haemoglobin switch is accelerated and could add to the severity of the fetal hypoxaemia before birth by increasing P_{50} (Robinson et al 1979).

Lung maturation

To the clinician, the process of maturation is exemplified by the lung and this is open to pharmacological manipulation. In the second half of pregnancy, the alveoli of the lungs develop and their walls are invaded by capillaries. At the same time, two distinct types of alveolar cells are recognized: the type 1 cells that form the future thin wall for gas exchange and the type 2 cells that secrete surfactant. In late pregnancy the volume of liquid in the alveoli exceeds the functional residual volume of the lung postnatally (Harding et al 1993). The maturation of the lung has been followed by measuring its distensibility and early maturation can be induced by cortisol, thyroid hormones and prolactin (Liggins et al 1988, Schellenberg et al 1988). Maturation induced by this combination is superior to that induced by cortisol alone (Liggins et al 1988, Schellenberg et al 1988). These classic animal experiments have now been followed by clinical trials of betamethasone and thyrotropin releasing hormone (TRH) (Liggins et al 1988a, Morales et al 1989, Jikihara et al 1990, Ballard et al 1992) and other trials are nearing completion (Australian Clinical Trial of Betamethasone and TRH, ACTOBAT). The evidence available from all the clinical trials leads to the very convincing conclusion that the use of corticosteroids is firmly established (Crowley

1989). Data is now accumulating to suggest that TRH may be a valuable addition, but ACTOBAT may cause some revision of this view (Crowther & Grant 1993, Crowther et al 1995). Therefore pharmacological maturation of the lung should be considered when preterm delivery is necessary because of fetal growth restriction.

Hepatic maturation

Many years ago, Alfred Jost demonstrated that the prepartum deposition of liver glycogen depends on the fetal pituitary and adrenal glands. In a number of species, this occurs over the last 10–20% of pregnancy (Jones 1982, Jones & Rolph 1985). The deposition of liver glycogen is maintained in the growth-restricted guinea-pig fetus even in the presence of severe hypoglycaemia (Lafeber et al 1984, Jones et al 1988). Thus an important store of nutrients is maintained in the growth-restricted fetus and is available for immediate mobilization after birth. However, the total quantity available is less since the liver is relatively small in the growth-restricted animals compared with fetal weight.

Glucose concentrations are also maintained after birth by endogenous production of glucose by gluconeogenesis. In many species this does not occur prenatally and it has been suggested that cord clamping is essential to allow gluconeogenesis to occur in sheep (Warnes et al 1977). Endogenous production of glucose only occurs in the normally growing fetus in sheep with low maternal blood glucose. This glucose production contributes a significant proportion of glucose turnover in the growth-restricted fetus; however, this may be by glycogenolysis or gluconeogenesis (Owens et al 1989a). The enzymes required for the latter are induced in late pregnancy by cortisol and this induction does not occur if the cortisol rise is prevented (Fowden et al 1993).

In gene knockout studies in mice, deletion of the paternally derived IGF-II gene results in a failure of fetal and placental growth with normal growth rate of the pup after birth (DeChiara et al 1990). This suggests that the paternally derived IGF-II gene is required for placental growth and function. Recent evidence has been obtained to show that the IGF-II gene in the human placenta is imprinted and that the active IGF-II gene is derived from the father (Giannoukakis et al 1993). The liver is a significant source of the insulin-like growth factors in fetal blood and these can act on the placenta. Normally in late pregnancy in sheep, there is a reduction in the expression of mRNA for IGF-II by the liver caused by the prepartum rise in cortisol (Li et al 1993). As noted earlier, IGF-I concentrations in the growth-restricted fetus are low, but the concentrations of IGF-II, although maintained until late in pregnancy, decrease earlier than in normally growing fetuses (Owens et al 1994). This early reduction in the concentration of IGF-II in the growth-restricted fetus may be due to the higher cortisol and, as a result, may

withdraw trophic support from the placenta at a time when compensatory processes would be beneficial to the small fetus.

Gut growth and maturation

Survival postnatally requires that there is a sufficient absorptive area in the gut since the prenatal stores (liver glycogen and brown fat) will only sustain the neonate for a short time. In the peripartum period, there is rapid growth and development of the gut. In the first few days postnatally there is a great increase in the length of the gut combined with an increase in the height of the villi of the small intestine. Cortisol greatly reduces cell proliferation time in the gut (Trahair & Harding 1987). In growth restriction of the fetus, the weight and length of the gut is reduced. The small intestine is disportionately reduced in all its layers (Avila et al 1989). In some species the period for catch-up growth postnatally is limited to the early neonatal period. Presumably in the human neonates, there is sufficient catch-up growth of the gut since most growth-restricted infants show complete catch-up in body size (Albertssonwikland et al 1993).

Brain growth and maturation

Disproportionate growth of the fetus results in a high brain weight to body weight ratio, a phenomenon known as brain sparing. However, this is rarely complete and a reduction in brain size is common. The parts of the brain most severely affected are those growing rapidly when the constraint to growth is maximal. In experimental growth restriction, there are many changes to the fine structure of the brain (Bisignano & Rees 1988, Rees et al 1988). As noted earlier, the odds ratio for cerebral palsy is increased by intrauterine growth restriction, especially when delivery is delayed to late gestation (Blair & Stanley 1990, 1992). There are other long-term sequelae since learning difficulties are more common in children who were growth restricted prenatally and especially so if they also were born prematurely (Abel-Smith & Knight-Jones 1990). Evoked responses have been used to investigate the maturation of the brain of infants and studies of the auditory evoked potential show that the growth-restricted neonate has earlier maturation of this response. However, later there is a reversal with the child who was restricted in utero lagging behind normally grown children (Henderson-Smart et al 1991).

MANAGEMENT OF GROWTH ACCELERATION AND RESTRICTION

It has already been emphasized that it is better to attempt to prevent growth acceleration or restriction by education or counselling before pregnancy (Table 6.3). Few comments relating to growth acceleration will be made and

Table 6.3 Management of intrauterine growth acceleration or restriction

---

Prevention
  Education
  Pre-pregnancy counselling
Minimize the effects of medical conditions
Early confirmation of pregnancy
Dating and morphology scan
Screen for neural tube defects and Down's syndrome
Monitor fetal growth
  Symphysial–fundal height
  Ultrasound
Monitor fetal well-being
  Fetal movement counting
  Hormonal tests of fetoplacental function
  Cardiotocography
  Umbilical artery flow velocity waveforms (waveforms in other fetal vessels)
  Uterine arterial flow velocity waveforms
  Umbilical blood flow
  Cordocentesis
Modification of lifestyle
  Stopping work
  Bedrest
Timing of delivery
  Well-being judged from monitoring
  Growth versus prematurity
Method of delivery
  Spontaneous
  Induction
  Elective Caesarean section
Assessment of the infant
Follow-up of the child

---

most of this section will relate to growth restriction. However, the general principles often are the same for both extremes of growth. Management after growth restriction has been detected should include attempts to modify factors which may compromise the fetus. In the past much importance was given to hormonal measurements such as oestriol and placental lactogen, but in recent years these have largely been abandoned in favour of dynamic or biophysical measurements, especially cardiotocography, biophysical profile or Doppler measurements of flow velocity waveforms. It has to be stated that this switch owes more to a process of myth and fashion (Stirrat 1988) than to a rigorous evaluation of each test. All these tests have been introduced to detect the fetus at risk for asphyxia because of its association with an adverse outcome. It is important to remember that these tests are indirect measures of asphyxia and an even more indirect assessment of the neurological state of the fetus. The indirect nature of the link to this important long-term outcome has recently been highlighted. There is no clear agreed definition of birth asphyxia and the difficulties of reaching a clinically operational definition has led to a proposal to drop the term birth asphyxia and to use terms which can be defined (Blair 1993). The response of the animal fetus to acute or acute-on-chronic hypoxia has been reviewed recently (Rurak 1993).

Maternal movement counting gained popularity in the 1970s and 1980s. Initial clinical trials found that maternal movement counting followed by cardiotocography and ultrasound examination of the fetus reduced perinatal mortality (Neldham 1980). However, the control group in this study had a higher than expected rate of intrapartum stillbirth. The most widely used form of recording the woman's perception of fetal movement was the Cardiff-Count-to-Ten chart. This had a disadvantage that it could take up to 12 hours to complete. Alternative tests include counting for fixed periods or an individualized approach in which the woman determined the normal pattern of movements of her fetus and reported any significant reduction. The latter method had the advantage that there were fewer false alarms (Grant & Hepburn 1984). The large multicentre trial of over 68 000 women conducted by Grant and his colleagues failed to show that recording fetal movements was of benefit. The policy of recording fetal movements would have to be used by 1250 women to prevent one stillbirth, but an adverse effect was just as likely. This was also true for women with at-risk pregnancies (Grant et al 1989). This result is combined with anxiety in about 23 % of women caused by the requirement to fill in the form. Draper et al (1986) indicates that this form of assessment of the fetus should be abandoned. An inquiry about fetal movements may still be justified.

Antenatal cardiotocography does not have greater support from randomized trials (Neilson 1993). Indeed it fails on three counts to satisfy the requirements for an adequate test of fetal well-being, particularly when it is related to later outcome. These criteria have been highlighted for intrapartum monitoring and include the lack of precision with poor intra- and inter-observer agreement, lack of correlation with long-term outcomes and doubt about the causal relationship between the two (Paneth et al 1993). There have been many studies since Trimbos & Keirse (1978) demonstrated that eyeballing fetal heart rate traces in the antenatal period or in labour is an inadequate form of assessment whether it is done by perinatologists (Gagnon et al 1993) or by any member of the midwifery or medical staff in a tertiary unit (Freemantle et al 1993). In an attempt to improve this situation a computerized analysis of antenatal heart rate recordings that provides advantages over the visual assessment has been developed (Dawes 1991). This method improves the quality of the record and reduces the recording time. The analysis concentrates attention on heart rate variability for which visual assessment is particularly unreliable (Dawes et al 1992; Fig. 6.2). Large trials of computer-assisted assessment of antenatal cardiotocography should be completed with clearly defined intervention criteria.

It is also pertinent to note that the studies to date suggest that most clinicians seek reassurance more than

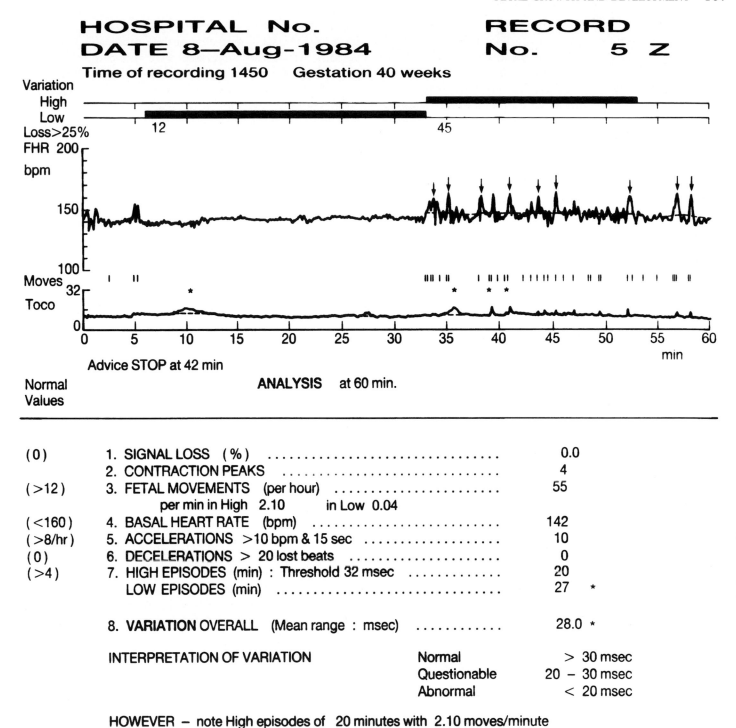

HOSPITAL No.

DATE 8—Aug—1984

RECORD No. 5 Z

Time of recording 1450   Gestation 40 weeks

Variation
High
Low
Loss>25%

FHR 200 bpm

150

100

Moves
Toco

Advice STOP at 42 min

Normal Values   **ANALYSIS** at 60 min.

(0)	1. SIGNAL LOSS (%)	0.0
	2. CONTRACTION PEAKS	4
(>12)	3. FETAL MOVEMENTS (per hour)	55
	per min in High 2.10 in Low 0.04	
(<160)	4. BASAL HEART RATE (bpm)	142
(>8/hr)	5. ACCELERATIONS >10 bpm & 15 sec	10
(0)	6. DECELERATIONS > 20 lost beats	0
(>4)	7. HIGH EPISODES (min) : Threshold 32 msec	20
	LOW EPISODES (min)	27 *
	8. **VARIATION** OVERALL (Mean range : msec)	28.0 *

INTERPRETATION OF VARIATION

Normal	> 30 msec
Questionable	20 – 30 msec
Abnormal	< 20 msec

HOWEVER – note High episodes of 20 minutes with 2.10 moves/minute

Fig. 6.2 Example of a normal fetal heart rate (FHR) record at term illustrating an unusually long episode of low heart rate variation (attributed to quiet sleep) during the first 33 min. Thereafter an episode of high variation began, accompanied by fetal movements and identified by the computer, which advised the nurse to stop recording 7 min later (after 40 min). The average length of such computerized records, required to identify normal episodes of high variation in frequency, was 15 min (Dawes et al 1985). Note the absence of signal loss; the monitor was Hewlett-Packard 8040 using autocorrelation and interfaced to a small microprocessor. The range of FHR variation is derived from the pulse intervals in ms (e.g. 11.5 ms in low episodes; 48.7 ms in high episodes). Reproduced with acknowledgements to Geoffrey Dawes.

look for abnormal findings in these recordings. The antenatal cardiotocogram only provides an assessment of the state of the fetus at the time when the test is undertaken and it should not be regarded as a test where its inter-mittent performance would provide useful prognostic information (Neilson 1993). Lumley has emphasized that the value, if any, of this investigation will only be realized when clinicians face up to these uncomfortable results

(Lumley 1988). Others have argued that there is a danger of 'throwing the baby out with the fetal monitoring' and pleaded for trials with sufficient power to address these uncomfortable conclusions (Henderson-Smart 1991). This debate is not likely to be quickly resolved but it is useful to remember that abnormal cardiotocographic findings can be present in growth-restricted humans (Trimbos & Keirse 1977) and sheep (Robinson et al 1985) for prolonged periods before acidaemia or asphyxia ensue. However, these decelerative traces could be present when the brain is slowing its growth or even being damaged by these intermittent events (Williams et al 1993). The margin of safety for this is not known.

In order to improve the detection of the fetus at risk, Manning and his colleagues developed the biophysical profile. Fetal movements, fetal breathing movements, fetal tone, volume of amniotic fluid and the non-stressed cardiotocogram are all used to construct a score evaluating fetal well-being (Manning et al 1990). Although there have been no large randomized trials of this combination for the assessment of fetal well-being, Manning and others have described the outcome for large numbers of fetuses with a wide variety of maternal and fetal problems. Generally, it may be concluded that a normal biophysical profile is associated with a very low perinatal mortality. Each component of the test has been compared with the growth of the fetus and the positive predictive accuracy is disappointingly low for fetal growth restriction (Manning et al 1990). In addition, the test is expensive in terms of both skilled operators and equipment.

The measurement of flow velocity waveforms in fetal and maternal blood vessels using Doppler ultrasound has gained recent attention. A more rigorous approach has been taken in its evaluation. The first measurements of flow velocity waveforms included a comment that abnormal waveforms were present in the growth-restricted fetus (Fitzgerald & Drumm 1977, McCallum et al 1978). A fuller description of this association was provided some years later (Erskine & Ritchie 1985, Trudinger et al 1985). Later studies showed that absence or reversal of the diastolic component is associated with growth restriction, haemorrhage, necrotizing enterocolitis and perinatal death (Hackett et al 1987, Malcolm et al 1991). It has been suggested that these abnormal waveforms are associated with obliteration of small arteries (the resistance vessels) of the tertiary villi of the placenta (Giles et al 1985). The abnormal flow velocity waveforms can be reproduced in the sheep fetus by chronic (Trudinger et al 1987b) infusions of microspheres into the umbilical vessels. Mathematical modelling of the umbilical circulation confirms that a high proportion of the resistance vessels need to be obliterated before there are significant changes in the flow velocity waveforms (Thompson & Stevens 1989). Together these studies provide a sound basis of the physi-

ology underpinning this test of fetal well-being. The first randomized trial of the value of the umbilical arterial flow velocity waveforms suggested that the test is a useful addition to the range of tests of fetal welfare (Trudinger et al 1987a). Since then a number of trials have been completed and in a recent overview, reporting abnormal waveforms is associated with a reduction in the number of perinatal deaths (Neilson 1993). However, abnormal waveforms are only useful in at-risk pregnancies and are not a useful screening test for low-risk pregnancies. Flow velocity waveforms obtained from other vessels, including the uterine artery, need further evaluation before being used routinely in clinical practice.

Acute and chronic experiments in the fetal sheep have shown that the fetus redistributes its cardiac output in response to hypoxia to essential organs such as the brain, heart, adrenal glands and placenta (Dawes 1968). Analysis of Doppler waveforms shows that this also occurs in the human fetus with growth restriction (Wladimiroff et al 1986, 1988). It has also been suggested that this pattern of flow to essential organs is only seen in the fetus with asymmetrical growth restriction and not in those with symmetrical restriction (Al-Ghazali et al 1989). There are significant correlations between abnormal flow velocity waveforms and blood gases and lactate concentrations obtained by cordocentesis (Bilardo & Nicolaides 1988, Ferrazzi et al 1988) or at Caesarean section (Tyrell et al 1989). Fetuses with absence of end-diastolic flow velocity waveforms are likely to be growth restricted and to have chronic hypoxia (Gudmundsson et al 1990). It has been suggested that cordocentesis may help to decide if the fetus has acidosis when cardiotocography (Pearce & Chamberlain 1987) and/or waveforms (Bilardo & Nicolaides 1988) are abnormal but it is unnecessary if both the heart rate and waveforms are normal (Pardi et al 1993).

The association between fetal hypoxia and abnormal waveforms has prompted investigation of the effects of hyperoxia on the fetus. Short term administration of 60% oxygen to the mother reverses the increased resistance to flow in the aorta and increases it in the internal carotid artery (Adruini et al 1989). It has been proposed that this may be used as a test to identify the fetus that will become distressed in labour if it cannot respond to the hyperoxia (Arduini et al 1989). The slow return of the circulation to the low carotid arterial resistance may partly account for the increased number of heart rate decelerations after hyperoxia (Bekedam et al 1991). Long-term treatment with maternal hyperoxia is discussed below.

Long-term follow-up of children from pregnancies with abnormal Doppler studies has not been possible yet. However, a lower developmental score has been found in children who had acidosis in fetal blood obtained by cordocentesis (Soothill et al 1992). A poorer outcome in a high risk obstetric population was more strongly associated with an abnormal heart rate pattern than with an abnormal Doppler result. This electively delivered group showed more developmental and growth delay than spontaneously delivering term or preterm babies (Todd et al 1992).

SPECIFIC TREATMENTS

Maternal malnutrition may be the commonest cause of fetal growth restriction, particularly in parts of the developing world. Dietary intervention has been noted earlier and generally a disappointing effect on birthweight has been reported (Rush 1989). For a more detailed review of treatment of growth restriction by augmentation of nutrient supply see Harding & Charlton (1989, 1990). The recently introduced technique of cordocentesis has identified nutritional and other deficiencies in the growth-restricted fetus. However, before selected supplementation is offered for any of these, its value will need to be established in randomized trials. For example, it has recently been suggested that maternal hyperoxia may have a role (Nicolaides et al 1987, Battaglia et al 1992). Maternal hyperoxia increases fetal blood Po_2 and reduced perinatal mortality in a small clinical trial. Larger trials are required before this is widely adopted as an option for treatment of the growth-restricted fetus and its use would have to be compared with preterm delivery or keeping the fetus in utero until other signs of compromise indicate delivery.

Doppler flow velocity waveforms have been used to detect placental insufficiency as an indicator for low-dose aspirin therapy. Aspirin therapy was associated with an increase in both birthweight and placental weight providing that there was still significant forward flow in diastole (Trudinger et al 1988). A similar improvement in birthweight was also found in women with a history of severe fetal growth restriction who were treated with low-dose aspirin (Wallenberg & Rotmans 1987). The results of a large randomized trial (CLASP) of low-dose aspirin do not support use of low-dose aspirin outside further clinical trials which would have to be for indications other than growth restriction or pre-eclampsia unless a method for identifying women at risk of early onset pre-eclampsia is found. This would provide a stimulus for a new trial that may be justified.

TIMING AND MODE OF DELIVERY

There are still many unresolved issues concerning the best time to deliver the growth-restricted fetus. When extreme prematurity offers a dismal prognosis then it is appropriate to test new and/or expensive interventions which may prolong pregnancy. For most, a balance between the fetal and maternal conditions and fetal maturity remain the cornerstone of timing of delivery. Improvements in neonatal care and the introduction of corticosteroids and artificial surfactant (Soll 1993) to improve lung function have encouraged the perinatologist to deliver the fetus earlier, before there is evidence of impending fetal death. Waiting for evidence of fetal compromise of the severely growth restricted fetus certainly has little place after 36 weeks. Earlier intervention may also be considered if it is considered unlikely that the fetus will continue to grow, particularly after 32 weeks. This leaves a difficult period between 26 and 31 weeks when each decision will be made on a complex set of factors. Late genetic diagnosis plays an increasingly important role by identifying those fetuses with chromosomal abnormalities who will not benefit from operative delivery. While chorionic villous biopsy is successful at this age, it can occasionally provide the first clue of placental mosaicism. Cordocentesis has an advantage that in addition to karyotyping, the fetal acid–base status may be obtained. This will also allow counselling of the woman and her partner about the prognosis for their child.

These difficult problems require a coordinated approach by a team comprising an obstetrician, a subspecialist in maternal-fetal medicine and a neonatologist. When a malformation requiring surgery after birth is present, prenatal discussion with the appropriate paediatric surgeon or physician can help the woman and her family prepare for this. It is imperative that the obstetrician provides continuity of care for the woman through this difficult period. Postnatally, this coordinating role is usually undertaken by the neonatologist.

FOLLOW-UP

No discussion of growth restriction is complete without emphasizing the continuing need for long-term follow-up studies. Many of these will have to continue into adult life given the remarkable epidemiological studies of the association of low birthweight with adult diseases. It will also be important to follow-up children born after use of experimental therapies, however funding constraints often make this difficult, if not impossible. In addition to the follow-up of selected disease categories, population studies as exemplified by those of cerebral palsy have much to offer.

Acknowledgements

I wish to thank Dr Caroline Crowther for critical comment and Glenys King and Meg Brodtmann for help in the preparation of this manuscript. Our experimental work has been generously supported by the NH&MRC and the Ramaciotti Foundation. I am indebted to Professor D.P. Davies for reminding me of Pierre Budin's book.

REFERENCES

Abel-Smith A E, Knight-Jones E B 1990 The abilities of very low-birthweight children and their classroom controls. Developmental Medicine and Child Neurology 32: 590

Aherne W, Dunhill M S 1966 Quantitative aspects of placental structure. Journal of Pathology and Bacteriology 91: 123

Ahlsten G, Cnattingus S, Lindmark G 1993 Cessation of smoking during pregnancy improves foetal growth and reduces infant morbidity in the neonatal period. A population-based study. Acta Paediatrica Scandinavica 82: 177

Al-Ghazali W, Chita S K, Chapman M G, Allen L D 1989 Evidence of redistribution of cardiac output in asymmetrical growth retardation. British Journal of Obstetrics and Gynaecology 96: 697

Albertssonwikland K, Wennergren G, Wennergren M, Vilvergsson G, Rosberg S 1993 Longitudinal follow-up of growth in children born small for gestational age. Acta Paediatrica Scandinavica 82: 438

Anderson G D I, Blidner N, McClemont S, Sinclair J C 1984 Determinants of size at birth in a Canadian population. American Journal of Obstetrics and Gynecology 150: 236

Arbuckle T E, Wilkins R and Sherman G J 1993 Birth weight centiles by gestational age in Canada. Obstetrics and Gynecology 81: 39–48

Arduini D, Rizzo G, Mancuso S, Romanini C 1988 Short-term effects of maternal oxygen administration on blood flow velocity waveforms in healthy and growth-retarded fetuses. American Journal of Obstetrics and Gynecology 159: 1077

Arduini D, Rizzo G, Mancuso S, Romanini C 1989 Fetal hemodynamic response to acute maternal hyperoxygenation predicts fetal distress in intrauterine growth retardation. British Medical Journal 298: 1561

Arngrimsson R, Björnsson S, Geirsson R T, Björnsson H, Walker J J, Snaedal G 1990 Genetic and familial predisposition to eclampsia and pre-eclampsia in a defined population. British Journal of Obstetrics and Gynaecology 97: 762

Avila C G, Harding R, Rees S, Robinson P M 1989 Small intestine development in the growth retarded fetal sheep. Journal of Pediatric Gastroenterology and Nutrition 8: 507

Ballard R A, Ballard P L, Creasy R K et al 1992 Respiratory disease in very-low-birthweight infants after prenatal thyrotropin-releasing hormone and glucocorticoid. Lancet 339: 510

Barker D J P (ed) 1992 The fetal and infant origins of adult disease. British Medical Journal, London

Barlow D P, Stoger R, Herrmann B G, Saito K, Schweifer N 1991 The mouse insulin-like growth factor type-2 receptor is imprinted and closely linked to the Tme locus. Nature 349: 84

Bastian H 1992 Confined, managed and delivered. British Journal of Obstetrics and Gynaecology 99: 92

Battaglia C, Artine P G, D'Ambrogio G, Galli P A, Serge A, Genazzani A R 1992 Maternal hyperoxygenation in the treatment of intrauterine growth retardation. American Journal of Obstetrics and Gynecology 167: 430

Bekedam D S, Mulder E J H, Snijders R J M, Visser G H A 1991 The effects of maternal hyperoxia on fetal breathing movements, body movements and heart rate variation in growth retarded fetuses. Early Human Development 27: 223

Belizan J M, Vilar J, Nardin J C, Malmud J, de Vinca L S 1978 Diagnosis of intrauterine growth retardation by a simple clinical method: measurement of uterine height. American Journal of Obstetrics and Gynecology 131: 643

Bilardo C M, Nicolaides K H 1988 Cordocentesis in the assessment of the small-for-gestational age fetus. Fetal Therapy 3: 24

Bisignano M, Rees S 1988 The effects of intrauterine growth retardation on synaptogenesis and mitochondrial formation in the cerebral and cerebellar cortices of fetal sheep. International Journal of Developmental Neuroscience 6: 453

Blair E 1993 A research definition for 'birth asphyxia'? Developmental Medicine and Child Neurology 35: 449

Blair E, Stanley F 1990 Intrauterine growth retardation and spastic cerebral palsy. I. Association with birthweight for gestational age. American Journal of Obstetrics and Gynecology 162: 229

Blair E, Stanley F 1992 Intrauterine growth and spastic cerebral palsy. II. The association with morphology at birth. Early Human Development 28: 91

Bonds D R, Gabbe S G, Kumar S, Taylor T 1984 Fetal weight/placental weight ratio and perinatal outcome. American Journal of Obstetrics and Gynecology 149: 195

Boyd P A, Scott A 1985 Quantitative structural studies on human placentas associated with pre-eclampsia, essential hypertension and intrauterine growth retardation British Journal of Obstetrics and Gynaecology 92: 714

Boyd P A, Scott A, Keeling J W 1986 Quantitative structural studies on placentas from pregnancies complicated by diabetes mellitus. British Journal of Obstetrics and Gynaecology 93: 31

Brosens I A 1988 The utero-placenta vessels at term — the changes in the distribution and extent of physiological changes. Trophoblast Research 3: 61

Budin P 1907 The nursling. Coxton, London

Butler N R, Alberman E D 1969 Perinatal mortality: the second report of the 1958 British Perinatal Mortality Survey. Livingstone, Edinburgh

Butler N R, Bonham 1963 Perinatal problems: the first report of the 1958 British Perinatal Mortality Survey. Livingstone, Edinburgh

Calvert J P, Crean E E, Newcombe R G, Pearson J F 1982 Antenatal screening by measurement of symphysis-fundus height. British Medical Journal 285: 846

Cetin I, Marconi A M, Bozzetti P et al 1988 Umbilical amino acid concentrations in appropriate and small for gestational age infants: a biochemical difference present in utero. American Journal of Obstetrics and Gynecology 158: 120

Cetin I, Corbetta C, Sereni L P et al 1990 Umbilical amino acid concentrations in normal and growth-retarded fetuses sampled in utero by cordocentesis. American Journal of Obstetrics and Gynecology 162: 253

Cetin I, Marconi A M, Corbetta C, Sereni L P, Battaglia F C, Pardi G 1991 Fetal–maternal amino acid relationship in normal and intrauterine growth retarded (IUGR) pregnancies. Placenta 12: 377(abstr)

Chamberlain G, Phillip E, Howlett B, Masters K 1978 British births 1970 vol 2: obstetric care. Heinemann Medical, London

Chamberlain P F, Manning F A, Morrison I, Harman C R, Lange I R 1984 Ultrasonic evaluation of amniotic fluid volume II. The relationship of marginal or decreased amniotic fluid volume to perinatal outcome. American Journal of Obstetrics and Gynecology 150: 245

Chamberlain R, Chamberlain G, Howlett B, Claireaux A 1975 British births 11970 vol 1: the first week of life. Heinemann Medical, London

Chesley L C, Cooper D W 1986 Genetics of hypertension in pregnancy: possible single gene control of pre-eclampsia and eclampsia in the descendants of eclamptic women. British Journal of Obstetrics and Gynaecology 93: 898

Clapp J F III, Rizk K H 1992 Effect of recreational exercise on midtrimester placental growth. American Journal of Obstetrics and Gynecology 167: 1518

CLASP (Collaborative Low-dose Aspirin Study in Pregnancy) Collaborative Group 1994 CLASP: a randomised trial of low-dose aspirin for the prevention and treatment of pre-eclampsia among 9364 women. Lancet 343: 617–627

Cnattingus S, Haglund B, Meirik O 1988 Cigarette smoking as a risk factor for late fetal and early perinatal death. British Medical Journal 297: 258

Cnattingus S, Forman M R, Berendez H W, Graubard B I, Isolato L 1993 Effect of age, parity and smoking on pregnancy outcome: a population-based study. American Journal of Obstetrics and Gynecology 168: 16

Comney J O O, Fitzhardinge P M 1979 Handicap in the preterm small-for-gestational age infant. Journal of Paediatrics 94: 779

Cooper D W, Hill J A, Chesley L C, Bryans C I 1988 Genetic control of susceptility to eclampsia and miscarriage. British Journal of Obstetrics and Gynaecology 95: 644

Crombleholme T M, Harrison M R, Golbus M S et al 1990 Fetal intervention in obstructive uropathy. Prognostic indicators and efficacy of intervention. American Journal of Obstetrics and Gynecology 162: 1239

Crowley P 1989 Promoting pulmonary maturity. In: Chalmers I,

Enkin M, Keirse M J N C (eds) Effective care in pregnancy and childbirth. Oxford University Press, Oxford, p 746

Crowther CA, Grant A 1993 Antenatal thyrotropin-releasing hormone (TRH) prior to preterm delivery. In: Enkin M W, Keirse M J N C, Renfrew M J, Neilson J P (eds) Cochrane database of systematic reviews, record 04749, Cochrane updates on disk. Update Software, Oxford

Crowther C A, Hiller J, Haslam R, Robinson J S 1995 Australian Collaborative Trial of Antenatal Thyrotrophin Releasing Hormone (ACTOBAT) for the prevention of neonatal distress. Lancet (Submitted)

Dawes G S 1968 Foetal and neonatal physiology. Year Book Medical Publications/Wiley, Chicago

Dawes G S 1991 Computerised measurement of heart rate variation antenatally and in labour. In: Bonnar J (ed) Recent advances in obstetrics and gynaecology. Churchill Livingstone, London, p 57

Dawes G S, Lobb M, Moulden M, Redman C W G, Wheeler T 1992 Antenatal cardiotocogram quality and interpretation using computers. British Journal of Obstetrics and Gynaecology 99: 791

DeBarro T M, Owens J, Earl C R, Robinson J S 1992 Nutrition during early/mid pregnancy interacts with mating weight to affect placental weight in sheep. Australian Society for Reproductive Biology, Adelaide (abstr)

DeChiara T M, Efstatiadis A, Robertson E J 1990 A growth-deficiency phenotype in heterozygous mice carrying an insulin-like growth factor II gene disrupted by targetting. Nature 345: 78

Divon M Y, Chamberlain P F, Sipos L, Mannind F A, Platt L D 1986 Identification of the small for gestational age fetus with the use of gestational age-independent indices of fetal growth. American Journal of Obstetrics and Gynecology 155: 1197

Draper J, Field S, Thomas H, Hare M J 1986 Womens' views on keeping fetal movement charts. British Journal of Obstetrics and Gynaecology 93: 334

Dunn P 1985 A perinatal growth chart for international reference. Acta Paediatrica Scandinavica 319 (suppl): 180

Dunn P M 1981 Variations of fetal growth: some causes and effects. In: van Assche F A, Robertson W B (eds) Fetal growth retardation. Churchill Livingstone, Edinburgh, p 79

Ebrahim G J 1984 Care of the newborn. British Medical Journal 289: 899

Economides D L, Nicolaides K H 1990 Metabolic findings in small-for-gestational-age fetuses. Contempory Reviews in Obstetrics and Gynaecology 2: 75

Economides D L, Nicolaides K H, Gahl W A, Bernardini I, Evans M I 1989 Plasma amino acids in appropriate and small for gestational age fetuses. American Journal of Obstetrics and Gynecology 161: 1219

Economides D L, Crook D, Nicolaides K H 1990 Hypertriglyceridemia and hypoxemia in small-for-gestational-age fetuses. American Journal of Obstetrics and Gynecology 162: 382

Erskine R L A, Ritchie J W K 1985 Umbilical artery blood flow characteristics in normal and growth-retarded fetuses. British Journal of Obstetrics and Gynaecology 92: 605

Faichney G J, White G A 1987 Effects of maternal nutrition on fetal growth. Australian Journal of Biological Science 40: 365

Ferrazzi E, Pardi G, Bauscaglia M et al 1988 The correlation of biochemical monitoring versus umbilical flow velocity measurements in the human fetus. American Journal of Obstetrics and Gynecology 159: 1081

Fisher C C, Garrett W, Kossoff G 1975 Placental aging monitored by gray scale echography. American Journal of Obstetrics and Gynecology 24: 483

Fisk N M, Ronderos-Dumit D, Solani A, Nicolini, Vaughan J, Rodeck C H 1991 Diagnostic and therapeutic transabdominal amnioinfusion in oligohydramnios. Obstetrics and Gynecology 78: 270

Fitzgerald D E, Drumm J E 1977 Non-invasive measurement of human fetal circulation using ultrasound, a new method. British Medical Journal 2: 1450

Fowden A L, Mijocvic J, Silver M 1993 The effect of cortisol on hepatic and renal gluconeogenesis enzyme activities in the sheep fetus during late gestation. Journal of Endocrinology 137: 213

Freemantle J, Crowther C A, O'Callaghan S, Broom T, Eckert K, Robinson J S 1993 Antenatal cardiotocography: visual assessment by medical and midwifery staff compared with computerised analysis.

Australian Perinatal Society 9: A19

Fryburg J S, Diamo M S, Yang-Feng T L, Mahoney M J 1993 Follow-up of pregnancies complicated by placental mosiacism diagnosed by chorionic villous sampling. Prenatal Diagnosis 13: 481

Gagnon R, Campbell K M, Hunse C 1993 A comparison between visual and computer analysis of antepartum fetal heart rate tracings. American Journal of Obstetrics and Gynecology 168: 842

Gardosi J, Chang A, Kaylan B, Sahota D, Symonds E M 1992 Customised antenatal growth charts. Lancet 339: 283

Gennser G, Persson P-H 1986 Biophysical assessment of placental function. Clinics in Obstetrics and Gynaecology 13: 521

Giannoukakis N, Deal C, Paquette J, Goodyer C G, Polychronakos C 1993 Paternal imprinting of the human IGF2 gene. Nature Genetics 4: 98

Giles W, Trudinger B J, Baird P J 1985 Fetal umbilical artery flow velocity waveforms and placental resistance: pathological correlation. British Journal of Obstetrics and Gynaecology 92: 31

Godfrey K M, Redman C W, Barker D J P, Osmond C 1991 The effect of maternal anaemia and iron deficiency on the ratio of fetal weight to placental weight. British Journal of Obstetrics and Gynaecology 98: 886

Grannum P A T, Berkowitz R L, Hobbins J C 1979 The ultrasonic changes in the maturing placenta. American Journal of Obstetrics and Gynecology 133: 915

Grant A, Hepburn M 1984 Merits of an individualized approach to fetal movement counting compared with fixed-time and fixed-number methods. British Journal of Obstetrics and Gynaecology 91: 1087

Grant A, Elbourne D, Valentin L, Alexander S 1989 Routine formal fetal movement counting and risk of antepartum late death in normally formed singletons. Lancet ii: 345

Gruendwald P 1963 Chronic fetal distress and placental insufficiency. Biology of the Neonate 5: 215

Gudmundsson S, Lindblad A, Marsal K 1990 Cord blood gases and absence of end-diastolic blood velocities in the umbilical artery. Early Human Development 24: 231

Hackett G A, Campbell S, Gamsu H, Cohen-Overbeek T, Pearce J M F 1987 Doppler studies in the growth retarded fetus and prediction of neonatal necrotising enterocolitis, haemorrhage and neonatal morbidity. British Medical Journal 294: 13

Hales C N, Barker D J P, Clark P M S et al 1991 Fetal and infant growth and impaired glucose tolerance at age 64. British Medical Journal 303: 1019

Hall M, Chng P K 1982 Antenatal care in practice. In: Enkin M W, Chalmers I (eds) Effectiveness and satisfaction in antenatal care. Heinemann, London, p 60

Harding J E, Charlton V 1989 Treatment of the growth retarded fetus by augmentation of substrate supply. Seminars in Perinatology 13: 211

Harding J E, Charlton V 1990 Experimental nutritional supplementation for intrauterine growth retardation. In: Harrison M R, Golbus M S, Filly R A (eds) The unborn patient. W B Saunders, Philadelphia, p 598

Harding R, Miller A A, Hooper S B 1993 Determinants of fetal lung expansion and lung growth in the ovine fetus. XXXII Congress of the International Union of Physiological Sciences (abstract 129.1)

Harvey D, Prince J, Bunton J, Parkinson C, Campbell S 1982 Abilities of children who were small-for-gestational-age babies. Pediatrics 69: 296

Henderson-Smart D 1991 Throwing the baby out with the fetal monitoring? Medical Journal of Australia 154: 576

Henderson-Smart D, Pettigrew A G, Edwards D A, Jiang Z D 1991 Brain stem auditory evoked responses: physiological and clinical issues. In: Hanson M (ed) The fetal and neonatal brainstem. Cambridge University Press, Cambridge, p 211

Henry I, Bonaiti-Pellie C, Chehensse V et al 1991 Uniparental paternal disomy in a genetic cancer-predisposing syndrome. Nature 351: 665

Hepburn M, Rosenberg K 1986 An audit of the detection and management of small-for-gestational age babies. British Journal of Obstetrics and Gynaecology 93: 212

Hoogland H J, deHaan J, Martin C B 1980 Placental size during early pregnancy and fetal outcome: a preliminary report of a sequential ultrasonographic study. American Journal of Obstetrics and Gynecology 138: 441

Hughes A B, Jenkins D A, Newcombe R G, Pearson J F 1987 Symphysis–fundus height, maternal height, labor pattern, and mode of delivery. American Journal of Obstetrics and Gynecology 156: 644

Jackson M R, Mayhew T M, Haas J D 1987 The volumetric composition of human term placentae: altitude, ethinic and sex differences in Bolivia. Journal of Anatomy 152: 173

Jackson M R, Mayhew T M, Haas J D 1988 Of the factors which contribute to the thinning of the villous membrane in human placentae at high altitude. I. Thinning and regional variation in the thickness of trophoblast. Placenta 9: 1

Jackson M R, Mayhew T M, Scott P A 1992 Quantitative description of the elaboration and maturation of villi from 10 weeks to term. Placenta 13: 357

Jikihara H, Sawada Y, Imai S et al 1990 Maternal administration of thyrotropin-releasing hormone for prevention of neonatal respiratory distress syndrome. In: Proceedings of the 6th Congress of the Federation of Asia-Oceania Perinatal Societies, Perth, p 87

Jones C T 1982 Development of metabolism in the fetal liver. In: Jones C T (ed) Biochemical development of the fetus and neonate. Elsevier Biomedical Press, Amsterdam, p 249

Jones C T, Rolph T P 1985 Metabolism during fetal life: a functional assessment of metabolic development. Physiological Reviews 65: 357

Jones C T, Harding J E, Gu W, Lafeber H N 1988 Placental metabolism and endocrine effects in relation to the control of fetal and placental growth. In: Jensen A, Kunzel W (eds) The endocrine control of the fetus. Physiological and pathological aspects. Springer-Verlag, Berlin, p 213

Joyce T 1990 The dramatic increase in the rate of low birthweight in New York City: an aggregate time-series analysis. American Journal of Public Health 80: 682

Kalousek D K, Langlois S, Barrett I et al 1993 Uniparental disomy for chromosome-16 in humans. American Journal of Human Genetics 52: 8

Khong T Y 1991a Acute atherosis in pregnancies complicated by hypertension, small-for-gestational-age infants and diabetes mellitus. Archives of Pathology and Laboratory Medicine 115: 722

Khong T Y 1991b The Robertson–Brosens–Dixon hypothesis — evidence for a role of the haemochorial placentation in pregnancy success — commentary. British Journal of Obstetrics and Gynaecology 98: 1195

Khong T Y, De Wolf F, Robertson W B, Brosens I 1986 Inadequate maternal vascular response to placentation in pregnancies complicated by pre-eclampsia and small-for-gestational age infants. British Journal of Obstetrics and Gynaecology 93: 1049

Knight D B, Liggins G C, Wealthall S R 1994 A randomized trial of antepartum thyrothrophin-releasing hormone and beta methasone in the prevention of respiratory disease in preterm infants. American Journal of Obstetrics and Gynecology 171: 11–16

Kusin J A, Kardjati S, Houtkooper J M, Renqvist U H 1992 Energy supplementation during pregnancy and postnatal growth. Lancet 340: 623

Lafeber H N, Rolph T P, Jones C T 1984 Studies on the growth of the fetal guinea pig. The effects of ligation of the uterine artery on organ growth and development. Journal of Developmental Physiology 6: 440

Li J, Saunders J C, Gilmour R S, Silver M, Fowden A 1993 Insulin-like growth factor-II messenger ribonucleic acid expression in fetal tissues of the sheep during late gestation: effects of cortisol. Endocrinology 132: 2083

Liggins G C, Schellenberg J C, Manzai M, Kitterman J A, Lee C C 1988 Synergism of cortisol and thyrotropin-releasing hormone in lung maturation in fetal sheep. Journal of Applied Physiology 65: 1880

Lindhard A, Nielsen P V, Mouritsen L A, Zacheriassen A, Sorensen H V, Roseno H 1990 The implications of introducing the symphysial–fundal height-measurement. A prospective randomised controlled trial. British Journal of Obstetrics and Gynaecology 97: 675

Low J A, Galbraith R S, Muir D, Killen H, Pater B, Karchmar J 1982 Intrauterine growth retardation: a study for long-term morbidity. American Journal of Obstetrics and Gynecology 142: 670

Lubchencho L O, Hansman C, Dressler M, Boyd B 1963 Intrauterine growth as estimated from liveborn birthweight data at 24 to 42 weeks of gestation. Pediatrics 32: 793

Lumley J 1988 Does continuous intrapartum fetal monitoring predict long-term neurological disorders? Paediatric and Perinatal Epidemiology 2: 299

Lumley J 1991 Stopping smoking — again. British Journal of Obstetrics and Gynaecology 98: 847

Lumley J, Correy J, Newman N, Curran J 1985 Cigarette smoking, alcohol consumption in Tasmania 1981–2. Australian and New Zealand Journal of Obstetrics and Gynaecology 25: 33

MacArthur C, Newton J R, Knox E G 1987 Effect of anti-smoking health education on infant size: a randomised controlled trial. British Journal of Obstetrics and Gynaecology 94: 295

McBurney R D 1947 Undernourished full-term infant: case report. Western Journal of Surgery, Obstetrics and Gynecology 55: 363

McCallum W D, Williams C S, Napel S, Daigle R E 1978 Fetal blood velocity waveforms. American Journal of Obstetrics and Gynecology 132: 425

McCrabb G J, Egan A R, Hosking B J 1992 Maternal undernutrition during mid-pregnancy in sheep: variable effects on placental growth. Journal of Agricultural Science 118: 127

Malcolm G, Ellwood D, Devonald K, Beilby R, Henderson-Smart D 1991 Absent or reversed end diastolic flow velocity in the umbilical artery and necrotising enterocolitis. Archives of Diseases in Childhood 66: 805

Manning F A, Morrison I, Harman C R, Mentigcoglou S M 1990 The abnormal fetal biophysical profile score. V. Predictive accuracy according to score composition. American Journal of Obstetrics and Gynecology 162: 918

Mayhew T M, Jackson M R, Haas J D 1990 Oxygen diffusive conductances of human placentae from term pregnancies at low and high altitudes. Placenta 11: 493

Milner R D G, Richards B 1974 An analysis of birth weight by gestational age of infants born in England and Wales, 1967 to 1971. Journal of Obstetrics and Gynaecology of the British Commonwealth 81: 956

Molteni R A, Stys S J, Battaglia F C 1978 Relationship of fetal and placental weight in human beings: fetal/placental weight ratios at various gestational ages and birth weight distributions. Journal of Reproductive Medicine 21: 327

Morales W J, O'Brien W F, Angel J L, Knuppel R A, Sawai S 1989 Fetal lung maturation: the combined use of corticosteroids and thyrotropin-releasing hormone. Obstetrics and Gynecology 73: 111

Naeye R L 1965 Malnutrition: probable cause of fetal growth retardation. Archives of Pathology 79: 284

Neilson J P 1993 Routine Doppler ultrasound scanning in unselected pregnancies. In: Enkin M W, Keirse M J N C, Renfrew M J, Neilson J P (eds) Cochrane database of systematic reviews, review 07357, Cochrane Updates on Disk. Update Software, Oxford

Neilson J P 1993 Cardiotocography for antepartum fetal assessment. In: Chalmers I (ed) Oxford database of perinatal trials, Version 1.3, Disk Issue 8, Autumn 1992, record 3881

Neilson J P, Whitfield C R, Aitchison T C 1980 Screening for the small-for-dates fetus: a two-stage ultrasonic examination schedule. British Medical Journal 1: 1203

Neldham S 1980 Fetal movements as an indicator of fetal wellbeing. Lancet i: 1222

Nicolaides K H, Campbell S, Bradley R J, Bilardo C M, Soothill P W, Gibb D 1987 Maternal oxygen therapy for intrauterine growth retardation. Lancet i: 942

Northern Region 1984 Collaborative survey of perinatal mortality report 1982. Newcastle upon Tyne, Northern Regional Health Authority

Ounsted M, Moar V A, Scott A 1982 Growth in the first four years: IV. Correlations with parental measures in small-for-dates and large-for-dates babies. Early Human Development 7: 357

Ounsted M, Moar V A, Cockburn J, Redman C W G 1984 Factors associated with the intellectual ability of children born to women with high risk pregnancies. British Medical Journal 288: 1038

Owens J A 1991 Endocrine and substrate control of fetal growth: placental and maternal influences and insulin-like growth factors. Reproduction Fertility and Development 3: 501

Owens J A, Falconer J, Robinson J S 1987a Effect of restriction of placental growth on oxygen delivery to and consumption by the pregnant uterus and fetus. Journal of Developmental Physiology 9: 137

Owens J A, Falconer J, Robinson J S 1987b Effect of restriction of placental growth on fetal and utero-placental metabolism. Journal of Developmental Physiology 9: 225

Owens J A, Falconer J, Robinson J S 1989a Glucose metabolism in pregnant sheep when placental growth is restricted. American Journal of Physiology 257: R350

Owens J A, Owens P C, Robinson J S 1989b Experimental fetal growth retardation: metabolic and endocrine aspects. In: Gluckman P D, Johnston B M, Nathanielsz P W (eds) Advances in fetal physiology: reviews in honor of G C Liggins. Perinatology Press, Ithaca, p 263

Owens J A, Kind K L, Carbone F, Robinson J S, Owens P C 1994 Circulating insulin-like growth factor-I and II in fetal blood and substrates in fetal sheep following restriction of placental growth. Journal of Endocrinology 140: 5

Paneth N, Bommarito M, Stricker J 1993 Electronic fetal monitoring and later fetal outcome. Clinical Investigative Medicine 16: 159

Pardi G, Cetin I, Marconi A M et al 1993 Diagnostic value of blood sampling in fetuses with growth retardation. New England Journal of Medicine 328: 692

Patterson R M, Hayashi R H, Cavazos D 1983 Ultrasonographically observed early placental maturation and perinatal outcome. American Journal of Obstetrics and Gynecology 147: 773

Pearce M, Chamberlain G V P 1987 Ultrasonically guided percutaneous umbilical blood sampling in the management of intrauterine growth retardation. British Journal of Obstetrics and Gynaecology 94: 318

Persson P-H 1989 Fetal growth curves. In: Sharp F, Fraser R B, Milner RDG (eds) Fetal growth, Proceedings of the 20th Study Group. RCOG, London, p 13

Persson, P-H, Kullander S 1983 Long-term experience of general ultrasound screening in pregnancy. American Journal of Obstetrics and Gynecology 146: 942

Persson P-H, Grennert L, Gennser G 1978 Impact of maternal and fetal factors on the normal growth of the biparietal diameter. Acta Obstetricia et Gynecologica Scandinavica 78 (suppl): 21

Peters T J, Golding J, Butler N R, Fryer J G, Lawrence C J, Chamberlain G V P 1983 Plus ca change: predictors of birthweight in two national studies. British Journal of Obstetrics and Gynaecology 90: 1040

Power C 1994 National trends in birth weight: implications for future adult disease. British Medical Journal 308: 1270

Proud J, Grant A M 1987 Third trimester placental grading by ultrasonography as a test of fetal wellbeing. British Medical Journal 294: 1641

Quaranta P R, Currell R, Redman C W G, Robinson J S 1981 Prediction of small-for-dates infants by measurement of symphysial-fundal height. British Journal of Obstetrics and Gynaecology 88: 115

Raman L 1987 Maternal nutritional status influencing intrauterine growth. In: Maeda K (ed) The fetus as a patient. Elsevier, Amsterdam, p 221

Rantakallio P 1985 A 14-year follow-up of children with normal and abnormal birth weight for their gestational age. Acta Paediatrica Scandinavica 74: 62

Rees S, Bocking A D, Harding R 1988 Structure of the fetal sheep brain in experimental growth retardation. Journal of Developmental Physiology 10: 211

Robertson W B, Khong T Y, Brosens I, De Wolf F, Sheppard B L, Bonnar J 1986 The placental bed biopsy: review from three European centers. American Journal of Obstetrics and Gynecology 155: 401

Robinson J S 1979 Growth of the fetus. British Medical Bulletin 35: 137

Robinson J S, Kingston E J, Jones C T, Thorburn G D 1979 Studies on experimental growth retardation in sheep. The effect of removal of endometrial caruncles on fetal size and metabolism. Journal of Developmental Physiology 1: 379

Robinson J S, Falconer J, Owens J A 1985 Intrauterine growth retardation: clinical and experimental. Acta Paediatrica Scandinavica Supplement 319: 135

Rodesch F, Simon P, Donner C, Jauniaux E 1992 Oxygen measurements in endometrial and trophoblastic tissues during early pregnancy. Obstetrics and Gynaecology 80: 283

Rurak D W 1993 Fetal oxygenation, carbon dioxide homeostasis and acid-base balance. In: Harding R, Thorburn G D (eds) Textbook of fetal physiology. Oxford University Press, Oxford, p 131

Rush D 1989 Effects of changes in protein and calorie intake during pregnancy on the growth of the human fetus. In: Chalmers I, Enkin M, Keirse MJNC (eds) Effective care in pregnancy and childbirth. Oxford University Press, Oxford p 255

Russell J K 1982 Early teenage pregnancy. Churchill Livingstone, Edinburgh

Schellenberg J C, Liggins G C, Manzai M, Kitterman J A, Lee C C 1988 Synergistic hormonal effects on lung maturation in fetal sheep. Journal of Applied Physiology 65: 94

Soll R F 1993 Prophylactic administration of any surfactant. In: Enkin M W, Keirse M J N C, Renfrew M J, Neilson J P (eds) Cochrane database of systematic reviews, review 05664, Cochrane updates on disk. Update Software, Oxford

Soothill P W, Nicolaides K H, Campbell S 1987 Prenatal asphxia, hyperlacticaemia, hypoglycaemia, and erythroblastosis in growth retarded fetuses. British Medical Journal 294: 1051

Soothill P W, Ajayi R A, Campbell S et al 1992 Relationship between fetal acidemia at cordocentesis and subsequent neurodevelopment. Ultrasound in Obstetrics and Gynecology 2: 80

Stirrat G M 1988 Risk arising during pregnancy. In: James D K, Stirrat G M (eds) Pregnancy and risk: the basis for rational management. John Wiley, Chichester, p 813

Stoger R, Kubicka P, Lui C G, et al 1993 Maternal-specific methylation of the imprinted mouse IGF2r locus identifies the expressed locus as carrying the imprinting signal. Cell 73: 61

Taylor P, Coulthard A C, Robinson J S 1984 Symphysial–fundal height from 12 weeks' gestation. Australian and New Zealand Journal of Obstetrics and Gynaecology 24: 189

Teasdale F 1984 Idiopathic intrauterine growth retardation: histomorphometry of the human placenta. Placenta 5: 83

Thompson R S, Stevens R J 1989 Mathematical model for interpretation of Doppler velocity waveform indices. Medical and Biological Engineering and Computing 27: 269

Thorpe-Beeston J G, Nicolaides K H, Snijders R J M, Felton C V, McGregor M C A M 1991 Thyroid function in small for gestational age fetuses. Obstetrics and Gynecology 77: 701

Todd A L, Trudinger B J, Cole M J, Cooney G H 1992 Antenatal tests of fetal welfare and development at age 2 years. American Journal of Obstetrics and Gynecology 167: 66

Trahair J F, Harding R 1987 Development of structure and function of the alimentary tract in fetal sheep. In: Nathanielsz P W (ed) Animal models in fetal medicine 7. Perinatology Press, Ithaca New York, p 1

Trimbos J B, Keirse M J N C 1977 Non-specific decelerations in the fetal heart rate during high risk pregnancies. British Journal of Obstetrics and Gynaecology 84: 732

Trimbos J B, Keirse M J N C 1978 Observer variability in assessment of antepartum cardiotocograms. British Journal of Obstetrics and Gynaecology 85: 900

Trudinger B J, Cook C M 1985 Umbilical and uterine artery flow velocity waveforms in pregnancy associated with major fetal abormality. British Journal of Obstetrics and Gynaecology 92: 666

Trudinger B J, Giles W B, Cook C M, Bombardieri J, Collins L 1985 Fetal umbilical artery flow velocity waveforms and placental resistance: clinical correlations. British Journal of Obstetrics and Gynaecology 92: 23

Trudinger B J, Cook C M, Giles W B, Conelly A, Thompson R S 1987a Umbilical artery flow velocity waveforms in high-risk pregnancy. Randomised controlled trial. Lancet 24: 188

Trudinger B J, Stevens D, Conelly A et al R S 1987b Umbilical artery flow velocity waveforms and placental resistance: the effects of embolization of the umbilical circulation. American Journal of Obstetrics and Gynecology 157: 1443

Trudinger B J, Cook C M, Thompson R S, Giles W B, Connelly A 1988 Low-dose aspirin therapy improves fetal weight in umbilical placental insufficiency. American Journal of Obstetrics and Gynaecology 159: 681

Tyrell S, Obaid A H, Lilford R J 1989 Umbilical artery Doppler velocimetry as a predictor of fetal hypoxia and acidosis at birth. Obstetrics and Gynecology 74: 332

van Assche F A, De Prins F, Aerts L, Verjans M 1977 The endocrine pancreas in the small-for-dates infants. British Journal of Obstetrics and Gynaecology 84: 751

Veille J C, Hanson R, Sivakoff, Hoen H, Ben-Ami M 1993 Fetal cardiac size in normal intrauterine growth retarded and diabetic pregnancies. American Journal of Perinatology 10: 275

Vilar J, Belizan J M 1982 The relative contribution of prematurity and fetal growth retardation to low birthweight in developing and developed societies. American Journal of Obstetrics and Gynecology 143: 793

Vilar J, Cogswell M, Kestler E, Castillo P, Menedez R, Repke J T 1992 Effect of fat and fat-free mass deposition during pregnancy on birth weight. American Journal of Obstetrics and Gynecology 167: 1344

Waldenstrom U, Axelsson O, Nilsson S et al 1988 The effect of routine one-stage ultrasound screening in pregnancy: a randomised controlled trial. Lancet ii: 585

Wallenberg H C S, Rotmans N 1987 Prevention of idiopathic fetal growth retardation by low-dose aspirin and dipyridamole. American Journal of Obstetrics and Gynecology 157: 1230

Warnes D, Ballard J, Seamark R F 1977 The appearance of gluconeogenesis at birth in the sheep. Activation of the pathway associated with blood oxygenation. Biochemical Journal 162: 627

Williams C E, Mallard C, Tan W, Gluckman D 1993 Pathophysiology of perinatal asphyxia. Clinical Perinatalology 20: 305

Wladimiroff J W, Campbell S 1974 Fetal urine production rates in normal and complicated pregnancies. Lancet i: 151

Wladimiroff J W, Tonge H M, Stewart P A 1986 Doppler ultrasound assessment of cerebral blood flow in the human fetus. British Journal of Obstetrics and Gynaecology 93: 471

Wladimiroff J W, Noordam M J, van den Wijngaard J A G W, Hop W C J 1988 Fetal internal carotid and umbilical artery blood flow velocity waveforms as a measure of fetal wellbeing in intrauterine growth retardation. Pediatric Research 24: 609

Wolf H, Oosting H, Treffers P E 1987 Placental volume measurement by ultrasonography: evaluation of the method. American Journal of Obstetrics and Gynecology 156: 1191

Wolf H, Oosting H, Treffers P E 1989 A longitudinal study of the relationship between fetal and placental growth as measured by ultrasound. American Journal of Obstetrics and Gynecology 161: 1140

World Health Organization 1961 Public health aspects of low birthweight. Technical Report Series No. 217. WHO, Geneva

Yudkin P L, Aboualfa M, Eyre J A, Redman C W G, Wilkinson A R 1987a Influence of elective preterm delivery on birthweight and head circumference standards. Archives of Disease in Childhood 62: 24

Yudkin P L, Wood L, Redman C W G 1987b Risk of unexplained stillbirth at different gestational ages. Lancet i: 1192

Zhang B, Chan A 1992 Teenage pregnancy in South Australia. Australian and New Zealand Journal of Obstetrics and Gynaecology 31: 291

7. Maternal physiology in pregnancy

Iain R. McFadyen

Maternal adaptation to a conception starts before implantation. As pregnancy progresses each system and every organ is affected but to different degrees and at different rates. Similarly recovery from these changes is not uniform: some systems return to their non-pregnant state within days, others may take 6 months and a few never do revert to their nulliparous condition. The quality and degree of adaptation varies from person to person, being affected both by genetic factors in the mother and in her fetus, and by environmental differences between individuals. If adaptation is not wholly physiological it may predispose to or produce overt pathology. If it is physiological the changes in the mother may be interpreted as pathology by the mother or her attendants. The proper practice of obstetrics requires knowledge of the whole range of normality and of the consequences of physiological adaptation.

MATERNAL CHARACTERISTICS WHICH AFFECT ADAPTATION

Gravidity is the most important determinant of the mother's response. Inadequate physiological changes are most likely in first pregnancies but the maternal reaction may also be affected by her age, obstetric history, overt or covert illness (acute or chronic), and the present or earlier environment. One or more previous normal pregnancies are likely to ensure that adaptation to the current pregnancy will be normal and complete. Many of the changes of pregnancy disappear after delivery but reappear during subsequent pregnancies. Others do not and they may be important in determining the response to the conceptus. Changes in uterine vessels and possibly in the maternal immune response are permanent and help to ensure satisfactory adaptation. First pregnancies are less physiological than subsequent ones; this is suggested by the reduced mean birthweight (Thomson et al 1968), increased rate of complications and raised perinatal mortality in primigravidae.

A first pregnancy need not go to term to have a beneficial effect: spontaneous abortion of the first pregnancy ensures that mean birthweight in subsequent pregnancies is similar to that of other multiparous women (Billewicz & Thomson 1973, Alberman et al 1980). Therapeutic termination has a similar effect (WHO Task Force 1979). A previous spontaneous abortion also protects against pregnancy-induced hypertension but, paradoxically, not so completely as one which is therapeutically aborted or which reaches viability (MacGillivray 1958, Beck 1985, Strickland et al 1986). More abortions do not confer additional protection. Curiously, however, increasing gravidity increases the risk of spontaneous abortion (Naylor & Warburton 1979).

Maternal age influences adaptation to pregnancy. Women can conceive in any decade from the first to the sixth; it may not be calendar age so much as the number of years following menarche or even those preceding the menopause which is important. The probability of conceiving an aneuploid fetus is possibly determined by the interval between conception and the menopause (Brook et al 1984). Spontaneous abortion and an empty gestation sac are both more frequent at the extremes of reproductive age (McFadyen 1985). Before the menarche, increase in pelvic size is slower than increase in height. After the menarche growth in height continues for only 2 years whereas pelvic diameter continues to enlarge for 5–12 years (Moerman 1982). By the time women reach 18, the age of the menarche and pelvic capacity are not well related, but among younger girls those who have an early menarche are shorter and have a smaller pelvis than those who start to menstruate when they are older. This difference is not of great clinical significance in most societies but if a girl conceives when she is in her early teens she is not only small but her pelvis will be even less capacious than would be expected from her height so that if she survives the pregnancy the chances of her sustaining a vesicovaginal fistula are high (McFadyen 1962, Tahzib 1983). Nature may be partly on her side, however, for among a group of Nigerian girls who were pregnant at 13–16 years, more than half grew 2–16 cm in height during the pregnancy; this reduced the proportion who had mechanical problems in labour (Harrison 1985). The rest of her body is less likely to adapt satisfactorily to the pregnancy. In every society, pregnancy-induced hypertension is commoner in young mothers (Stearn 1963, Harrison 1985). It is not a situation in which youngest is best: 18–25 years of age is probably the period for optimal physiological adaptation (Baird & Thomson 1969).

The older woman has other problems. Her development is complete but the physiological changes of ageing or concurrent disease may prevent the development of a totally healthy pregnancy although only a minority exhibit frank pathology. She may have developed habits with cumulative effects; for example, the higher risk of retarded fetal growth in women of 35 or more who smoke (Chattinguis et al 1985) may be a consequence of the effects of tobacco on her cardiovascular system. Increasing age raises the possibility of fetal chromosome anomalies and of dizygotic twins (Campbell et al 1974). After the age of 35 blood vessels become less flexible (Roach & Burton 1957) and with increasing age both systolic and diastolic blood pressures rise (MacGillivray et al 1969). In the childbearing age group this is rarely of clinical significance but it is worth remembering that at any age a primigravida with a normal pregnancy has a higher blood pressure than a multigravida (Christianson 1976).

Many diseases are covert in the childbearing ages; abnormalities of carbohydrate metabolism, bacteriuria, chronic renal disease, hypertension and many other disorders may be undetected before conception, yet affect the mother's reaction to pregnancy. Treatment of disease may also modify reactions. Many women are on long-term treatment with steroids, non-steroidal analgesics, drugs affecting the adrenergic system or other drugs which can affect their mechanisms of adaptation. Treatment of involuntary infertility with gonadotrophins or other drugs may have an effect, but little is known about this apart from an increased rate of abortion (Australian In Vitro Fertilisation Collaborative Group 1985). Many of these women are however poor reproducers who can be recognized by their history of recurrent abortion or other obstetric problems as being less likely to respond physiologically to the stimulus of pregnancy (Gibson 1973).

Social class and reproductive performance are related: the lower the social class the worse is pregnancy outcome. Since adaptation and outcome are also related, it is likely that social class does affect how well the mother adapts, but there is little direct evidence for this. Physiological

investigations and reference ranges of normality do not often define the social class of the population on which they are based. Young age at first conception, high parity which depletes stores, smoking, inappropriate diet, not knowing what care and advice is available—all are associated with lower social class and may affect adaptation. Even the effect of smoking is social class-related (Rush & Cassano 1983). While reduced birthweight is found in smokers of all classes, increased perinatal mortality is present only in smokers of classes III, IV and V. Studies of the non-pregnant may, however, be relevant to the mechanism of the effects of social class on maternal adaptation. Iron stores are frequently low in lower social class women, and cell-mediated immune responses are less effective in iron deficiency (Jacobs 1977). Other less well defined deficiencies may also affect adaptation. Fibrinogen levels in the blood are raised in lower social class men and women (Markowe et al 1985). Raised fibrinogen increases viscosity which in pregnancy is associated with poor results. More observations such as these could be illuminating but would be better done during pregnancy.

Heavy work may also affect adaptation. Certainly in pregnancy the respiratory system does not respond to increasing workloads as well as in the non-pregnant (Artal et al 1986), but in both pregnant sheep and women training increases physical work capacity (Errkkola 1976) and uterine blood flow during exercise (Curet et al 1976). Africans who work hard adopt methods which are economical in energy use (Thomson & Baird 1967, Maloiy et al 1986). Such satisfactory dynamic adaptation may reflect good physiological adjustment to pregnancy, but only indirectly. Raised blood pressure at conception affects adaptation and at age 36 (an age relevant to childbearing) hypertension is more common in lower than upper social classes (Wadsworth et al 1985). Although many data such as these suggest that there is a social class effect on maternal adaptation to pregnancy, accurate and specific information is incomplete.

The effects of social class and of ethnic origin are not always clearly differentiated. In part this is due to the difficulty of allocating one ethnic group to another's social classification. If an Asian husband was a qualified accountant before moving to the UK where he runs a shop, what is his real social class? Religion may also be associated with differences in traditions and practices; in diet there are variations which could affect birthweight and other measures of adaptation. Intermarriage between close relatives reduces mean birthweight (Rao & Imbari 1977). Hindus have lighter babies than Europeans, even when the weights are adjusted for maternal size and the other variables relevant to birthweight (McFadyen et al 1984). This is not due to calorie deficiency as both groups have equal intake from different diets. Essential nutrients can be in short supply or the balance of constituents may be relevant. High fibre content reduces blood oestrogen (Hughes 1986), which is associated with delay in sexual maturation. Dietary differences may also account for the wide range of twinning rates among neighbouring rural Africans (Nylander 1978). Migration unavoidably alters environmental factors which are relevant to maternal health, and frequently leads to gradual alterations in diet and social behaviour. Whatever the mechanism, migration appears also to affect maternal adaptation. For example, mean birthweight falls in Jewish women who move from North Africa to Israel; the longer they live in Israel the more it falls (Yudkin et al 1983).

Ethnic variations also influence some basic physiological differences. Nigerians have a smaller non-pregnant blood volume than Europeans, so that while an increase of 1270 ml during pregnancy is a 55% increase (Harrison 1966), it is considerably less than occurs in Europeans. Negroid peoples may not have a developed renal dopamine response to sodium as it is not required in warm and humid climates (Lee 1981) but the relevance of this and other differences to pregnancy has not been fully explored. Some features of other communities have however been examined in detail. While Indian Asians have lipid changes in pregnancy which are almost identical with those of whites (Rouse et al 1985a), the Asians require a higher level of insulin in the blood to maintain the same blood sugar (Rouse et al 1985b). Asians have a lower blood pressure but a similar pattern of change during pregnancy to Europeans. Vegetarian Asians have low serum vitamin B_{12} levels without suffering ill effects from it possibly because of an effective enterohepatic circulation of the vitamin (Abraham et al 1985). This wide range of ethnic similarities and differences is relevant to the construction of reference ranges and to the recognition that normality is not the same for each race or even for racial subgroups.

The number of fetuses in the uterus determines the extent of many adaptive changes. While electrolyte concentrations, osmolality and other indices of the *milieu intérieur* are the same in single and multiple pregnancy, the increase in blood volume is 30% greater with twins and 50% greater with quadruplets. Plasma volume increases proportionately more with twins than singletons so haemodilution is greater (Fullerton et al 1965, Rovinsky & Jaffin 1965, MacGillivray et al 1971). Total body water increase is greater in twins, even in the first trimester, so that weight gain is increased by more than that of the additional conceptus. Cardiac output, glomerular filtration rate, uterine blood flow and tidal volume increases are greater than in singletons. Mothers carrying twins have more potential stresses on almost all of their systems than mothers of singletons.

GENERAL EFFECTS OF PREGNANCY ON THE MOTHER

Pregnancy affects each system, and some in several ways. The substance common to every system is water and this increases from early pregnancy. The mean total increase is about 8.5 litres although there is wide individual variation. It is one of the few adaptations in which there is no difference between primigravid and multiparous women (Hytten et al 1966). The greater the increase in total body water, the more likely is the mother to become oedematous and clinically detectable oedema appears in half of all pregnancies. Since oedema in otherwise normal pregnancies is associated with increased birthweight and reduced perinatal mortality (Thomson et al 1967) it is an index of good physiological adaptation. The increase in body water deduced from the amount calculated to be present in the fetus, amniotic fluid, placenta and maternal tissues is 2.5–3 litres short of the actual increase. The deficit is due partly to oedema fluid and partly to increased hydration of the connective tissue ground substance. This leads to laxity and swelling of connective tissue and consequent changes in joints which occur mainly in the last trimester and are not related to maternal age. It is, however, more marked in those having second than first babies (Calguneri et al 1982). These joint changes, together with the postural changes consequent on the alteration in the centre of gravity, produce much of the backache and other aches which are so common in pregnancy. The symphysis pubis may become very lax and extremely painful (especially during walking) but this has physiological benefit, because as it occurs the capacity of the pelvis increases (Abramson et al 1934). Generalized tissue swelling produces corneal swelling and intraocular pressure changes, gingival oedema and the common and persistent symptoms arising in the cranial sinuses resulting from their increased vascularity (Fabricant 1960). It may also produce tracheal oedema which can lead to problems with anaesthesia if intubation is required, and the carpal tunnel syndrome often develops.

Extra energy is required during pregnancy to fuel the growth of the conceptus and for the increased work which the mother must do because she is pregnant. The total requirement has been calculated to be 80 000 kcal, of which 36 000 is for maintenance metabolism (Hytten & Leitch 1971). This estimate may be too high. Studies in the Gambia (Lawrence et al 1984) and in Scotland (Durnin 1985, Illingworth et al 1987) suggest that the additional energy required for a successful pregnancy is 13 000–20 000 kcal. The difference between the calculated and observed requirements arises because the calculation assumes a steady increase in resting metabolic rate which does not occur. Among the well nourished, or those whose diet has been supplemented, there is little change in the first 10 weeks of pregnancy; a gradual rise from then until 36 weeks of 50–100 kcal/day and an increase of 200–300 kcal/day in the final 4 weeks. All this occurs with no change in maternal activity, or at most a slight reduction close to term (Durnin 1985). In rural Africans with a low food intake, resting metabolism falls in the first 2 weeks and may not return to prepregnancy levels until 25–30 weeks. In these women, the total energy cost of pregnancy may be as little as 1000 kcal but this is associated with low birthweight (Lawrence et al 1984).

Weight gain in pregnancy is usually in the range of 10–12 kg. It comprises increases in maternal body water, fat and other tissues but at term 40% of the weight gained is in the fetus, amniotic fluid, placenta and uterus (Hytten 1980). The rate of weight gain is fairly steady throughout pregnancy and in the last trimester the mean is about 0.4 kg/week. The total gained during pregnancy is slightly greater in younger women, and possibly in primigravidae than in multigravidae but the difference is not large enough to affect the clinical significance of weekly weight gain. Overall weight gain has a positive association with birthweight (Simpson et al 1965), with low weight gain being associated with light babies. There may be a fall in weight during the first trimester because of nausea and vomiting, but this is usually made up quickly from about 15 weeks.

While the physiology of early morning sickness is uncertain it is associated with a satisfactory outcome for the pregnancy. Those who report vomiting to their doctor are less likely to abort or have a preterm or stillborn child (Klebanoff et al 1985). Other common reasons for failure to gain weight in physiological amounts are dieting, vomiting due to oesophageal reflux or diarrhoea. Excessive weight gain is sometimes a consequence of reducing or stopping smoking (Hofstetter et al 1986).

Fat deposition accounts for about 3.5 kg of weight gain. It accumulates in the abdominal wall, upper back, hips and thighs. Fat deposition is most rapid between 20 and 30 weeks (Taggart et al 1967) and is possibly less in those who have generalized oedema. The other tissues which contribute to weight gain are shown in Figure 7.1.

Diurnal, circadian and other rhythms change but there is no consistent pattern. In normotensive pregnancy the blood pressure has a 24-hour periodicity initially but after 30 weeks this shortens to 20 hours (Ruff et al 1982). Sodium excretion shows two patterns: in the ambulant, it peaks at night (Kalousek et al 1969) whereas in the recumbent, it peaks near the middle of the day (Lindheimer et al 1973). Another rhythm which changes in many women is sleep. Insomnia is common but there are often good reasons for this, including nocturia, excessive fetal movements or feeling too hot because of peripheral vasodilatation. Insomnia can also be a sign of depression.

Baroreceptors and other sensing mechanisms are reset to aid physiological adaptation. Osmoregulation uses the same arginine vasopressor (AVP) mechanism as in the non-pregnant woman but the threshold for AVP secretion and thirst is set 6–8 mosmol/kg lower (Davison et al 1984). The volume-sensing mechanism is also reset (Davison 1984), as is that for respiratory regulation.

Adrenoceptors may increase in number during pregnancy. Animal experiments suggest that α-receptor re-

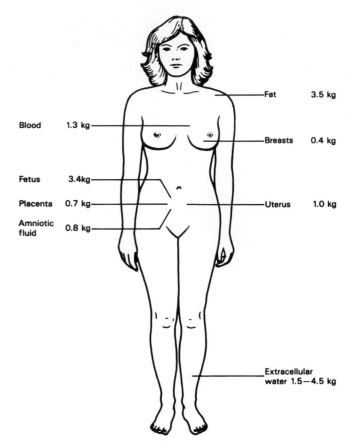

Fig. 7.1 The tissues which form the major part of weight gain in pregnancy (after Hytten 1980). There is considerable variation; the range in normal pregnancy is from 0 to 23 kg. Mean weight gain in primigravidae is 12.5 kg.

sponsiveness increases with oestrogens and β-receptor with progesterone (Roberts et al 1977). While this occurs in the human uterus it does not occur in all tissues, for example in human platelets (Roberts et al 1986).

The fetoplacental unit produces hormones which affect the mother. Renin, human placental lactogen, oestrogens, progesterone and others pass into the maternal circulation and exert their activity. Fetal excretion across the placenta may contribute to serum levels in the mother's blood. Some of the plasma proteins which bind and transport hormones, drugs and other substances in the circulation increase during pregnancy. For example, total globulin increases but albumin remains unchanged. Thyroxine-binding globulin increases from increased hepatic synthesis (Dowling et al 1960). Hormone binding also varies: aldosterone is not tightly bound, so its rising concentration in plasma during pregnancy probably implies increasing biological activity. Desoxycorticosterone levels are also raised in the plasma but the compound binds avidly to globulin. Nevertheless, secretion is increased enough to produce normal free desoxycorticosterone levels in plasma which will be metabolically active (Nolten et al 1979).

Plasma aldosterone rises within 2 weeks of conception; by mid-pregnancy it is 3–5 times the non-pregnant level and by 36 weeks it is 8–10 times that level (Weir et al 1975). This balances the rise in plasma progesterone from the placenta and the normal pregnancy increase in glomerular filtration rate, both of which promote sodium loss and potassium retention (Sundsfjord 1971). Both progesterone and oestrogen increase plasma renin substrate, which reaches 2–3 times the non-pregnant level at 30 weeks, so that the renin–angiotensin–aldosterone activation balances the sodium-losing volume-reducing effect of progesterone. Plasma angiotensin II increases to twice normal non-pregnant levels within 2 weeks of conception (Weir et al 1975). If this very active vasopressor compound was not antagonized the maternal blood pressure would rise quickly. It does not in normal pregnancy, due to increased synthesis of the vasodilators prostaglandin E_2 (PGE_2) and prostacyclin (PGI_2), which also have an antiaggregatory effect on platelets (Bolton et al 1981, Broughton Pipkin et al 1982). The effects of PGI_2 are balanced by the vasoconstrictor and aggregatory thromboxane. It is by the maintenance of equilibrium between changes such as these that the physiology of normal pregnancy is maintained (Fig. 7.2). If equilibria are upset pathology appears. Pathological processes are complex: reduction in production of PGE_2 and PGI_2 would lead not only to vasoconstriction and increased platelet aggregation but because their vasodilator and natriuretic effects on the kidney would also be reduced, glomerular filtration would be reduced and sodium retained. Fortunately, most systems have a large reserve of

normal function and can maintain the correct balance of adaptive changes necessary for a healthy normal pregnancy.

METABOLISM

Pregnancy is hyperlipidaemic and glucosuric. These physiological changes in lipid and carbohydrate metabolism are accompanied by related alterations in amino acids. Together they increase the availability of glucose for the fetus (its preferred source of energy) while the mother utilizes lipids. These metabolic modifications start soon after conception, increase and become most marked in the second half of pregnancy coinciding with increasing fetal requirements for growth. The uterus and placenta also require carbohydrate, fat and amino acids for work as well as for structure.

Carbohydrate

Glucose passes freely across the placenta so its increased availability in the maternal circulation is of direct benefit to the fetus. Glucose also passes freely across the glomerulus. Normally the quantity in the filtered urine does not exceed the capacity of the tubule to reabsorb it but in pregnancy the increase in the glomerular filtration rate means that the tubular threshold is exceeded frequently; if the urine of pregnant women is tested sufficiently often glycosuria will be detected in 50 per cent (Lind & Hytten 1972). Accompanying the glycosuria are other apparent abnormalities. As pregnancy progresses insulin sensitivity changes. In the first half it increases and in the second half it decreases. In the first half fasting glucose levels are lower, and the increase in blood glucose following a carbohydrate load is not so great as in the non-pregnant (Lind et al 1973). This increased sensitivity stimulates glycogen synthesis and storage, deposition of fat and transport of amino acids into cells. It also produces a fall in glycosylated haemoglobin which because glycosylation takes some weeks, does not occur until early in the middle trimester but then is maintained until term: the reduction is from 7.4 per cent of haemoglobin in early pregnancy to 6.55 per cent at term (Lind & Cheyne 1979). After 20 weeks resistance to the action of insulin develops progressively and plasma levels rise: a carbohydrate load produces a higher rise in plasma insulin than earlier, to three to four times the pre-pregnant level (Phelps et al 1981), but the plasma glucose level also rises to higher levels than before 20 weeks and the rise lasts for longer: the peak of a glucose tolerance test is then at 60 rather 30 minutes and the return to fasting levels is delayed (Fig. 7.3). Despite these high and prolonged rises in postprandial plasma glucose the fasting level in late pregnancy remains below the non-pregnant (Lind et al 1973, Phelps et al 1981) even though the basal endogenous glucose production rises by 30 per cent during pregnancy

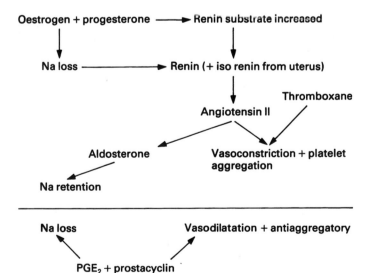

Fig. 7.2 Blood pressure in pregnancy is maintained within the normal range by a balance between mechanisms which affect the circulation. This scheme helps to explain why aspirin is effective in preventing low birthweight in pre-eclampsia, but it is incomplete. Plasma α-natriuretic peptide, calcitonin gene-related peptide and other physiological substances are also relevant to cardiovascular control.

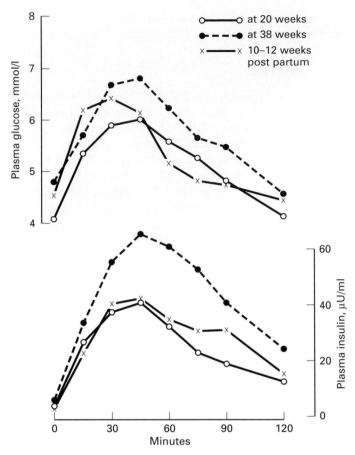

Fig. 7.3 The response of plasma glucose and plasma insulin to an oral load of glucose at 20 and 38 weeks, and 10–12 weeks post-partum (after Lind et al 1973). Fasting glucose is reduced before 20 weeks and raised thereafter as is the maximum glucose level reached. Plasma insulin shows a similar pattern.

(Catalano et al 1992). Fasting plasma insulin levels reach their maximum at around 32 weeks but the decrease in sensitivity to its action persists until delivery. This reduces maternal utilization of glucose and induces glycogenolysis and gluconeogenesis as well as the utilization of lipids as energy sources. One consequence of these changes is the rapid development of ketosis by the pregnant woman, especially during the hard work of labour. The resistance to the action of insulin is not due to increases in glucagon or growth hormone; nor is there any alteration in the absorption of glucose from the gut or in the half-life of insulin (Lind et al 1977). It may be a consequence of increased levels of human placental lactogen (hPL), oestrogen and progesterone. Oestrogen increases cortisol binding globulin which stimulates the adrenal to produce sufficient cortisol to produce insulin resistance. Progesterone increases the level of serum insulin without altering the concentration of glucose; hPL stimulates insulin release and inhibits glucose uptake (Kim & Felig 1971). Ethnicity or diet, or both may be relevant. Vegetarian Hindu Indians have lower serum hPL and higher serum glucose than Europeans (Hutchins 1982). Well-nourished African women have the same increase in insulin sensitivity as Europeans early in pregnancy but do not develop insulin resistance in the second half of pregnancy (Fraser 1981). While there may be inherent metabolic differences between races, diet is also relevant. The increase in plasma glucose following a glucose load is reduced by regular consumption of the vegetable karela (bitter gourd) which is eaten by many Indians (Leatherdale et al 1981). If the carbohydrate intake is restricted to pulses the postprandial rise in blood sugar is less than that which follows the ingestion of bread, pasta or similar foods (Jenkins et al 1980). Obesity in any ethnic group is relevant; fasting insulin is raised, insulin response is greater and glucose disposal is slower in the overweight (Freinkel et al 1985, Farmer et al 1992). Although ethnicity and other factors modify the changes in carbohydrate metabolism which occur during pregnancy, they remain beneficial to the fetus provided they remain physiological.

Amino acids

Amino acids are required by both mother and fetus for growth and for energy. The plasma concentration of most amino acids falls during pregnancy. This starts in the second half of the menstrual cycle and continues into the pregnancy (Cox & Calame 1978) and until the third trimester. The decrease is greater than that produced by physiological haemodilution. It is most marked in the gluconeogenic amino acids such as alanine. Following a meal the amino acid levels rise but not so much as in the non-pregnant and for a shorter time (Phelps et al 1981). In part this may be due to transport across the placenta: also increased insulin response during pregnancy may accelerate the uptake of amino acids by the mother for gluconeogenesis.

Pregnancy is an anabolic state so urea synthesis is reduced possibly due to decreased hepatic extraction of circulating amino acids (McGarrity et al 1949, Kalhan et al 1982). Protein breakdown which occurs with fasting is reduced (De Benoist et al 1985). The concentrations of proteins in the maternal serum fall markedly: by 20 weeks the total protein concentration has fallen from 7.0 g to 6.0 g per 100 ml. Most of this is due to the fall in serum albumin from 3.5 g to 2.5 g per 100 ml; gobulins may even rise by 0.2 g per 100 ml. The fall in albumin concentration reduces the colloid osmotic pressure in the plasma, which is one of the factors predisposing to oedema in pregnancy. The total albumin concentration of the blood falls in the first trimester and continues to do so until at least 36 weeks, the total fall being 22 per cent. The rate of synthesis of albumin increases between 12 and 28 weeks so that its intravascular mass increases by 19 per cent (Studd 1975, Whittaker & Lind 1993).

Lipids

Normal pregnancy is hyperlipaemic. All lipid levels are raised but the greatest increase is in triglyceride-rich components. Plasma concentrations tend to underestimate the magnitude of the total increase because plasma volume doubles during pregnancy. As with glucose and amino acids there is loss from the maternal circulation into and across the placenta so the changes in intermediate metabolism are more complex than simple alterations in plasma levels. There are different patterns of increase; some lipid levels rise to three or four times the pre-pregnant level, some hardly at all; some peak by mid-pregnancy and some not until 36 weeks. After delivery the plasma levels return to normal but this may take 6 months for some lipids, and is affected by whether or not the mother breastfeeds and by the use of oral contraceptives.

Early in pregnancy fat is deposited but from mid pregnancy it is used as a source of energy, mainly by the mother so that glucose is available for the growing fetus. There is considerable variation in the amount of fat which is laid down, there being a trend towards thin women gaining more than those who are obese, and primigravidae more than multigravidae (Hytten 1991), but 3.3 kg in the first 15 weeks is physiological (Clapp et al 1988). The increase in triglycerides and VLDL-cholesterol, however, is positively correlated with the mother's Quetelet index (Knopp et al 1982). It is related to gravidity but not to maternal age (Potter & Nestel 1979). The absorption of fat from the intestine is not directly altered during pregnancy but the reduction in intestinal motility may allow more time for the absorption of fat. The enterohepatic circulation is reduced with increased excretion of cholesterol in the bile (Kern et al 1981). These changes are controlled by the balance of maternal hormones. The increased insulin sensitivity of early pregnancy increases the activity of lipoprotein lipase (LPL) so fat is deposited, but as insulin secretion increases and resistance develops fat mobilization is activated through increased tissue lipase and maintained by oestriol, oestradiol, progesterone and hPL, but not by human chorionic gonadotrophin (hCG) (Desoye 1981, Knopp et al 1986). Although general lipoprotein lipase activity decreases after mid pregnancy the LPL concentrations in the uterus and in the placenta increase, as they do in the mammary tissue. Part of the increase in VLDL during pregnancy may be a consequence of the reduction in hepatic lipase and LPL so that clearance of VLDL is reduced (Kinnunen 1980, Herrera et al 1987) although the hypertriglyceridaemia is principally due to increased entry of triglyceride-rich lipoprotein into the circulation (Knopp et al 1982).

Total plasma cholesterol falls by 5% early in pregnancy, reaching its lowest point at 6–8 weeks. There is considerable individual variation in this as in all lipid changes in pregnancy. Following the initial fall there is a progres-

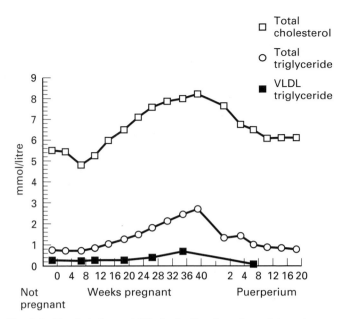

Fig. 7.4 Total cholesterol falls in the first 8 weeks and then rises progressively to term. Triglycerides do not show the initial fall but rise progressively to term (after Darmady & Postle 1982, Knopp et al 1982).

sive rise to term (Fig. 7.4). Total cholesterol increases by 24–206%; in VLDL it is raised by 36% and in LDL by 50–90%. In HDL cholesterol is raised by 10–23% at term having risen to 30% in mid gestation and then fallen. Triglyceride concentrations are raised by 90–570% at term (Warth et al 1975, Darmady & Postle 1982, Knopp et al 1982, Ordovas et al 1984). The increase in triglyceride is mainly in VLDL and LDL; HDL triglyceride does increase by 30% at the end of the second trimester, the rise then stops and the accompanying rise in HDL cholesterol is reversed although HDL protein is not reduced. The fall in HDL is in HDL 2 and not in HDL 3 since it is HDL 3 which accepts free cholesterol from cells. This cholesterol is esterified and transferred into the core of the particle which increases its content of lipids so that it is transformed into HDL 2. The level of HDL 2 indicates the flux of cholesterol through HDL 3. This requires the enzyme LCAT and apoprotein A-I: apoprotein A-II modulates the reaction. Apoprotein A-I levels rise during pregnancy; those of apo-II do not. LCAT activity increases during pregnancy; that of apo-II does not. The increase in LCAT activity is only by 20–25%; this occurs in the last trimester of pregnancy coinciding with the maximal increase of triglyceride and VLDL levels and the decline in HDL 2 (Ordovas et al 1984, Wallentin & Fahraeus 1986). The esterification of cholesterol continuously decreases from the 14th until the 28th week, accompanying the rise in cholesterol and LDL. These changes may be due to an increased turnover of cholesterol and VLDL with reduction in removal of cholesterol from lipoprotein, giving an increased supply of cholesterol to most tissues. The fall in HDL 2 from 28 weeks coincides with a steep rise in VLDL (Fahraeus et al 1985). Plasma fasting triglycerides peak at 36 weeks, at this point being 2–4 times the non-pregnancy level. The VLDL content of triglyceride cholesterol also peaks at 36 weeks. Steroid production by the placenta in late pregnancy may be 500 mg or more in 24 hours which is equivalent to 50% of the daily synthesis of steroids in the non-pregnant so that demand for cholesterol may then exceed supply and account for the fall in late pregnancy. An additional factor in this fall may be the increasing LPL activity in the uterus and in the mammary tissues at that time.

The hyperlipidaemia of normal pregnancy is not athero-genic even though lipid levels move well into the anxiety zone because the pattern of increase is not that of athero-genesis. Although lipoprotein(a) increases until 22 weeks it then falls steadily until it reaches non-pregnant levels at term (Zechner et al 1986). Apoprotein A-I rises but A-II does not change, apoprotein B does rise but propor-tionately less than apoprotein A-I or HDL 3, LDL is rich in triglyceride but poor in apoprotein (Montes et al 1984, Rosing et al 1989): these are different from atherogenic alterations in lipids (Miller et al 1990). Pregnancy may, however, unmask pathological hyperlipidaemia although it does not always do so (Montes et al 1984). The lipid changes of pregnancy may be exaggerated in women with pre-existing hypercholesterolaemia even when they are on an appropriate diet (Potter & Nestel 1979). Diet during pregnancy does not affect the increase in lipid (Hasen et al 1964) but there are ethnic variables. Lipid concentrations are lower in black-skinned North Americans than in white-skinned, and they are higher in white-skinned individuals than in other ethnic groups in the USA (Knopp et al 1982).

Birthweight, placental weight and maternal weight gain are directly related to VLDL, triglyceride levels at the end of pregnancy (Whaley et al 1966, Jiminez et al 1988) and inversely to apoprotein A-I and A-2 (Knopp et al 1985). Birthweight is negatively correlated with the levels of triglycerides in the umbilical vein. Cord blood lipids are one-half or one-quarter of maternal levels (Cajal et al 1985). The umbilical venous levels of cholesterol, triglycerides, HDL cholesterol and apoprotein A-I are all higher than those in the umbilical artery.

After delivery plasma free fatty acids fall to non-pregnant levels within 3 days but LDL and apoprotein B are still raised at 20 weeks (Montes et al 1984, Ordovas et al 1984). Total triglycerides begin to fall within 2 weeks and continue to do so. There is great variation in the time taken for triglycerides to return to non-pregnant levels, part of this depending on whether or not the mother is lactating. In those who are lactating the fall takes about 6 weeks, whereas it takes around 18 weeks in those who never established lactation (Darmady & Postle 1982). Prolactin is relevant to this since it increases mammary LPL activity (Zinder et al 1987) so that, along with intrinsic synthesis of fatty acids (Hachey et al 1989), the mother can secrete 250–400 calories per day into the milk as lipids. HDL cholesterol too is significantly higher in lactating mothers (Knopp et al 1985). Total cholesterol is raised after delivery in all mothers; unlike the rise during pregnancy it can be reduced by dieting (Potter & Nestel 1979). The fractional rate of removal of cholesterol from lipoproteins by CETP and LCAT rises and is still above pre-pregnant values at 8 weeks (Wallentin & Fahraeus 1986). The slow fall in LDL may be a conse-quence of low oestradiol levels in the puerperium, VLDL being converted to LDL (Fahreus et al 1985). As with the increase in pregnancy, the variation in return to pre-pregnant levels is not only between individuals but also between individual lipids.

Lipid peroxidation and free radicals

Lipids undergo peroxidation in all tissues as part of normal cellular function. The site of the process is the cell membrane where polyunsaturated fats are peroxidized. This occurs during the synthesis of prostacyclin, thrombox-ane and other metabolites. In physiological amounts these stimulate cyclo-oxygenase, but in excess they inhibit both this enzyme and prostacyclin synthase so that prostacyclin synthesis is reduced. Thromboxane produc-tion is not affected since thromboxane synthase is not affected by the excess of lipid peroxides (Warso & Lands 1983). Excessive free radical activity also damages cell membranes. This occurs both locally and at a distance because plasma lipoprotein may also undergo peroxida-tion and be transported to vulnerable tissues within the few minutes' half-life of the peroxides. Such damaging effects of free radical activity are contained in normal pregnancy by vitamin E which is a free radical scavenger and by other substances in maternal blood or within her cells. Plasma proteins and uric acid buffer free radicals but more specific antagonists are extracellular plasma thiols and ceruloplasmin, and within red cells lysate thiols and superoxide dismustase.

In normal pregnancy lipid peroxide levels rise in step with the general rise in lipids, indicating that the rate of peroxidation is not increased (Wickens et al 1981, Maseki et al 1981). Peroxidation products may plateau or fall towards term (Uotila et al 1991). As the peroxide levels rise so do those of vitamin E and other antioxidants: this rise is proportionately greater than that of peroxides so physiological activities are protected (Cranfield et al 1979, Wang et al 1991, Wisdom et al 1991). Lipid peroxidation is active in the placenta also, increasing with gestation (Diamant et al 1980); there too antioxidant defences are required to protect both mother and fetus from free radical activity since the placenta contains high concentrations of unsaturated fats.

INDIVIDUAL SYSTEMS

Cardiovascular

Cardiac output increases during pregnancy. The rise has started by the time of the first missed period (Clapp 1985), and at least 60% of the total rise during the pregnancy has occurred by 8–10 weeks (Walters et al 1966, Capeless & Clapp 1989, Robson et al 1989b). The increase in cardiac output is due to an increase of 10% in stroke volume and in pulse rate of 10–15% per minute, and is accompanied by enlargement of the left ventricle. There is generalized enlargement of the heart, probably due to increased venous filling. The heart also changes position: with the rise in the level of the diaphragm it rises and is displaced anterolaterally which alters the electrocardiogram and may mimic ischaemic heart disease. There is no change in central venous pressure or pulmonary wedge pressure (Clark et al 1989). The cardiac changes are, however, accompanied by dilatation of the peripheral resistance vessels and of the peripheral veins due to relaxation of vascular smooth muscle (Pickles et al 1989). There is considerable individual variation. The increase in distensibility of veins in fingers is greater in women who have varicose veins than in those who do not (McCauseland et al 1961). The overall increase may be considerable (Goodrich & Wood 1964) or small (Duncan 1967). The average woman has a fall in peripheral resistance (mean arterial pressure/cardiac output) from 1700 dyn/s/cm^{-5} before pregnancy, to 980 dyn/s/cm^{-5} in mid pregnancy, rising to 1200–1300 dyn/s/cm^{-5} towards term (Pyorala 1966).

The predisposition of pregnant women to develop varicose veins of the legs, vulva, rectum and pelvis is a consequence of the increased distensibility and increased pressure in their veins. The reduction in venous flow is compounded by the pressure of the enlarging uterus on the inferior vena cava and other veins. This produces a general dilatation since the plexus of veins around the vagina, uterus, bladder and rectum anastomose with each other. The superior rectal vein is part of the portal system and has no valves: consequently the considerable pressure within this system is communicated to the pelvic veins and, in particular, produces haemorrhoids. In labour, cardiac output rises by 30% during each contraction with an increase in stroke volume but no rise in heart rate (Hendricks 1958). The increase is less in the lateral than in the supine position because the supine position interferes less with flow to the heart between contractions for the uterus is not compressing the inferior vena cava

(Less et al 1967). Blood expressed from the uterus by each contraction produces a rise in central venous pressure of 3–5 mmHg and largely accounts for the increase in cardiac output. Arterial pressure increases by 10–20 mmHg following this increase in central venous pressure and with the peripheral vasoconstriction which starts with every contraction (Herbert et al 1958). The effort of pushing in the second stage raises both cardiac output and blood pressure even higher in many women. The normotensive healthy cardiovascular system can cope with these changes but cardiac disease or hypertensive disease in addition may produce progressive or sudden deterioration.

Severe illness may be mimicked by these physiological changes. Early or mid-systolic functional murmurs develop in many women; these cannot be differentiated during pregnancy from those due to significant cardiac or valvular pathology. They may be very loud along the left edge of the sternum, develop during mid-pregnancy and disappear a few days after delivery. Some of these arise in the mammary vessels (Tabatznik et al 1960) and others are functional (Cutforth & MacDonald 1966). They are due not only to the increased cardiac output and change in configuration of the heart but also to the physiological haemodilution which occurs in pregnancy. Their importance is that healthy women have to be treated as potential cardiac problems during pregnancy and the puerperium until these functional murmurs disappear as the cardiovascular system returns to normal.

Haemodilution is not due to a fall in total circulating haemoglobin because the red cell mass increases progressively during pregnancy by about 18% in women not given iron supplements and by 30% in those who are supplemented (Hytten & Leitch 1971). The plasma volume, however, increases by 50% in healthy women (Pirani et al 1973, Whittaker & Lind 1993) so that there is an apparent haemodilution. This is greater in multigravid than in primigravid women and in multiple than in single pregnancies. It is positively associated with birthweight (Hytten & Paintin 1963) and the increase is less marked in poor reproducers who recurrently abort or have low birthweight children (Gibson 1973). The advantages of the increase in circulating volume are that it helps to compensate for the increased blood flow to the uterus and other organs and it reduces the viscosity of the blood (Baum 1966) which improves capillary flow. Apparent anaemia may therefore be a sign of excellent physiological adjustment to pregnancy while a high haemoglobin may be a sign of pathology.

Measurement of the circulating blood volume is not practical clinically, but a useful assessment can be made from Coulter counter measurements. In this context, the most important are the packed cell volume (PCV) and the mean cell volume (MCV). The MCV is steady or rises in normal pregnancy from 82–84 fl in the first trimester to 86–100 fl or more at term (Taylor & Lind 1976, Chanarin et al 1977), being greatest in those who are iron-supplemented. Thus in those who have a normal MCV at the start of pregnancy and a normal increase during it, a PCV of 36 or less early in pregnancy, falling to 32 in the third trimester is a sign of normality and a haemoglobin of 9 g/dl in these circumstances would be within normal limits. On the other hand, a PCV of 40 early in pregnancy which does not fall below 38 is likely to be a sign of unsatisfactory physiological change and a haemoglobin of 14.5 g/dl would actually represent a warning signal of a risk pregnancy with a reduced plasma volume. Both the actual values and the pattern of change are significant in this assessment (Fig. 7.5).

The output from the heart is not distributed in the same way in the pregnant woman as in the non-pregnant woman. There is peripheral vasodilatation, with a rise in temperature of the hands and feet which is greater in smokers than non-smokers (Ashton 1975). While flow to the uterus and kidneys also rises, that to the brain does not (McCall 1949) nor does flow to the liver (Munnell & Taylor 1947, Laaks et al 1971).

Blood pressure does not rise with the increase in cardiac output. While the systolic pressure remains almost constant, the diastolic pressure falls during the first trimester and reaches its lowest level at 16–20 weeks, the mean fall being 15 mmHg or possibly more; after that it rises again to reach its early pregnancy level by term (MacGillivray et al 1969). These observations were made on women who were sitting. If the blood pressure is taken with the mother supine, 70% have a fall in blood pressure of at least 10% and in 8% it falls by 30–50% (Holmes 1960). The supine position leads to compression of the inferior vena cava at its bifurcation (Lees et al 1967) and of the aorta from the level of the first lumbar vertebra to its bifurcation (Bieniarz et al 1968) by the uterus once it has enlarged sufficiently to do so. Late in pregnancy the uterus may completely obliterate the lumen at the level

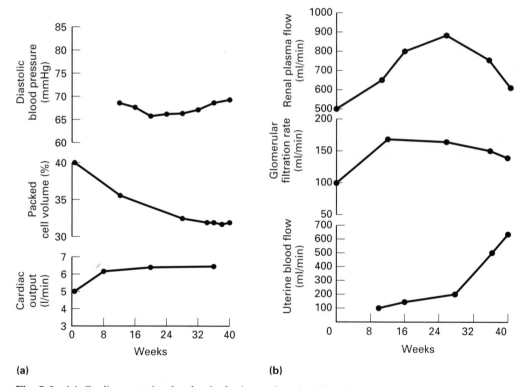

(a)   **(b)**

Fig. 7.5 **(a)** *Cardiac output* is related to body size so there is wide variation at the beginning of pregnancy but in the average woman it is 5 l/min. During pregnancy cardiac output increases by 1.5–3 l/min, most of this occurring in the first trimester. Changes in cardiac output are independent of changes in blood volume (Rovinsky & Jaffin 1965).
  Packed cell volume: with haemodilution the packed cell volume decreases progressively in normal pregnancy until around 34 weeks, and then rises slightly. If the woman takes oral iron during the pregnancy the packed cell volume is 0.5–3% higher.
  Diastolic blood pressure falls early in pregnancy, the lowest levels being at 16–20 weeks, then rising to term. The values shown here are for multigravid women with singleton pregnancies: in primigravid mothers mean diastolic pressure is 1–3 mmHg higher at all gestational ages (Christianson 1976). Systolic pressure shows a similar pattern but the later increase is less.
  (b) *Uterine blood flow* is 12–15 ml/100 g conceptus throughout pregnancy. As the myometrium and its contents enlarge total flow increases. Intervillous flow near term is 65–120 ml/100 g placenta/min.
  Glomerular filtration rate and renal plasma flow: both increase during pregnancy but while the glomerular filtration rate remains raised for the whole of the pregnancy renal plasma flow falls in the third trimester.

of the bifurcation. This reduces flow to the right heart which is partly compensated for by increased systemic vascular resistance. If this compensatory mechanism is inadequate, blood pressure falls. This fall is less marked once the fetal head engages (Holmes 1960, Lees et al 1967). That most women show only a fall in blood pressure and do not develop the supine hypotensive syndrome is due to collateral venous return to the heart via the paravertebral veins and azygos vessels (Kerr et al 1964) and to the uterine venous return via the ovarian veins which also bypasses the constricted inferior vena cava (Bieniarz et al 1969). The fall in blood pressure in the remainder of women is not consistent: it may be marked if they have an illness and is particularly important if there is shock. Obstetric intervention may unintentionally have a similar effect: placing a pregnant woman in the lithotomy position may reduce her cardiac output by 17% (Vorys et al 1961). These postural effects emphasize the necessity for standardizing the technique of measuring blood pressure in the management of individual patients or in epidemiological comparisons. Not only must the mother be relaxed at rest with the correct size of cuff properly placed on her arm, but she should be sitting or semi-recumbent with the cuff at the level of the left atrium. A standardized technique produces consistent clinically useful information.

The structure of the vessels of the uterus undergoes considerable modification during pregnancy, influencing the distribution of blood flow. Before conception, flow to the uterus is almost completely via the uterine arteries, but during pregnancy the ovarian arteries make a 20–30% contribution in 70% of women and are particularly likely to do so if the pregnancy is multiple (Bieniarz et al 1969). In a few mothers, arteries in the round ligaments which flow from the external iliacs supply the myometrium and may join the uteroovarian anastomosis. During pregnancy, the uterine arteries dilate so that their diameter is 1.5 times that in the non-pregnant woman; the arteries which stem from them become three times as wide and the arcuate arteries which supply the placenta become 10 times as wide (Bieniarz et al 1969). The spiral arteries supplying the placenta also dilate due to physiological alterations in their structure and can reach 30 times their prepregnancy diameter.

A total of 100–150 spiral arteries supply the intervillous space. On average, there is one per 2 cm^2 of the placental bed, but they cluster so distribution is uneven (Brosens & Dixon 1966). Each placental cotyledon is supplied by at least one spiral artery. Two or three of these rise from each radial artery. Before conception they lie coiled in the myometrium and basal layers of the endometrium which are not shed at menstruation. They are muscular vessels, well able to respond to vasoactive stimuli. During pregnancy the majority of the spiral arteries in the placental bed lose this ability and dilate as a consequence

of trophoblastic invasion, dilatation being progressive as they approach the placenta (Ramsey et al 1976). Non-villous trophoblast invades the interstitial tissues of the decidua and myometrium in the first 10 weeks of the pregnancy (Robertson et al 1975, Pijnenborg et al 1983). This trophoblast extends from the decidua into the walls of the spiral arteries producing distintegration of the smooth muscle. A wave of trophoblastic invasion starts at 10 weeks and is complete by 16 weeks. It is villous trophoblast and extends down the lumen of the decidual portion of the vessel (Robertson et al 1975). A second wave of endovascular trophoblastic invasion occurs at 16–22 weeks and extends more deeply to involve the myometrial portions of the spiral (but not the basal) arteries. This increases the capacity of the spiral arteries and reduces or abolishes their capacity to respond to vasoactive stimuli (Robertson et al 1967, Moll et al 1975, Zuspan et al 1981). A proportion of arteries do not undergo these physiological changes, particularly at the periphery of the placental bed (Pijnenborg et al 1981, Khong et al 1987).

Failure of physiological change is found in the myometrial segments of the spiral arteries in pre-eclampsia and intrauterine growth retardation, which means that in these abnormal states these vessels can still respond to vasoactive stimuli and reduce flow to the intervillous space. This failure of normal adaptation is associated with maternal serum uric acid levels of 300 μmol/l or more (McFadyen et al 1986) which helps to explain the clinical value of this measurement.

Uterine blood flow increases progressively during pregnancy. At 34–40 weeks mean uterine flow in a singleton pregnancy is 500–600 ml/min but there is a wide range which is partly dependent on the method of measurement used (Assali et al 1953, Browne 1954, Blechner et al 1974). Variation is also due to gestational age and to birthweight; flow is directly proportional to birthweight (Wootton et al 1977). The intervillous space receives 84–90% of the uterine flow near term; the myometrium and decidua receive the remainder (Makowski et al 1968, Lees et al 1971). The myometrium underlying the placenta has a flow 2.5 times as great as that of the rest of the myometrium and this does not change between mid and late pregnancy (Jansson 1969).

Flow in the arcuate and radial arteries during normal pregnancy is high with low resistance. There is a considerable fall in resistance after 20 weeks, although later in pregnancy this falls only slowly (Trudinger et al 1985). In abnormal pregnancies in which the spiral arteries show unsatisfactory or incomplete physiological changes, resistance remains relatively high and flow remains low.

Flow into the intervillous space is from the openings of the spiral arteries situated under the centre of the placental cotyledons (Freese 1968). A bolus of blood emerges and spreads through the spaces between the villi. Some passes into the intervillous space of adjacent cotyledons but most leaves through veins around the artery. In the monkey (whose uterine blood supply is similar to the human) not all spiral arteries supply blood at the same time so that blood flow through them is intermittent (Martin et al 1964). Closure of these vessels may be due to myometrial contraction, but contraction of the vessel itself at the endometrial–myometrial junction is probably the commoner explanation.

Monkey spiral arteries do not undergo the physiological changes found in human pregnancy; this makes such intermittence in the human unlikely, although possible in pregnancies with incomplete physiological vascular changes. Pressure and oxygen content are highest at the centre of the cotyledonary intervillous space and fall towards its periphery (Reynolds et al 1968). In the human, mean intervillous flow at 35–42 weeks is 140 ml/100 ml intervillous blood/min (Kaur et al 1980).

The pressure within the spiral arteries is 70–80 mmHg; in the intervillous space 5–10 mmHg and in the veins draining placenta and uterine wall 6–8 mmHg (Browne 1954, Boyd & Hamilton 1970). During labour, the pressure within the intervillous space rises to four times its resting level (Eastman 1958) so arterial flow to it slows. At the beginning of a contraction blood is expelled from the uterus but the rise in intramyometrial pressure then closes the veins. Arterial flow continues and the volume of the intervillous space may be increased (Borell et al 1965).

The vascular system of the placental bed is less well developed in first pregnancies than in later pregnancies, so flow is less in first than in subsequent pregnancies (Becker 1948). In some women, one or both ascending uterine arteries divides into two branches so that the anterior and posterior arcuate arteries arise from separate vessels. This may reduce uterine blood flow for it is certainly associated with an increased rate of abortion and unsuccessful pregnancy (Burchell et al 1978).

Compression and displacement of the aorta by the pregnant uterus diminishes placental perfusion, but this returns to normal if the mother lies on her side (Abitbol 1976). The diminution is in intervillous rather than in myometrial flow (Kauppila et al 1980). The myometrium normally receives about 10% of uterine blood flow and this is not affected by the mother's position. If she lies supine, however, intervillous flow falls by 20%. This suggests that there is a regulatory mechanism whereby the myometrium can respond to reduced perfusion.

The kidney can maintain its blood flow despite changes in perfusion pressure, probably by altering the tone of afferent and efferent arterioles. Whether or not the uterus can do the same is uncertain. Certainly in anaesthetized sheep (Greiss 1966, Ladner et al 1970) or rats (Bruce 1973) uterine blood flow is directly related to cardiac output but if this falls below a critical pressure (25–40 mmHg in sheep), uterine flow is reduced considerably more than

is cardiac output. In sheep which are not anaesthetized and have been made hypertensive, the uterus may be able to autoregulate its flow (Brinkman 1975). The sheep uterus and placenta are different from the human while the rabbit has a haemochorial circulation similar to the human. The rabbit can autoregulate uterine flow in response to hypertension or hypotension provided the blood pressure does not fall below a mean arterial pressure of 40 mmHg: if this occurs renal flow is maintained but uterine flow falls (Venuto et al 1976). Human myometrial flow falls if the mother is alarmed but quickly recovers (Browne 1954), a response which protects the placenta.

In animals, myometrial flow is maintained even if placental flow is reduced by hypotension (Novy et al 1975). In hyperoxia, however, both flows are reduced, protecting the fetus against unduly high levels of oxygen (Karlsson & Kjellmer 1974). Whether or not human pregnancy possesses a similar differential response by the myometrium and placental bed is not known. While intervillous flow is dependent on a balance between prostacyclin and thromboxane (Makila et al 1986), more peripheral vessels are controlled by a combination of humoral and nervous influences. Their site may affect their response. Uterine arteries contract more strongly than myometrial when stimulated by prostaglandins but both respond equally to noradrenaline and vasopressin (Maigaard et al 1985). It is therefore possible that different vessels respond differently to stress. The extent to which physiological changes in the spiral arteries are essential for alteration in the uterine circulation is not known. Possibly in those without physiological changes the spiral vessels contract when blood pressure rises but whether or not they relax when blood pressure falls, and so help to maintain placental perfusion, remains to be established.

The venous system gradually becomes more distensible as pregnancy progresses. The mean increase is 50% (McCauseland et al 1961) but there is considerable variation. Some women have an inherited predisposition to venous laxity and are more likely to develop varicose veins in pregnancy (Reagan & Folse 1971). Those with varicose veins in pregnancy have more distensible veins than those who do not (McCauseland et al 1961). The pressure within leg veins also rises. In the legs, venous pressure rises from 9 cmH$_2$O early in pregnancy to 24 cmH$_2$O at term (McLennan 1943). Flow through the veins slows as the pressure rises, being halved by term (Wright et al 1950). The increase in pressure is due to mechanical obstruction of venous return by the pressure of the uterus on the iliac veins and inferior vena cava. The intervillous pressure is 10 mmHg and that at the confluence of the iliac veins is 16 mmHg. Venous flow from the uterine veins which occurs maximally during a uterine contraction (Bieniarz et al 1969), intermittently reduces flow in the legs. This also produces intermittent rises in central venous pressure of 2.0–4.6 mmHg (Colditz & Josey 1970) with rises during Braxton Hicks contractions being 4–10 cm saline (Palmer & Walker 1949).

Respiratory system

While the lungs effect gas exchange for the mother, the placenta does it for the fetus. Effective exchange of CO_2 from fetus to mother requires the P_{CO_2} to be higher in the fetus than in the mother. Resetting the maternal respiratory centre achieves this. During pregnancy the threshold at which the respiratory centre is stimulated is reduced. A rise of 1 mmHg in maternal P_{CO_2} increases the mother's ventilation by 6 l/min instead of by the 1.5 l/min this would produce when she is not pregnant (Prowse & Gaensler 1965). This change depends on increased tidal volume but not on increased respiratory rate. The mechanics of breathing also change in pregnancy. The shape of the chest changes, with the lower ribs flaring outwards and the level of the diaphragm rising by 4 cm (Thomson & Cohen 1938). Diaphragmatic movement is increased and costal breathing reduced in pregnancy (McGinty 1938). These changes rotate the heart forwards and alter the electrocardiogram signal.

The pulmonary alterations in pregnancy increase tidal volume by 200 ml and vital capacity by 100–200 ml (Eng et al 1975). Thus less air is left in the lungs at the end of expiration, so less expired air is mixed with the next inspiration and the CO_2 gradient favourable for the fetus is maintained. The maternal P_{CO_2} is reduced to 4 kPa or lower, while fetal P_{CO_2} is 6 kPa. The reduction in threshold of the respiratory centre is probably a progesterone effect (a similar pattern of increased respiration is found in women treated with large doses of progestogens for endometrial carcinoma), with the raised level of oestrogen increasing the centre's sensitivity (Wilbrand et al 1959). These influences combine to make the pregnant woman prone to dyspnoea and dizzy spells (Gilbert & Auchincloss 1966). The woman whose respiratory centre is set to an alveolar P_{CO_2} of 4.7 kPa when she is not pregnant may well become dyspnoeic when alveolar P_{CO_2} falls to 4 kPa during pregnancy. The higher her normal P_{CO_2}, the more likely she is to develop dyspnoea at rest when pregnant. Exercise has an exaggerated effect on such dyspnoeic women. The P_{CO_2} can be reduced to 2 kPa or lower, producing cerebral arteriospasm and dizziness. Even without such extreme changes, pregnant women produce a less effective response than non-pregnant women to work (Artal et al 1986). Exercise is safe for a healthy mother with a normally grown fetus, and has benefits. Both her pulse rate and oxygen consumption are raised in proportion to the severity of the exercise: provided the pulse rate does not rise above 150–160 per minute there is little risk (Williams et al 1988). There is little effect on the blood pressure or temperature (Tuffnall et al 1990) nor is

there an increase in uterine contractions with activities involving only the upper part of the body although there may be with whole-body exercise (Durak et al 1990). Myometrial, placental and umbilical flow may be affected, but there is no agreement about the extent of this. A transient reduction in flow occurring during exercise may produce a compensatory increase in placental size and weight, and in birthweight (Clapp & Rizk 1992). Even if there is a reduction in flow it does not harm the healthy fetus whose heart rate and its variability rises with exercise (Hauth et al 1982, Tuffnell et al 1990). Another positive effect of exercise is to raise plasma β-endorphin: this is maintained in labour and reduces the maternal perception of pain (Varrassi et al 1989). Anaesthesia is affected by these physiological changes. If the normally hyperventilating pregnant patient hypoventilates under general anaesthesia, she requires less inhalational agents than are required by a woman who is not pregnant (Schnider 1981). The cardiovascular and respiratory changes of pregnancy do not have deleterious effects during air travel (Huch et al 1986).

Genital tract

The uterus consists of smooth muscle arranged in bundles which are 100 μm in diameter. Before conception the uterus weighs about 100 g and is pear-shaped, measuring $10 \times 5 \times 2.5$ cm. During pregnancy, it grows initially by hyperplasia of the myometrium and later by hypertrophy and stretching of the cells (Csapo et al 1965, Marshall 1973). By 20 weeks it weighs 300–400 g and by term 1100 g, almost completely filling the abdominal cavity (Hytten & Cheyne 1969). The individual cells lengthen from 50 μm in their non-pregnant state to 200–600 μm at term. In the first half of pregnancy, the muscle cells in the fundus are stretched to 70–90% of the optimal length for contraction. By term they have reached 90–100% of the optimal length and those in the lower segment are also close to their optimal length for isometric contraction (Wood 1964). The connective, elastic, and other tissue components of the uterus also grow during pregnancy. The cervix contains more fibrous and less muscular tissue than the body of the uterus. Only 10% of uterine muscle fibres are in the cervix (Danforth 1954, Schwalm & Dubrawsky 1966). This helps to explain the fundal dominance of uterine contraction. The uterine body and the cervix also differ in their content of glycogen, actomyosin, prostaglandins and other substances related to their activity.

The myometrium is a functional syncytium. In labour myometrial cells are coupled by low resistance pathways (gap junctions) so that the wave of contraction can pass rapidly through the organ (Marshall 1973). The myometrium is arranged in three layers which interdigitate and interconnect with a characteristic pattern. The external layer is thin and passes longitudinally over the

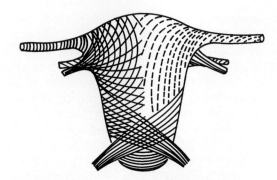

Fig. 7.6 The innermost longitudinal layer of muscle fibres is shown on the left and the outer circular layers on the right. These layers extend into the Fallopian tube, round ligament, and supporting structures of the uterus.

fundus, extending into the round and transverse cervical ligaments and into the vault of the vagina (Fig. 7.6). The middle layer is thick; it runs downwards and inwards from the fundus interlacing with muscle bundles from the other side and is the main muscle mass involved with parturient uterine contractions. The internal layer is thin and runs obliquely under the endometrium, forming sphincters around the openings of the Fallopian tubes and the cervix (Youssef 1958). The muscular spirals of the uterine vessels tend to uncoil as pregnancy progresses. The shape of the uterine cavity changes during pregnancy. Initially pear-shaped, it becomes spherical at about 20 weeks and elongates thereafter to term, although more slowly after 32 weeks (Gillespie 1950). Not only does this alter the shape of the cavity but it reduces the tension in the uterine wall, which becomes thinner towards term.

Spontaneous contractions of the myometrium occur from 20 weeks. They increase intrauterine pressure by 10–15 cmH$_2$O and may improve the circulation within the uterus. Such spontaneous uterine activity is greater in multiple than in singleton pregnancies (Newman et al 1986) and increases in strength and frequency up to term. It also facilitates the formation of the lower uterine segment by stretching and thinning the cervix between the anatomical and the histological internal os (Danforth 1947). There may also be dilatation of the cervix, the degree of which is related to the time of onset of labour, although this is far from absolute. If the cervix is completely uneffaced and closed at 42 weeks it may indicate a degree of uterine dysfunction or raise doubts about the calculated gestational age.

Although the uterus can function in a partially or totally denervated state, it does have afferent and efferent nerve supplies. There is an afferent pathway from uterus to hypothalamus (Ferguson 1941). Cervical cerclage may interrupt this reflex and so prevent abortion. Ferguson's reflex, by which distension of the cervix and vagina stimulates release of oxytocin (Fitzpatrick 1961, Dawood et al 1978), may in turn stimulate prostaglandin production in the myometrium (Flint et al 1975). Epidural analgesia, by blocking this reflex and preventing oxytocin release, may prolong the second stage of labour (Bates et al 1985). The cervix (internal os and isthmus) and uterine vessels are well supplied with adrenergic nerves (Owman et al 1967) while cholinergic nerves are confined to the blood vessels of the cervix (Coupland 1962). Adrenergic receptors in the myometrium have both α and β activity but near term the β activity is dominant.

The cervix undergoes characteristic changes both in early and late pregnancy. Early in the first trimester, the squamous epithelium of the ectocervix becomes hyperactive and occasionally the changes are so marked as to mimic carcinoma in situ. The endocervical epithelium also proliferates and grows out over the ectocervix. Being vascular, this tissue produces the clinical appearance of cervical erosion, a normal physiological response to the hormonal changes in pregnancy. Being mucus-secreting tissue, this proliferation adds to the physiological vaginal discharge which may become heavy enough to be noticed by the mother. These secretions within the endocervical canal produce the antibacterial mucus plug of the cervix.

Towards the end of the pregnancy, the cervical collagen network is disorganized and the amount of collagen within the cervix is reduced to one-third of the non-pregnant amount. The quantity of elastin is unchanged but there is marked accumulation of glycosaminoglycans and water (Buckingham et al 1962). These factors bring about the changes of cervical ripening. The duration of spontaneous labour is inversely proportional to the concentration of collagen in the cervix at the beginning of dilation (Uldbjerg et al 1983). The cervix contains prostaglandin receptors, more for PGE$_2$ than for PGF$_{2\alpha}$. These do not appear to increase during pregnancy. The cervical stroma can synthesize eicosanoids but the relationship between these and the outcome of pregnancy or labour has yet to be established.

The round ligaments increase in length, muscular content and diameter during pregnancy. In labour contraction of the ligaments pulls the uterus forward so that the expulsive force is directed as much into the pelvis as possible. During pregnancy the ligaments may contract spontaneously or in response to movement of the uterus (Mahran & Ghaleb 1964). This may produce pain in either iliac fossa, close to the site of insertion of the ligament into the uterus where it enters the internal inguinal ring or between these two points.

The vaginal epithelium also hypertrophies and its connective tissues undergo changes similar to those in the cervix. With this hypertrophy, the quantity of glycogen-containing cells shed into the vagina increases. Doderlein's bacilli convert this into lactic acid which produces an acid environment of pH 4.0–5.0 (Hanna et al 1985). This discourages the growth of most pathogens but yeasts thrive in it.

Endocrine system

The maternal endocrine system is modified during pregnancy by the addition of the fetoplacental unit. This produces human chorionic gonadotrophin, human placental lactogen and other unique hormones which affect the mother's endocrine organs directly or indirectly. The placenta also contains steroid metabolic pathways which are absent in the non-pregnant woman, but the capacity for the production of oestrogens and other hormones is underused before conception and can cope with the revised demands of pregnancy (Slaunwhite et al 1973). Raised oestrogen levels increase the production of the globulins which bind thyroxine, corticosteroids and the sex steroids. This increases the total plasma content of these hormones but does not necessarily raise the amount which is free in the plasma and is physiologically active. It may however be a readily available store and a protective mechanism which prevents exposure of the fetus to harmful quantities of hormones (Soloff et al 1974). Raised levels would also be required if binding sites on target organs were increased.

The psyche alters during pregnancy and, at least in part, this is a hormonal effect. Progesterone produces tiredness and dyspnoea and can also produce depression. Many pregnant women, however, are almost euphoric—a side-effect of corticosteroids. The changing balance of hormones may affect the function of the hypothalamus and higher centres. Some hypothalamic functions continue normally but the level at which feedback control is set can alter. Dexamethasone does not suppress adrenocorticotrophic hormone (ACTH) secretion as effectively as in the non-pregnant woman (Nolton & Rueckert 1981), which results from the control being set at a higher level. It may also be due to the secretion of placental ACTH (Genazzani et al 1975), to a fetal contribution to the level of maternal cortisol which regulates the hypothalamic response (Fenel et al 1980), or to suppression of pituitary ACTH secretion by progesterone or oestrogen (Carr et al 1979). Not only is the psyche affected by pregnancy, the whole system of endocrine control undergoes perturbation.

Pituitary gland

The pituitary gland increases in weight by 30% in first pregnancies and by 50% in subsequent conceptions (Rasmussen 1934). Even this normal increase can produce headache. It also increases the gland's sensitivity to haemorrhage, a feature which is accentuated by the lack of a direct arterial supply to the anterior pituitary (Fig. 7.7). Since blood is delivered via a portal system, in which the pressure is lower than the systemic arterial pressure, the effects of any hypotension will be greater in the anterior pituitary circulation; hypotension may be aggravated by

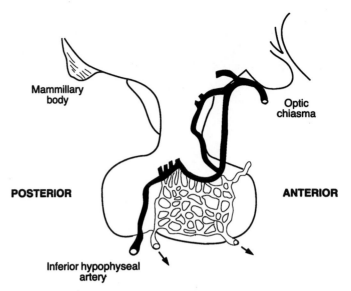

Fig. 7.7 The posterior pituitary has a direct arterial blood supply from the inferior hypophyseal artery. The anterior pituitary has no direct arterial supply. Blood reaches the anterior pituitary only after it has passed through the hypothalamus. The superior hypophyseal arteries divide into capillaries in the hypothalamus which drain directly into vessels in the anterior pituitary, where they become vascular sinusoids among the secretory cells of the anterior pituitary. There is also an anastomosis between the superior and inferior hypophyseal arteries from which vessels pass into the anterior pituitary. These portal systems are the route for hypothalamic-releasing factors to reach the anterior pituitary. Its trophic hormones enter the general circulation by veins which pass from the gland into the dural venous sinuses.

thrombotic tendencies or necrotic swelling (Sheehan & Stanfield 1961). Since the posterior pituitary has a direct arterial supply, its function is rarely permanently affected by hypotension.

The increase in weight of the pituitary is not due to an increase in the number or size of all cells. While the prolactin-secreting cells do increase, the number of growth hormone-secreting cells is reduced (Golubuff & Ezrin 1969), their secretion possibly being suppressed by high levels of cortisol or human placental lactogen. Plasma prolactin begins to rise within a few days of conception and by term may be 10–20 times as high as in the non-pregnant woman (see Ch. 10). The secretion of other anterior pituitary hormones may be unchanged or reduced. Thyroid-stimulating hormone secretion is not different from that in the non-pregnant woman (except that it is possibly lower in the first trimester) and it responds normally to thyrotropin-releasing hormone from the hypothalamus (Kannan 1973). There is, however, a blunted response of follicle-stimulating hormone to gonadotrophin-releasing hormone (GnRH). This shows a progressive decrease, finally leading to no response, 3 weeks after ovulation (Jeppsson et al 1977). The luteinizing hormone response also disappears but not until some weeks after the loss of GnRH response (Miyake et al 1977). This blunting of GnRH response may be due to human chorionic gonadotrophin, as it starts to rise before oestrogen levels rise, and before progesterone or prolactin rises significantly (Miyake et al 1977). ACTH also shows a subnormal response to glucocorticoid deprivation and metyrapone and to ACTH produced by the placenta (Genazzani et al 1975). A reduced rate of cortisol clearance (Migeon et al 1957, Beitins et al 1973) would also account for the increased response of cortisol and 17-hydroxycorticosterone (17-OHCS) to ACTH while urinary 17-OHCS and ketosteroid are unchanged (Jailer et al 1959). ACTH does not cross the placenta.

Adrenal gland

Adrenal cortical metabolism in pregnancy is closely related to the fetoplacental unit. The placenta passes oestrogens and other hormones into the maternal circulation; the cortisol which passes from fetus to mother may affect her blood levels and their rate of change. The kidneys may produce DOC (deoxycorticosterone) (Winkel et al 1980).

The maternal adrenal glands do not enlarge during pregnancy but there is an increase in width of the zona fasciculata, with histological changes there suggesting increased secretion (Whiteley & Stoner 1957). Plasma cortisol and other corticosteroids increase progressively from 12 weeks to term, reaching 3–5 times their non-pregnant levels (Gemzell 1953, Wintour et al 1978). The half-life of cortisol in the plasma is prolonged (Migeon et al 1957) and its metabolic clearance rate is reduced. This is associated with a rise in transcortin levels to 2–3 times above the non-pregnant level at term. The proportion of unbound cortisol does not change significantly during pregnancy, partly because the rising concentration of progesterone fills 10% of binding sites (Dunn et al 1981). There is no change in glucocorticoid receptor numbers in the cells during pregnancy (Nolten et al 1981) but again the high levels of progesterone may compete for binding sites. Other corticosteroids show similar patterns during normal pregnancy (Wintour et al 1978).

Thyroid

The thyroid increases in size during pregnancy. A frank goitre may develop due to increased blood flow and hyperplasia of the follicular tissue (Stoffer et al 1957). Clearance of iodide from the plasma by the thyroid increases (Aboul-Khair et al 1964) unless the diet has a high iodine content (Dworkin et al 1966). Renal clearance of iodine doubles by the end of the first trimester and then remains constant for the rest of the pregnancy (Man et al 1969). During pregnancy, thyroid-binding globulin levels also double but other thyroid-binding proteins do not increase. The result of these changes is that while free plasma triiodothyronine (T3) and thyroxine (T4) remain at the non-pregnant level or fall (Franklyn et al 1983), the mother remains euthyroid.

Long-acting thyroid-stimulating hormone, human thyroid-stimulating immunoglobulin and T4 all cross the placenta but in normal pregnancy the quantities are not sufficient to produce ill effects on the fetus. Iodide crosses the placenta and satisfies fetal requirements. Thyrotrophin-releasing hormone also crosses the placenta but thyroid-stimulating hormone does not.

Parathyroid

Parathormone levels are raised in pregnancy (Pitkin 1975), increasing calcium absorption by the mother and thus offsetting loss across the placenta to the fetus. Neither calcitonin nor parathormone cross from mother to fetus. By term, serum parathormone is higher in the mother but calcitonin is higher in the fetus (Somaan et al 1975), encouraging the deposition of bone in the fetus.

Pancreas

The size of the islets of Langerhans and the number of β cells increase during pregnancy, as does the number of receptor sites for insulin (Puavilai et al 1982). The serum level of insulin rises during the second half of pregnancy; its response to a glucose load is a greater increase than in the non-pregnant woman but blood sugar does not fall in proportion—it is less (Spellacy et al 1965, Lind et al 1968). This resistance to the action of insulin which appears during normal pregnancy may be due to the presence of human placental lactogen, prolactin, or other pregnancy hormones; it is not a consequence of changes in hepatic utilization or in peripheral sensitivity to insulin, which remain at non-pregnant levels (Kuhl et al 1981, Cowett 1985). As pregnancy advances the resistance increases. One practical effect of this and other physiological changes in pregnancy is that the upper limit of normal blood sugar in a glucose tolerance test increases from 7.5 mmol/l in the second trimester to 9.6 mmol/l in the third trimester (Hatem et al 1988).

Glucagon levels are slightly raised during pregnancy, but not to the same extent as insulin. A glucose load suppresses glucagon further in pregnant than in non-pregnant women (Metzger et al 1973).

The cells in the blood

The circulating red cell mass increases by 20–30% during pregnancy; the maximum rise occurs in those who take oral iron. From the non-pregnant level of 1400 ml it can rise in singleton pregnancy by 240 ml in those who do not take iron supplements and by 400 ml in those who do (Pritchard et al 1960). In women expecting twins the increase is about 680 ml and in triplets 900 ml. The rise is due to an increase in the number and size of red cells, which have a normal 120-day lifespan (Pritchard

& Adams 1960). It is accompanied by an increase in the reticulocyte count to 2% or more (Pritchard & Adams 1960, Trail 1975). In pregnant women not taking iron, red cell volume shows an increase from 82–85 to 87–88 fl, whereas in those supplemented with iron, with or without folic acid, it rises to 88–90 fl (Taylor & Lind 1976, Chanarin et al 1977). These are mean changes, but by the third trimester some individuals may have red cells of 100 fl or more yet no abnormality in their bone marrow. A possible advantage of these large red cells would be better transport of oxygen and carbon dioxide. A disadvantage would be reduced deformability of the cells in the capillary circulation although the raised fibrinogen concentration in pregnancy may counteract this tendency (Rampling & Sirs 1972). Erythrocyte deformability does decrease during normal pregnancy (Wilson et al 1986). It falls to about half of the non-pregnant value by 16 weeks and then returns to non-pregnant deformability by term.

The increased size of the red cells could be due in part to the fall in plasma oncotic pressure leading to increased red cell uptake of water. It could also be due to release of relatively immature cells from the marrow, which tend to be large. The marrow is hyperplastic with an increase in immature erythyroid precursors (De Leeuw et al 1966). The concentration of fetal haemoglobin (HbF) increases by 1–2% during pregnancy, due to an increase in the number of red cells containing HbF which are also large (Popat et al 1977). Iron is incorporated more quickly into pregnancy cells than it is in the non-pregnant woman (Pritchard & Adams 1960). The physiological mechanisms producing the increase in circulating haemoglobin are not yet clear. Although plasma erythropoietin rises during pregnancy the reticulocyte count increases and the iron stores decrease before this rise occurs (Howells et al 1986). Human placental lactogen and other hormones which increase early in pregnancy probably have erythropoietic actions.

That the marrow is able to respond so actively in normal pregnancy is surprising. While the 10 or more periods of menstruation which are suppressed contribute 250 mg of iron saved toward the cost of conception, this does not balance the 300–500 mg required for the increase in maternal haemoglobin or the 500 mg required for fetus and placenta (Scott 1962). This deficit could be compounded by reduction in iron absorption and by the loss of folic acid and other nutrients in the urine. Maternal stores of these are, however, usually adequate for normal adaptation to pregnancy. Some of these are quickly replenished after delivery, but it may take months for iron stores to return to normal. Frequent pregnancies can prevent this replenishment, especially if diet is inadequate; this may produce anaemia in multigravida.

If the mother has a haemoglobinopathy, her haematological responses to pregnancy may be modified. Those with beta-thalassaemia trait have a smaller increase in their red cell mass because of the disorder of haemoglobin synthesis (Schuman et al 1973). This is not improved by iron supplementation unless there are other signs of iron deficiency.

The white cells do not show a uniform pattern of change during pregnancy. The number of eosinophils, basophils, and monocytes in each millilitre of blood does not change significantly during pregnancy (Cruikshank 1970, Pitkin & Witte 1979), but with the increase in circulating volume the total numbers of these cells are increased. Neutrophil numbers rise in the first trimester and continue to do so until about 30 weeks, after which their count remains steady: the mean value they reach is 6.8×10^9/l, but there is a wide range which may reach 20×10^9/l in normal pregnancy. Neutrophil metabolic activity increases (Poloshuk et al 1970), as does phagocytic function (Mitchell 1966). Lymphocyte counts do not change but their function is suppressed. This renders the pregnant woman more susceptible to viral infections, malaria and leprosy (Duncan 1980).

The erythrocyte sedimentation rate rises early in pregnancy due to the increase in fibrinogen and other physiological changes: 100 mm in an hour is not uncommon in normal pregnancy.

Platelet count and platelet volume remain within the normal non-pregnant range in the majority of pregnancies even though platelet survival is reduced (Wallenberg & Van Kessel 1978). In 8–10% of normal pregnancies, however, the platelet count falls below 150×10/l without ill effects on the fetus or neonate (Burrows & Kelton 1990, Ahmed et al 1993). This probably is a consequence of physiological increased fibrinolysis within the uteroplacental circulation to maintain blood flow (Gerbasi et al 1990). Platelet reactivity is increased in the second and third trimesters and does not return to normal until 12 weeks after delivery (Louden 1992).

The kidney and urinary tract

Early in pregnancy the mother is aware of changes in her urinary tract. Increased frequency of micturition is one of the commonest symptoms in the first trimester and frequently persists for the remainder of the pregnancy. Nocturia is physiological later in pregnancy. Passing urine even four times during the night is within normal limits (McFadyen et al 1973). Polydipsia by day aggravates the tendency to nocturia, as does the transfer of fluid from oedematous tissue into the general circulation when lying recumbent in bed. Fetal movements and the insomnia which is so common in pregnancy also contribute to nocturia. Stress incontinence occurs frequently during normal pregnancy, resulting from relaxation of the bladder supports (Francis 1960). The urethra normally elongates during pregnancy but this does not occur in those who develop stress incontinence (Iosif & Uemsten 1981).

Bladder tone decreases and its capacity increases progressively during pregnancy but there is no residual urine after micturition (Muellner 1939). Despite the relaxation of ureters and bladder, ureteric reflux is very uncommon in normal pregnancy (Mattingly & Borkowf 1978), although it may appear during an episode of urinary tract infection (Bumpus 1924). The protection against ureteric reflux is proliferation of Waldeyer's sheath around the ureter where it passes through the bladder wall (Baird 1935).

Progressive dilatation and kinking of the ureters is found in over 90% of pregnant women and may appear as early as 6 weeks (Baird 1935). It is more marked in multiparous than primigravid women and is accompanied by a slowing of flow of urine down the ureter, perhaps by 4–6 times (Baird 1935). It is not accompanied by a decrease in ureteric tone or contractions (Rubi & Sala 1968, Mattingly & Borkowf 1978). Dilatation is greater on the right than the left due to dextrorotation of the uterus and does not extend below the pelvic brim (Dure-Smith 1970); it is due to a combination of physical obstruction by the pregnant uterus (as may occur with other large masses rising out of the pelvis) and the effects of pregnancy hormones (Hundley et al 1935, Van Wagenen & Jenkins 1948). Ureteric dilatation extends up to the calyces. Kidneys are enlarged by this, by increased glomerular size, and by increased interstitial fluid. Their length increases by 1 cm (Bailey & Rolleston 1971) and their weight by 20% (Sheehan & Lynch 1973).

Renal function changes early in pregnancy (Fig. 7.5b). Renal plasma flow increases from early in the first trimester, reaching 30–50% above non-pregnant levels by 20 weeks and remaining at that level until 30 weeks, when it starts to decline slowly although at term it is still above non-pregnant levels (Davison & Dunlop 1980). The glomerular filtration rate (GFR) also begins to increase soon after conception, reaching 60% above non-pregnant levels by the 16th week of gestation and remaining there for the remainder of the pregnancy (Davison 1974, 1978). The initial rise in GFR appears to be due to the rise in cardiac output but subsequently there is a fall in the resistance of the efferent glomerular arteriole (Dal Canton et al 1982). The agents which effect these changes may be intrarenal prostacyclin, angiotensin II, parathyroid hormone or prolactin. The reduction in plasma albumin concentration which occurs early in pregnancy and remains until term tends to increase GFR by reducing the oncotic pressure within the glomerular capillaries.

Tubular function also changes during pregnancy. While the tubules are presented with increased quantities of urine because of the increased GFR, they also lose some of their reabsorptive capacity. Glucose (Davison & Hytten 1974), uric acid (Dunlop & Davison 1977), amino acids (Hytten & Cheyne 1969) and other substances are not so completely reabsorbed as in the non-pregnant woman.

There is an increase in protein loss (possibly due to increased GFR) of up to 300 mg in a 24-hour period.

The plasma osmolality at which arginine vasopressin secretion is stimulated falls by 10 mosmol during pregnancy (Davison et al 1984). Renal handling of water is otherwise similar to that in the non-pregnant state, although more sensitive to maternal posture. The excretion of water in the upright position is reduced more in the pregnant than the non-pregnant woman and is also reduced by moving from lateral recumbent to supine position (Lindheimer & Weston 1969). Women who had prolonged lateral recumbency and then changed to upright had retention of sodium for 72 hours (Lindheimer et al 1973). Sitting also affects excretion of water load. In this position pregnant women have greater diuretic response than the non-pregnant and this difference is greater early in pregnancy than it is toward term (Hytten & Klopper 1963). Posture also affects circadian rhythms of sodium excretion. Recumbent pregnant women have maximal excretion in the middle of the day whereas women who are active tend to have maximum excretion at night (Kalousek et al 1969), which tends to aggravate nocturia.

Renal retention of sodium is the factor determining increased water retention in pregnancy. The mother and conceptus increase their sodium content by 500–900 nmol due to increased reabsorption by the renal tubules. Progesterone increases sodium excretion but its increase during pregnancy is balanced by the effects of increased aldosterone, mineralocorticoids and prostaglandins. It may be the increased progesterone which helps to conserve 350 nmol potassium during pregnancy.

The hyperventilation of pregnant women produces a mild alkalaemia (arterial pH 7.44) with a decrease in plasma bicarbonate. Renal bicarbonate absorption and hydrogen ion excretion are unchanged in pregnancy so that pregnant women are at a disadvantage if there is a sudden metabolic acidosis.

These changes in renal function may be beneficial in healthy pregnancy, but the alterations in normal values in blood and urine which they produce must be recognized as part of the physiological adaptation to normal pregnancy if clinical care is to be based on a clear understanding of what is, and is not, normal.

Gastrointestinal system

Taste often alters early in pregnancy and the change can occur even before a period has been missed. It may be a metallic taste, similar to that experienced in liver disease, a loss of taste for something usually enjoyed or a craving for a food or other substance not normally eaten, such as wall plaster. Such cravings (pica) may be an expression of nutritional lack but many have no such potentially therapeutic effect. Some are potentially hazardous. Eating mothballs is not uncommon; this may produce a fetal haemolytic anaemia. Many cravings are concealed by the mother and may be discovered only after delivery.

Salivary secretion is usually within the normal non-pregnant range (Marder et al 1972) but is occasionally excessive although it is more of a nuisance to the mother than a threat to her fluid balance. Gastric secretion is reduced (Murray et al 1957). So is the motility of the stomach and it used to be considered to cause delayed emptying, particularly in labour (Davison et al 1970) with the risk of regurgitation during the induction of anaesthesia. It is now widely recognized that intrapartum changes in gastric emptying are entirely the result of analgesic drug administration. Nevertheless, the whole intestinal tract has decreased motility: this may be the explanation for increased absorption of water and salt (Parry et al 1970) and other substances. Gut transit time returns to non-pregnant levels in the third trimester (O'Sullivan & Bullingham 1984). The increase in water absorption produces a tendency to constipation, although oral iron may also contribute. Another symptom, so common that many mothers do not complain of it, is heartburn—reflux, producing regurgitation of acid mouthfuls with retrosternal or epigastric pain. This is a consequence of increased intragastric pressure without concomitant increase in tone of the oesophageal cardiac sphincter (Lind et al 1968). It is greater in heavier patients (Brock-Utne et al 1981). There may also be reflux of bile into the stomach due to pyloric incompetence (Atlay et al 1978) which responds to treatment with aluminium hydroxide rather than magnesium sulphate. The underlying mechanism may be increased progesterone or decreased concentrations of the hormonal peptide motilin (Christofides et al 1982).

Although the gallbladder increases in size and empties more slowly during pregnancy (Gerdes & Boyden 1938), there is no change in the constitution of the bile. Hepatic function does, however, increase during pregnancy (Davis et al 1973). Plasma globulin and fibrinogen concentrations increase despite the diluting effect of the increase in plasma volume. Albumin concentration falls by 22% but the synthetic rate rises so that the total albumin mass increases by 19%, plateauing at 28 weeks (Whittaker & Lind 1993).

While hepatic blood flow does not change the velocity patterns in the hepatic vein flatten (Kurmanavicius et al 1993). This may be due in part to the cholestasis which is almost physiological in pregnancy. There is stasis of bile in dilated biliary canaliculi but no cellular necrosis or alteration in the secretion of bile (Adlercreutz et al 1967). It may be associated with generalized pruritus which responds to treatment with cholestyramine, very rarely does it produce jaundice: it is, however, associated with raised postprandial serum glucose (Wojcicka-Jagodzinska et al 1989). The cholestasis is probably a hormonal effect since it also occurs in users of oral contraceptives and postmenopausal hormone replacement. Real hepatic malfunction may be falsely suggested by reddening of the palms or by the appearance of spider naevi. Serum alkaline phosphatase levels rise during pregnancy but this is largely due to the placental production of an isoenzyme. This is another example of physiological changes leading to apparent pathology and requiring caution in the interpretation of laboratory results.

Maternal handling of many drugs alters during pregnancy (Cummings 1983). Renal clearance is speeded up, reducing the effective dose of many antibiotics elsewhere in the body. Plasma binding may change, as may intestinal absorption. Hepatic metabolism is not usually affected. The mechanisms for the fall in plasma levels of phenytoin of those on treatment or the doubling of the half-life of caffeine, have not been established. Whatever the reason for these differences they are very relevant to treatment with phenytoin during pregnancy or in advising about coffee drinking.

Skin

The most obvious change in the skin is pigmentation in some areas. The development of a linea nigra and darkening of the nipple and areola are almost universal, although the depth of pigmentation varies in different people and different races. Facial chloasma is almost as common. All are due to increased secretion of pituitary melanocyte-stimulating hormone (Ances & Pomerantz 1974). A suntan acquired during pregnancy lasts longer than any other. Spider naevi are also common and some reddening of the palms is found in most mothers. Both are oestrogen effects. The striae which develop on the abdomen, breasts and elsewhere are a response to increased circulating corticosteroids (Poidevin 1959). There is generalized vasodilatation to assist in losing the extra heat produced by maternal, placental and fetal metabolism.

Fingernails grow more quickly during pregnancy (Hillman 1960). Hair does not but the rate at which hair is shed is reduced (Lynfield 1960). The excess which is retained is lost in the puerperium, to the consternation of many mothers, who worry that they may be going bald. Subcutaneous fat increases but the generalized increase in skinfold thickness is due to oedema and increased vascularity (Taggart et al 1967). Intensely itchy papules sometimes appear during normal pregnancy—pregnancy prurigo—and disappear spontaneously either before or after delivery (Nurse 1968); there does not appear to be underlying pathology.

AFTER DELIVERY

Maternal metabolism and anatomy do not necessarily return to their nulliparous state even after a normal first pregnancy and delivery. Skin striae and pigmentation become less obvious but persist. Maternal weight often remains 1 kg or more above the preconception weight—more if the woman does not breastfeed (Stallabrass & Huntingford, personal communication). Menstruation may be longer or heavier; uterine vascularization frequently is permanently increased. Sensing system settings may be permanently altered; if the osmoreceptors return to a higher level than before pregnancy this may account for the greater increase in circulating volume found in later pregnancies (Davison et al 1981). Most systems of the body do however return close to their prepregnancy state.

The rate of return is not uniform. Carbohydrate metabolism is close to prepregnant levels within 24 hours of delivery but it may take months for iron stores to recover. Cardiac output is back to normal within 2 weeks, venous distensibility within 3–12 weeks but stroke volume not until 24 weeks after delivery (McCauseland et al 1961, Robson et al 1987). Cervical erosions may persist for a year (McLaren 1952) while circulating volume reverts within days. These data are not academic since a cervical erosion found at the 6-week postnatal visit is not abnormal and a haemoglobin estimation the day after delivery is an accurate reflection of the maternal situation (Taylor et al 1981). Joint changes may take 3–5 months to return to normal (Abramson et al 1934). The rate of involution is dependent on whether or not the mother is breastfeeding.

Some changes are peculiar to this period rather than a loss of adaptation. In one-third of women who have had normotensive pregnancies, diastolic blood pressure rises to 90 mmHg or more 48 hours after delivery (Brown 1958). Oestrogen formation falls, remaining low during breastfeeding (Bonnar et al 1975), and may produce vaginal atrophy (Hytten & Lind 1973). White cell count rises to 20×10^9 or more (Gibson 1937, Taylor et al 1981). Thyroid function is frequently altered, possibly in as many as one-fifth of mothers. This may be asymp-tomatic or produce overt hyperthyroidism or hypothyroidism, but often only lassitude (How & Bewsher 1978, Fung et al 1988). Almost always function returns to normal spontaneously, but this may take 6 months. Although the puerperium is defined as the 6 weeks which follow delivery it takes considerably longer than this for all the physical and psychological changes of pregnancy to return as close to their previous state as they will do. Repeated childbearing at short intervals may prevent this ever happening.

CONCLUSION

Women prepare for pregnancy in the luteal phase of the menstrual cycle. If conception occurs these changes persist: the fall in plasma amino acids continues (Cox & Calame 1978), as does the reduction in maternal $P\text{co}_2$ (Goodland & Romerrenke 1952). Adaption starts before embedding. Although all systems are affected there is not a uniform pattern of change. The cardiovascular and renal modifications are established in the first trimester and plateau or decrease in the third trimester. Alternatives in other systems may appear later in pregnancy and increase to term, while metabolic modification is continuous. Age, race and other factors may affect the extent or pattern of adaption: multiple pregnancy adds another dimension. Most changes benefit the fetus, sometimes to the discomfort of the mother, but some (such as the general relaxation of smooth muscle) may be a side-effect rather than a purposeful adaption. The totality of adaptation explains many of the common signs and symptoms of normal pregnancy. The obstetrician who is aware of the maternal changes which are physiological interprets laboratory results appropriately and can reassure the anxious mother that apparent pathology is not abnormal. Recognition of physiology defines pathology and determines clinical care from conception until at least 6 months after delivery.

REFERENCES

Abitbol M M 1976 Aortic compression by the pregnant uterus. New York State Journal of Medicine 76: 1470–1475

Aboul-Khair S A, Crooks J, Turnbull A C, Hytten F E 1964 The physiological change in thyroid function during pregnancy. Clinical Science 27: 195–207

Abraham R, Campbell Brown M, Haines A P et al 1985 Diet during pregnancy in an Asian community in Britain—energy, protein, zinc, copper, fibre and calcium. Human Nutrition: Applied Nutrition 39a: 23–35

Abramson D, Roberts S M, Wilson P D 1934 Relaxation of the pelvic joints in pregnancy. Surgery, Gynecology and Obstetrics 58: 595–613

Adlercreutz H, Svanborg A, Anberg A 1967 Recurrent jaundice in pregnancy. I. A clinical and ultrastructural study. American Journal of Medicine 42: 335–340

Ahmed Y, Van Iddekinge B, Paul C, Sullivan M H F, Elder M G 1993 Retrospective analysis of platelet numbers and volumes in normal pregnancy and in pre-eclampsia. British Journal of Obstetrics and Gynaecology 100: 216–220

Alberman E, Roman E, Pharoah P O D, Chamberlain G 1980 Birth weight before and after a spontaneous abortion. British Journal of Obstetrics and Gynaecology 87: 275–280

Ances I G, Pomerantz S H 1974 Serum concentrations of B-melanocyte-stimulating hormone in human pregnancy. American Journal of Obstetrics and Gynecology 119: 1062–1065

Artal R, Wiswell R, Roman Y, Dorey F 1986 Pulmonary responses to exercise in pregnancy. American Journal of Obstetrics and Gynecology 154: 378–383

Ashton H 1975 Cigarette smoking in pregnancy—differences in circulation between smokers and non-smokers. British Journal of Obstetrics and Gynaecology 82: 868–881

Assali N S, Douglas R A, Baird W W et al 1953 Measurement of uterine blood flow and uterine metabolism: IV Results in normal pregnancy. American Journal of Obstetrics and Gynecology 66: 248–253

Atlay R D, Weekes A R L, Entwistle G D, Parkinson D J 1978 Treating heartburn in pregnancy: comparison of acid and alkali mixtures. British Medical Journal 2: 919–920

Australian In Vitro Fertilisation Collaborative Group 1985 High incidence of preterm births and early losses in pregnancy after in vitro fertilisation. British Medical Journal 291: 1160–1163

Bailey R R, Rolleston G L 1971 Kidney length and ureteric dilatation in the puerperium. Journal of Obstetrics and Gynaecology of the British Commonwealth 78: 55–61

Baird D 1935 The upper urinary tract in pregnancy and puerperium, with special reference to pyelitis of pregnancy. Journal of Obstetrics and Gynaecology of the British Empire 42: 733–774

Baird D, Thomson A M 1969 General factors underlying perinatal mortality rates. In: Butler M R, Alberman E D (eds) Perinatal problems. Livingstone, Edinburgh, pp 16–35

Bates R G, Helm C W, Duncan A, Edmonds D K 1985 Uterine activity in the second stage of labour and the effect of epidural analgesia. British Journal of Obstetrics and Gynaecology 92: 1246–1250

Baum R S 1966 Viscous forces in neonatal polycythemia. Journal of Pediatrics 69: 975

Beck I 1985 Incidence of pre-eclampsia in first full-term pregnancies preceded by abortion. Journal of Obstetrics and Gynaecology 6: 82–84

Becker J G 1948 Aetiology of eclampsia. Journal of Obstetrics and Gynaecology of the British Empire 55: 756–765

Beitins I Z, Bayard F, Angus J G et al 1973 The metabolic clearance rate, blood production, interconversion and transplacental passage of cortisol and cortisone in pregnancy near term. Pediatric Research 7: 509–519

Bieniarz J, Crottogini J J, Curuchet E et al 1968 Aortocaval compression by the uterus in late human pregnancy. American Journal of Obstetrics and Gynecology 100: 203–217

Bieniarz J, Yoshida T, Romero-Salinas G et al 1969 Aortocaval compression by the uterus in late human pregnancy. IV Circulatory homeostasis by preferential perfusion of the placenta. American Journal of Obstetrics and Gynecology 103: 19–31

Billewicz W Z, Thomson A M 1973 Birthweights in consecutive pregnancies. Journal of Obstetrics and Gynaecology of the British Commonwealth 80: 491–498

Blechner J N, Stenger V G, Prystowsky H 1974 Uterine blood flow in women at term. American Journal of Obstetrics and Gynecology 120: 633–638

Bolton P J, Jogee M, Myatt L, Elder M G 1981 Maternal plasma 6-oxo-prostaglandin F1 alpha levels throughout pregnancy: a longitudinal study. British Journal of Obstetrics and Gynaecology 88: 1101–1103

Bonnar J, Franklin M, Nott P N, McNeilly A S 1975 Effect of breast-feeding on pituitary–ovarian function after childbirth. British Medical Journal 4: 82–84

Borell U L F, Fernstrom I, Ohlson L, Wiquist N 1965 Influence of uterine contractions on the utero-placental blood flow at term. American Journal of Obstetrics and Gynecology 93: 44–57

Boyd J D, Hamilton W J 1970 In: The human placenta. Heffer, Cambridge, p 271

Brinkman C R 1975 Renal hypertension and pregnancy in the sheep. I. behaviour of uteroplacental vasomotor tone during mild hypertension. American Journal of Obstetrics and Gynecology 121: 931–937

Brock-Utne J G, Dow T G B, Dimopoulos G E et al 1981 Gastric and lower oesophageal sphincter (LOS) pressures in early pregnancy. British Journal of Anaesthesia 53: 381–384

Brook J D, Gosden R G, Chandley A C 1984 Maternal ageing and aneuploid embryos—evidence from the mouse that biological and not chronological age is the important factor. Human Genetics 66: 41–45

Brosens I, Dixon H G 1966 The anatomy of the maternal side of the placenta. Journal of Obstetrics and Gynaecology of the British Commonwealth 73: 357–363

Broughton Pipkin F, Hunter J C, Turner S R, O'Brien P M S 1982 Prostaglandin E_2 attenuates the pressor response to angiotensin II in pregnant subjects but not in non-pregnant subjects. American Journal of Obstetrics and Gynecology 142: 166–176

Brown F J 1958 Aetiology of pre-eclamptic toxaemia and eclampsia. Fact and theory. Lancet i: 115–120

Browne J C M 1954 Utero-placental circulation. Cold Spring Harbor Symposia on Quantitative Biology, vol XIX. Long Island Biological Association, New York

Bruce N W 1973 The distribution of blood flow to the reproductive organs of rats near term. Journal of Reproduction and Fertility 46: 359–362

Buckingham J C, Selden R, Danforth D 1962 Connective tissue changes in the cervix during pregnancy and labour. Annals of the New York Academy of Sciences 97: 733–741

Bumpus H C 1924 Urinary reflux. Journal of Urology 12: 341–346

Burchell R C, Creed F, Rasoulpour M, Whitcomb B 1978 Vascular anatomy of the human uterus and pregnancy wastage. British Journal of Obstetrics and Gynaecology 85: 698–706

Burrows R F, Kelton J G 1990 Thrombocytopenia at delivery: a prospective survey of 6715 deliveries. American Journal of Obstetrics and Gynecology 162: 731–734

Cajal J R, Pocovi M, Jiminez D et al 1985 Plasma lipids, apolipoproteins A and B in maternal and umbilical vessels in term pregnancies. Artery 13: 32–40

Calguneri M, Bird H A, Wright V 1982 Changes in joint laxity occurring during pregnancy. Annals of Rheumatic Disease 41: 126–128

Campbell D M, Campbell A J, MacGillivray I 1974 Maternal characteristics of women having twin pregnancies. Journal of Biosocial Science 6: 463–470

Capeless E L, Clapp J F 1989 Cardiovascular changes in early phase of pregnancy. American Journal of Obstetrics and Gynecology 161: 1449–1453

Carr B R, Parker C R, Madden J D et al 1979 Plasma levels of adrenocorticotropin and cortisol in women receiving oral contraceptive steroid treatment. Journal of Clinical Endocrinology and Metabolism 49: 346–349

Catalano P M, Tyzbir E D, Wolfe R R, Roman N M, Amini S B, Sims E A H 1992 Longitudinal changes in basic hepatic glucose production and suppression during insulin infusion in normal pregnant women. American Journal of Obstetrics and Gynecology 167: 913–919

Chanarin I, McFadyen I R, Kyle R 1977 The physiological macrocytosis of pregnancy. British Journal of Obstetrics and Gynaecology 84: 504–508

Chattinguis S, Axelsson O, Eklund G, Lindmark G 1985 Smoking, maternal age and fetal growth. Obstetrics and Gynecology 66: 449–452

Christianson R E 1976 Studies on blood pressure during pregnancy. I Influence of parity and age. American Journal of Obstetrics and Gynecology 125: 509–513

Christofides N D, Ghatei M A, Bloom S R, Borberg C, Gillmer M D G 1982 Decreased plasma motilin concentrations in pregnancy. British Medical Journal 285: 1453–1454

Clapp J F 1985 Maternal heart rate in pregnancy. American Journal of Obstetrics and Gynecology 152: 659–660

Clapp J F, Rizk K H 1992 Effect of recreational exercise on midtrimester placental growth. American Journal of Obstetrics and Gynecology 167: 1518–1521

Clapp J, Seaward B L, Sleamaker R H, Hiser J 1988 Maternal physiologic adaptations to early human pregnancy. American Journal of Obstetrics and Gynecology 159: 1456–1460

Clark S L, Cotton D B, Lee W et al 1989 Central hemodynamic assessment of normal term pregnancy. American Journal of Obstetrics and Gynecology 161: 1439–1442

Colditz R B, Josey W E 1970 Central venous pressure in supine position during normal pregnancy. Obstetrics and Gynecology 36: 759–772

Coupland R E 1962 Histochemical observations on the distribution of cholinesterase in the human uterus. Journal of Obstetrics and Gynaecology of the British Commonwealth 69: 1041–1043

Cowett R M 1985 Hepatic and peripheral responsiveness to a glucose infusion in pregnancy. American Journal of Obstetrics and Gynecology 153: 272–279

Cox B D, Calame D P 1978 Changes in plasma amino acid levels during the human menstrual cycle and in early pregnancy: a preliminary report. Hormone and Metabolic Research 10: 428–430

Cranfield L M, Gollan J L, White A G, Dormandy T L 1979 Serum antioxidant activity in normal and abnormal subjects. Annals of Clinical Biochemistry 16: 299–306

Cruikshank J M 1970 The effects of parity on the leucocyte count in pregnant and non-pregnant women. British Journal of Haematology 18: 531–537

Csapo A, Erdos T, De Mattos C R et al 1965 Stretch-induced uterine growth, protein synthesis and function. Nature 207: 1378–1379

Curet L B, Orr J A, Raukin J H G, Ilugloed T 1976 Effect of exercise on cardiac output and distribution of uterine blood flow in pregnant ewes. Journal of Applied Physiology 40: 725–728

Cutforth R, MacDonald C B 1966 Heart sounds and murmurs during pregnancy. American Heart Journal 71: 741–747

Dal Canton A, Conte G, Esposito C et al 1982 Effects of pregnancy on glomerular dynamics: micropuncture study in the rat. Kidney International 22: 608–612

Danforth D N 1947 The fibrous nature of the uterine cervix, and its relation to the isthmic segment in gravid and non-gravid uteri. American Journal of Obstetrics and Gynecology 53: 541–560

Danforth D N 1954 The distribution and functional activity of the cervical musculature. American Journal of Obstetrics and Gynecology 68: 1261–1270

Darmady J M, Postle A D 1982 Lipid metabolism in pregnancy. British Journal of Obstetrics and Gynaecology 89: 211–215

Davis M, Simmons C J, Dordoni B, Maxwell J O, Williams R 1973 Induction of hepatic enzymes during normal human pregnancy. Journal of Obstetris and Gynaecology of the British Commonwealth 80: 690–694

Davison J M 1974 Changes in renal function and other aspects of homeostasis in early pregnancy. Journal of Obstetrics and Gynaecology of the British Commonwealth 81: 1003

Davison J M 1978 Changes in renal function in early pregnancy in women with one kidney. Yale Journal of Biology and Medicine 51: 347–352

Davison J M 1984 Renal haemodynamics and volume homeostasis in pregnancy. Scandinavian Journal of Clinical and Laboratory Investigation 44: 15–27

Davison J M, Dunlop W 1980 Renal hemodynamics and tubular function in normal human pregnancy. Kidney International 18: 152–161

Davison J M, Hytten F E 1974 Glomerular filtration during and after pregnancy. Journal of Obstetrics and Gynaecology of the British Commonwealth 81: 588–595

Davison J M, Vallotton M B, Lindheimer M D 1981 Plasma osmolality and urinary concentration and dilution during and after pregnancy: evidence that lateral recumbency inhibits maximal urinary concentrating ability. British Journal of Obstetrics and Gynaecology 88: 472–479

Davison J M, Gilmore E A, Durr J, Robertson G L, Lindheimer M D 1984 Altered osmotic thresholds for vasopressin secretion and thirst in human pregnancy. American Journal of Physiology 246: F105–F109

Davison J S, Davison M C, Hay D M 1970 Gastric emptying time in late pregnancy and labour. Journal of Obstetrics and Gynaecology of the British Commonwealth 77: 37–41

Dawood M Y, Raghavan K S, Pociask C, Fuchs F 1978 Oxytocin in human pregnancy and parturition. Obstetrics and Gynecology 51: 138–143

De Benoist B, Jackson A A, Hall J St E et al 1985 Whole-body protein turnover in Jamacian women during pregnancy. Human Nutrition Clinical Nutrition 39C: 167–179

De Leeuw N K M, Loevenstein L, Hsieh Y S 1966 Iron deficiency and hydremia in normal pregnancy. Medicine (Baltimore) 45: 291–315

Diamant S, Kissilewitz R, Diamant Y 1980 Lipid peroxidation system in human placental tissue: general properties and the influence of gestational age. Biology of Reproduction 23: 776–781

Dowling J T, Freinkel N, Ingbar S H 1960 The effect of oestrogens upon the peripheral metabolism of thyroxine. Journal of Clinical Investigation 39: 1119–1123

Duncan D L 1967 Some aspects of the interpretation of mineral balances. Proceedings of the Nutrition Society 26: 102

Duncan M E 1980 Babies of mothers with leprosy have small placentae, low birthweight and grow slowly. British Journal of Obstetrics and Gynaecology 87: 471–476

Dunlop W, Davison J M 1977 The effect of normal pregnancy upon the renal handling of uric acid. British Journal of Obstetrics and Gynaecology 84: 13–21

Dunn J F, Nisula B C, Robard D 1981 Transport of steroid hormone: binding of 21 endogenous steroids to both testosterone-binding globulin and corticosteroid-binding globulin in human plasma. Journal of Clinical Endocrinology and Metabolism 53: 58–68

Durak E P, Jovanovic-Peterson L, Peterson C M 1990 Comparative evaluation of uterine response to exercise on five aerobic machines. American Journal of Obstetrics and Gynecology 162: 754–756

Dure-Smith P 1970 Pregnancy dilatation of the urinary tract: the iliac sign and its significance. Radiology 96: 545–549

Durnin J V G A 1985 Is nutritional status endangered by virtually no extra intake during pregnancy? Lancet ii: 823–825

Dworkin H J, Jacquez J A, Beierwaltes W H 1966 Relationship of iodine ingestion to iodine excretion in pregnancy. Journal of Clinical Endocrinology and Metabolism 26: 1329–1342

Eastman N J 1958 Hemodynamics of uterine contraction. American Journal of Obstetrics and Gynecology 76: 981–982

Eng M, Butler J, Bonica J J 1975 Respiratory function in pregnant obese women. American Journal of Obstetrics and Gynecology 123: 241–245

Errkkola R 1976 The influence of physical training during pregnancy on physical work capacity and circulatory parameters. Scandinavian Journal of Clinical and Laboratory Investigation 36: 747–754

Fabricant N D 1960 Sexual functions and the nose. American Journal of Medical Science 239: 498–502

Fahraeus L, Larsson-Cohn U, Wallentin L 1985 Plasma lipoproteins including high density lipoprotein subfractions during normal pregnancy. Obstetrics and Gynecology 66: 468–472

Farmer G, Hamilton-Nicol D R, Sutherland H W et al 1992 The ranges of insulin response and glucose tolerance in lean, normal, and obese women during pregnancy. American Journal of Obstetrics and Gynecology 167: 772–777

Fencl M de M, Stillman R J, Cohen J, Tulchinsky D 1980 Direct evidence of sudden rise in fetal corticoids late in human gestation. Nature 287: 225–226

Ferguson J K W 1941 A study of the motility of the intact uterus at term. Surgery, Gynecology and Obstetrics 73: 359–366

Fitzpatrick R J 1961 Blood concentration of oxytocin in labour. Journal of Endocrinology 22: XIX–XXX

Flint A P F, Forsling M L, Mitchell M D, Turnbull A C 1975 Temporal relationship between changes in oxytocin and prostaglandin F levels in response to vaginal distension in the pregnant and puerperal ewe. Journal of Reproduction and Fertility 43: 551–554

Francis W J A 1960 The onset of stress incontinence. Journal of Obstetrics and Gynaecology of the British Commonwealth 67: 899–903

Franklyn J A, Sheppard M C, Ramsden D B 1983 Serum free thyroxine and free triodothyronine concentrations in pregnancy. British Medical Journal 287: 394

Fraser R B 1981 The normal range of the OGTT in the African female: pregnant and non-pregnant. East African Medical Journal 58: 90–95

Freese U E 1968 The uteroplacental vascular relationship in the human. American Journal of Obstetrics and Gynecology 101: 8–16

Freinkel N, Metzger B E, Phelps R L, Dooley S L, Ogata E S 1985 Gestational diabetes mellitus. Heterogeneity of maternal age, weight, insulin secretion, HLA antigens, and islet cell antibodies and the impact of maternal metabolism on pancreatic B-cell and somatic development in the offspring. Diabetes 34 (suppl 2): 1–7

Fullerton W T, Hytten F E, Klopper A I, McKay E 1965 A case of quadruplet pregnancy. Journal of Obstetrics and Gynaecology of the British Commonwealth 72: 791–796

Fung H Y M, Kologlu M, Collinson K et al 1988 Postpartum thyroid dysfunction in Mid Glamorgan. British Medical Journal 296: 241–244

Gemzell C A 1953 Blood levels of 17 hydroxycorticosteroids in normal pregnancy. Journal of Clinical Endocrinology 13: 898–901

Genazzani A R, Fraioli F, Hierlimann J et al 1975 Immunoreactive ACTH and cortisol plasma levels during pregnancy. Detection and partial purification of corticotropin-like placental hormone: the human chorionic corticotropin (hCC). Clinical Endocrinology 4: 1–14

Gerbasi F R, Bottoms S, Farag A, Mammen E 1990 Increased intravascular coagulation associated with pregnancy. Obstetrics and Gynecology 75: 385–389

Gerdes M M, Boyden E A 1938 The rate of emptying of the human gall-bladder in pregnancy. Surgery, Gynecology and Obstetrics 66: 145–149

Gibson A 1937 On leucocyte changes during labour and the puerperium. Journal of Obstetrics and Gynaecology of the British Empire 44: 500–509

Gibson H M 1973 Plasma volume and glomerular filtration rate in pregnancy and their relation to differences in fetal growth. Journal of Obstetrics and Gynaecology of the British Commonwealth 80: 1067–1074

Gilbert R, Auchincloss J H 1966 Dyspnea of pregnancy—clinical and physiological observations. American Journal of Medical Science 252: 270–276

Gillespie E C 1950 Principles of uterine growth in pregnancy. American Journal of Obstetrics and Gynecology 59: 949–959

Goluboff L G, Ezrin C 1969 The effect of pregnancy on the somatotroph and the prolactin cell of the human adenohypophysis. Journal of Clinical Endocrinology 29: 1533–1538

Goodland R L, Rommerenke W T 1952 Cyclic fluctuations of the alveolar carbon dioxide tension during the normal menstrual cycle. Fertility and Sterility 3: 394–399

Goodrich S M, Wood J E 1964 Peripheral venous distensibility and velocity of venous blood flow during pregnancy and during oral contraceptive therapy. American Journal of Obstetrics and Gynecology 90: 740–744

Greiss F C 1966 Pressure-flow relationship in the gravid uterine vascular bed. American Journal of Obstetrics and Gynecology 96: 41–46

Hachey D L, Silber G H, Wong W W et al 1989 Human lactation. 2. Endogenous fatty acid synthesis by the mammary gland. Pediatric Research 25: 63–68

Hanna N F, Taylor-Robinson D, Kalodiki-Karamanoli M, Harris J R, McFadyen I R 1985 The relation between vaginal pH and the microbiological status in vaginitis. British Journal of Obstetrics and Gynaecology 92: 1267–1271

Harrison K A 1966 Blood volume changes in normal pregnant Nigerian women. Journal of Obstetrics and Gynaecology of the British Commonwealth 73: 717–721

Harrison K A 1985 Childbearing, health and social priorities: a survey of 22 774 consecutive hospital births in Zaria, Northern Nigeria. British Journal of Obstetrics and Gynaecology (suppl 5): 1–119

Hasen A E, Wiese H F, Adam D J D et al 1964 Influence of diet on blood serum lipids in pregnant women and newborn infants. American Journal of Clinical Nutrition 15: 11–17

Hatem M, Anthony F, Hogston P, Rowe D J F, Dennis K J 1988 Reference values for 75 g oral glucose tolerance test in pregnancy. British Medical Journal 296: 676–678

Hauth J C, Gilstrap L C, Widmer K 1982 Fetal heart rate activity before and after maternal jogging during the third trimester. American Journal of Obstetrics and Gynecology 142: 545–547

Hendricks C H 1958 The hemodynamics of a uterine contraction. American Journal of Obstetrics and Gynecology 76: 969–974

Herbert C N, Banner E A, Watkin K G 1958 Variations in the peripheral circulation during pregnancy. American Journal of Obstetrics and Gynecology 76: 742–744

Herrera E, Gomez-Coronado D, Lasuncion M A 1987 Lipid metabolism in pregnancy. Biology of the Neonate 51: 70–77

Hillman R W 1960 Fingernail growth in pregnancy. Relations to some common parameters of the reproductive process. Human Biology 32: 119–124

Hofstetter A, Schutz Y, Jequier E, Wahren J 1986 Increased 24-hour energy expenditure in cigarette smokers. New England Journal of Medicine 314: 79–82

Holmes F 1960 Incidence of the supine hypotensive syndrome in late pregnancy. Journal of Obstetrics and Gynaecology of the British Empire 67: 254–258

How J, Bewsher P D 1978 Thyroid disease and pregnancy. British Medical Journal 2: 1568–1569

Howells M R, Jones S E, Napier J A F, Saunders K, Cavill I 1986 Erythropoiesis in pregnancy. British Journal of Haematology 64: 595–599

Huch R, Baumann H, Fallenstein G, Schneider K T M, Holdener F, Huch A 1986 Physiologic changes in pregnant women and their fetuses during jet air travel. American Journal of Obstetrics and Gynecology 154: 996–1000

Hughes R E 1986 Dietary fibre may retard uterus development. Human Nutrition: Clinical Nutrition 40C: 81–86

Hundley W P, Walton J M, Hibbits J T et al 1935 Physiologic changes occurring in the urinary tract during pregnancy. American Journal of Obstetrics and Gynecology 30: 625–649

Hutchins J 1982 Physiological and biochemical responses in normal pregnancy in Indian and European subjects. In: McFadyen I R, MacVicar J (eds) Obstetric problems of the Asian community in Britain, 1st edn. Royal College of Obstetricians and Gynaecologists, London, pp 89–98

Hytten F E 1980 Weight gain in pregnancy. In: Hytten F E, Chamberlain G V P (eds) Clinical physiology in obstetrics. Blackwell, Oxford, pp 193–233

Hytten F E 1991 Weight gain in pregnancy. In: Hytten F, Chamberlain G (eds) Clinical physiology in obstetrics, 2nd edn. Blackwell Scientific Publications, Oxford, p 174

Hytten F E, Cheyne G A 1969 The size and composition of the human pregnant uterus. Journal of Obstetrics and Gynaecology of the British Commonwealth 76: 400–403

Hytten F E, Klopper A I 1963 Response to a water load in pregnancy. Journal of Obstetrics and Gynaecology of the British Commonwealth 70: 811–816

Hytten F E, Leitch I 1971 The physiology of human pregnancy, 2nd edn. Blackwell Scientific Publications, Oxford

Hytten F E, Lind T 1973 Diagnostic indices in pregnancy. CIBA-Geigy, Basle

Hytten F E, Paintin D B 1963 Increase in plasma volume during normal pregnancy. Journal of Obstetrics and Gynaecology of the British Commonwealth 70: 402–407

Hytten F E, Thomson A M, Taggart N 1966 Total body water in normal pregnancy. Journal of Obstetrics and Gynaecology of the British Commonwealth 73: 553–561

Illingworth P J, Jung R T, Howie P W, Isles T E 1987 Reduction in postprandial energy expenditure during pregnancy. British Medical Journal 294: 1573–1576

Iosif S, Uemsten U 1981 Comparative urodynamic studies of continent and stress incontinent women in pregnancy and in the puerperium. American Journal of Obstetrics and Gynecology 140: 645–650

Jacobs A 1977 Disorders of iron metabolism. In: Hoffbrand A V, Brain M E, Hirsh J (eds) Recent advances in haematology, vol 2. Churchill Livingstone, Edinburgh, pp 1–26

Jailer J W, Christy N P, Longson D et al 1959 Further observations on adrenal cortical function during pregnancy. American Journal of Obstetrics and Gynecology 78: 1–10

Jansson I 1969 ^{133}Xenon clearance in the myometrium of pregnant and non-pregnant women. Acta Obstetricia et Gynecologica Scandinavica 48: 302–321

Jenkins D K J, Wolever T M S, Taylor R H, Barker H M, Fielden H 1980 Exceptionally low blood glucose response to dried beans: comparison with other carbohydrate foods. British Medical Journal 281: 578–580

Jeppsson S, Rennevik G, Thorell J I 1977 Pituitary gonadotrophin secretion during the first weeks of pregnancy. Acta Endocrinologica 85: 177–188

Jiminez D M, Pocovi M, Ramon-Cajal J, Romero M A, Martinez H, Grande F 1988 Longitudinal study of plasma lipids and lipoprotein cholesterol in normal pregnancy and puerperium. Gynecologic and Obstetric Investigation 25: 158–164

Kalhan S C, Tserng K-Y, Gilfillan C et al 1982 Metabolism of urea and glucose in normal and diabetic pregnancy. Metabolism 31: 824–833

Kalousek G, Hlavacek C, Nedoss B, Pollek V E 1969 Circadian rhythms of creatinine and electrolyte excretion in healthy pregnant women. American Journal of Obstetrics and Gynecology 103: 856–867

Kannan V 1973 Plasma thyrotropin and its response to thyrotropin releasing hormone in normal pregnancy. Obstetrics and Gynecology 42: 547–549

Karlsson K, Kjellmer I 1974 The influence of asphyxia on uterine blood flow. Journal of Perinatal Medicine 2: 170–176

Kauppila A, Koskinen M, Puolakka J, Twimala R, Kuikka J 1980

Decreased intervillous and unchanged myometrial blood flow in supine recumbency. Obstetrics and Gynecology 55: 203–205

Kaur K, Joppila P, Kuikka J, Luotola H, Ioivanen J, Rekonen A 1980 Intervillous blood flow in normal and complicated late pregnancy measured by means of an intravenous ^{133}Xe method. Acta Obstetricia et Gynecologica Scandinavica 59: 7–10

Kern F, Everson G T, DeMark B et al 1981 Biliary lipids, bile acids, and gallbladder function in the human female: effects of pregnancy and the ovulatory cycle. Journal of Clinical Investigation 1981: 1229–1242

Kerr M G, Scott D B, Samuel E 1964 Studies of the inferior vena cava in late pregnancy. British Medical Journal 1: 532–533

Khong T Y, Liddell H S, Robertson W B 1987 Defective haemochorial placentation as a cause of miscarriage: a preliminary study. British Journal of Obstetrics and Gynaecology 94: 649–655

Kim Y J, Felig P 1971 Plasma chorionic somatomammotropin levels during starvation in mid-pregnancy. Journal of Clinical Endocrinology and Metabolism 32: 864–867

Kinnunen P K J, Unnerus H-A, Ranta T, Ehnholm C, Nikkila E A, Seppala M 1980 Activities of post-heparin lipase and hepatic lipase during pregnancy and lactation. European Journal of Clinical Investigation 10: 469–474

Klebanoff M A, Koslowe P A, Kaslow R, Rhoads G G 1985 Epidemiology of vomiting in early pregnancy. Obstetrics and Gynecology 66: 612–616

Knopp R H, Berglin R O, Wahl P W, Walden C E, Chapman M, Irvine S 1982 Population-based lipoprotein lipid reference values for pregnant women compared to nonpregnant women classified by sex hormone usage. American Journal of Obstetrics and Gynecology 143: 626–637

Knopp R H, Bergelin R O, Wahl P W, Walden C E 1985 Relationships of infant birth size to maternal lipoproteins, apoproteins, fuels, hormones, clinical chemistries, and body weight at 36 weeks gestation. Diabetes 34 (suppl 2): 71–77

Knopp R H, Warth M R, Charles D et al 1986 Lipoprotein metabolism in pregnancy, fat transport to the fetus, and the effects of diabetes. Biology of the Neonate 50: 297–317

Kuhl C, Holmes P J, Faber P K 1981 Hepatic insulin extraction in human pregnancy. Hormonal Metabolism Research 13: 71–72

Kurmanavicius J, Huch A, Huch R 1993 Blood flow velocity waveforms in the maternal hepatic vein during pregnancy. Journal of Maternal-Fetal Investigation 3: 169–173

Laaks L, Ruotsalainen P, Punnonen R, Maatela J 1971 Hepatic blood flow during late pregnancy. Acta Obstetricia et Gynecologica Scandinavica 50: 175–178

Ladner C, Brinkman C R, Weston P, Assali N S 1970 Dynamics of uterine circulation in pregnant and non-pregnant sheep. American Journal of Physiology 218: 257–263

Lawrence M, Lawrence F, Lamb W H, Whitehead R G 1984 Maintenance energy cost of pregnancy in rural Gambian women and influence of dietary status. Lancet ii: 363–365

Leatherdale B A, Panesar R K, Sing G, Atkins T W, Bailey C J, Bignell A H C 1981 Improvement of glucose tolerance due to Monnordica charantia (Karela). British Medical Journal 282: 1823–1827

Lee M R 1981 The kidney fault in essential hypertension may be a failure to mobilize renal dopamine adequately when dietary sodium chloride is increased. Cardiovascular Reviews and Reports 2: 785–789

Lees M H, Hill J D, Ochsner A J, Thomas C L, Novy M J 1971 Maternal placental and myometrial blood flow of the rhesus monkey during uterine contractions. American Journal of Obstetrics and Gynecology 110: 68–81

Lees M M, Scott D B, Kerr M G, Taylor S H 1967 The circulatory effects of recumbent postural change in late pregnancy. Clinical Science 32: 453–465

Lind J F, Smith A M, McIver D K et al 1968 Heartburn in pregnancy—a manometric study. Canadian Medical Association Journal 98: 571–575

Lind T, Cheyne G A 1979 Effects of normal pregnancy upon the glycosylated haemoglobins. British Journal of Obstetrics and Gynaecology 86: 210–213

Lind T, Hytten F E 1972 The excretion of glucose during normal pregnancy. Journal of Obstetrics and Gynaecology of the British Commonwealth 79: 961–965

Lind T, Bell S, Gilmore E, Huisjes H J, Schally A V 1977 Insulin disappearance rate in pregnant and non-pregnant women, and in non-pregnant women given GHRIH. European Journal of Clinical Investigation 7: 47–50

Lind T, Billewicz W Z, Brown G 1973 A serial study of changes occurring in the oral glucose tolerance test during pregnancy. Journal of Obstetrics and Gynaecology of the British Commonwealth 80: 1033–1039

Lindheimer M D, Weston P V 1969 Effects of hypotonic expansion on sodium, water and urea excretion in late pregnancy: the influence of posture on these results. Journal of Clinical Investigation 48: 947–950

Lindheimer M D, DelGreco F, Ehrlich E N 1973 Postural effects on Na and steroid excretion and serum renin activity during pregnancy. Journal of Applied Physiology 35: 343–348

Louden K A 1992 Platelets and platelet behaviour in normal and hypertensive pregnancy. Clinical and Experimental Hypertension Part B—Hypertension in Pregnancy B11: 91–116

Louden K A, Broughton Pipkin F, Heptinstall S, Fox S C, Mitchell J R A, Symonds M 1990 A longitudinal study of platelet behaviour and thromboxane production in whole blood in normal pregnancy and the puerperium. British Journal of Obstetrics and Gynaecology 97: 1108–1114

Lynfield Y L 1960 Effect of pregnancy on the human hair cycle. Journal of Investigative Dermatology 35: 323–327

MacGillivray I 1958 Some observations on the incidence of pre-eclampsia. Journal of Obstetrics and Gynaecology of the British Empire 65: 536–539

MacGillivray I, Rose G A, Rowe B 1969 Blood pressure survey in pregnancy. Clinical Science 37: 395–407

MacGillivray I, Campbell D M, Duffus G M 1971 Maternal metabolic response to twin pregnancy in primigravidae. Journal of Obstetrics and Gynaecology of the British Commonwealth 78: 530–536

Mahran M, Ghaleb H A 1964 The physiology of the human round ligament. Journal of Obstetrics and Gynaecology of the British Commonwealth 71: 374–378

Maigaard S, Forman A, Anderson K E 1985 Different responses to prostaglandin $F_{2\alpha}$ and E_2 in human extra- and intramyometrial arteries. Prostaglandins 30: 599–607

Makila U M, Jouppila P, Kirkinen P, Viinikka L, Ylikorkala O 1986 Placental thromboxane and prostacyclin in the regulation of placental blood flow. Obstetrics and Gynecology 68: 537–540

Makowski E L, Meschia G, Droegemudler W, Battaglia F C 1968 Distribution of uterine blood flow in the pregnant sheep. American Journal of Obstetrics and Gynecology 101: 409–412

Maloiy G M O, Heglund N C, Prager L M, Cavagna G A, Taylor C R 1986 Energetic cost of carrying loads: have African women discovered an economic way? Nature 319: 668–669

Man E B, Reid W A, Hellegers A E, Jones W S 1969 Thyroid function in human pregnancy. III. Serum thyroxine-binding pre-albumin (TBPAT) and thyroxine-binding globulin (TBG) of pregnant women aged 14 through 43 years. American Journal of Obstetrics and Gynecology 103: 328–347

Marder M Z, Wotman S, Mandel I D 1972 Salivary electrolyte changes during pregnancy. I. Normal pregnancy. American Journal of Obstetrics and Gynecology 112: 233–236

Markowe H L J, Marmot M G, Shipley M J et al 1985 Fibrinogen: a possible link between social class and coronary heart disease. British Medical Journal 291: 1312–1314

Marshall J M 1973 In: Morris H J, Hertig A T, Abell M R (eds) The physiology of the myometrium in the uterus. Williams & Wilkins, Baltimore, pp 89–109

Martin C B, McGaughey H S, Kaiser I H, Donner M W, Ramsey E M 1964 Intermittent functioning of the uteroplacental arteries. American Journal of Obstetrics and Gynecology 90: 819–823

Maseki M, Nishigaki I, Hagihara M, Tomoda Y, Yagi K 1981 Lipid peroxide levels and lipid serum content of serum lipoprotein fractions of pregnant subjects with and without pre-eclampsia. Clinica Chimica Acta 155: 155–161

Mattingly R F, Borkowf H I 1978 Clinical implications of ureteric reflux in pregnancy. Clinics in Obstetrics and Gynaecology 21: 863–873

McCall M L 1949 Cerebral blood flow and metabolism in toxemias of pregnancy. Surgery, Gynecology and Obstetrics 89: 715–720

McCauseland A M, Hyman C, Winsor T, Trotter A D 1961 Venous distensibility during pregnancy. American Journal of Obstetrics and Gynecology 81: 472–478

McFadyen I R 1962 Vesico-vaginal fistula. A series of 27 cases. British Medical Journal 2: 1717–1720

McFadyen I R 1985 Missed abortion, and later spontaneous abortion, in pregnancies clinically normal at 7–12 weeks. European Journal of Obstetrics and Gynecology and Reproductive Biology 20: 381–384

McFadyen I R, Eykyn S J, Gardner N H N et al 1973 Bacteriuria in pregnancy. Journal of Obstetrics and Gynaecology of the British Commonwealth 80: 385–405

McFadyen I R, Campbell Brown M, Abraham R, North W R S, Harris A P 1984 Factors affecting birthweight in Hindus, Moslems and Europeans. British Journal of Obstetrics and Gynaecology 91: 968–972

McFadyen I R, Price A B, Geirsson R T 1986 The relation of birth weight to histological appearances in vessels of the placental bed. British Journal of Obstetrics and Gynaecology 93: 476–481

McGarrity W J, McHenry H B, Van Wyck H B et al 1949 An effect of pyridoxine on blood urea in human subjects. Journal of Biological Chemistry 178: 511–516

McGinty A P 1938 The comparative effect of pregnancy and phrenic nerve interruption on the diaphragm and their relation to pulmonary tuberculosis. American Journal of Obstetrics and Gynecology 35: 237–241

McLaren H C 1952 The involution of the cervix. British Medical Journal 1: 347–352

McLennan C 1943 Antecubital and femoral venous pressure in normal and toxemic pregnancy. American Journal of Obstetrics and Gynecology 45: 568–591

Metzger B E, Daniel R R, Frienkel N et al 1973 The role of glucagon in gestational diabetogenesis. Clinical Research 21: 887–891

Migeon C J, Bertrand J, Wall P E 1957 Physiological disposition of 4-C-14 cortisol during late pregnancy. Journal of Clinical Investigation 36: 1350–1362

Miller M, Mead L A, Kwiterovich P O, Pearson T A 1990 Dyslipidemias with desirable plasma total cholesterol levels and angiographically demonstrated coronary artery disease. American Journal of Cardiology 65: 1–5

Mitchel G W 1966 The role of the phagocyte in host–parasite interactions. IV. The phagocytic activity of leucocytes in pregnancy and its relationship to urinary tract infections. American Journal of Obstetrics and Gynecology 96: 687–695

Miyake A, Tanizawa O, Toshihiro A, Kurachi K 1977 Pituitary responses in LH secretion to LHRH during pregnancy. Obstetrics and Gynecology 49: 549–551

Moerman M L 1982 Growth of the birth canal in adolescent girls. American Journal of Obstetrics and Gynecology 143: 528–532

Moll W, Kunzel W, Herberger J 1975 The haemodynamic implications of hemochorial placentation. European Journal of Obstetrics, Gynecology and Reproductive Biology 5: 67–71

Montes A, Walden C E, Knopp R H, Cheung M, Chapman M B, Albers J J 1984 Physiologic and supraphysiologic increases in lipoprotein lipids and apoproteins in late pregnancy and postpartum. Possible markers for the diagnosis of "Prelipemia". Arteriosclerosis 4: 407–417

Muellner S R 1939 Physiological bladder changes during pregnancy and the puerperium. Journal of Urology 41: 691–695

Munnell G W, Taylor H C 1947 Liver blood flow in pregnancy—hepatic vein catheterization. Journal of Clinical Investigation 26: 952–955

Murray F A, Erskine J P, Fielding J 1957 Gastric secretion in pregnancy. Journal of Obstetrics and Gynaecology of the British Empire 64: 373–378

Naylor A F, Warburton D 1979 Sequential analysis of spontaneous abortion. II. Collaborative study data show that gravidity determines a very substantial rise in risk. Fertility and Sterility 31: 282–286

Newman R B, Gill P J, Katz M 1986 Uterine activity during pregnancy in ambulatory patients: comparison of singleton and twin gestations. American Journal of Obstetrics and Gynecology 154: 530–531

Nolten W E, Rueckert P A 1981 Elevated free cortisol level in pregnancy: possible regulatory mechanisms. American Journal of Obstetrics and Gynecology 139: 492–498

Nolten W E, Lindheimer M D, Oparil S et al 1979 Desoxycorticosterone in normal pregnancy. II. Cortisol-dependent fluctuations in free plasma desoxycorticosterone. American Journal of Obstetrics and Gynecology 133: 644–648

Nolten W E, McKenna M V, Rueckert P A, Ehrlich E N 1981 Inhibition of 3H-dexamethasone binding to lymphocytes in vitro: relevance to the apparent development of refractoriness to cortisol in pregnancy. Clinical Research 29: 760a

Novy M J, Thomas C L, Lees M H 1975 Uterine contractility and regional blood flow responses to oxytocin and prostaglandin E_2 in pregnant rhesus monkeys. American Journal of Obstetrics and Gynecology 122: 419–433

Nurse D S 1968 Pregnancy prurigo: a study of 40 cases. Australian Journal of Dermatology 9: 258–261

Nylander P P S 1978 Causes of high twinning frequencies in Nigeria. Proceedings of Clinical and Biological Research 246: 35–43

Ordovas J M, Pocovi M, Grande F 1984 Plasma lipids and cholesterol esterification rate during pregnancy. Obstetrics and Gynecology 63: 20–25

O'Sullivan G M, Bullingham R E S 1984 The assessment of gastric acidity and antacid effect in pregnant women by a non-invasive radiotelemetry technique. British Journal of Obstetrics and Gynaecology 91: 973–978

Owman C, Rosenbren E, Sjoberg N O 1967 Adrenergic innervation of the human female reproductive organs: a histochemical and chemical investigation. Obstetrics and Gynecology 30: 763–773

Palmer A J, Walker A H C 1949 The maternal circulation in normal pregnancy. Journal of Obstetrics and Gynaecology of the British Empire 56: 537–547

Parry E, Shields R, Turnbull A C 1970 The effect of pregnancy on the colonic absorption of sodium, potassium and water. Journal of Obstetrics and Gynaecology of the British Commonwealth 77: 616–619

Perez V, Gorodisch S, Casavilla F, Maratto C 1971 Ultrastructure of human liver at the end of normal human pregnancy. American Journal of Obstetrics and Gynecology 110: 428–431

Phelps R L, Metzger B E, Hare J W, Freinkel N 1981 Carbohydrate metabolism in pregnancy. XVII. Diurnal profiles of plasma glucose, insulin, free fatty acids, triglycerides, cholesterol, and individual amino acids in late normal pregnancy. American Journal of Obstetrics and Gynecology 140: 730–736

Pickles C J, Brinkman C R, Stainer K, Cowley A J 1989 Changes in peripheral venous tone before the onset of hypertension in women with gestational hypertension. American Journal of Obstetrics and Gynecology 160: 678–680

Pijnenborg R, Bland J M, Robertson W B, Dixon G, Brosens I 1981 The pattern of interstitial trophoblast invasion of the myometrium in early human pregnancy. Placenta 2: 303–316

Pijnenborg R, Bland J M, Robertson W B, Brosens I 1983 Uteroplacental arterial changes related to interstitial trophoblast migration in early human pregnancy. Placenta 4: 397–414

Pirani B B K, Campbell D M, MacGillivray I 1973 Plasma volume in normal first pregnancy. Journal of Obstetrics and Gynaecology of the British Commonwealth 80: 884–887

Pitkin R M 1975 Calcium metabolism in pregnancy: a review. American Journal of Obstetrics and Gynecology 121: 724

Pitkin R M, Witte D L 1979 Platelet and leukocyte counts in pregnancy. Journal of the American Medical Association 242: 2696–2699

Poidevin L O S 1959 Striae gravidarum. Their relation to adrenal cortical hyperfunction. Lancet ii: 436–439

Poloshuk W Z, Diamant Y Z, Zuckerman H, Sadousky E 1970 Leukocyte alkaline phosphatase in pregnancy and the puerperium. American Journal of Obstetrics and Gynecology 107: 604–609

Popat N, Wood W G, Weatherall D J, Turnbull A C 1977 Pattern of maternal F-cell production during pregnancy. Lancet ii: 377

Potter J M, Nestel P J 1979 The hyperlipidemia of pregnancy in normal and complicated pregnancies. American Journal of Obstetrics and Gynecology 133: 165–170

Pritchard J A, Adams R H 1960 Erythrocyte production and destruction during pregnancy. American Journal of Obstetrics and Gynecology 79: 750–755

Pritchard J A, Wiggins K M, Dickey J C 1960 Blood volume changes in pregnancy and the puerperium. I. Does sequestration of red blood cells accompany parturition? American Journal of Obstetrics and Gynecology 80: 956–963

Prowse C M, Gaensler E A 1965 Respiratory and acid base changes during pregnancy. Anaesthesiology 26: 381–392

Puavilai G, Drogny E C, Domont L A, Bauma G 1982 Insulin receptors and insulin resistance in human pregnancy: evidence for a post receptor defect in insulin action. Journal of Clinical Endocrinological Metabolism 54: 247–253

Pyorala T 1966 Cardiovascular response to the upright position during pregnancy. Acta Obstetricia et Gynecologica Scandinavica 45 (suppl 5): 1–116

Rampling M, Sirs J A 1972 The interactions of fibrinogen and dextrans with erythrocytes. Journal of Physiology (London) 223: 199–212

Ramsey E M, Houston M L, Harris J W S 1976 Interactions of the trophoblast and maternal tissues in three closely related primate species. American Journal of Obstetrics and Gynecology 124: 647–652

Rao P S S, Imbari S G 1977 Inbreeding effects on human reproduction in Tamil Kadu of South India. Annals of Human Genetics 41: 87–98

Reagan B, Folse R 1971 Lower limb venous dynamics in normal persons and children of patients with varicose veins. Surgery, Gynecology and Obstetrics 132: 15–18

Reynolds S R M, Freese U E, Bieniarz J, Caldeyro-Barcia R, Mendez-Bauer C, Escarcena L 1968 Multiple simultaneous intervillous space pressures recorded in several regions of the hemochorial placenta in relation to functional anatomy of the fetal cotyledon. American Journal of Obstetrics and Gynecology 102: 1128–1134

Roach M R, Burton A C 1957 The reason for the shape of the distensibility curves of arteries. Canadian Journal of Biochemistry and Physiology 35: 681–687

Roberts J M, Insel P A, Goldflien R, Goldflien A 1977 The effect of progesterone and/or estradiol on uterine contractility and β-adrenergic receptor number. Gynecologic Investigation 8: 56

Roberts J M, Lewis V, Mize N, Tsuchiya A, Starr J 1986 Human platelet α-adrenergic receptors and responses during pregnancy: no change except that with differing hematocrit. American Journal of Obstetrics and Gynecology 154: 206–210

Robertson W B, Brosens I, Dixon H G 1967 The pathological response of the vessels of the placental bed to hypertensive pregnancy. Journal of Pathology and Bacteriology 93: 481–592

Robertson W B, Brosens I, Dixon G 1975 Uteroplacental vascular pathology. European Journal of Obstetrics, Gynecology and Reproductive Biology 5: 47–65

Robson S C, Hunter S, Moore M, Dunlop W 1987 Haemodynamic changes during the puerperium: a Doppler and M-mode echo cardiographic study. British Journal of Obstetrics and Gynaecology 94: 1028–1039

Robson S C, Hunter S, Boys R J, Dunlop W 1989a Hemodynamic changes in twin pregnancy. A Doppler and M-mode echocardiographic study. American Journal of Obstetrics and Gynecology 161: 1273–1278

Robson S C, Hunter S, Boys R J, Dunlop W 1989b Serial study of factors influencing changes in cardiac output during human pregnancy. American Journal of Physiology 256 (Heart Circ Physiol): H1060–1065

Rosing U, Samsioe G, Olund A, Johansson B, Kallner A 1989 Serum levels of Apolipoprotein A-I, A-II and HDL-cholesterol in second half of pregnancy and in pregnancy complicated by pre-eclampsia. Hormone and Metabolic Research 21: 276–382

Rouse K A, Montague W, MacVicar J 1985a Carbohydrate metabolism during pregnancy in groups of women with differing perinatal mortality rates. Journal of Obstetrics and Gynaecology 6: 24–27

Rouse K A, Montague W, MacVicar J 1985b Cholesterol and triglyceride metabolism during pregnancy in women of different ethnic origins and dietary habits. Journal of Obstetrics and Gynaecology 6: 28–31

Rovinsky J J, Jaffin H 1965 Cardiovascular hemodynamics in pregnancy. I. Blood and plasma volumes in multiple pregnancy. American Journal of Obstetrics and Gynecology 93: 1–13

Rubi R A, Sala N L 1968 Ureteral function in pregnant women. III. Effect of different positions and fetal delivery upon uterine tonus. American Journal of Obstetrics and Gynecology 101: 230–237

Ruff S C, Mitchell R H, Murnaghan G A 1982 Long term variations of blood pressure rhythms in normotensive pregnancy and pre-eclampsia. In: Sammour M, Symonds M, Zuspan F, El-Tomi N (eds) Pregnancy hypertension. Ain Shams University Press, Cairo, pp 129–143

Rush D, Cassano P 1983 Relationship of cigarette smoking and social class to birth weight and perinatal mortality among all births in Britain, 5–11 April 1970. Journal of Epidemiology and Community Health 37: 249–255

Schnider S M 1981 Choice of anaesthesia for labour and delivery. Obstetrics and Gynecology 58: 245–345

Schuman J E, Tanser C L, Peloquin R, De Leeuw N K M 1973 The erythropoietic response to pregnancy in B-thalassaemia minor. British Journal of Haematology 25: 249–260

Schwalm H, Dubrawsky V 1966 The structure of the musculature of the human uterus—muscles and connective tissue. American Journal of Obstetrics and Gynecology 94: 391–404

Scott J M 1962 Anaemia in pregnancy. Postgraduate Medical Journal 38: 202–213

Sheehan H L, Lynch J B 1973 In: Pathology of toxaemia of pregnancy. Churchill Livingstone, Edinburgh, p 47

Sheehan H L, Stanfield J P 1961 The pathogenesis of postpartum necrosis of the anterior lobe of the pituitary gland. Acta Endocrinologica 37: 479–510

Simpson J, Jameson E, Dickhams D, Glover R 1965 Effect of size of cuff bladder on accuracy of measurement of indirect blood pressure. American Heart Journal 70: 208–215

Slaunwhite W R Jr, Kirdani R Y, Sandberg A A 1973 Metabolic aspects of oestrogens in man. In: Magoun H W, Hall V E (eds) Handbook of physiology, vol II. American Physiology Society, Washington DC, p 485

Soloff M S, Swartz T L, Steinberg A H 1974 Oxytocin receptors in the human uterus. Journal of Clinical Endocrinology and Metabolism 38: 1052–1056

Somaan N A, Anderson G D, Adam-Mayne M E 1975 Immunoreactive calcitonin in the mother, neonate, child and adult. American Journal of Obstetrics and Gynecology 121: 622

Spellacy W N, Gaetz B Z, Ells J 1965 Plasma insulin in normal mid pregnancy. American Journal of Obstetrics and Gynecology 92: 11–15

Stearn R H 1963 The adolescent primigravida. Lancet ii: 1083–1085

Stoffer R P, Koeneke I A, Chesky V E, Hellwig C A 1957 The thyroid in pregnancy. American Journal of Obstetrics and Gynecology 74: 300–308

Strictland D M, Guzick D S, Cox K, Gant N F, Rosenfield C R 1986 The relationship between abortion in the first pregnancy and development of pregnancy-induced hypertension in the subsequent pregnancy. American Journal of Obstetrics and Gynecology 154: 146–148

Studd J 1975 The plasma proteins in pregnancy. Clinics in Obstetrics and Gynecology 2: 285–291

Sundsfjord J A 1971 Plasma renin activity and aldosterone excretion during prolonged progesterone administration. Acta Endocrinologica 67: 483–490

Tabatznik B, Randall T W, Hearsch C 1960 The mammary souffle in pregnancy and lactation. Circulation 22: 1069

Taggart N R, Holliday R M, Billewicz W Z, Hytten F E, Thomson A M 1967 Changes in skinfolds during pregnancy. British Journal of Nutrition 21: 439–444

Tahzib F 1983 Epidemiological determinants of vesico-vaginal fistulas. British Journal of Obstetrics and Gynaecology 90: 387–391

Taylor D J, Lind T 1976 Haematological changes during normal pregnancy: iron induced macrocytosis. British Journal of Obstetrics and Gynaecology 83: 760–767

Taylor D J, Phillips P, Lind T 1981 Puerperal haematological indices. British Journal of Obstetrics and Gynaecology 88: 601–606

Thomson B, Baird D 1967 Some impressions of child-bearing in a tropical area. Part II. Pre-eclampsia and low birth weight. Journal of Obstetrics and Gynaecology of the British Commonwealth 74: 499–509

Thomson K J, Cohen M E 1938 Studies on the circulation in pregnancy. II. Vital capacity observations in normal pregnant women. Surgery, Gynecology and Obstetrics 66: 591–597

Thomson A M, Hytten F E, Billewicz W Z 1967 The epidemiology of oedema during pregnancy. Journal of Obstetrics and Gynaecology of the British Commonwealth 74: 1–10

Thomson A M, Billewicz W Z, Hytten F E 1968 The assessment of fetal growth. Journal of Obstetrics and Gynaecology of the British Commonwealth 75: 903–916

Trail L M 1975 Reticulocytes in healthy pregnancy. Medical Journal of Australia 2: 205–206

Trudinger B J, Giles W B, Cook C M 1985 Uteroplacental blood flow velocity-time waveforms in normal and complicated pregnancy. British Journal of Obstetrics and Gynaecology 92: 39–45

Tuffnell D J, Buchan P C, Albert D, Tyndale-Biscoe S 1990 Fetal heart rate responses to maternal exercise, increased maternal temperature and maternal circadian variation. Journal of Obstetrics and Gynaecology 10: 387–391

Uldbjerg N, Ekman G, Malmstrom A, Olsson K, Ulmsten U 1983 Ripening of the human uterine cervix related to changes in collagen, glycosaminoglycans, and collagenolytic activity. American Journal of Obstetrics and Gynecology 147: 662–666

Uotila J, Tuimala R, Aarnio T et al 1991 Lipid peroxidation products, selenium-dependent glutathione peroxidase and vitamin E in normal pregnancy. European Journal of Obstetrics and Gynecology 42: 95–100

Uotila J T, Tuimala R J, Aarnio T M, Pyykko K A, Ahotupa M O 1993 Findings on lipid peroxidation and antioxidant function in hypertensive complications of pregnancy. British Journal of Obstetrics and Gynaecology 100: 270–276

Van Wagenen G, Jenkins R H 1948 Pyeloureteral dilatation or pregnancy after death of the fetus: an experimental study. American Journal of Obstetrics and Gynecology 56: 1146–1151

Varrassi G, Bazzano C, Edwards W T 1989 Effects of physical activity on maternal plasma B-endorphin levels and perception of labour pain. American Journal of Obstetrics and Gynecology 160: 707–712

Venuto R C, Cox J W, Stein J H, Ferris T F 1976 The effect of changes in perfusion pressure on uteroplacental blood flow in the pregnant rabbit. Journal of Clinical Investigation 57: 938–944

Vorys N, Ulberg J C, Hanusek G E 1961 The cardiac output changes in various positions in pregnancy. American Journal of Obstetrics and Gynecology 82: 1312–1321

Wadsworth M E J, Cripps H A, Midwinter R E, Colley J R T 1985 Blood pressure in a national birth cohort at the age of 36 related to social and familial factors, smoking, and body mass. British Medical Journal 291: 1534–1538

Wallenberg H C T, Van Kessel P H 1978 Platelet lifespan in normal pregnancy as determined by a non radioisotopic technique. British Journal of Obstetrics and Gynaecology 85: 33–37

Wallentin L, Fahraeus L 1986 Cholesterol esterification rate and its relation to lipoprotein levels in normal human pregnancy. Journal of Laboratory and Clinical Medicine 107: 216–220

Walters W A W, MacGregor W G, Hills M 1966 Cardiac output at rest during pregnancy and the puerperium. Clinical Science 30: 1–11

Wang Y, Walsh S W, Guo J, Zhang J 1991 The imbalance between thromboxane and prostacyclin in preeclampsia is associated with an imbalance between lipid peroxides and vitamin E in maternal blood. American Journal of Obstetrics and Gynecology 165: 1695–1700

Warso M A, Lands W E M 1983 Lipid peroxidation in relation to prostacyclin and thromboxane physiology and patho-physiology. British Medical Bulletin 39: 277–280

Warth M R, Arky R A, Knopp R H 1975 Lipid metabolism in pregnancy. III. Altered lipid composition in intermediate, very low, low and high density lipoprotein fractions. Journal of Clinical Endocrinology and Metabolism 41: 649–655

Weir R J, Brown J J, Fraser et al 1975 Relationship between plasma renin substrate, angiotensin II, aldosterone, and electrolytes in normal pregnancy. Journal of Clinical Endocrinology 40: 108–115

Whaley W H, Zuspan E P, Nelson G H 1966 Correlation between maternal and fetal plasma levels of glucose and free fatty acids. American Journal of Obstetrics and Gynecology 94: 419–421

Whiteley H J, Stoner H B 1957 The effect of pregnancy on the human adrenal cortex. Journal of Endocrinology 14: 325–334

Whittaker P G, Lind T 1993 The intravascular mass of albumin during human pregnancy: a serial study in normal and diabetic women. British Journal of Obstetrics and Gynaecology 100: 587–592

WHO Task Force 1979 Spontaneous and induced abortion. Technical Report Series 110, 461. WHO, Geneva

Wickens D, Wilkins M H, Lunec J, Ball G, Dormandy T L 1981 Free-radical oxidation (peroxidation) peroxidation products in plasma in normal and abnormal pregnancy. Annals of Clinical Biochemistry 18: 158–162

Wilbrand U, Porath C H, Mathaes P, Jaster R 1959 Der Einfluss der Ovariaesteroide auf die Funktion des Atemzentrums. Archiv für Gynäkologie 191: 507–511

Williams A, Reilly T, Campbell I, Sutherst J 1988 Investigation of changes in responses to exercise and in mood during pregnancy. Ergonomics 31: 1539–1549

Wilson S, Todd A S, Taylor D J 1986 Erythrocyte deformability during and after normal pregnancy. Journal of Obstetrics and Gynaecology 6: 244–247

Winkel C A, Simpson E R, Milewich L, MacDonald P C 1980 Deoxycorticosterone biosynthesis in human kidney: potential for formation of a potent mineralo-corticosteroid in its site of action. Proceedings of the National Academy of Sciences (USA) 77: 7069–7073

Wintour E M, Coghlan J P, Oddie C J, Scoggins B A, Walters W A W 1978 A sequential study of adrenocorticosteroid level in human pregnancy. Clinical Experience of Pharmacology and Physiology 5: 399–403

Wisdom S J, Wilson R, McKillop J H, Walker J J 1991 Antioxidant systems in normal pregnancy and in pregnancy-induced hypertension. American Journal of Obstetrics and Gynecology 165: 1701–1704

Wojcicka-Jagodzinska J, Kuczynska-Sicinska J, Czajkowski K, Smolarczyk R 1989 Carbohydrate metabolism in the course of intrahepatic cholestasis in pregnancy. American Journal of Obstetrics and Gynecology 161: 959–964

Wood C 1964 Physiology of uterine contractions. Journal of Obstetrics and Gynaecology of the British Commonwealth 71: 360–373

Wootton R, McFadyen I R, Cooper J E 1977 Measurement of placental blood flow in the pig and its relation to placental and fetal weight. Biology of the Neonate 31: 333–338

Wright H P, Osborn S B, Edmonds D G 1950 Changes in the rate of flow of venous blood in the leg during pregnancy measured with radioactive sodium. Surgery, Gynecology and Obstetrics 90: 481–486

Youssef A F 1958 The uterine isthmus and its sphincter mechanism, a radiographic study. American Journal of Obstetrics and Gynecology 75: 1305–1332

Yudkin P K, Harlap S, Baras M 1983 High birth weight in an ethnic group of low socio-economic status. British Journal of Obstetrics and Gynaecology 90: 291–296

Zechner R, Desoye G, Schweditsch M O, Pfeiffer K P, Kostner G M 1986 Fluctuations of plasma lipoprotein-a concentrations during pregnancy and post-partum. Metabolism 35: 333–336

Zinder O, Mendelson C R, Blancette-Mackie E J et al 1987 Lipoprotein lipase and uptake of chylomicron triacyl-glycero and cholesterol by perfused rat mammary tissue. Biochimica et Biophysica Acta 431: 526–537

Zuspan F P, O'Shaughnessy R W, Vinsel J, Zuspan M 1981 Adrenergic innervation of uteric vasculature in human term pregnancy. American Journal of Obstetrics and Gynecology 139: 678–680

8. Immunology of pregnancy

Peter M. Johnson

INTRODUCTION

The relatively young discipline of immunology originates essentially from the first effective immunization performed by Edward Jenner in 1796 with cowpox vaccination for protection against smallpox. It has since consistently attracted a small band of talented scientists, including some of the best known names in medicine—Pasteur, Metchnikoff, von Behring, Ehrlich, Bordet, Landsteiner, Medawar, Burnet, Jerne, Dausset and Milstein to name a few from the roll-call along this historic road. Indeed, immunology has gained a lion's share of Nobel prizes and now spread its wings to encompass a wide spectrum from basic science to applied medicine; it has thus become of relevance to most medical subdisciplines.

Against this historical backdrop, there has been a tremendous explosion of advances in immunology over the past 30–40 years, seemingly at an ever-increasing pace. The subject has become diversified into specialized fields (immunohistochemistry, immunogenetics, immunopathology and immunotherapy), each now including detail that would have daunted the pioneers of the 19th and early 20th centuries. Separate identification of T and B lymphocytes only became established 25 years ago, since when an ever-increasing complexity of lymphocyte subsets has been characterized using cell marker or cell function analyses. Many of the recent exciting observations in immunology need time to be distilled into simple cogent dogma before being applied to relevant allied areas, such as pregnancy.

The immunology of pregnancy, although potentially a vast topic, still remains somewhat of an outsider. With the one remarkable exception of immunoprophylaxis for rhesus haemolytic disease of the newborn (see Ch. 20), it is only in the past 20 years that relevant factual information has accumulated (Claman 1993, Dondero & Johnson 1993, Johnson 1993a, b). Because concepts and technical capabilities in immunology are so fast-moving, our scope of application will certainly accelerate in the coming years. The foundations of our understanding of immunological involvement in clinical and pathological events associated with pregnancy rest with the body of knowledge gained in studying essential immunobiological events in normal pregnancy. Two broad areas can be identified:

1. The embryo acquires its genetic information from both parents and hence, in outbred populations such as man, represents a foreign tissue graft (allograft), known colloquially as *Nature's transplant*. Immunologists have been intrigued to identify the multifactorial immunoregulatory mechanisms contributing normally to successful evasion of any maternal immune rejection in utero, hence allowing viviparous reproduction.

2. The fetus, and indeed neonate, develop facets of the immune system progressively to achieve full immunocompetence. Various interactions occur between the maternal and fetal immune systems within the intrauterine environment, including selective transfer of maternal IgG across the placenta, whereby the fetus passively acquires antibody immunity prior to exposure to the non-sterile extrauterine environment at parturition. In specific instances, unusual maternal–fetal immunological interactions may lead to a disorder of pregnancy itself with possible effects on the pregnant woman or her baby. Alternatively, since an immunological component is apparent in many, if not most, disease

states, in certain situations this can influence outcome in any concomitant pregnancy.

This chapter attempts to develop basic and clinical fetomaternal immunobiology, but first an introductory outline of the essential elements of the immune system is presented (see also Stites & Terr, Roitt et al 1993).

BASIC IMMUNOLOGY

Leukocytic cells

The average adult has about 10^{12} lymphoid cells; the lymphoid system as a whole represents 2% of total body weight. Mature antigen-specific lymphocytes can be divided into two major groups:

1. *B cells* express surface immunoglobulins acting as specific antigen receptors and are the precursors of plasma cells which secrete immunoglobulins (antibodies), they constitute 5–15% of the circulating lymphoid pool.
2. *T cells* differentiate in the thymus and include many important subpopulations, defined either functionally or by cell surface marker analysis. These include *helper, regulatory, cytotoxic* and *memory* T cells, whose functions in orchestrating the immune response by direct action or controlling mechanisms are synonymous with their generic name. All mature T cells express a specific cell surface dimeric molecule (the T-cell receptor) that, like an immunoglobulin molecule, has both a constant and a variable region and acts as a specific antigen receptor.

During early maturation, both B and T lymphocytes develop their cell surface receptor for antigen so that each cell is then committed to a single antigenic specificity for its entire lifespan. A third group of lymphocytes, less well defined, does not express specific antigen receptors or markers of either B or T cells. These *null* cells are of bone marrow origin, are usually granulated and may express cell surface receptors for the Fc region of IgG. They include antibody-dependent cellular cytotoxic (ADCC) cells which can lyse target cells via antibodies bound to the cell surface, and also the majority of *natural killer* (NK) cells which lyse various tumour or virally infected cell targets in an antigen non-specific manner. This third population may also include cells with other, less overt, biological properties—possibly including cells with a natural suppressor function (Maier et al 1986), whose relationship to regulatory T cells may be analogous to that between NK and cytotoxic T cells. Indeed, the granulated null lymphoid cell population may play a particularly important role in regulating immune responses.

Finally, macrophages and other phagocytic cells are also important because they act both as antigen-presenting cells (APC) processing antigenic molecules for appro-priate presentation to specific lymphocytes and also in a phagocytic capacity removing debris following local immunological or inflammatory reactions.

Cytokines

Cytokines are antigen-non-specific soluble intercellular signalling proteins produced by activated immune and other cells that act locally to mediate or modify the function of cells. The affected target cells may be neighbouring cells or those producing the cytokine in question themselves; in either case, they will express a specific cell membrane receptor that binds the particular cytokine. Binding of cytokine to a cell results in the intracellular transmission of a signal that will most often activate certain cell genes and thus alter cell function. Most cytokines are able to bind to more than one cell type and are pleiotropic (multifunctional), which means that their regulatory function may differ according to the cell type to which they are bound. Typical functions of cytokines include controlling T and B lymphocyte activation and may, in certain circumstances, include inhibition of other cytokines (Stites & Terr 1991, Roitt et al 1993).

The nomenclature of cytokines is complex and confusing, reflecting the heterogeneous nature of the effects displayed. Included under the broad umbrella are interleukins, interferons and certain cell growth factors. Of particular note are the following:

1. *Interleukin-1 (IL-1)*, a T lymphocyte-activating factor produced mostly by macrophages but also many other cell types, which also promotes a variety of other pyrogenic and cell proliferative sequelae.
2. *Interleukin-2 (IL-2)*, previously known as T-cell growth factor, a polypeptide hormone produced by activated T cells and essential for long-term growth of T cells, B cells and NK cells.
3. *Interleukin-4 (IL-4)*, a similar polypeptide hormone produced by certain activated T cells and important in triggering antibody-directed immune responses.
4. *Interleukin-6 (IL-6)*, produced by many cell types and has a wide multifunctional activity as an acute phase protein in inflammation.
5. *Interleukin-10 (IL-10)*, previously known as cytokine synthesis inhibiting factor, is produced by certain activated T cells and acts to suppress cytotoxic T-cell responses and macrophage cytokine production.
6. *Interferons*, a family of related cytokines produced by many cell types following activation or infection and which act on neighbouring cells to inhibit cell or viral growth, increase human leucocyte antigen (HLA) expression, activate macrophages, NK cells or cytotoxic T cells, and suppress antibody-directed immune responses.
7. *Tumour necrosis factor (TNF)*, produced by

macrophages and activated lymphocytes: participates widely in inflammatory responses acting on endothelial cells, neutrophils and other cells as well as, under certain conditions, being toxic to some tumour cells.

8. *Colony stimulating factors,* family of mostly leucocyte-derived cytokine glycoproteins that regulate bone marrow production and proliferation of cells along the mononuclear phagocyte pathway.

Major histocompatibility complex

The major histocompatibility complex (MHC) is located on the short arm of chromosome 6 and represents a gene cluster occupying about 1/3000th of the total genome (Stites & Terr 1991, Roitt et al 1993). It was originally identified because cell surface histocompatibility antigens (HLA antigens) encoded within the MHC genetic region play a central role in transplantation rejection. It is now also recognized that MHC proteins direct fundamental cellular interactions in the immune response, and also that the genes for several other biologically important proteins lie within this region. HLA antigens are encoded by multiple loci within MHC and express a remarkable degree of genetic polymorphism, with up to 60 closely related alternative genes (alleles) that could be inherited at any individual HLA gene locus. This pool of multiple alleles creates a vast genetic variability and, although some HLA alleles are more common than others, the likelihood of any two unrelated individuals being HLA-identical is extremely remote. HLA alleles are inherited within intact sets (haplotypes) containing all the MHC genes, one from each parent in an orderly Mendelian fashion. There is codominant expression of maternally and paternally inherited HLA antigens.

It has been convenient to divide HLA antigens into two broad classes based on biochemical and functional similarities. Thus, the products of the HLA-A, -B and -C loci are called class I MHC antigens; each is a 43–46 000 dalton glycoprotein associated non-covalently at the cell surface with a non-polymorphic polypeptide called β_2-microglobulin (12 000 daltons) encoded by a gene on chromosome 15. These class I MHC antigens are carried by nearly all nucleated cells in varying amounts, and are essential cell surface recognition molecules identified by cytotoxic T cells. There are also numerous closely related gene loci immediately distal to the main MHC region that have sometimes been termed class I-like or class IV (Jordan et al 1985). There are at least 17 such loci and, although the majority are pseudogenes or fragments, a small number are intact genes capable of translation into protein. These include the HLA-E, -F and -G genes. It is thought that human class I-like MHC genes are most analogous to a region defined for the murine MHC and termed *Qa/Tl* genes; these have a gene structure and

association with β_2-microglobulin similar to regular class I MHC genes, but express less genetic polymorphism and have a restricted tissue distribution; their biological functions are unknown.

Class II MHC antigens (HLA-DP, -DQ and -DR) are cell surface glycoproteins composed of a 32–35 000 dalton (α) chain together with a related 27–30 000 dalton (β) chain; both are encoded within the centromeric region of the MHC and both may carry allelic determinants. Class II MHC antigens display a restricted tissue expression (B cells, monocytes and macrophages, activated T cells and certain epithelia) and are essential as cell surface recognition molecules presenting antigen to helper T cells. The concept that cytotoxic and helper T cells do not bind free antigen but only recognize antigen in association with class I or II MHC antigens, respectively, on cell surfaces has become a central dogma in modern immunology (Zinkernagel & Doherty 1979).

The genetic region between class I and II encodes a closely knit group of genes for certain of the complement proteins—those for factor B (Bf), the complement protein C2 and the tandem genes for the complement protein C4 (C4A and C4B). This region is sometimes known as the class III MHC region. Other genes, not necessarily of direct immunological interest, are also found in this area; these include the tandem genes for the enzyme 21-hydroxylase (21-OHA and 21-OHB) as well as the genes for TNF. In addition, it has recently become recognized that the class II and III MHC region also included genes (*lmp* and *tap* genes) that encode essential cytoplasmic proteins involved in the intracellular processing and transport of antigenic peptides prior to presentation to T cells.

CELLULAR AND ANTIBODY TRANSFER BETWEEN MOTHER AND FETUS

It is well established that fetal red cells can be detected in maternal blood, particularly after delivery, but there is also a progressive rise in fetal red cells entering maternal circulation during the third trimester (Woodrow & Finn 1968). Transplacental haemorrhage can result in rhesus isoimmunization and, more rarely, immunological sensitization to other blood group antigens or platelet antigens has been described. Similarly, some passage of leucocytes into maternal blood occurs, which may sensitize the mother to fetal (paternally inherited) HLA. The prevalence of detection of antibodies against paternal leucocytes will depend on the specificity and sensitivity of assay technique, although 10–20% of women may develop cytotoxic antibody in primiparous pregnancy and up to 50% of women in multiparous pregnancy (Ahrons 1971). Indeed, multiparous sera are the usual source for serological tissue typing reagents. It is known that the presence of these HLA antibodies from previous pregnancies or prior blood transfusions (or, indeed, their absence) does not prejudice the immunological viability of the pregnancy (Jazwinska et al 1987). However, the nature of the fetal leucocytes which sensitize the mother is unknown; these could be Hofbauer cells, other tissue cells or blood leucocytes from fetomaternal haemorrhage.

Transplacental trafficking of sensitized lymphocytes from mother to fetus has been difficult to assess other than when associated with a subsequent abnormality. For example, chimerism has been found in occasional children with severe combined immunodeficiency and runting shown in experimental animals following adoptive transfer to the mother of hyperimmune cells specific for the fetal MHC antigens (Hunziker & Wegmann 1986). The conclusion from studies using cell labelling techniques is that small numbers of maternal erythrocytes may enter the fetus but that leucocytes are generally excluded (Hunziker et al 1984).

Immunoglobulins of the IgG class are selectively transported across the human placenta from maternal blood within the intervillous spaces. The initial molecular event is specific recognition by receptors on the surface of placental syncytiotrophoblast microvilli that bind the Fc region of IgG—Fcγ receptors (Johnson & Brown 1981). Protected cellular transfer of IgG then occurs within intracellular endocytotic vesicles prior to release into placental tissue and subsequent movement into the lumen of fetal stem vessels to confer passive immunity to the fetus. Significant transplacental passage of maternal IgG to fetal circulation commences around the 20th to 22nd week of gestation and all four subclasses of IgG (IgG1, 2, 3 and 4) are actively transferred from mother to fetus, although it has been suggested that IgG2 transfer may lag very slightly behind the others; there is no selective transport of any other immunoglobulin class or plasma protein.

THE SURVIVAL OF THE FETAL ALLOGRAFT

Background

Medawar (1953) proposed various hypotheses to account for mammalian viviparity as a unique example of successful transplantation; these theories created a fundamental basis from which most modern investigations have been derived. Medawar's hypotheses included the following:

1. The conceptus is not immunogenic and therefore does not evoke an immunologic response. However, it is now known that the conceptus itself does express MHC antigens in pregnancy and, for example, that maternal antifetal HLA antibodies are a common occurrence.
2. Pregnancy alters the immune response. It is now accepted that pregnant women are not non-specifically immunosuppressed since normally they neither succumb to systemic or local infection in pregnancy nor, in experimental animals, do they accept

mismatched tissue allografts (including, for example, paternal skin grafts or ectopic fetal tissue grafts). Nevertheless, more subtle alterations to antigen-specific responses remain possible.
3. The uterus is an immunologically privileged site. However, other foreign tissue allografts placed within the uterus will be rejected, even in hormonally primed animals, albeit often after a longer time than tissue grafts at other sites. This emphasizes the unique status of the fetal graft, as do observations in experimental animals that grafts placed at other privileged sites, such as the brain, anterior chamber of the eye or the testis, do not induce transplantation immunity yet are nevertheless rejected if the host has been pre-immunized—unlike the situation for intrauterine pregnancy (Beer & Billingham 1976).
4. The placenta is an effective immunological barrier between mother and fetus. This has been discussed above, and it is also pertinent to remember that both the lymphatic and vascular systems remain essentially distinct for both mother and fetus, in contrast to direct contact in most examples of clinical transplantation. Together with the effect of endometrial decidualization, this may lead to a slight immunological quarantining effect.

Current concepts on the riddle of the fetal allograft acknowledge multifactorial mechanisms, discussed below.

Human leucocyte antigen expression at fetomaternal interfaces

Because of the extensive genetic polymorphism, nearly all human pregnancies involve fetomaternal MHC disparity. Since HLA molecules are the focus of both regulatory and cytotoxic immune responses, the maternal–fetal immunogenetic enigma is central to our understanding of the immunology of pregnancy. It is trophoblast in its various differentiated forms which forms the sole and continuous fetal tissue interface with both maternal blood and decidual tissue. The extensive interfaces between fetal trophoblast and maternal tissues are anatomically complex (see Ch. 4), and it is important to view trophoblast as acting in response to a variety of differentiation signals at these sites. Hence, anatomically defined trophoblast subpopulations may express distinct cell surface antigen phenotypes (Bulmer & Johnson 1985).

It has been consistently established that there is no detectable expression of classical polymorphic class I (HLA-A, -B, -C) or class II (HLA-DP, -DQ, -DR) MHC alloantigens by human trophectoderm and chorionic villous trophoblast through gestation (Hunt et al 1987, Johnson 1992, Roberts et al 1992). However, there is normal development of class I and, later in gestation, class II MHC antigens on non-trophoblastic cells in extraembryonic tissues. The remarkable absence of regular HLA transplantation antigen expression on placental trophoblast is undoubtedly of pivotal significance in protecting this vital tissue from effective maternal immune recognition or cytotoxic cell attack.

This observation explains why there is no rejection response to trophoblast placed under the kidney capsule in experimental animals, unlike for other foreign tissues placed adjacent to trophoblast at this ectopic site (Simmons & Russell 1967). Also, trophoblastic cellular elements continuously break away from the implantation site during human pregnancy, pass into the uterine vein, lodge eventually in the lung and mostly degrade (Thomas et al 1959, Attwood & Park 1961, Kozma et al 1986); this process occurs without provoking any inflammatory or immunological rejection response. It is unknown whether the continuous deportation of villous trophoblastic elements into maternal blood induces a form of systemic immunological tolerance to fetal trophoblast antigens in the mother. However, during the second half of pregnancy, these exfoliated elements will carry the heat-stable placental-type alkaline phosphatase (PLAP) isoenzyme which itself expresses significant genetic polymorphism (McLaughlin & Johnson 1984, Webb et al 1985). Maternal immunity to paternally inherited fetal PLAP alleles has never been described in pregnancy and hence as yet unidentified mechanisms may exist to enable the mother to tolerate these fetal trophoblast antigens but not other polymorphic antigens expressed by non-trophoblastic fetal cells, such as HLA-A, -B or -DR.

Since MHC molecules regulate the T cell immune response, HLA-negative villous trophoblast also may not be recognized by cellular antiviral or other foreign antigen responses. There is some attraction for this concept. Thus, trophoblast in cell culture may have an unusual resistance to cytotoxic effector cells (Clark & Chaouat 1986). In addition, human trophoblast has been shown to contain endogenous retrovirus-like particles and antigenic activity as well as express retrovirus-like RNA-directed DNA polymerase activity; also, it may be involved in the antibody response to retroviruses observed in some pregnancy sera (Johnson et al 1990).

Our understanding of the molecular genetics of how fetal trophoblast exceptionally fails to transcribe regular HLA molecules is still in its infancy, as is the determination of factors that might influence this unusual example of gene regulation (Head et al 1987, Hunt et al 1987). It may require the development of uncontaminated homogeneous trophoblast cell lines to test mechanistic models, although this approach has not yet achieved full success (Loke et al 1986). Thus, at present, it is unknown whether normal human trophoblast can ever be induced to express such transplantation target antigens.

Although trophoblast does not express regular class I MHC alloantigens, extravillous cytotrophoblast populations do express an antigenically related molecule that is not a classical HLA-A or -B antigen (Redman et al 1984, Bulmer & Johnson 1985). This is a class I-like MHC molecule that has been identified as HLA-G and is further discussed below in the section on immunoregulation in pregnancy.

Fetal protection from maternal IgG antibody

Fcγ receptors are also abundant on non-trophoblastic cells within the placental villous stroma, notably macrophages (Hofbauer cells) and fetal stem vessel endothelium. Unlike syncytiotrophoblast Fcγ receptors, the non-trophoblastic placental Fcγ receptors do not bind native IgG but instead have specificity for aggregated or antigen-complexed IgG (Johnson & Brown 1981). This selective binding has been termed the placental sink, since these high avidity Fcγ receptors are thought to act as an extensive filter, sequestering soluble immune complexes formed locally between fetal antigens and any corresponding maternal IgG antibody transported across trophoblastic tissue (Johnson et al 1980). This protective mechanism may be expected to be essential since any such deleterious IgG antibodies and immune complexes, if allowed to penetrate further than extraembryonic tissue, could potentially have catastrophic consequences on the fetus for the development of its own immunological capacity. The trapping of a significant amount of maternal IgG as immune complexes within placental tissue is evident from the extensive immunopathology involving immunoglobulin and complement deposition within normal term placentae (Faulk & Johnson 1977, Johnson et al 1977).

Several situations involving specific antibodies illustrate this phenomenon. Firstly, maternal IgG autoantibodies that are organ-specific and do not have their corresponding autoantigen accessible within the placenta, such as in Graves' thyrotoxicosis or myasthenia gravis, would not form immune complexes and not be retained within placental tissue. These IgG antibodies would be expected to reach the fetus; that this can indeed occur is shown by clinical reports of transient neonatal manifestations of the corresponding autoimmune disease (Scott 1976). Secondly, maternal IgG antibodies to fetal HLA are not uncommon in pregnancy and, following transfer across HLA-negative syncytiotrophoblast, these antibodies would then bind to HLA-positive non-trophoblastic cells within chorionic villi; soluble complexes would be removed onto macrophage and endothelial Fcγ receptors. This process is remarkably efficient in negating maternal antifetal HLA antibodies access to cord blood. Thus, such antibodies with specificity for the present pregnancy are detected in placental eluates but not in neonatal sera (Jeannet et al 1977), whereas the converse is the case for any maternal anti-HLA antibody without specificity for the present pregnancy that may have arisen from a previous pregnancy or blood transfusion (Doughty & Gelsthorpe 1976). Finally, this concept cannot be directly applied to rhesus antigens because these are not expressed in the placenta other than on erythrocytes. Thus, fetal red cell haemolysis by native maternal IgG antibody will occur prior to retention of any antibody on endothelial Fcγ receptors for immune complexes although endothelial cell damage does occur in placentae from cases of maternal–fetal rhesus incompatibility (Jones & Fox 1978).

Immunoregulation in pregnancy

The discussion above describes passive mechanisms for protection of the fetal graft. Current concepts also emphasize a variety of active mechanisms induced by pregnancy-associated events involving production of specific immunological factors or immunoregulatory proteins.

Trophoblast membrane molecules

Human cytotrophoblast populations in the placental bed and chorion leave express class I MHC-type molecules that are unreactive with antibodies to the relevant fetal HLA-A or -B polymorphic tissue-type expected from the paternal genotype (Redman et al 1984). The general rule in normal pregnancy of complete HLA-negativity for all syncytial and villous trophoblast, and expression only of an unusual class I-type MHC molecule by extravillous cytotrophoblast, appears also to hold for pregnancy disorders such as ectopic pregnancy, hydatidiform mole and choriocarcinoma (Earl et al 1985, Bulmer et al 1988). Difficulties in separation of invasive fetal extravillous trophoblast from the complex cellular constitution of HLA-positive maternal decidual tissues has hindered more precise biochemical studies. However, observations from choriocarcinoma cell lines and from baboon placentae have indicated the unusual class I-type MHC antigen to be a 39–40 000 dalton molecule associated with β_2-microglobulin and of limited polymorphism (Stern et al 1987).

It has now been shown that this class I-type MHC molecule selectively expressed by extravillous cytotrophoblast is HLA-G (Ellis et al 1990, Kovats et al 1990, Risk & Johnson 1990). HLA-G is a structural homologue of the classical class I MHC alloantigens (HLA-A, B, C) but shows less genetic variability (polymorphism); whether there is functional homology remains to be determined, e.g. whether HLA-G can present antigenic peptide to cytotoxic T cells and whether HLA-G-restricted T cells are indeed selected in the thymus for survival. Although HLA-G protein or mRNA transcripts may be expressed at lower levels by certain other fetal cells, it is clear that strong HLA-G expression may have evolved in humans for a reason related to the immunogenetics of pregnancy. Since it is expressed at maternal-facing surfaces prior

to establishment of full fetal T-cell immunocompetence, the biological drive for HLA-G expression could be in the context of cognate interaction with the maternal immune system, either to provide T-cell immunosurveillance of fetal tissue at risk of infection or, more probably, for fetal signalling of maternal immunoregulatory responses.

A separate molecular system expressed by both trophoblast and leucocytes was originally identified using rabbit antisera and termed the trophoblast-leucocyte common or cross-reactive (TLX) antigen system. Monoclonal antibodies have since been produced that recognize protein antigens of this family and which exhibit a size heterogeneity between individuals (Stern et al 1986). It has now been shown that this antigen is indeed a cell surface complement regulatory protein called membrane cofactor protein (MCP) or CD46 (Purcell et al 1990). MCP is strongly expressed by all trophoblast populations and by the preimplantation embryo (Roberts et al 1992). The gene for MCP is located on chromosome 1 as part of a multigene family encoding structurally related complement regulatory proteins. MCP is an intrinsic-acting protein that binds C3b and C4b, rather like a cell surface scavenger identifying these components for proteolytic inactivation by a component called factor I. A related complement regulatory protein encoded within the same multigene family is decay accelerating factor (DAF) or CD55. This protein also acts at the level of C3b and C4b and is strongly expressed by trophoblast cell subpopulations, as is a third cell surface complement regulatory protein called membrane attack complex inhibitory factor or CD59 which acts to inhibit the terminal membrane attack complex of complement (C5–C9) (Holmes et al 1992). The strong trophoblastic expression of these complement regulatory proteins at the fetal tissue interface with maternal blood and endometrium would have the effect of negating complement-mediated damage to trophoblast subsequent to complement activation following either maternal antibody attack or local restructuring events and haemostatic alterations.

Together with control of HLA expression, the selective expression of certain trophoblast membrane molecules (summarized in Table 8.1) is thought to contribute to

Table 8.1 HLA and complement regulatory protein expression by trophoblast cell populations

	Extravillous cytotrophoblast	Syncytiotrophoblast	Villous cytotrophoblast
HLA-A, B alloantigens	–	–	–
HLA-G	+	–	–
Class II MHC antigens	–	–	–
MCP (CD46)	+	+	+
DAF (CD55)	+	+	+
CD59	+	+	+

the innate resistance of fetal trophoblast to cytolysis by maternal complement or cytotoxic cells (Johnson 1993a).

Maternal antibody responses

Pregnancy sera have been reported to contain molecules, including many pregnancy-associated proteins and steroidal hormones, which non-specifically inhibit a wide variety of in vitro assays of T lymphocyte proliferation or function (Rocklin et al 1976, Bissenden et al 1980, Stimson 1983, Stites et al 1983). Since extrauterine immunocompetence is not prejudiced in pregnancy, attention has focused on pregnancy-induced maternal antibodies that may serve a more specific blocking function (Lancet Editorial 1983). It is an attractive concept that such blocking antibodies could influence maternal cell-mediated immunity to the fetus. There are several candidates that, individually or together, may contribute to blocking antibody activity in pregnancy.

Although anti-HLA-A and -B antibodies can be detected in many multiparous sera, serological data have shown the majority of reactivity to be directed against broadly shared class I MHC antigenic determinants rather than single specific HLA tissue-type antigens (Konoeda et al 1986). Furthermore, up to 20% of multiparous sera contains antibodies reactive only with activated T cells and not ascribable to classical class I or II MHC antigen specificities (Johnson & Stern 1986). Antibodies to class II MHC antigens can block stimulator function in MLR assays; however, they are infrequent in pregnancy and may not arise until late in gestation when class II MHC antigens are eventually expressed in extraembryonic tissues (Redman et al 1984).

Other pregnancy-induced antibodies that could contribute to an immunoregulatory function include less well defined systems, such as non-cytotoxic antibodies that block Fcγ receptors of B cells (Power et al 1986) and also autoanti-idiotypic antibodies reactive with maternal T-cell receptors for paternal HLA (Suciu-Foca et al 1983); idiotypic determinants are unique antigenic determinants characteristic of the specific variable region of individual immunoglobulin or T-cell receptor molecules (Roitt et al 1993). It should be borne in mind, however, that laboratory procedures for these in vitro blocking antibody assays are technically complex and difficult to repeat. Furthermore, results with pregnancy sera in any one assay system will not necessarily be of clinical usefulness. For example, it is attractive to postulate an anti-trophoblast antibody response in normal pregnancy, although this has not yet been convincingly demonstrated by laboratory assay and remains a matter of some controversy. Thus, the relative importance of blocking antibody to the immunological viability of an on-going pregnancy remains to be defined, and it is still possible that this may be no more than a consequence of pregnancy rather than

of fundamental biological importance for the maintenance of that pregnancy.

Maternal cellular responses

There is little consistent evidence for intrinsic non-specific depression of in vitro responses of maternal peripheral blood lymphocytes to foreign antigens or mitogens (Gusdon 1976, Loke 1978), although there have been reports of impaired specific lymphocyte blastogenic responses to various micro-organisms, including cytomegalovirus (Gehrz et al 1981a,b); this could be due to increased environmental exposure or an inadequate immune response associated with hormonal changes in pregnancy. The consensus is that there is no significant change in the balance between helper and regulatory (suppressor) T cells in peripheral blood (Moore et al 1983). More important is whether maternal cell-mediated sensitization to paternally inherited fetal antigens commonly occurs in a manner analogous to maternal anti-HLA antibody production. It has been shown that circulating cytotoxic effector T cells specific for paternal lymphocytes may occur only rarely in normal pregnancy (Sargent et al 1987).

Events at maternal–fetal interfaces may be of particular importance in controlling maternal cellular or humoral sensitization to fetal antigens. Endometrial tissue undergoes cellular changes in pregnancy with hormonal alterations leading to the decidual reaction and with invasion by fetal trophoblast. Extensive numbers of leucocytes can also be highlighted in decidua (Bulmer & Sunderland 1984). A proportion are class II MHC-positive macrophages, often found closely associated with extravillous cytotrophoblast; these may serve essential phagocytic functions and provide a defence to infection in the presence of local immunosuppression, allowing fetal graft survival (Bulmer & Johnson 1984). However, the major leucocytic component in early pregnancy decidua has been characterized as unusual non-T non-B lymphocytes that phenotypically and morphologically resemble NK cells, although they do not express such strong NK cell activity as peripheral blood NK cells (Bulmer et al 1991). These cells express many, but not all, of the markers of mature NK cells, and could be a form that is in arrested maturation which might otherwise become involved in the removal of flawed or otherwise doomed embryos. Evidence has been presented that selective HLA-G expression by trophoblast might protect it from any NK-type cell attack (Deniz et al 1994). These NK-like endometrial leucocytes are clearly hormonally regulated in their appearance and also occur in any decidualized tissue in ectopic pregnancy. Finally, B cells and polymorphonuclear leucocytes are uncommon in the endometrium, and mature T cells are a consistent feature but become relatively less of the total number of leucocytes when other immunological cell types increase in the secretory phase or early pregnancy

Table 8.2 Immunological cell populations in the human endometrium

	Proliferative phase	Secretory phase	First-trimester decidua	Term decidua
NK-like cells	+	++	+++	+
T cells	+	+	+	+
B cells	–	–	–	–
Macrophages	+	+/++	++	++

(Johnson 1993a). The relative occurrence of immunological cell populations in the human endometrium is shown in Table 8.2.

Local cellular production within uteroplacental tissues of various factors shown to have immunomodulatory properties, albeit sometimes only at supraphysiological levels, may together give some bias towards non-specific immunosuppression at maternal–fetal interfaces (Stimson 1983, Stites et al 1983, Anderson & Yunis 1985); these would include progesterone and other steroids, pregnancy-associated proteins, prostaglandins, polyamines, interferons and, possibly, soluble HLA molecules. There is also evidence that some decidual leucocytes may act as regulatory cells through the generation of a soluble factor which impairs IL-2-dependent lymphocyte responses (Clark et al 1988). However, investigations with heterogeneous decidual or placental cell populations can be difficult to interpret, and the exact nature and cellular sources(s) of decidual suppressor factors await clarification by functional studies with homogeneous cell preparations (Nakayama et al 1985). Nevertheless, there is general support favouring local decidual production of potent factors which inhibit IL-2 activity (Nicholas & Panayi 1986). This could provide a cocoon of an appropriate form of non-specific immunosuppression in the pregnant uterus since a requirement for IL-2 is a common denominator for the generation of cytotoxic T cell or NK cell responses; any failure of this mechanism could potentially lead to an IL-2-dependent cytotoxic attack against fetal tissue.

Two additional concepts are also worth mentioning. Firstly, the placental syncytiotrophoblastic surface is rich in a specific receptor for the iron-transport plasma protein, transferrin, which effectively lines the intervillous blood space and acts as the initial molecular recognition step in the transfer of iron from mother to fetus (Webb et al 1985). However, since transferrin-bound iron is also an essential growth factor for lymphocyte proliferation, any rapidly dividing lymphocyte within intervillous spaces would need to compete for binding transferrin with the excess expression of transferrin receptors on the surrounding syncytiotrophoblastic tissue (Johnson et al 1980). Secondly, an alternative biological role for decidual leucocytes has been considered—that fetal trophoblast may be dependent on leucocyte-derived growth factors (lymphokines) for its development (Athanasakis et al

1987, Wegmann 1987). Thus, local maternal leucocyte activity could be beneficial to trophoblastic growth and function by a paraimmunological mechanism. CSFs are the cytokines which have attracted most interest in this role, and it is of note that syncytiotrophoblast unusually expresses the specific receptors for many different cytokines on its surface (Hampson et al 1993).

IMMUNOLOGICAL IDENTIFICATION OF TROPHOBLAST

The syncytiotrophoblast plasma membrane expresses numerous protein components (Webb et al 1985), although much less detail is known about the surface of cytotrophoblast populations. However, the development and application of monoclonal antibodies has identified many cellular antigens that, taken together, constitute the characteristic cellular antigenic phenotype of different trophoblast populations in the chorionic villous tissue (Fig. 8.1), placental bed and surrounding chorion laeve (Bulmer & Johnson 1985). This approach, based on a panel of monoclonal antibodies, has been useful for the immunohistological identification of trophoblast and non-trophoblastic cell types in abnormal pregnancies (Earl et al 1985, Bulmer et al 1988) as well as for identification of cell types within isolated placental cell cultures (Loke et al 1986).

Certain monoclonal antibodies recognize cell surface antigens with a relatively restricted tissue distribution other than expression by trophoblast; several are also abnormally expressed by various tumour cells and can be described under a generic term of oncotrophoblast antigens, e.g. PLAP, which has proven to be of some value as a tumour marker in ovarian carcinoma and seminoma

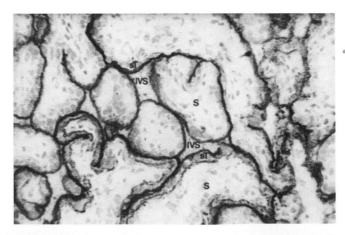

Fig. 8.1 Indirect immunoperoxidase staining of a cryostat section of normal term chorionic villous tissue using the murine H317 monoclonal antibody to placental alkaline phosphatase (PLAP) followed by peroxidase-conjugated anti-mouse immunoglobulin. Note the intense staining for PLAP on the apical surface of syncytiotrophoblast. sT = syncytiotrophoblast; S = villous stroma; IVS = intervillous space.

(McLaughlin & Johnson 1984). However, WHO workshops have screened selected monoclonal antibodies and confirmed the elusive nature of an entirely trophoblast-specific membrane antigen represented on all human trophoblast populations (Anderson et al 1987 and in preparation).

There are two major thrusts for this line of research. Firstly, a monoclonal antibody recognizing a cell surface antigen entirely specific for fetal trophoblast, in concert with a fluorescence-activated cell sorter, could potentially provide a means for isolating from peripheral blood any trace numbers of the extensive amount of fetal trophoblastic cells that are detached from the implantation site and enter the uterine vein (100–200 000 cells per day are oft-quoted figures). This could enable prenatal genetic diagnosis by a minimally invasive technique in situations where there was a sensitive probe analysis available for the inherited disease gene or polyploidy. However, this approach has yet to reach maturity because the numbers of fetal trophoblastic cells that cross the lung barrier into peripheral blood may be infinitesimally small in early pregnancy and also there may be intravascular uptake of trophoblastic cell membrane fragments by maternal cells which would then contaminate any subsequent separation of fetal cells.

Secondly, a specific trophoblast cell surface antigen, expressed very early in gestation but not represented in any other normal adult or fetal tissue, could be engineered to form the basis for future development of a birth control (contragestational) vaccine. Such a target antigen would only be expressed at a defined anatomic site, initially in small amounts and exclusively following conception. The approach fits into a wider development programme for birth control vaccines aimed primarily to meet a developing world requirement and is analogous to that established for very early interruption of pregnancy by prior vaccination against a synthetic peptide representing the C-terminal portion of the β-chain of human chorionic gonadotrophin, a secreted protein hormone of trophoblast. This strategy has achieved an effective repeatable contragestational effect of limited duration in baboons (Stevens 1986), and a WHO-sponsored clinical trial to assess safety and immunogenicity in sterilized women has been completed (Jones et al 1988). A phase II study for efficacy of fertility control in fertile women volunteers is currently in progress.

CLINICAL ASPECTS OF PREGNANCY IMMUNOLOGY

Recurrent spontaneous abortion

Recent evidence has focused attention towards a possible immunological background for a proportion of patients suffering repeated early fetal loss. This is usually identified by three or more consecutive confirmed unexplained first-trimester spontaneous abortions and sometimes divided into two groups:

1. No live births or pregnancy exceeding 28 weeks' gestation (primary abortion).
2. A single live birth or pregnancy of at least 28 weeks' gestation preceding the unbroken series of pregnancy losses (secondary abortion).

Cytogenetic, anatomical endocrinological, infectious and other medical causes (e.g. diabetes) that could contribute to recurring fetal loss will have been ruled out by both clinical and laboratory investigation, including karyotypic analyses, hysterosalpingogram, thyroid function tests and cervical cultures. Immunotherapeutic studies would exclude women with a history of aneuploidic pregnancy loss, detectable serum antinuclear or lupus anticoagulant auto-antibody (see later section), clinical evidence of auto-immune disease or an abnormal full blood count. Thus, these women fall into an, as yet, unexplained group of recurrent spontaneous abortion patients. Their selection is essentially one of exclusion of other causes and clearly it is unjustified to assume a single common mechanism for all cases of unexplained recurrent spontaneous abortion.

Investigation

Whilst animal models of recurrent fetal loss have been described which are responsive to immunotherapeutic procedures (Clark et al 1987), there is little histopathological evidence in humans of immune-mediated attack in the placenta of an abortus (Fox 1978). Nevertheless, it has been proposed that defects within immunoregulatory responses normally resultant from fetomaternal immunological interactions might lead to occasional women suffering RSA because of failure in immune adaptation in early pregnancy (Mowbray & Underwood 1985, Johnson et al 1986, Clark et al 1987). This could involve either intrinsic maternal hyporesponsiveness (which would be partner-non-specific) or absent maternal recognition due to repeated maternal–fetal allelic identity of a relevant genetically polymorphic antigen (which would be partner specific).

What evidence in man is there no support this conjecture? Some work has pointed towards greater parental HLA sharing than expected by chance (Thomas et al 1985, McIntyre et al 1986), although this does not achieve statistical significance at all centres (Johnson et al 1988b, 1993b). Healthy neonates can be completely HLA-identical with their mother (Jazwinska et al 1987) and, conversely, completely HLA-mismatched pregnancies often occur in donor oocyte motherhood; hence there is no gross correlation between fetomaternal HLA disparity and pregnancy outcome. It is clear that parental HLA sharing is of uncertain statistical significance and, more importantly, of neither diagnostic nor prognostic significance (Johnson 1993b). In addition, a significant trend towards increased female HLA-B and C4 locus homozygosity has been described in RSA women, as well as increased prevalence of certain unusual HLA haplotypes, although this does not necessarily involve the majority of patients (Johnson & Ramsden 1988, Johnson et al 1988b). The cumulative immunogenetic data in recurrent spontaneous abortion, although inconsistent between centres, could nonetheless reflect a subtle genetic variation within MHC or the presence of an MHC-linked gene which influences intrauterine prenatal selection. Other studies of serum lymphocytotoxic antibodies, tissue-reactive autoantibodies, total serum IgE levels and circulating T-cell populations also have not identified a major subgroup of unexplained recurrent spontaneous abortion patients that clearly correlates with either the previous clinical history (primary or secondary recurrent spontaneous abortion) or outcome in a subsequent pregnancy (Johnson & Ramsden 1988, Johnson et al 1988b). Thus, these parameters do not assist prediction of clinical behaviour.

There are indications that other pregnancy-induced lymphocyte-reactive antibodies, detected by functional blocking activity in various laboratory assays, are absent in recurrent spontaneous abortion women during pregnancies which abort (Rocklin et al 1976, Beer et al 1985, Power et al 1986, Takakuwa et al 1986). In addition, hyporesponsiveness of maternal lymphocytes reacting to paternal cells has been described in recurrent spontaneous abortion (Beer et al 1985, McIntyre et al 1986), although it is unclear whether this inconsistent observation identifies an intrinsic cellular hyporesponsiveness or action of serum factors within the cell culture assay (Johnson 1993b). Nevertheless, these findings formed the original basis for immunization with paternal or third-party unmatched leucocytes as immunotherapy in unexplained recurrent spontaneous abortion (Beer et al 1985, McIntyre et al 1986).

Immunotherapy

Although the cell source (paternal or third-party leucocytes), timing, dose (up to 5×10^8 cells) and route of administration (intravenous, intradermal, subcutaneous) has varied between centres, initial open studies have indicated favourable reproductive outcome following leucocyte immunization and describe successful pregnancies occurring in 70–90% of cases. Patient referral and selection varies between centres, some of which exclude lymphocytotoxic antibody-positive patients partly because of a risk of anaphylactic reaction and also because its presence indicates that at least one particular maternal–fetal immunological interaction has occurred. One randomized control trial has shown a 78% pregnancy success following immunization with paternal leucocytes compared with 37% following administration of control autologous (maternal)

leucocytes (Mowbray et al 1985). However, two more recent randomized controlled studies have demonstrated no statistically significant benefit of paternal leucocyte immunization in recurrent spontaneous abortion and the control groups achieved pregnancy success outcome figures of approximately 70% (Cauchi et al 1991, Ho et al 1991). Indeed, these figures are close to those reported in untreated retrospective and prospective epidemiological studies and, since placebo effects are undoubtedly strong in immunotherapeutic studies in unexplained recurrent spontaneous abortion, current opinion is leaning towards only a very small proportion that might possibly be helped by such intervention (Johnson 1993b).

Although convenient, repeated immunization of healthy immunocompetent women with viable leucocytes should be approached with clinical caution and considered at present only within research centres with appropriate multidisciplinary interests. Thus, concomitant sensitization to fetal HLA or other leucocyte antigens may occur and could be associated with an increased risk of intra-uterine growth retardation and, at least theoretically, entry of any maternal immune cells could cause fetal engraftment in rare cases leading to graft-versus-host disease (Lancet Editorial 1983, Beer et al 1985, Johnson & Ramsden 1988). Concomitant sensitization to blood group or platelet antigens can also compromise a subsequent pregnancy, although leucocyte immunization may be given with anti-Rh(D) immunoglobulin cover. In addition, transfusion-related risks have to be considered, including viral (e.g. cytomegalovirus or human immuno-deficiency virus) transmission by viable leucocytes. Congenital cytomegalovirus is the commonest infective cause of fetal malformation and hence the cytomegalovirus immune status of recurrent spontaneous abortion couples is relevant when considering leucocyte immunization during the periconception period (Radcliffe et al 1988). Thus, although an attractive approach, it is imperative to remember that detailed assessment as well as long-term follow-up of recurrent spontaneous abortion patients following leucocyte immunization is required before this controversial issue is finally settled.

Alternative approaches may also require further exploration (Johnson et al 1988a). Indeed, central questions focus on the most rational and safe approach to immunotherapy. Further placebo-controlled or comparative studies need to be undertaken to assess accurately the efficacy of active immunotherapy, particularly since similar claims have been made in favour of supportive psychotherapy (Stray-Pedersen & Stray-Pedersen 1984). Equally, attention needs to be directed towards improvements in laboratory identification of women from within the undoubted clinical heterogeneity of unexplained recurrent spontaneous abortion who may benefit from an immunotherapeutic approach. Since immunization is not an insignificant procedure, this is urgently required to improve patient selection and to avoid unnecessarily offering false hope in this area with substantive emotive pressures. At present, active immunotherapy presupposes the development of a relevant immunoregulatory response—which has been elusive to identification by laboratory assays (as indeed has been the consistent identification of laboratory parameters characteristic of trophoblast survival in normal pregnancy). Thus, the exact mechanism of action could involve direct cellular, antibody or cytokine stimulation effects.

Leucocyte immunization may increase apparent fertility and twinning rates (Mowbray, personal communication), hence introducing the question whether immunotherapy could influence very early pregnancy events. More than 30% of all conceptions are lost during the peri-implantation period, many of which are due to cytogenetic or implantation defects. It is difficult to envisage immunological (as distinct, for example, from hormonal) events acting so immediately in response to pregnancy, although factors have been described in very early pregnancy with apparent in vitro immunoregulatory properties. Antisperm antibodies have been reported in unexplained infertility and contrasting results may depend on the precise assay procedure employed (Haas 1987); there is some doubt, however, as to the strength of their biological effect in vivo in women other than in extreme cases of immunological infertility. Nevertheless, since the early embryo might express some of the same surface antigens as spermatozoa, there could be an inter-relationship between embryotoxic and antisperm antibodies in certain cases of recurring occult or early fetal loss (Haas et al 1986). This may be more pronounced in a subgroup of secondary recurrent spontaneous abortion women associated with the development of antibody responses, including lymphocytotoxic and trophoblast-reactive antibodies (McIntyre et al 1986).

Autoimmunity and pregnancy

Childbearing women may be affected by various connective tissue diseases which are themselves linked with particular antibody or HLA patterns, as well as a multifactorial background including genetic and environmental factors (Scott 1984). Some correlation is emerging between fetal and neonatal effects and particular types of maternal autoantibody.

Antiphospholipid antibodies

Antiphospholipid antibodies (APA) autoantibodies are directed against negatively charged phospholipids and are found in various myeloproliferative disorders, acute infections and connective tissue disease, including 15–20% of systemic lupus erythematosus (SLE) patients; APA can occur as IgM or IgG, or both. They are associated with a syndrome that may involve a history of thrombotic episodes, thrombocytopenia and intrauterine fetal death, although additional features can occasionally include

neurological complaints and livedo reticularis. Only a small fraction (up to 10%) of all recurrent spontaneous abortion patients will have significant APA levels. Women with APA need not necessarily have clinical evidence of connective tissue disease at the time of investigation (Scott 1984, Lubbe & Liggins 1985).

APA exert a complicated effect on the coagulation system which led to a rather enigmatic definition as lupus anticoagulant antibody. Thus, in contrast to an association with thromboembolic events in vivo, APA in fresh plasma paradoxically prolong phospholipid-dependent coagulation times in vitro (including the activated partial thromboplastin or kaolin-cephalin clotting times) even when the plasma is mixed with an equal quantity of normal plasma (Scott 1984). APA are also frequently associated with a biologically false positive Venereal Disease Research Laboratories serological test for syphilis. The most promising immunological test for APA so far has been immunoassay of antibody reactive with cardiolipin, a particular mixture of negatively charged phospholipids. This has proved to be a sensitive, if not entirely specific, method for APA detection applied to pregnancy monitoring (Lockshin et al 1985). Low transient levels of anticardiolipin antibodies can occur in many asymptomatic women, but repeated screening in pregnancy is advised for APA-negative women with a history of thrombotic episodes and fetal loss. The conclusions from application of these various assays point to an overlapping family of antiphospholipid autoantibodies, including lupus anticoagulant; these are actively acquired and it is unknown whether they can result from a form of immunological autosensitization in a previous pregnancy (Johnson 1993b).

There is a correlation between maternal APA and recurrent intrauterine death in all three trimesters of pregnancy. APA can bind to cell surface phospholipids of a variety of cell types, including platelets, vascular endothelial cells and, possibly, trophoblastic cells. There may also be an overlap between APA and lymphocytotoxic antibodies found in SLE subgroups of secondary recurrent spontaneous abortion patients (McIntyre et al 1986). The mechanism of action of APA in recurring fetal death might include platelet damage with increased adhesiveness, interference with the phospholipid part of the prothrombin activator complex and inhibition of prostacyclin (PGI_2) production by vascular tissues, leading to decidual vasculopathy and placental infarction; prostacyclin is a potent vasodilator and inhibitor of platelet aggregation (Branch et al 1985). A recent advance in understanding how APA may induce pathological changes has been the discovery that these antibodies in recurrent spontaneous abortion bind to to phospholipids via a cofactor protein, β_2 glycoprotein 1, which is a phospholipid-binding plasma protein also known as apolipoprotein H (Chamley et al 1991, McNeil et al 1991).

Therapeutic doses of heparin anticoagulation, high-dose intravenous immunoglobulin or prednisone with low-dose aspirin, compatible with maintenance of maternal health in pregnancy have been reported to correct the serological detection of APA with subsequent achievement of healthy offspring in many but not all pregnancies (Lubbe & Liggins 1985, McIntyre et al 1986). However, comparative randomized therapeutic trials have not been completed, and it is clear that therapy is not always needed for patients without other risk factors (Lockwood et al 1989). Treatment with prednisone and low-dose aspirin may not completely alleviate the underlying pathophysiology, and a high incidence of pre-eclamptic toxaemia and intrauterine growth retardation has been observed (Branch et al 1985). In addition, a postpartum maternal syndrome of pleuropulmonary disease, fever and cardiac manifestation has been described (Kochenour et al 1987).

Anti-Ro(SS-A) antibodies

Systemic lupus erythematosus (SLE) sera may contain a bewildering array of autoantibodies against nucleic acids, nucleoproteins, cell surface antigens and phospholipids. One particular IgG autoantibody to a soluble ribonucleoprotein, anti-Ro(SS-A), is found in approximately 25% of SLE patients and 50% of patients with Sjögren's syndrome (Scott 1984). Anti-Ro(SS-A) antibodies are associated with photosensitive cutaneous lesions and renal damage, usually in mild SLE; they have also been reported in asymptomatic ANA-negative women. Similar neonatal lupus-like skin lesions may occur in offspring of SLE mothers due to passively acquired maternal autoantibody; there may also be haemolytic anaemia and thrombocytopenia, although the most dramatic association of anti-Ro(SS-A) antibodies is with congenital complete heart block (Scott et al 1983). This lesion is permanent, whilst other neonatal symptoms are transient. The strong association suggests that transplacental passage of maternal anti-Ro(SS-A) or related antibodies is involved in pathological events causing this permanent sequela for the fetus in utero, whilst there is no evidence of a related pathological effect in the mother herself; this could involve either direct action on fetal cardiac tissues or the IgG anti-Ro(SS-A) autoantibody being a marker of a coincidental pathogenetic agent that is transferred to the fetus in pregnancy.

Immune thrombocytopenic purpura

Immune thrombocytopenic purpura (ITP) can have an insidious onset and may only be diagnosed following exclusion of other possible causes for thrombocytopenia. The maternal disease is characterized by destruction of circulating platelets by *autoantibodies*, although these IgG antibodies can also cross the placenta and cause transitory neonatal thrombocytopenia in around 45% of cases.

Maternal risk is mainly from bleeding at the time of parturition. It should be distinguished from the rarer *isoimmune* neonatal thrombocytopenia, which follows placental transfer of maternal IgG antibody resultant from isoimmunization with fetal platelets; the platelet antigen to which these antibodies are directed (PLA-1) is common in the general population, and hence the majority of mothers are positive for this antigen and do not produce antibodies. Testing of maternal and neonatal platelets will determine whether the maternal antibody is reactive with platelets from both individuals (due to autoimmunity) or only the neonate (due to isoimmunization).

Maternal therapy for ITP may involve corticosteroids to reduce the antibody level. Plasmapheresis and, latterly, high doses of intravenous immunoglobulin have also been used in extreme cases with some success. Several mechanisms, which may act singly or in concert, have been proposed to explain the effect of high-dose intravenous immunoglobulin: these include transient blockade of Fcγ receptors on cells in the reticuloendothelial system, protection of platelets by non-specific coating with IgG, antiviral therapy, suppression of antibody production and anti-idiotypic immunoregulatory effects.

Pemphigoid gestationis

Pemphigoid gestationis is an uncommon bullous skin disorder induced only by pregnancy, including molar pregnancies with no fetus or fetal circulation. The diagnosis of pemphigoid gestationis (previously termed herpes gestationis) centres on immunopathological demonstration of C3 complement component deposition at the basement membrane zone of skin. A complement-fixing autoantibody which binds to this site is also found in pemphigoid gestationis sera; it is thought that this may be induced by placental antigens abnormally provoking an immune response which is cross-reactive with skin (Holmes et al 1983). There is a strong association with HLA-DR3 and -DR4, as well as with the HLA-A1, B8, DR3 haplotype, which could reflect an immunogenetic susceptibility to autoimmune reactions. Pemphigoid gestationis usually recurs with subsequent pregnancies; occasional subsequent unaffected pregnancies are associated either with a change of sexual partner or complete HLA-DR compatibility between mother and fetus, indicative of the importance of a paternal genetic component (Holmes et al 1983). The nature of the provoking placental antigen is unknown; nevertheless, pemphigoid gestationis appears to be a rare but fascinating example of a detectable immune response to a placental antigen associated with subsequent pathology.

Blood group incompatibilities

Blood group incompatibility is the most clinically

significant isoimmunization that can occur in pregnancy and results from leakage of fetal cells into maternal circulation, mostly at parturition. Any maternal IgG antibody can cross into the fetus in a subsequent pregnancy and provoke haemolysis which may result in severe anaemia, jaundice, hydrops and fetal death. Rhesus isoimmunization is discussed in depth in Chapter 35. The use of anti-Rh(D) to prevent sensitization demonstrates specific antibody-mediated immune suppression, probably by accelerating removal of fetal Rh(D)-positive erythrocytes in the spleen before the maternal immune system becomes sensitized. Antibodies in the ABO system are nearly always of the IgM type and hence do not cross into the fetal compartment. However, other blood group incompatibilities, notably of the Kell system, can occasionally cause neonatal haemolysis (Beal 1979). Maternal iso-antibodies to Lewis and other blood group antigens may also develop in pregnancy, although these do not cause haemolytic disease of the newborn because fetal red cells express insufficient antigen on their surface (Beal 1979). Maternal antineutrophil antibodies, resulting from iso-immunization, and which may cause a neonatal neutropenia, have also been described but are extremely rare.

Pre-eclamptic toxaemia

Numerous concepts have been proposed to account for the pathogenesis of pre-eclamptic toxaemia (PET), and further consideration of hypertension in pregnancy is given in Chapter 24. An immunological explanation based on fetomaternal compatibility has gained particular attention since the clinical picture fits with that which might be expected in an immune response. Thus, PET is a disorder of the second half of pregnancy, more common in primigravidae, and previous pregnancy or pre-immunization may be protective; an impaired or absent beneficial maternal immunoregulatory response in primigravidae could be counteracted by prior blood transfusion or more frequent preconceptual exposure to sperm or seminal antigens (Redman 1980, Need et al 1983). However, available immunological data now give, at best, inconclusive support (Johnson 1993b).

The placenta is of central importance, since PET can occur in a complete molar pregnancy in the absence of fetal tissue or circulation and it regresses immediately on placental removal. Endovascular cytotrophoblast invasion into spiral arteries in the placental bed is decreased in PET, resulting in inadequate physiological changes and failure to form uteroplacental arteries. These histopathological changes do not show evidence of cellular immune attack on trophoblast or appear to involve a contribution from the decidual leucocyte component (Fox 1978, Khong 1987). Serum APA may be found in a proportion of cases with severe early-onset PET without symptomatic autoimmune disease (Branch et al 1989); this could re-

flect an immunopathological relationship with endothelial cell activation. Immunoglobulin, complement and fibrin deposits in decidual vessels (Kitzmiller & Benirschke 1973) may be the effect of occluded blood flow, rather than the cause; analogous results described in chorionic villous tissue (Sinha et al 1984) may have resulted from placental ischaemia, and similar necrotic foci have also been identified in placentae from insulin-dependent diabetic and healthy mothers. Hence, thee are no sustained data favouring an immune response to fetal trophoblast antigens in PET. Conversely, several wisps of evidence have been put forward to support a reduced maternal response in PET. Thus, a decreased prevalence of pregnancy-induced antibodies to paternal HLA (Jenkins et al 1977) and an abnormal mixed lymphocyte reaction between parents in pre-eclamptic pregnancy (Sargent et al 1982) have been claimed. However, other studies have shown no difference for antigen- or mitogen-stimulated lymphocyte responses between PET and uncomplicated pregnancy (Alanen & Lassila 1982) and there appears to be little concordance of information in the literature on cell-mediated immunity in PET.

There is evidence that PET is a familial disorder with a possible single recessive gene determination (Chesley & Cooper 1986). It is not associated with any particular HLA or blood group antigens, although a weak association with maternal HLA homozygosity has been reported (Redman 1980). A putative role for an as yet ill-defined maternal–placental genetic interaction is supported by other observations: thus, PET occurs more frequently in situations with increased placental mass (including multiple gestation) and in fetal triploidy (Redman 1980). The relevance of a male genetic factor in PET merits further investigation since it has now been shown that heritable paternal rather than maternal imprinting of the genome is necessary for the normal development of trophoblast and extraembryonic membranes (Reik et al 1987). Hence, this could also be related to unusual presentations of PET occurring with hydatidiform mole. Opinion on whether placental antigens or the fetal genetic component appears more relevant in the pathogenesis of PET may be moving towards genetic rather than immunological interpretation.

Gestational trophoblastic disease

Complete hydatidiform moles lack a fetus and have a diploid nuclear genome entirely of paternal genetic (androgenetic) origin; hence, they are completely mismatched with the maternal host (Kajii & Ohama 1977). Partial moles are associated with the presence of a fetus and are usually triploid, the extra haploid component being paternal (Lawler & Fisher 1987a). Choriocarcinoma may follow normal term delivery, molar pregnancy or non-molar abortion; it is often associated with a local mononuclear cell response (Fox 1978). Both hydatidiform mole and choriocarcinoma are discussed in detail in Chapter 31, although points of immunological relevance are highlighted here.

Because trophoblast may be both proliferative and invasive in normal early pregnancy, the distinction between normal and malignant trophoblast can be unclear; nevertheless, trophoblastic neoplasms are of interest because they represent the only naturally occurring examples of genetically foreign (allogeneic) tumours (Loke 1978). Fetal trophoblast antigen expression in both molar pregnancy and choriocarcinoma obeys the same general pattern according to morphological and anatomical classification as for normal pregnancy (Bulmer et al 1988). This phenotypic heterogeneity in choriocarcinoma highlights the extensive differentiation into cellular subgroups that occurs for malignant trophoblast. The unusual granulated lymphoid cells found in normal pregnancy decidua are also found in molar pregnancy but not in uterine tissue in choriocarcinoma, suggesting that these cells are associated with decidualization rather than presence of fetal trophoblast (Bulmer et al 1988).

High serum levels of antipaternal HLA antibodies may be found in trophoblastic neoplasia (Shaw et al 1979, Lawler & Fisher 1987b). This introduces the question as to how these women may become sensitized, since trophoblast lacks classical HLA-A or -B antigens. In the case of a complete mole lacking a fetus or fetal blood cells, the immunogenic source may be stromal cells of the chorionic villi (Lawler & Fisher 1987b).

Choriocarcinoma may be associated with a small increase in HLA compatibility between patient and spouse although a higher risk is associated with the ABO system. Thus, there is an increased preponderance in group A women, particularly with a group O partner, and women with ABO-compatible partners appear to be protected from subsequent development of a trophoblastic tumour following evacuation of a mole (Bagshawe et al 1971, Lawler & Fisher 1987b). How ABO antigens could influence postmolar trophoblastic proliferation is immunologically obscure, since trophoblast does not express ABO blood group antigens, and direct immunological sensitization is clearly not involved, but could instead include the action of a separate gene linked to the ABO system.

REFERENCES

Ahrons S 1971 HL-A antibodies: influence on the human foetus. Tissue Antigens 1: 121–128

Alanen A, Lassila O 1982 Cell-mediated immunity in normal pregnancy and pre-eclampsia. Journal of Reproductive Immunology 4: 349–354

Anderson D J, Yunis E J 1985 The elusive immunosuppressive factors of pregnancy. American Journal of Reproductive Immunology and Microbiology 9: 91–92

Anderson D J, Johnson P M, Alexander N J, Jones W R, Griffin P D 1987 Monoclonal antibodies to human trophoblast and sperm antigens: report of two WHO-sponsored workshops. Journal of Reproductive Immunology 10: 231–257

Athannasakis A, Bleachley R C, Paetkau V, Guilbert L, Barr P J, Wegmann T G 1987 The immunostimulatory effect of T cells and T cell lymphokines on murine fetally-derived placental cells. Journal of Immunology 138: 37–44

Attwood H O, Park W O 1961 Embolism to the lungs by trophoblast. Journal of Obstetrics and Gynaecology of the British Commonwealth 68: 611–617

Bagshawe K D, Rawlins G, Pike M, Lawler S D 1971 ABO blood-groups in trophoblastic neoplasia. Lancet i: 553–557

Beal R W 1979 Non-rhesus (D) blood group isoimmunisation in obstetrics. Clinics in Obstetrics and Gynaecology 6: 493–508

Beer A E, Billingham R E 1976 The immunobiology of mammalian reproduction. Prentice-Hall, New Jersey

Beer A E, Semprini A E, Xiaoyn Z, Quebbeman J F 1985 Pregnancy outcome in human couples with recurrent spontaneous abortion: HLA antigen profiles, HLA antigen sharing, female serum MLR blocking factors and paternal leucocyte immunization. Experimental and Clinical Immunogenetics 2: 137–153

Bissenden J G, Ling N R, MacKintosh P 1980 Suppression of mixed lymphocyte reactions by pregnancy serum. Clinical and Experimental Immunology 39: 195–202

Boyd P A, Lindenbaum R H, Redman C W G 1987 Pre-eclampsia and trisomy 13: a possible association. Lancet ii: 425–427

Branch D W, Scott J R, Kochenour N K, Hershgold E 1985 Obstetric complications associated with the lupus anticoagulant. New England Journal of Medicine 313: 1322–1326

Branch D W, Andres R, Digre K B, Rote N S, Scott J R 1989 The association of antiphospholipid antibodies with severe pre-eclampsia. Obstetrics and Gynecology 73: 541–545

Bulmer J N, Johnson P M 1984 Macrophage populations in the human placenta and amniochorion. Clinical and Experimental Immunology 57: 393–403

Bulmer J N, Johnson P M 1985 Antigen expression by trophoblast populations in the human placenta and their possible immunobiological relevance. Placenta 6: 127–140

Bulmer J N, Sunderland C S 1984 Immunohistological characterisation of lymphoid cell populations in the early human placental bed. Immunology 52: 349–357

Bulmer J N, Johnson P M, Sasagawa M, Takeuchi S 1988 Immunohistochemical studies of fetal trophoblast and maternal decidua in hydatiform mole and choriocarcinoma. Placenta 9: 183–200

Bulmer J N, Morrison L, Ritson A 1991 Leucocytes in human decidua: investigation of surface markers and function. Colloque INSERM 212: 188–196

Cauchi M N, Lim D, Young D E, Kloss M, Pepperell R J 1991 Treatment of recurrent aborters by immunization with paternal cells—a controlled trial. American Journal of Reproductive Immunology 25: 16–17

Chamley L W, Pattison M S, McKay E J 1991 Cofactor-dependent and cofactor-independent anticardiolipin antibodies. Thrombosis Research 61: 291–299

Chesley L C, Cooper D W 1986 Genetics of hypertension in pregnancy: possible single gene control of pre-eclampsia and eclampsia in the descendants of eclamptic women. British Journal of Obstetrics and Gynaecology 93: 898–908

Claman H N 1993 The immunology of human pregnancy. Totowa, New Jersey: Humana Press

Clark D A, Chaouat G 1986 Characterisation of the cellular basis for the inhibition of cytotoxic cells by murine placenta. Cellular Immunology 102: 43–51

Clark D A, Croy B A, Wegmann T G, Chaouat G 1987 Immunological and para-immunological mechanisms in spontaneous abortion: recent insights and future directions. Journal of Reproductive Immunology 12: 1–12

Clark D A, Falbo M, Rowley R B, Banwatt D, Stedromska-Clark J 1988 Active supression of host-versus-graft reaction in pregnant mice. IX. Soluble supressor activity obtained from alloppregnant mouse decidua that blocks cytolytic effector response to IL-2 is related to transforming growth factor β. Journal of Immunology 141: 3833–3840

Deniz G, Christmas S E, Brew R, Johnson P M 1994 Phenotypic and functional differences between CD3⁻ decidual and peripheral blood leukocytes. Journal of Immunology 152: 4255–4261

Dondero F, Johnson P M (eds) 1993 Reproductive immunology, second symposium, vol 97. New York: Raven Press

Doughty R W, Gelsthorpe K 1976 Some parameters of lymphocyte antibody activity through pregnancy and further eluates of placental material. Tissue Antigens 8: 43–48

Earl U, Wells M, Bulmer J N 1985 The expression of major histocompatibility complex antigens by trophoblast in ectopic tubal pregnancy. Journal of Reproductive Immunology 8: 13–24

Ellis S A, Palmer M S, McMichael A 1990 Human trophoblasts and the choriocarcinoma cell line. BeWo express a prenatal class I molecule. Journal of Immunology 144: 731–735

Faulk W P, Johnson P M 1977 Immunological studies of human placentae: identification and distribution of proteins in mature chorionic villi. Clinical and Experimental Immunology 27: 365–375

Fox H 1978 Pathology of the placenta. Saunders, London

Gehrz R C, Christianson W R, Linner K M, Conroy M M, McCue S A, Balfour H H 1981a Cytomegalovirus-specific humoral and cellular immune responses in human pregnancy. Journal of Infectious Diseases 143: 391–395

Gehrz R C, Christianson W R, Linner K M, Conroy M M, McCue S A, Balfour H H 1981b A longitudinal analysis of lymphocyte proliferative responses to mitogens and antigens during human pregnancy. American Journal of Obstetrics and Gynecology 140: 665–670

Gusdon J P 1976 Maternal immune responses in pregnancy. In: Scott J S, Jones W R (eds) Immunology of human reproduction. Academic Press, London, pp 103–125

Haas G G 1987 How should sperm antibody tests be used clinically? American Journal of Reproductive Immunology and Microbiology 15: 106–111

Haas G G, Kubota K, Quebbeman J F, Jijon A, Menge A C, Beer A E 1986 Circulating anti-sperm antibodies in recurrently aborting women. Fertility and Sterility 45: 209–215

Hampson J, McLaughlin P J, Johnson P M 1993 Low affinity receptors for TNFα, interferon-and GM-CSF are expressed on human placental syncytiotrophoblast. Immunology 79: 485–490

Head J R, Drake B L, Zuckermann F A 1987 Major histocompatibility antigens on trophoblast and their regulation: implications in the maternal–fetal relationship. American Journal of Reproductive Immunology and Microbiology 15: 12–18

Holmes R C, Black M M, Jurecka W et al 1983 Clues to the aetiology and pathogenesis of herpes gestationis. British Journal of Dermatology 109: 131–139

Holmes C H, Simpson K L, Okada H et al 1992 Complement regulating proteins at the feto-maternal interface during human placental development: distribution of CD59 by comparison with membrane cofactor protein (CD46) and decay accelerating factor (CD55). European Journal of Immunology 22: 1579–1585

Ho H-N, Gill T J, Hsieh H-J, Jiang J-J, Lee T-Y, Hsieh C-Y 1991 Immunotherapy for spontaneous abortions in a Chinese population. American Journal of Reproductive Immunology 25: 10–15

Hunt J S, Andrews G K, Wood G W 1987 Normal trophoblasts resist induction of class I HLA. Journal of Immunology 138: 2481–2487

Hunziker R D, Wegmann T G 1986 Placental immunoregulation. CRC Critical Reviews in Immunology 6: 245–285

Hunziker R D, Gambel P, Wegmann T G 1984 Placenta as a selective barrier to cellular traffic. Journal of Immunology 133: 667–671

Jazwinska E C, Kilpatrick D C, Smart G E, Liston W A 1987 Feto-maternal HLA compatibility does not have a major influence on human pregnancy except for lymphocytotoxin production. Clinical and Experimental Immunology 68: 116–122

Jeannet M, Werner C, Ramirez E, Vassalli P, Faulk W P 1977 Anti-HLA, anti-human 'Ia-like' and MLC blocking activity of human placental IgG. Transplantation Proceedings 9: 1417–1422

Jenkins D M, Need J, Rajah S M 1977 Deficiency of specific HLA antibodies in severe pregnancy pre-eclampsia/eclampsia. Clinical and Experimental Immunology 27: 485–486

Johnson P M 1992 Immunology of human extraembryonic fetal membranes. In: Coulam C B, McIntyre J A, Faulk W P (eds) Immunological obstetrics. Philadelphia: WW Norton, pp 177–188

Johnson P M 1993a Reproductive and maternofetal relations. In: Lachmann P J, Peters D K, Rosen F S, Walpol M J (eds) Clinical aspects of immunology, 5th edn. Oxford: Blackwell Science, pp 755–767

Johnson P M 1993b Reproductive immunopathology. In: Lachmann P J, Peters D K, Rogers F S, Walpol M J (eds) Clinical aspects of immunology, 5th edn. Oxford: Blackwell Science, pp 2137–2152

Johnson P M, Brown P J 1981 Fcγ receptors in the human placenta. Placenta 2: 355–370

Johnson P M, Ramsden G H 1988 Immunology of recurrent miscarriage. In: Johnson P M (ed) Baillière's clinical immunology and allergy, vol 2. Ballière Tindall, London, pp 607–624

Johnson P M, Stern P L 1986 Antigen expression at human maternal–fetal interfaces. In: Cinader B, Miller R G (eds) Progress in immunology VI. Academic Press, Orlando, pp 1056–1069

Johnson P M, Natvig J B, Ystehede U A, Faulk W P 1977 Immunological studies of human placentae: the distribution and character of immunoglobulins in chorionic villi. Clinical and Experimental Immunology 30: 145–153

Johnson P M, Brown P J, Faulk W P 1980 Immunobiological aspects of the human placenta. In: Finn C A (ed) Oxford reviews in reproductive biology, vol 2. Oxford University Press, Oxford, pp 1–40

Johnson P M, Chia K V, Risk J M 1986 Immunological question marks in recurrent spontaneous abortion. In: Clark D A, Croy B A (eds) Reproductive immunology 1986. Elsevier Biomedical, Amsterdam, pp 239–246

Johnson P M, Chia K V, Hart C A, Griffith H B, Francis W J A 1988a Trophoblast membrane infusion for unexplained recurrent miscarriage. British Journal of Obstetrics and Gynaecology 95: 342–347

Johnson P M, Chia K V, Risk J M, Barnes R M R, Woodrow J C 1988b Immunological and immunogenetic investigation of recurrent spontaneous abortion. Disease Markers 6: 163–171

Johnson P M, Lyden T W, Mwenda J M 1990 Endogenous retroviral expression in the human placenta. American Journal of Reproductive Medicine 23: 115–120

Jones C J P, Fox H 1978 An ultrastructural study of the placenta in materno–fetal rhesus incompatibility. Virchows Archiv Pathologische Anatomie und Histologie 379: 229–241

Jones W R, Bradley J, Judd S J et al 1988 Phase I clinical trial of a World Health Organization birth control vaccine. Lancet i: 1295–1298

Jordan B R, Caillol D, Damotte M et al 1985 HLA class I genes: from structure to expression, serology and function. Immunological Reviews 85: 73–92

Kajii T, Ohama K 1977 Androgenetic origin of hydatidiform mole. Nature 268: 633–634

Khong T Y 1987 Immunohistologic study of the leukocytic infiltrate in maternal uterine tissues in normal and pre-eclamptic pregnancies at term. American Journal of Reproductive Immunology and Microbiology 15: 1–8

Kitzmiller J L, Benirschke K 1973 Immunofluorescent study of placental bed vessels in pre-eclampsia of pregnancy. American Journal of Obstetrics and Gynecology 115: 248–251

Kochenour N K, Branch D W, Rote N S, Scott J R 1987 A new postpartum syndrome associated with antiphospholipid antibodies. Obstetrics and Gynecology 69: 460–468

Konoeda Y, Terasaki P I, Wakisaka A, Park M S, Mickey M R 1986 Public determinants of HLA indicated by pregnancy antibodies. Transplantation 41: 253–259

Kovats S, Main E K, Librach C, Stubbleline M, Fisher S J, DeMars R 1990 A class I antigen, HLA-G, expressed in human trophoblasts. Science 248: 220–223

Kozma R, Spring J, Johnson P M, Adinolfi M 1986 Detection or syncytiotrophoblast in maternal peripheral and uterine veins using a monoclonal antibody and flow cytometry. Human Reproduction 5: 335–336

Lancet Editorial 1983 Maternal blocking antibodies, the fetal allograft, and recurrent abortion. Lancet ii: 1175–1176

Lawler S D, Fisher R A 1987a Genetic studies in hydatidiform mole with clinical correlations. Placenta 8: 77–88

Lawler S D, Fisher R A 1987b Immunogenicity of hydatidiform mole. Placenta 8: 195–199

Lockshin M D, Druzin M L, Goei S et al 1985 Antibody to cardiolipin as a predictor of fetal distress or death in pregnant patients with systemic lupus erythematosus. New England Journal of Medicine 313: 152–156

Lockwood C J, Romero R, Feinberg R F, Clyne L P, Coster B, Hobbins J C 1989 The prevalence and biologic significance of lupus anticoagulant and anticardiolipin antibodies in a general obstetric population. American Journal of Obstetrics and Gynecology 161: 369–373

Loke Y W 1978 Immunology and immunopathology of the human foetal-maternal interaction. Elsevier/North Holland, Amsterdam

Loke Y W, Butterworth B H, Margetts J J, Burland K 1986 Identification of cytotrophoblast colonies in cultures of human placental cells using monoclonal antibodies. Placenta 7: 221–231

Lubbe W F, Liggins G C 1985 Lupus anticoagulant and pregnancy. American Journal of Obstetrics and Gynecology 153: 322–327

Maier T, Holda J H, Claman H N 1986 Natural suppressor (NS) cells: member of the LGL regulatory family. Immunology Today 7: 312–315

McIntyre J A, Faulk W P, Nichols-Johnson V R, Taylor C G 1986 Immunologic testing and immunotherapy in recurrent spontaneous abortion. Obstetrics and Gynecology 67: 169–175

McLaughlin P J, Johnson P M 1984 A search for human placental-type alkaline phosphatases using monoclonal antibodies. In: Stigbrand T, Fishman W H (eds) Human alkaline phosphatases. Alan R Liss, New York, pp 67–75

McNeil H P, Chesterman C N, Krilis S A 1991 Immunology and clinical importance of antiphospholipid antibodies. Advances in Immunology 49: 193–230

Medawar P B 1953 Some immunological and endocrinological problems raised by the evolution of viviparity in vertebrates. Symposium of the Society of Experimental Biology 7: 320–328

Moore M P, Carter N P, Redman C W G 1983 Lymphocyte subsets defined by monoclonal antibodies in human pregnancy. American Journal of Reproductive Immunology 3: 161–164

Mowbray J F, Underwood J L 1985 Immunology of abortion. Clinical and Experimental Immunology 60: 1–7

Mowbray J F, Gibbings C, Liddell H, Reginald P W, Underwood J L, Beard R W 1985 Controlled trial of treatment of recurrent spontaneous abortion by immunisation with paternal cells. Lancet i: 941–943

Nakayama E, Asano S, Kodo H, Miwa S 1985 Suppression of mixed lymphocyte reaction by cells of human first trimester pregnancy endometrium. Journal of Reproductive Immunology 8: 25–31

Need J A, Bell B, Meffin E, Jones W R 1983 Pre-eclampsia in pregnancies from donor inseminations. Journal of Reproductive Immunology 5: 329–338

Nicholas N S, Panayi G S 1986 Inhibition of interleukin-2 production by retroplacental sera; a possible mechanism for human fetal allograft survival. American Journal of Reproductive Immunology and Microbiology 9: 6–11

Power D A, Mather A J, MacLeod A M, Lind T, Catto G R D 1986 Maternal antibodies to paternal B lymphocytes in normal and abnormal pregnancy. American Journal of Reproductive Immunology and Microbiology 10: 10–13

Purcell D F J, McKenzie I F C, Lublin D M et al 1990 The human cell surface glycoproteins HuLy-m5, membrane cofactor protein (MCP) of the complement system, and trophoblast-leukocyte common (TLX) antigen are CD46. Immunology 70: 155–161

Radcliffe J J, Hart C A, Francis W J A, Johnson P M 1986 Immunity to cytomegalovirus in women with unexplained recurrent spontaneous abortion. American Journal of Reproductive Immunology and Microbiology 12: 103–105

Redman C W G 1980 Immunological aspects of eclampsia and pre-eclampsia. In: Hearn J P (ed) Immunological aspects of reproduction and fertility control. MTP Press, Lancaster, pp 83–103

Redman C W G, McMichael A J, Stirrat G M, Sunderland C A, Ting L A 1984 Class I major histocompatibility antigens on human extravillous cytotrophoblast. Immunology 52: 457–468

Reik W, Collick A, Norris M L, Barton S C, Surani M A 1987 Genomic imprinting determines methylation of parental alleles in transgenic mice. Nature 328: 248–251

Risk J M, Johnson P M 1990 Northern blot analysis of HLA-G expression by BeWo human choriocarcinoma cells. Journal of Reproductive Immunology 18: 199–203

Roberts J M, Taylor C T, Melling G C, Kingsland C R, Johnson P M 1992 Expression of the CD46 antigen, and absence of class I MHC antigen, on the human oocyte and preimplantation embryo. Immunology 75: 202–205

Rocklin R E, Kitzmiller J L, Carpenter C B, Garovoy M R, David J R 1976 Maternal–fetal relation: absence of an immunologic blocking factor from the serum of women with chronic abortions. New England Journal of Medicine 295: 1209–1213

Roitt I M, Brostoff J, Male D K 1993 Immunology, 3rd edn. Churchill Livingstone, Edinburgh/Gower Medical Publishing, London

Sargent I L, Redman C W G, Stirrat G M 1982 Maternal cell-mediated immunity in normal and pre-eclamptic pregnancy. Clinical and Experimental Immunology 50: 601–609

Sargent I L, Arenas J, Redman C W G 1987 Maternal cell-mediated sensitisation to paternal HLA may occur, but is not a regular event in normal human pregnancy. Journal of Reproductive Immunology 10: 111–120

Scott J S 1976 Pregnancy: nature's experimental system. Transient manifestations of immunological disease in the child. Lancet i: 704–706

Scott J S 1984 Connective tissue disease antibodies and pregnancy. American Journal of Reproductive Immunology 6: 19–24

Scott J S, Maddison P J, Taylor P V, Esscher E, Scott O, Skinner R P 1983 Connective-tissue disease, antibodies to ribonucleoprotein, and congenital heart block. New England Journal of Medicine 309: 209–212

Shaw A R E, Dasgupta M K, Kovithavongs T et al 1979 Humoral and cellular immunity to paternal antigens in trophoblastic neoplasia. International Journal of Cancer 24: 586–593

Simmons R L, Russell P S 1967 Immunologic interactions between mother and fetus. Advances in Obstetrics and Gynecology 1: 38–58

Sinha D, Wells M, Faulk W P 1984 Immunological studies of human placentae: complement components in pre-eclamptic chorionic villi. Clinical and Experimental Immunology 56: 175–184

Stern P L, Beresford N, Thompson S, Johnson P M, Webb P D, Hole N 1986 Characterization of the human trophoblast-leukocyte antigenic molecules defined by a monoclonal antibody. Journal of Immunology 137: 1604–1609

Stern P L, Beresford N, Friedman C I, Stevens V C, Risk J M, Johnson P M 1987 Class I-like M H C molecules expressed by baboon placental syncytiotrophoblast. Journal of Immunology 138: 1088–1091

Stevens V C 1986 Current status of anti-fertility vaccines using gonadotrophin immunogens. Immunology Today 7: 369–374

Stimson W H 1983 The influence of pregnancy-associated serum proteins and steroids on the maternal immune response. In: Wegmann T G, Gill T J III (eds) Immunology of reproduction. Oxford University Press, New York, pp 281–301

Stites D P, Bugbee S, Siiteri P K 1983 Differential actions of progesterone and cortisol on lymphocyte and monocyte interaction during lymphocyte activation—relevance to immunosuppression in pregnancy. Journal of Reproductive Immunology 5: 215–228

Stites D P, Terr A I (eds) 1991 Basic and clinical immunology, 7th edn. Appleton & Lange, Norwalk, Connecticut

Stray-Pedersen B, Stray-Pedersen S 1984 Etiologic factors and subsequent reproductive performance in 195 couples with a prior history of habitual abortion. American Journal of Obstetrics and Gynecology 148: 140–146

Suciu-Foca N, Reed E, Rohowsky C, Kung P, King D W 1983 Anti-idiotypic antibodies to anti-HLA receptors induced by pregnancy. Proceedings of the National Academy of Sciences (USA) 80: 830–831

Takakuwa K, Kanazawa K, Takeuchi S 1986 Production of blocking antibodies by vaccination with husband's lymphocytes in unexplained recurrent aborters: the role in successful pregnancy. American Journal of Reproductive Immunology and Microbiology 10: 1–9

Thomas L, Douglas G W, Carr M C 1959 The continual migration of syncytial trophoblast from the fetal placenta into the maternal circulation. Transactions of the Association of American Physicians 72: 140–148

Thomas M L, Harger J H, Wagener D K, Rabin B S, Gill T J III 1985 HLA Sharing and spontaneous abortion in humans. American Journal of Obstetrics and Gynecology 151: 1053–1058

Webb P D, Evans, P W, Molloy C M, Johnson P M 1985 Biochemical studies of human placental microvillous plasma membrane proteins.

American Journal of Reproductive Immunology and Microbiology 8: 113–117

Wegmann T G 1987 Placental immunotrophism; maternal T cells enhance placental growth and function. American Journal of Reproductive Immunology and Microbiology 15: 67–70

Woodrow J C, Finn R 1968 Transplacental haemorrhage. British Journal of Haematology 12: 297–309

Zinkernagel R M, Doherty P C 1979 MHC-restricted cytotoxic cell studies on the biological role of polymorphism restriction, specificity, function and responsiveness. Advances in Immunology 27: 51–70

Normal pregnancy

9. Prepregnancy care

Geoffrey Chamberlain

Antenatal care is now a well established feature of all maternity services. Both consumers and professionals see the advantage of such services and in almost a hundred years the system has been modified many times to include advances in knowledge about mother and baby. When regular antenatal examinations were suggested in 1901, however, this was thought a strange innovation. Why should normal pregnant women subject themselves to scrutiny and examination by doctors and midwives? Surely this was an intrusion upon the freedom of women and an unnecessary use of professional time. It was further argued that since having a baby was a natural event, there should be no need to interfere in pregnancy—although, somewhat illogically, it has been recognized for some years that obstetricians and midwives often had to interfere in labour. During the 20th century antenatal care slowly became accepted so that by 1925, 30% of women who delivered in England and Wales were going to such clinics and 95% by 1945. Now, less than 2% of women who deliver have not had some antenatal care and the system has been accepted as the norm.

Similar arguments are now being advanced against prepregnancy care which has been in existence for less than 30 years. The concept was not codified until the late 1970s, when workers in the UK and USA began to suggest guidelines and establish special clinics to see women who wanted advice and occasionally treatment before embarking on pregnancy.

THE EXTENSION OF ANTENATAL CARE

Prepregnancy care is the logical precursor of antenatal care. Since it occurs before pregnancy, it allows a wider series of choices for the couple than may be available once pregnancy begins.

For early pregnancy problems, there are only two options: to continue the pregnancy or to terminate it. Pregnancy termination is a profound step for any couple and for many it is unacceptable; for them there is no alternative to continuing with the pregnancy, whatever the problem and its risks.

For the same couple attending in the prepregnancy stage, a series of options can be offered. In some cases, the effects on the mother and fetus of her chronic disease (or the drugs used to treat this disease) can be more precisely delineated and the exact risks calculated and explained. Although the drug regimen may be teratogenic, it may be possible, in consultation with her physician, temporarily to discontinue medication to allow an interval when pregnancy can be achieved and the embryo established safely; after the first trimester of pregnancy drug therapy might be restarted, since by this time the risk of teratogenesis would be greatly reduced.

In many countries, adoption is still a possibility and may be another option.

If there is a problem with the women's partner being incompatible with the chances of a successful outcome to pregnancy, artificial insemination by donor may be considered. For instance, in severe rhesus sensitization, a decision could be made to use semen from a rhesus-negative donor if the natural partner is homozygous rhesus-positive and if there is otherwise little chance of the woman producing a healthy infant. Alternatively, extra-corporeal fertilization of donor oocytes may be considered an acceptable alternative by society.

After full discussion, a couple can be advised of the risks of the mother or child being affected by an inherited disorder in the next pregnancy. The couple may consider these odds to be so high they do not wish to start a pregnancy and therefore will continue with effective contraception or even decide on male or female sterilization.

All these options are available at discussion in the

163

prepregnancy clinic; it is too late to consider them once pregnancy has started.

The importance of the first visit of a pregnant woman for early antenatal care is stressed. A few women with previous problems may see an obstetrician at 6 or 7 weeks' gestation, but the vast majority do not attend a booking clinic until 11–13 weeks of pregnancy. The avowed purposes of early antenatal care are:

1. To ensure that the mother avoids exposure to teratogens in early pregnancy.
2. To perform an increasing number of investigations which exclude fetal abnormality. These used to be done in mid trimester but soon will be at the end of the first trimester (e.g. ultrasound diagnosis of Down's syndrome).
3. To check basic measurements such as maternal blood pressure and weight before pregnancy.
4. To introduce the pregnant mother to the system of medical and social benefits sufficiently early for her to receive most help from them.

Some of these aspects would be better done in the prepregnancy phase. In most instances, by the time a pregnant woman arrives at a booking clinic for antenatal care, fetal organogenesis is complete and it is too late to give advice about avoiding teratogens. The woman's blood pressure may not be basal if the booking visit is in the second trimester, since many women can reduce their normal diastolic pressure by 5–10 mmHg. Advice about the obstetric future and measures to be taken is better given at a prepregnancy clinic.

It was with these ideas in mind that the author started one of the first hospital-based prepregnancy clinics at Queen Charlotte's Hospital on 9 January 1978 (Chamberlain 1980). Since then, many of the aims of prepregnancy care have changed and the subject is now quite properly generally considered to be one of general health education.

ASPECTS OF PREPREGNANCY CARE

When a couple consult a doctor for prepregnancy care, he or she can be helpful to them in a very short time if properly prepared. To do this most effectively, the tangled skein of treads affecting mother and baby in pregnancy must be unravelled. The doctor must distinguish clearly between those aspects which are unchangeable and those which can be modified; he or she must explain this clearly to the couple, pointing out those factors which are already fixed and cannot be altered.

Fixed features include:

1. The *age* of the woman and sometimes that of her partner.
2. The woman's *parity*.
3. If parous, her *past obstetric performance*.
4. The couple's *socioeconomic class*.
5. The *race* of each partner.
6. The *genetic* and *biological background* of both.

Other influences affecting the fetus or pregnant woman are variable; these are the ones for which prepregnancy counselling can be most effective. Features which might be changed include:

1. *Tobacco* and *alcohol* consumption—twin scourges of modern society.
2. *Nutrition* before and in pregnancy.
3. *Maternal diseases*, existing before the pregnancy.
4. *Drug treatments* being given for pre-existing disease.
5. The levels of *exercise* and *stress* during pregnancy.

Another important feature of prepregnancy consultations is the recognition of complications arising from a previous pregnancy or delivery and advising about the risk of recurrence in the present pregnancy. Many obstetricians consider this should be a part of postnatal care. After the previous pregnancy, those who looked after the woman should have considered all the data about any problems that had occurred and discussed with the woman and her partner the risk of further problems in future pregnancies. However, hospital postnatal clinics are rapidly diminishing and postnatal care is being passed to general practitioners who may not have either all the information about what happened or the expertise to advise about the implications. People tend to erase unhappy events from their memories which reduces the potential benefit of postnatal discussion. It is therefore of some value to reconsider the previous pregnancy problem at some later time. In practice, this forms the basis of much prepregnancy counselling in hospital clinics.

FIXED FACTORS IN PREPREGNANCY CARE

Age

Maternal age has a distinct influence on outcome. For a few years after the menarche, and before menopause, ovulation is irregular, probably because of fluctuations in hormone secretion (Table 9.1). In the premenopausal phase, in the latter part of reproductive life, intercourse tends to be less frequent and this, combined with irregular ovulation, leads to the low fertility rate characteristic of the climacteric.

In addition, in the older woman oocytes, which have been present all her life, have aged and there is an increase in chromosomal abnormalities such as Down's syndrome. The incidence increases after the age of 35 and especially so after 40 years. Other variations or abnormalities are commoner in the older mother, such as

Table 9.1 The proportion of anovular and normal cycles at different quinquennia of reproductive life

Age group (years)	Number of cycles studied	Anovular cycles (%)	Normal cycles (%)
< 15	268	52	16
16–20	495	34	28
21–25	287	17	60
26–30	418	6	85
31–35	822	7	87
36–40	640	4	83
41–45	275	11	70
46–50	67	13	50

Data do not add up to 100% because the variable proportion of cycles with ovulation but with a short luteal phase are not in either column.

monozygotic twins, hydatidiform moles and the presence of a single umbilical artery.

A further feature of increased maternal age is diminished flexibility of the ligamentous and muscular system. In such women, in consequence, pregnancy is a greater burden than in younger women and increased rest is needed earlier in pregnancy. If warned before pregnancy, the woman can make plans to adjust her lifestyle at home and at work; being forewarned, arrangements can often be made more easily than in mid-pregnancy. Despite these theoretical remarks, in many western societies the shift of first births from 25–29 to 30–34 years continues as women wish to establish a place in their careers before starting a family.

States associated with the increased ageing processes of life will obviously have a higher incidence in the later reproductive years. Hence, conditions such as essential hypertension and diabetes increase in relative frequency. It is wise to warn the prospective mother aged over 35 years that she may have to think of reducing or even giving up paid employment at an earlier stage than her younger contemporaries. If this advice is given at a prepregnancy clinic the mother is less disappointed than if she first hears of this during pregnancy. There is a sliding scale of probable complications which are worse after the age of 40 and these have to be freely discussed at the prepregnancy clinic.

Parity

In many ways the effects of parity on pregnancy are similar to those of age. The relationship is obvious, for a woman will obviously be older when she delivers her third child than when she had her second. However, some aspects are associated mainly with increased parity alone. In most societies the risks of increasing parity do not appear until four or five children have been born. In subsequent pregnancies there are increased risks of uterine laxity, fetal malpresentation and postpartum haemorrhage

for the mother and accidents of birth, such as cord prolapse, for the fetus.

Past obstetric history

Many women attending a prepregnancy clinic who have had problems in their previous obstetrical experience want information about the chances of recurrence and must be informed accurately by the prepregnancy counsellor.

The progress and outcome of any previous pregnancy must be obtain in some detail. If the woman is attending the same hospital the information should be in the hospital records but if she attends another unit, it is wise to write to the hospital where she was previously confined to obtain details from her records, unless a very full summary is available. It would have been best if the advice was given by her previous obstetrician at the time of postnatal examination but this is often not done.

Prepregnancy counsellors must be willing to listen to much irrelevant materials. It is essential to allow the couple to talk about what is central to their anxiety. They have normally mulled the problem over in their minds so that it may have been exaggerated and had additional blemishes added. The counsellor should dissect out enough to know what actually happened in pregnancy or labour and offer helpful, prospective advice. The chances of a problem recurring should be based on data relevant to the couple. There is little point referring to publications, however well written and statistically sound, which are concerned with different populations. A good example is the problem of fibroids in pregnancy. Much of the literature refers to American black women, who often develop fibroids at an earlier age than do white women. In most published series, women were dealt with under the American medical system which has very different treatment approaches from the National Health Service.

The recurrent risk rates of common conditions should be known. Some of them are more reassuring once looked at fully. For example, a common problem is a series of previous spontaneous abortions. On the whole, textbooks and conventional wisdom imply a steeply increasing risk of recurrence as the number of previous abortions inveighs but data produced by Warburton & Fraser (1964; Table 9.2) indicate that, in general, the risk of recurrent abortion does not increase greatly after the first. Although the studied number of women having three or four abortions is small, the chances of successful pregnancy seem to be good and a reasonably optimistic assessment can be given. Women who have had more than one previous abortion can be told genuinely that if there was no obvious cause for the spontaneous abortion, the chances of a normal term pregnancy are about two in three.

Nayler & Warburton (1979) have further fractionated the risk of spontaneous abortion in relation to live

Table 9.2 Risk of recurrent abortion in relation to number of previous abortions (Warburton & Fraser 1964)

Number of previous abortions	Number of succeeding pregnancies examined	Abortions (%)
0	5432	12.3
1	1403	23.7
2	385	36.2
3	21	32.2
4	58	25.9

Table 9.3 Risk of spontaneous abortion in relation to past obstetrical history (adapted from Naylor & Warburton 1974)

Past obstetric history	Risk of spontaneous abortion (%)
L	13
LL	14
LLL	14
A	23
AA	36
AAA	33
AL	19
LA	27
ALL	21
LAL	23
LLA	29
AAL	36
ALA	18
LAA	27
ALLL	19
LALL	19
LLAL	34

L = live birth; A = abortion.

pregnancies in multiparae (Table 9.3) among 14 000 reproductive histories. These data show that the risk of a repeated abortion relates not just to the number of previous abortions but to the closeness of any previous abortions in pregnancy order. An examination of 275 couples who had one or more first-trimester miscarriages in Glasgow (Cox et al 1992) showed previously unsuspected or poorly controlled medical conditions in 11 only and only a few had abnormal investigations for antibodies.

Similar data can be obtained by the prepregnancy doctor about the major forms of congenital abnormalities, problems associated with cervical incompetence, preterm delivery, polyhydramnios, multiple pregnancy, pre-eclampsia and intrauterine growth retardation. A review of many of these is given by Howie (1986).

The best advice to give a woman with a previous obstetric problem is to discuss the problem with the obstetrician who will be supervising her next pregnancy. There is much variation in obstetricians' opinions and in their intervention rates after previous events; the couple should consult him or her and feel happy about the proposed management. However, a general indication can be given at the prepregnancy clinic and the doctor there may act as a catalyst or mediator, stimulating the woman to approach her obstetrician, or helping her do so if she is hesitating. It is important at the prepregnancy clinic that no firm rules should be laid down which might clash later with other ideas on treatment. One should avoid giving absolute answers because unforeseen circumstances in later pregnancy may completely alter management.

Socioeconomic class

In the UK socioeconomic class is assessed from the Registrar General's classification of male occupations. The use of the husband's occupation to label socioeconomic class may seem chauvinistic but it is because male occupations still offer a wider range of gradation than do female activities. Female employment tends to group round the home (housewife) and posts connected with secretarial work. In most epidemiological studies nowadays, the partner's post is accepted for a permanent partner who has a job which can be used for classification. When women marry out of their social class, some at the upper boundaries of a socioeconomic class group—the more intelligent and the taller—migrate upwards at marriage but fewer marry into a lower class. Hence the partner's socioeconomic class is a good approximation of the woman's status.

Socioeconomic class represents a marker indicating a most important group of aspects of the woman's youth such as nutrition, diseases, education, attitudes to medical care and genetic inheritance. All these factors influence the woman's obstetric performance. Good correlation and gradients exist between socioeconomic groups and the prevalences of many types of congenital abnormality, and reduced birthweight. Both preterm labour and intrauterine growth retardation are measures of fetal and neonatal outcome and are increased with socioeconomic deprivation. Many of the differences between perinatal mortality rates in different regions of the country are influenced more by the socioeconomic structure of the population than by the provision of medical care and facilities.

Some personal habits are related to socioeconomic status. Cigarette smoking in excess occurs in the same lower socioeconomic groups who have higher rates of preterm labour and intrauterine growth retardation. It may not therefore be correct to say that cigarette smoking causes low birthweight babies; it may be causal, but could very well simply be an associated factor.

No woman can resign from her assigned socioeconomic class, but she can overcome adverse influences. She can, for example, reduce or stop smoking or alcohol consumption, and improve her diet and approach to exercise.

Race

Race again is a marker of a couple's genetic background

and will include factors of varying relevance in differing countries of the world. The differences may be:

1. In the genetics of their race.
2. In the upbringing of the woman or her partner in their youth in another country.
3. In the nutrition of that country.
4. In the schooling and educational standards.
5. In the diseases endemic to that country.

Many immigrants from the West Indies and the Indian subcontinent lived in a very different environment during the earlier years of their lives. Conversely, a black woman born in Tooting, London, and living there all her life may suffer problems relating to the genetics of her race but her pregnancy outcome will be similar to those of any other woman brought up in the environment of south London. Many immigrant families such as West Indians integrate well with their host communities and share their background. Other groups, such as those from Pakistan, tend to live in close communities which reduce the influence of surrounding communities; here, the original nutritional, educational and attitudinal influences may be strong, even when the woman has been born in this country.

Thalassaemia and certain haemoglobinopathies are well known to be associated with race (see Ch. 15). Inherited haemoglobin defects can cause problems for the mother because of increased haemopoiesis in pregnancy, even in those women who are heterozygous or carriers. Prenatal diagnosis of whether or not the fetus is affected may be of vital importance in deciding on further management. It is therefore important to check before pregnancy both for the thalassaemia status and for the presence of abnormal haemoglobins in those who come from races at high risk; this can lead to proper advice for couples on the chances of the problems affecting their potential offspring, and how to predict these problems in future pregnancies.

Genetic background

Some couples are already aware of familial or medical histories which raise worries about the health of their future children. If any condition discussed at a prepregnancy clinic has an obvious genetic background, it is wise to seek the help of a clinical geneticist. In the UK there are regional genetic centres providing a service for counselling and risk assessment for families with known genetic disease. The prepregnancy adviser will be wise to consult early. Clinical genetics is a rapidly expanding subject; those who are experts at genetics can give correct authoritative advice at once. This avoids the series of conflicts and doubts which can be set up in the minds of the couple following incorrect advice given earlier by well meaning but less well informed doctors.

Many conditions not previously considered to have a genetic component can now be shown to have a chromosomal element amongst the multifactorial modes of inheritance. For example, asthma and pre-eclampsia may be shown to fall into this category in the near future. In consequence, the larger prepregnancy clinics should have easy access to genetic counselling and do some work in parallel, with the geneticist attending the prepregnancy consultation clinics.

The geneticist may wish to perform karyotyping of potential parents. This will be useful if a potential or known medical condition with chromosome flagging is present in either parent, in the family, or if a previous baby has been shown to have as chromosomal abnormality. Otherwise it may be necessary to karyotype the fetus in the next pregnancy. This may be performed in cells obtained by transcervical chorionic villus sampling (CVS) at 8–10 weeks, at transabdominal CVS at 12–14 weeks or by amniocentesis at 13–17 weeks with culture of amnion cells of fetal origin. As well as the simple light microscopic examination of chromosomes on which karyometric studies have been based for 30 years, the new potential of DNA recombinant technology is allowing many more diagnoses to be made; this subject is well reviewed by Weatherall & Higgs (1982).

At the prepregnancy clinic it is wise to advise couples with chromosomally based problems which are not currently capable of being treated against undergoing irrevocable sterilization of either partner. The surge of advance in DNA technology is so rapid that treatments may well be available in 5 years' time which will effectively treat conditions which we can at present only diagnose and cannot treat. The subject is dealt with in detail in Chapter 15.

VARIABLE FACTORS IN PREPREGNANCY CARE

Cigarette smoking

One of the important contributions which prepregnancy counselling can make to pregnancy relates to the effects of cigarette smoking. In the UK, 37% of women were smoking in pregnancy (Office of Population and Census Surveys 1981) whilst about 30% of the women of the same age group in the USA smoked (Moore 1980); in Australia and New Zealand the proportion was also about 30% (Hill & Gray 1982). The potential effects of prepregnancy advice were shown when Sexton & Hebel (1984) found that 11% of pregnant women who had previously smoked stopped before becoming pregnant following counselling. In the British Births 1970 study (Chamberlain et al 1975), 42% of women were still smoking at the end of pregnancy, but 59% had been smoking before pregnancy; therefore 17% of the 17 000 women had given up during or before pregnancy.

Effects of smoking

Cigarette smoking can affect fertility by decreasing ovulation (Vessey et al 1978); Mattison (1982) showed that smoking diminished male sperm penetrating capacity and was associated with a higher percentage of abnormal sperms than in non-smokers. The risk of spontaneous abortion in early pregnancy is about twice as high in smokers as among non-smokers (Kline et al 1983). This may result partly from an increased number of abnormal embryos, with which smoking is associated.

Meyer et al (1976) showed a relative risk of preterm labour of 1.5 times greater for smokers than for non-smokers. The same authors assessed the perinatal deaths in their series and considered that about 10% of all such deaths could be attributed to maternal smoking.

As with all findings in the perinatal mortality field, there are no simple straightforward cause-and-effect relationships, but smoking may be associated with other variables such as anaemia, previous low birthweight, high parity and low socioeconomic status. Moore (1980) found the risk ratio for babies born with a birthweight below 2500 g to be 1.9 times greater for smokers than for non-smokers. His analysis in *Public Health Reports* also showed increased risks of spontaneous abortion of 1.7 times and perinatal deaths of 1.2 times greater.

The relationship between congenital abnormalities and smoking is complex. Butler & Alberman (1969) found no difference in the incidence of congenital abnormalities amongst the smoking population of the National Birthday Trust Perinatal Mortality Survey. Most studies, however, have shown a relative risk of abnormalities—some are as high as 2.3 times greater for the smoker than for the non-smoker (Himmelberger et al 1978). These were also related to other factors such as pregnancy history and maternal age. There was in addition a firm association with preterm labour.

Perhaps the most marked associations with cigarette smoking are reduced length of pregnancy and low birthweight. The birthweight effect can be seen in the National Birthday Trust study, British Births 1970 (Chamberlain et al 1975). The mean birthweight of infants born to smokers was 3200 g, while those babies of mothers who had never smoked weighed on average 3376 g—a difference of birthweight of 170 g at term. While babies seemed to be small for dates whatever the length of pregnancy at birth, the effect was greatest after 36 weeks.

Superficially, some women might think that a baby of slightly reduced birthweight would ensure an easier labour. Reduced birthweight is not the only fetal effect of tobacco. There is also delay in maturation which may be serious for the child's future development. Children of mothers who smoke cigarettes in pregnancy have a deficit in reading ability and educational testing standards up to the age of 11. Persuading a potential mother to stop smoking before pregnancy starts is perhaps the best present she can give her future child.

Mechanisms

The cause of deficient birthweight among smoking mothers is unknown. It may be due to the action of nicotine constricting the placental bed blood vessel flow. Secondly, since carbon monoxide (found in tobacco smoke) binds preferentially to fetal haemoglobin excluding oxygen, the higher fetal carboxyhaemoglobin levels probably reduce oxygen delivery to fetal tissues. Thirdly, smoking may have a direct toxic effect on the syncytiotrophoblast, reducing the transfer of amino acids and other nutrients (Browne 1989).

Prepregnancy care

Prepregnancy advisers should warn women about the increased risks of smoking in pregnancy. There is a graduated fetal response to maternal inhaled cigarette smoke and there is no cutoff point below which it can be said not to affect the fetus. The only advice is no smoking in the lead-up time to pregnancy.

More difficult is the problem of passive smoking. In theory, if a non-smoking woman lives in the atmosphere of her husband's cigarette smoke, the fetus could receive a tertiary effect of the smoke. But concentrations are very low and firm evidence on this is not yet clear.

Alcohol

Alcohol is a fetal teratogen in early gestation and also has effects on fetal growth throughout the whole of pregnancy. Like cigarette smoking, there seems to be no critical dose and if a woman seeking pregnancy is already concerned, she should be advised not to drink any alcohol at all. At the other end of the scale is binge drinking, with a large amount of alcohol being consumed on one occasion. These are two different alcohol-related problems to pregnancy and prepregnancy counsellors should be prepared to address themselves to either.

Extent of the problem

The extent of women's drinking in the prepregnancy age group is difficult to assess. Little (1976) reported a poor correlation between questions about alcohol intake asked by the obstetrician at the antenatal clinic and answers obtained by skilled interviewers. In consequence, estimates obtained by questioning at antenatal clinics may under-represent the problem. Wright et al (1983) found 44% of a west London population of women attending for antenatal care admitted taking alcohol. Cox et al (1992) examined 1075 women's records at their prepregnancy clinic in Glasgow, finding that 74% were occasional alcohol users with 1% drinking heavily (more than 20 units a week). Newman (1986) reported 54% of a Tasmanian population drinking, while even higher levels were found in a recent study in Dundee examining a population of women attending for antenatal care (Sulaiman et al 1988). Using questionnaires and gamma glutamine transferase activity, they showed that, before realizing they were pregnant, more than 90% of the women drank alcohol. In the first 4 months of pregnancy the proportion consuming alcohol reduced by 56%; 58% of women who drank were consuming less than 50 g of alcohol a week before pregnancy while 19% took over 100 g a week. In the Dundee study, after adjustment for the effects of the other variables, an alcohol intake of more than 120 g per week was significantly related to a shorter gestational age and a lower Apgar score at 5 minutes. The Dundee study was unable to show a detectable effect on fetus or neonate of a maternal alcohol consumption below 100 g a week.

Mechanism

Alcohol is a tissue poison and probably affects the growing fetus at the time of maximum cell division. However, for many years the effects have been so gradual that people have not noticed. Smoking has received its reprobation because of the very obvious effects on the lung where most of the tobacco smoke goes. If alcohol ingestion produced cancer of the stomach, people would be much more willing to believe that it was a major problem. Its effect on organs like the brain is gradual and long-term; this allows doubt about the effects of alcohol taken in pregnancy to develop in the minds of the observers.

The effect of maternal alcohol on an unborn child is even more remote. It has been known for many years that alcohol can affect the fetus for the placenta is no barrier to alcohol; it is distributed in the fetus in direct proportion to the water content of the tissues so that organs with a high proportion of water, such as the fetal brain, are particularly exposed to the potentially harmful effects of alcohol. Since the blood alcohol clearance rate of the fetus at term is only half that of the mother, the fetal compartments maintain higher levels for longer than do the maternal compartments. Lemoine et al (1968) showed that among infants born to alcoholic mothers, the effect on the fetus relates to the maturation of fetal liver enzymes in the second trimester of pregnancy. In the first trimester, alcohol is handled as though the fetus is another body compartment of the mother while in the second trimester, alcohol effects may be modified by maturing fetal liver enzymes.

Many women reduce alcohol intake spontaneously when they realize they are pregnant, possibly because of a fear of affecting the baby. Raised oestrogen levels may play a part by removing the desire to drink alcohol, a phenomenon noted amongst women taking combined oral contraception as well as those in early pregnancy.

Fetal alcohol syndrome

The fetal alcohol syndrome is a group of neonatal features characterized in association with higher alcohol drinking. On the basis of 245 cases, the Fetal Alcohol Study Group (Majewski 1981) has defined the criteria outlined in Table 9.4.

Growth retardation is symmetrical, indicating an early intrauterine influence rather than late malnutrition. There is a lack of catch-up growth after delivery.

The face is used as a characteristic area by those who diagnose the condition. In many ways it is reminiscent of those in children born with Cornelia Lang syndrome, or of babies of mothers with phenylketonuria. The diagnosis is not very specific but the baby with true fetal alcohol syndrome has microphthalmia with short palpebral features, prominent epicanthic folds and often a squint. There is a short, retroussé nose and the whole mid-face seems squashed or frog-like. The philtrum is not well formed and the upper lip is thin. Ears may be low-set (as they are in so many conditions) and rotated posteriorly.

Milder degrees of alcohol consumption may produce more subtle effects on the fetus. About 20% of children born to mothers who had drunk heavily in pregnancy but did not have the full diagnostic criteria of a fetal alcohol syndrome have been shown by Shawitz et al (1980) to be generally small, with a low IQ, hyperactive behaviour and failing to progress at school.

Other hazards

Alcohol consumption in early pregnancy relates to

Table 9.4 Characteristics of the fetal alcohol syndrome

Characteristic facial features
  Microcephaly
  Microphthalmia
  Short palpebral fissures
  Poorly developed philtrum
  Narrow vermilion border of upper lip

Central nervous system involvement
  Mental retardation
  Developmental delay
  Hyperactivity
  Neurological abnormality

Intrauterine growth retardation
  Less than tenth percentile for gestational age of:
    Birthweight
    Length
    Head circumference

embryonic morbidity. Moderate alcohol intake has been associated with increased spontaneous abortion rates, even adjusting for maternal age, previous abortions, the stage of gestation and smoking habits. It has been reported that there is a two-times increased risk of spontaneous abortion with as little as two drinks a week (Kline et al 1980). Wright et al (1983) examined 900 pregnancies in London. Women were classified as heavy drinkers (more than 10 drinks a week), moderate drinkers (5–10 drinks a week) or light drinkers (less than 5 drinks a week). The heavy drinking group had a two times greater risk factor of having a low birthweight baby, compared with those in the light-risk group.

Binge drinking

Binge drinking is harder to document but may be the real associate of the fetal alcohol syndrome, as excessive alcohol intake may impair the transfer of nutrients across the placenta at crucial stages in the development of the fetus.

Other variables such as caffeine and nicotine need to be assessed separately from alcohol intake, for high consumption of these three drugs commonly goes together.

Advice

Prepregnancy advice is difficult in this field. On the one hand, there are authoritative groups such as the Royal College of Psychiatrists (1982) who advised no alcohol intake in the prepregnancy phase or during pregnancy. This measure is draconian and may drive women who are used to alcohol into other abuses. The Dundee study indicated that moderate to light drinking had little effect on fetal health (Sulaiman et al 1988). The more studies produced, the more difficult it is to be dogmatic, but it may be that a high blood alcohol concentration achieved in a given episode of binge drinking has more serious effects on the fetus than the background daily average. If one of these peaks of alcohol consumption happened to correspond with a critical time of embryo development, it could be important. The detrimental effect of binge drinking may be more important than a constant low rate of social drinking.

Nutrition

If we believe that *we are what we eat* then we should logically concur that *the fetus is what its mother eats*. Generally, what people eat is decided by their appetite more than any other single factor. In pregnancy itself, many myths exist about the amount that should be eaten. The Victorian idea of eating for two has probably been overcome in the western world but it still exists in many developing countries. In its place has come the myth of supplementation with vitamin and trace elements, an idea of the 1930s which still persists in some western societies.

If a woman is eating a normal diet, she is almost certainly providing enough of nutrients for her fetus to develop and grow normally. A major aspect of nutrition is the energy balance. During pregnancy a woman takes in about 2400 kcal/day in order to satisfy her energy needs. Assuming this comes from a mixed diet, it will contain more than enough of all the other constituents required in nutrition. For instance, there will be more than 10 g of protein a day; most of the vitamin and all the mineral requirements will be provided. Hence, if a good mixed diet is taken to the level at which a woman feels she needs it, there is no need for any supplementation or manipulation of the diet. This obviously does not apply to women who are having unusual diets, such as vegans or those with intestinal absorption diseases, but they are a small minority.

Different nutrients are handled in different ways and the nutritional needs of pregnancy should be seen to be aimed at a common purpose rather than manipulated by a common mechanism. Hence, it is meddlesome for us to interfere, changing complex patterns by supplementing perceived needs such as certain vitamins, proteins or even iron and folate. In the prepregnancy period, general advice is that a diet should contain less fatty meats, sugar and salt and more proteins, vegetables, cereals and fibre. This would provide most of the protein need, the energy requirements and more vitamins and minerals that women require. In the western world, nutrition is rarely deficient in a person taking a non-fad diet.

Nutritional status does have an effect upon ovulation and readers are referred to a good review by Warren (1983). If fat stores are low, menarche is delayed, ovulation is infrequent and may even stop. When fat stores are replaced in normal women, there is usually a return of normal pituitary ovarian activity. When consulting a prepregnancy counsellor, a couple's diet should be reviewed to ensure that it provides adequate amounts of protein, vitamins and mineral-containing foods. There is little point in supplementing vitamins if the diet is normal; additional minerals are rarely needed.

There are organizations which believe that many pregnancy problems are due to lack of vitamins or minerals. They place much emphasis on the international standards of requirements for pregnant women. Such recommendations are very suspect. They usually advise quantities greatly in excess of the needs of the body, even in pregnancy. To compare this poor database with measurements of the mineral content of various body fluids or hair merely compounds confusion. There is little evidence that the mineral content of any of these fluids or tissues relates to the correct tissue content, except in severe deficiencies. Further, to add extra minerals to the diet does not of necessity mean they will be absorbed, and even if they are, they may not be metabolized along usual pathways. Finally, there is little evidence that exogenous administration of minerals to correct levels in peripheral tissues is of help in prepregnancy care, or improves fetal or neonatal outcome; such attempts are generally dismissed by recognized nutritionists.

One aspect of a potential vitamin deficiency has received much publicity in the prepregnancy sphere. Several reports have been published about women who, having previously had a baby with a neural tube defect, have taken mixed vitamin supplements in early pregnancy and are claimed to have a lower risk of having a subsequent baby born with central nervous system abnormalities (Smithells et al 1983). In order to ensure the availability of these vitamins in very early pregnancy, the vitamin supplements had to be started in the prepregnancy time. These studies were not designed to distinguish which of the micronutrients were effective; in some cases the doses used were higher than physiological. Such has been the concern that the Medical Research Council has mounted a multicentre randomized controlled trial to test the potential benefit of folate and multivitamins independently; this is proceeding at the moment and should be finished in the early years of the next decade. Even if the study does show improvement and a lowering of risk amongst those women in the trial, it does not automatically mean that normal women who have never given birth to a baby with a neural tube defect would also benefit from receiving vitamins. It is important that the prepregnancy counsellor advises couples that there is no proven benefit from taking vitamins unless there is a need for them. The argument that vitamins can do no harm but might do some good is a false one. Clinical syndromes of hypervitaminosis have been described for most vitamins.

At the prepregnancy clinic, advisers can persuade individuals to avoid any persistent dietary excesses so that when they do become pregnant, they can easily adopt a healthy diet and provide all the appropriate nutrition for the growing fetus.

Pre-existing medical diseases

Women who have chronic disease from their youth are often anxious about the possible effects of the disease on pregnancy. Mostly, the fears are about the effects of the disease on the fetus but the prepregnancy counsellor should also remember the potential effects of the pregnancy on the disease. Women may consult the physician who is in charge of their particular disease but he or she may not be very experienced about its management in pregnancy. It therefore needs an obstetrician or physician who has looked after this condition in pregnancy to give advice at a prepregnancy clinic on the dual aspects of the disease affecting the pregnancy, and of pregnancy affecting the disease. A further aspect is the pharmacological therapy of any disease, which can be of more serious import to the fetus than the condition itself; this should be carefully considered.

Generally, women in the childbearing years are fit and

Table 9.5 Some long-term medical conditions in women attending the prepregnancy clinic at St George's Hospital from 1989 to 1992

Cardiac diseases
  Rheumatic mitral stenosis
  Rheumatic aortic incompetence
  Congenital diseases
    Eisenmenger's syndrome
    Fallot's tetralogy
    Aortic coarctation
  Women with artificial heart valves
  Supraventricular tachycardia

Hypertension
  Essential hypertension
  Renal hypertension

Respiratory diseases
  Asthma
  Sarcoidosis
  Cystic fibrosis
  Bronchiectasis

Haemorrhagic diseases
  Thrombocytopenia purpura
  von Willebrand's disease
  Leukaemia
  Deep vein thrombosis
  Pulmonary embolism

Urinary diseases
  Renal stone
  Renal failure
  Acute nephritis
  Chronic nephritis
  Stress incontinence
  Time incontinence

Connective tissue diseases
  Lupus erythematosus
  Rheumatoid arthritis

Endocrine problems
  Diabetes
  Hyperthyroidism
  Hypothyroidism
  Addison's disease
  Congenital adrenal hyperplasia
  Carcinoma of the breast

Neurological conditions
  Epilepsy
  Multiple sclerosis
  Peripheral neuritis

only a few have any long-term illnesses. Table 9.5 shows the conditions present in women who have attended the author's prepregnancy clinic in a 3-year period. In a review of a Glasgow prepregnancy clinic in the 1980s, Cox et al (1992) reported that 240 of 1075 women attending suffered from a chronic disease.

The prepregnancy advice for women whith these conditions is well reviewed by de Swiet (1994) who considers all the diseases occurring in this age group and their therapies.

Stress

This word is one of the four hangovers left in modern medicine from Victorian times when doctors were mainly concerned with symptoms. Words such as shock, miasma, pyrexia or toxaemia have been replaced by terms based more scientifically on the underlying pathophysiology of the various disorders. Stress is still recognized in modern medicine, however, having effects at most times of life. It would be surprising therefore if it did not affect early pregnancy, but its effects remain difficult to quantify.

In the prepregnancy clinic, the subject of stress is often raised by couples as a potential cause of problems. They see the economic and work stresses to which women are subjected in the 1980s as a potential cause of problems and expect doctors to understand what they are talking about. Sometimes the questions relate to specific stresses such as previous pregnancy loss in relation to future pregnancies (Barnett et al 1983). Unfortunately they are usually much more general and vague and the importance of psychosocial stress as a cause of pregnancy pathology has now become inflated to an entirely unrealistic level in the minds of many lay people. The *Schedule of Recent Experiences* is a commonly used questionnaire to measure stress but its questions are very tightly phrased and do not allow much variation within the experience expressed. *Life Event Scales* may be useful for acute phenomena but are poor at measuring more chronic problems such as an unsatisfactory marriage or living beyond available means.

The prepregnancy counsellor's advice should avoid adding to stress. For example, if a woman has for many years had a glass of sherry before dinner or a glass of wine with her meals, unnecessary stress might be induced by advising her to cut out all alcohol to achieve a normal pregnancy result. Prepregnancy care is a sensitive area; badly done it can cause more harm than good.

Najman et al (1983) consider that altered neuroendocrine functions resulting from stress may influence fertility. Norbeck & Tilden (1983) have reported increased pregnancy complications after life stresses in the year preceding pregnancy. In such women, continuing stress may be associated with preterm delivery and with increased need for analgesia in labour. A comprehensive review has been written by Haddad (1989), while the lasting influence of women's emotions in pregnancy on the subsequent development of the child is addressed by Wolkind (1981). The fact that there is still too little evidence in the field to answer these questions should be borne in mind when giving advice in the prepregnancy period.

Work

Couples attending a prepregnancy clinic are often concerned about the potential effect of work done by the female partner on future pregnancy. This problem has increased in the last decade because more women are working out of the home and more women are working later in pregnancy. There is no barrier at 28 weeks of pregnancy and many women work up to even 38 or 39 weeks.

There are two main reasons for this. First, many women, particularly in social classes I and II, wish to advance their careers by promotion and this is best done between the ages of 25 and 35, which are also the childbearing years. In consequence, career and childbearing may compete. Secondly, most young couples nowadays entering marriage have a double income and their whole lifestyle depends upon this. With the poor maternity allowances in this country, giving up work because of pregnancy carries an almost unacceptable financial penalty.

When discussing the problems of women's work, couples must appreciate early that every woman works at home and although there may be fewer hazards there, the physical work is as great or greater than when working outside. There are no rest rooms or facilities for days off; often there are other children or the couple's parents to be looked after (Kapadia & Chamberlain 1995).

As well as doing their own housework, many women take on additional paid work outside the house. In only a small proportion does this involve specific environmental hazards of a chemical, physical or biological nature. For example, female anaesthetists, radiologists and teachers are at higher risk, respectively, from contact with inhalant gases, from X-rays or from children with rubella. Any known hazards should be identified and avoided. A careful history must be taken about the mother's work and if the counsellor is uncertain about any risk, enquiries should be made through the health and safety officers or the relevant trade union. A good introduction to the problem of chemical hazards is the comprehensive review by Barlow & Sullivan (1982).

From time to time, particular aspects become a source of many questions and public interest increases. Working during pregnancy at visual display units was a source of anxiety for five years. Whilst it is hard to prove a negative, so many studies have now indicated they are associated with no harm to pregnant women that 'statements to the contrary are not soundly based'. This quotation and a good review of the whole subject is provided by Blackwell & Chang (1988). An important form of work in western countries among women in social classes I and II are the increased loads in leisure when athletic exercise can easily lead to a degree of physical activity well beyond any endured in house or paid work. Extremes of physical work could result in lower blood flow through the spiral arteries to the placental bed. This change is exaggerated in women with complicated pregnancies where there could be malperfusion already in the afferent blood supply, for example in pre-eclampsia. Social sports cause no problems to normal pregnant women and their fetuses but extreme competitive sports should be avoided.

As well as specific hazards that cause anxiety, many

couples need to be reminded that the effects of fatigue and boredom at work—whether paid or unpaid—are important. The first by Mamelle et al (1984) looked at the harder-to-measure indices of boredom, noise and the effects of standing jobs, and also examined physical work in the open air, as opposed to that done sitting at desks. They were able to correlate low birthweight and preterm labour with an increasing number of fatigue measures. Because of the difficult nature of isolating any one factor, particularly those relating to socioeconomic class and age, regression analysis was carried out for these and for parity, ethnic origin, past obstetric history and pathology in the current pregnancy. The various factors found at work, especially mental stress and environmental conditions leading to boredom and tiredness, still showed an association with a bad obstetric outcome. Multivariant analysis of selected subsets of female textile workers in Anhui, China by Xiping Xu et al (1994) showed adjusted odds ratios for preterm birth was 2.0 (95% CI 1.1–3.4) and for low birthweight 2.1 (95% CI 1.1–4.1). Other workers using different methods of analysis do not confirm these associations with hard work (e.g. Klebanoff et al 1990). A wide review of the whole subject of the effect of work in pregnancy has been recently published by Chamberlain (1993).

In giving advice at the prepregnancy clinic, the obstetrician must be careful to avoid causing undue worry. A balance is needed in deciding between the hazards that might exist at work compared with the boredom or dissatisfaction which could result from stopping work. For many women, getting out of the house during the day is important; they enjoy meeting others at work and doing non-stressful work. It is inadvisable for prepregnancy counsellors to be too didactic. It is probably safest to concentrate on women with previous obstetric problems such as preterm labour or low birthweight babies to try to ensure that they are not subjecting themselves to inadvisable levels to work, travel or stress. There is a little evidence that if such women did less strenuous work in late pregnancy they would have a better chance of continuing pregnancy for longer and having a baby of a reasonable size. It is less sure however if the baby's birthweight is increased or the length of gestation prolonged that the infant will automatically enter the level of perinatal mortality or morbidity of the heavier or longer pregnancy group, independent of the condition causing the hazard.

WIDER PREPREGNANCY CARE

Full prepregnancy care should be set out like an archery target. In the centre is the prepregnancy clinic acting as the apex of a series of levels of prepregnancy care. It is staffed by an obstetrician, considering precise medical conditions or past obstetric problems, and is essential for those who have such problems. The next ring of the target is a slightly less intense level where prepregnancy care can be given in groups. Advice can be given to five or six couples who attend the contraceptive clinic, for example, and who may wish to ask questions or develop further consultations from this. The prepregnancy workers on this level answer general questions about health and diet and perform checks on haemoglobin, rhesus or rubella status and haemoglobinopathies. Such a clinic is well run by a trained midwife who can deal with six to eight couples in the course of an evening, referring to the specialist clinic problems which she feels need more consultation.

In the outer zone of the target of prepregnancy care, personnel may go out to youth clubs and schools to talk to young people before pregnancy is imminent. This may influence them and also allows them to consider their reproductive future. Such dissemination of simple information about functions can also be helped by the use of the mass media, including radio and television, for these have more influence than the written word in some segments of the population.

All this is prepregnancy care; whilst consultant obstetricians may see the obvious advantages of the formal clinic setting to which they are used, they must also be prepared to take themselves out to the community and to the public, so influencing attitudes at the times when they are being formed.

REFERENCES

Barlow S, Sullivan F 1982 Reproductive hazards of industrial chemicals. Academic Press, London
Barnett B, Harma B, Parker G 1983 Life event scales for obstetric groups. Psychosomatic Research 27: 313–320
Blackwell R, Chang A 1988 Visual display units and pregnancy. British Journal of Obstetrics and Gynaecology 95: 446–453
Browne A 1989 Placental transfer of amino acids. Contemporary Reviews in Obstetrics and Gynaecology 1: 22–28
Butler N, Alberman E 1969 Perinatal problems. Livingstone, London
Chamberlain G 1980 The prepregnancy clinic. British Medical Journal 281: 29–30
Chamberlain G 1993 Work in pregnancy. American Journal of Industrial Medicine 23: 559–573

Chamberlain R, Chamberlain G, Haslett B, Claireaux A 1975 British births 1970. Heinemann Medical, London, p 19
Cox M, Whittle M, Kingdom J, Ryan G 1992 Prepregnancy counselling experience from 1075 cases. British Journal of Obstetrics and Gynaecology 99: 873–876
de Swiet M 1986 Pre-existing medical disease. In: Chamberlain G, Lumley J (eds) Prepregnancy care. John Wiley, Chichester
de Swiet M 1994 Medical disorders in obstetrical practice. Blackwell Scientific, Oxford
Haddad A 1989 Anxiety in pregnancy. Contemporary Reviews in Obstetrics and Gynaecology 2: 123–133
Hill D J, Gray N 1982 Patterns of tobacco smoking in Australia. Medical Journal of Australia 1: 23–25

Himmelberger D, Brown B, Cohen E 1978 Cigarette smoking during pregnancy. American Journal of Epidemiology 108: 470–479

Howie P 1986 Past obstetrical performance. In: Chamberlain G, Lumley J (eds) Prepregnancy care. John Wiley, Chichester

Kapadia & Chamberlain G 1995 Women at work: In: Cox R, Edwards F, McCallum (eds) Fitness for work. Oxford Medical Publications, Oxford, pp 338–356

Klebanoff M, Shiono P, Cavey J 1990 The effects of physical activity during pregnancy on preterm delivery and low birthweight. American Journal of Obstetrics and Gynecology 163: 1450–1456

Kline J, Shrout P, Stein Z, Zusser M, Warburton D 1980 Drinking during pregnancy and spontaneous abortion. Lancet ii: 176–179

Kline J, Levine B, Shrout P, Steil L, Susser M, Warburton D 1983 Maternal smoking and trisomy among spontaneously aborted conceptions. American Journal of Human Genetics 35: 421–431

Lemoine P et al 1968 Les enfants de parents alcooliques. Ouest Medicine 21: 476–482

Little R 1976 Alcohol consumption during pregnancy. Annals of the New York Academy of Sciences (USA) 273: 588–592

Majewski F 1981 Alcohol embryopathy. Neurobehavioral Toxicology and Teratology 3: 129–144

Mamelle N, Lauarmon B, Lazer P 1984 Prematurity and occupational activity during pregnancy. American Journal of Epidemiology 19: 309–322

Mattison D 1982 The effects of smoking on fertility. Environmental Research 28: 410–433

Meyer M B, Jones B, Jonassen J 1976 Perinatal events and maternal smoking in pregnancy. American Journal of Epidemiology 103: 464–476

Moore E 1980 Women and Health. Public Health Reports

Najman J, Keepling J, Chang A, Morrison J, Western P 1983 Employment, unemployment and the health of pregnant women. New Doctor 8: 8

Nayler A, Warburton D 1979 Segmented analysis of spontaneous abortion. Fertility and Sterility 31: 282–286

Newman N 1986 In: Chamberlain G, Lumley J (eds) Prepregnancy care. John Wiley, Chichester

Norbeck J, Tilden V 1983 Life stress, social support and emotional disequilibrium in complications of pregnancy. Health, Society and Behaviour 24: 30–46

Office of Population and Census Surveys 1981 General household survey 81/1. HMSO, London

Royal College of Psychiatrists 1982 Alcohol and alcoholism. Bulletin of the Royal College of Psychiatrists of London 6: 69

Sexton M, Hebel J 1984 A clinical trial of change of maternal smoking. Journal of the American Medical Association 251: 911–915

Shawitz S, Cohen D, Shawitz B 1980 Behaviour and learning defects in children born to alcoholic mothers. Journal of Pediatrics 96: 972–982

Smithells et al 1983 Further experiences in vitamin supplementation for prevention of neural tube defect recurrences. Lancet i: 1027–1031

Steel J, Johnston F 1986 Prepregnancy management of the diabetic. In: Chamberlain G, Lumley J (eds) Prepregnancy care. John Wiley, Chichester

Sulaiman N, Florey C, Taylor D, Ogston S 1988 Alcohol consumption in Dundee primigravidas. British Medical Journal 296: 1500–1503

Vessey M, Weight N, McPherson K, Wiggins P 1978 Fertility after stopping different methods of contraception. British Medical Journal 1: 265–267

Warburton D, Fraser F 1964 Spontaneous abortion risks in man. American Journal of Human Genetics 16: 1–25

Warren M 1983 Effects of undernutrition on reproductive function. Endocrinology Review 4: 363–377

Weatherall D, Higgs J 1982 Application of genetic engineering techniques to the study of haemoglobinopathies. Hospital Update 8: 927–933

Wolkind S 1981 Prepregnancy emotional stress—effects on the fetus. Psychological and social study. Academic Press, London, pp 177–194

Wright J T et al 1983 Alcohol consumption, pregnancy and low birthweight. Lancet i: 663–665

Xiping X U, Min Ding, Baoluo L, Chistiani D 1994 Association of rotating shiftwork with preterm birth and low birth weight among never smoking women textile workers in China. Occupational and Environmental Medicine 51: 470–474

10. Antenatal care

Marion H. Hall

Material in this chapter contains contributions from the first edition and we are grateful to the previous author for the work done.

INTRODUCTION

Throughout the world, a great many women deliver their babies with little or no antenatal care. In the developed world, however, professional expertise is widely available, and there can be no doubt that the use of antenatal care is one factor in the very low maternal and perinatal mortality and morbidity rates prevailing in Western countries compared with those in developing areas. However, demographic differences, higher standards of living, better general health of the population, sophisticated care for delivery and the neonatal period are also important, and the contribution of antenatal care can be estimated only after careful scrutiny and analysis.

One major difficulty is that it is relatively easy to find out what proportion of women received no care, or to count how many visits or episodes of care most woman had, but since it is not known what number of visits is necessary or sufficient (and of course the appropriate number may vary with women's needs) it is difficult to define minimum care. Even more important than the number of visits is the *content* of care (Report of the Public Health Service Expert Panel on the Content of Prenatal Care 1989, Rooney 1992) but with so many components of care it is not straightforward to define what is appro-priate as a total package for individual women or groups of women.

The concept of antenatal care enjoys universal appro-bation, but although some individual interventions have been fully investigated there remains a lack of clarity about the objectives, the necessary components, and the effectiveness and efficiency of care. This was neatly ex-pressed in the Short Report (1980): 'while we unhesi-tatingly accept the often reiterated aim of antenatal care as a means of reducing perinatal and neonatal mortality, what exactly antenatal care consists of, and how it works has been less clear to us.'

This lack of clarity may be illustrated by considering Bradford Hill's list of factors which must be scrutinized before inferring cause and effect (Doll 1992). Does antenatal care improve health outcomes for mother and baby? An impressively strong consistent and coherent *association* between good outcomes and frequent visits is typically reported in retrospective comparisons of women receiving care and other groups (Committee to Study the Prevention of Low Birthweight 1985, Wilson et al 1992), but such comparisons are invariably flawed by selection bias as the women not receiving care (either historical controls, pregnant women in settings where care is not widely available, or women who do not know of it or do not wish to avail themselves of it) will often have poorer health status and different behaviour from treated groups. The concept of a *biological gradient* (in which outcomes would be progressively better the more care/intervention the women received) is not really applicable to antenatal care for two reasons. First, pregnancies of short gestation length (with poorer neonatal outcomes) are bound to have fewer antenatal visits even if they participate in a full pro-gramme of care. Secondly, very frequent visits (e.g. daily) would clearly be intrusive and may cause unnecessary intervention. *Biological plausibility* is possible for some measures, e.g. identification and treatment of rhesus isoimmunization, but difficult to envisage for the vast majority of antental visits where no abnormality is detected and no treatment given. No experimental evidence is available on random assignment of women to receive or not receive care, and it is doubtful whether such a proposal would receive ethical approval. A further important factor influencing inference of causality of benefit by care is that there may be a conflict between the welfare of the mother and the fetus. The various health professionals involved (midwives, general practitioners, obstetricians) may differ as to how good outcomes should be defined (House of Commons Health Committee 1992). Also the views of women themselves both as individuals and as expressed by organizations may not accord with professional views, but are certainly in principle valid (Report of a Working Group prepared by the Director of Research and Development of the NHS Management Executive 1993). A logistic problem is that some outcomes (such as the health in adult life of the offspring of the pregnancy) cannot be measured until many decades later (Barker et al 1993, Blair & Stanley 1993).

It is clearly desirable that care should be *appropriate* as defined by the Director of Research and Development Working Group. It should do more good than harm with women's views incorporated into measurements of good and harm and it should be delivered efficiently so that resources are not wasted. To the extent that it is possible programmes of care will be evaluated in this chapter against this yardstick.

DIAGNOSIS OF PREGNANCY

History

Although a few women do experience vaginal bleeding in pregnancy and therefore fail to recognize their condition, the vast majority have amenorrhoea from the last menstrual period (LMP) until after the birth of the baby. The convention is to estimate that there will on average be 280 days (40 weeks) from the first day of the LMP and midwives and obstetricians measure the length of the pregnancy from the first day of the LMP because it is convenient to do so, although of course the pregnancy would more accurately be considered as starting on the day of conception (usually day 14 of the menstrual cycle).

When menstrual data only is being used to calculate the expected date of delivery it is of course necessary to take account of whether the woman is certain of the date of the LMP, whether the LMP was of the same duration and nature as her usual periods, and whether it came at the expected time. Attention to the regularity of the cycle is also necessary as conception occurs 14 days before the first day of the next expected period, rather than 14 days after the first day of the LMP. Similarly, if the woman has recently been using combined oestrogen/progestogen oral contraception and has conceived while using the pill or in the first cycle following cessation, then the expected date of delivery will probably be more than 280 days from the LMP, but cannot be calculated from the menstrual data.

If pregnancy results from assisted reproduction or artificial insemination, or from an isolated act of coitus, a very accurate estimate can be made.

Symptoms

Although amenorrhoea is expected, it is not necessarily the first observation that the woman makes. She may have nausea with or without vomiting, from about the date of the missed period. She may notice breast enlargement and tenderness from about 6 weeks' gestation and enlargement and pigmentation of the areola later on. Urinary frequency is also common. While none of these symptoms is specific to pregnancy they may in fact alert the woman to the fact that she is pregnant, and can be of value in assessment of early pregnancy problems such as ectopic pregnancy and miscarriage.

Signs

Some clinical signs can be noted, although they are difficult to quantify. Breast enlargement, tension and venous distension are particularly obvious in a primigravida. Also bimanual examination in early pregnancy, if indicated, will show a soft cystic globular uterus with enlargement consistent with the duration of pregnancy and may be used to assess whether there is any gross discrepancy between the uterine size and menstrual data and to assess in the case of an unwanted pregnancy whether vaginal termination will be possible. However routine vaginal examination at booking may not be necessary (O'Donovan et al 1988).

Pregnancy tests

Most women in Britain do themselves confirm pregnancy by using a pregnancy test purchased at a pharmacist. Many general practitioners will also offer such testing on request and while there is no evidence of clinical benefit from routine testing it does seem to meet a need perceived by women. When women in the reproductive age group have pain with or without amenorrhoea, modern pregnancy tests are invaluable in the early exclusion or suspicion of ectopic pregnancy.

What is being tested is the β subunit of human chorionic gonadotrophin (hCG), a glycoprotein produced by the developing placenta shortly after implantation. This can be detected in maternal serum or urine by using a monoclonal antibody to the hCG antigen (thus eliminating cross-reaction with other gonadotrophins). The complex formed by the hCG with the antibody can then be measured often using polyclonal antibody to hCG.

Quantitative testing is useful when monitoring women with trophoblastic disease or when managing ectopic pregnancy medically, but qualitative testing is used simply to diagnose pregnancy. Modern pregnancy tests are available to detect as little as 25–50 iu/ml hCG and while testing may be more reliable when performed by technicians or other trained staff, tests are available commercially with clear instructions that most women can follow. Tests can be done as early as 2–3 days before the missed period and as a result may be read by 1 minute after adding urine to the slide kit. False negatives may occur if the test is done too early or with very dilute urine, but there should not be any false positives unless hormones are being administered.

Ultrasonic scanning

Although early ultrasound scanning can diagnose pregnancy once a gestation sac is present, it is not generally used simply to diagnose pregnancy, but:

a. to confirm, if it is suspected that the pregnancy may be ectopic, that it is in fact intrauterine;
b. to confirm that there is a fetal heart where there is a previous history of miscarriage;
c. to diagnose multiple pregnancy;
d. to estimate gestational age.

It had been thought that routine ultrasonic scanning would, by improving the precision of dating, reduce the rate of induction of labour, but a recent meta-analysis of four large randomized controlled trials (Buchner & Schmidt 1993) has refuted that claim. Early scanning as a routine is therefore not effective in improving outcome and may be restricted to women with particular indications (previous ectopic, previous miscarriage, family history of twins, etc.) However, it has become fashionable to offer this test and women and their husbands or partners often expect or request it. This demand may decline following recent (very tentative) reports of possible harmful effects (Salvesen et al 1993).

Although there is no apparent benefit from routine scan dating in terms of induction practice, it has been argued that it is essential to improve the sensitivity and specificity of serum screening for fetal chromosome anomaly (Wald et al 1992). However this proposal was based on very small numbers and has not been economically evaluated. Gardosi & Mongelli (1993) have argued that only about 14% of women having serum screening would benefit from scan dating.

Because ultrasound scanning measures the size of the fetus, not the gestational age, and because biological variation in size increases as gestation advances, scan dating becomes progressively less accurate. However, it can still be useful up to about 20 weeks of gestation if there is no reliable menstrual data or if the menstrual data conflicts with clinical findings. Proponents of routine scanning have, therefore, argued that a scan around 18–20 weeks' gestation can clarify the gestational age as well as identifying structural anomalies of the fetus. Prenatal diagnosis is discussed in Chapter 15, but it seems that the case of mid-trimester scanning must be made on the basis of its value for anomaly detection rather than for dating.

Radiological examination

Advanced pregnancy may very occasionally be accidentally diagnosed on X-ray or magnetic resonance imaging, but these tests would not be suitable as a method of choice for diagnosis.

GESTATION AT BOOKING

The consultation with a midwife, family doctor or obstetrician at which antenatal care starts is considered as the main booking visit, although women may be referred by one professional to another. It can of course be argued that advice and care should begin before the woman is pregnant at all (see Ch. 9), but this is not always practicable as so many pregnancies are unplanned.

How early in pregnancy should care begin? Numerous studies have reported on better outcomes in women who book early, but there are many obvious confounding factors and Thomas et al (1991) concluded that early booking was not in fact advantageous. However, since it is not necessarily obvious to women whether they are in a group which would benefit from early booking, it is probably best to continue to advise that the first consultation should be in the first trimester. Women who can benefit from early assessment will include:

1. Those who may be offered an early scan as discussed earlier.
2. Those with a history of second-trimester miscarriage who can be offered cerclage.
3. Those with a previously unexplored history of genetic disease who may need detailed advice and testing.
4. Those with serious medical disorders who may need discussion of the hazards of pregnancy and adjustment of drug therapy or other treatment.
5. Women who have not yet had advice on nutrition, use of medicines, substance abuse, including cigarette smoking, and any need for adjustment to patterns of work.

IDENTIFICATION OF RISK AT BOOKING

The purpose of the initial consultation after assessment of gestational age as discussed earlier is to identify risk factors relating to the individual woman so that preventive or remedial intervention can be discussed, to initiate routine investigations and to discuss any problems that the woman may have.

The principles involved in risk assessment are discussed in detail by Golding & Peters (1988) and the techniques of decision analysis by Thornton et al (1992). Unfortunately, many pregnancy risk factors are of low sensitivity and specificity but combination into scoring systems is not particularly helpful (Alexander & Keirse 1989) and it is usual therefore to consider each risk factor separately so that an appropriate intervention can be planned.

Maternal age

Maternal age is considered a problem when the woman is very young and thus at greater risk of preterm labour (Committee on Prevention of Low Birthweight 1985). Women older than 30 are also at risk of preterm birth and also of smallness for gestational age (Cnattingius et al 1992). Booking for confinement in a specialist unit is therefore advised but successful preventive measures have not been identified.

Maternal size

The extremes of maternal height, weight and weight for height are associated with different problems. Short women (less than 1.52 m in the UK) may not have reached their genetic potential skeletal size and are more likely to require operative or instrumental delivery (Hall & Chng 1982), whereas very thin women (less than 50 kg) may be at risk of having a fetus which is small for dates (Carr-Hill & Pritchard 1985). Obese women on the other hand are at increased risk of developing pregnancy-induced hypertension. This cannot be prevented but can be identified early by frequent blood pressure checks.

Social factors

Deprivation is certainly a risk factor for poor obstetric outcome, but this is much less marked in the UK where all women have access to antenatal care (Paterson & Roderick 1990) than in the USA (Brown 1988) where they do not.

Medical history and examination

The identification of significant medical conditions is clearly necessary and is discussed in Chapters 21–26. Routine full medical examination at booking used to be customary and may well have been indicated when many women had previously undiagnosed problems. However, it has not been the subject of recent evaluation. A minimum would be to check the blood pressure and analyse the urine. Proteinuria at booking may point to renal disorder, glycosuria to carbohydrate intolerance, and ketosis to hyperemesis needing antiemetic and/or intravenous fluid therapy.

Previous obstetric history

In developed countries high parity is so uncommon that it is impossible to be sure whether grand multiparity is still a significant risk factor. Primiparity is a risk factor for preterm delivery and pregnancy-induced hypertension; neither can usually be prevented, but plans can be made for closer surveillance.

Most pregnant women in developed countries are in their second or third pregnancies and in this group previous obstetric history is an excellent predictor of subsequent events. Miscarriage is commoner in women with previously unsuccessful pregnancies (Regan et al 1989) but cannot unfortunately be prevented. Preterm labour has a tendency to recur, with a three-fold risk in women who have had one previous preterm birth compared to those with a previous term birth (Bakketeig & Hoffman 1981, Carr-Hill & Hall 1985). Few successful interventions are known except cerclage for selected cases (MRC/RCOG Working Party on Cervical Cerclage 1993). Pre-eclampsia is commoner in first pregnancies, but in second pregnancies is more likely to occur in those who have had the condition before (Campbell et al 1985). The questions as to whether low-dose aspirin is a successful prophylactic treatment is still under evaluation. Previous smallness for gestational age of the fetus is a risk factor for recurrence of the same condition but it is increasingly recognized that this observation is of very limited practical use since isolated smallness for gestational age is more morbid than when it is a recurrent condition (Bakketeig & Hoffman 1983, Skjoerven et al 1988). Third stage complications also tend to recur (Hall et al 1985b) but this is relevant to antenatal care only in as much as it should be discussed and booking for specialist care recommended. The significance of a previous perinatal death (or serious morbidity) depends on the cause, which should be carefully investigated.

It should be noted that for all of the above conditions, the attributable risk is low, i.e. most cases occur in low-risk women because they are more numerous. Thus, even if there was a successful intervention it could only have a limited impact if applied to those women. Also even if careful risk assessment is made at booking, many women develop problems during the antenatal period, and the rate at which this occurs seems not to vary with the stringency of the initial assessment (Hall 1992).

ROUTINE INVESTIGATIONS

The following investigations are usually advised at booking:

1. Full blood count (because iron deficiency anaemia or folic acid deficiency anaemia can be treated without problems). Routine haematinic supplementation is not however of proven value (Mahomed & Hytten 1989). Full blood count is repeated at least once in the third trimester.

2. Haemoglobin electrophoresis in women of African, Asian or Mediterranean origin (to detect haemoglobinopathy which will need specialist referral).

3. Blood group and antibody checks are necessary in each pregnancy since Rhesus-negative women will certainly need anti-D in the puerperium and perhaps also in the antenatal period. Also immunization may have occurred since the last pregnancy, sometimes causing haemolytic anaemia in the fetus and also making it difficult to cross-match blood. In Rhesus-negative women antibody checks are repeated in the third trimester.

4. Hepatitis B surface antigen is checked mainly to make immunization available to the neonate, but also to alert clinical and laboratory staff to the risk of infection, especially if the woman is E antigen positive.

5. VDRL checks are usual (although syphilis is extremely rare), because congenital syphilis is such a serious condition and can be prevented by antibiotic therapy.

6. Rubella immunity is checked so that non-immune women can be offered immunization in the puerperium. Also, such women might be advised to try to avoid exposure to young children who might be infectious.

A number of other checks are currently under evaluation—cystic fibrosis screening, which might be offered by the *step-wise* method where all carriers and their relatives are informed of their status even if there is a minimal risk to the fetus, and the *couple* method where information is given only if both members of the couple are carriers. Testing for human immunodeficiency virus (HIV) status is not currently offered on an attributable basis to mothers unless they are at high risk, since anonymous screening suggests a low prevalence in most areas. Some other screening tests (e.g. for toxoplasmosis) have been evaluated and thought not to be appropriate in the UK at the moment. In general, the widespread or routine use of tests suitable for high-risk women is not helpful (Mason et al 1993).

EDUCATION

The goals and ideology of antenatal educators vary widely and may not necessarily correspond to those of people expecting babies, but will usually include promotion of healthy behaviour in pregnancy, hazard avoidance and preparation for parturition, parenthood and breast feed-ing. Group teaching in classes is usually offered, but not always well attended, and because it is recognized that those who do not attend may be those most in need of information and support, informal discussion during home visits or clinic visits may be offered instead. It goes without saying that all tests and procedures should be explained and discussed, and never performed without consent.

Scientific evaluation of education programmes is very difficult as participants are very rarely randomly assigned, except to very specific interventions, and a wide range of other sources of information may be differentially utilized. A good example is the problem of cigarette smoking which is known to be harmful in pregnancy in relation to a wide variety of outcome measures (Poswillo & Alberman 1992). Many people know this, and will have stopped smoking prior to, or in the early stages of pregnancy. The question for antenatal education is whether any additional women can be assisted to stop smoking by specific interventions. The evidence is that a small but significant proportion of those targeted do stop using tobacco but it has not yet been demonstrated convincingly that there is any evidence of improvement in outcomes such as low birthweight, preterm delivery or perinatal death (Lumley 1993). A further question is whether resources used for such a relatively ineffectual intervention might be better spent in other fields (Shipp et al 1992).

Rational resource use requires a great deal of further research into antenatal education, but it will be particularly important in this field to make sure that the agenda of the expectant parents is being addressed. This is likely to require qualitative as well as quantitative studies.

TREATMENT OF SYMPTOMS

Some of the symptoms specifically attributable to pregnancy itself do not usually have a serious health impact, e.g. leg cramps, constipation; some are usually only of moderate severity, e.g. nausea and vomiting, heartburn, urinary infection, but can result in severe dehydration and liver failure, oesophageal abrasions and pyelonephritis respectively. It is usual therefore to offer pharmaceutical treatment at an early stage, to make women feel better and to avert progression of pathology. Available treatments are summarized by Bracken et al (1989).

ROUTINE CARE THROUGHOUT PREGNANCY

How frequently should pregnant women be seen, and should they all be seen at the same frequency, irrespective of risk?

The most important issue in the planning of routine care for pregnant women without specific medical conditions is whether to try to treat (or screen) the whole population as advocated by Rose (1992) in the context of ill health in general, or whether to target resources upon those with risk factors. Since most antenatal care does not meet the stringent criteria proposed by Holland (1993), or Mant & Fowler (1990) and as screening may be harmful (Marteau 1989, 1993) the approach of targeting high-risk individuals has been widely advocated (Chamberlain 1978, Hall et al 1980, Marsh 1982, RCOG 1982, Hall et al 1985a, Report of the Public Health Service Expert Panel on the Content of Prenatal Care 1989, Bull 1990, House of Commons Health Committee 1992). However, the inertia of a system which has been in place since 1929 has rendered change very difficult to achieve, as evidenced by a recent survey in Scotland which showed little discrimination in the delivery of care between high- and low-risk women (Tucker et al 1994).

When success for intervention in low-risk women, or across the board, is claimed, as it has been for preterm delivery preventive measures (Rumeau-Rouquette 1986, Alexander et al 1991) or for antenatal care in general (Hulsey et al 1991), the comparison groups are often historical or geographical controls or non-compliers, and the conclusions therefore not robust.

Schedules of care

Schedules of care should not be rigid, but should be designed to meet the needs of individual women (House of Commons Health Committee 1992). Care intended to deal with women's *complaints* and their need for information and reassurance, should be at a frequency determined largely by the woman herself, i.e. she should be able to make an appointment when she wishes, as other citizens do. Care of women *with complications* or those determined to be at high risk of complications should be focused on the problems identified, with validated interventions, which should not harm the false positives, who have been identified by tests or screening programmes, but who do not have any pathology.

Asymptomatic problems

Routine care for low-risk women can be justified to identify problems which are asymptomatic at least in their early stages. These are malpresentation, growth disorders and pre-eclampsia.

Malpresentation

Unless preterm labour has occurred, malpresentation (usually breech) is of no clinical significance until the last month of the pregnancy, since external cephalic version reduces the rate of breech presentation only if performed at term (Hofmeyr 1989). One routine late pregnancy visit should suffice for this purpose and for assessment of the station of the head if that is presenting (Fig. 10.1).

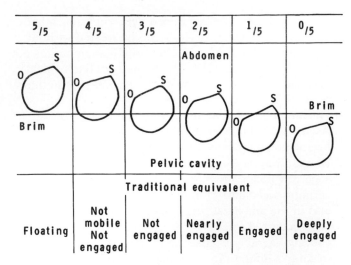

Fig. 10.1 Relationship of fetal head to pelvis assessed in fifths palpable above the brim. This is measured abdominally by the amount of occiput (O) and sinciput (S) felt.

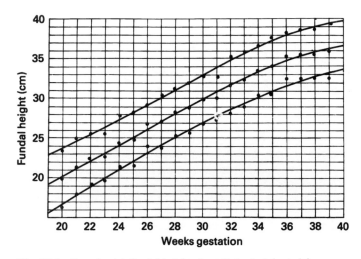

Fig. 10.2 Symphysial–fundal height chart (± 1SD). Adapted from Quarawa et al (1981).

Growth retardation

Failure to grow adequately is usually defined as being small for gestational age, though this may be caused by a number of other factors and may fail to include some cases of growth failure. The identification and management of this condition is discussed in Chapter 17. It is mentioned here merely to indicate that identification by fundal height measurement (Fig. 10.2) and/or maternal weight gain assessment (Dimperio et al 1992, Lancet Leading Article 1991) would not require more than three routine visits. Routine fetal movement counting is not helpful in the prediction of growth retardation (Grant & Elbourne 1989).

Pre-eclampsia

Pre-eclampsia remains a major cause of maternal death

(Duley 1992). Essential hypertension will be evident at booking and care planned. Certain groups of women are at higher risk (primigravidae, those with previous pre-eclampsia, multiple pregnancy, obese women, women with family history of hypertension, and women with very high weight gain), but low-risk women need only four or five visits to screen for previously undiagnosed hypertension (Hall & Campbell 1992). The gain from additional routine visits would be negligible and the marginal cost very high.

Postmaturity

The question as to whether postmaturity should be managed by induction or conservatively is controversial (Hannah 1993), but postmaturity would always be agreed as needing a specialist assessment.

By defining the main objective of each visit, a rational schedule of basic care for low-risk women can be proposed and defended on the basis that there is no evidence of better outcomes in settings where much more frequent care is offered or delivered (Blondel et al 1985, Mascarenhas et al, 1992). An example of a basic schedule is shown in Table 10.1. Additional visits for blood pressure assessment would be needed for primigravidae or multigravidae with previous pre-eclampsia, e.g. at 30, 36 and 40 weeks.

CASE RECORDS

Because care may have to be delivered by more than one health professional, it is important that there should be some standardization of case record design, with a structured database, so that items of information can be quickly found in an emergency. Structured records also facilitate complete history taking. The suggested content of the record is outlined in the RCOG Medical Audit Unit Second Bulletin (1991).

There is good evidence from randomized controlled trials (Reid & Garcia 1989) that for the pregnant woman to carry the record herself promotes good communication, empowers the woman, and does not lead to an increase in the rate of missing records.

Table 10.1 Minimum care for normal multigravidae

Gestation (weeks)	Main purpose of visit
12	History and examination, gestation assessment Risk identification and advice
16–18	Serum screening and/or scan for fetal anomaly Baseline weight, BP, urinalysis
26	Fundal height, weight, BP, urinalysis
34	Fundal height, weight, BP, urinalysis
38	Fundal height, malpresentation, weight, BP, urinalysis
41–42	Postmaturity assessment

ORGANIZATION OF CARE

In the UK three main professional groups are involved in the delivery of antenatal care—midwives, general practitioners and specialist obstetricians. However, the fragmented distribution of care between them seems to be the subject of a territorial dispute (House of Commons Health Committee 1992) and is certainly not seen by woman as providing the continuity they would desire (Hall et al 1985a). Continuity of care is not only desired by women, but may, by utilizing accumulated knowledge, rationalize resource use as has been demonstrated in the primary care field (Hjortdahl & Borchgrevink 1991).

Because obstetric complications are rare, specialists with the expertise to deal with them cannot undertake routine care for healthy women (Keirse 1989) but should be involved in discussions with midwives and general practitioners about what complications or problems would require referral for specialist care. There is no good evidence on whether one or more visits to a specialist during pregnancy actually improves process or outcome. This topic is the subject of an ongoing randomized controlled trial in nine centres in Scotland, funded by the Chief Scientist Organization of the Scottish Office Home and Health Department. Previous case control work (Klein et al 1983) and a small randomized controlled trial (Flint & Poulengeris 1987) suggest that predominantly primary care results in less intervention and some other advantages.

There is no scientific evidence which would allow an informed opinion on which type of primary care is to be preferred for low-risk women (or indeed for collaborating with specialists in the care of high-risk women). Because general practitioners rarely engage in intrapartum care, the House of Commons Health Committee proposed, in the interests of improving continuity, that they should no longer engage in antenatal care. However, this ignores the fact that in a stable population they usually provide care 'from the cradle to the grave' and will therefore have some advantages in providing care in pregnancy. In any event, although most deliveries are conducted by midwives, it is not yet the case that this is usually a midwife already known to the woman, and although many models of team midwifery are currently being tried and evaluated, the extent to which they can provide continuity between antepartum and intrapartum care, and whether this is very important to women, remains to be seen (McVicar et al 1993). Although general practitioner fund holders do not at present purchase maternity care, they often manage practice-attached midwives, and there must be scope for collaboration between general practitioners and midwives in the provision of care. The average general practitioner in Scotland will have an annual case load of between 20 and 30 pregnant women. Flint & Poulengeris (1987) estimated that a team of five midwives could look after 500 low-risk women per annum, but this has not been confirmed outside research studies. Some studies have shown potential economic benefits from an increase in domiciliary care (Twaddle & Harper 1992) but this was not confirmed in randomized controlled trials in France (Blondel & Breart 1992).

One way of assessing whether the primary/secondary interface is working well would be to look carefully at women transferred, who seem to be a high-risk group, either because specialist care does harm by unnecessary intervention (Tew 1985, 1986) or because primary carers refer women too late (Bryce et al 1990) or because a high-risk group had been correctly selected (Russell 1985). Some studies report very high transfer rates (McVicar et al 1993).

CONCLUSION

In spite of the fact that routine antenatal care for all women has been in place for over 60 years, there are many controversial areas in the provision of care. Nevertheless there are many developments such as increasing use of meta-analysis of randomized controlled trials to evaluate interventions and inform practice, and welcome attention to the views and values of women themselves, which should result in better care in the near future, provided that the essential matter of the content and validity of care is not bypassed in a headlong rush towards changing structures. Some suggestions on how to audit care are described elsewhere (Hall 1993).

REFERENCES

Alexander S, Keirse M 1989 Formal risk scoring during pregnancy. In: Chalmers I, Enkin M, Keirse M J N C (eds) Effective care in pregnancy and childbirth, Oxford University Press, Oxford

Alexander G R, Weiss J, Hulsey T C, Papierri K E 1991 Preterm birth prevention: an evaluation of programs in the United States 1991. Birth 18: 160–169

Bakketeig L S, Hoffman H J 1981 Epidemiology of preterm birth: results from a longitudinal study of births in Norway. In: Elder M G, Hendricks C H (eds) Preterm labour. Butterworths International Medical Review, London

Bakketeig L S, Hoffman H J 1983 The tendency to repeat gestational age and birthweight in successive births related to perinatal survival. Acta Obstetricae Gynecologicae Scandinavica 62: 385–392

Barker D J P, Lukeman P D, Godfrey K M, Harding J E, Owens J A, Robinson J S 1993 Fetal nutrition and cardiovascular disease in adult life. Lancet 341: 9938–9941.

Blair E, Stanley F 1993 When can cerebral palsy be prevented? The generation of causal hypotheses by multivariate analysis of a case controlled study. Paediatric and Perinatal Epidemiology 7: 272–301

Blondel B, Breart G 1992 Home visits for pregnancy complications and management of antenatal care: an overview of three randomised controlled trials. British Journal of Obstetrics and Gynaecology 99: 283–286

Blondel B, Pusch D, Schmide E 1985 Some characteristics of antenatal care in 13 European countries. British Journal of Obstetrics and Gynaecology 92: 565–569

Bracken M, Enkin M, Campbell H, Chalmers I 1989 Symptoms in pregnancy: nausea and vomiting, heartburn, constipation, and leg cramps. In: Chalmers I, Enkin M and Keirse M J N C (eds) Effective care in pregnancy and childbirth. Oxford University Press, Oxford

Brown S 1988 Prenatal care: reaching mothers, reaching infants. Washington DC, National Academy Press

Bryce F D, Clayton J K, Rand R J, Bigg I, Farquharson D I M, Jones S E 1990 General practitioner obstetrics in Bradford. British Medical Journal 300: 725–727

Buchner H C, Schmidt J G 1993 Does routine ultrasound scanning improve outcome in pregnancy: meta-analysis of various outcome measures. British Medical Journal 307: 13–17

Bull M J V 1990 Maternal and fetal screening for antenatal care. British Medical Journal 300: 1118–1120

Campbell D M, MacGillivray I, Carr-Hill R 1985 Pre-eclampsia in a second pregnancy. British Journal of Obstetrics and Gynaecology 92: 131–140

Carr-Hill R, Hall M H 1985 The repetition of spontaneous preterm labour. British Journal of Obstetrics and Gynaecology 92: 921–928

Carr-Hill R, Pritchard C 1985 The development and exploration of empirical birthweight standards. Macmillan Press, London

Chamberlain G 1978 A re-examination of antenatal care. Proceedings of the Royal Society of Medicine 71: 662–668

Cnattingius S, Forman M R, Berendes H W, Isotalo L 1992 Delayed childbearing and risk of adverse perinatal outcome. Journal of American Medical Association 268: 886–890

Committee to Study the Prevention of Low Birthweight 1985 Preventing low birthweight. Division of Health Promotion and Disease Prevention, Institute of Medicine, National Academy Press, Washington DC

Dimperio D L, Frentzen B H, Cruz A C 1992 Routine weighing during antenatal visits. British Medical Journal 304: 460

Doll R 1992 Sir Austin Bradford Hill and the progress of medical science. British Medical Journal 305: 1521–1526

Duley L 1992 Maternal mortality associated with hypertension of pregnancy in Africa, Asia, Latin America and the Caribbean. British Journal of Obstetrics and Gynaecology 9: 547–553

Flint C, Poulengeris P 1987 The 'Know Your Midwife' Report— London. C Flint, 49 Peckarman's Wood, Sydenham Hill, London SE26 6RZ

Gardosi J, Mongelli M 1993 Risk assessment adjusted for gestational age in maternal serum screening for Down's syndrome. British Medical Journal 306: 1509–1511

Golding J, Peters T J 1988 Quantifying risk in pregnancy. In: James D K, Stirratt G M (eds) Pregnancy and risk: the basis for rational management. John Wiley, Chichester

Grant A, Elbourne D 1989 Fetal movement counting to assess fetal well being. In: Chalmers I, Enkin M, Keirse M J N C (eds) Effective care in pregnancy and childbirth. Oxford University Press, Oxford

Hall M H 1992 The content and process of antenatal care. In: Chamberlain G, Zander L (eds) Pregnancy care in the 1990s. Parthenon Publishing Group, Carnforth, Lancs

Hall M H 1993 Audit of antenatal care. Fetal and Maternal Medicine Review 5: 19–28

Hall M H, Campbell D M 1992 Cost effectiveness of present programmes for detection of asymptomatic hypertension in relation to the severity of hypertension and proteinuric hypertension. International Journal of Technology. Assessment in Health Care 8 (suppl 1): 75–81

Hall M H, Chng P K 1982 Antenatal care in practice. In: Enkin M, Chalmers I (eds) Effectives and satisfaction in antenatal care. Spastics International Medical Publications, Heinemann, London

Hall M H, Chng P K, MacGillivray I 1980 Is routine antenatal care worthwhile? Lancet ii: 78–80

Hall M H, Macintyre S, Porter M 1985a Antenatal care assessed. Aberdeen University Press, Aberdeen

Hall M H, Halliwell R, Carr-Hill R A 1985b Concomitant and repeated happenings in the third stage of labour. British Journal of Obstetrics and Gynaecology 92: 732–738

Hannah M E 1993 Post term pregnancy: should all women have labour induced? A review of the literature. Fetal and Maternal Medicine Review 5: 3–17

Hjortdahl P, Borchgrevink C F 1991 Continuity of care: influence of general practitioner's knowledge about their patients on use of resources in consultations. British Medical Journal 303: 1181–1184

Hofmeyr G J 1989 Breech presentation and abnormal lie in late pregnancy. In: Chalmers I, Enkin M, Keirse M J N C (eds) Effective care in pregnancy and childbirth. Oxford University Press, Oxford

Holland W W 1993 Screening: reasons to be cautious. British Medical Journal 306: 1222–1223

House of Commons Health Committee 1992 Second Report on the Maternity Services. HMSO, London

Hulsey T C, Patrick C H, Alexander G R, Ebeling M 1991 Prenatal care and prematurity—is there an association in uncomplicated pregnancies? Birth 18: 146–150

Keirse M J N C 1989 Interaction between primary and secondary care during pregnancy and childbirth. In: Chalmers I, Enkin M, Keirse M J N C (eds) Effective care in pregnancy and childbirth. Oxford University Press, Oxford

Klein M, Lloyd I, Redman C, Glow M, Turnbull A C 1983 A comparison of low risk pregnant women booked for delivery in two systems of care—shared care (consultant) and integrated general practitioner unit. II. Labour and delivery management and neonatal outcome. British Journal of Obstetrics and Gynaecology 90: 123–128

Lancet Leading Article 1991 Maternal weight gain in pregnancy. Lancet 338: 415

Lumley J 1993 Strategies for reducing smoking in pregnancy. In: Enkin M W, Keirse M J N C, Refnrew M J, Neilson J P (eds) Pregnancy and childbirth module. Cochrane database of systematic reviews: Review No 3312, 27.4.93. Published through Cochrane Updates on Disk, Oxford Update Software, Spring 1993

McVicar J, Dobbie G, Owen-Johnstone L, Jagger C, Hopkins M, Kennedy J 1993 Simulated home delivery in hospital: a randomised controlled trial. British Journal of Obstetrics and Gynaecology 100: 316–323

Mahomed K, Hytten F 1989 Iron and folate supplementation in pregnancy. In: Chalmers I, Enkin M, Keirse M J N C (eds) Effective care in pregnancy and childbirth. Oxford University Press, Oxford

Mant D, Fowler G 1990 Mass screening theory and ethics. British Medical Journal 300: 916–918

Marsh G N 1982 New programme of antenatal care in general practice. British Medical Journal 291: 646–648

Marteau T M 1989 Psychological costs of screening. British Medical Journal 299: 527

Marteau T M 1993 Psychological consequences of screening for Down's syndrome. British Medical Journal 307: 146–147

Mascarenhas L, Eliot B W, Mackenzie I Z 1992 A comparison of perinatal outcome, antenatal and intrapartum care between England and Wales, and France. British Journal of Obstetrics and Gynaecology 99: 955–958

Mason G C, Lilford R J, Porter J, Nelson E, Tyrell S 1993 Randomised comparison of routine versus highly selective use of Doppler ultrasound in low risk pregnancies. British Journal of Obstetrics and Gynaecology 100: 103–133

MRC/RCOG Working Party on Cervical Cerclage 1993 Final Report of the Medical Research Council/Royal College of Obstetricians and Gynaecologists, Multicentre randomised trial of cervical cerclage. British Journal of Obstetrics and Gynaecology 100: 516–523

O'Donovan P, Gupta J K, Savage J, Thomson J G, Lilford R J 1988 Is routine antenatal booking vaginal examination necessary for reasons other than cytology if ultrasound examination is planned? British Journal of Obstetrics and Gynaecology 95: 556–559

Paterson C, Roderick P 1990 Obstetric outcome in homeless women. British Medical Journal 301: 263–266

Poswillo D, Alberman E 1992 Effects of smoking on the fetus, neonate and child. Oxford University Press, Oxford

Quaranta P, Currell R, Redman C W G R et al 1981 Prediction of small for dates infants by measurement of symphysial–fundal height. British Journal of Obstetrics and Gynaecology 88: 115–119

RCOG Medical Audit Unit Second Bulletin 1991 RCOG, London

RCOG 1982 Report of Working Party on Antenatal and Intrapartum Care. RCOG, London

Regan L, Braude P R, Trembath P L 1989 Influence of past reproductive performance on risk of spontaneous abortion. British Medical Journal 299: 541–545

Reid M, Garcia J 1989 Women's view of care during pregnancy and childbirth. In: Chalmers I, Enkin M, Keirse M J N C (eds) Effective care in pregnancy and childbirth, Oxford University Press, Oxford

Report of the Public Health Service Expert Panel on the Content of Prenatal Care 1989 Caring for our future: the content of prenatal care. Public Health Service, Department of Health and Human Service, Washington DC

Report of a Working Group prepared for the Director of Research and Development of the NHS Management Executive 1993 What do we mean by appropriate health care? Quality in Health Care 2: 117–123

Rooney C 1992 Antenatal care and maternal health: how effective is it? Maternal Health and Safe Motherhood Programme Division of Family Health. World Health Organization, Geneva

Rose G 1992 The strategy of preventive medicine, Oxford University Press, Oxford

Russell D 1985 Place of birth and perinatal mortality. Journal of the Royal College of General Practitioners 35: 587–588

Rumeau-Rouquette C 1986 Evolution of preterm birth rate and prevention in France. In: Papiernik E, Breart G, Spira N (eds) Prevention of preterm birth. INSERM, Paris

Salvesen K A, Batten L J, Eik-nes S H, Hugdahl K, Bakketeig L 1993 Routine ultrasonographny in utero and subsequent handedness and neurological development. British Medical Journal 304: 159–164

Shipp M, Cronghan-Minihane M S, Petioti D B, Washington A E 1992 Estimation of the break-even point for smoking cessation programs in pregnancy. American Journal of Public Health 82: 383–390

Short Report 1980 Second Report from the Social Services Committee, Session 1979–80. Perinatal and neonatal mortality session, vol 1. HMSO, London

Skjoerven R, Wilcox A J, Russell D 1988 Birthweight and perinatal mortality of second births conditional on weight of the first. International Journal of Epidemiology 17: 830–838

Tew M 1985 Place of birth and perinatal mortality. Journal of the Royal College of General Practitioners 35: 390–394

Tew M 1986 Do obstetric interventions make birth safer? British Journal of Obstetrics and Gynaecology 93: 659–675

Thomas P, Golding J, Peters T J 1991 Delayed antenatal care: does it affect pregnancy outcome? Social Science Medicine 32: 715–723

Thornton J G, Lilford R J, Johnson N 1992 Decision analysis in medicine. British Medical Journal 304: 1099–1103

Tucker J S, Howie P W, Florey C D U V, McIlwaine G, Hall M H 1994 Is antenatal care apportioned according to obstetric risk? Journal of Public Health Medicine 16: 60–70

Twaddle S, Harper M 1992 Economic evaluation of daycare in the management of hypertension in pregnancy. British Journal of Obstetrics and Gynaecology 99: 459–463

Wald N J, Kennard A, Densen J W, Cuckle H S, Chard T, Butler L 1992 Antenatal maternal serum screening for Down's syndrome: results of a demonstration project. British Medical Journal 305: 391–394

Wilson A L, Munmsen D P, Schubot D B, Leonardson G, Stevens D C 1992 Does perinatal care decrease the incidence and cost of neonatal intensive care admissions? American Journal of Perinatology 9: 281–284

11. Endocrinological and metabolic assessment of early pregnancy

J. G. Grudzinskas

Table 11.1   Major fetal, trophoblast and decidual proteins identified in early pregnancy

Fetal
Alphafetoprotein (AFP)
Fetal antigen 1 (FA-1)
Fetal antigen (FA-2)

Trophoblast
Human chorionic gonadotrophin (hCG)
Schwangerschaftsprotein 1 (SP1)
Human placental lactogen (hPL)
Pregnancy-associated plasma protein A (PAPP-A)
Placental protein 5 (PP5)

Decidual endometrial
Insulin-like growth factor binding protein (IGF-BP; α-1 PEG; PP12)
Progesterone-dependent endometrial protein (PEP; α-2 PEG; PP14; AUP)

INTRODUCTION

The detection of human chorionic gonadotrophin (hCG) in maternal blood or urine is the basis of pregnancy diagnosis by biochemical methods, since hCG is observed from the time of implantation. More recently, the systematic examination of the placenta, decidua and maternal blood has led to the identification of a new generation of proteins which may be used in the diagnosis of early pregnancy and its failure (Table 11.1). For example, measurements of Schwangerschaftsprotein 1 (SP1) can be used in the biochemical diagnosis of pregnancy (Grudzinskas et al 1977), and recent reports have described consistently depressed levels of pregnancy-associated plasma protein A (PAPP-A) in early pregnancy failure and in association with Down's syndrome in the first trimester (Westergaard et al 1985, Brambati et al 1991, 1993a,b, Wald et al 1992a, Muller et al 1993). Furthermore, the recent detection of secretory proteins of decidual/endometrial origin holds the promise of the first non-invasive indices of function of these tissues. This chapter deals with the clinical application of measurement of hormones and proteins of fetal, maternal and placental origin in normal and abnormal early pregnancy.

DIAGNOSIS OF PREGNANCY

The early diagnosis of pregnancy depends on the detection of hCG in maternal urine, or 1–2 days earlier in blood. The current developments in assay technology have contributed to the resolution of problems of potential non-specific results (Chard 1992). In clinical practice a single estimation of hCG should only be considered indicative of pregnancy if it is greater than 25 iu/l or if a lower level of hCG is seen to increase twofold at an interval of 3 days (Jones et al 1983). If hCG has been administered in the luteal phase, estimations should be delayed until clearance of the exogenous hCG has occurred, possibly postponing the diagnosis by up to 14 days. In this circumstance, assays for other proteins of placental origin, namely SP1, may be appropriate. Other pregnancy-associated proteins, such as human placental lactogen (hPL), PAPP-A and placental protein 5 (PP5), are not serious contenders as diagnostic tests since they do not appear in the maternal blood until after 6 weeks of amenorrhoea. Finally, hCG results immediately after implantation should be interpreted with care; the earlier the diagnosis is made, the less likely is the outcome to

Table 11.2 Pregnancy outcome in relation to time of diagnosis

Time of diagnosis	Likelihood of normal outcome (%)
Preimplantation	25–30
Postimplantation	43–60
Six weeks' amenorrhoea	85–90
Second trimester	95
Third trimester	98

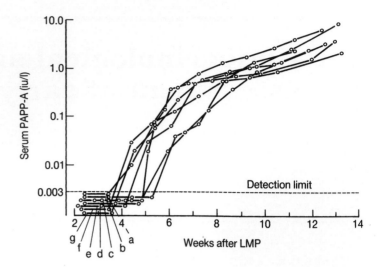

Fig. 11.2 Serum levels of pregnancy-associated plasma protein A in seven women during early normal pregnancy. From Chemnitz et al (1986).

be normal (Table 11.2) given the very high rate of spontaneous pregnancy failure in the periimplantation period (see below).

It may be desirable to restrict the use of the most sensitive hCG tests to specific clinical situations (e.g. subfertility or suspected ectopic gestation) rather than increasing the availability of diagnosis at this early stage of pregnancy in the normal population.

ENDOCRINOLOGY AND METABOLISM OF NORMAL EARLY PREGNANCY

The apparent trigger for synthesis of hCG by the conceptus is implantation. The stimulus for the production of other placental products, such as hPL, SP1 and PAPP-A, is unclear but is likely to include implantation and other as yet unrecognized events. SP1 secretion into the maternal circulation appears likely to be simultaneous with implantation and the trends in blood concentration seem to parallel the growth rate curve of functioning trophoblast (Grudzinskas et al 1977, Lenton et al 1981, Ahmed & Klopper 1985; Fig. 11.1). In normal pregnancy this pattern contrasts with that of hCG, but is similar to hPL, PAPP-A and PP5. The synthesis of SP1, at least for the initial weeks of pregnancy, seems to be independent of the presence of an embryo or fetus, and also of the site of implantation, as seen in women with ectopic gestation. In normal pregnancy the doubling times for hCG and SP1 are quite similar; concentrations of hCG and SP1

double in 2–3 days in the first 6 weeks of pregnancy (Lenton et al 1981).

The disappearance rates of these molecules after removal of the placenta are also equivalent: 40–60 hours. There is not a large literature on hPL in early pregnancy, and this hormone is not considered to be useful as a pregnancy test (Letchworth 1976). Blood levels of hPL increase as pregnancy advances, and have a relationship to functioning trophoblast mass. Circulating PAPP-A can be detected in the maternal circulation consistently 28 days after conception in singleton pregnancies, but the relatively late appearance of this molecule in the peripheral blood also precludes it from use as a primary diagnostic test for pregnancy (Chemnitz et al 1986; Fig. 11.2). PAPP-A levels increase throughout gestation with a mean doubling time of 4.9 days during the first trimester; the disappearance rate after removal of the placenta is several days (Sinosich et al 1988).

The production of oestradiol and progesterone is transferred from the corpus luteum of pregnancy to the fetoplacental unit in the middle of the first trimester (Klopper 1985). The synthesis of fetal proteins such as alphafetoprotein (AFP) by embryonal endodermal tissues is reflected by an increase in circulating levels during the first trimester; substantial amounts of AFP are detected consistently after 10 weeks' gestation (Olajide et al 1989). Synthesis of the secretory proteins of the endometrium may parallel the morphological changes which this tissue undergoes (Bell 1986).

Insulin-like growth-factor-binding protein of stromal cell origin is consistently seen in the maternal blood in the latter half of the first trimester. These changes are preceded by a dramatic increase in amniotic fluid IGP BPI levels late in the first trimester, a three-fold order of change of magnitude and being seen in the 8–11 gestational week

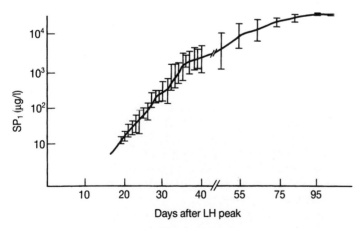

Fig. 11.1 Mean serum levels of Schwangerschaftsprotein 1 in nine women during early normal pregnancy. From Lenton et al (1981).

interval (Wathen et al 1993). Serum levels reach a peak in the second trimester (Wang et al 1991). By contrast, the trends in blood levels of progestogen-dependent endometrial protein (PEP) bear a striking similarity to hCG.

CONTROL OF SYNTHESIS AND SECRETION

The mechanisms which control the synthesis of proteins of trophoblastic origin are poorly understood; uteroplacental perfusion probably plays a major role, influencing synthesis and secretion according to the law of mass action (Chard & Grudzinskas 1985). Nevertheless, it is possible to draw some conclusions on the possible effects of the ovary, the embryo and the endometrium. Firstly, following successful intrauterine pregnancy in women participating in embryo donation programmes, pregnancy seems to be independent of ovarian support as synthetic oestrogens and progestogens are required only for the first 8–9 weeks of the pregnancies of women with ovarian failure, or after bilateral oophorectomy (Lutjen et al 1984). Secondly, whereas depressed levels of some trophoblastic proteins and hormones are seen when complications of early pregnancy become evident clinically, the initiation of synthesis and secretion appears to be unrelated to the presence of the embryo, as evidenced in blighted ovum and hydatidiform mole.

Thirdly, the site of implantation and presumably the interaction between the trophoblast and decidualized endometrium seem to be of minor relevance for the majority of the substances considered here, at least in the earliest days of pregnancy. Serum levels of trophoblastic hormones and proteins have been consistently depressed in ectopic gestation, but the abnormalities in synthesis have varied widely, the earliest and greatest difference being seen for PAPP-A (Sinosich et al 1985). Finally, with the possible exception of PAPP-A in Cornelia de Lange syndrome, gross structural fetal congenital abnormalities are not related to changes in circulating hormones or proteins in either direction (Westergaard et al 1983). Furthermore, normal pregnancy has been reported in women with an apparent absence of hPL and SP1. However, depressed serum PAPP-A and elevated free β subunit hCG levels are seen in the first trimester in fetal aneuploidy, in particular Down's syndrome (Brambati et al 1991, 1993a, b, 1994, Spencer et al 1992, Wald et al 1992a, Muller et al 1993). Gross elevations of hCG and SP1 in amniotic fluid have been reported in pregnancies complicated by Meckel's syndrome, but these changes are not reflected in the maternal circulation (Heikinheimo et al 1982). By contrast, the metabolism of progesterone and oestrogen in pregnancy is well described, and the dramatic changes in ovarian hormones observed in early pregnancy, given the work of Lutjen and his colleagues (1984), are presumably part of the maternal response to pregnancy rather than a primary phenomenon.

This also seems to be the case for the major secretory protein of pregnancy endometrium PP14, which was originally thought to be progesterone dependent. Low PP14 levels seen in pregnant women following ovum donation suggest that PP14 synthesis is due to a complex interaction between corpus luteum and the endometrium, with the possibility of the corpus luteum as the major source of PP14 being raised (Johnson et al 1993a).

COMPLICATIONS OF EARLY PREGNANCY

Early pregnancy failure

The chances of a woman desirous of pregnancy producing a viable offspring in any one ovarian cycle is approximately 25%. Detailed studies using sensitive biochemical tests confirm these conclusions; the findings are remarkably similar whether ovulation and pregnancy have occurred spontaneously, or whether they resulted from an in-vitro fertilization–embryo transfer (IVF–ET) programme (Table 11.3).

The incidence of clinically obvious miscarriage is 10–15%, whether fertilization occurred in vivo or in vitro. Estimates of the incidence of this phenomenon vary from 8 to 55%. The meticulous work of Hertig et al (1952), together with the calculations of Roberts & Lowe (1975), stimulated these studies. Differences in clinical study design, assay techniques, and populations account for the discordance in the current data; one of the major issues is the specificity of the substances measured as an index of trophoblastic activity. In this respect, hCG measurements must still be considered as superior to those of SP1 (unless hCG has been given therapeutically). By contrast, ultrasonic findings such as uterine distension or a gestational sac cannot be considered as specific signs of pregnancy.

Threatened and spontaneous miscarriage

Circulating levels of hormones and proteins of fetal, placental and maternal origin have been used to predict

Table 11.3 Studies on subclinical and clinical miscarriage

Reference	Method	Pregnancy loss (%)
Hertig et al (1952)	Histology	43
Block (1976)	hLH	37.5
Braunstein et al (1977)	hCG	15
Chartier et al (1979)	hCG	30
Miller et al (1980)	hCG	43
Edmonds et al (1982)	hCG	62
Edwards & Steptoe (1983)	hCG	25–35
Jones et al (1983)	hCG	33
Whittaker et al (1983)	hCG	20
Wilcox et al (1985)	hCG	24
Seppala et al (1979a)	SP1	Not stated
Ahmed & Klopper (1983)	SP1	Not stated

hLH = human luteinizing hormone; hCG = human chorionic gonadotrophin; SP1 = Schwangerschaftsprotein 1 the outcome in women with vaginal bleeding in early pregnancy (Niven et al 1972, Nygren et al 1973, Garoff & Seppala 1975, Kunz & Keller 1976, Braunstein et al 1978, Damber et al 1978, Jovanovic et al 1978, Schultz-Larsen & Hertz 1978, Joupilla et al 1979, Masson et al 1983a,b, Salem et al 1984). Ultrasound examination has revolutionized this practice, and some of these tests are probably obsolete if fetal life can be demonstrated by ultrasound (Joupilla et al 1980a,b, Hertz et al 1980). Nevertheless, a proportion of patients in whom fetal heart action has been demonstrated will spontaneously miscarry. We have examined serum levels of hPL, SP1, PAPP-A, progesterone, oestradiol, AFP and pregnancy-zone protein (PZP) in this situation (Westergaard et al 1985). In the 108 patients in whom the history and clinical findings were indicative of threatened miscarriage, ultrasound revealed a fetal heart action in 77, whereas examination during the first week of study gave no clearcut evidence of fetal life in the remaining 31 patients. Ultrasound scans were done at weekly intervals of 3 weeks and every 2 weeks thereafter, unless otherwise indicated by vaginal bleeding. Maternal venous blood was obtained at each ultrasound scan, and samples obtained within 24 hours of miscarriage were excluded from analysis.

Spontaneous miscarriage occurred in 42 pregnancies, 31 of which showed no sign of fetal heart action on repeated scan examination. In the remaining 11 patients, the fetal heart action was observed repeatedly until miscarriage occurred. The predictive value of an abnormal level in the sample obtained at presentation was greatest for PAPP-A, particularly if there was scan evidence of fetal life (54%). When all abnormal results were considered, the predictive value was highest for AFP and PAPP-A.

The differences between the indices, both in single and serial samples, were less if the ultrasound findings were not included. The sensitivity was highest for PAPP-A levels, regardless of whether the first sample (64%) or all samples (89%) were considered, in patients with ultrasound evidence of a live fetus. The predictive value of a normal test was comparable for all variables if the first sample was considered. However, when serial samples were considered and ultrasound demonstrated a live fetus, the highest value (99%) was for PAPP-A estimations.

The relative risk of miscarriage was highest for depressed levels of PAPP-A, being at least three times greater than that calculated for the other biochemical indices at clinical presentation if the fetus was alive, and 5–10 times greater if all samples were considered, regardless of the ultrasound findings. All the 11 women who had evidence of a live fetus but subsequently miscarried had depressed PAPP-A levels. In the sera obtained from these patients, PAPP-A levels were abnormal at least 4 weeks before miscarriage in four patients and in every sample obtained in the other seven (Fig. 11.3). In contrast, the levels of the other substances measured generally remained within the normal range—the only exception was AFP.

This study examined the value of biochemical tests relative to ultrasound. Firstly, only abnormal PAPP-A levels distinguished those pregnancies which miscarried from those which did not, even when there was ultrasonic evidence of fetal heart action at the time of blood sampling. Secondly, depressed PAPP-A levels were seen several weeks before spontaneous miscarriage in some

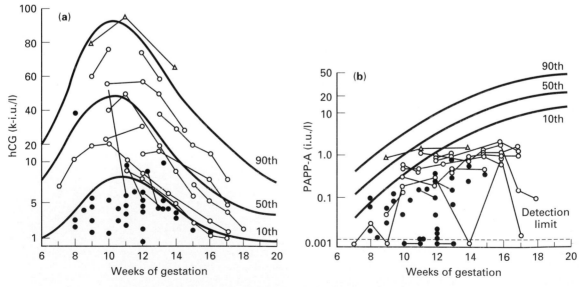

Fig. 11.3 Serum levels of human chorionic gonadotrophin (**a**) and pregnancy-associated plasma protein A (**b**) in 42 women with spontaneous abortion. Heavy lines represent the 10th, 50th and 90th centiles of the normal range. ● = No ultrasonic evidence of fetal heart action; ○ = ultrasonic evidence of heart action; △ = twin pregnancy with live fetuses. WHO reference material for pregnancy proteins 78/610. From Westergaard et al (1985).

patients. Thirdly, if the heart action was not evident ultrasonically on repeated examination, depressed or abnormal levels of placental hCG, SP1, hPL, oestradiol, PAPP-A, AFP and progesterone were consistently seen. Fourthly, if miscarriage occurred after the detection of fetal heart action, the levels of these molecules were generally in the normal range, the sole exception being PAPP-A. Finally, if the heart action was detected and the serum PAPP-A levels were normal, the chance of a normal outcome for that pregnancy was in excess of 98%.

ANEMBRYONIC PREGNANCY

Failure of development of the embryo makes it possible to examine the contribution of the growing conceptus to the control of protein and hormone synthesis by trophoblastic tissue. This condition can be diagnosed using ultrasound if an embryo is not apparent in a gestational sac of greater than 3 ml (7 weeks' gestation) (Stabile et al 1989). Levels of placental hormones and proteins are low or normal. Serum AFP levels are usually within the normal range, suggesting that an embryo has been present at some stage and that the term anembryonic pregnancy is in fact a misnomer (Stabile et al 1989). Mean serum levels of hCG have also been shown to be depressed at 4 weeks' gestation in a group of patients studied prospectively at a subfertility clinic who subsequently were shown to have blighted ovum; mean levels of maternal PAPP-A, oestradiol and progesterone fell some 3 weeks later (Yovich et al 1986). Regardless of the pathogenesis of this condition these and other data confirm that a deviation from the normal rise in blood levels of hCG is highly suggestive of failed pregnancy at a time before ultrasound can provide useful information (i.e. in the absence of an embryonic heart action) (Johnson et al 1993a).

ECTOPIC PREGNANCY

The improved image resolution, ease of use and patient acceptability of transvaginal ultrasound (TVS) has revolutionized the management of women suspected of ectopic pregnancy, permitting the correct diagnosis in as many as 90% before life-threatening haemorrhage from tubal rupture occurs if hCG is detected (Cacciatore et al 1990). The definitive diagnosis can be made by observing the embryonic heart action outside the uterus in up to 21% of women at 6–7 weeks' gestation (Bohm-Velez et al 1990), but hormonal tests must be considered prior to this time to make the diagnosis of pregnancy and to establish the normality of the pregnancy (Stabile 1992, Johnson et al 1993c).

A woman who has a positive pregnancy test and in whom the diagnosis of ectopic pregnancy cannot further be made or excluded on clinical grounds should have an ultrasonic examination by the transvaginal route. If this is not diagnostic, the circumstances may permit other tests such as quantitative hCG estimations, a level of 500–1000 iu/l (1st IRP) being associated with the transvaginal ultrasonic observation of a gestational sac in a normal intrauterine pregnancy a few days after the missed period. A second quantitative hCG estimation after 48 hours, demonstrating a normal doubling time, may provide further reassurance that the pregnancy is not likely to miscarry or is not ectopic (Check et al 1992). Using this approach, Kadar et al (1981) demonstrated that 15% of normal intrauterine pregnancies will also appear abnormal (false positives) and 13% of ectopic pregnancies would not initially be identified (false negatives). Although most abortions are diagnosed clinically, those that present prior to 6 weeks' gestation may cause diagnostic difficulties with ectopic pregnancy. If serial measurements of hCG over a 48-hour period reveal a disappearance rate (half-life) of less than 1.4 days, then the patient is most likely to miscarry and is best managed expectantly. A half-life of greater than 7 days (plateauing hCG levels) was almost always associated with ectopic pregnancy in the study of Kadar & Romero (1988).

A single or serial measurement of serum progesterone may be useful in distinguishing between normal and abnormal pregnancy. Whereas this can be considered in women who have conceived after spontaneous ovulation, it certainly cannot after controlled ovarian hyperstimulation for assisted conception procedures when very high serum progesterone levels are seen (Fig. 11.4; Lower et al 1993). The practical issue in modern practice is really whether serum progesterone estimations provide information in addition to that afforded by TVS (Grudzinskas & Stabile

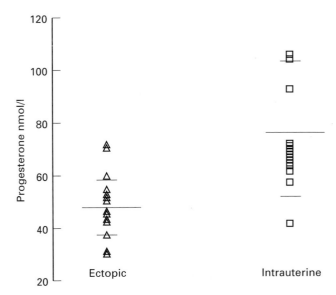

Fig. 11.4 Serum progesterone levels in women with asymptomatic ectopic pregnancy 14–16 days after conception in relation to levels in women matched for serum hCG levels, gestational age who ovulated and conceived spontaneously (Lower et al 1993).

1993), as the problem lies in distinguishing between spontaneous abortion and ectopic pregnancy and no single progesterone value reliably predicts the presence or absence of ectopic pregnancy (Gelder et al 1991). Interesting findings are seen in endometrial secretory proteins, other placental proteins such as PAPP-A and immunoreactive renin levels in women with ectopic pregnancy, but the speed and simplicity of performance of these assays are still not at the same level as for hCG (Meunier et al 1991, Stabile 1992). Perhaps in women at risk of ectopic pregnancy because of known tubal disease, assisted conception procedures or history of ectopic pregnancy, prospective testing using biochemical markers before TVS can provide useful information either for reassurance or to facilitate early detection.

TROPHOBLASTIC DISEASE

The syncytiotrophoblast in hydatidiform mole maintains its ability to synthesize hormones and proteins, and although this capacity is reduced for hPL and steroids, it is considerably greater for hCG.

As the risk of development of choriocarcinoma and subsequent poor prognosis is higher in women in the presence of excessive hCG secretion in gestational trophoblast tumours (Newlands 1983), various centres have evaluated measurements of proteins specifically synthesized by trophoblastic tissue (e.g. SP1, PP5 and PAPP-A) in this context. In untreated hydatidiform mole reduced levels of PAPP-A have been observed in women prior to treatment, whereas elevated levels of circulating SP1 and PP5 are seen (Fig. 11.5, Tsakok et al 1983). High SP1 levels may be predictive of subsequent malignant change but these observations require confirmation. In patients with extensive choriocarcinoma, serum SP1 levels are usually lower than in benign disease and circulating PP5 cannot be detected (Seppala et al 1979b, Lee et al 1981, 1982, Soma et al 1981). Although the place of hCG estimation in the monitoring of women with this disease is firmly established, estimations of the new trophoblastic-specific proteins may give further insight into the pathogenesis of this condition.

Than & colleagues (1988) observed high serum concentrations of PP14 in patients prior to treatment for hydatidiform mole, falling rapidly after evacuation. Circulating PP14 was not seen in women with choriocarcinoma.

BIOCHEMICAL SCREENING FOR FETAL ANEUPLOIDY

Maternal serum measurements of analytes such as AFP, hCG and its β subunit and unconjugated oestriol (uE₃) in the second trimester can detect at least twice as many women with Down's syndrome fetuses for the same number of amniocenteses if maternal age is used for

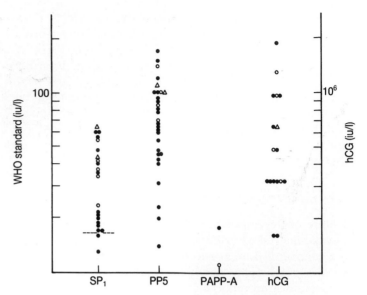

Fig. 11.5 Circulating Schwangerschaftsprotein 1 (SP1), placental protein 5 (PP5), pregnancy-associated plasma protein A (PAPP-A) and human chorionic gonadotrophin (hCG) in 31 patients with gestational trophoblastic tumours before treatment. ● = Hydatidiform mole; ○ = choriocarcinoma; △ = patient with lung metastases; dashed line = 16.5 iu/l WHO standard 78/610. Levels of proteins (SP1, PP5 and PAPP-A) < 10 iu/l or hCG < 100 000 iu/l are not shown. From Tsakok et al (1983).

screening (Wald et al 1992b, Muller et al 1993; see Ch. 12). Recent studies in the first trimester have reported low maternal serum PAPP-A levels in women with Down's syndrome fetuses (Brambati et al 1991, 1993a,b, Wald et al 1992a) as well as elevated serum free β hCG subunit levels (Spencer et al 1992, Brambati et al 1993b). The discrimination in serum PAPP-A levels between normal and affected fetuses is only seen in the first trimester (Cuckle et al 1992), the sensitivity in the first trimester being as high as 65% (Figs 11.6, 11.7).

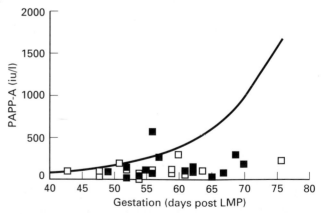

Fig. 11.6 Maternal serum PAPP-A levels in pregnancies with chromosome anomalies. The curve is the median value of PAPP-A in normal pregnancies given by $\log_e$ (PAPP-A) = 0.5115 + 0.0911 (days). ■ = Chromosome anomalies; □ = Down's syndrome.

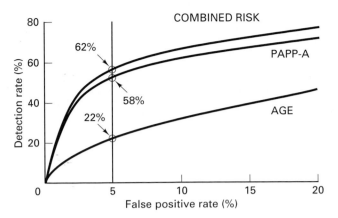

Fig. 11.7 Sensitivity vs false positive rates (received-operator characteristic (ROC) curves) applying various cut-off levels of PAPP-A, age and combined risks to the general population. The false-positive rate is the proportion of the normal population that have a positive test and is equivalent to 1-specificity.

FUTURE DEVELOPMENTS

Ultrasonic examination has contributed substantially to precise assessment of early pregnancy. Nevertheless, hCG estimations are still the mainstay of the diagnosis of early pregnancy and, when used in conjunction with ultrasound, provide valuable clinical information prior to 6 weeks' gestation. After detection of the embryonic heart action at 6–7 weeks' gestation, only PAPP-A measurements seem to provide useful information concerning spontaneous miscarriage. Biochemical screening for aneuploidy, in particular Down's syndrome, is now possible in the first trimester, the most sensitive markers being depressed serum PAPP-A and elevated free β hCG subunit levels.

The diagnosis of ectopic gestation is largely dependent on awareness of a possible pregnancy-related disorder. Maternal PAPP-A or progesterone measurements, used in conjunction with hCG, may increase diagnostic accuracy in this condition.

The identification of the ability of the endometrium and decidua to synthesize secretory proteins which can be measured in the uterine lumen and peripheral blood encourages their inclusion into the reproductive axis as active rather than passive participants. Since these tissues produce hormones, lipids and proteins which act locally and distally, it is possible to consider the endometrium/decidua as an endocrine organ (Healey & Hodgen 1983, Bell 1986, Fay & Grudzinskas 1991). The ability to measure these substances, in particular insulin-like growth-factor-binding protein and progestogen-dependent endometrial protein, may provide not only a non-invasive test of endometrial function in the assessment of fertility, but also an index of endometrial/decidual function in the earliest days and weeks of pregnancy.

REFERENCES

Ahmed A G, Klopper A 1983 Diagnosis of early pregnancy by assay of placental proteins. British Journal of Obstetrics and Gynaecology 90: 604–611

Ahmed A G, Klopper A 1985 Concomitant secretion of Schwangerschaftsprotein and human chorionic gonadotrophin following conception. Clinical Endocrinology 23: 677–681

Bell S C 1986 Secretory endometrial and decidual proteins: studies on clinical significance of a maternally derived group of pregnancy associated serum proteins. Human Reproduction 1: 129–143

Bell S C 1988 Synthesis and secretion of proteins by the endometrium. In: Chapman M, Grudzinskas G, Chard T (eds) Implantation. Springer, London, pp 95–118

Bellman O, Tebbe J, Lang N, Baur M P 1980 Determination of SP1 and hPL for predicting perinatal asphyxia. In: Klopper A, Genazzani A, Crosignani P G (eds) The human placenta: proteins and hormones. Academic Press, London, pp 99–108

Block S K 1976 Occult pregnancy. Obstetrics and Gynecology 48: 365–368

Bohm-Velez M, Mendelson E B, Freimains M J 1990 Transvaginal sonography in evaluating ectopic pregnancy. Seminars in Ultrasound CT MR 11: 44–58

Brambati B, Lanzani A, Tului L 1991 Ultrasound and biochemical assessment of first trimester pregnancy. In: Chapman M, Grudzinskas J G, Chard T (eds) The embryo: normal and abnormal development and growth. Springer Verlag, Berlin, pp 181–194

Brambati B, Macintosh M C M, Teisner B et al 1993a Low maternal serum levels of pregnancy associated plasma protein A (PAPP-A) in the first trimester in association with abnormal fetal karyotype. British Journal of Obstetrics and Gynaecology 100: 324–326

Brambati B, Tului L, Bonacchi I, Shrimanker K, Suzuki Y, Grudzinskas J G 1993b Serum PAPP-A and free β hCG are first trimester screening markers for Down's syndrome. Human Reproduction 8 (suppl 1): 183

Brambati B, Tului L, Bonnacchi I, Suzuki Y, Shrimanker K, Grudzinskas J G 1994 Biochemical screening for Down's syndrome in the first trimester. In: Grudzinskas J G, Chard T, Chapman M, Cuckle H (eds) Screening for Down's syndrome. Cambridge University Press, Cambridge, pp 275–284

Braunstein G D, Karow W G, Gentry W D, Wade M E 1977 Subclinical spontaneous abortion. Obstetrics and Gynecology 50: 415–445

Braunstein G D, Karow W G, Gentry W C, Rasor I, Wade M M 1978 First trimester chorionic gonadotrophin measurements as an aid in the diagnosis of early pregnancy disorders. American Journal of Obstetrics and Gynecology 143: 25–32

Cacciatore B, Stenman U K, Yostalo P 1990 Diagnosis of ectopic pregnancy by vaginal ultrasonography in combination with a discriminatory serum hCG level of 1000 IU/L (IRP). British Journal of Obstetrics and Gynaecology 97: 904–908

Chapman M G, Bolton A E, Mellows H, Grudzinskas J G 1984 Anembryonic pregnancy—a prospective study of placental biochemical parameters. Proceedings of the 5th International Congress of Placental Proteins, Annecy, France, p 102

Chard T 1992 Pregnancy tests: a review. Human Reproduction 7: 701–710

Chard T, Grudzinskas J G 1985 Placental and pregnancy-associated proteins: control mechanisms and clinical application. In: Bischof P, Klopper A (eds) Proteins of the placenta. Karger, Basel, pp 104–113

Chartier M M, Roger N, Barrat J, Michelon B 1979 Measurement of plasma hCG and BhCG in the late luteal phase. Evidence of the occurrence of spontaneous menstrual abortions in infertile women. Fertility and Sterility 31: 134–137

Check J, Weiss R M, Lurie D 1992 Analysis of serum human chorionic gonadotrophin levels in normal singleton, multiple and abnormal pregnancies. Human Reproduction 7: 1176–1180

Chemnitz J, Tornehave D, Teisner B, Poulsen H K, Westergaard J G

1984 The localisation of pregnancy proteins (hPL, SP1 and PAPP-A) in intra- and extrauterine pregnancies. Placenta 5: 489–494

Chemnitz J, Folkersen J, Teisner B et al 1986 Comparison of different antibody preparations against pregnancy-associated plasma protein A (PAPP-A) for use in localisation and immunoassay studies. British Journal of Obstetrics and Gynaecology 93: 111–118

Cuckle H, Lilford R J, Teisner B, Holding S, Chard T, Grudzinskas J G 1992 Pregnancy associated plasma protein A in Down's syndrome. British Medical Journal 305: 425

Damber M G, von Schoultz B, Solheim F, Stigbrand T, Carlstrom K 1978 Prognostic value of the pregnancy zone protein during early pregnancy in spontaneous abortion. Obstetrics and Gynecology 51: 677–681

Edmonds D K, Lindsey K S, Miller J R, Williamson E, Wood P J 1982 Early embryonic mortality in women. Fertility and Sterility 38: 447–453

Edwards R G, Steptoe P C 1983 Current status of in vitro fertilisation and implantation of human embryos. Lancet ii: 1265–1269

Fay T N, Grudzinskas J G 1991 Human endometrial peptides: a review of their potential role in implantation and placentation. Human Reproduction 6: 1311–1326

Garoff L, Seppala M 1975 Prediction of fetal outcome in threatened abortion by maternal serum placental lactogen and alphafetoprotein. American Journal of Obstetrics and Gynecology 121: 257–261

Gelder M S, Boots L R, Younger J B 1991 Use of a single random progesterone value as a diagnostic aid for ectopic pregnancy. Fertility and Sterility 55: 497–500

Grudzinskas J G, Stabile I 1993 Ectopic pregnancy: are biochemical tests at all helpful? British Journal of Obstetrics and Gynaecology 100: 508–510

Grudzinskas J G, Gordon Y B, Jeffrey D, Chard T 1977 Specific and sensitive determination of pregnancy specific beta-1 glyco-protein by radioimmunoassay. Lancet i: 333–335

Grudzinskas J G, Westergaard J G, Teisner B 1985 Pregnancy-associated plasma protein A in normal and abnormal pregnancies. In: Bischof P, Klopper A (eds) Proteins of the placenta. Karger, Basel, pp 184–197

Grudzinskas J G, Westergaard J G, Teisner B 1986 Biochemical assessment of placental function: early pregnancy. Clinics in Obstetrics and Gynaecology 13: 553–569

Grudzinskas J G, Stabile I, Campbell S 1988 Early pregnancy failure: biochemical and biophysical assessment. In: Beard R W, Sharp F (eds) Early pregnancy loss: mechanisms and treatment. Peacock Press, Ashton-under-Lyme, pp 183–192

Healey D L, Hodgen G 1983 Endocrinology of the endometrium. Obstetric and Gynaecological Survey 38: 509–530

Heikinheimo M, Wahlstrom T, Aula P, Seppala M 1982 Pregnancy specific beta-1 glycoprotein in amniotic fluid. In: Grudzinskas J G, Teisner B, Seppala M (eds) Pregnancy proteins: biology, chemistry and clinical application. Academic Press, Sydney, pp 215–221

Hertig A T, Rock J, Adams E C, Menkin E C 1952 Thirty-four fertilized human ova, good, bad and indifferent recovered from 210 women of known fertility. Pediatrics 23: 202–211

Hertz J B, Mantoni M, Svenstrup B 1980 Threatened abortion studied by estradio-17-beta in serum and ultrasound. Obstetrics and Gynecology 55: 324–328

Huisjes J J 1984 Spontaneous abortion. In: Lind T (ed) Current review in obstetrics and gynaecology. Churchill Livingstone, Edinburgh, pp 132–136

Johnson M R, Brookes A, Norman-Taylor J Q et al 1993a Serum placental protein 14 levels in the first trimester of ovum donation pregnancies. Human Reproduction 8: 485–487

Johnson M R, Riddle A F, Sharma V, Collins W P, Nicolaides K H, Grudzinskas J G 1993b Placental and ovarian hormones in anembryonic pregnancy. Human Reproduction 8: 112–115

Johnson M R, Riddle A F, Irvine R et al 1993c Corpus luteum failure in ectopic pregnancy. Human Reproduction 8: 1491–1495

Jones H W, Acosta A A, Andrews M C et al 1983 What is pregnancy? A question for in vitro fertilisation. Fertility and Sterility 40: 728–733

Joupilla P, Tapanainen J, Huhtaniemi I 1979 Plasma hCG levels in patients with bleeding in the first and second trimesters of pregnancy. British Journal of Obstetrics and Gynaecology 86: 343–349

Joupilla P, Seppala M, Chard T 1980a Pregnancy-specific beta-1 glycoprotein in complications of early pregnancy. Lancet i: 667–668

Joupilla P, Huhtaniemi I, Tapanainen J 1980b Early pregnancy failure: study by ultrasonic and hormonal methods. Obstetrics and Gynecology 55: 42–47

Jovanovic L, Dawood M Y, Landesmann R, Saxena B B 1978 Hormonal profile as a prognostic index of early threatened abortion. American Journal of Obstetrics and Gynecology 130: 274–278

Kadar N 1983 Ectopic pregnancy. In: Studd J (ed) Progress in obstetrics and gynaecology, vol 3. Churchill Livingstone, Edinburgh, pp 305–323

Kadar N, Romero R 1988 Further observations on serial hCG patterns in ectopic pregnancy and abortions. Fertility and Sterility 50: 367–370

Kadar N, Caldwell B V, Romero R 1981 A method for screening for ectopic pregnancy and its indication. Obstetrics and Gynecology 58: 162–166

Klopper A 1985 Steroids in pregnancy. In: Shearman R P (ed) Clinical reproductive endocrinology. Churchill Livingstone, Edinburgh, pp 209–223

Kunz J, Keller P J 1976 hPL, oestradiol, progesterone and AFP in patients with threatened abortion. British Journal of Obstetrics and Gynaecology 83: 640–644

Lee J N, Salem H T, Al-Ani A T M et al 1981 Circulating concentrations of specific placental proteins (human chorionic gonadotrophin, pregnancy-specific beta-1 glycoprotein and placental protein 5) in untreated gestational trophoblastic tumours. American Journal of Obstetrics and Gynecology 39: 702–704

Lee J N, Salem H T, Chard T, Huang S C, Ouyang P C 1982 Circulating placental proteins (hCG, SP1 and PP5) in trophoblastic disease. British Journal of Obstetrics and Gynaecology 89: 69–72

Lenton A E, Grudzinskas J G, Gordon Y B, Chard T, Cooke I D 1981 Pregnancy specific beta-1 glycoprotein and chorionic gonadotrophin in early pregnancy. Acta Obstetricia et Gynecologica Scandinavica 60: 489–492

Letchworth A T 1976 Human placental lactogen assay as a guide to fetal wellbeing. In: Klopper A (ed) Plasma hormone assays in evaluation of fetal wellbeing. Churchill Livingstone, Edinburgh, pp 147–173

Lower A M, Yovich J L, Hancock C, Grudzinskas J G 1993 Is luteal function maintained by factors other than human chorionic gonadotrophin in early pregnancy? Human Reproduction 8: 645–648

Lutjen C, Trounson A, Leeton J, Findlay J, Wood C, Renou P 1984 The establishment and maintenance of pregnancy using in-vitro fertilisation and embryo donation in a patient with primary ovarian failure. Nature 307: 174–175

Masson G M, Anthony F, Wilson M S, Lindsay K 1983a Comparison of serum and urine hCG levels with SP1 and PAPP-A levels in patients with first-trimester vaginal bleeding. Obstetrics and Gynecology 61: 223–226

Masson G M, Anthony F, Wilson M S 1983b Value of Schwangerschaftsprotein 1 (SP1) and pregnancy associated plasma protein (PAPP-A) in the clinical management of threatened abortion. British Journal of Obstetrics and Gynaecology 90: 146–149

Meunier K, Mignot T M, Maria B, Guichard A, Zorn J R, Cedard L 1991 Predictive value of active renin assay for the diagnosis of ectopic pregnancy. Fertility and Sterility 55: 432–435

Miller J F, Williamson E, Glue J, Gordon Y B, Grudzinskas J G, Sykes A 1980 Fetal loss after implantation. Lancet ii: 554–556

Muller F et al 1993 Serum PAPP-A levels are depressed in women with fetal Down syndrome in early pregnancy. Prenatal Diagnosis 13: 633–636

Newlands E S 1983 Treatment of trophoblastic disease. In: Studd J (ed) Progress in obstetrics and gynaecology, vol 3. Churchill Livingstone, Edinburgh, pp 158–174

Niven P A R, Landon J, Chard T 1972 Placental lactogen levels as a guide to outcome of threatened abortion. British Medical Journal iii: 799–801

Nygren K G, Johansson E D G, Wide L 1973 Evaluation of the prognosis of threatened abortion from the peripheral levels of plasma progesterone, estradiol and human chorionic gonadotrophin. American Journal of Obstetrics and Gynecology 116: 916–922

Olajide F, Kitau M J, Chard T 1989 Maternal serum AFP levels in the first trimester of pregnancy. European Journal of Obstetrics, Gynecology and Reproductive Biology 30: 123–128

Pittaway D E, Wentz A C, Maxon W S, Herbert C, Daniell J, Fleischer A C 1985 The efficacy of early pregnancy monitoring with serial chorionic gonadotrophin determinations and realtime ultrasonography in an infertile population. Fertility and Sterility 44: 190–194

Roberts C J, Lowe C R 1975 Where have all the conceptions gone? Lancet i: 498–499

Salem H T, Ghaneimah S A, Shabaan M M, Chard T 1984 Prognostic value of biochemical tests in the assessment of fetal outcome in threatened abortion. British Journal of Obstetrics and Gynaecology 91: 382–385

Schultz-Larsen P, Hertz J B 1978 The predictive value of pregnancy specific beta-1 glycoprotein in threatened abortion. European Journal of Obstetrics, Gynecology and Reproductive Biology 8: 253–257

Seppala M, Ronnberg L, Ylostalo P, Joupilla P 1979a Early detection of implantation by pregnancy specific beta-1 glycoprotein secretion in an infertile woman treated by artificial insemination and human chorionic gonadotrophin. Fertility and Sterility 32: 608–609

Seppala M, Wahlstrom T, Bohn H 1979b Circulating levels and tissue localisation of placental protein 5 (PP5) in pregnancy and trophoblastic disease: absence of PP5 expression in the malignant trophoblast. International Journal of Cancer 24: 6–10

Sinosich M J 1988 Biological role of pregnancy-associated plasma protein A in human reproduction. In: Bischof P, Klopper A (eds) proteins of the placenta. Karger, Basel, pp 158–184

Sinosich M J, Ferrier A, Teisner B et al 1988 Pregnancy-associated plasma protein: fact, fiction, future. In: Chapman M, Grudzinskas G, Chard T (eds) Implantation. Springer, London, pp 45–82

Soma H, Kikuchi M, Takayama M et al 1981 Concentrations of SP1 and beta-hCG in serum and cerebrospinal fluid and concentrations of hCG in urine in patients with trophoblastic tumour. Archives of Gynecology 230: 321–327

Spencer K, Macri J N, Aitken D A, Connor J M 1992 Free beta (hCG) is a first trimester marker for fetal trisomy. Lancet 339: 1480

Stabile I 1992 Diagnosis and management of ectopic pregnancy. In: Stabile I, Grudzinskas J G, Chard T (eds) Spontaneous abortion. Springer Verlag, London, pp 159–179

Stabile I, Olajide F, Grudzinskas J G 1989 Maternal serum alphafetoprotein levels in anembryonic pregnancy. Human Reproduction 4: 204–205

Than G N, Tatra G, Szabo D G, Csaba K, Bohutt E 1988 Beta lactoglobulin homologue placental protein 14 (PP14) in serum of patients with trophoblastic disease and non trophoblastic gynaecological pregnancy. Archives of Gynaecology 243: 131–137

Tsakok F T M, Koh M, Ratnam S S et al 1983 Pregnancy associated proteins in trophoblastic disease. British Journal of Obstetrics and Gynaecology 90: 483–486

Wald N J, Cuckle H S, Densem W et al 1988 Maternal screening for Down's syndrome in early pregnancy. British Medical Journal 2: 883–887

Wald N J, Cuckle H S, Stone R et al 1992a First trimester concentrations of pregnancy associated plasma protein A and placental protein 14 in Down's syndrome. British Medical Journal 305: 28

Wald N J, Kownard A, Densem J, Cuckle H S, Chard T, Butler L 1992b Antenatal maternal serum screening for Down's syndrome: result of a demonstration project. British Medical Journal 305: 391–394

Wang H S, Perry L A, Kanisius J, Iles R K, Holly J M P, Chard T 1991 Purification and assay of insulin-like growth factor-binding protein-1: measurement of circulating levels throughout pregnancy. Journal of Endocrinology 128: 161–168

Ward R H T, Grudzinskas J G, Bolton A E et al 1985 Fetoplacental products as a prognostic guide following chorionic villus sampling. In: Fraccaro M, Simoni G, Brambati B (eds) First trimester diagnosis. Springer-Verlag, Berlin, pp 73–76

Wathen N C, Egembah S, Campbell D J, Farkas A, Chard T 1993 Levels of insulin-like growth factor binding protein-1 increase rapidly in amniotic fluid from 11 to 16 weeks gestation. Journal of Endocrinology 137: R1–R4

Westergaard J G, Chemnitz J, Teisner B et al 1983 Pregnancy-associated plasma protein A—a possible marker in the classification and diagnosis of Cornelia de Lange syndrome. Prenatal Diagnosis 3: 225–232

Westergaard J G, Teisner B, Sinosich M J, Madsen L T, Grudzinskas J G 1985 Does ultrasound examination render biochemical tests obsolete in the prediction of early pregnancy failure? British Journal of Obstetrics and Gynaecology 92: 77–83

Whittaker P G, Taylor A, Lind T 1983 Unsuspected pregnancy loss in healthy women. Lancet i: 1126–1127

Wilcox A J, Weinberg C R, Wehmann R E, Armstrong E G, Canfield R E, Nisula B C 1985 Measuring early pregnancy loss: laboratory and field methods. Fertility and Sterility 44: 366–374

Yovich J L, McColin J C, Willcox D L, Grudzinskas J G, Bolton A E 1986 The prognostic value of beta hCG, PAPP-A, oestradiol and progesterone in early human pregnancies and the effect of medroxy progesterone acetate. Australia and New Zealand Journal of Obstetrics and Gynaecology 26: 59–64

12. Biochemical detection of neural tube defects and Down's syndrome

Nicholas J. Wald

Material in this chapter contains contributions from the first edition and we are grateful to the previous author for the work done.

Neural tube defects and Down's syndrome are two of the most common serious congenital malformations. Antenatal screening can identify nearly all pregnancies with open neural tube defects and about two-thirds of pregnancies with Down's syndrome. Screening for these conditions is an important part of antenatal care in many countries. The diagnosis of neural tube defects relies on detailed ultrasound examination of the fetus and biochemical examination of amniotic fluid; the diagnosis of Down's syndrome relies on examining the chromosome pattern (karyotype) in fetal cells obtained from amniocentesis or chorionic villus sampling. Screening is carried out because the medical risks or the financial costs of the diagnostic procedures preclude them being offered routinely to all women and so selection is needed. The purpose of antenatal screening is to identify women who are at sufficiently high risk of having one or the other abnormality to justify a diagnostic procedure and to do so in a simple and equitable manner.

DEFINITION OF SCREENING TERMS

A number of terms used in screening, such as detection rate, false-positive rate and likelihood ratio, are defined in the short glossary at the end of this chapter.

NEURAL TUBE DEFECTS

Birth prevalence

In the UK the birth prevalence of neural tube defects in

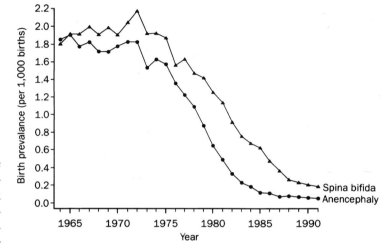

Fig. 12.1 Birth prevalence of anencephaly and spina bifida (without anencephaly) in England and Wales from 1964 to 1991.

the absence of antenatal diagnosis and selective abortion is about 3–4 per 1000 births. Figure 12.1 shows the birth prevalence corrected for under-reporting. Between 1965, when few affected pregnancies were terminated, and 1991 when an antenatal screening programme for neural tube defects had been established for some years, the birth prevalence of anencephaly fell by 98% (there were 1335 affected births in 1965 and 22 in 1991) and the birth prevalence of spina bifida without anencephaly fell by 93% (1395 affected births in 1965 and 103 in 1991). The actual numbers will be somewhat higher due to under-reporting; the numbers adjusted for under-reporting in 1991 were 27 births with anencephaly and 118 births with spina bifida alone.

The most important cause of neural tube defects is a lack of dietary folic acid; with adequate dietary folic acid approximately three-quarters of neural tube defect pregnancies can be prevented (Expert Advisory Group 1992, Wald 1993).

There are genetic as well as environmental determinants of neural tube defects. It has been long recognized that the risk of a fetal neural tube defect is increased about ten-fold among women who previously had one affected pregnancy, about 20-fold among women who had two affected pregnancies, and about 40-fold among those who had three. These women are at sufficiently high risk to justify amniocentesis and a detailed ultrasound examination without first carrying out a screening test.

In spite of these high risks of recurrence, 95% of affected pregnancies arise in women who have not previously had a neural tube defect pregnancy. It is primarily to these women that screening for open neural tube defects is offered.

Natural history

An important distinction, from the point of view of screening and antenatal diagnosis, is whether the lesion is open or closed. An open lesion is one in which neural tissue is exposed or covered by a thin transparent membrane. A closed lesion is one in which the neural tissue is completely covered by skin or a thick opaque membrane. The type of lesion has an important influence on biochemical screening because the pathophysiological basis of the screening test is leakage of alpha-fetoprotein (AFP) from the fetus into the amniotic fluid and then into the maternal circulation. Leakage does occur with open lesions, which can usually be detected. Anencephaly is always an open lesion, and 80–90% of spina bifida cases are open. Closed lesions, which do not allow this leakage, are not associated with high levels in amniotic fluid or maternal serum and therefore escape detection.

Anencephaly is a fatal condition. Infants born with open spina bifida have a poor prognosis, with a 36% 5-year survival rate (Althouse & Wald 1980). Among this group of 5-year survivors, 82% were severely handicapped and 10% were moderately handicapped. They had, on average, spent over half a year in hospital and had, on average, six surgical operations by the age of five. Closed spina bifida has a somewhat better prognosis. The 5-year survival rate was 60%, and among these survivors, about one-third were severely handicapped and another third moderately handicapped.

Screening

AFP screening has a minor role in the detection of anencephaly since this is readily detected by ultrasound (though AFP screening will also detect nearly all cases) and AFP screening should not be expected to detect *closed* spina bifida. AFP screening is intended for *open* spina bifida. The separation between maternal serum AFP levels in pregnancies with open spina bifida and unaffected pregnancies is greatest at 17 weeks of pregnancy. Screening is therefore best done around this time. To allow for the increase in the concentration of maternal serum AFP in the second trimester of pregnancy, it is convenient to express all AFP values as a multiple of the normal median (MoM) at the relevant gestational age. By using laboratory-specific medians, allowance is also made for systematic differences between laboratories. The use of the median as a measure of central tendency (the middle value at a given week of pregnancy, when all the values are arranged in ascending order) is preferred to the mean value because it is not influenced by occasional outlying values. Maternal serum AFP values are therefore usually expressed in MoMs.

In the Fourth UK Collaborative AFP Study (Wald & Cuckle 1982b) serum AFP data on pregnancies with and without neural tube defects were combined in 3-week groups and separate estimates of the means and standard deviations of the distributions in these periods were calculated. This led to abrupt changes in the median MoM values for, say, open spina bifida, from one 3-week period to the next. This was artificial, and to avoid the problem revised parameters for each week of gestational age have been estimated and published (Wald et al 1992a). Table 12.1 shows the detection rate and screening false-positive

Table 12.1 Maternal serum AFP screening at 15–20 weeks' gestation: detection rate for open spina bifida and false-positive rate according to method of estimating gestational age used to calculate MoM value and AFP cut-off level. Timing of test based on dates

| AFP (MoM) | Detection rate (%) | | | | | | False-positive rate (%) |
| | Gestation (completed weeks) | | | | | | 15–20 weeks |
	15	16	17	18	19	20	
	Dates used to estimate gestation to calculate MoM values						
≥ 2.0	67	77	81	80	76	66	6.8
≥ 2.5	57	67	72	72	67	55	2.4
≥ 3.0	48	59	64	64	58	46	0.9
	Biparietal diameter used to estimate gestation to calculate MoM values						
≥ 2.0	81	88	91	90	88	80	5.8
≥ 2.5	73	82	85	85	81	72	1.9
≥ 3.0	65	75	79	79	74	64	0.6

Detection and false-positive rates estimated using parameters of distributions from Wald et al (1992a). (AFP MoM values not adjusted for maternal weight.)
MoM = multiple of the median for unaffected pregnancies of the same gestational age.

rate for open spina bifida according to AFP cut-off level, gestational age and method of determining gestational age, either dates (time since first day of last menstrual period) or biparietal diameter (BPD) estimated using an ultrasound examination. At 17 weeks' gestation, using an AFP cut-off level of 2.5 MoM or greater, the detection rate for open spina bifida is 85% with a false-positive rate of 1.9% using a BPD to estimate gestational age. Using dates the detection rate is 72% for a 2.4% false-positive rate. Figure 12.2 shows the distribution of maternal serum AFP in unaffected and open spina bifida pregnancies at 17 weeks' gestation based on dates, with gestational age estimated by dates or ultrasound BPD to calculate the AFP MoM value. Improved performance of screening when gestational age is estimated from an ultrasound BPD arises in two ways. First, there is a small effect because ultrasound increases the precision of estimating gestational age and so reduces the variance of AFP at a given gestation. Second, because spina bifida fetuses tend to have small BPDs, they are, on average, credited with a less advanced gestational age than is the case. This error turns out to be advantageous, since it leads to AFP MoM values being higher when based on a BPD measurement than when based on dates—on average, 43% higher (Wald et al 1980). This has a large effect on increasing spina bifida detection rates and also, incidentally, leads to the detection of some cases of closed spina bifida because ultrasound increases the MoM value in these cases as well.

Maternal serum AFP levels decrease on average with increasing maternal weight (Haddow et al 1981, Wald et al 1981), probably due to dilution of fetal AFP in the maternal circulation, the extent of dilution being greater in the larger plasma volume of heavier women than in that of lighter women. A simple method of adjusting AFP values for maternal weight is to divide the observed MoM value by the expected MoM value for a given weight. Adjusting AFP values in this way will reduce the variance of maternal serum AFP in affected and unaffected pregnancies and so tend to reduce the extent of overlap in the distributions shown in Figure 12.2. The effect is small; the detection and false-positive rates at an AFP cut-off level of 2.5 MoM with maternal weight adjustments are 72% and 2.2% with dates and 86% and 1.4% with scan.

Anterior abdominal wall defects

The two anterior abdominal wall defects gastroschisis and exomphalos are associated with increased maternal serum AFP levels—on average about four times higher than expected for exomphalos and about seven times higher for gastroschisis (Fig. 12.3) (Palomaki et al 1988). Table 12.2 shows the detection rate and false-positive rate for exomphalos and gastroschisis for various AFP cut-off levels. At AFP cut-off levels of 2.5 MoM, over 99% of pregnancies with gastroschisis would be detected and the detection rate for exomphalos would be 71%.

Statistical considerations

Before judging the value of a screening or diagnostic test, two questions need to be answered:

1. What is the detection rate at any given cut-off level and what is the corresponding false-positive rate?
2. What is the average risk of being affected (or having an affected pregnancy) for individuals with results equal to or greater than any given cut-off level?

Before interpreting an individual's results, a further question needs to be answered; namely

3. What is the specific risk of being affected (or having an affected pregnancy) for an individual with a particular test result?

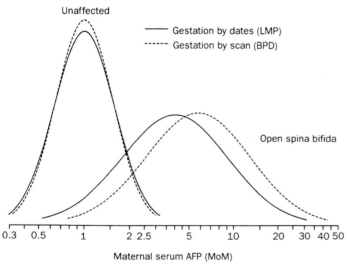

Fig. 12.2 Distribution of maternal serum alpha-fetoprotein (AFP) levels in pregnancies with open spina bifida and pregnancies without neural tube defects (unaffected) at 17 weeks of gestation with gestational age estimated by dates (from first day of last menstrual period) and by an ultrasound (fetal biparietal diameter measurement). MoM = Multiple of the median for unaffected pregnancies of the same gestational age.

Table 12.2 Detection rates and false-positive rates for anterior abdominal wall defects acording to maternal serum AFP (15–22 weeks' gestation)

AFP (MoM)	Detection rate (%)		False-positive rate (%)
	Exomphalos	Gastroschisis	
≥ 2.0	78	>99	6.48
≥ 2.5	71	>99	2.25
≥ 3.0	65	99	0.81
≥ 3.5	60	97	0.31

Derived from parameters in Palomaki et al (1988).
MoM = multiple of the median for unaffected pregnancies of the same gestational age.

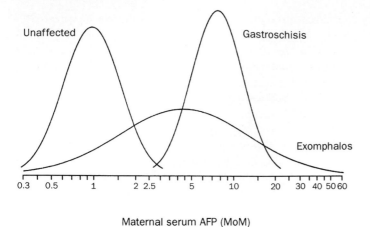

Fig. 12.3 The distributions of maternal serum alphafetoprotein in unaffected pregnancies and pregnancies with abdominal wall defects (exomphalos and gastroschisis). Parameters of distributions from Palomaki et al (1988) and Wald et al (1992a).

The method of calculating these estimates is illustrated for open spina bifida and maternal serum AFP using an AFP value of 2.5 MoM.

The open spina bifida *detection rate* and *false-positive rate* can be estimated approximately by examining the AFP distributions in affected and unaffected pregnancies and judging what proportion of each distribution lies to the right of 2.5 MoM (shaded in Fig. 12.4). To estimate the proportions, it is only necessary to know the mean and standard deviation of each distribution (Table 12.3); these define each of the distributions uniquely. The two proportions are then determined by calculating how many standard deviations 2.5 MoM is away from each of the

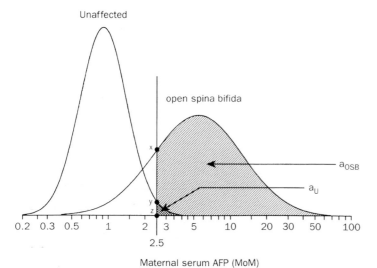

Fig. 12.4 Distribution of maternal serum alphafetoprotein (AFP) levels in unaffected and open spina bifida pregnancies showing a cut-off level of 2.5 MoM. The likelihood ratio (see text) for open spina bifida is: (i) AFP ≥ 2.5 MoM is a_{OSB}/a_u; (ii) AFP = 2.5 MoM is xy/yz. MoM = Multiple of the median for unaffected pregnancies of the same gestational age.

Table 12.3 Mean and standard deviation of maternal serum AFP ($\log_{10}$ MoM) in singleton pregnancies with and without spina bifida

	Gestation estimated by:	
	Dates	Scan (BPD)
Open spina bifida		
Mean		
15 completed weeks	0.4581	0.6134
16 completed weeks	0.5579	0.7132
17 completed weeks	0.6063	0.7617
18 completed weeks	0.6034	0.7567
19 completed weeks	0.5491	0.7044
20 completed weeks	0.4434	0.5987
21 completed weeks	0.2864	0.4417
22 completed weeks	0.0779	0.2333
Standard deviation		
15–22 weeks	0.3535 (0.3507*)	0.3489 (0.3429*)
Closed spina bifida (15–22 weeks)		
Mean	0.0000	0.1553
Standard deviation	0.1986 (0.1936*)	0.1902 (0.1789*)
Unaffected pregnancies (15–22 weeks)		
Mean	0.0000	0.0000
Standard deviation	0.1986 (0.1936*)	0.1902 (0.1789*)

*Adjusted for maternal weight.
MoM = multiple of the median for unaffected pregnancies of the same gestational age.

respective means and looking up these values in tables of the Gaussian distribution. This is done in steps 1–6 in Table 12.4. The same procedure can be used for any cut-off level.

The average risk of having an open spina bifida pregnancy for women with a positive screening result using a cut-off level of 2.5 MoM is estimated by determining the ratio of the shaded areas in Figure 12.4 (spina bifida divided by unaffected), which is the detection rate divided by the false-positive rate (in our example, 85% divided by 1.8% = 47 shown as step 6 in Table 12.4). This ratio is called the likelihood ratio and it is the number of times that a woman with a positive result is more likely to have a spina bifida pregnancy compared with women in general. The likelihood ratio is used to multiply the background birth prevalence of open spina bifida expressed as an odds. For example, if the background prevalence were 2 per 1000 births, expressed as odds this would be 2 : 998. Multiplying 2 : 998 by 47 yields 94 to 998, which, expressed as a probability, is about 9% or 1 in 12.

To determine the *specific risk of having an open spina bifida pregnancy for a particular woman with a given AFP level*, the calculation is similar except that the likelihood ratio is the ratio of the *heights* of the distribution curves for affected and unaffected pregnancies (spina bifida divided by unaffected) at the given AFP value (xz divided by yz in Fig. 12.4 at 2.5 MoM) instead of the ratio of the *areas*. This calculation is given in Table 12.4 in steps 7–9; the likelihood ratio is 2.8 for a woman with an AFP level of exactly 2.5 MoM. If, as before, the background prevalence of open spina bifida births is 2 : 998, her odds

Table 12.4 Maternal serum AFP screening for open spina bifida at 17 completed weeks of pregnancy (estimated from a biparietal diameter measurement): illustration of the calculation of (1) the detection rate (DR), false-positive rate (FPR) and likelihood ratio (LR) for women with maternal serum AFP levels ⩾ 2.5 MoM (steps 1–6) and (2) the likelihood ratio for a woman with an AFP level of exactly 2.5 MoM (steps 1–3 and 7–9)

Steps	Open spina bifida	Unaffected pregnancies
1. Convert 2.5 into log$_{10}$	0.3979	0.3979
2. Subtract mean from Table 12.2	0.379–0.7617 = –0.3638	0.3979 – 0.0 = 0.3979
3. Divide by SD from Table 12.2 to determine Z	–0.3638/0.3489 = –1.04	0.3979/0.1902 = 2.09
4. Look up Z in table of normal distribution*	0.1492	0.9817
5. Subtract from 1.0 and multiply by 100% to determine DR and FPR	(1 – 0.1492) × 100% = 85%	(1 – 0.9817) × 100% = 1.8%
6. Divide DR by FPR to determine LR for ⩾ 2.5 MoM	47 (LR)	
7. Look up Z in table of heights of normal distribution†	0.2323	0.0449
8. Divide by SD from Table 12.2 to determine heights of the AFP distributions	0.2323/0.3489 = 0.6658	0.0460/0.1902 = 0.2419
9. Divide heights to determine LR for 2.5 MoM	2.8 (LR)	

*The table will give the area under the distribution to the left of [Z], i.e. ignoring any minus sign. If Z is negative look up [Z] and subtract from 1.
†This table will give the height of the standardized distribution (assuming SD = 1) at [Z], i.e. ignoring any minus sign.
MoM = multiple of the median for unaffected pregnancies of the same gestational age.

of having an affected pregnancy become approximately 6 : 998 (2.8 × 2 : 998), which, expressed as a probability is 6/(998 + 6), about 0.6% or 1 in 170.

Diagnosis

The main biochemical diagnostic tests for open neural tube defects are amniotic fluid AFP measurement and amniotic fluid acetylcholinesterase (AChE) measurement. The AChE test is usually performed by polyacrylamide gel electrophoresis, a qualitative test. A result is positive if there is an AChE band in the gel that migrates to the same position as the AChE in cerebral spinal fluid and the band is inhibited by the specific AChE inhibitor given the code name BW284C51. An alternative assay (Rasmussen-Loft et al 1990) based on an immunoassay performs well but has not been shown to perform better than the gel electrophoresis test. The Second Report of the Collaborative Acetylcholinesterase Study (Wald et al 1989) showed that AChE measurement was a better diagnostic test than AFP. The study was based on 32 642 women with singleton pregnancies, including 428 with open spina bifida and 238 with anencephaly, who had an amnio-

centesis at 13–24 weeks' gestation. The AChE test yielded a detection rate for open spina bifida of 99% (95% confidence interval, 98–100%), 98% for anencephaly (95% confidence interval, 96–100%) and a false-positive rate of 0.34% (95% confidence interval, 0.28–0.40%) excluding miscarriage, intrauterine death and serious fetal abnormalities. Comparable rates for amniotic fluid AFP as a diagnostic test were less favourable, yielding a lower detection rate and a higher false-positive rate—e.g. 85% and 0.36% respectively.

Although AChE is a better diagnostic test than AFP, almost as high a detection rate can be achieved by restricting AChE measurement to women with AFP levels exceeding 2 MoM (about 5%) with the advantage of reducing the corresponding false-positive rate (see Table 12.5, column headed 'any reason' for the amniocentesis, 0.06% compared to 0.34% with a small change in detection, 97% compared to 99%). Table 12.5 also shows the performance according to whether the amniocentesis is performed on account of a raised maternal serum AFP level or for other reasons, and whether the amniotic fluid sample was clear. Blood contamination of amniotic fluid is an important cause of false-positive results. Fortunately

Table 12.5 Open spina bifida detection rates and false-positive rates according to reason for amniocentesis and quality of amniotic fluid sample

Test policy	Amniocentesis for high serum AFP — All AF samples DR (%) n = 344	FPR (%) n = 5557	Clear* AF samples DR (%) n = 298	FPR (%) n = 4785	Amniocentesis for other reasons — All AF samples DR (%) n = 84	FPR (%) n = 25 896	Clear* AF samples DR (%) n = 76	FPR (%) n = 24 223	Any reason — All AF samples DR (%) n = 428	FPR (%) n = 31 453	Clear* AF samples DR (%) n = 374	FPR (%) n = 29 008
A. AChE alone	99	0.56	99	0.23	96	0.29	96	0.15	99	0.34	99	0.16
B. AFP alone†	90	1.5	91	1.3	92	0.23	92	0.11	90	0.46	91	0.30
C. AChE if AF-AFP ⩾ 2.0 MoM	97	0.40	98	0.19	95	0.09	95	0.03	97	0.06	95	0.03

*Clear sample is one that is not visibly blood stained.
†Using gestation specific AF-AFP cut-off levels; 3.0 MoM (13–15 weeks); 3.5 (16–18); 4.0 (19–21); 45 (22–24).
n = number of pregnancies; AFP = alphafetoprotein; AChE = acetylcholinesterase; AF = amniotic fluid; MoM = multiple of the median for unaffected pregnancies of the same gestational age.

this is rare. Among clear (not blood-stained) samples the selective AChE testing policy (C in Table 12.5) yields a detection rate of 98% with a false-positive rate of 2 per 1000 (0.19%) among women having an amniocentesis on account of a high serum AFP screening test.

The reason for the higher amniotic fluid AFP false-positive rate in women with a high serum AFP level is that there is an association between maternal serum and amniotic fluid AFP. The higher AChE false-positive rate is less easily explained but may be due to an association between high amniotic fluid AFP and the presence of amniotic fluid AChE.

The diagnosis of spina bifida using ultrasound to visualize the fetal spine is effective. In specialist centres the detection rate has been estimated to be 87% with a false-positive rate of 1.2% (Cuckle & Wald 1992)—a performance similar to diagnosis based on amniotic fluid biochemical analysis. The main medical cost of a biochemical diagnosis is the risk of fetal loss due to amniocentesis. The best estimate of this is from the randomized trial of amniocentesis reported by Tabor and her colleagues (1986). An excess risk of 1.0% is cited. If the fetal loss rate in women randomized to the control group is subtracted from the rate in women allocated to the control group, the excess risk is 0.78% (95% confidence interval 0.04–1.53%). If an adjustment is made for cytogenetically abnormal fetuses that were terminated but would otherwise have miscarried, the estimate would be 0.87 with wide confidence intervals (0.08–1.58%). In terms of diagnostic accuracy it is best to use both ultrasound and amniocentesis; only if a woman chooses to forego the extra accuracy (and knows this) would it be reasonable to abandon the amniocentesis. If the spina bifida birth prevalence were 1 per 1000, then from Table 12.1, women with serum AFP levels greater than or equal to 2.5 MoMs at 17 weeks based on a BPD measurement have a 1 : 22 odds (85/1.9 × 1 : 1000) of having an affected pregnancy. Using the detection and false-positive rates applicable when gestation is estimated by ultrasound (Table 12.1), a positive scan diagnosis will increase the odds to $(1 \times 87\%)$: $(22 \times 1.2\%)$ or 3 : 1; one out of every four positives would be a false-positive. It would therefore be wise to confirm the diagnosis with an amniocentesis which would correct most of the false-positives. If the diagnostic scan examination were negative the odds would be reduced to $[1 \times (100 - 87\%)]$: $[22 \times (100 - 1.2\%)]$ or 1 : 167 which is still six times greater than the odds prior to screening. The best policy is the one in which amniocentesis and ultrasound are used as complementary diagnostic investigations. This yields a detection rate of 95%, a false-positive rate of less than 0.1% and an overall fetal loss rate (mainly due to amniocentesis) of 0.8% (Table 12.6).

DOWN'S SYNDROME

Birth prevalence

Figure 12.5 shows the birth prevalence of Down's syndrome in the absence of antenatal screening and selective abortion. The estimates are derived by applying the maternal age-specific prevalence to the distribution of maternal ages among maternities from 1974 to 1987. In 1991 the estimate was 1.4 per 1000. The figure also shows estimates for the proportion of Down's syndrome births identified through antenatal diagnosis as derived from the National Cytogenetic Down's Syndrome Register. In 1991 38% of Down's syndrome pregnancies were identified in this way.

The cytogenetic abnormality in an affected individual with Down's syndrome is the presence in the cells of three copies of chromosome 21, instead of two. The third copy arises from failure of two chromosome 21s to separate (non-dysjunction) at the first or second meiotic division. Usually this occurs in the female germ cell, but

Table 12.6 Comparison of three policies in the diagnosis of open spina bifida among women with raised maternal serum alphafetoprotein (AFP) levels

Diagnostic policy	Detection rate (%)	False-positive rate (%)	Fetal loss rate per 1000 women with unaffected pregnancies due to		
			Diagnostic error	Amniocentesis	Both
Ultrasonography only	87	1.2	12	0	12
Amniocentesis only	97	0.4	4	8	12
Ultrasonography and amniocentesis[†]	95[‡]	<0.1[§]	<1	8	<9

Based on Wald & Cuckle (1992).
*From the Copenhagen randomized study (Tabor et al 1986), subtracting the fetal loss rate in women allocated to the control group from the rate in women allocated to the amniocentesis group.
†Ultrasonographic examination is repeated if it is negative but the amniotic fluid results are positive; a final positive result is one in which both the ultrasonographic examination and amniotic fluid results are positive.
‡Assumes four out of five of cases missed by ultrasonographic examination are detected upon re-examination after a positive amniotic fluid result is known (as found in Richards et al 1988 and Drugan et al 1988).
§Assumes that at least three out of four of amniotic fluid false-positives will be corrected by ultrasonographic examination; in fact the proportion is likely to be greater, but data on this are lacking.

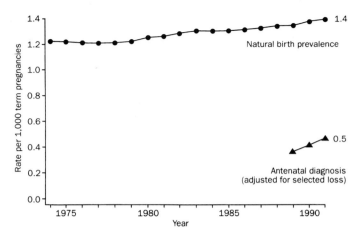

Fig. 12.5 Estimated birth prevalence of Down's syndrome in England and Wales from 1974 to 1991 in the absence of antenatal diagnosis and selective abortion (natural birth prevalence) and reported prevalence of antenatal screening.

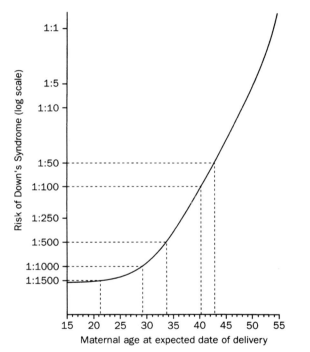

Fig. 12.6 Risk of a Down's syndrome birth according to maternal age at expected date of delivery. Based on Cuckle et al (1987).

Table 12.7 Risk of a Down's syndrome term pregnancy according to maternal age, in years and months at the expected date of delivery

Years	Completed months			
	0	3	6	9
15	1 : 1580	1 : 1579	1 : 1577	1 : 1576
16	1 : 1575	1 : 1574	1 : 1572	1 : 1570
17	1 : 1569	1 : 1567	1 : 1565	1 : 1563
18	1 : 1561	1 : 1558	1 : 1556	1 : 1553
19	1 : 1550	1 : 1547	1 : 1543	1 : 1540
20	1 : 1536	1 : 1532	1 : 1527	1 : 1523
21	1 : 1518	1 : 1512	1 : 1506	1 : 1500
22	1 : 1494	1 : 1487	1 : 1480	1 : 1472
23	1 : 1463	1 : 1455	1 : 1445	1 : 1435
24	1 : 1425	1 : 1414	1 : 1402	1 : 1390
25	1 : 1376	1 : 1363	1 : 1348	1 : 1333
26	1 : 1317	1 : 1300	1 : 1283	1 : 1264
27	1 : 1245	1 : 1225	1 : 1205	1 : 1183
28	1 : 1161	1 : 1138	1 : 1115	1 : 1090
29	1 : 1065	1 : 1040	1 : 1014	1 : 978
30	1 : 960	1 : 932	1 : 905	1 : 877
31	1 : 848	1 : 820	1 : 791	1 : 763
32	1 : 734	1 : 706	1 : 678	1 : 650
33	1 : 623	1 : 596	1 : 570	1 : 544
34	1 : 518	1 : 494	1 : 470	1 : 446
35	1 : 424	1 : 402	1 : 381	1 : 360
36	1 : 341	1 : 322	1 : 304	1 : 287
37	1 : 270	1 : 254	1 : 239	1 : 225
38	1 : 212	1 : 199	1 : 187	1 : 175
39	1 : 164	1 : 154	1 : 144	1 : 135
40	1 : 126	1 : 118	1 : 111	1 : 103
41	1 : 97	1 : 90	1 : 84	1 : 79
42	1 : 73	1 : 69	1 : 64	1 : 60
43	1 : 56	1 : 52	1 : 48	1 : 45
44	1 : 42	1 : 39	1 : 36	1 : 34
45	1 : 31	1 : 29	1 : 27	1 : 25
46	1 : 24	1 : 22	1 : 20	1 : 19
47	1 : 17	1 : 16	1 : 15	1 : 14
48	1 : 13	1 : 12	1 : 11	1 : 10
49	1 : 9.5	1 : 8.8	1 : 8.1	1 : 7.5

From Cuckle & Wald (1990) and derived from the formula for risk given in Cuckle et al (1987), namely $P = 0.000627 + e^{-16.2395 + (0.286 \times MA)}$ where the risk of having Down's syndrome is 1: $(1 - P) / P$ and MA is maternal age in completed years, derived by subtracting 5.5 months from the age in years and completed months and expressing the result as a decimal, before substitution in the formula. For example, 27 y and 8 m = 27 y 2.5 m in completed years and months or 27.21 as a decimal.

maternal age alone as the basis for selecting women for a diagnostic amniocentesis. More recently, age and serum markers have been used together and offered as a screening test to pregnant women of all ages.

A previous pregnancy with a fetus with Down's syndrome increases the risk of a recurrence. This increased prior risk is taken into account when calculating the risk based on the serum concentrations. If the previous fetus had a non-inherited form of Down's syndrome, the risk of having a further Down's syndrome pregnancy still depends largely on maternal age but it is higher than if the previous pregnancy was not associated with Down's syndrome. The risk of a recurrence can be estimated as

sometime it occurs in the male germ cell. The cause of the non-dysjunction is not known and so the cause of Down's syndrome remains unknown, but it is recognized that the risk of Down's syndrome increases with maternal age, and to a small extent paternal age. Figure 12.6 shows the relationship between the risk of a Down's syndrome birth in relation to maternal age at the expected date of delivery, highlighting the maternal age corresponding to five specified risks. Table 12.7 shows the precise risk estimates. Until serum markers for Down's syndrome were discovered, screening was based on using advanced the age-specific risk plus an additive component (0.42% at mid trimester and 0.34% at term). If the previous fetus had an inherited form of Down's syndrome, the recurrence risk is much higher than the age-specific risk at most ages. On average, the resultant risk is about 10% plus the age-specific risk, but expert genetic advice is needed in individual cases.

Natural history

Over 50% of Down's syndrome fetuses are miscarried during the first trimester of pregnancy (Creasy & Crolla 1974). Between about 15 weeks of pregnancy and term, an estimated 23% cent of Down's syndrome pregnancies miscarry (Cuckle & Wald 1990). Infants with Down's syndrome are usually severely mentally retarded and they may have associated physical congenital abnormalities affecting the heart (about 35%), gastrointestinal tract, eyes and ears. The main burden of care arises from the fact that people with Down's syndrome are dependent on others and require considerable personal supervision throughout their lives. The expectation of life is about 50 years (Oster et al 1975, Masaki et al 1981, Baird & Sadovnick 1988). Most adults with Down's syndrome develop neurological changes in their brain typical of Alzheimer's disease, neuritic plaques and neurofibrillary tangles (Dalton 1982, Kolata 1985). The amyloid polypeptide of Alzheimer's disease is coded by a gene on chromosome 21 (Goldgaber et al 1987) and the polypeptide is found in adults with Down's syndrome (Glenner & Wong 1984, Masters et al 1985).

Screening

Screening for Down's syndrome by selecting women for an amniocentesis on the basis of advanced maternal age is not very effective because only a small proportion of affected pregnancies occur in older women. With the discovery of serum markers for Down's syndrome it has become possible to carry out serum screening for this disorder. The principal early second-trimester markers are AFP, unconjugated oestriol (uE$_3$) and human chorionic gonadotrophin (hCG) which, with age, form the basis of the *triple test*. On average, AFP and uE$_3$ levels are reduced by about 25% in pregnancies with Down's syndrome and hCG levels are about double. Figure 12.7 shows the distribution of the three markers at 15–22 weeks of pregnancy. The best way to use the information on maternal age and the three serum markers is to estimate each woman's risk of having an affected pregnancy from the four variables, taking appropriate account of the correlations that exist between them. In this way, the risk estimate becomes a new composite screening variable. Women with a risk above a specified cut-off level are

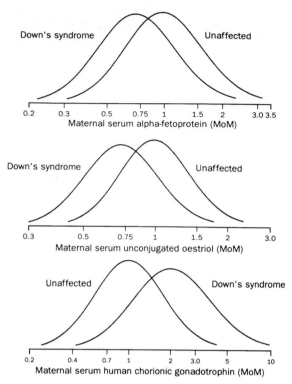

Fig. 12.7 Gaussian relative frequency distributions of maternal serum alphafetoprotein, unconjugated oestriol and human chorionic gonadotrophin in women with fetuses with Down's syndrome and with unaffected fetuses at 15–20 weeks' gestation. Log scale derived from parameters in Wald et al (1994b).

designated screen-positive and those with a lower risk are designated screen-negative. To estimate a woman's risk of having a fetus with Down's syndrome the following equation is used:

$$\text{Test specific risk} = \text{likelihood ratio} \times \text{age specific risk}$$

For one test, the likelihood ratio, as was illustrated in the example with spina bifida, is the factor by which a woman's risk of having an affected fetus is increased above the rate that would have been expected without the test. As before, it is numerically equal to the ratio of the heights of the distribution curves shown in Figure 12.4. If two or more tests are used and the tests are independent (so that among either affected or unaffected pregnancies the value of one test is not related to the value of the other), the likelihood ratios for the two tests are combined by simple multiplication so that if for AFP the given result yields a likelihood ratio of 3 and for hCG the likelihood ratio is 4, the combined likelihood ratio for the two test results would be 12. In practice, the tests are not completely independent (one test shows some association with the other) so the combined likelihood ratio is somewhat less than the product of the two, the reduction being dependent on the correlation between the two.

The triple test

Table 12.8 shows the likelihood ratio for specified combinations of AFP, uE$_3$ and hCG. Tables 12.6 and 12.7 can be used to interpret a serum screening result using the triple test. The woman's age-specific risk from Table 12.7 is multiplied by the likelihood ratio from Table 12.8, corresponding to her set of serum results to yield her test-specific risk estimate.

Figure 12.8 shows the distributions of risk in affected and unaffected pregnancies based on maternal age, AFP, uE$_3$ and hCG with gestation based on dates (LMP) and scan (BPD). The figure gives a clear impression of the performance of screening. For example, with a risk cut-off level of 1 : 250 (so that all women with a risk of 1 : 250 or greater are regarded as screen-positive) 59% of pregnan-

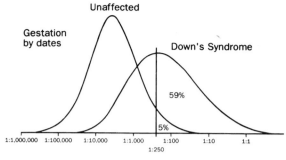

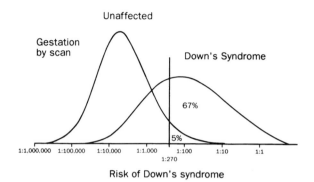

Fig. 12.8 Distribution of risk of Down's syndrome at term in affected and unaffected pregnancies using maternal age, serum alphafetoprotein, unconjugated oestriol and human chorionic gonadotrophin at 15–20 weeks' gestation (log scale). The upper part of the figure shows the distribution with gestational age estimated using dates (time since first day of last menstrual period); the lower part of the figure shows the distribution with gestational age estimated by ultrasound (using the fetal biparietal diameter measurement). In both parts of the figure, cut-off levels have been selected to yield a 5% false-positive rate.

Table 12.8 Estimates of the likelihood ratio for specified combinations of maternal serum alphafetoprotein (AFP), unconjugated oestriol (uE$_3$) and total human chorionic gonadotrophin (hCG) at 15–22 weeks of gestation

hCG (MoM)	uE$_3$ (MoM)	AFP (MoM)						
		0.4	0.5	0.8	1.0	1.25	2.0	2.5
0.40	0.50	0.50	0.24	0.047	0.020	0.0086	0.0013	0.0005
	0.80	0.57	0.31	0.083	0.042	0.0021	0.0042	0.0019
	1.00	0.55	0.33	0.10	0.054	0.02	0.0067	0.0032
	1.25	0.49	0.32	0.11	0.065	0.037	0.010	0.0051
	2.00	0.33	0.24	0.12	0.079	0.052	0.019	0.011
0.50	0.50	0.83	0.42	0.092	0.042	0.019	0.0031	0.0013
	0.80	0.77	0.45	0.13	0.072	0.037	0.0085	0.0040
	1.00	0.67	0.42	0.15	0.084	0.047	0.012	0.0062
	1.25	0.55	0.37	0.15	0.092	0.055	0.017	0.0092
	2.00	0.30	0.24	0.13	0.092	0.063	0.026	0.017
0.80	0.50	2.3	1.35	0.38	0.20	0.099	0.021	0.0096
	0.80	1.4	0.95	0.36	0.22	0.13	0.037	0.020
	1.00	1.0	0.73	0.32	0.21	0.13	0.044	0.025
	1.25	0.69	0.53	0.27	0.19	0.13	0.059	0.030
	2.00	0.25	0.27	0.15	0.12	0.10	0.051	0.036
1.00	0.50	3.8	2.3	0.73	0.40	0.22	0.052	0.025
	0.80	1.9	1.3	0.58	0.37	0.23	0.075	0.042
	1.00	1.2	0.94	0.47	0.32	0.21	0.081	0.049
	1.25	0.77	0.62	0.36	0.26	0.19	0.083	0.054
	2.00	0.22	0.21	0.17	0.14	0.12	0.070	0.053
1.25	0.50	6.3	4.0	1.4	0.83	0.47	0.13	0.065
	0.80	2.6	1.9	0.92	0.62	0.41	0.15	0.090
	1.00	1.5	1.2	0.68	0.49	0.35	0.15	0.095
	1.25	0.85	0.72	0.47	0.37	0.28	0.14	0.094
	2.00	0.20	0.20	0.18	0.16	0.14	0.10	0.076
2.00	0.50	17	13	5.8	3.8	2.4	0.84	0.48
	0.80	4.67	3.9	2.4	1.9	1.4	0.65	0.44
	1.00	2.27	2.0	1.5	1.2	0.96	0.53	0.38
	1.25	1.0	1.0	0.84	0.74	0.62	0.40	0.31
	2.00	0.16	0.18	0.21	0.21	0.21	0.18	0.16
2.50	0.50	28	22	11	7.7	5.20	2.0	1.25
	0.80	6.2	5.5	3.9	3.1	2.43	1.3	0.92
	1.00	2.7	2.6	2.1	1.8	1.54	0.96	0.73
	1.25	1.1	1.2	1.1	1.0	0.92	0.66	0.54
	2.00	0.15	0.17	0.22	0.24	0.2502	0.25	0.23

Parameters of distributions from Wald et al (1994b). MoM = multiple of the median for unaffected pregnancies of the same gestational age.

cies with Down's syndrome and 5% of unaffected pregnancies are designated positive, that is, the detection rate is 59% and the false-positive rate 5%. If gestation is based on scan a risk cut-off of 1 : 270 yields the same false-positive rate but a higher detection rate (67%). Lowering the risk cut-off level increases both the detection rate and the false-positive rate, and raising it will decrease them.

The quadruple test

One of the serum markers, hCG, has two independently synthesized subunits, designated α and β. A proportion of the total concentration of each subunit exists in the free form. The measurement of the two subunits has been shown to improve the performance of screening. The median free β-hCG level in affected pregnancies was, in one study (Wald et al 1994b), found to be 2.22 MoM. The median free α-hCG level in the same dataset was 1.31 MoM. Both were significantly higher than the levels in unaffected pregnancies. Table 12.9 shows the detection rate corresponding to specified false-positive rates (and

Table 12.9 Detection rate corresponding to specified false-positive rates (and the false-positive rate corresponding to specified detection rates) with gestational age based on dates and an ultrasound scan examination using different combinations of AFP, uE₃, total hCG, free β-hCG and free α-hCG

Maternal age with	Dates gestation						Scan gestation					
	Detection rate (%) for a false-positive rate of			False-positive rate (%) for a detection rate of			Detection rate (%) for a false-positive rate of			False-positive rate (%) for a detection rate of		
	1%	5%	9%	30%	50%	70%	1%	5%	9%	30%	50%	70%
Nil	15	30	38	5	19	45	15	30	38	5	19	45
AFP	18	35	45	3.4	12	29	18	36	45	3.3	12	29
AFP, uE₃	23	44	54	1.9	7.2	20	29	51	62	1.1	4.6	14
AFP, total hCG	31	54	65	0.9	3.9	12	33	58	68	0.8	3.2	10
AFP, free β-hCG	29	54	65	1.1	4.1	11	31	57	68	0.9	3.5	10
AFP, free α-hCG, free β-hCG	35	59	68	0.6	2.9	9.9	45	67	76	0.2	1.5	6.1
AFP, uE₃, total hCG	36	59	68	0.6	2.9	9.9	45	67	76	0.2	1.5	6.1
AFP, uE₃, free β-hCG	35	59	68	0.7	2.9	9.5	45	67	76	0.3	1.5	6.1
AFP, uE₃, free α-hCG, free β-hCG	42	65	74	0.3	1.8	7.0	51	72	79	0.1	0.9	4.4

Based on parameters in Wald et al (1994b).

the false-positive rate corresponding to specified detection rates) with gestational age based on dates and an ultrasound scan examination using different combinations of AFP, uE₃, total hCG, free β-hCG and free α-hCG. Table 12.9 shows an increase in detection as a result of adding different serum markers. Due to the high correlation between total hCG and free β-hCG (correlation coefficient 0.9), there is no advantage in measuring both these markers together, and so combinations including them are not shown in the table. Using the standard triple test with gestational age based on dates (AFP, uE₃, and total hCG), the detection rate for a 5% false-positive rate is 59%; using an ultrasound scan to estimate gestational age the detection rate is 67%. Measuring the free hCG subunits instead of total hCG yields estimates of 65% and 72% respectively for the same false-positive rate. Adjusting the values of the serum markers for maternal weight increases the detection rates by about 1%.

Choice of combination of markers

If three serum markers were used, the best combination would be free β-hCG, uE₃ and free α-hCG, yielding a 62% detection rate for a 5% false-positive rate. If three serum markers were used, of which one was serum AFP (retained as a screening test for open neural tube defects), the best combination would be AFP with either: (1) free β-hCG and free α-hCG, (2) free β-hCG and uE₃ or (3) total hCG and uE₃, each yielding a detection rate of 59% for a 5% false-positive rate, 3% less than the combination which excluded AFP. If ultrasound is routinely used to estimate gestational age, combinations of markers should include uE₃. As the marker that changes the most in concentration with increasing gestation, uE₃ is the one that will yield the greatest improvement in screening performance with increases in the precision of gestational age estimation.

If a laboratory can manage performing the four biochemical tests at an acceptable cost, four-marker screening is the best option. Table 12.10 shows the detection rate, false-positive rate and the odds of being affected given a positive result according to the risk cut-off level for different combinations of screening markers and according to the method of estimating gestational age (dates or from a BPD or crown–rump length ultrasound measurement). At a risk cut-off level of 1 : 300 using the four serum markers, for example, the detection rate is 65% and the false-positive rate 5.1% with an odds of being affected given a positive result of 1 : 60. If scan is used to estimate gestational age the same risk cut-off level would yield a detection rate of 70% for a 4.5% false-positive rate, with an odds of being affected given a positive result of 1 : 49.

Use of ultrasound to estimate gestational age in a woman with a positive screening test for Down's syndrome

A woman with a positive screening test for Down's syndrome is usually referred for a dating scan if she has not already had one. This will tend to reduce her risk of Down's syndrome because one of the reasons for having a positive result is overestimated gestational age. By reducing the estimate of gestational age, her AFP and uE₃ levels will be increased and her hCG result decreased when expressed in MoMs. With the triple test, all this will tend to reduce her risk estimate. With the quadruple test, the position is somewhat different since α-hCG increases with gestation and is raised in Down's syndrome pregnancies. The increase in risk due to gestational age overestimation will therefore be somewhat reduced with the quadruple test. With either test, the net effect is to reduce the number of false-positives, and also lessen the number of true-positives, that is, some women with affected pregnancies originally classified as positive will now be

Table 12.10 Down's syndrome detection rate (DR), false-positive rate (FPR) and the odds of being affected given a positive result (OAPR) according to risk cut-off level and combination of screening markers. Gestational age estimated by dates with no adjustment for maternal weight

Risk ≥	Maternal age, AFP:-														
	With free β-hCG			With free α- and free β-hCG			uE$_3$ and free β-hCG			With uE$_3$ and total hCG			With free α- and free β-hCG and uE$_3$		
	DR (%)	FPR (%)	OAPR	DR (%)	FPR (%)	OAPR	DR (%)	FPR (%)	OAPR	DR (%)	FPR (%)	OAPR	DR (%)	FPR (%)	OAPR
Gestational age estimated by dates (LMP)															
1 in 100	30	1.1	1 : 28	37	1.2	1 : 25	37	1.2	1 : 25	42	1.7	1 : 30	45	1.3	1 : 22
1 in 150	39	2.1	1 : 42	45	2.2	1 : 37	46	1.7	1 : 31	50	2.8	1 : 43	53	2.2	1 : 32
1 in 200	45	3.2	1 : 54	52	3.3	1 : 48	52	3.3	1 : 49	55	3.9	1 : 55	58	3.1	1 : 41
1 in 250	51	4.5	1 : 67	56	4.3	1 : 59	57	4.4	1 : 60	59	5.1	1 : 67	62	4.1	1 : 51
1 in 300	57	5.9	1 : 80	61	5.5	1 : 70	61	5.5	1 : 70	63	6.4	1 : 79	65	5.1	1 : 60
1 in 350	60	7.1	1 : 90	64	6.5	1 : 78	64	6.6	1 : 80	65	7.5	1 : 88	68	6.0	1 : 68
1 in 400	63	8.2	1 : 99	66	7.6	1 : 88	66	7.7	1 : 89	68	8.7	1 : 99	70	6.9	1 : 76
1 in 450	67	9.9	1 : 114	69	8.8	1 : 98	69	8.9	1 : 99	70	9.9	1 : 108	72	7.9	1 : 84
1 in 500	69	10.8	1 : 116	71	9.9	1 : 107	71	10.0	1 : 109	72	11.0	1 : 118	74	8.8	1 : 92
1 in 550	71	12.0	1 : 130	73	10.9	1 : 115	72	11.0	1 : 117	74	12.1	1 : 127	75	9.7	1 : 100
Gestational age estimated by scan (BPD or CRL)															
1 in 100	34	1.3	1 : 28	39	1.3	1 : 25	49	1.3	1 : 21	52	1.6	1 : 24	54	1.3	1 : 18
1 in 150	42	2.3	1 : 41	48	2.3	1 : 37	56	2.2	1 : 31	58	2.7	1 : 35	60	2.1	1 : 27
1 in 200	49	3.4	1 : 53	54	3.3	1 : 47	60	3.1	1 : 39	63	3.6	1 : 45	65	2.9	1 : 35
1 in 250	55	4.6	1 : 64	58	4.4	1 : 58	64	4.0	1 : 48	66	4.6	1 : 54	68	3.7	1 : 42
1 in 300	59	5.7	1 : 75	62	5.5	1 : 68	67	4.9	1 : 57	69	5.6	1 : 62	70	4.5	1 : 49
1 in 350	63	6.9	1 : 85	65	6.5	1 : 76	69	5.8	1 : 64	71	6.6	1 : 71	72	5.3	1 : 56
1 in 400	66	8.2	1 : 96	68	7.6	1 : 86	71	6.7	1 : 72	73	7.5	1 : 79	74	6.1	1 : 63
1 in 450	69	9.3	1 : 105	70	8.6	1 : 94	73	7.5	1 : 79	75	8.4	1 : 87	76	6.9	1 : 70
1 in 500	71	10.4	1 : 114	73	9.8	1 : 103	75	8.4	1 : 87	76	9.2	1 : 93	77	7.6	1 : 76
1 in 550	72	11.5	1 : 123	74	10.6	1 : 110	76	9.3	1 : 94	77	10.2	1 : 101	78	8.3	1 : 82

Based on parameters in Wald et al (1994b).
LMP = last menstrual period; BPD = biparietal diameter; CRL = crown–rump length.

classified as negative. This is a serious adverse effect of such a revision of gestational age and to reduce such false-negatives it is sensible to avoid reclassifying a positive screening result as negative unless the estimate of gestational age has been changed substantially, say by more than 2–3 weeks. Even then, occasionally a true-positive will be missed. It is better for screening programmes to rely on a routine dating scan prior to the interpretation of the screening result. This will completely avoid the problem and also improve the performance of screening.

Other markers for Down's syndrome

Pregnancy-specific β-1 glycoprotein (SP1), dehydro-epiandrosterone sulphate (DHEAS) and progesterone have been found to be associated with Down's syndrome (Wald et al 1989, Cuckle et al 1990). The performance, however, is relatively poor. Urea-resistant neutrophil alkaline phosphatase (Cuckle et al 1990) has a good discriminatory performance but it is still a research technique and requires further development and confirmation before routine use in screening. The assay is unfortunately not robust and relies on subjective interpretation.

First-trimester screening for Down's syndrome

A number of biochemical markers in maternal serum have been proposed for first-trimester screening for Down's syndrome. The most promising four are pregnancy-associated plasma protein A (PAPP-A), the free β subunit of hCG, uE$_3$ and AFP. An analysis of the published literature suggests that about two-thirds of affected pregnancies can be detected for a 5% false-positive rate if the four markers are used in combination with maternal age and assumed to be independent measures of risk (Wald et al 1994c). This is a level of performance that would be similar to second-trimester screening. It is, however, a tentative estimate because of the assumption of independence and the possibility of publication bias in the reporting of small preliminary studies. Further research is needed before such screening is introduced.

The timing of antenatal diagnosis by means of chorionic villus sampling should be delayed until 11 weeks of pregnancy because of the risk of causing limb defects. Screening, if shown to be justified, should not, therefore, be performed before about 9 or 10 weeks of pregnancy.

OTHER FACTORS RELEVANT TO SCREENING FOR NEURAL TUBE DEFECTS AND DOWN'S SYNDROME

Twins and diabetics

Table 12.11 shows the median value for AFP, uE$_3$, hCG free α-hCG and free β-hCG in twin pregnancies and

Table 12.11   The median, 10th and 90th centile AFP, uE$_3$, hCG, free α-hCG and free β-hCG (MoM) in twin pregnancies and pregnancies associated with insulin-dependent diabetes mellitus

Marker	Centile			Significantly different in specified group than in control
	10th	Median	90th	
Twin pregnancies				
AFP*	1.33	2.13	3.51	Yes
uE$_3$*	1.03	1.67	2.41	Yes
hCG*	0.87	1.84	3.76	Yes
free α-hCG[†]	1.16	1.66	2.59	Yes
free β-hCG[‡]	0.82	1.90	4.44	Yes
Insulin-dependent diabetes mellitus				
AFP[§]	0.34	0.77	1.39	Yes
uE$_3$[§]	0.59	0.92	1.26	Yes
hCG[§]	0.43	0.95	1.87	No
free α-hCG[‖]	0.53	0.86	1.47	Yes
free β-hCG[‖]	0.38	0.96	2.16	No

MoM = multiple of the median for unaffected pregnancies of the same gestational age.
*Taken from Wald et al (1991).
[†]Taken from Wald & Densem (1994b).
[‡]Taken from Wald & Densem (1994a).
[§]Taken from Wald et al (1992b).
[‖]Taken from Wald et al (1994a).

pregnancies associated with insulin-dependent diabetes mellitus together with the 10th and 90th centile. All five markers are raised in twin pregnancies and AFP, uE$_3$ and free α-hCG levels are significantly lower than in women without insulin-dependent diabetes mellitus, though only AFP and possibly free α-hCG to any material extent. Adjustment for AFP is needed in diabetic pregnancies; the case for adjustment with the other four markers is less clear. In screening programmes for neural tube defects or Down's syndrome, adjustment is carried out by dividing the appropriate marker MoM value in a twin pregnancy or diabetic pregnancy by the corresponding medians for twin or diabetic pregnancies, as appropriate. This will, in expectation, yield a similar false-positive rate in twin and diabetic pregnancies as in singleton non-diabetic pregnancies. Screening in twin pregnancies poses a special problem because of the presence of two fetuses, one usually being unaffected. There is a reasonable reluctance to act on a positive screening result and perform an amniocentesis or consider a termination of an unaffected co-twin in the event of a positive diagnosis, so many centres will regard the discovery of a twin pregnancy as an indication to avoid screening.

Ethnic group

Table 12.12 summarizes the data on ethnic group. AFP values are, on average, 20% higher for blacks compared with whites, and total hCG 15% higher, total free β-hCG values are 9% higher and free α-hCG 8% lower. The levels of uE$_3$ are similar. AFP and free β-hCG are similar in Asians and whites, while uE$_3$, total hCG and free α-

Table 12.12   Serum markers in black and Asian women compared to white women at 15–22 weeks of gestation

Marker	Ratio of median in blacks to median in whites (95% CI)	Ratio of median in Asians to median in whites (95% CI)
AFP	1.20 (1.18–1.22)	1.03 (1.02–1.05)
uE$_3$	1.00 (0.98–1.01)	1.11 (1.09–1.13)
hCG	1.15 (1.12–1.18)	1.12 (1.10–1.15)
free α-hCG	0.92 (0.89–0.96)	1.11 (1.01–1.22)
free β-hCG	1.09 (1.01–1.18)	0.99 (0.84–1.15)

CI = confidence interval.
Taken from Wald et al (1995).

hCG appear to be somewhat raised. Weight adjustment had little influence on the results relating to blacks, but tended to decrease the values in Asians because Asian women are, on average, lighter than white women. At present it is reasonable to adjust for ethnic group in respect of AFP and hCG in blacks and in respect of AFP and hCG in Asians. This could be done by dividing the observed serum marker levels by the ratio of the median MoMs for blacks (or Asians) compared to whites. Alternatively, race-specific normal medians could be used without adjusting individual values.

Within-person fluctuations in marker levels

Most of the variance of the serum markers in a given week of pregnancy is due to differences between individuals and between pregnancies; only a relatively small proportion of the variance is due to assay. For example, with AFP the assay accounts for 14% of the variance and the within-person AFP fluctuations account for 17% (Wald & Cuckle 1982a). This means that there is little advantage in performing a repeat test. In open spina bifida screening, if a repeat test is performed only on women with high levels, there will be a substantial reduction in the false-positive rate but this will also lead to a reduction in the detection rate. It is best to adopt a 'no repeat test' policy; it has the advantage of simplicity and the avoidance of delay in making a diagnosis at the time when the women concerned, having been told that they have a positive AFP screening test, are particularly anxious.

In Down's syndrome screening, if all women had a repeat test a week or two later the detection rate would increase by about 4% (Cuckle et al 1994), not large enough to justify a routine policy of repeat testing in view of the extra cost and delay.

Policies of repeating the test in women with a high risk of Down's syndrome would reduce the false-positive rate but would also reduce the detection rate. The reclassification of true-positives to false-negatives associated with such policies is, as it is for the ultrasound revision of gestational age in screen-positive women, a serious adverse effect which should be avoided.

Maternal weight

Table 12.13 shows the median marker level according to quintile of maternal weight. It extends the observations made on AFP (see above) to the other markers. As with AFP, the marker levels are adjusted by taking the observed MoM value and dividing this by the expected MoM value derived from a regression of the observed MoM value on maternal weight based on local data. Maternal weight has a small effect on Down's syndrome screening performance. The effect is small because adjustment alters the MoM value of all the markers in the same direction which has opposite effects on the risk of Down's syndrome derived from total hCG (free α or free β) on the one hand and from AFP and uE_3 on the other. There is a tendency for, say, an increase in hCG MoM (increased risk) to be counteracted by an increase in AFP and uE_3 MoM (decreased risk).

Smoking

The median AFP level in women who smoked cigarettes was 3% greater than in non-smokers (95% confidence interval, 2–4%), 3% less for uE_3 (95% confidence interval, 2–4%), and 23% less for hCG (95% confidence interval, 22–24%). In spite of the relatively large difference in hCG levels, adjusting all three serum markers used for Down's syndrome screening for the effect of maternal smoking has a small effect on overall screening performance and is not worthwhile (Palomaki et al 1993). There is also a suggestion that the birth prevalence is lower in smokers than non-smokers. This needs confirmation and, if true and of any consequence, the difference would need to be allowed for in screening.

Computer-assisted test interpretation

Serum screening for Down's syndrome relies on the use of several variables simultaneously to determine the risk of Down's syndrome in each woman. Women are screen-positive if their risk lies above a cut-off that is specified by the user and entered into the computer program; they are screen-negative if it falls below the specified cut-off. Such risk estimation can be performed by computer-assisted test interpretation and allows the risk estimate to take account of other factors such as maternal weight, ultrasound measures of gestational age, ethnic origin, diabetic status, multiple pregnancy and repeat samples which can affect the interpretation of the test. Figure 12.9 gives an example of a computer-assisted test interpretation report from a 20-year-old woman with a positive screening result.

Wolfson Institute of Preventive Medicine
The Medical College of St Bartholomew's Hospital
Tel: 0171-982-6293

NEURAL TUBE DEFECT AND DOWN'S SYNDROME SCREENING 21-MAR-94

Surname	:	DOE
Forename(s)	:	Jane
ID Code	:	142857
Date of Birth	:	01–04–72
LMP	:	28–11–93
Date of Sample	:	18–03–94
Doctor	:	Dr A Jones
Report Address	:	General Hospital London SW1

CLINICAL DETAILS AND TEST RESULTS

Previous NTD	:	None
Previous Down's	:	None
Insulin-dependent diabetes	:	None
Maternal Age at EDD	:	20 years
Scan Measure	:	BPD
Gestation at Date of Sample	:	15 weeks 5 days (by dates) 16 weeks 3 days (by scan)
Gestation used	:	Scan estimate
Weight	:	56 kg
Ethnic origin	:	Not specified
MS-AFP Level	:	21 iu/mL; 0.66 MoM
MS-uE3 Level	:	3 nmol/L; 0.65 MoM
MS-hCG Level	:	61.4 iu/mL; 1.86 MoM

INTERPRETATION

Screening Result	:	*** SCREEN POSITIVE ***
Reason	:	Increased risk of Down's syndrome
Risk of Down's	:	1 in 190 (at Term)
Comment	:	The risk of Down's is greater than that expected from the maternal age alone (1 in 1500)

A screen positive result indicates an increased risk of having a pregnancy with Down's syndrome or a neural tube defect. However, most women with positive screening results will not have an affected pregnancy.

Table 12.13 Marker level (MoM) according to quintile of maternal weight

	Quintile of maternal weight				
Marker	1 ($n = 191$)	2 ($n = 185$)	3 ($n = 175$)	4 ($n = 178$)	5 ($n = 179$)
AFP	1.16	1.07	1.04	0.93	0.83
uE_3	1.01	1.00	1.04	0.99	0.92
hCG	1.13	1.09	0.98	0.91	0.84
free α-hCG	1.09	1.08	0.99	0.97	0.88
free β-hCG	1.15	1.09	1.04	0.90	0.85
Mean weight (kg)	51.0	57.7	63.0	69.0	79.5

Taken from Wald et al (1995).
n = number of women; MoM = multiple of the median for unaffected pregnancies of the same gestational age.

Fig. 12.9 Specimen of a computer-assisted test interpretation report from a 20-year-old woman with a positive screening result (patient and doctor details are fictitious).

TRISOMY 18

The median AFP, uE$_3$ and hCG levels in pregnancies with trisomy 18 have recently been reported from a collaborative study to be 0.65, 0.43 and 0.36 respectively. Using a risk cut-off level of 1 in 350 at term an estimated 60% of cases of trisomy 18 would be detected for a 0.2% false-positive rate, with an odds of being affected given a positive result of about 1 : 25.

Diagnosis

Diagnosis is based on a fetal karyotype, either based on chorionic villus sampling or amniocentesis. A new technique, fluorescent in situ hybridization (FISH), uses probes to identify specific DNA sequences on chromosome 21. In trisomy 21, three signals are seen, instead of two (Ward et al 1993). The method has not been shown to be sufficiently reliable to replace the conventional karyotype (Palomaki et al 1994).

PLANNING A SCREENING PROGRAMME

There are several practical issues that need to be considered when setting up a serum screening programme for Down's syndrome and neural tube defects. These include the choice of tests, assay method, risk cut-off, provision of counselling services, and coordination of the programme with the clinical and laboratory staff. In centres in which serum AFP screening is already being performed for open

neural tube defect, the system is already partly set up and so can be extended relatively easily.

It is important that the screening programme is directed and coordinated with counselling available and continuing education for the staff. As with many other screening services this is an area that can fail—often the different parts of the screening programme act in isolation without anyone who has overall responsibility. Provided the right structure is set in place, with a named person responsible for the programme who has the necessary managerial authority to match the responsibility, serum screening for Down's syndrome can be implemented without difficulty. The challenge is not scientific or technical, it is managerial.

Glossary

Screening is the systematic application of a test or inquiry, to identify individuals at sufficient risk of a specific disorder to benefit from further investigation or direct preventive action, among persons who have not sought medical attention on account of symptoms of that disorder.

The **detection rate** (or **sensitivity**) of a screening test is the proportion of affected individuals with positive results.

The **false-positive rate** is the proportion of unaffected individuals with a positive result. The **specificity** of a test is the complement of the false-positive rate (specificity = 1 – false-positive rate).

The **Odds of being Affected given a Positive Result** is the ratio of the number of affected to unaffected individuals among those with positive test results. The **predictive value positive** is the odds of being affected given a positive result expressed as a proportion or percentage.

The **prevalence** of a disease is the number of cases of a disorder present at a point in time in a defined population (e.g. at birth). The **incidence** of a disease is the number of new cases occurring in a specified period of time in a defined group.

REFERENCES

Althouse R, Wald N 1980 Survival and handicap of infants with spina bifida. Archives of Disease in Children 55: 845–850
Baird P A, Sadovnick A D 1988 Life expectancy in Down syndrome adults. Lancet ii: 1354–1356
Creasy M R, Crolla J A 1974 Prenatal mortality of trisomy 21 (Down's syndrome). Lancet i: 473
Cuckle H S, Wald N J 1990 Screening for Down's syndrome. In: Lilford R J (ed) Prenatal diagnosis and prognosis. Butterworths, Guildford, pp 67–92
Cuckle H S, Wald N J 1992 Complementary use of biochemical tests and ultrasonography for detection of neural tube defects and down syndrome: diagnosis. In: Chervenak F A, Isaacson G, Campbell S (eds) Ultrasound in obstetrics and gynaecology. Little Brown & Co, Boston, pp 1145–1150
Cuckle H S, Wald N J, Thompson S G 1987 Estimating a woman's risk of having a pregnancy associated with Down's syndrome using her age and serum alpha-fetoprotein level. British Journal of Obstetrics and Gynaecology 94: 387–402
Cuckle H S, Wald N J, Densem J W, Royston P 1990 The effect of smoking in pregnancy on maternal serum alpha-fetoprotein, unconjugated oestriol, human chorionic gonadotrophin, progesterone and dehydroepiandrosterone sulphate levels. British Journal of Obstetrics and Gynaecology 97: 272–276
Cuckle H, Densem J, Wald N 1994 Repeat maternal serum testing in multiple marker Down's syndrome screening programmes. Prenatal Diagnosis 14: 603–607
Dalton A J 1982 A prospective study of Alzheimer's disease in Down's syndrome. Paper presented at a meeting of the International

Association of the Scientific Study of Mental Deficiency, Toronto. (Cited in Pueschel S M 1982 Health concerns in persons with Down syndrome. In: Pueschel S M, Tingey C, Rynders J E, Crocker A C, Cructer D M (eds) New perspectives in Down syndrome. Brookes, Baltimore, pp 113–133)
Drugan A, Zador I E, Syner F N, Sokol R J, Sacks A J, Evans M I 1988 A normal ultrasound does not obviate the need for amniocentesis in patients with elevated serum alpha-fetoprotein. Obstetrics and Gynecology 72: 627–630
Expert Advisory Group 1992 Folic acid and the prevention of neural tube defects. UK Department of Health, London
Glenner G G, Wong W C 1984 Alzheimer's disease and Down's syndrome: sharing of a unique cerebrovascular amyloid fibril protein. Biochemical and Biophysical Research Communications 122: 1131–1135
Goldgaber D, Lerman M I, McBride O W, Saffiotti V, Gajdusek D C 1987 Characterisation and chromosomal localisation of a cDNA encoding brain amyloid of Alzheimer's diseases. Science 235: 877–880
Haddow J E, Kloza E M, Knight G J, Smith D E 1981 Relationship between maternal weight and serum alpha-fetoprotein concentration during the second trimester. Clinical Chemistry 27: 133–134
Kolata G 1985 Down syndrome—Alzheimer's linked. Science 230: 1152–1153
Masaki M, Higurashi M, Iijima K et al 1981 Mortality and survival for Down syndrome in Japan. American Journal of Human Genetics 33: 629–639
Masters C L, Simms G, Weinman N A, Multhaup G, McDonald B L,

Neyreuther K 1985 Amyloid plaque core protein in Alzheimer's disease. Proceedings of the National Academy of Science USA 822: 4245–4249

Oster J, Mikkelsen M, Nielsen A 1975 Mortality and life-table in Down's syndrome. Acta Paediatrica Scandinavica 64: 322–326

Palomaki G E, Hill L E, Knight G J, Haddow J E, Carpenter M 1988 Second trimester maternal serum alpha-fetoprotein levels in pregnancies associated with gastroschisis and omphalocele. Obstetrics and Gynecology 71: 906

Palomaki G E, Knight G J, Haddow J E, Canick J A, Wald N J, Kennard A 1993 Cigarette smoking and levels of maternal serum alpha-fetoprotein, unconjugated estriol and hCG: impact on Down syndrome screening. Obstetrics and Gynecology 81: 675–678

Palomaki G E, Bradley L A, Haddow J E 1994 A new approach to analyzing fluorescence in-situ hybridization data for rapid detection of aneuploidy in amniocytes. Journal of Medical Screening 1: 96–97

Rasmussen-Loft A G, Nanchahal K, Cuckle H S et al 1990 Amniotic fluid acetylcholinesterase in the antenatal diagnosis of open neural tube defects and abdominal wall defects: a comparison of gel electrophoresis and a monoclonal antibody immunoassay. Prenatal Diagnosis 10: 449–459

Richards D S, Seeds J W, Katz V L, Lingley L H, Albright S G, Cefalo R C 1988 Elevated maternal serum alpha-fetoprotein with normal ultrasound: is amniocentesis always appropriate? A review of 26 069 screened patients. Obstetrics and Gynecology 71: 203–207

Tabor A, Philip J, Madsen M, Bang J, Obel E B, Norgaard Pederson B 1986 Randomised controlled trial of genetic amniocentesis in 4606 low-risk women. Lancet i: 1287–1293

Wald N 1993 Folic acid and the prevention of neural tube defects. Maternal nutrition and pregnancy outcome. In: Keen C L, Bendich A, Willhite C C (eds) Annals of the New York Academy of Sciences 678: 112–129

Wald N J, Cuckle H S 1982a Survival of infants with open spina bifida in relation to maternal serum alpha-fetoprotein level. Third Report of the UK Collaborative Study on Alpha-Fetoprotein in Relation to Neural-tube Defects. British Journal of Obstetrics and Gynaecology 89: 3–7

Wald N J, Cuckle H S 1982b Estimating an individual's risk of having a fetus with open spina bifida and the value of repeat alpha-fetaprotein testing. Fourth Report of the UK Collaborative Study on Alpha-Fetoprotein in Relation to Neural-tube Defects. Journal of Epidemiology and Community Health 36: 87–95

Wald N, Cuckle H 1992 Antenatal screening and diagnosis. In: Elwood J M, Little J, Elwood J H (eds) The epidemiology and control of neural tube defects. Oxford University Press, Oxford, pp 711–726

Wald N J, Densem J W 1994a Maternal serum free β-human chorionic gonadotrophin levels in twin pregnancies: implications for screening for Down's syndrome. Prenatal Diagnosis 14: 319–320

Wald N J, Densem J W 1994b Maternal serum free α human chorionic gonadotrophin levels in twin pregnancies: implications for screening for Down's syndrome. Prenatal Diagnosis 14: 717–719

Wald N, Cuckle H, Boreham J, Stirrat G 1980 Small biparietal diameter of fetuses with spina bifida: implications for antenatal screening. British Journal of Obstetrics and Gynaecology 87: 219–221

Wald N J, Cuckle H, Boreham J, Terzian E, Redman C 1981 The effect of maternal weight on maternal serum alpha-fetoprotein levels. British Journal of Obstetrics and Gynaecology 88: 1094–1096

Wald N J, Cuckle H S, Nanchahal K 1989 Amniotic fluid acetylcholinesterase measurement in the prenatal diagnosis of open neural tube defects. Second Report of the Collaborative Acetylcholinesterase Study. Prenatal Diagnosis 9: 813–829

Wald N, Cuckle H, Wu T, George L 1991 Maternal serum unconjugated oestriol and human chorionic gonadotrophin levels in twin pregnancies: implications for screening for Down's syndrome. British Journal of Obstetrics and Gynaecology 98: 905–908

Wald N J, Cuckle H S, Densem J W, Kennard A, Smith D 1992a Maternal serum screening for Down's syndrome: the effect of routine ultrasound scan determination of gestational age and adjustment for maternal weight. British Journal of Obstetrics and Gynaecology 99: 144–149

Wald N J, Cuckle H S, Densem J W, Stone R B 1992b Maternal serum unconjugated oestriol and human chorionic gonadotrophin levels in pregnancies with insulin-dependent diabetes: implications for screening for Down's syndrome. British Journal of Obstetrics and Gynaecology 99: 51–53

Wald N J, Densem J W, Cheng R, Collishaw S 1994a Maternal serum free α and free β human chorionic gonadotrophin in pregnancies with insulin dependent diabetes mellitus: implications for screening for Down's syndrome. Prenatal Diagnosis 14: 835–837

Wald N J, Densem J W, Smith D, Klee G G 1994b Four marker serum screening for Down's syndrome. Prenatal Diagnosis 14: 707–716

Wald N J, Kennard A, Smith D 1994c First trimester biochemical screening for Down's syndrome. Annals of Medicine 26: 23–29

Wald N J, Smith D, Kennard A, Densem J W, Watt H 1995 Serum markers for Down's syndrome in different ethnic groups. (in preparation)

Ward D E, Gersen S L, Carelli M P et al 1993 Rapid prenatal diagnosis of chromosomal aneuploidies by fluorescence in situ hybridization: clinical experience with 4500 specimens. American Journal of Human Genetics 52: 854–865

13. Biophysical diagnosis of fetal abnormalities

J. Malcolm Pearce

INTRODUCTION

Since Professor Ian Donald introduced ultrasound into obstetrics in the late 1950s vast improvements have been made in electronics so that equipment is now cheaper and easy to use. This together with the fact that examinations may be repeated and are apparently without hazard (Royal College of Obstetricians and Gynaecologists 1984) has revolutionized obstetrics. Confirmation or determination of gestational age, monitoring of fetal growth (see Ch. 6) and the assessment of the biophysical aspects of fetal well-being (see Ch. 14) are well known examples of the use of ultrasound antenatally.

Antenatal diagnosis of many fetal structural abnormalities is possible only by ultrasound and its availability in the last decade has allowed many women to continue through pregnancy knowing that their fetus would not be handicapped by the same abnormality as a previous baby. The use of ultrasound to complement amniocentesis, chorion villus sampling, fetoscopy and direct umbilical cord needling is discussed in Chapter 15. This chapter will consider ultrasound in its unique role as both a screening and a diagnostic test for fetal abnormalities.

GENERAL PRINCIPLES OF DIAGNOSIS AND MANAGEMENT

The images displayed on the television monitor of an ultrasound machine are essentially computer reconstructions based on echoes reflected from tissue junctions and discontinuities within tissues. They are two-dimensional pictures and the skill of the ultrasound operator comes from interpreting these in a three-dimensional fashion and from avoiding incorrect interpretations due to artefacts. Unlike conventional X-rays or computer tomography, ultrasound produces many artefactual appearances to trap the novice operator.

The diagnosis of fetal abnormalities is made in one of three ways (Campbell & Pearce 1984):

1. By direct visualization of a structural defect, for example the absence of the fetal skull vault in anencephaly.
2. By demonstrating disproportionate size or growth of a particular fetal part, for example, the short limbs in cases of dwarfism.
3. By recognition of the effect of an anomaly on an adjacent structure, for example the presence of posterior urethral valves which may be diagnosed by the consequent dilatation of the renal tract.

The widespread use of ultrasound to confirm gestational age and for the early diagnosis of multiple pregnancy has led to the diagnoses of many abnormalities being made in the first half of pregnancy. In this respect ultrasound examination performed in the routine setting by ultrasonographers, doctors or midwives is best seen as a screening test. If an abnormality is suspected at this examination facilities should be available for an early referral to an operator who is able to make a definitive diagnosis. As fetal abnormalities are often multiple the entire fetus should be examined carefully by ultrasound and if the diagnosed abnormality is known to be associated with chromosome anomalies then karyotyping either by amniocentesis or directly from leucocytes in the fetal blood (see Ch. 15) should also be offered. It therefore behoves the doctor carrying out diagnostic ultrasound examinations to be fully aware of the associations of individual abnormalities and to keep abreast of the management of such conditions.

Having arrived at a definitive diagnosis there are then three options open to the parents:

1. The pregnancy may be terminated. In November 1992 the changes in the law made by the Human Fertilisation and Embryology Act (1990) came into force. The 1967 Abortion Act was modified such that termination at any stage of pregnancy is legal if it is necessary to save the life of the mother, or to prevent grave permanent injury to her mental or physical health, or if there is a substantial risk that if the child were born 'it would suffer from any such physical or mental abnormalities as to be seriously handicapped'.

   The law does not define 'seriously handicapped' and therefore the interpretation is left to the counselling doctors and the parents. Each doctor undertaking prenatal diagnosis will have to reach their own ethical and moral stance. A reasonable starting point for considering late termination of pregnancy is to decide if it would have been offered had the abnormality been diagnosed at 18–20 weeks' gestation. Termination of pregnancy for handicap will continue to be controversial and this even more so for third-trimester terminations. Debate can be kept to a minimum by ensuring that the counselling is performed by at least two consultants and allowing the parents a thinking period. Additional support during this time from counselling midwives is invaluable. Finally, the termination should be notified immediately; it is easy for the forms to go astray as these patients do not normally go through the same channels as the first-trimester terminations.

2. The pregnancy may be allowed to continue with continuing ultrasound surveillance. Many abnormalities do not carry a threat to the life of the fetus and usually do not deteriorate in utero. An example of this is pelviureteric junction obstruction. In such cases continued monitoring with appropriate measurements will determine if the condition is worsening. If deterioration does occur then the options are usually premature delivery or possibly in utero surgery. Again a balanced judgement should be made, assisted by the free use of amniocentesis to determine the lecithin : sphingomyelin ratio and to assay for phosphatidylglycerol to help in management. In general the obstetrician and his paediatric colleagues should lean towards early delivery with subsequent appropriate management rather than attempting intervention in utero.

3. Prenatal therapy or surgery. This is only available at present for a few conditions and should only be carried out by people who are expert at intrauterine manipulation. Where such manoeuvres are available, they are discussed under the specific diagnosis.

The decision as to which line of management to adopt is difficult and should be made by a multidisciplinary team. The parents should obviously be involved to the extent of their understanding but the timing of delivery and discussion of the long-term treatment and prognosis should be done in conjunction with a neonatologist and a paediatric surgeon, if appropriate. Furthermore although most obstetricians involved in prenatal diagnosis by ultrasound became amateur geneticists by necessity, the now widespread availability of clinical geneticists means their help should be sought.

Terminating pregnancies complicated by fetal abnormalities is best performed by extra-amniotic prostaglandin infusion or prostaglandin pessaries as dilatation and evacuation or intra-amniotic instillations often renders the tissue unsuitable for diagnosis. Terminations performed after 22 weeks carry the risk of the child being born alive so an invasive procedure such as the intracardiac injection of air or potassium should be considered. Consent should be sought for a post-mortem examination; although consent is only legally required if the fetus is more than 24 weeks' gestation, it must be remembered that the parents will still consider this fetus as a baby. The parents should also be given a chance to see and hold the baby after it has been suitably clothed. A consent form of the type shown in Figure 13.1 should also be provided for parents who wish to bury or cremate their baby. In addition, whether consent is given for post-mortem or not the following investigations should be carried out before the fetus is sent fresh to the mortuary.

1. Blood should be obtained by direct cardiac puncture for karyotyping.
2. The fetus should be X-rayed.
3. The baby should be photographed. This should be done by the hospital photographer and should include a full facial view, a view of the whole body and of any

St. George's Hospital
Medical School

UNIVERSITY OF LONDON
Patron: Her Majesty the Queen

DEPARTMENT OF OBSTETRICS
AND GYNAECOLOGY

CRANMER TERRACE
LONDON SW17 0RE

Tel: 01-672 1255 Ext. 4175
Telex: 945291 SAGEMS G

Professor G. V. P. Chamberlain
Mr. J. M. Pearce
Dr. T. R. Varma
Dr. C. Wilson
Mr. A. G. Amias
Mr. S. L. Stanton
Mrs. U. Lloyd

To: A local undertaker

Dear Sir

Re: The baby of Mr & Mrs Smith

This is to confirm that I was present at the birth of baby Smith who was born before 24 weeks gestation without signs of life. I should be grateful if you would give the parents your assistance in burying/cremating their baby.

Yours faithfully

Fig. 13.1 A specimen consent form to allow burial or cremation of a fetus born before 24 weeks' gestation without signs of life.

obvious abnormalities. These photographs should be available for the geneticist. If a Polaroid camera is used do not stand closer than the 1 m minimum focusing distance. The parents should be offered a photograph of their baby suitably dressed. If they refuse it should be carefully filed in case they later change their minds.

4. The placenta should be sent fresh for histology.

Ideally the post-mortem should be carried out by a trained perinatal pathologist and if intracranial abnormalities are suspected the brain should be fixed by perfusion before it is cut.

ULTRASOUND AS A SCREENING TEST

Ultrasound in the first half of pregnancy has been shown to be superior to bimanual pelvic examination in early pregnancy (Campbell 1974) and to X-rays for maturity in later pregnancy (Robinson et al 1979) in the assessment of gestational age in patients with unknown dates. Controversy still exists as to whether ultrasound examination in the first half of pregnancy should be reserved for those patients in whom there is doubt about the validity of their last menstrual period or whether it should be a matter of routine. Evidence from a study based on historical controls (Grennert et al 1978) and from a prospective non-randomized study (Warsof et al 1983) is in favour of routine ultrasound. Meta-analysis (Neilson 1993) demonstrates a reduction in the number of inductions for apparent post-term pregnancy and supports the concept that ultrasound measurements are more accurate at predicting the date of delivery and hence reduce the number of patients who exceed 42 weeks's gestation. Only one study, however (Eik-Nes et al 1984), shows a benefit from this. This is to be expected, as it would need a very large study to demonstrate the significance of reducing the number of people who exceed 42 weeks' gestation from 12 to 6%. What is certain, however, is that the use of ultrasound reduces the number of babies who are born unexpectedly premature after induction of labour (Chapman et al 1979). Apart from establishing gestational age, routine ultrasound examination in early pregnancy is very accurate at diagnosing multiple gestations (Grennert et al 1978, Persson et al 1978, Warsof et al 1983) and in localizing the placenta. Placental localization is worthwhile at this time as over 95% of the population will have a fundal placenta which will not become a placenta praevia.

With the widespread use of ultrasound, pregnant women and their attendants are coming to expect to deliver babies free from any structural abnormalities. With increasing litigation against health care practitioners it is important to realize what can reasonably be expected from the average ultrasonographer in the exclusion of abnormalities.

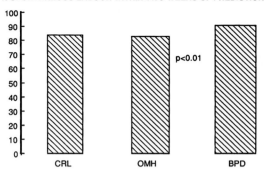

Fig. 13.2 A comparison of ultrasound parameters with optimal menstrual history in predicting the date of delivery of a mature fetus. CRL = Crown–rump length; OMH = optimal menstrual history; BPD = biparietal diameter.

Timing of the first ultrasound examination

Many ultrasound departments have now recognized the value of scanning the patient at 16–20 weeks' gestation (Warsof et al 1983). Practitioners of ultrasound know that examining the anatomy of the fetus is a great deal easier at 18 weeks' than at 16 weeks' gestation. Figure 13.2 demonstrates that in predicting the date of delivery routine ultrasound is superior to optimal menstrual dates up to about 22 weeks' gestation. Since most obstetricians will not be more than 4 weeks out in estimating gestation age in the first half of pregnancy, ultrasound planned at 18 weeks' gestation is unlikely to be performed at more than 22 weeks.

If ultrasound examinations are performed in the first trimester and crown–rump length is measured, there is little hope of diagnosing major structural abnormalities with the possible exception of anencephaly, unless transvaginal ultrasound is used.

What abnormalities may be diagnosed at the time of routine ultrasound?

Table 13.1 illustrates the diagnosis made at King's

Table 13.1 Prenatal diagnosis made at the time of routine early ultrasound (from Campbell & Pearce 1984)

Detected	Missed
6 Anencephaly	
6 Spina bifida	
5 Hydrocephaly	
1 Microcephaly	1 Microcephaly
1 Encephalocele	
1 Holoprosencephaly	
2 Omphaloceles	
1 Duodenal atresia	
1 Obstructive uropathy	
1 Renal agenesis	1 Renal agenesis
4 Fetal tumour	1 Single atrium
	1 Pulmonary atresia
	1 Hypertrophic cardiomyopathy

$n = 11\,664$.

College Hospital from routine early ultrasound (Campbell & Pearce 1984). It is important to realize that although the majority of the examinations were carried out by ultrasonographers, they worked in a department where referral for the diagnosis of fetal abnormalities was common and so were exposed to ultrasonically diagnosed anomalies much more frequently than the average ultrasonographer. If the ultrasound examinations for 3000 patients are carried out by two or three ultrasonographers, each can only expect to see three or four abnormalities a year. Since many of the abnormalities are subtle they may be overlooked.

Despite this it is reasonable to expect all ultrasonographers to diagnose such gross conditions as anencephaly and not to miss masses attached to the fetus such as cystic hydromata or omphaloceles. Cystic dilatation or masses within the fetal abdomen or chest are usually easily detectable and after a few months of training all ultrasonographers should be able to spot reduced amniotic fluid volume in the first half of pregnancy. Oligohydramnios at this stage has an extremely poor outcome and should encourage the ultrasonographer to look in detail for associated abnormalities or to refer the patient to an appropriate centre.

In order to achieve such diagnoses a mental checklist is necessary for every ultrasound examination. Even a routine examination to confirm gestational age which lasts for only 10–15 minutes should involve the ultrasonographer following a checklist similar to that given in Table 13.2.

The question of what measurements should be made at routine examination is debatable. Most would believe that the minimum should be measurement of the bi-parietal diameter and of the fetal femur length. If both of these agree with the postmenstrual age derived from the first day of the last menstrual period no further measurements are necessary. If the measurements differ from the menstrual dates and, more particularly, if the measurements differ from each other then it is necessary to measure the fetal head circumference and abdominal circumference (or area). A value judgement should be made on these measurements and the fetal gestational age confirmed or altered as appropriate. If there is a discrepancy between the measurements of the femur and the fetal head then the possibility of microcephaly, spina bifida or dwarfism should be considered. Despite the fact that 80% of babies with spina bifida have large cerebral ventricles at 18 weeks' gestation, the fetal head is often reduced in size (Roberts & Campbell 1980, Wald et al 1980) and therefore a small fetal head compared with other measurements should lead to a detailed examination of the fetal spine.

The value of routine ultrasound in low-risk pregnancies has recently been questioned by the publication of the RADIUS trial (Ewigman et al 1993). Figure 13.3 illustrates how the 15 530 women who were randomized were recruited. Of concern is the large number of women who were excluded or ineligible as most were excluded because they had a clinical reason for an ultrasound examination. The authors concluded that amongst the randomized women the detection of congenital abnormalities had no effect on perinatal outcome. The prevalence of major abnormalities in this trial was 2.3% and the detection

Table 13.2 A specimen checklist for use at routine ultrasound examination in early pregnancy

Anatomy	Measurement
Number of fetuses	
Beating fetal heart(s)	
Fetal head	Biparietal diameter
Intact cerebral vault	Head circumference
Normal shape	
Normal ventricles	VH ratio
Normal cerebellum	
Normal spine	
Longitudinal view	
Transverse view of each vertebra	
Normal chest, appearance	
Four-chamber view of heart	
Intact abdominal wall	Abdominal circumference
Single stomach bubble	
Normal kidneys	
Normal bladder	
Limbs	Femur length
Amniotic fluid volume	
(subjective impression)	
Placental site	
Three vessels in cord	

VH = ventricular hemisphere

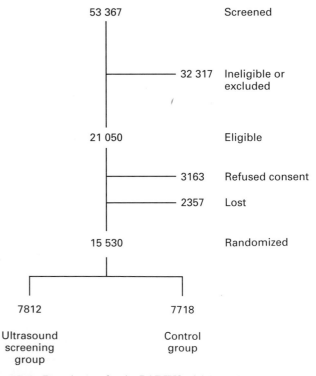

Fig. 13.3 Recruitment for the RADIUS trial (modified from Ewigman et al 1993).

rate in the ultrasound group was 35% (versus 10% in the control group). However, 52% (34/65) of cases were not detected until after 24 weeks' gestation (the upper limit of abortion in most states in the USA). This poor detection rate contrasts strongly with the European experience, which reports detection rates of about 80% (see Table 13.1). This has been criticized in that results come from centres of excellence but detection rates of over 70% have been reported from the Helsinki Ultrasound Trial (Saari-Kemppainen et al 1990) and from a British district general hospital (Chitty et al 1991). In this latter trial 72/87 (83%, 95% confidence intervals of 73–90%) of lethal or severely disabling abnormalities were detected before 24 weeks' gestation. The RADIUS trial has large numbers and so it will heavily bias meta-analyses, a fault of this type of overview.

Should screening for neural tube defects be by serum alpha-fetoprotein or ultrasound?

This is a question which at present cannot clearly be answered. It depends largely upon the following factors:

The prevalence of neural tube defects

If the upper confidence limit on maternal serum alpha-fetoprotein (MSAFP) is set at 2.5 times the multiple of the median (2.5 MoM) as recommended by the UK Collaborative Study (1977) then approximately 2% of all pregnant women screened will be positive. If the prevalence of neural tube defects (NTD) is 5 per 1000 then for every 5000 deliveries 100 women will require further investigations in order to detect 25 NTD. This is obviously an extremely good balance particularly if the further investigation is detailed ultrasound, rather than amniocentesis. If, however, the incidence of NTD is only 1 per 1000, then only 5 of the 100 positive-screened women will have an abnormality and the test becomes less acceptable.

It is not surprising therefore that many areas where there is a low prevalence of NTD have stopped screening by MSAFP (Standing et al 1981). The arguments for not screening by MSAFP are further strengthened if the diagnostic test is amniocentesis, which probably carries at least 1 in 50 risk of miscarrying a normal pregnancy (see Ch. 33).

The incidence of NTD is falling (Owens et al 1981) and in future screening for all by means of ultrasound will probably be routine, except where MSAFP is measured as part of a Down's screening test.

The quality of the local ultrasound

Many hospitals have now opted to spend valuable resources on ultrasound machinery and technicians rather than on screening by MSAFP. If routine ultrasound for establishing gestational age is delayed until 18 weeks' gestation then it is not unreasonable to expect to diagnose

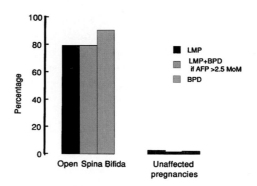

Fig. 13.4 The effect of ultrasound estimation of gestation on the specificity of alpha-fetoprotein screening. AFP = Alpha-fetoprotein; BPD = biparietal diameter; LMP = last menstrual period.

all anencephaly and at least 80% of cases of spina bifida at that time. Although the diagnosis of spina bifida by ultrasound requires a degree of skill, at least 80% of all such babies will have enlarged cerebral ventricles or a lemon-shaped head (Nicolaides et al 1986) at the 18 weeks' ultrasound and this is much more readily recognizable and diagnosed by direct measurements. This compares favourably with the direct diagnosis of spina bifida by ultrasound (UK Collaborative Report 1977).

Ideally all patients should be screened by means of a routine ultrasound and also by MSAFP. The interpretation of MSAFP should be made on the gestational age estimated from the ultrasound examination (Fig. 13.4). A combination of the two tests should be expected to detect more than 90% of all NTD with no concomitant increase in the false positive rate.

What to tell the patient thought to be carrying an abnormal fetus at the time of routine ultrasound

As a general rule ultrasound scanning is a joyous occasion for the parents and if the operator takes time to point out the baby on the screen it can improve the woman's compliance with antenatal advice (Campbell et al 1982). Thoughtless comments or reports, or unnecessary recall for further examination may however create anxiety and stress. This is more so when an anomaly is suspected.

If the operator is confident of the diagnosis then the parents should probably be told but without embarking on management discussions (Lind 1986). Early referral to the obstetrician is essential. The situation is more complex when an abnormality is only suspected. Patients are extremely sensitive to a variation in routine (Furness 1987) and will commonly ask: 'Is my baby normal?' The choice of approach lies between the following:

1. Telling the truth. This involves telling the patient what is suspected and arranging a definitive scan, preferably immediately or certainly within 48 hours. This approach is extremely helpful to the person performing the second scan as the patient will have recovered from the initial shock of a possible

abnormality and be more capable of comprehending the options offered once the diagnosis is established.

2. Telling the patient that a particular measurement cannot be obtained because of fetal position or that the placenta cannot be accurately localized. This approach may provoke less anxiety.

The referring obstetrician must retain the prerogative of deciding which lines of management to discuss with the patient, and each hospital should have its own policy on what to tell patients. Probably the best situation occurs when one obstetrician performs the definitive scan and, with the prior agreement of all the other referring obstetricians, performs the necessary counselling.

DIAGNOSTIC ULTRASOUND EXAMINATION FOR FETAL ABNORMALITIES

Table 13.3 indicates patients who should be offered detailed ultrasound examination. Although this examination has often been called high-resolution ultrasound, most modern ultrasound equipment is capable of producing the images necessary to make the diagnosis. The diagnosis is extremely operator-dependent and in good centres accurate diagnosis can be made in 99% of cases with a false negative rate of under 1% (Campbell & Pearce 1984).

Diagnosis of structural fetal abnormalities comes from a sound knowledge of normal fetal anatomy which can only be gained with experience. As the fetus has a limited way in which it can express abnormalities, once it is recognized that the anatomy is abnormal the differential diagnosis is not too difficult. Well over 50% of fetal abnormalities are craniospinal.

THE DIAGNOSIS OF SPECIFIC ABNORMALITIES

Craniospinal abnormalities

Figure 13.5 is an ultrasound picture of a transverse section of a fetal head on which the biparietal diameter is usually measured. Figure 13.6 is a pathological section

Table 13.3 Reasons for referral for detailed ultrasound examination (from Chudleigh & Pearce 1992)

Raised maternal serum alpha-fetoprotein
Patients undergoing amniocentesis
Patients with a personal or family history of a structural anomaly
Patients with a personal or family history of a chromosome anomaly that has a structural marker
Oligohydramnios
Polyhydramnios
Maternal diabetes mellitus
Patients in preterm labour, especially with a breech presentation
Multiple gestation
Patients exposed to teratogens in early pregnancy
Patients with suspicious findings on ultrasound
Patients with symmetrically small fetuses

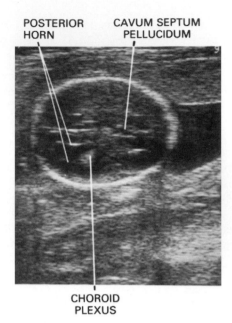

Fig. 13.5 Transverse section of a fetal head on which the biparietal diameter is measured. From Chudleigh & Pearce (1992).

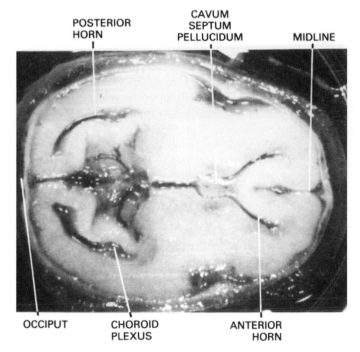

Fig. 13.6 Pathological specimen of a fetal head taken at the same level as Figure 13.5. From Chudleigh & Pearce (1992).

taken at the same level and demonstrates how well the ultrasound image echoes the intracranial anatomy. The main reasons for referral for detailed examination to exclude craniospinal abnormalities are a raised maternal alpha-fetoprotein, previous history of an affected infant or, more recently, because of abnormality suspected at the time of routine ultrasound examination.

Figure 13.7 illustrates an anencephalic fetus; this is an

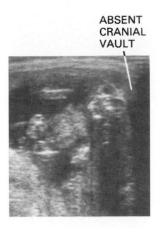

Fig. 13.7 Anencephalic fetus. The absence of the fetal cranial vault is readily appreciated. From Chudleigh & Pearce (1992).

easy diagnosis to make with ultrasound if due care is taken. The main reason for overlooking the diagnosis is because inability to measure the biparietal diameter is wrongly attributed to fetal position. In order to measure correctly the biparietal diameter, the fetal head needs to be in an occipitotransverse position, that is with the midline echo from the fetal brain at right angles to the ultrasound beam. Failure to achieve such a measurement should lead to the patient being re-scanned 1 week later. Patients should never have gestation estimated on the basis of femur length measurement alone because unless the fetal head is seen in the correct position all chance of examining the intracranial anatomy is lost. As long as these patients are recalled (this only refers to about 10%) such abnormalities should not be overlooked.

Figure 13.5 also illustrates the lateral cerebral ventricles. These should be easily visible on the same transverse section as is used to measure the biparietal diameter. With experience it is easy to recognize hydrocephaly or, more strictly, ventriculomegaly, as at this stage the head circumference is not usually large while the lateral ventricles are. Normality can be confirmed by measuring ventricular hemisphere ratio. This is usually done for both the anterior and posterior horns and plotted on an appropriate chart. Figure 13.8 illustrates a case of hydrocephaly; Figure 13.9 is a nomogram of the anterior horn ventricular hemisphere ratio together with cases of proven hydrocephaly. As can be seen, all cases of hydrocephaly had measurements well outside the confidence intervals.

Ventricular dilatation does not usually increase the biparietal diameter or head circumference measurement before 24 weeks' gestation and in cases of spina bifida associated with hydrocephaly these measurements may even be small for gestational age (Roberts & Campbell 1980, Wald et al 1980). In the UK the most common cause of ventriculomegaly in early pregnancy is spina bifida. A careful examination should therefore be made of the fetal spine.

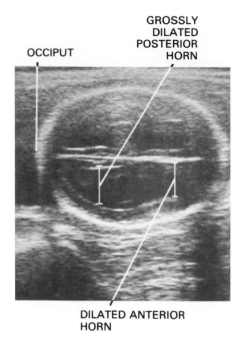

Fig. 13.8 Hydrocephaly. The section is the same as Figure 13.5 but the massive dilatation of the ventricles can be readily appreciated. From Chudleigh & Pearce (1992).

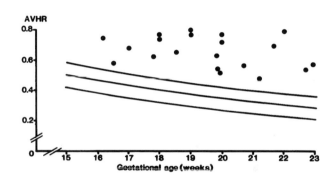

Fig. 13.9 Nomogram of the anterior ventricular hemisphere ratio (AVHR) together with proven cases of hydrocephaly.

Isolated hydrocephaly is uncommon. In early pregnancy the condition may be due to aqueduct stenosis, occasionally inherited as a sex-linked condition, but more commonly of unknown aetiology; it carries a recurrence risk of about 1 in 30. In general, isolated hydrocephaly tends to be more severe than hydrocephaly associated with spina bifida. In the USA this condition is more common than NTD and intrauterine drainage by means of ventrioculo-amniotic shunting has been attempted (Birnholz & Frigoletto 1981). Initially this was by means of ultrasonically guided puncture of the cerebral ventricles but this failed to stop fluid re-accumulating and latter a rubber shunt with a one-way valve was introduced which could be inserted under ultrasound guidance. The results in 41 fetuses were reported in 1986 (Report of the International Fetal Surgery Registry) and are summarized in

Table 13.4 Outcome of intrauterine therapy for hydrocephaly (from Report of International Fetal Surgery Registry 1986)

7 Deaths
  4 procedure-related
  3 from coexisting anomalies
12 Normal infants
  All had aqueduct stenosis as the cause of the hydrocephaly
  These were 43% of all cases of aqueduct stenosis
4 Mild/moderate handicap
  Developmental delay
  Developmental quotients < 80
18 Severe handicap
  Developmental quotients < 60
  5 cortical blindness
  3 fits
  2 spastic displegia

Table 13.4. It is apparent from this table that the outcome in all these babies was extremely poor and the procedure has now largely been abandoned.

Hydrocephaly in the first half of pregnancy may also be associated with abnormal kidneys (Meckel's syndrome). This condition is usually fatal and is inherited in an autosomal recessive fashion.

Mild dilatation of the cerebral ventricles causes serious concern. Having carefully excluded a coexisting abnormality serious consideration should be given to obtaining a fetal karyotype. If karyotyping is normal and there is no evidence of a recent TORCH virus infection, then patients can be given a favourable prognosis. Ultrasound examination should be carried out fortnightly to assess the growth of the fetal head and to determine if the degree of ventricular dilatation is worsening. Very occasionally a cause will be found for this, as in Figure 13.10 which

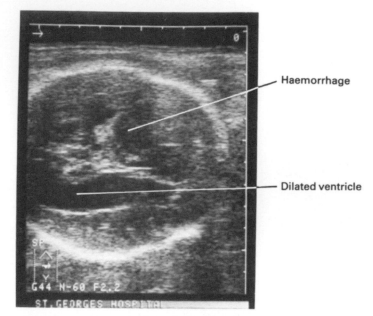

Fig. 13.10 Oblique section of a fetal head at 34 weeks' gestation illustrating mild dilatation of the ventricles due to a periventricular haemorrhage.

illustrates a prenatal periventricular haemorrhage of unknown aetiology. Figure 13.11 illustrates the postnatal scan of this baby, who demonstrates no neurological abnormality.

Having determined that the ventricles are of normal size, the skull vault should be carefully examined looking for the defect of an encephalocele (Fig. 13.12). These are rare lesions and constitute less than 1% of all NTD. They range in size from a small bony defect without

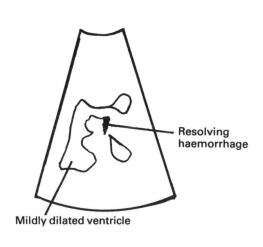

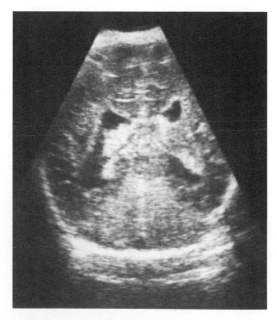

Fig. 13.11 Postnatal scan of the fetus illustrated in Figure 13.10 demonstrating the resolving haemorrhage together with mild dilatation of the ventricles. Courtesy of Professor Neil McIntosh.

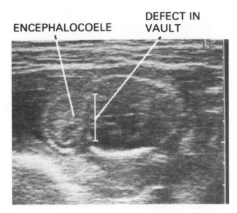

Fig. 13.12 Encephalocele.

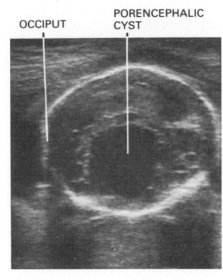

Fig. 13.14 Porencephalic cyst; end-result of a periventricular haemorrhage which burst out into the fetal brain. In this case the asphyxial insult to the fetus was maternal status epilepticus. From Chudleigh & Pearce (1992).

brain tissue in the herniated meninges to a major vault defect in which there are large amounts of brain in the herniated sac, usually called exencephaly. The prognosis depends on how much brain tissue there is within the lesion (Lorber 1967); the more extruded the brain, the worse the prognosis. In severe lesions the fetal head measurements usually indicate microcephaly. Encephaloceles may be occipital, parietal or frontal in origin although occipital encephaloceles are by far the most common. The lesion is easy to diagnose but has been confused with cystic hygroma. Clear guidelines on the differential diagnosis have been given by Pearce et al (1991); essentially there is always a vault defect in the presence of an encephalocele. Encephaloceles are rarely associated with elevated MSAFP levels as the lesions are skin-covered.

Whilst examining the fetal head, the cerebral ventricles should be further examined for the presence of cysts. Figure 13.13 illustrates a choroid plexus cyst. Most are

thought to be developmental and will usually disappear by 24 weeks' gestation (Chudleigh et al 1984). Choroid plexus cysts are associated with chromosomal abnormalities in about 1 in 250 cases (Chitty & Chudleigh, MRC study, personal communication). Other brain cysts are rare; that seen in Figure 13.14 is a porencephalic cyst which resulted from maternal asphyxia due to status epilepticus. Prognosis in these cases is difficult as world experience is limited but such an extensive cyst was felt to have a poor outcome.

Finally before leaving the fetal head the posterior fossa should be examined for abnormalities which, although uncommon, generally have a poor prognosis. Figure 13.15 illustrates normal cerebellar hemispheres which are

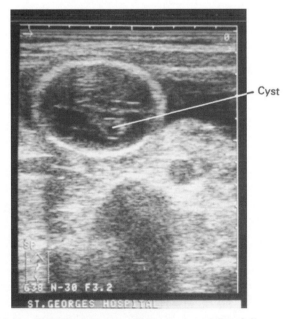

Fig. 13.13 Choroid plexus cyst. This cyst was small and disappeared by 24 weeks' gestation.

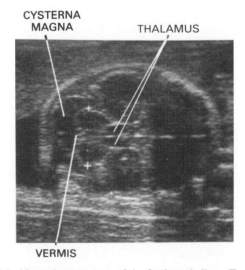

Fig. 13.15 Normal appearance of the fetal cerebellum. From Chudleigh & Pearce (1992).

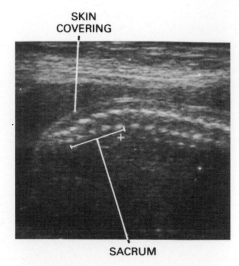

Fig. 13.16 Longitudinal section of a normal fetal spine. The skin covering can be seen along the entire length of the spine. From Chudleigh & Pearce (1992).

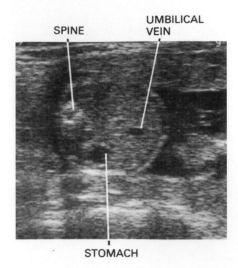

Fig. 13.17 The appearance of a normal vertebra viewed in transverse section. From Chudleigh & Pearce (1992).

dumb-bell shaped. Absence of the cerebellum is usually associated with trisomies but may also be associated with spina bifida, microcephaly or hydrocephaly. The Arnold–Chiari malformation may lead to a change in the shape of the fetal head which looks more like a lemon than a rugby ball. Enlargement of the fourth ventricle constitutes the Dandy–Walker malformation which may readily be diagnosed by ultrasound (Dempsey & Hobbs 1981). Absence of all or part of the cerebellum is also easily diagnosed by ultrasound.

Examination of the fetal spine requires some care and must never be done in one single view. Figure 13.16 shows a normal spine seen in longitudinal section; the skin covering the whole length of the spine can clearly be seen. This view alone, however, can lead to grave errors and each vertebra should be examined in transverse section. The typical normal vertebra is illustrated in Figure 13.17; Figure 13.18 illustrates the abnormality seen in cases of spina bifida. The term *spina bifida* refers to the bony abnormality and Figure 13.19 illustrates the correct terminology for other abnormalities.

Ultrasound diagnosis of spina bifida has advantages over the diagnosis made by means of amniotic fluid alpha-fetoprotein levels. Ultrasound will confirm that the cause of the raised maternal serum or amniotic fluid alpha-fetoprotein is a spina bifida. In addition the type of lesion can be determined; the separate strands of neural tissue that exist in the meningomyelocele are visible with careful scanning. The association of hydrocephaly with the lesion can be readily determined and the parents can be given a sensible prognosis based on that proposed by Lorber (1972). Table 13.5 lists the criteria used in determining the prognosis.

Patients with a normal fetus but a raised MSAFP can be strongly reassured at the end of the detailed ultrasound

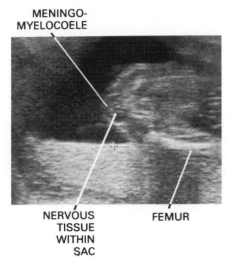

Fig. 13.18 Transverse section of the spine in cases of spina bifida. Compare with Figure 13.17. From Chudleigh & Pearce (1992).

examination and should be shown their baby on the screen as this significantly reduces anxiety levels (Tsoi et al 1987). This is preferable to the wait necessitated by laboratory analysis of amniotic fluid alpha-fetoprotein. Many patients who have a raised MSAFP and undergo amniocentesis are told: 'If you do not hear in 2 weeks, everything is normal'. They have high anxiety levels throughout their pregnancy (Fearn et al 1982) even after hearing the subsequent normal result.

Patients with a normal fetus and a raised MSAFP have a higher incidence of intrauterine growth retardation and preterm delivery. They should therefore be subsequently managed by serial measurements and Doppler ultrasound waveforms from the uterine arteries may have a prognostic role (Robson et al 1994).

Diagnosis of microcephaly by ultrasound may be

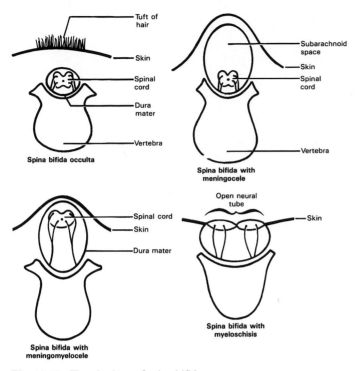

Fig. 13.19 Terminology of spina bifida.

Table 13.5 Predicting outcome of spina bifida diagnosed before 26 weeks' gestation

Feature	Favourable	Unfavourable
Hydrocephaly	Absent or mild	Severe
Spine	Not deformed	Deformed
Lesion	Closed	Open
	Meningocele	Meningomyelocele
Number of vertebrae involved*	Less than 2	More than 2
Associated anomalies (rare—5%)	No	Yes

*If more than two lumbosacral vertebrae are involved there will be bowel and bladder sphincter problems.

extremely difficult and is one of the abnormalities that will almost always be over-looked at the time of routine ultrasound in the first half of pregnancy. The primary defect in microcephaly is in brain growth, but since brain growth determines head growth (Warkany 1975) the skull is also small. Microcephalic infants are nearly always severely abnormal intellectually and, as brain growth appears to affect stature, the infants are often underweight. Amongst the better known causes for microcephaly are rubella infections in the first trimester, cytomegalovirus and toxoplasmosis infections, severe irradiation, maternal addiction to heroin and other drugs, for example the hydantoin syndrome. A few cases are associated with an autosomal mode of inheritance. In the absence of an obvious cause the recurrence rate appears to be about 1 in 30.

A reduced rate of head growth may be due to intrauterine growth retardation or microcephaly. Growth rates must

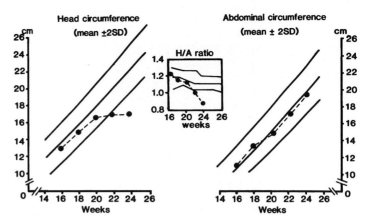

Fig. 13.20 Biparietal diameter and head/abdominal (H/A) ratio measurements in the case of microcephaly. Note that diagnosis was not made until almost 24 weeks' gestation.

therefore be related to the size of the abdominal circumference and the femur length. The diagnosis by ultrasound is not easy and nearly always relies on serial measurements (Fig. 13.20). It is not possible to make the diagnosis of microcephaly on an isolated measurement unless the head measurements are at least three standard deviations below those expected for gestational age whilst the abdominal circumference and femur are appropriate. The diagnosis of microcephaly in women who have had a previously affected infant may be delayed as late as 24 weeks' gestation. Late termination of pregnancy is usually strongly requested by all patients with this diagnosis following a previously abnormal child.

Rare abnormalities of the fetal head are usually easy to recognize. Holoprosencephaly is the presence of a single centrally placed cerebral ventricle and may be associated with midline abnormalities of the fetal face. Hydranencephaly is complete absence of the cerebral hemispheres thought to be due to failure of carotid arteries to cannulate. It is easily recognized on ultrasound as the cerebral vault contains only fluid. Abnormalities of the fetal head shape are rare, apart from the well recognized dolichocephalic shape of the head of the breech presentation.

Fetal tumours

The commonest reason for referral in this category is because of a suspicious finding on routine ultrasound. The two most common fetal tumours are cystic hygroma and sacrococcygeal teratoma. The latter is easy to diagnose in that the fetal spine is obviously normal and the tumour is apparent (Fig. 13.21). These teratomas are benign in two-thirds of patients (Donnelan & Swenson 1968) but there are no antenatal characteristics which allow the prediction of the nature so all such patients should be delivered by Caesarean section as these teratomas are associated with dystocia.

Fetal cystic hygroma is almost always associated with

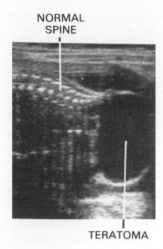

Fig. 13.21 Longitudinal view of the fetal spine demonstrating a sacrococcygeal teratoma.

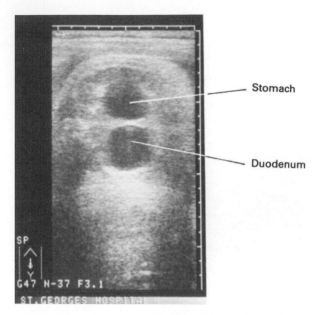

Fig. 13.22 Transverse section of the fetal abdomen illustrating a double bubble sign associated with duodenal atresia.

Turner's syndrome. The outcome of pregnancies associated with Turner's syndrome has been reviewed (Connor 1986, Pearce 1992). These reviews also dealt with the question of what to tell parents who have an incidental diagnosis of Turner's syndrome based on amniocentesis. The natural history of Turner's syndrome based on ultrasound findings in the mid-trimester is poor (Chervenak et al 1983, Pearce et al 1985). This is because most coexist with chylothorax and ascites and these findings carry a grave prognosis (Chervenak et al 1983). The finding of a cystic hygroma should therefore warrant karyotyping and detailed fetal echocardiography. In many of these pregnancies intrauterine death occurs but in the absence of a chromosome abnormality or ascites the outlook is favourable and the cystic hygroma may be dealt with surgically after delivery.

Gastrointestinal anomalies

Bowel obstruction above the ileum in the fetus usually results in polyhydramnios due to failure of absorption of swallowed amniotic fluid. Excess of amniotic fluid is the usual reason for referral for detailed ultrasound. Bowel obstruction such as duodenal atresia is easy to recognize as it presents a classical appearance known as the double bubble sign (Fig. 13.22). These lesions are readily amenable to surgery but as up to one-third are associated with Down's syndrome, karyotyping should be considered before a prognosis is given. Oesophageal atresia may be suspected because of the presence of polyhydramnios and the absence of a stomach bubble on repeated examinations. Colonic obstruction in Hirschsprung's disease or anal atresia may be detected by ultrasound because of distended loops of descending colon. Such diagnoses, however, are not usually made until the third trimester. Meconium peritonitis is usually recognizable prenatally

because of the intense intra-abdominal calcification that it excites and although it is nearly always associated with cystic fibrosis, it may result from maternal antidepressant therapy (such as lithium and tricyclic antidepressants).

One of the more unusual causes of raised MSAFP is an omphalocele or a gastroschisis. These conditions are easy to diagnose on ultrasound and can usually be differentiated. Omphaloceles are due to a midline defect in the abdominal wall, through which the peritoneal sac containing the liver and varying amounts of small bowel bulges (Fig. 13.23). The most common variety is due to failure of the physiological hernia to return at 9 weeks' gestation.

More severe abnormalities may also occur and may be associated with midline defects involving the bladder (ectopia vesicae) or the thorax and heart (ectopia cordis). Approximately half of all fetuses with an omphalocele will have associated cardiac or chromosome abnormalities. Karyotyping and detailed cardiac ultrasound are therefore important before providing a prognosis. As a general guideline the outlook for a fetus that has both an omphalocele and a cardiac abnormality (usually the tetralogy of Fallot) is poor, whereas if the omphalocele is an isolated defect surgical repair after birth has an excellent prognosis. There is conflicting evidence in the literature as to the best mode of delivery but the problem often solves itself as the condition is often associated with polyhydramnios and an unstable lie. If, however, the pregnancy does continue to term there seems to be no overwhelming reason to deliver by Caesarean section as the peritoneal sac is often toughened by exposure to amniotic fluid.

Gastroschisis is a much less common condition than

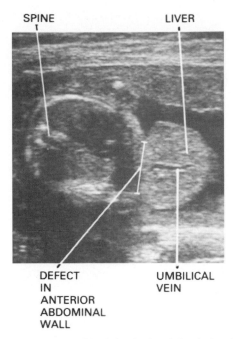

Fig. 13.23 Omphalocele. The defect in the abdominal wall is clearly seen and the liver bulges through this defect. From Chudleigh & Pearce (1992).

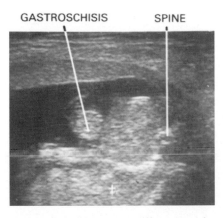

Fig. 13.24 Gastroschisis. This can be differentiated from an omphalocele by the presence of a normal umbilical vein within the fetal abdomen. From Chudleigh & Pearce (1992).

omphalocele; the insertion of the umbilical cord into the abdominal wall is intact, but usually to the right and somewhat lower than the umbilicus, and the small bowel can be seen to be extruded (Fig. 13.24). Counselling of patients is best done in conjunction with the paediatric surgeon but in general an encouraging prognosis can be given. The abdominal wall defect is usually small and the bowel can be readily replaced. The only caveat, however, is that the extruded small bowel does not have a peritoneal covering and may therefore become oedematous, matted and stenosed at the site of the extrusion. This may necessitate extensive resection of bowel with con-

comitant long-term intravenous feeding and malabsorption syndromes.

Diaphragmatic herniae may be diagnosed prenatally as cystic spaces seen within the chest. The outcome of such lesions is poor and up to one-third of such babies die antenatally. Overall some 85% of antenatally diagnosed diaphragmatic hernia cases will die and in 15% there will be an associated chromosomal anomaly. As yet there are no well-recognized ultrasonic markers of neonatal death, which is usually from pulmonary hypoplasia. The condition deteriorates after birth due to the child swallowing air, distending the bowel in the chest which leads to increased displacement of the neonatal heart. This is perhaps one of the conditions which may in future be treated with fetal surgery. Experimental work in monkeys (Harrison 1983) has demonstrated that if the diaphragmatic hernia is reduced by mid-pregnancy the fetal lungs continue to grow. It is possible to consider opening the uterus, temporarily removing the fetus, correcting the hernia and replacing the fetus. Diaphragmatic herniae are usually isolated defects, and do not tend to recur in future pregnancies.

Renal tract abnormalities

Normal fetal kidneys are clearly seen from 18 weeks' gestation (Fig. 13.25). The fetal bladder is also easily visible at this time and this, together with a normal amount of amniotic fluid, is an added reassurance of good renal function. The diagnosis of renal agenesis, however, is extremely difficult. This is because it is based on the absence of renal echoes, the absence of bladder-filling and severe

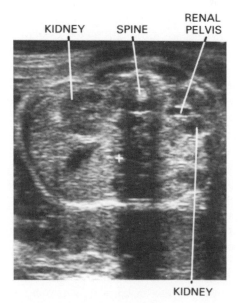

Fig. 13.25 Transverse section of the fetal abdomen demonstrating both kidneys. From Chudleigh & Pearce (1992).

Table 13.6 Outcome of oligohydramnios before 26 weeks' gestation

Finding	Percentage
Urinary tract anomalies	39
Renal agenesis	
Urethral valves	
Urethral atresia	
Infantile polycystic kidneys	
Multicystic kidneys	
Other structural anomalies	7
Cardiac	
Neural tube	
Chromosomal anomalies	7
Structurally normal fetus	7
Spontaneous abortion	
Intrauterine death	13
Neonatal death	14
Alive and well	13

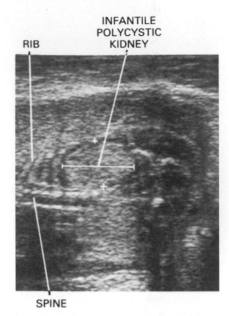

Fig. 13.26 Infantile polycystic kidneys. The kidneys take on an unusually bright appearance because of microcysts within them. From Chudleigh & Pearce (1992).

oligohydramnios. Visualization of kidneys is difficult due to lack of amniotic fluid and the inability to see one kidney which usually lies in the shadow produced by the spine. Furthermore perirenal fat or large adrenal glands may mimic the renal shadow. The difficulty in making the diagnosis of renal agenesis is widely recognized (Kierse & Meeran 1978, Hobbins et al 1979, Pearce & Campbell 1983) and the diagnosis should only be made by an experienced ultrasonographer. If there is doubt it is perhaps best to err on the side of caution but extreme oligohydramnios in the first half of pregnancy carries a very poor prognosis (Table 13.6).

Polycystic disease of the kidneys is divided into infantile and adult types. The infantile variety shows an autosomal recessive pattern of inheritance and is almost always associated with death from renal failure in early childhood. Patients referred for detailed ultrasound to exclude infantile polycystic disease usually have a past history of an affected child. Since the disease process tends to recur if bilateral cystic disease of the kidneys is seen in the current fetus it is safe to assume the diagnosis and offer a poor prognosis. Infantile polycystic kidneys may well be missed at the time of routine ultrasound, however, as the cysts are usually microscopic and interpretation of the pattern requires skill (Fig. 13.26).

Obstructive uropathy is the term applied to anatomical or physiological obstruction in any part of the urinary tract. In the fetus such conditions show a wide spectrum of pathological, clinical and ultrasonical features. Those with the most favourable prognosis present as the pelviureteric junction obstruction. The diagnosis is readily made by demonstrating an enlarged renal pelvis (Fig. 13.27). The condition may be bilateral although it is not uncommon for it to be expressed unilaterally in utero.

The large majority of these fetuses need only frequent monitoring and as the condition is usually an isolated defect, a good prognosis can be given to the parents. Although the insertion of nephrostomy tubes in utero has

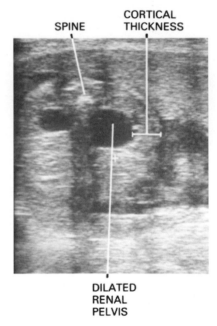

Fig. 13.27 Pelviureteric junction obstruction. From Chudleigh & Pearce (1992).

been described the author has never found it necessary. Pelviureteric junction obstruction is now considered as a series of acute obstructions, rather than a chronic obstruction. The management of these children has changed over the last few years and in the absence of grade IV reflux (reflux of urine into the renal pelvis at the time of micturition) or of hypertension, long-term monitoring seems to be all that is necessary.

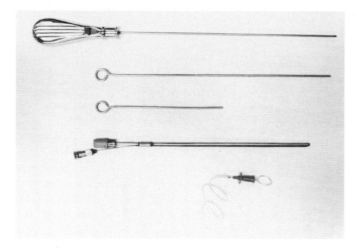

Fig. 13.28 Vesicoamniotic shunt set (Rocket Ltd, UK). The catheter is a double pigtail catheter. One end is inserted into the fetal bladder and the other remains in the amniotic fluid cavity.

Table 13.7 Outcome of vesicoamniotic shunt (73 fetuses) (from Report of the International Fetal Surgery Registry 1986)

Outcome	Number (percentage)
Elective termination	11 (15)
Abnormal chromosomes	6
Renal dysplasia	5
Other abnormalities	5
Deaths	32 (44)
Pulmonary hypoplasia	27
Chronic renal failure	1
Associated anomalies	1
Procedure-related	3
Survivors	30 (41)
Chronic renal failure	2
Cloacal syndrome	1

The other end of the spectrum of obstructive uropathy is of complete urethral stenosis. This condition presents ultrasonically as a complete absence of amniotic fluid together with gross dilatation of the renal tract. In addition the kidneys are often small and of increased echogenicity, suggesting severe dysplasia. The outcome is inevitably fetal demise and no therapy can be offered.

Posterior urethral valves occur exclusively in male infants and cause varying degrees of dilatation of the renal tract. It is in this group of babies that in utero surgery by means of suprapubic catheterization (the vesicoamniotic shunt; Fig. 13.28) may perhaps alter the outcome. The condition is diagnosed by dilated bladder and renal pelves in a male fetus. Before considering vesicoamniotic shunting, detailed ultrasound should be carried out to exclude other abnormalities. Approximately 25% of these babies will have a chromosome abnormality so at the time of insertion of the shunt, blood should be taken from the umbilical cord for karyotyping. Inserting the shunt should be regarded as a diagnostic test. The following lines of management are suggested depending upon initial results:

1. If the karyotype is abnormal, termination of pregnancy should be offered.
2. If the urinary sodium is more than 80 mmol/l or the vesicoamniotic shunt is not working, termination should be offered. Severely dysplastic kidneys seem unable to conserve sodium. It is easy to determine if the shunt is working because the amount of amniotic fluid should rapidly increase. If this does not occur then most babies die from pulmonary hypoplasia.
3. If the fetus is chromosomally normal and the amniotic shunt is working, weekly ultrasound examination should be preformed to determine fetal growth, bladder volume and size, and amniotic fluid volume.

The shunts are relatively small and have a tendency to become blocked but may be replaced. If the shunt blocks after 32 weeks' gestation fetal lung maturity should be assessed by measurement of amniotic fluid lecithin : sphingomyelin ratio and phosphatidyl glycerol. If the fetus is mature, delivery is preferable to inserting a further shunt. Table 13.7 illustrates the outcome for these fetuses.

Limb reduction deformities

All fetal long bones can easily be measured on ultrasound but measurement may be time-consuming due to fetal movements. Nomograms are available for all the long bones (Queenan et al 1980). Tables 13.8 and 13.9 illustrate the ultrasound findings in cases of dwarfism together with its common associations. All lethal forms of dwarfism are associated with early shortening of the limb bones, readily recognizable before 22 weeks' gestation. Less than lethal conditions commonly result in slow growth which may not be apparent until later in pregnancy. This is best seen in achondroplastic fetuses. Homozygous achondroplasia leads to severe early limb reduction and usually results in death after birth because of reduced size of the

Table 13.8 Ultrasonic features of lethal limb reduction deformities

Syndrome	Limbs	Other features
Achondrogenesis	Severe micromelia	Polyhydramnios Hydrops
Thanatophoric dwarfism	Severe micromelia	Megalocephaly Small chest Polyhydramnios Absent corpus
Jeune's syndrome	Severe micromelia	Polydactyly Dysplastic kidneys
Camptomelic dwarfism	Severe micromelia Bowed tibia	Polyhydramnios Macrocephaly Cardiac defects Cleft palate

Table 13.9 Ultrasonic features of less than lethal limb reduction deformities

Syndrome	Limbs	Other features
Achondrogenesis	Micromelia—onset after mid-pregnancy	Mild hydrocephaly
Hypochondroplasia	Micromelia—onset after mid-pregnancy	
Acromesomelic dwarfism	Micromelia with more distal than proximal limb reduction	
Ellis-van Creveld syndrome	Micromelia—onset after mid-pregnancy	Polydactyl ASD
Diastrophic dwarfism	Late-onset micromelia Flexion deformities	
Cleidocranial dysostosis	Late-onset micromelia	Absent clavicles Hypomineralized skull

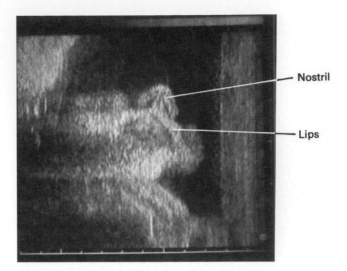

Fig. 13.29 Frontal view of a normal fetal face. The fetal lips and nostrils are clearly visible.

fetal chest, whereas heterozygous achondroplasia tends not to show deviation in fetal growth until well after 24 weeks' gestation (Filly & Golbus 1983).

In addition to dwarfism, hypomineralization due to conditions such as achondrogenesis, hypophosphatasia and osteogenesis imperfecta can be recognized on ultrasound. The genetics of osteogenesis imperfecta is difficult and at least four types are described. In the most severe degree, intrauterine fractures can be diagnosed. Isolated limb deformities are easily missed at the time of routine ultrasound but with care amelia, phocomelia and amputation deformities can be detected. Likewise, abnormalities of fetal fingers and toes can be determined in the second trimester but examination is extremely time-consuming. If the structural abnormalities being sought of the hands or fingers are not clearly seen and are markers for a more severe syndrome, fetoscopy should be considered.

Rocker bottom feet can be recognized on ultrasound with experience and postural deformities such as talipes can also be detected.

Facial abnormalities

Full frontal views of the face, and views of the face in profile, are possible with ultrasound. Abnormalities of the face are therefore recognizable and may be associated with various syndromes. For example, the arrhinencephaly cyclops syndrome is usually detected by the presence of a single, abnormal orbit. Soft tissues of the face are more difficult to visualize (Fig. 13.29) but with care, harelip and cleft palate may also be diagnosed.

Cardiac abnormalities

These constitute the second most common group of abnormalities and occur in approximately 8 per 1000 live births. Half of these defects however are small, self-correcting or easily correctable defects but one-quarter of all children born with congenital heart disease die of their defect; in over half of this group, death occurs in the first year of life.

The prenatal diagnosis of cardiac lesions may therefore lead to termination of pregnancy for lesions which carry a high mortality. More optimistically, recognizing the defect during pregnancy leads to the baby being transferred in utero to be born in a hospital with the appropriate cardiac facilities to offer early surgery.

Although detailed diagnosis is time-consuming and demands clear understanding of cardiac anatomy, many major structural abnormalities can be diagnosed from the simple four-chamber view (Fig. 13.30). If this view is extended to show the origin of the aorta from the left ventricle to the pulmonary outflow tract from the right ventricle, most major abnormalities can be excluded by 24 weeks' gestation. Interested readers should consult Allan (1986).

Structural markers of chromosomal abnormalities

Recently, minor structural abnormalities have been associated with chromosomal anomalies (Benacerraf 1991, Nicolaides et al 1992). Table 13.10 lists the described markers and the possible risk of an associated chromosomal anomaly. The risk appears to be additive (Nicolaides et al 1992) but we are unsure that they are independent of maternal age and like all screening tests their presence or absence should not refute another screening test such as the triple test. Overall, it is believed that some 85% of fetuses with Down's syndrome will demonstrate a minor marker, such as a nuchal fat pad (Fig. 13.32).

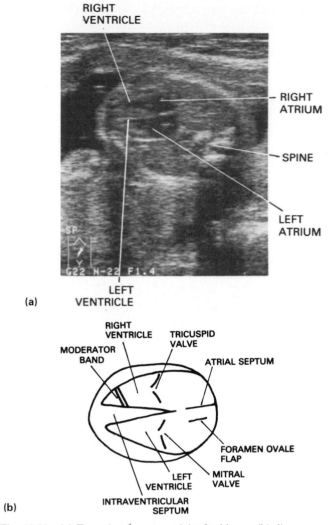

(a)

(b)

Fig. 13.30 (a) Four-chamber view of the fetal heart; (b) diagram to illustrate the normal anatomy. From Chudleigh & Pearce (1992).

Table 13.10 Structural markers suggestive of associated chromosomal abnormalities

Markers	Karyotype	Probable risk
Agenesis of corpus callosum	Trisomy 13	5%
Cardiac abnormalities	Trisomies 13, 18, 21 Triploidy	15%
Choroid plexus cysts	Trisomy 18, 21	0.5%
Clasped/overlapping fingers	Trisomy 18	?
Clinodactyly	Trisomy 21	?
Cystic hygromata	45X	95%
	Trisomy 21, 18, 13	4%
Diaphragmatic hernia	Trisomy 21, 18 Deletions	15%
Dilated ureters	Trisomy 18, 21	30%
Duodenal atresia (Fig. 13.23)	Trisomy 21	30%
Holoprosencephaly	Trisomy 18, 21	90%
Lateral facial cleft	Trisomy 18	<1%
Median facial cleft	Trisomy 13, 21	50%
Microcephaly	Deletions	?
Bilateral multicystic dysplastic kidneys	Trisomy 18	?
Non-immune hydrops	45X	?
Non-immune hydrops with cystic hygromata	45X	99%
Nuchal fat pad (Fig. 13.32)	Trisomy 21, 45X	?
Low obstructive uropathy	Trisomy 18, 13, 21	20%
Omphalocele (Fig. 13.23)	Trisomy 13, 18	30%
Radial aplasia/ aplasia of the thumb	Trisomy 13	90%
Rocker bottom feet	Trisomy 13	50%
Sandal gap	Trisomy 21	?
Single umbilical artery (Fig. 13.32)	Trisomy 18, 21	5%
Syndactyly/polydactyly	Trisomy 13 Triploidy	?

Note: figures are best estimates from the literature. Those markers with a '?' probably have a low association and on their own probably do not warrant karyotyping.

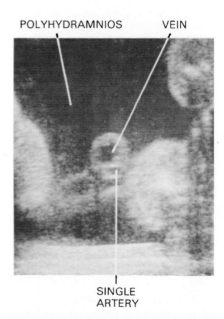

Fig. 13.31 A single umbilical artery. From Chudleigh & Pearce (1992).

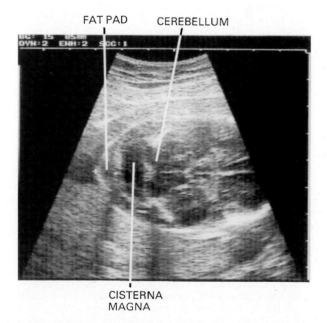

Fig. 13.32 An enlarged nuchal fat pad of 7.8 mm (upper limit of normal = 5 mm) associated with Down's syndrome.

CONCLUSIONS

Ultrasound examination is now routine in most pregnancies. Its primary aim in early pregnancy is to confirm or establish gestational age and to diagnose multiple pregnancies. Its use at this time should be regarded as a screening procedure for fetal anomalies, and with care, most major anomalies can be detected. In this role it may replace MSAFP in screening for NTD.

As a diagnostic instrument for women at high risk of fetal anomalies it is extremely accurate. The subsequent management of fetal anomalies diagnosed necessitates sensitive communication between the parents, the perinatal obstetrician, neonatologist and paediatric surgeon. Final counselling also requires the expertise of the geneticist and the perinatal pathologist.

REFERENCES

Allan L D 1986 Manual of fetal echocardioagraphy. MTP Press, New York

Bakketieg L S, Eik-Nes S H, Jacobsen G et al 1984 Randomised controlled trial of ultrasonographic screening in pregnancy. Lancet ii: 207–211

Benacerraf B R 1991 Prenatal sonography of autosomal trisomies. Ultrasound in Obstetrics and Gynaecology 1: 66–75

Bennett N Y, Little G, Dewhurst J, Chamberlain G V P 1982 Predictive value of ultrasound measurement in early pregnancy: a randomised controlled trial. British Journal of Obstetrics and Gynaecology 89: 338–341

Birnholz J C, Frigoletto A 1981 In utero decompression of obstructive hydrocephalus. New England Journal of Medicine 304: 1021–1023

Campbell S 1974 Fetal growth. In: Beard R W, Nathanielsz P W (eds) Fetal physiology and medicine, 1st end. Saunders, London, pp 271–301

Campbell S, Pearce J M F 1984 The prenatal diagnosis of fetal structural anomalies by ultrasound. Clinics in Obstetrics and Gynaecology 10: 475–506

Campbell S, Reading A E, Cox D N et al 1982 Ultrasound scanning in pregnancy; the short term effects of early real time scans. Journal of Psychosomatic Obstetrics and Gynaecology 1: 57–61

Chapman M, Sheat J H, Furness E T, Jones W R 1979 Routine ultrasound screening in early pregnancy. Medical Journal of Australia 2: 62–63

Chervenak F A, Isaacson G, Blakemore K J 1983 Fetal cystic hygroma. Cause and natural history. New England Journal of Medicine 309: 822–825

Chitty L S, Hunt G H, Moore J, Lobb M O 1991 Effectiveness of routine ultrasonography in detecting fetal structural abnormalities in a low risk population. British Medical Journal 303: 1165–1169

Chudleigh P, Pearce J M F 1992 Obstetric ultrasound: how, why and when, 2nd edn. Churchill Livingstone, Edinburgh

Chudleigh P, Pearce J M F, Campbell S 1984 The prenatal diagnosis of transient cysts of the fetal choroid plexus. Prenatal Diagnosis 4: 135–137

Connor J M 1986 Prenatal diagnosis of the Turner syndrome; what to tell the parents. British Medical Journal 293: 711–712

Dempsey P J, Hobbs H J 1981 The in utero diagnosis of the Dandy–Walker syndrome. Journal of Clinical Ultrasound 9: 403–405

Donnelan W A, Swenson O I 1968 Benign and malignant sacrococcygeal teratomas. Surgery 64: 834–836

Eik-Nes S H, Okland O, Aure J C, Ulstein M 1984 Ultrasound screening in pregnancy: a randomised controlled trial. Lancet: 1347

Ewigman B G, Crane J P, Frigoletto F D et al 1993 Effect of prenatal ultrasound screening on prenatal outcome. New England Journal of Medicine 329: 821–827

Fearn J, Hibbard B M, Laurence K M, Roberts A 1982 Screening for neural tube defects and maternal anxiety. British Journal of Obstetrics and Gynaecology 89: 218–221

Filly R A, Golbus M S 1983 Ultrasonography of the normal and abnormal fetal skeleton. In: Callan P W (ed) Ultrasonography in obstetrics and gynaecology. Saunders, Philadelphia, pp 81–96

Furness M E 1987 Reporting obstetric ultrasound. Lancet i: 675–676

Grennert L, Persson P-H, Gennser G 1978 Benefits of ultrasound screening of a pregnant population. Acta Obstetricia et Gynecologica Scandinavica (suppl) 78: 5–14

Harrison M R 1983 Prenatal management of the fetus with a correctable defect. In: Callan P W (ed) Ultrasonography in obstetrics and gynaecology. Saunders, Philadelphia, pp 177–192

Hobbins J C, Grannum P A T, Berkowitz R L 1979 Ultrasound in the diagnosis of congenital abnormalities. American Journal of Obstetrics and Gynecology 134: 331–338

Kierse M J N C, Meeran R H 1978 Antenatal diagnosis of Potter's syndrome. Obstetrics and Gynecology (suppl) 52: 64–67

Lind T 1986 Obstetric ultrasound: getting good vibrations. British Medical Journal 299: 576–577

Lorber J 1967 The prognosis of occipital encephalocoeles. Developmental Medicine and Child Neurology (suppl) 13: 75–79

Lorber J 1972 Spina bifida cystica. Archives of Disease in Childhood 47: 854–873

Neilson J P 1993 Routine ultrasound in early pregnancy. In: Enkin M W, Keirse M J N C, Renfrew M J, Neilson J P (eds) Pregnancy and childbirth module. Cochrane Database of Systematic Reviews: Review No: 03872 9 June 1993. Published through 'Cochrane Updates on Disk'. Oxford: Update Software, Disk Issue 2.

Nicolaides K H, Snijders R J M, Gosden C M et al 1992 Ultrasonographically detectable markers of fetal chromosomal abnormalities. Lancet 340: 704–707

Owens J R, McAllister E, Harris F, West L 1981 19 Year incidence of neural tube defects in area under constant surveillance. Lancet ii: 1032–1034

Pearce J M 1992 Turner's syndrome. Maternal and Child Health 17: 365–369

Pearce J M F, Campbell S 1983 The prenatal diagnosis of fetal urinary tract anomalies. In: Rodeck C H, Nicolaides K H (eds) Prenatal diagnosis. Proceedings of the 11th Study Group of the Royal College of Obstetricians and Gynaecologists, London, pp 313–324

Pearce J M F, Griffin D, Campbell S 1985 The differential prenatal diagnosis of cystic hygromata and encephalocoele by ultrasound examination. Journal of Clinical Ultrasound 13: 317–320

Persson P-H, Grennert L, Gennser G, Kullander S 1978 On improved outcome of twin pregnancies. Acta Obstetricia et Gynecologica Scandinavica 58: 3–7

Queenan J T, O'Brien G B, Campbell S 1980 Ultrasound measurements of fetal limb bones. American Journal of Obstetrics and Gynecology 138: 297–301

Report of the International Fetal Surgery Registry 1986 New England Journal of Medicine 315: 336–340

Roberts A B, Campbell S 1980 Fetal head measurements of spina bifida. British Journal of Obstetrics and Gynaecology 87: 927–931

Robinson H P, Sweet E M, Adam A H 1979 The accuracy of radiological estimates of gestation age using fetal crown rump length measurements by ultrasound as a basis for comparison. British Journal of Obstetrics and Gynaecology 82: 702–710 ·

Robson M, Hamid R, McParland P, Pearce J M 1994 Doppler ultrasound of the uteroplacental circulation in the prediction of pregnancy outcome in women with raised maternal serum alpha-fetoprotein. British Journal of Obstetrics and Gynaecology 101: 481–484

Royal College of Obstetricians and Gynaecologists 1984 Report of the RCOG working party on routine ultrasound examination in pregnancy. RCOG, London

Saari-Kemppainen A, Karjalainen O, Ylostalo P, Heinonen O P 1990 Ultrasound screening and perinatal mortality: controlled trial of systematic one-stage screening in pregnancy. Lancet 336: 387–391

Standing S J, Brindle M J, MacDonald A P, Lacey R W 1981 Maternal alpha-fetoprotein screening: two years' experience in a low risk district. British Medical Journal 283: 705

Tsoi M M, Hunter M, Pearce J M F, Chudleigh P, Campbell S 1987 Ultrasound scanning in women with raised serum alpha-fetoprotein: short term psychological effect. Journal of Psychosomatic Research 31: 35–39

UK Collaborative Study 1977 Alphafetoprotein in relation to neural tube defects. Lancet i: 1323–1332

Wald N, Cuckle H, Boreham J 1980 Biparietal diameter measurements in fetuses with spina bifida. British Journal of Obstetrics and Gynaecology 87: 219–221

Wald N, Cuckle H, Boreham J 1982 Effect of estimating gestational age by ultrasound cephalometry on the specificity of alphafetoprotein screening for open neural tube defects. British Journal of Obstetrics and Gynaecology 89: 1050–1053

Warkany J 1975 Congenital malformations. Year Book Medical Publishers, New York, p 237

Warsof S L, Pearce J M F, Campbell S 1983 The present place of routine ultrasound screening. Clinics in Obstetrics and Gynaecology 10: 445–458

14. Fetal assessment in the third trimester: biophysical methods

Naren B. Patel   Philip Owen

Material in this chapter contains contributions from the first edition and we are grateful to the previous authors for the work done.

CARDIOTOCOGRAPHY

Introduction

Obstetricians have long looked for antenatal tests that would identify the fetus at risk of intrauterine hypoxia and death. Ideally such a test should not only be reliable, but performed easily and repeatedly. The result should be available immediately and the cost should be minimal. While many biochemical tests, such as estimations of oestriol and placental lactogens, have been carried out in the past, these are poor predictors of fetal outcome (Varma 1981).

Currently, the most commonly used antenatal test of fetal well-being is cardiotocography—either the contraction stress test which is popular in the USA or the non-stress test used widely in Europe. The sophisticated equipment needed for fetal heart rate recording and the significance of the various changes that occur in heart rate are the results of many years of observations and research.

Historical perspective

Marsac, a French obstetrician, was probably the first to observe the fetal heart sounds (Pinkerton 1976). On 22 December 1822, Jean Alexander Le Jumeau, Vicomte de Kergaradec, read his monograph 'Memoir sur l'auscultation appliquee a l'etude de la grossesse' in the Royal Academy of Medicine in Paris. He recognized the distinct fetal tones and sounds which he thought were from the umbilical cord and the placenta. In 1833, Kennedy, an obstetrician in Dublin, published his monograph on obstetrical auscultation. Von Hoefft in 1836 described the normal range of fetal heart rate and the fact that the rate de-

creased with gestational age. Hohl (1833) and Huter (1862) thought that tachycardia was associated with fetal compromise and maternal fever. Kennedy (1833) thought that the most ominous fetal heart signs were 'slowness of its return following a contraction'. With further evaluation of the fetal heart the importance of auscultation throughout labour was stressed by Schwartz (1858) and Von Winckel (1893).

The introduction of continuous fetal heart rate recording using the averaging technique developed by Hon & Lee (1963) in the 1960s and 1970s changed the pattern of monitoring in labour (Hon 1972). However, it was Hammacher (1962, 1966) who not only developed the first antenatal cardiotocograph equipment with the phonocardiograph but also reported on the fetal heart rate characteristics associated with fetal compromise in the antepartum period. Kubli et al (1969) noted the association of late decelerations, baseline tachycardia and loss of variability with fetal compromise associated with pathological pregnancies. For monitoring the fetus antenatally the contraction stress test (CST) began to be evaluated in the USA while the non-stress test (cardiotocography; CTG) was being used in Europe.

Methodology

Antenatal cardiotocography employs external (indirect) methods of monitoring the fetal heart rate. The signals obtained are often small, sometimes discontinuous and constantly shifting, and therefore, the qualities of tracing are often not as good as those obtained by direct methods, such as the fetal scalp electrode used during labour. Three techniques have been evaluated to obtain fetal heart recordings antenatally—phonocardiography, fetal electrocardiography and ultrasound Doppler cardiography.

Phonocardiography

In phonocardiography the signal is obtained by pressing a microphone on the maternal abdomen and the natural

231

fetal heart sounds are amplified and converted into electrical signals. Theoretically this should allow the fetal heart signal to be identified clearly, however in practice sound generated by the placenta, umbilical vessels and maternal intra-abdominal vessels are also picked up by the abdominal microphone which may mask the fetal heart sounds.

Due to the presence of additional unwanted sound, a system of signal filtration is required to produce a fetal heart rate signal free of artefacts. The clinical usefulness of this method in recording the fetal heart sounds has been looked at both antenatally and during the intrapartum period. The results indicate that there is a high incidence of poor tracings obtained using this method. The proportion of fetal heart rate tracings considered to be of good quality varies between 22% and 77% (Ruttgers & Kubli 1969, Saling 1969, Jauer et al 1976).

Clearly, although satisfactory recordings of the fetal heart rate may be obtained using this method, the recording is affected by many factors; it is found to be difficult to use in practice and has a high incidence of poor-quality tracings.

Fetal electrocardiography

By placing electrodes on the maternal abdominal wall it is possible to record the fetal ECG. However, the maternal ECG is also recorded; elimination of this maternal ECG complex requires electronic filtration of the signals and amplification of the fetal component before a clear fetal heart rate recording can be obtained.

With an abdominal fetal ECG, the fetal R waves of the fetal ECG complex are used as trigger signals. The potential of this part of the ECG signal varies throughout pregnancy.

From the 18th week of gestation until the 27th, the R-wave potential is high. Following this, there is a decline to a minimum potential at 30 weeks' gestation. Between 27 and 34 weeks' gestation it is impossible to obtain continuous fetal heart rate tracings in 70% of cases (Steer 1986). Thereafter the fetal R-wave potential increases until delivery. This variation is thought to be due to the effect of vernix caseosa altering the electrical resistance of the fetal skin (Wheeler et al 1978).

A number of studies have been reported during the antenatal period to determine the frequency with which satisfactory recordings of the fetal heart can be made. Direct comparison between different studies is difficult because of the imprecise assessment of tracings, which in most cases are simply divided into good, intermediate and poor quality. However, many groups have reported successful use of abdominal ECG to record the fetal heart, particularly when used in the last 4 weeks of pregnancy (Wheeler et al 1978, Keegan & Paul 1980). The newer equipment using noise reduction techniques may be more satisfactory (Jenkins 1984, Greene 1987, Jenkins et al 1986).

Ultrasound fetal cardiotocography

This is the most commonly used method for recording the fetal heart rate antenatally. It utilizes the physical principle of the Doppler effect in which sound waves hitting a moving object are reflected back at an altered frequency. Using this principle, the fast opening and closing of the fetal heart valves can be detected. Since they cause a definite ultrasound frequency shift, this physical movement can be used to generate well-defined trigger pulses.

Initially, the ultrasound transducers used consisted of a single transmitter and a single piezoelectric crystal receiver. This combination of narrow beam transducers had the disadvantage that the ultrasound beam required precise positioning to produce a good signal. Broad beam array transducers, consisting of several pairs of transmitters and receiver crystals, which detect the movement of a large area of the fetal heart wall and produced smaller, slower frequency shifts compared with those produced by the fetal heart valves themselves are a reliable method of recording the fetal heart (Bishop 1968, Solum 1980). However using ultrasound fetal cardiotocography with a broad beam transducer, true beat-to-beat variability of the fetal heart or short-term variability cannot be recorded accurately. Assessment of baseline variability is possible in clinical practice with good-quality recordings (Solum et al 1981).

In spite of the potential difficulties in obtaining recordings of suitable quality for analysis with Doppler ultrasound monitors, this method has become the most useful in clinical practice with good recordings being obtained relatively easily, independent of gestational age.

Some more recent machines incorporate the technique of autocorrelation, which uses the technique of processing the ultrasound signal with microprocessors. The advantage of autocorrelation is that a more precise calculation of the periodicity of the wave forms can be achieved (Steer 1986). The main disadvantage is that erroneous accelerations and decelerations may be recorded as a result of detection of the maternal pulse or resulting from transient variations in autocorrelation. These errors in recording can however be detected and eliminated by on-line computer analysis (Dawes et al 1990).

Physiology

Details of fetal cardiovascular physiology are fully dealt with in Chapter 6. A brief discussion follows with particular reference to the clinical relevance of the fetal heart rate changes.

The parasympathetic and sympathetic components of the autonomic nervous system control fetal cardiac behaviour. The regulation of fetal heart rate is also influenced by vasomotor centres, chemoreceptors and baroreceptors and cardiac autoregulation. Pathological events such as fetal hypoxia modify these influences and fetal cardiac responses. Minor changes in fetal blood gases do not produce a change in fetal heart rate (Wood et al 1979).

Baseline fetal heart rate

Fetal heart rate falls with increasing gestational age (Schifferle & Caldeyro-Barcia 1973) and also becomes more variable (Ruttgers et al 1972). The decrease in fetal heart rate is due to the development of vagal tone (Hon & Yeh 1969). Therefore the mean baseline fetal heart rate is a reflection of a balance of sympathetic and parasympathetic autonomic influences. The mean normal baseline fetal heart rate in late pregnancy is between 120 and 150 beats/min.

Rates between 100 and 120 beats/min are regarded as fetal bradycardia. If the variability is normal, it is usually a reflection of increased vagal tone. If observed spasmodically it may suggest cord compression. Persistent marked bradycardia is associated with congenital heart defects (Garite et al 1979) or represents complete heart block secondary to transplacentally acquired autoantibodies (Olah & Gee 1992). Baseline bradycardia is rarely associated with antepartum hypoxia (Young et al 1979) unless placental abruption is present.

A baseline tachycardia of over 160 beats/min is associated with maternal fever or chorioamnionitis; in the latter there may also be loss of variability. Kubli & Rutgers (1972) showed that with chronic fetal hypoxia the fetal heart rate is within the normal range, in contrast to the situation in acute or subacute fetal hypoxia where there is a baseline tachycardia present which may be due to an increase in the levels of catecholamines. Administration of beta-mimetic drugs such as ritodrine to the mother leads to a mild fetal tachycardia.

Fetal tachyarrhythmias are uncommon but are a potentially reversible cause of hydrops fetalis. Supraventricular tachycardia is commoner than atrial fibrillation although both may be intermittent, making prolonged examination necessary if a rhythm disturbance is suspected (Maxwell et al 1983, Hansmann et al 1991).

Fetal heart rate variability

Under normal physiological conditions the interval between each heart beat (beat-to-beat) is different and this is referred to as short-term variability; it increases with advancing gestational age (Goodlin 1977, Wheeler et al 1979). Long-term variability is due to the periodic changes in the direction and size of the changes from hypoxia resulting in oscillations around the mean baseline fetal heart rate. These oscillations occur approximately two to six times per minute. Short-term variability, normally of the order of 1–3 beats/min, cannot be identified visually (Wheeler et al 1979).

In addition to gestational age, heart rate variability is influenced by fetal sleep states, accelerations and decelerations (deHaan et al 1971, Romer et al 1979). Under normal physiological situations the fetal heart rate variability is the product of opposing sympathetic and parasympathetic influence on the heart. Several investigators have shown the relationship between reduced variability and chronic fetal hypoxia (Hammacher 1966, Kubli & Ruttgers 1972) and severe fetal hypoxia resulting in loss of variability (Dalton et al 1977). However, mild and early stages of hypoxia may also be associated with a reduction in fetal heart rate variability (Flynn et al 1979). Drugs that cause depression of the central nervous system, such as hypnotics and opiate alkaloids, are also associated with reduced fetal heart rate variability (Petrie et al 1978, Keegan et al 1979).

The fetus is known to undergo sleep–wake cycles of 60–70 minutes (Sterman 1967, Junge 1979). The quiet phase can average from 20 to 30 minutes. True wakefulness is associated with accelerations and increased fetal heart rate variability, while sleep cycles are associated with reduced variability. Motor and respiratory movements are similarly affected (Dalton et al 1977). Respiratory sinus arrhythmia is the change in heart rate in response to fetal breathing and can be detected by Doppler ultrasound (Brown et al 1992).

Sinusoidal pattern

This pattern is typically associated with an anaemic fetus as a result of rhesus sensitization or fetal exsanguination (Manseau et al 1972, Modanlouh et al 1977). Sinusoidal fetal heart rate pattern resembles a sine wave of fixed periodicity of 2–5 cycles/min usually with profound loss of short-term variability (Young et al 1980). Original publications describing this pattern of fetal heart rate all reported a very high perinatal loss (Kubli & Ruttgers et al 1972, Manseau et al 1972, Rochard et al 1976). However, apart from cases of rhesus sensitization, its usefulness in clinical management antenatally requires further evaluation.

In a prospective study, Murphy et al (1991) distinguished pseudo-sinusoidal patterns from sinusoidal ones on the basis of episodes of baseline oscillations of constant amplitude alternating with episodes of normal baseline reactivity. Such episodes are often associated with fetal sucking identified by real-time ultrasound (Giacomello et al 1987) and are not an indication for intervention.

Fetal heart rate accelerations

Accelerations are usually transient, of about 15–20 beats/min, and are invariably associated with fetal movement, external stimuli or uterine contractions. They are rarely present in the hypoxic fetus (Wood et al 1979). The presence of accelerations suggests intact fetal sympathetic activity and is therefore a major component in the evaluation of antenatal cardiotocography or non-stress tests (Fischer 1976, Paul & Millar 1978).

Fetal heart rate decelerations

Decelerations of a transient nature are a frequent occurrence. The non-recurring early or mildly variable type, in association with uterine activity or fetal movement, are usually associated with normal fetal outcome (Kidd et al 1985a). Late and recurrent decelerations are of hypoxic origin (Perar et al 1980, Kidd et al 1985a). Decelerations in the presence of loss of baseline variability are also associated with fetal hypoxia (Kubli & Rutgers 1972). Occasional late decelerations without any other abnormal fetal heart rate characteristics, such as loss of variability, are not an indication for intervention (Kidd et al 1985b). Marked decelerations may also result from the maternal supine hypotensive syndrome. Several publications have reported the association of repeated late decelerations and fetal death, particularly in high-risk cases (Visser & Huisjes 1977, Kubli et al 1978, Lenstrup & Falck-Larson 1979, Solum & Sjoberg 1980). Recurrent late decelerations, particularly in association with loss of heart rate variability, are a sign of a poor prognosis (Visser et al 1980).

Based on the physiology and pathophysiology of fetal heart rate, the following criteria could be used in the diagnosis of fetal hypoxia in the antepartum period.

Normal and abnormal antepartum fetal heart rate

A normal trace is one with a baseline of 120–160 beats/min with a variability of 5–25 beats/min, with at least two accelerations of an amplitude of 10–15 beats/min over a 15–20-minute interval. There should be no decelerations, except for an occasional sporadic mild variety. An abnormal fetal heart rate pattern is characterized by a marked baseline tachycardia (over 180 beats/min) or bradycardia (less than 100 beats/min). Furthermore, loss of variability and recurrent late or atypical decelerations are associated with fetal compromise; these are the most important features in the prognostic value of the test.

Performing non-stress cardiotocography

The pregnant woman should be comfortable either in a left lateral position or semirecumbent to avoid supine hypotension. The maternal blood pressure and pulse rate should be recorded prior to performing the test. An external ultrasound transducer for the recording of fetal heart rate and tocodynamometer for recording of uterine activity are attached to the maternal abdomen. The ultra-sound transducer is located to obtain the best fetal heart signal. The tocodynamometer is usually placed on the fundus of the uterus.

The recording is carried out over a period of 30 minutes. External stimulus by palpation or gentle movement of the fetus is performed if the non-stress test remains non-reactive (absence of fetal heart rate accelerations) after 20 minutes. Alternatively, other stimulatory tests such as an acoustic test as described by Luz (1979) are sufficient to wake the fetus. Maternal blood pressure and pulse are recorded at the end of a 30-minute period.

For clinical purposes the antenatal fetal heart rate patterns can be divided into:

1. normal
2. showing transient abnormality
3. suspicious
4. abnormal, requiring intervention.

The tracing is regarded as normal when the baseline is within normal range, has normal variability and when accelerations are present with fetal activity or uterine contractions (Fig. 14.1). Shallow spiked occasional decelerations are not an ominous sign.

A transient reduction in variability and lack of accelerations may be related to fetal sleep states or medication (Fig. 14.2). A fall in maternal blood pressure may also

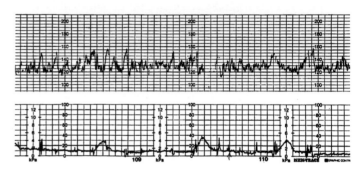

Fig. 14.1 Normal non-stress test showing fetal movement and uterine activity, normal fetal heart rate with normal long-term variability and accelerations.

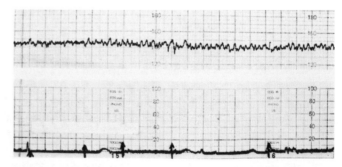

Fig. 14.2 Antenatal non-stressed fetal heart rate recording showing reduced long-term variability with no accelerations. Arrows are event markers during fetal movements. Tracing is an effect of sedative drugs.

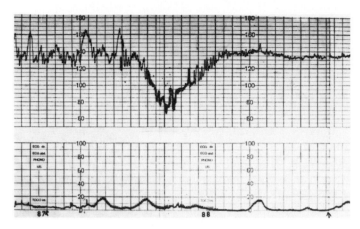

Fig. 14.3 Isolated marked late deceleration of fetal heart rate which had previously followed a normal reactive pattern. Tracing is of suspicious but doubtful significance and should be repeated.

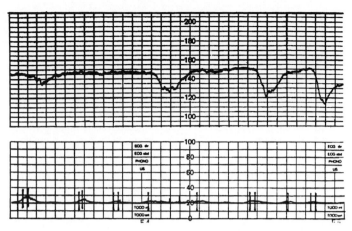

Fig. 14.5 Antenatal heart rate tracing showing loss of variability with recurrent decelerations following fetal movements. Tracing suggests fetal hypoxic state.

be the cause. Tests of fetal stimulation should be carried out in these situations.

Suspicious tests are associated with reduced fetal activity and reactivity. There may be reduced variability and accelerations may be absent. Sporadically occurring non-repeating late decelerations may occur in the presence of fetal activity and reactivity (Fig. 14.3). Similarly, mild repeated decelerations in the presence of accelerations are suspicious signs and require the test to be repeated. Minor deviations of baseline fetal heart rate and sinusoidal patterns require further evaluation.

Fetal heart rate tracings showing a marked reduction in variability and an absence of accelerations with isolated or recurrent decelerations should be regarded as abnormal (Figs 14.4, 14.5).

The need for a uniform method of interpretation of antenatal cardiotocography trace is obvious. It will make the test more comparable and the task of teaching staff in training easier. Various attempts have been made in the form of devising scoring systems. Kubli & Ruttgers (1972) described the first of these. Others followed and all are

based on the changes in the fetal heart rate as described by Schifferle & Caldeyro-Barcia (1973) and others. Each system has tried to modify or add to the original systems (Hammacher et al 1974, Fischer et al 1976, Krebs & Peters 1978, Pearson & Weaver 1978, Lyons et al 1979, Breart et al 1981). Some of these scoring systems did not include accelerations; the quantitative methods which include accelerations and decelerations have a better prognostic index in diagnosing fetal compromise (Garoff et al 1978, Wilken et al 1980).

The two most commonly used scoring systems in Europe are those devised by Fischer et al (1976) and Meyer-Menk et al (1976). They are similar and are based on a 10-point scoring system (Table 14.1). The simplified system by Pearson & Weaver (1978) does not take into account the variability of the fetal heart rate and is based on a 6-point scoring system. Trimbos & Keirse (1978) showed that the assessment of cardiotocographs using scoring systems improved the interobserver and intra-observer reliability compared to subjective assessment. Keirse & Trimbose (1980) found that using the Meyer-Menk scoring system there were no false-positives, in contrast to other systems in which the false-positive rate could be as high as 20%. Adis et al (1978) showed a strong correlation between cardiotocograph scores and umbilical artery pH (Fig. 14.6). However, when Flynn et al (1982) compared the Meyer-Menk/Fischer, the Cardiff and the Birmingham scoring systems with a subjective assessment of the cardiotocographs as either reactive or non-reactive, they found the subjective categorization to be superior to the scoring systems at predicting a range of measures of poor outcome.

Some of the American scoring systems have tried to simplify the interpretation further by only looking at acceleration patterns (Paul & Millar 1978, Schifrin et al 1979, Mandenhall et al 1980). As periods of non-reactive

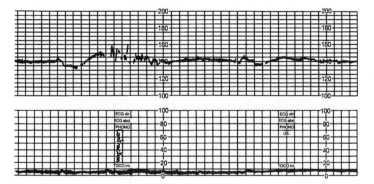

Fig. 14.4 Fetal heart rate with low-amplitude decelerations, complete loss of variability and no fetal reactivity. No fetal movements are marked. Tracing suggestive of severely abnormal state.

Table 14.1   Scoring system for interpretation of antenatal cardiotocography trace

Parameter	Score		
	0	1	2
Baseline level (beats/min)	$< 100, > 180$	$\geq 100, < 120; > 160; \leq 180$	$\geq 120, \leq 160$
Amplitude of fluctuation (4 beats/min)	≤ 5, sinusoidal	$> 5, \leq 10 \; (\geq 25)$	$> 10, < 25$
Frequency of fluctuation (cpm)	< 2, sinusoidal	$\geq 2, \leq 4$	> 4
Deceleration pattern with uterine contractions	Late deceleration pattern frequency $\geq 25\%$, marked variable pattern, severe supine syndrome	Late deceleration pattern frequency $< 25\%$, moderate or mild variable deceleration pattern, early deceleration pattern	Lack of deceleration, single mild variable, deceleration, dip 0
Acceleration with arousal test or fetal movements	Absolute lack of acceleration (negative response)	Atypical shape, no spontaneous acceleration	Acceleration with fetal movements (positive response)

A total of 10 points is optimal; 0 is the worst result: 8–10 points, normal; 5–7 points, prepathological or suspicious record; 0–4 points, pathological. From Meyer-Menk et al (1976).

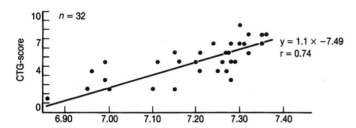

Fig. 14.6   Correlation between the cardiotocograph (CTG) score of the last antepartum record and the umbilical artery pH in 32 high-risk pregnancies with prelabour Caesarean section. From Adis et al (1978).

tracings in relation to fetal sleep–wake periods are common, further evaluation of tracings without accelerations becomes necessary.

Computer analysis of fetal heart rate recordings

The correct interpretation of the CTG is essential if clinical decision making is to be influenced appropriately. Poor intraobserver and interobserver reliability have been demonstrated when the individual components of tracings were assessed visually (Trimbos & Keirse 1978), although reliability was improved if observers were asked to classify recordings as either reactive or unreactive (Flynn et al 1982).

Computer analysis attempts to provide an objective and reproducible numerical evaluation of the fetal heart rate (FHR) recording. Attempts at computerized analysis were initially hampered by high signal loss resulting in failure times averaging 40% (Dawes et al 1981). However, by employing the technique of autocorrelation and with interactive advice to the operator, signal loss is dramatically reduced with resulting improvement in record keeping and saving of time (Dawes et al 1985, 1992).

Dawes et al (1981, 1982) have described a system of on-line microprocessor numerical analysis of the fetal pulse intervals which has been assessed in clinical practice. Cheng et al (1992) found close correlation between computer assessment and visual assessment of 100 CTG tracings performed antenatally although there were several episodes of computer misclassification of tracings as false-positive, but no false-negatives. By analysing umbilical cord blood following prelabour Caesarean section, Smith et al (1988) demonstrated that the reduced variation of suboptimal and decelerative traces was associated with fetal hypoxia and possible nutritional deprivation.

Recently, computerized FHR variation has been employed as a non-invasive test to evaluate the degree of fetal anaemia caused by rhesus alloimmunization (Economides et al 1992). A close correlation between fetal haematocrit and FHR variability exists and these initial findings warrant further investigation.

Clinical application

According to the Scottish stillbirth and neonatal death report (Cole 1985), 275 normally formed infants died before labour started; the majority of them weighed less than 2500 g. In an attempt to prevent these deaths, obstetricians have always looked for a reliable, quick test to identify fetuses who are at risk. Antepartum fetal heart rate monitoring has become widely accepted over the last few years, but the stillbirth rate still remains too high. The overall incidence of antepartum death is approximately 5 per 1000 singleton livebirths (Scottish Stillbirth and Neonatal Mortality Survey). In an unselected population the risk of antenatal fetal death rate is 1 in 1000 within 1 week of a normal cardiotocograph (Kubli et al 1978, Schifrin et al 1979).

The incidence of normal and pathological cardiotocographs in low- and high-risk obstetric populations varies, as shown in Table 14.2. In the management of 250 pregnancies with intrauterine growth retardation, Varma (1984) found that non-reactive cardiotocographs were significantly associated with adverse intrapartum factors and neonatal outcome. Similar findings have been reported by Lenstrup & Hasse (1985) in 454 high-risk pregnancies.

Table 14.2 Incidence of normal and pathological cardiotocography in low- and high-risk pregnancies

Cardiotocograph	Low risk ($n = 411$)	High risk ($n = 401$)
Normal	384 (93.5%)	311 (77.6%)
Suspect	22 (5.4%)	29 (7.2%)
Pathological	5 (1.1%)	61 (15.2%)

From Solum (1980).

Several other reports of a randomized trial in high-risk pregnancies do not support these findings (Brown et al 1982, Flynn et al 1982, Lumley et al 1983, Kidd et al 1985b). Most of these series however were not reporting on frequent fetal heart testing in high-risk pregnancies. In most cases the results were related to one or two isolated cardiotocographs prior to delivery or death of the fetus. Kubli would have quite rightly argued that the concept of antenatal fetal heart testing demands frequent testing, particularly in the compromised fetus, since the fetal heart rate changes occur in a progressive fashion with an increasing duration of low fetal activity periods (Halbertstadt 1981). However, in situations of acute hypoxia, fetal death may occur shortly after a normal reactive tracing is obtained. Freeman (1981) has shown that with frequent proper antenatal monitoring, the rate of fetal death can be reduced to 3.2/1000 in high-risk pregnancies. In terms of adverse intrapartum neonatal events the false negative rate varies from 2% to 20% (Rochard et al 1976, Keirse & Trimbose 1980, Weingold et al 1980). A normal tracing is therefore not reassuring in all cases but a pathological tracing relates closely to poor fetal outcome (Solum 1980). When an abnormal tracing is obtained in the very premature fetus, the consequences of intervening may be disasterous if the fetus is not acidotic (false-positive CTG) and additional methods of assessment should be employed such as Doppler or a biophysical profile.

As the natural course of chronic fetal hypoxia is slow, antenatal fetal heart rate monitoring if carried out once per week in low-risk pregnancies may be sufficient. However in high-risk cases, with placental insufficiency or maternal disease such as hypertension or diabetes, testing will need to be more frequent, even daily. The mode of delivery will be influenced by the severity of the abnormality and other clinical features. With completely unreactive tracings and late decelerations, the incidence of subsequent brain damage is near to 10%, particularly so in small-for-dates and preterm infants (Visser et al 1980).

Antenatal stress tests

Oxytocin challenge tests

The contraction stress test (CST) or oxytocin challenge test was developed by Kubli et al (1968) and remains more popular in the USA than Europe. The test is performed in the same manner as the non-stress test with the addition of an infusion of oxytocin if spontaneous uterine activity is not recorded after 20 minutes of testing. The infusion aims to provoke three uterine contractions within 10 minutes. A vast literature has accumulated concerning the CST (Freeman 1975, Schifrin et al 1975, Huddleston et al 1979, Staisch et al 1980, Lin et al 1981, Devoe 1984) in the management of high-risk pregnancies. The incidence of false-positive tests is between 5% and 10% with a similar range of hyperstimulation.

The correlation of a positive test with intrapartum events is poor (Paul & Millar 1978) and the test is invasive and time consuming. It has been recommended as a second-line test following equivocal non-stress cardiotocography (Keegan & Paul 1980).

Nipple stimulation tests

Nipple stimulation during human lactation insitutes a neurohypophyseal reflex resulting in the release of oxytocin (Cobo 1974). Stimulation of the nipples in late pregnancy produces a uterine contraction and this forms the basis of the nipple CST which is potentially cheaper, less invasive and less time consuming than the oxytocin CST. The technique has been evaluated and found to have a hyperstimulation rate around 4%, a failure rate of 4–15% and poor correlation with intrapartum events and neonatal outcome (Huddleston et al 1984, Lanke & Nemes 1984, Chayen et al 1985, Copel et al 1985). Curtis et al (1989) compared different methods of stimulation and found that using a breast pump or manual stimulation for up to 30 minutes was most effective in reducing the incidence of exaggerated contractions whilst optimizing the success rate.

Other tests

Vibroacoustic stimulation is a technique whereby an artificial larynx is applied over the uterus and an auditory stimulus created in order to provoke fetal heart rate accelerations when the tracing is initially non-reactive (Reid & Millar 1977). The test is considered negative if a fetal heart rate acceleration of 15 beats/min or more is evoked. The test cannot be reliably applied to the very immature fetus since there is no consistent response before 30–31 weeks' gestation (Zimmer & Divon 1993). A positive vibroacoustic test has been found to be highly sensitive in predicting a subsequent abnormal oxytocin CST and possessing similar positive predictive value for the development of intrapartum fetal distress as the oxytocin CST (Schiff et al 1992).

The fetal recoil test relies upon generating a fetal startle response following sound stimulation. A test is considered negative and re-assuring when a palpable fetal response occurs. In a series of 100 consecutive NST, a reassuring recoil test had a 98% positive predictive value for a subsequent reactive NST (Strong et al 1992). In a larger study of high-risk patients, Nyman et al (1992) found a sensitivity of 81% compared to a reactive NST and they suggest the test may have a place in the preliminary screening of at-risk pregnancies where resources are limited.

The light stimulation test is similarly designed to provoke a fetal response and involves exposing the fetus to a cold light source via an amnioscope (Peleg & Goldman 1980). The procedure is invasive and likely to be unacceptable to many.

Other developments include the introduction of a digital system for distant heart rate recording and subsequent rapid transmission by telephone to the hospital which overcomes any difficulties experienced by the patient in having to attend the clinic (Gough et al 1986). The complete recording of fetal heart rate carried out by the mother at home is transmitted to hospital in less than 30 seconds and stored on computer for later analysis. Preliminary reports are promising and the tracings obtained appear to be satisfactory (Fig. 14.7). The introduction of such a system can result in a reduction in hospital admissions and improved patient satisfaction (Moore & Sill 1990).

DOPPLER ULTRASOUND

Introduction

Investigation of the fetal cardiovascular and haemodynamic system has become a clinical reality with the advent of advanced ultrasound technology enabling precise evaluation of patterns of blood flow within the uterine, placental and even fetal circulations. Since the first report of the application of the Doppler principle to

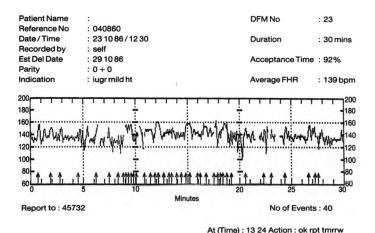

Fig. 14.7 Antenatal fetal heart rate tracing obtained using Huntley technology. Distant fetal monitor with home monitoring equipment. Compressed signal transmitted via telephone line.

the human fetal circulation (Fitzgerald & Drumm 1977), a large experience with this technique has been reported with respect to the prediction of the fetus at risk of developing growth retardation, antepartum and intrapartum asphyxia, perinatal mortality and neonatal morbidity. Many of the earlier studies employed relatively simple equipment in order to obtain and process signals from the umbilical circulation, whereas study of most of the fetal vessels requires expensive equipment and a degree of operator expertise.

Principles

Sound waves returning from a moving object (e.g. a column of erythrocytes) will have an altered frequency with respect to the incident beam and this difference or frequency shift is dependent upon the direction and velocity of the moving object. This phenomenon was first described by Johann Christian Doppler, an Austrian physicist after whom the Doppler effect is named (White 1982). The shifted frequencies obtained are not only directly proportional to the velocity of the moving blood cells but also proportional to the cosine of the angle of insonation (the angle between the ultrasound beam and the column of blood).

In order to calculate the amount of blood flowing in a vessel, accurate estimation of the angle of insonation and the diameter of the vessel must be possible. Significant errors in estimating these parameters together with errors in estimating fetal weight mean that the measurement of actual blood flow is not useful in clinical practice (Erskine & Ritchie 1985a). Alternatively, semiquantitative assessment of the flow velocity waveform (FVW) can be made and this has been widely adopted. The waveform obtained is the result of several different factors including fetal cardiac contraction force, density of blood, vessel wall elasticity and peripheral or downstream resistance (McDonald 1974). The fetal and umbilical circulations are typified by low resistance flow patterns demonstrating continuous forward flow where the velocity in diastole is inversely related to peripheral impedance (Olson & Cooke 1975; Fig. 14.8).

Although both systolic and diastolic frequencies are dependent upon the angle of insonation, ratios comparing the pulsatile or systolic element of the waveform to the continuous or diastolic element are independent of the angle, making this a useful index of changes in peripheral resistance (Stuart et al 1980). Alternatives to the S/D or A/B ratios include the Pulsatility Index and the Resistance Index (or Pourcelot Index) (Fig. 14.9). As the end-diastolic velocities decrease, all the indices rise and the changes in the values obtained correlate closely between the different indices (Thompson et al 1986). Theoretically, the Pulsatility Index is preferred since it can still quantify the FVW in the absence of diastolic flow, although in practice

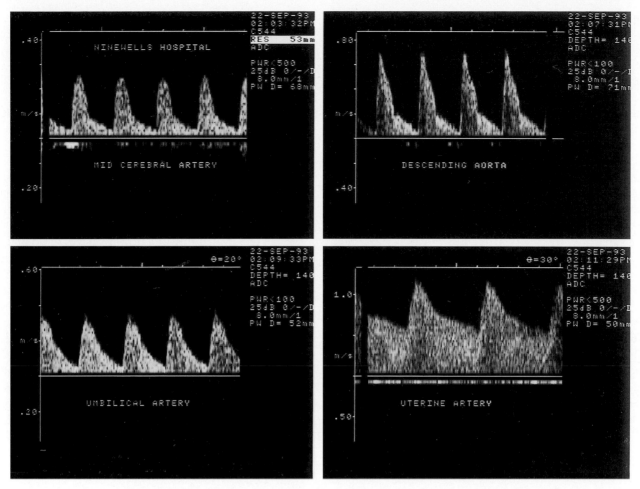

Fig. 14.8 Flow velocity waveforms obtained from the umbilical, fetal aortic and middle cerebral arteries and maternal uterine artery at 19 weeks' gestation. Courtesy of Dr A.D. Christie, Dundee. (Also reproduced in colour as plate 1, pp xvi.)

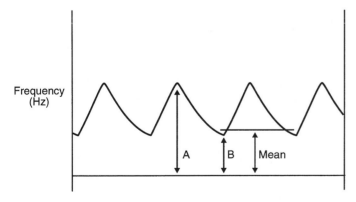

Fig. 14.9 Characteristics of the umbilical artery flow velocity waveform. A = Peak systolic frequency, B = end diastolic frequency. Pulsatility index = (A–B)/Mean; Resistance Index = (A–B)/A. From Mires et al (1990).

A/B ratios are commonly used whilst waveforms with absent end-diastolic flow (AEDF) are classified separately.

A variety of Doppler ultrasound methods exist, with three types being employed in clinical practice: continuous wave (CW), pulsed wave (PW) and colour flow mapping (CFM).

Continuous wave Doppler emits and receives an ultrasound beam continuously, has a low acoustic energy output and is relatively inexpensive. However, obtaining a FVW with CW Doppler is a blind technique and it cannot discriminate between signals from different locations which may result in mixed waveforms. Despite this, CW equipment has been widely employed in the study of the umbilical circulation where it produces results similar to those obtained by PW equipment (Brar et al 1989).

Pulsed wave Doppler differs in that pulses of ultrasound energy are emitted. By varying the time interval of the pulses it becomes possible to determine the distance of the signal origin from the transducer by range-gating. Combining PW Doppler with real-time ultrasound provides a Duplex system, with the obvious advantage that the vessel to be examined is positively identified before it is sampled.

Colour flow mapping is a further refinement of the Duplex system whereby two-dimensional flow images are superimposed on the real-time image. Special signal processing techniques permit colour coding of the direction of the flow with different degrees of shading according to the magnitude of the Doppler shift. Although the equipment necessary for CFM is expensive, it permits more precision in vessel location and identification including the fetal cerebral and renal circulations (Veille & Kanaan 1989).

Umbilical flow velocity waveform

The umbilical arteries were the first fetal vessels to be studied with Doppler ultrasound , the signals being readily obtained with CW Doppler (Fitzgerald & Drumm 1977). Subsequently, FVW from these vessels have been widely investigated in the hope that they would provide an appropriate test of fetal well-being in the complicated pregnancy and also as a screening test for the development of problems in the low-risk population. The ease with which signals can be obtained is reflected by good reproducibility in the measurement of the waveforms (Schulman et al 1984). FVW should be obtained with the mother lying at rest in a semirecumbent position during periods of fetal apnoea and quiescence since the impedance indices are modified by fetal breathing (Kopelaar & Wladimiroff 1992) and elevated fetal heart rates (Mires et al 1987).

Relationship of the flow velocity waveform to placental pathology

The umbilical artery FVW is characterized by continuous forward flow typical of a low resistance circuit, with a gradual fall in the resistance indices as gestation increases due to enlargement of the placenta with a corresponding expansion of its vascular tree (Stuart et al 1980). A reduction in end-diastolic velocity suggests increased resistance to blood flow originating in the placenta and this pattern is seen in pregnancies complicated by growth retardation and fetal compromise (Fleischer et al 1985, Erskine & Ritchie 1985b, Trudinger et al 1985).

Vascular abnormalities are known to be present in the placenta of the growth-retarded fetus (Sheppard & Bonnar 1976) and histological examination of placentas from pregnancies with abnormal FVW has revealed obliteration of tertiary stem villus arteries and deficient functional differentiation (Giles et al 1985, Hitschold et al 1993). It is possible to demonstrate a strong correlation between the percentage of obliterated placental vessels and the resistance to umbilical artery flow, providing an anatomical basis for the observed FVW changes seen in many complicated pregnancies (Fok et al 1990).

Placental pathology such as this would be expected to give rise to an abnormal fetal acid–base status through hypoxia. A relationship between very high impedance ratios and umbilical venous hypoxia and acidosis has been demonstrated by obtaining fetal blood at cordocentesis and at prelabour Caesarean section (Tyrrell et al 1989, Weiner 1990).

Clinical application of umbilical artery Doppler

Prediction of the small-for-gestational-age pregnancy

The detection of the small-for-gestational-age (SGA) and growth-retarded fetus remains one of the central goals in antenatal care, since it is well recognized that low birthweight is a risk factor for perinatal mortality and neurodevelopmental handicap (McIllwaine 1979, Taylor 1984). The availability of a non-invasive, rapid and reproducible test that identifies a placental vascular lesion led to the hope that umbilical FVW analysis would reliably identify the SGA baby which had been suggested by early Doppler studies (Erskine & Ritchie 1985b, Fleischer et al 1985, Trudinger et al 1985).

Many studies have subsequently confirmed the relationship between abnormal FVW and delivery of an SGA baby with sensitivities as high as 78% (Rochelson et al 1987a, Gaziano et al 1988, Schulman et al 1989) in preselected high-risk populations. However, such promising results have not been found by all studies with disappointing results found by many (Mulders et al 1987, van Vugt et al 1988, Chambers et al 1989, Hata et al 1989). Dempster et al (1989) found abnormal FVW ratios in only 41% of all SGA babies, concluding that whereas umbilical artery FVW analysis may be useful in identifying a group of SGA fetuses, it is insufficiently sensitive to be of value in identifying the individual small fetus.

When comparing Doppler with established ultrasound biometry, several studies have found estimated fetal weight and abdominal circumference measurements to be superior in correctly predicting the SGA fetus (Divon et al 1988, Chambers et al 1989, Miller & Gabert 1992), although the addition of Doppler to standard ultrasound biometry has been found to further improve diagnostic accuracy by increasing the specificity of the test (Berkowitz et al 1988a).

With the recognition that umbilical artery FVW analysis is of limited value in detecting the SGA pregnancy in high-risk populations, it is not surprising that it performs poorly as a screening test in low-risk populations where the prevalence of SGA and growth-retarded pregnancies is even lower. Beattie & Dornan (1989) employed a three-stage programme of examination at 28, 34 and 38 weeks in 2097 singleton pregnancies and found that abnormal impedance indices failed to adequately predict measures of poor fetal nutrition, hypoxia and the necessity for operative or instrumental intervention due to fetal distress. Umbilical FVW analysis lacks the necessary sensitivity to be an appropriate primary screening test for fetal smallness and poor perinatal outcome in the low-risk obstetric population (Bruinse et al 1989, Newnham et al 1990).

Prediction of the pregnancy compromised by hypoxia and acidosis

The performance of Doppler in predicting the SGA baby is disappointing , and it is in fact being used inappropriately for this purpose.

It is becoming increasingly appreciated that being SGA is not synonymous with being growth retarded and does not necessarily imply that there is an underlying pathology. By taking an arbitrary cut-off point of birthweight for gestational age (usually the tenth percentile), then many small, but normally grown babies are included amongst those who are of low birthweight as a consequence of inadequate placental nutrient and oxygen transfer. It is largely because of the heterogeneous nature of SGA babies that umbilical FVW analysis has proved to be disappointing in the identification of individual SGA pregnancies. This is one of the reasons behind the apparently conflicting results of different studies, since the criteria for inclusion in a study will significantly influence the predictive values obtained (Mires et al 1990).

It would be expected that Doppler studies would more readily detect pregnancies compromised by an impaired fetoplacental circulation and whilst there is an association between abnormal impedance indices and birthweight, the true association probably lies between impedance and compromise due to asphyxia, with birthweight being an intervening variable (Haddad et al 1988).

It is well recognized that pregnancies with abnormal FVW are at increased risk of several aspects of perinatal morbidity, including increased rates of preterm delivery, abnormal FHR in labour, operative delivery and admission to and duration of stay in neonatal units (Trudinger et al 1985, 1991, Berkowitz et al 1988b, Dempster et al 1989). In a blind prospective study of apparently growth retarded fetuses, Reuwer et al (1987) found that abnormal FVW reliably identified the distressed fetus, with the appearance of abnormal FVW preceding FHR abnormalities by at least 9 days. A similar relationship between abnormal FVW and antepartum late FHR decelerations was found by Bekedam et al (1990) when FVW abnormalities appeared before the decelerations in 27 of 29 intrauterine growth-retarded fetuses with a median duration of the interval being 17 days with a wide range of 0–60 days.

Umbilical artery FVW analysis appears to be a more sensitive predictor of fetal compromise than antepartum cardiotocography when compromise is taken to be a 5-minute Apgar score < 5 and/or birthweight < 10th percentile for gestation (Trudinger et al 1986). By comparing FVW analysis with the antepartum CTG in SGA fetuses, Almstrom et al (1992) found that the Doppler group experienced significantly fewer hospital admissions, inductions of labour and emergency Caesarean sections for fetal distress, although there were no differences in gestational age at delivery or Apgar scores.

Similar reductions in the rates of fetal distress in labour and emergency Caesarean section were found in a randomized controlled trial of FVW analysis by Trudinger et al (1987), leading them to conclude that the availability of Doppler results in more appropriate obstetrical decision making. Indeed, it has been suggested that cardiotocography may be unnecessary for monitoring the high-risk pregnancy when the FVW is normal (Jensen & Guimaraes 1991). The routine, rather than selective use of Doppler in high-risk pregnancies does not result in an iatrogenic increase in preterm delivery and does in fact reduce the frequency of depressed Apgar scores at birth and of serious neonatal morbidity (Tyrrell et al 1990).

Whereas an abnormal FVW appears to identify the SGA fetus at risk of perinatal hypoxia, for Doppler to be an appropriate test of fetal well-being, the finding of a normal FVW should be re-assuring by identifying the constitutionally small fetus not affected by placental pathology. Burke et al (1990) examined 179 ultrasonically diagnosed SGA pregnancies and found that of the 119 physically normal fetuses with normal flow, there was only one unfavourable outcome. Certainly, the presence of a normal Doppler study places the SGA fetus in a much lower risk category than those with an abnormal FVW (Rochelson et al 1987a). Whereas a normal Doppler result can be taken to be a re-assuring sign when monitoring the SGA fetus, it must be considered along with the other individual features of the pregnancy in order to optimize the outcome since a normal Doppler result does not exclude subsequent intrapartum fetal distress in all cases (Dempster et al 1988).

Extreme abnormalities of the flow velocity waveform

Extreme elevation of resistance to flow results in a FVW with no end-diastolic component or even reversal of flow in the umbilical artery. The frequency of absence of end-diastolic flow is low, between 3% and 7% in high-risk groups (Rochelson et al 1987a,b, Tyrrell et al 1990). Although they form only a small number, these pregnancies have a high incidence of hypoxia and acidosis in utero (Weiner 1990). In a series of 59 fetuses with umbilical absence of end-diastolic flow referred for assessment of severe growth retardation, cordocentesis revealed 25 to be hypoxic, five acidotic and 22 both acidotic and hypoxic with only seven fetuses with normal acid–base status (Nicolaides et al 1988). Unfortunately, knowledge of the acid–base status in utero does not discriminate between those fetuses who will die and those that will survive since values of pH, P_{O_2}, P_{CO_2} and base equivalents are similar in both survivors and non-survivors (Nicolini et al 1990).

Not surprisingly, fetuses with absence of end-diastolic flow have a poorer outcome than those with elevated ratios alone. Growth retardation and chronic hypoxia are almost invariably present, resulting in high rates of perinatal mortality (Rochelson et al 1987b, Brar & Platt 1988). Battaglia et al (1993) found a 60% perinatal mortality rate among 26 growth-retarded fetuses with absence of end-diastolic flow or reversed flow, highlighting the ominous nature of this class of FVW. This is further reflected in delivery being almost exclusively by Caesarean section for fetal distress and a significantly higher rate of abnormal neurological signs in the neonatal period compared with a group matched for gestational age with normal FVW (Weiss et al 1992).

The management of such cases must be individualized to take into account other obstetric features, particularly gestation and the confidence with which congenital and karyotypic abnormalities can be excluded. Absence of end-diastolic flow is not only seen in pregnancies complicated by maternal hypertension and abnormal placental function, but also in some pregnancies with lethal malformations and chromosomal disorders (Wenstrom et al 1991). Careful consideration should be given to detailed anatomical screening and obtaining a fetal karyotype before considering operative delivery in cases of absence of end-diastolic flow where maternal disease is not evident.

It is possible for end-diastolic velocities to re-appear with subsequent improvement in perinatal outcome, implying a possible future therapeutic avenue to reduce the hypothesized reversible spasm in the vessels of the placental villi (Brar & Platt 1989). In a preliminary study, Karsdorp et al (1992) were able to demonstrate a temporary return of end-diastolic flow in women undergoing circulatory volume expansion. In this preliminary study, neonatal outcome was improved by expansion and these results need to be evaluated by a larger randomized study.

Diabetic pregnancy

Diabetic pregnancies will continue to present management problems to the obstetrician as long as unexpected, third-trimester intrauterine fetal deaths are reported. Initial optimism concerning the usefulness of Doppler as an appropriate test of well-being in diabetic pregnancies has been tempered by more recent findings.

Bracero et al (1986) found a significant positive correlation between the FVW and maternal serum glucose and elevated resistance indices with increased number of stillbirths and neonatal morbidity. However, recent studies have found the A/B ratios of diabetic pregnancies to be independent of glycosylated haemoglobin concentration or mean glucose levels (Landon et al 1989, Johnstone et al 1992).

Whereas an abnormal FVW remains a predictor of antenatal compromise, the demonstration of a normal FVW does not exclude the possibility of fetal compromise and unexpected death in the diabetic pregnancy (Bradley et al 1988, Tyrrell 1988, Johnstone et al 1992). The explanation lies in the fact that fetal compromise is multifactorial in these pregnancies where a metabolic component may play a greater role in causing eventual fetal demise than borderline impairment of placental perfusion which may not be currently detectable.

Doppler studies of the fetal aorta

Flow velocity waveforms from the descending aorta in late pregnancy were first described by Eik-Nes et al (1980). In normal pregnancy the blood flow velocity profile remains above zero throughout the cardiac cycle with the presence of a notch in the waveform which coincides with closure of the aortic valve (Griffin et al 1984). There appears to be a small increase in end-diastolic velocities with advancing gestation, although this has not been found in all studies (Tonge et al 1983).

There is clearly an association between fetal growth retardation and an abnormal aortic FVW (Griffin et al 1984, Tonge et al 1986). The absence of end-diastolic flow has been found to precede abnormalities of the FHR in pregnancies complicated by hypertension, suggesting that aortic FVW analysis might have a role in fetal assessment (Jouppila & Kirkinen 1984).

Laurin et al (1987) examined the ability of a semiquantitative description of the aortic FVW, blood flow class, to predict fetal outcome in a group of 159 pregnancies suspected of growth retardation and found blood flow class to be superior to the pulsatility index and measurements of volume flow. A blood flow class indicating absence or reversal of diastolic flow was highly predictive of birthweight > 2 standard deviations below the gestation mean and a sensitive indicator of the need for operative delivery due to fetal distress.

Nevertheless, the aortic FVW may not be any better at predicting growth retardation and neonatal outcome than the umbilical FVW (Groenenberg et al 1991, Gudmundsson & Marsal 1991).

A close association between aortic mean velocity and abnormal acid–base status in utero exists in the growth-retarded fetus, implying that hypoxia results in peripheral vasoconstriction (Soothill et al 1986). Such a peripheral vasoconstriction, with associated reduction in visceral perfusion, partly explains the increased rate of necrotizing enterocolitis (NEC) experienced by growth-retarded fetuses with aortic absence of end-diastolic flow when compared to those with diastolic flow (Hackett et al 1987), since reduced blood flow in the superior mesenteric artery is believed to be a risk factor for NEC (Kempley et al 1991).

In addition to NEC, aortic absence of end-diastolic

flow is associated with a significantly greater risk of haemorrhage (pulmonary, gastrointestinal or intraventricular) and perinatal death, with only 15% of pregnancies experiencing an uncomplicated neonatal course (Hackett et al 1987). It is not surprising therefore that abnormal aortic FVW are associated with neurodevelopmental impairment in childhood (Marsal & Ley 1992).

Doppler studies of the fetal carotid and intracranial arteries

The advent of colour flow mapping has enabled the study of FVW in the vessels of the head and neck of the human fetus. The FVW of the carotid and cerebral arteries always displays forward flow in normal pregnancy with a small reduction in the impedance indices as gestation advances so that the brain is supplied by a low resistance vascular bed with increased perfusion towards term (Wladimiroff et al 1986). Caution must be exercised during cranial Doppler examination not to apply too much pressure over the fetal skull since raising the intracranial pressure in this way can alter the FVW (Vyas et al 1990a).

Studies of asphyxiated primate and lamb fetuses have demonstrated a redistribution of cardiac ouput, favouring the cardiac and cerebral circulations at the expense of the abdominal viscera and carcass (Behrman et al 1970, Cohn et al 1974). This brain-sparing effect is believed to exist in asymmetrical growth retardation where the infant's head size appears to be disproportionately large in relation to its wasted trunk. Such a pattern of growth retardation may be evident in infants with apparently normal birthweights for gestation and is associated with increased perinatal morbidity (Wilcox 1983, Patterson & Pouliot 1987).

A similar brain-sparing effect can be demonstrated in the human fetus whereby a reduction in the impedance indices of the carotid and cranial vessels is seen in growth retardation frequently associated with elevated impedance in the thoracic aorta and umbilical artery (Wladimiroff et al 1987, Lingman & Marsal 1989). By obtaining blood at cordocentesis in SGA fetuses, Vyas et al (1990b) examined the relationship between middle cerebral artery (MCA) FVW and acid–base status, demonstrating a positive relationship between the degree of hypoxia and reduction in FVW impedance. An abnormal MCA waveform identifies the SGA fetus at increased risk of an abnormal outcome (Echizenya et al 1989, Mari & Deter 1992). However, the MCA may not be suitable for serial monitoring since it reaches maximum dilatation with mild hypoxia only (Vyas et al 1990b, Arduini et al 1992).

Although cerebral FVW changes frequently precede FHR abnormalities (Kirkinen et al 1987, Satoh et al 1989), the interval may be as long as 2 weeks (Arduini et al 1992). The vasodilatory response of the cerebral circulation to hypoxia is not only a predictor of short-term morbidity but also points to an increased risk of neonatal neurological abnormalities (Rizzo et al 1989) which are possibly the result of cerebral ischaemia as reflected by increased carotid artery impedance in the neonatal period (Scherjon et al 1992).

Combining the results of fetal velocity waveform analysis from several fetal vessels

By combining the results of waveform indices from several fetal vessels it is possible to improve the prediction of growth retardation and hypoxia.

Internal carotid artery FVW analysis alone is not helpful in predicting growth retardation and is inferior to the umbilical artey FVW in this respect (Wladimiroff et al 1988) but the ratio between the pulsatility indices of the umbilical artery and internal carotid artery has a positive predictive value of over 80% for growth retardation (Arduini et al 1987). Similar improvements in the accuracy of predicting the SGA fetus and of adverse perinatal events can be obtained by combining MCA and umbilical artery FVW (Gramellini et al 1992). Bilardo et al (1990) studied the umbilical and fetal circulations in 41 SGA fetuses and correlated the FVW indices and ratios of indices with an asphyxia index derived from acid–base values at the time of cordocentesis. The best combined predictor of asphyxia was the aortic-carotid index, representing a mathematical summation of the aortic mean velocity and common carotid artery pulsatility index. A normal index was always associated with normal acid–base status whereas an abnormal result predicted an asphyxia index 1 standard deviation above the mean in 89% of cases.

FETAL MOVEMENT COUNTING

It is a well-established practice to enquire of mothers antenatally whether they are feeling regular and frequent fetal movements or not since continuing fetal activity is a reassuring, albeit crude, indicator of fetal well-being.

In an attempt to quantify maternally perceived fetal activity and relate it to perinatal performance, Pearson & Weaver (1976) developed the Cardiff Kick Chart whereby mothers recorded the time taken each day to feel ten movements. The results suggested that antepartum fetal demise was preceded by the cessation of fetal activity, giving rise to the hope that this would become a cheap and widely applicable method for the prevention of antepartum stillbirth.

The value of routine formal fetal movement counting has been addressed in two randomized trials to date. Neldam (1983) found that there was a significant reduction in fetal loss in the counting group but this was not found in the much larger multicentre trial of Grant et al (1989). Although not an effective method for assessing fetal well-being in the general obstetric population, the value of fetal movement counting remains to be assessed in pregnancies previously identified as being at risk of late antepartum stillbirth (Neilson 1993a). A further point of view is taken in Chapter 6.

FETAL BIOPHYSICAL PROFILE

Introduction

The biophysical profile (BPP) is a method of ascertaining antenatal fetal well-being by employing real-time ultrasound and cardiotocography. Originally described by Manning et al (1980), the BPP has been widely adopted and evaluated as a clinical tool in the prediction of antenatal fetal demise and perinatal morbidity and mortality.

The clinical basis for employing the BPP arises from the observation that combining several fetal parameters improves the predictive value of an abnormal test above that obtained by employing a single variable (Manning et al 1980, Baskett et al 1984). The original BPP assigned an arbitrary score of 0 or 2 according to the presence or absence of each of five variables (Table 14.3). A total score of 8 or 10 is considered normal, a score of 6 considered equivocal and an indication for repeat assessment, a score of 4 or less deemed abnormal and an indication for delivery according to the clinical circumstances.

Physiology

The physiological basis for using the BPP lies in the fact that coordinated fetal activities such as breathing and movement require an intact and therefore by implication non-hypoxic central nervous system. However, although

Table 14.3 Variables included in the biophysical profile

	Score
Non-stress test	
Reactive; at least 2 FHR accelerations > 15 bpm in a 20-minute period	2
Non-reactive; 1 FHR acceleration or nil	0
Fetal breathing movements	
FBM present; at least one episode of prolonged breathing (> 60 s) within 30-minute period	2
FBM absent; absence of above	0
Gross fetal body movements	
FM present; at least three discrete episodes of fetal movement within a 30-minute period	2
FM absent; < 3 or absence of movements	0
Fetal tone	
Normal; extremities and neck held in flexion. At least one episode of completed limb extension and flexion	2
Abnormal; extremities in extension. Fetal movement not followed by return to flexion	0
Amniotic fluid volume	
Normal; largest pocket of fluid > 1 cm in vertical diameter	2
Decreased; absence of above. Crowding of fetal parts	0
Total score	0–10

Reproduced with permission from Manning et al (1980).

hypoxia and acidosis are certainly responsible for producing abnormal fetal behaviour, other factors may be responsible and awareness of these influences is essential before inappropriate conclusions regarding fetal welfare are made.

The presence of different fetal behavioural states is well recognized (Nijhuis et al 1982) and the influence of this physiological variation should be appreciated when performing the BPP. Pillai & James (1990) found that the time taken to achieve a satisfactory BPP was strongly dependent on whether the fetus was in state 1F (quiet sleep), or states 2F and 4F (active states), with the recommendation that biophysical recording should be extended to at least 40 minutes before the BPP is considered suspicious.

Fetal breathing movements may be absent for up to 120 minutes in the healthy term fetus (Patrick et al 1980) and are influenced by gestation such that the time spent breathing increases from 12% at the start of the third trimester to 50% by the end (Fox et al 1979). Fetal breathing is inhibited by maternal cigarette smoking (Manning & Feyerabend 1976) and stimulated by maternal hyperglycaemia, necessitating the standardization of patient preparation before testing.

The amniotic fluid volume reflects chronic changes in intrauterine oxygenation whereas the other four variables are indicators of a more acute or current state.

Reduced liquor volume in chronic hypoxia is believed to be the result of a redistribution of fetal organ perfusion towards the brain and away from the abdominal viscera including the fetal kidneys. Doppler studies of the renal arteries of growth-retarded fetuses with reduced liquor have shown increased resistance to renal blood flow lending support to the hypothesis that impaired renal perfusion results in reduced fetal urine production and subsequent oligohydramnios (Nicolaides et al 1990, Arduini & Rizzo 1991).

Clinical application

Clinical testing of the BPP began with a prospective study of 216 high-risk patients where the test results were withheld and not allowed to influence clinical decision making (Manning et al 1980). The last result of each test variable prior to delivery was related to markers of fetal hypoxia and perinatal mortality (PNMR), with the result that the PNMR was zero when all variables were normal (score 10) and 600/1000 when all the variables were abnormal (score 0).

Baskett et al (1984) applied the BPP in the management of 2400 high-risk pregnancies and calculated the perinatal morbidity and mortality according to the most recent BPP score (Table 14.4).

False-negative outcomes (i.e. perinatal death within a week of a normal test) are recognized to occur (Watson et al 1991) but are very uncommon, with a normal BPP

Table 14.4 Distribution of BPP test scores and their relationship to perinatal morbidity and mortality in a high-risk population

BPP score	No.	Fetal distress (%)*	Apgar < 7 at 5 min (%)	Birthweight < 3rd centile	Perinatal death (%)
Normal (8–10)	1938 (97.1)	123 (7)	24 (1.2)	103 (5.3)	5 (0.3)
Equivocal (6)	34 (1.7)	7 (23.3)	1 (2.9)	10 (29.4)	2 (5.9)
Abnormal (0–4)	24 (1.2)	12 (66.7)	8 (33.3)	10 (41.7)	7 (29.2)

Reproduced with permission from Baskett et al (1984).
* Calculated for the 1811 fetuses who underwent labour.

being reassurring of fetal health. In a series of 19 221 referred high-risk pregnancies, there were only 14 deaths unrelated to major fetal anomalies, giving a false-negative rate of 0.72/1000 (Manning et al 1987a). However, the positive predictive value of an abnormal test for perinatal death has a high false-positive rate (i.e. abnormal score with normal outcome), resulting in the potential for unnecessary intervention and its associated maternal and neonatal morbidity (Baskett et al 1987).

There does appear to be a progressive evolution of changes in the BPP as intrauterine hypoxia and acidosis worsens. By examining the relationship between the results of BPP performed immediately prior to prelabour Caesarean section and subsequent umbilical artery acid–base values, Vintzileos et al (1991a) found that a non-reactive CTG and the absence of fetal breathing movements were the first manifestations of hypoxia and acidosis. Such a progression of changes whereby fetal movements and tone are the last of the variables to be affected has also been confirmed in growth-retarded fetuses undergoing cordocentesis (Ribbert et al 1990).

The original BPP does not take the composition of the score into account and this has formed the basis of several criticisms of Manning's original test. The arbitrary scoring system whereby each parameter is accorded the same importance means that an apparently abnormal score of 4 can be achieved by a number of combinations. If this is achieved by a reactive CTG and normal liquor volume then the fetus is not showing evidence of acute or chronic hypoxia, rather the low score is due to normal periodicity of fetal activity and intervention is not warranted (Vintzileos et al 1987a).

Modifications to Manning's original biophysical profile

There is inevitably an interdependence of the test variables and whilst most possible combinations can be seen, score composition is important when considering the test's predictive accuracy (Manning et al 1990). This has resulted in several modifications of the original BPP in order to rationalize the use of human and equipment resources without impairing test performance.

Fetal assessment based solely on real-time ultrasonographic examination has been proposed (Shah et al 1989) and Manning et al (1987b) have previously found that the CTG was unnecessary when all the ultrasound parameters were normal, thus reducing the use of the CTG to only 2.7% of 7851 tests. Although this is may be attractive with respect to saving time and patient convenience, the CTG is a long-established tool which is widely accepted and understood by obstetricians and is generally more available than the BPP.

By limiting the number of variables included in a test, the potential for error is reduced, time is saved and interpretation is simplified. Disregarding the presence or absence of fetal movements does not adversely influence the test performance (Devoe et al 1992). Walkinshaw et al (1992) found that a BPP comprising the CTG, amniotic fluid volume and fetal breathing movements performed as well as the full BPP in predicting acidosis at delivery in SGA infants. In fact, reducing the BPP further to include the CTG and ultrasound evaluation of amniotic fluid volume alone, with no additional biophysical assessment unless the CTG is unreactive, may be appropriate for routine clinical practice (Eden et al 1988). This is based on the fact that a reactive CTG reasonably excludes the possibility of fetal acidosis at the time of testing and the absence of FHR decelerations with an adequate liquor volume is reassurring regarding the exclusion of chronic hypoxia and the likelihood of a cord accident (Vintzileos et al 1987b, 1991b).

An extension of this is the creation of a two-tier approach to fetal biophysical assessment whereby the indication for assessment and periodic ultrasound growth are employed to influence the necessity, nature and frequency of fetal testing. By employing such an approach, a reduction in the workload of the CTG by > 60% and BPP by > 75% could be achieved when managing high-risk pregnancies (Mills et al 1990).

The biophysical profile in relation to Doppler ultrasound

In most obstetric units where biophysical profile scoring is being employed, it is unlikely to be utilized in isolation from Doppler studies of the uteroplacental circulation since the facilities for Doppler examination are usually present with modern ultrasonography equipment. The relationship between umbilical artery Doppler indices and the BPP in high-risk pregnancies has been studied. If the umbilical artery FVW is normal then there are no cases with persistently abnormal BPP scores and a persistently abnormal BPP is always associated with absent end-diastolic flow (Tyrrell et al 1990, James et al 1992). The umbilical artery FVW is superior to either the BPP or FHR variation analysis in predicting fetal distress in labour and acidosis at birth in SGA infants (Nordstrom et al 1989, Soothill et al 1993).

CONCLUSION

Antepartum fetal heart rate monitoring remains the most widely accepted diagnostic test for assessment of the fetus at risk of hypoxia. The non-stress test is most commonly employed and the various stress tests, particularly the oxytocin challenge test, whilst still used in certain countries, are rarely used in Europe now.

For monitoring an apparently normal pregnancy the non-stress test has been found to be lacking and is probably not cost effective. In designated high-risk pregnancies, the test is used serially and identifies fetuses at risk of hypoxia having normal outcome in 90% of cases, whilst a pathological test, particularly one where there is loss of variability with decelerations, is associated with fetal compromise in nearly all cases. However, the test needs to be performed frequently in order to identify the changing fetal heart rate pattern associated with hypoxia and interpretation is open to error.

Doppler ultrasound has enabled the obstetric sonographer to gain considerable insight into the understanding of the vascular changes underlying intrauterine hypoxia and growth retardation. Despite this being a relatively new technique, analysis of the umbilical waveform has been extensive. Analysis of waveforms obtained from other fetal vessels has demonstrated the progression of vascular changes occurring in the compromised fetus, but such studies require expensive equipment, highly trained personnel and are time consuming.

Although it is not appropriate to apply umbilical Doppler as a screening tool to an entire antenatal population, it is useful in clinical practice in differentiating constitutionally small fetuses from those at increased risk from placental dysfunction, enabling the obstetrician to make a more rational approach to patient management. Randomized trials of umbilical Doppler have generally demonstrated a reduction in perinatal mortality when the results are made available to the clinicians. This reduction in the incidence of perinatal death after correction for lethal malformation is of the order of 35% (Neilson 1993b).

The biophysical profile is potentially time consuming, labour intensive and has undergone many modifications since its original description. A major advantage of performing detailed ultrasound as part of fetal assessment is the detection of previously undiagnosed fetal anomalies which will influence pregnancy management. Although a normal test is very reassuring, determining abnormality with certainty may require prolonged scanning since fetal activity is prone to physiological fluctuations. Whilst recognizing that the number of women involved in randomized trials of the BPP is relatively small, the available results do not support its use as a test of fetal well-being in high-risk pregnancies (Neilson & Alfirevic 1993).

Where facilities exist, Doppler ultrasound is preferable to the BPP as a second-line test of fetal well-being since it is performed more easily and abnormalities of the FVW precede an abnormal BPP. It would appear reasonable to reserve comprehensive BPP scoring for those fetuses with an abnormal Doppler examination or a CTG which remains non-reactive after prolonged recording.

REFERENCES

Adis B, Wurth G, Stuke P 1978 Grundlagen und Ergebnisse fur die Beurtelung der Kardiotokographic mid eineum neuren CTG -score. Inaugural dissertation, Heildelberg

Almstrom H, Axellsson O, Cnattingius S et al 1992 Comparison of umbilical-artery velocimetry and cardiotocography for surveillance of small-for-gestational age fetuses. Lancet 340: 936

Arduini D, Rizzo G 1991 Fetal renal artery velocity waveforms and amniotic fluid volume in growth retarded and post-term fetuses. Obstetrics and Gynecology 77: 370

Arduini D A, Rizzo G, Romanini C, Mancuso S 1987 Fetal blood flow velocity waveforms as predictors of growth retardation. Obstetrics and Gynecology 70: 7

Arduini D, Rizzo G, Romanini C 1992 Changes of pulsatility index from fetal vessels preceding the onset of late decelerations in growth-retarded fetuses. Obstetrics and Gynecology 79: 605

Baskett T F, Gray J H, Prewett S J, Young L M, Allen A C 1984 Antepartum fetal assessment using a fetal biophysical profile score. American Journal of Obstetrics and Gynecology. 148: 630

Baskett T F, Allen A C, Gray J H, Young D C, Young L M 1987 Fetal biophysical profile and perinatal death. Obstetrics and Gynecology 70: 357

Battaglia C, Artini P G, Galli P A D, Ambrogio G, Droghini F, Genazzani R 1993 Absent or reversed end-diastolic flow in umbilical artery and severe intrauterine growth retardation. An ominous association. Acta Obstetrica Gynecologica Scandinavia 72: 167

Beattie R B, Dornan J C 1989 Antenatal screening for intrauterine growth retardation with umbilical artery Doppler ultrasonography. British Medical Journal 298: 631

Behrman R E, Lees M H, Peterson E N, de Lannoy C W, Seeds A E 1970 Distribution of the circulation in the normal and asphyxiated fetal primate. American Journal of Obstetrics and Gynecology 108: 956

Bekedam D J, Visser G H A, van der Zee A G J, Snijders R J M, Poelmann-Weesjes 1990 Abnormal velocity waveforms of the umbilical artery in growth retarded fetuses; relationship to antepartum late heart rate decelerations and outcome. Early Human Development 24: 79

Berkowitz G S, Chitkara U, Rosenberg J et al 1988a Sonographic estimation of fetal weight and Doppler analysis of umbilical artery velocimetry in the prediction of intrauterine growth retardation; a prospective study. American Journal of Obstetrics and Gynecology 158: 1149

Berkowitz G S, Mehalek K E, Chitkara U, Rosenberg J, Cogswell C, Berkowitz R L 1988b Doppler umbilical velocimetry in the prediction of adverse outcome in pregnancies at risk for intrauterine growth retardation. Obstetrics and Gynecology 71: 742

Bilardo C, Nicolaides K H, Campbell S 1990 Doppler measurements of fetal and uteroplacental circulations; relationship with umbilical venous blood gases measured at cordocentesis. American Journal of Obstetrics and Gynecology. 162: 115

Bishop E H 1968 Ultrasonic fetal monitoring. Clinical Obstetrics and Gynecology 11: 1154

Bracero L, Shulman H, Fleischer A, Farmakides G, Rochelson B 1986 Umbilical artery velocimetry in diabetes and pregnancy. Obstetrics and Gynecology 68: 654

Bradley R J, Brudenell J M, Nicolaides K M 1988 Chronic fetal hypoxia in diabetic pregnancy. British Medical Journal 296: 790

Brar H S, Platt L D 1988 Reverse end-diastolic flow on umbilical artery velocimetry in high-risk pregnancies; an ominous finding with adverse pregnancy outcome. American Journal of Obstetrics and Gynecology 159: 559

Brar H S, Platt L D 1989 Antepartum improvement of umbilical artery velocimetry; does it occur? American Journal of Obstetrics and Gynecology 160: 36

Brar H S, Madearis A L, deVore G R, Platt L D 1989 A comparative study of fetal umbilical velocimetry with continuous and pulsed wave Doppler ultrasonography in high-risk pregnancies; relationship to outcome. American Journal of Obstetrics and Gynecology 160: 375

Breart G, Coupil F, Legrand H et al 1981 Antepartum fetal heart rate monitoring. A semi-quantitative evaluation of the 'non-stress' fetal heart rate. European Journal of Obstetrics, Gynecology and Reproductive Biology 11: 227

Brown J S, Gee H, Olah K S, Docker M F, Taylor E W 1992. A new technique for the identification of respiratory sinus arrhythmia in utero. Journal of Biomedical Engineering 14: 263

Brown V A, Sawers R S, Parsons F J, Duncan S L B, Cooke I D 1982 The value of antenatal cardiotocography in the management of high risk pregnancy: a randomised control trial. British Journal of Obstetrics and Gynaecology. 98: 716

Bruinse H W, Sijmons E A, Reuwer P J 1989 Clinical value of screening for fetal growth retardation by Doppler ultrasound. Journal of Ultrasound in Medicine. 8: 207

Burke G, Stuart B, Crowley P, Scanaill S N, Drumm J 1990 Is intra-uterine growth retardation with normal umbilical artery blood flow a benign condition ? British Medical Journal 300: 1044

Chambers S E, Hoskins P R, Haddad N G, Johnstone F D, McDicken W N , Muir B B 1989 A comparison of fetal abdominal circumference measurements and doppler ultrasound in the prediction of small for dates babies and fetal compromise. British Journal of Obstetrics and Gynaecology. 96: 803

Chayen B, Scott E, Cheung C, Perera C, Schiffer M A 1985 Contraction stress test by breast stimulation as part of antepartum monitoring. Acta Obstetrica et Gynecologica Scandinavica 64: 3

Cheng L C, Gibb D M F, Ajayi R A, Soothill P W 1992 A comparison between computerised (mean range) and clinical visual cardiotocographic assessment. British Journal of Obstetrics and Gynaecology 99: 817

Cobo E 1974 Neuroendocrine control of milk ejection in women. In: Josimovich J F, Renaulds M, Cobo E (eds) Lactogenic hormones, fetal nutrition and lactation. Wiley, New York, p 433

Cohn H E, Sacks E J, Heymann M A, Rudolph A M. 1974 Cardiovascular responses to hypoxemia and acidemia in fetal lambs. American Journal of Obstetrics and Gynecology 120: 817

Cole S 1985 Perinatal mortality survey. Information Services Division, Edinburgh

Copel J A, Otis C S, Stewart I, Rosetti C, Weiner S 1985 Contraction stress testing with nipple stimulation. Journal of Reproductive Medicine 30: 465

Curtis P, Evens S, Resnick J, Thompson C J, Rimer R, Hisley J 1989 Patterns of uterine contractions and prolonged uterine activity using three methods of breast stimulation for contraction stress tests. Obstetrics and Gynaecology. 73: 631

Dalton K J, Dawes G C, Patrick J E 1977 Diurnal, respiratory and other rhythms of fetal heart rate in lambs. American Journal of Obstetrics and Gynaecology. 127: 414

Dawes G S, Visser G H A, Goodman J D S, Venene D H 1981 Numerical analysis of the human fetal heart rate; the quality of ultrasound records. American Journal of Obstetrics and Gynaecology 141: 43

Dawes G S, Houghton R S, Redman C W G 1982 Base line in human fetal heart records. British Journal of Obstetrics and Gynaecology 89: 270

Dawes G S, Redman C W G, Smith J H 1985 Improvements in the registration and analysis of fetal heart rate records at the bedside. British Journal of Obstetrics and Gynaecology 92: 317

Dawes G S, Moulden M, Redman C W G 1990 Limitations of fetal heart rate monitors. American Journal of Obstetrics and Gynaecology 162: 170

Dawes G S, Lobb M M, Oulden M, Redman C W G, Wheeler T 1992 Antenatal cardiotocogram quality and interpretation using computers British Journal of Obstetrics and Gynaecology 99: 791

deHaan J, Bemmel J H, von Veth A F L et al 1971 Quantitative evaluation of FHR patterns. European Journal of Obstetrics and Gynecology 3: 95

Dempster J, Mires G J, Taylor D J, Patel N B 1988 Fetal umbilical artery flow velocity waveforms; prediction of small for gestational age infants and late decelerations in labour. European Journal of Obstetrics, Gynecology and Reproductive Biology 29: 21

Dempster J, Mires G J, Patel N, Taylor D J 1989 Umbilical artery velocity waveforms; poor association with small for gestational age babies. British Journal of Obstetrics and Gynaecology 96: 692

Devoe L D 1984 Clinical features of the reactive positive contraction stress test. Obstetrics and Gynaecology 63: 523

Devoe L D, Alaaeldin A Y, Gardner P, Dear C, Murray C 1992 Refining the biophysical profile with a risk-related evaluation of test performance. American Journal of Obstetrics and Gynecology 167: 346

Divon M Y, Guidetti D A, Braverman J J, Oberlander E, Langer O, Merkatz I R 1988 Intrauterine growth retardation—a prospective study of the diagnostic value of real-time sonography combined with umbilical artery flow velocimetry. Obstetrics and Gynecology 72: 611

Echizenya N, Kagiya A, Tachizaki T, Saito Y 1989 Significance of velocimetry as a monitor of fetal assessment and management. Fetal Therapy 4: 188

Economides D L, Selinger M, Ferguson J, Bowell P J, Dawes G S, Mackenzie I Z 1992 Computerized measurement of heart rate variation in fetal anaemia caused by rhesus allo-immunisation. American Journal of Obstetrics and Gynecology 167: 689

Eden P D, Seifert L S, Kodack L D, Trofatter K F, Killam A P, Gall S A 1988 A modified biophysical profile for antenatal fetal surveillance. Obstetrics and Gynecology 71: 365

Eik-Nes S H, Marsal K, Person P H, Ulstein M K 1980 Ultrasonic measurements of blood flow in human fetal aorta and umbilical vein. In: Dawes G S (ed) Proceedings of the 7th Conference on Fetal Breathing and Other Measurements, Oxford, pp 1–8

Erskine R L A, Ritchie J W K 1985a Quantitative measurement of fetal blood flow using Doppler ultrasound. British Journal of Obstetrics and Gynaecology 92: 600

Erskine R L A, Ritchie J W K 1985b Umbilical artery flow charateristics in normal and growth retarded fetuses. British Journal of Obstetrics and Gynaecology 92: 605

Fischer W M (ed) 1976 Kardiotokography. Geburtshilfe. Thieme, Stuttgart

Fischer W M, Stude J, Brandl H 1976 Ein Vorschlag zur Beurteilung des antepartalen Kardiotokogramms. Zeitschrift fur Perinatologie 180: 117

Fitzgerald D E, Drumm J E 1977 Non-invasive measurement of human fetal circulation using ultrasound; a new method. British Medical Journal 2: 1450

Fleischer A, Schulman H, Farmakides G, Bracero L, Blattner P, Randolph G 1985 Umbilical artery velocity waveforms and intrauterine growth retardation. American Journal of Obstetrics and Gynecology 151: 502

Flynn A M, Kelly J, O'Connor M 1979 Unstressed antepartum cardiotocography in the management of the fetus suspected of growth retardation. British Journal of Obstetrics and Gynaecology 86: 106

Flynn A M, Kelly J, Matthews K, O'Connor M, Viegas O 1982 Predictive value of an observer variability. British Journal of Obstetrics and Gynaecology 89: 434

Fok R Y, Pavlova Z, Benirschke K, Paul R H, Platt L D 1990 The correlation of arterial lesions with umbilical artery Doppler velocimetry in the placentas of small-for-dates pregnancies. Obstetrics and Gynecology 75: 578

Fox H E, Inglis J, Steinbrecher M 1979 Fetal breathing movements in uncomplicated pregnancies. I. Relationship to gestational age. American Journal of Obstetrics and Gynecology 134: 544

Freeman R K 1975 The use of the OST for antepartum clinical evaluation of utero-placental function. American Journal of Obstetrics and Gynecology 121: 481

Freeman R 1981 Antepartum fetal heart rate. Rate monitoring lecture. In: The World Symposium of Perinatal Medicine, San Francisco

Garite T J, Linzee M E, Freeman R K, Dorchester W 1979 FHR patterns and fetal distress in fetuses with congenital anomalies. Obstetrics and Gynecology 53: 716

Garoff L, Vansellow H, von Hagen C, Grothe W, Ruttgers H, Kubli F 1978 Evaluation of 6000 antepartum CTG according to the previously published CTG code. Lecture presented to the 6th European Congress of Perinatal Medicine, Vienna

Gaziano E, Knox E G, Wager G P, Bendel R P, Boyce D J, Olson J 1988 The predictability of the small for gestational age infant by real time ultrasound derived measurements combined with pulsed Doppler umbilical artery velocimetry. American Journal of Obstetrics and Gynecology 158: 1431

Giacomello F, Ticconi C, Baschieri L 1987 Sinusoidal-like fetal heart rate pattern; real-time ultrasound may help in the differential diagnosis Acta Obstetrica et Gynecologica Scandinavica 66: 713

Giles W B, Trudinger B J, Baird P J 1985 Fetal umbilical artery flow velocity waveforms and placental resistance; pathological correlation. British Journal of Obstetrics and Gynaecology 92: 31

Goodlin R C 1977 Fetal cardiovascular responses to distress. A review. Obstetrics and Gynaecology 49: 371

Gough N A G, Dawson A A J, Tomins T J 1986 Antepartum fetal heart rate recording and subsequent fast transmission by a distributed microprocessor based dedicated system. International Journal of Biomedical Computing 18: 61

Gramellini D, Folli M C, Raboni S, Vadora E, Merialdi A 1992 Cerebral-umbilical Doppler ratio as a predictor of adverse perinatal outcome. Obstetrics and Gynecology 79: 416

Grant A M, Elbourne D R, Valentin L, Alexander S 1989 Routine formal fetal movement counting and risk of antepartum late death in normally formed singletons. Lancet ii: 345

Greene K R 1987 The ECG waveform. Bailliere's Clinical Obstetrics and Gynaecology 1: 131

Griffin D, Bilardo K, Masini L, Diaz-Recasens A, Pearce J M, Willson K, Campbell S 1984 Doppler blood flow waveforms in the descending aorta of the human fetus. British Journal of Obstetrics and Gynaecology 91: 997

Groenenberg I A, Baerts W, Hop W C, Wladimiroff J W 1991 Relationship fetal cardiac and extracardiac Doppler flow velocity waveforms and neonatal outcome in intra-uterine growth retardation. Early Human Development 26: 185

Gudmundsson S, Marsal K 1991 Blood velocity waveforms in the fetal aorta and umbilical artery as predictors of fetal outcome; a comparison. American Journal of Perinatology 8: 1

Hackett G A, Campbell S, Gamsu H, Cohen-Overbeek T, Pearce J F 1987 Doppler studies in the growth retarded fetus and prediction of neonatal necrotizing enterocolitis, haemorrhage and neonatal morbidity. British Medical Journal 294: 13

Haddad N G, Johnstone F D, Hoskins P R, Chambers S E, Muir B B, McDicken W N 1988 Umbilical artery Doppler waveform in pregnancies with uncomplicated intrauterine growth retardation. Gynaecological and Obstetrical Investigation 26: 206

Halberstadt E 1981 Zeitdauer und Assagekraft des antepartelen CTG. Perinatal Magazine 8

Hammacher K 1962 Neue Metode zur selecktiven Registrierung der fetalen Herzschlagfrequenz. Geburtshilfe und Frauenheilkunde 22: 1542

Hammacher K 1966 Fruherkennung intrauteriner Gefahrenzustand durch Elektophonokardiographie und Tokographie. In: Elert R, Huter K (eds) Die Parophylaxe fruhkindlicher Hirnschaden. Thieme, Stuttgart

Hammacher K, Brudell R E, Gaudenzp R, Grandi D E P, Richter R 1974 Kardiotocographischer Nachweis einer fetalen Gefahrdung mit einen CTG score. Gynaekologische Rundschau 14: 61

Hansmann M, Gembruch U, Bald R, Manz Redel D A 1991 Fetal tachyarrhythmias; transplacental and direct treatment of the fetus—a report of 60 cases. Ultrasound in Obstetrics and Gynecology 1: 162

Hata K, Katoh S, Senoh D et al 1989 Umbilical artery velocity waveforms are not valid indices for assessing growth retardation in utero. International Journal of Gynecology and Obstetrics 29: 25

Hitschold T, Weiss E, Beck T, Huntefering H, Berle P 1993 Low target birthweight or growth retardation? Doppler flow velocity waveforms and histometric analysis of fetoplacental vascular tree. American Journal of Obstetrics and Gynecology 168: 1260

Hohl A F 1833 Die geburtschilfliche Exploration. Theil I, Halle, p 34

Hon E H 1972 The present status of electronic monitoring of the human fetal heart. International Journal of Gynaecology and Obstetrics 10: 191

Hon E H, Lee S T 1963 Noise reduction in fetal electrocardiography. 2. Averaging techniques. American Journal of Obstetrics and Gynecology 135: 609

Hon E H, Yeh S Y 1969 Electronic evaluation of fetal heart rate. X. The fetal arrhythmia index. Medical Research Engineering 8: 14

Huddleston J F, Sutcliffe G, Kerry F E, Flowers C E 1979 Oxytocin challenge test for antepartum fetal assessment. American Journal of Obstetrics and Gynecology 135: 609

Huddleston J F, Sutcliffe G, Robinson D 1984 Contraction stress test by intermittent nipple stimulation. Obstetrics and Gynecology 63: 669

Huter V 1862 Uber dem Fotalpuls Monatz. Geburtskunde Frauenkrankheiten XVIII (suppl)

James D K, Parker M J, Smoleniec J S 1992 Comprehensive fetal assessment with three ultrasonographic characteristics. American Journal of Obstetrics and Gynecology 166: 1486

Jauer P C, Heinrich J, Koepck E, Hopp H, Seidenschnur G 1976 Vergleichende Untersuchungen zur Frage der Wertigkeit der Impulsaufnahmeverfahren der vorgeburtlichen Kardiotokographie. Zentralblatt fur Gynaekologie 98: 990

Jenkins H 1984 A study of the intrapartum fetal electrocardiogram using a real-time computer. Thesis, Nottingham University

Jenkins H M L, Symonds E M, Kirk D L, Smith P R 1986 Can fetal electrocardiography improve the prediction of intrapartum fetal acidosis? British Journal of Obstetrics and Gynaecology 93: 6

Jensen O H, Guimaraes M S 1991 Prediction of fetal outcome by Doppler examination and by the non-stress test. Acta Obstetrica et Gynecologica Scandinavica 70: 271

Johnstone F D, Steel J M, Haddad N G, Hoskins P R, Greer I A, Chambers S 1992 Doppler umbilical artery flow velocity waveforms in diabetic pregnancy. British Journal of Obstetrics and Gynaecology 99: 135

Jouppila P, Kirkinen P 1984 Increased vascular resistance in the descending aorta of the human fetus in hypoxia. British Journal of Obstetrics and Gynaecology 91: 853

Junge H D 1979 Behavioural state related heart rate and motor activity patterns in the newborn infant and the fetus antepartum. I. Technique, illustration of recordings and general results. Journal of Perinatal Medicine 7: 85

Karsdorp V H M, van Vugt J M G, Dekker G A, van Geijn H P 1992 Reappearance of end-diastolic velocities in the umbilical artery following maternal volume expansion; a preliminary study. Obstetrics and Gynecology 80: 679

Keegan K A, Paul R H 1980 Antepartum fetal heart rate testing, IV. The non-stress test as a primary approach. American Journal of Obstetrics and Gynecology 136: 75

Keegan K A, Paul R H, Brouissard P M, McCart T, Smith M A 1979 Antepartum fetal heart rate testing. III. The effect of phenobarbital on the non-stress test. American Journal of Obstetrics and Gynecology 133: 579

Keirse M C, Trimbose J M 1980 Assessment of antepartum cardiotocograms in high risk pregnancy. British Journal of Obstetrics and Gynaecology 87: 261

Kempley S T, Gamsu H R, Vyas S, Nicolaides K 1991 Effects of intrauterine growth retardation on postnatal visceral and cerebral blood flow velocity. Archives of Diseases of Childhood 66: 1115

Kennedy E 1833 Observations of obstetrical auscultation on obstetrical auscultation. Dublin

Kidd L C, Patel N B, Smith R 1985a Non-stress antenatal cardiotocography — a prospective blind study. British Journal of Obstetrics and Gynaecology 92: 1152

Kidd L C, Patel N B, Smith R 1985b Non-stress antenatal cardiotocography — a prospective randomised clinical trial. British Journal of Obstetrics and Gynaecology 92: 1156

Kirkinen P, Muller R, Huch R, Huch A 1987 Blood flow velocity waveforms in human fetal intracranial arteries. Obstetrics and Gynecology 70: 617

Koppelaar I, Wladimiroff J W 1992 Quantitation of breathing-related modulation of umbilical arterial and venous flow velocity waveforms in the normal term fetus. European Journal of Obstetrics, Gynaecology and Reproductive Biology 45:177

Krebs H B, Petres R E 1978 Clinical application of a scoring system for evaluation of antepartum fetal heart rate monitoring. American Journal of Obstetrics and Gynecology 130: 765

Kubli F, Ruttgers H 1972 Semi-quantitative evaluation of antepartum fetal heart rate. International Journal of Gynaecology and Obstetrics 10: 182

Kubli F W, Kaeser O, Hinselman M 1968 Diagnostic management of chronic placental insufficiency. In: The fetal placental unit. Excerpta Medica, Amsterdam

Kubli F W, Hon E H, Khazin A F, Takemura H 1969 Observations on heart rate and pH in the human fetus during labour. American Journal of Obstetrics and Gynecology 104: 1190

Kubli F, Ruttgers H, von Hagens C, Vansclow H 1978 Antepartum FHR monitoring. In: Beard R W, Campbell S (eds) Current status of FHR monitoring and ultrasound in obstetrics. RCOG, London

Landon M B, Gabbe S G, Bruner J P, Ludmir J 1989 Doppler umbilical artery velocimetry in pregnancy complicated by insulin-dependent diabetes mellitus. Obstetrics and Gynecology 73: 961

Lanke R R, Nemes J M 1984 Use of nipple stimulation to obtain contraction stress test. Obstetrics and Gynaecology 623: 345

Laurin J, Marsal K, Persson P-H, Lingman G 1987 Ultrasound measurement of fetal blood flow in predicting fetal outcome. British Journal of Obstetrics and Gynaecology 94: 940

Lenstrup C, Falck-Larson J 1979 Cardiotocogram in fetuses at risk. Ugeskrift for Laeger 1141: 1485

Lenstrup C, Hasse N 1985 Predictive value of antepartum fetal heart rate non-stress test in high risk pregnancy. Acta Obstetricia et Gynecologica Scandinavica 64: 133

Lin C, Devoe L, River P, Moawa D, Moawa A 1981 Oxytocin challenge test in intrauterine growth retardation. American Journal of Obstetrics and Gynecology 140: 282

Lingman G, Marsal K 1989 Non-invasive assessment of cranial blood circulation in the fetus . Biology of the Neonate 56: 129

Lumley J, Lester A, Anderson I, Renou P, Wood C 1983 A randomised trial of weekly cardiotocography in high risk obstetric patients. British Journal of Obstetrics and Gynaecology 90: 1018

Luz N P 1979 Auditory evoked response. In: Scientific exhibitin monograph. VIIII World Congress of Gynaecology and Obstetrics, Tokyo

Lyons E R, Blysma-Howel L M, Shamshee S, Toll M E 1979 Scoring system for non-stress antepartum FHR monitoring. American Journal of Obstetrics and Gynecology 133: 242

Mandenhall H W, O'Leary J A, Phillips K O 1980 The non-stress test: the value of a single acceleration in evaluating the fetus at risk. American Journal of Obstetrics and Gynecology 136: 87

Manning F A, Feyerabend C 1976 Cigarette smoking and fetal breathing movements. British Journal of Obstetrics and Gynaecology 83: 262

Manning F A, Platt L D, Sipos L 1980 Antepartum fetal evaluation; development of a fetal biophysical profile. American Journal of Obstetrics and Gynecology 136: 787

Manning F A, Morrison I, Harman C R, Lange I R, Menticoglou S

1987a Fetal assessment based on fetal biophysical profile scoring; experience in 19 221 referred high-risk pregnancies II. American Journal of Obstetrics and Gynecology 157: 880

Manning F A, Morrison I, Lange I R, Harman C R, Chamberlain P 1987b Fetal biophysical profile scoring; selective use of the nonstress test. American Journal of Obstetrics and Gynecology 156: 709

Manning F A, Morrison I, Harman C R, Menticoglou S M 1990 The abnormal fetal biophysical profile score V. Predictive accuracy according to score composition. American Journal of Obstetrics and Gynecology 162: 918

Manseau P, Vaquier J, Chavinine J, Sureau C 1972 Le rythme cardiaque foetal 'sinocoidal'. Aspect evocatur de souffrance foetal au cours de la grosse. Journal of Gynecology, Obstetrics and Reproductive Biology 1: 343

Mari G, Deter R L 1992 Middle cerebral artery flow velocity waveforms in normal and small-for-gestational age fetuses. American Journal of Obstetrics and Gynecology 166: 1262

Marsal K, Ley D 1992 Intra-uterine blood flow and postnatal neurologic development in growth retarded fetuses. Biology of Neonate 62: 258

Maxwell D J, Crawford D C, Curry P V M, Tynan M J, Allan L D 1983 Obstetric importance, diagnosis and management of fetal tachycardias. British Medical Journal 297: 107

Meyer-Menk W, Ruttgers H, Boos R, Wurth G, Eddis B, Kulbi F 1976 A proposal for a new matter of CTG evaluation. In: Abstracts of the 5th European Congress of Perinatal Medicine in Uppsala. Armquist and Wiksel, Stockholm, p 138

McDonald D A 1974 Blood flow in arteries, 2nd edn. Edward Arnold, London

McIlwaine G M, Howat R C L, Dunn F, MacNaughton M C 1979 The Scottish Perinatal Mortality Survey. British Medical Journal 2: 1103

Miller J M, Gabert H A 1992 Comparison of dynamic image and pulsed Doppler ultrasonography for the diagnosis of the small for gestational age fetus. American Journal of Obstetrics and Gynecology 166:1820

Mills M S, James D K, Slade S 1990 Two-tier approach to biophysical assessment of the fetus. American Journal of Obstetrics and Gynecology. 163: 12

Mires G J, Dempster J, Patel N B, Crawford J W 1987 The effect of fetal heart rate on umbilical artery flow velocity waveforms. British Journal of Obstetrics and Gynecology 94: 665

Mires G J, Patel N, Dempster J 1990 Review; the value of fetal umbilical artery flow velocity waveforms in the prediction of adverse fetal outcomes in high risk pregnancies. Journal of Obstetrics and Gynecology 10: 261

Modanlouh D, Freeman R K, Braly P, Rasmussen S B 1977 A simple matter of fetal and neonatal heart rate beat to beat variability quantitation; preliminary report. American Journal of Obstetrics and Gynecology 127: 861

Moore K H, Sill R. 1990 Domicilliary fetal monitoring in a district maternity hospital. Australian and New Zealand Journal of Obstetrics and Gynaecology 30: 36

Mulders L G, Wijn P F F, Jongsma H W, Hein P R 1987 A comparative study of three indices of umbilical blood flow in relation to the prediction of growth retardation. Journal of Perinatal Medicine 15: 3

Murphy K W, Russell V, Collins A, Johnson P 1991 The prevalence, aetiology, and clinical significance of pseudo-sinusoidal fetal heart rate patterns in labour. British Journal of Obstetrics and Gynaecology 98: 1093

Neilson J P 1993a Routine formal fetal movement counting. In: Enkin M W, Keirse M J N C, Renfrew M J, Neilson J P (eds) Pregnancy and childbirth module. Cochrane Database of Systematic Reviews. Review No 04364 April, Oxford

Neilson J P 1993b Doppler ultrasound (all trials) In: Enkin M W, Keirse M J N C, Renfrew M J, Neilson J P (eds) Pregnancy and childbirth module. Cochrane Database of Systematic Reviews. Review No.07337 February, Oxford

Neilson J P, Alfirevic Z 1993 Biophysical profile for antepartum fetal assessment. In: Enkin M W, Keirse M J N C, Renfrew M J, Neilson J P (eds) Pregnancy and childbirth module. Cochrane Database of Systematic Reviews; Review No. 07432. April, Oxford

Neldam S 1983 Fetal movements as an indicator of fetal well-being. Danish Medical Bulletin 30: 274

Newnham J P, Patterson L L, James I R, Diepeeven D A, Reid S E 1990 An evaluation of the efficacy of Doppler flow velocity waveform analysis as a screening test in pregnancy. American Journal of Obstetrics and Gynecology 162: 403

Nicolaides K H, Bilardo C M, Soothill P W, Campbell S 1988 Absence of end diastolic frequencies in umbilical artery; a sign of fetal hypoxia and acidosis. British Medical Journal 297: 1026

Nicolaides K H, Peters M T, Vyas S, Rabinowitz R, Rosen D J D, Campbell S 1990 Relation of rate of urine production to oxygen tension in small for gestational age fetuses. American Journal of Obstetrics and Gynecology 162: 387

Nicolini U, Nicolaidis P, Fisk N M et al 1990 Limited role of fetal blood sampling in prediction of outcome in intrauterine growth retardation. Lancet 336: 768

Nijhuis J G, Prechtl H F R, Martin C B, Bots R S G M 1982 Are there behavioural states in the human fetus? Early Human Development 6: 177

Nordstrom U L, Patel N B, Taylor D J 1989 Umbilical artery waveform analysis and biophysical profile. A comparison of two methods to identify compromised fetuses. European Journal of Obstetrics, Gynecology and Reproductive Biology 30: 241

Nyman N, Arulkumaran S, Jakobsson J, Westgren M 1992 Vibroacoustic stimulation in high-risk pregnancies; maternal perception of fetal movements, fetal heart rate and fetal outcome. Journal of Perinatal Medicine 20: 267

Olah K S, Gee H 1992 Fetal heart block associated with maternal anti-Ro(SS-A) antibody-current management. A review. British Journal of Obstetrics and Gynaecology 98: 751

Olson R M, Cooke J P 1975 Human carotid artery diameter and flow by a non-invasive technique. Medical Instruments 9: 99

Paul R H, Millar F C 1978 Antepartum FHR monitoring. Klinische Obstetrische und Gynaekologie 21: 375

Patrick J, Campbell K, Carmichael L 1980 Patterns of human fetal breathing during the last ten weeks of pregnancy. Obstetrics and Gynecology 65: 24

Patterson R M, Pouliot M R 1987 Neonatal morphometrics and perinatal outcome; who is growth retarded ? American Journal of Obstetrics and Gynecology 157: 691

Pearson J F, Weaver J B 1976 Fetal activity and fetal wellbeing; an evaluation. British Medical Journal 1: 1305

Pearson J F, Weaver J B 1978 A six point scoring system for antenatal cardiotocographs. British Journal of Obstetrics and Gynaecology 85: 321

Peleg T, Goldman J 1980 Fetal heart rate acceleration and response to light stimulation as a clinical measure of fetal well being. A preliminary report. Journal of Perinatal Medicine 8: 38

Perar J T, Kuueger T R, Harris J L 1980 Fetal oxygen consumption and mechanisms of heart rate response during artifically produced late decelerations of fetal heart rate in sleep. American Journal of Obstetrics and Gynecology 136: 478

Petrie R H, Yeh S Y, Manata Y et al 1978 The effect of drugs on fetal FHR variability. American Journal of Obstetrics and Gynecology 130: 294

Pillai M, James D 1990 The importance of the behavioural state in biophysical assessment of the term human fetus. British Journal of Obstetrics and Gynaecology 97: 1130

Pinkerton J H M 1976 Fetal auscultation—some aspects of its history and evolution. Journal of the Irish Medical Association 69: 363

Reid J, Miller F 1977 Fetal heart rate acceleration in response to acoustic stimulation as a measure of fetal wellbeing. American Journal of Obstetrics and Gynecology 129: 512

Reuwer P J H M, Sijmons E A, Rietman G W, van Tiel M W M, Bruinse H W 1987 Intrauterine growth retardation; prediction of perinatal distress by Doppler ultrasound. Lancet i: 415

Ribbert L S M, Snijders R J M, Nicolaides K H, Visser G H A 1990 Relationship of fetal biophysical profile and blood gas values at cordocentesis in severely growth-retarded fetuses. American Journal of Obstetrics and Gynecology 163: 569

Rizzo G, Arduini D, Luciano R et al 1989 Prenatal cerebral Doppler ultrasonography and neonatal neurologic outcome. Journal of Ultrasound in Medicine 8: 237

Rochard F, Chiforene B, Gone-Poponpil F, Legrand H, Blottiere J, Sureau C 1976 Non stress fetal heart rate monitoring in the antepartum period. American Journal of Obstetrics and Gynecology 126: 699

Rochelson B L, Schulman H, Fleischer A et al 1987a The clinical significance of Doppler umbilical artery velocimetry in the small for gestational age fetus. American Journal of Obstetrics and Gynecology 156: 1223

Rochelson B, Schulman H, Farmakides G et al 1987b The significance of absent end-diastolic velocity in umbilical artery velocity waveforms. American Journal of Obstetrics and Gynecology 156: 1213

Romer V M, Heinzl S, Peters F E, Mietzner S, Bruhl G, Heening P 1979 Auscultation frequency in baseline FHR in the last 30 minutes of labour. British Journal of Obstetrics and Gynaecology 86: 472

Ruttgers H, Kubli F 1969 Kontinuierliche Registrierung von fetaler Herzfrequenz bie gleichzeitiger Wehenschreibung. II Probleme der Instrumentierung. Gynakologie 2: 82

Ruttgers H, Kubli F, Haler U, Bachmann M, Grunder E 1972 Die antepartale fetal Herzfrequnz. Zeitschrift fur Geburtshilfe und Perinatologie 176: 294

Saling E 1969 Verbesserung der apparativen Herzschlagregisdrierung beim Feten unter der Geburt. Fortschritte der Medizin 87: 777

Satoh S, Koyanagi T, Fukuhara M, Hara K, Nakano H 1989 Changes in vascular resistance in the umbilical and middle cerebral arteries in the human intra-uterine growth-retarded fetus, measured with pulsed Doppler ultrasound. Early Human Development 20: 213

Scherjon S A, Kok J H, Oosting H, Wolf H, Zondervan H A 1992 Fetal and neonatal cerebral circulation; a pulsed Doppler study. Journal of Perinatal Medicine 20: 79

Schiff E, Lipitz S, Sivan E, Barkai G, Mashiach S 1992 Acoustic stimulation as a diagnostic test; comparison with the oxytocin challenge test. Journal of Perinatal Medicine 20: 275

Schifrin B, Lapidus M, Geetis De, Leviton N A 1975 Contraction stress test for antepartum evaluation. Obstetrics and Gynecology 45: 433

Schifrin B, Foy G, Amato J, Kates R, McKenna J 1979 Routine FHR monitoring in the antepartum period. Obstetrics and Gynecology 54: 21

Schifferle P, Caldeyro-Barcia R 1973 Effects of atropine and beta adrenergic drugs on the heart rate of the human fetus. In: Boreus L (ed) Fetal pharmacology. Raven, New York, pp 259–279

Schulman H, Winter D, Farmakides G et al 1989 Pregnancy surveillance with Doppler velocimetry of uterine and umbilical arteries. American Journal of Obstetrics and Gynecology 160: 192

Schwartz H 1858 Die vorzeitigen Atembewgungen, Leipzig

Shah D M, Brown J E, Salyer S L, Fleischer A C, Boehm F H 1989 A modified scheme for biophysical profile scoring. American Journal of Obstetrics and Gynecology 160: 586

Sheppard B L, Bonnar J 1976 The ultrastructure of the arterial supply of the human placenta in pregnancy complicated by fetal growth retardation. British Journal of Obstetrics and Gynaecology 83: 948

Smith J H, Anand K J S, Cotes P M et al 1988 Antenatal fetal heart rate variation in relation to the respiratory and metabolic status of the compromised human fetus. British Journal of Obstetrics and Gynaecology 95: 980

Solum T 1980 Antenatal cardiotocography methods, interpretation and clinical application. Acta Obstetricia et Gynecologica Scandinavica (suppl 96)

Solum T, Sjoberg N O 1980 Antenatal cardiotocography and intrauterine death. Acta Obstetricia et Gynecologica Scandinavica 59: 481

Solum T, Ingemarsson I, Nygren A 1981 The accuracy of ultrasonic fetal cardiotocography. Journal of Perinatal Medicine 9 (suppl): 54

Soothill P W, Nicolaides K H, Bilardo C M, Campbell S 1986 Relation of fetal hypoxia in growth retardation to mean blood velocity in the fetal aorta. Lancet i: 1118

Soothill P W, Ajayi R A, Campbell S, Nicolaides K H 1993 Prediction of morbidity in small and normally grown fetuses by fetal heart rate variability, biophysical profile score and umbilical artery Doppler studies. British Journal of Obstetrics and Gynaecology 100: 742

Staisch K J, Wesleg J R, Barshore L A 1980 Blind oxytocin challenge test and perinatal outcome. American Journal of Obstetrics and Gynecology 138: 399

Steer P J 1986 Evaluation of cardiotocographs. DHSS scientific and technical branch. British Medical Journal 292: 827

Sterman M B 1967 The relationship of intrauterine fetal activity to maternal sleep state. Experiments in Neurology (suppl) 19: 98

Strong T H, Jordan D L, Marden D W 1992 The fetal recoil test. American Journal of Obstetrics and Gynecology 567: 1382

Stuart B, Drumm J, Fitzgerald D E, Duignan N M 1980 Fetal blood velocity waveforms in normal pregnancy. British Journal of Obstetrics and Gynaecology 87: 780

Taylor D J 1984 Low birthweight and neurodevelopmental handicap. Clinical Obstetrics and Gynecology 11: 525

Thompson R S, Trudinger B J, Cook C M 1986 A comparison of Doppler ultrasound waveform indices in the umbilical artery 1. Indices derived from the maximum velocity waveform. Ultrasound in Medicine and Biology 12: 835

Tonge H M, Struyk P C, Custers P ,Wladimiroff J W 1983 Vascular dynamics in the descending aorta of the human fetus in normal late pregnancy. Early Human Development 9: 21

Tonge H M, Wladimiroff J W, Noordam M J, van Kooten C 1986 Blood flow velocity waveforms in the descending fetal aorta; comparison between normal and growth-retarded pregnancies. Obstetrics and Gynecology 67: 851

Trimbos J M, Keirse M J N C 1978 Observer variability in the assessment of antepartum cardiotocograms. British Journal of Obstetrics and Gynaecology 85: 900

Trudinger B J, Giles W B, Cook C M, Bombardieri J, Collins L 1985 Fetal umbilical artery flow velocity waveforms and placental resistance; clinical significance. British Journal of Obstetrics and Gynaecology 92: 23

Trudinger B J, Cook C M, Jones L, Giles W B 1986 A comparison of fetal heart rate monitoring and umbilical artery waveforms in the recognition of fetal compromise. British Journal of Obstetrics and Gynaecology 93: 171

Trudinger B J, Cook C M, Giles W B, Connelly A , Thompson R S 1987 Umbilical artery flow velocity waveforms in high-risk pregnancy. A randomised, controlled trial. Lancet: 188

Trudinger B J, Cook C M, Giles W B et al 1991 Fetal umbilical artery waveforms and subsequent neonatal outcome. British Journal of Obstetrics and Gynaecology 98: 378

Tyrrell S N 1988 Doppler studies in diabetic pregnancy. British Medical Journal 296: 428

Tyrrell S N, Obaid A H, Lilford R J 1989 Umbilical artery Doppler velocimetry as a predictor of fetal hypoxia and acidosis at birth. Obstetrics and Gynecology 74: 332

Tyrrell S N, Lilford R J, Macdonald H N, Nelson E J, Porter J, Gupta J K 1990 Randomized comparison of routine versus highly selective use of Doppler ultrasound and biophysical scoring to investigate high-risk pregnancies. British Journal of Obstetrics and Gynaecology 97: 909

van Vugt J M G, Ruissen K J, Schouten H J A, Theunissen M, Hoogland H J, de Haan J 1988 Umbilical artery blood velocimetry; a prospective longitudinal study in search of the intrauterine growth retarded fetus. Early Human Development. 18: 59

Varma T R 1981 Clinical experience in non-stressed antepartum cardiotocography in high risk pregnancies. International Journal of Gynaecology and Obstetrics 19: 433

Varma T R 1984 Unstressed antepartum cardiotocography in the management of pregnancy complicated by intrauterine growth retardation. Acta Obstetricia et Gynecologica Scandinavica 63: 129

Veille J C, Kanaan C 1989 Duplex Doppler ultrasonographic evaluation of the fetal renal artery in normal and abnormal fetuses. American Journal of Obstetrics and Gynecology 161: 1502

Vintzileos A M, Campbell W A, Nochimson D J, Weinbaum P J 1987a The use and misuse of the fetal biophysical profile. American Journal of Obstetrics and Gynecology 156: 527

Vintzileos A M, Gaffney S E, Salinger L M, Campbell W A, Nochimson D J 1987b The relationship between fetal biophysical profile and cord pH in patients indergoing cesarean section before onset of labour. Obstetrics and Gynecology 70: 196

Vintzileos A M, Fleming A D, Scorza W E et al 1991a Relationship between fetal biophysical activities and umbilical cord blood gas values. American Journal of Obstetrics and Gynecology 165: 707

Vintzileos A M, Campbell W A, Rodis J F, McLean D A, Fleming

A D, Scorza W E 1991b The relationship between fetal biophysical assessment, umbilical artery velocimetry and fetal acidosis. Obstetrics and Gynecology 77: 622

Visser G H A, Huisjes H J 1977 Diagnostic value of the unstressed antepartum cardiotocogram. British Journal of Obstetrics and Gynaecology 84: 321

Visser G H A, Redman C W G, Huisjess J, Turnbull A C 1980 Non-stress antepartum heart rate monitoring; implications of decelerations after spontaneous contraction. American Journal of Obstetrics and Gynecology 138: 429

Von Hoefft H 1836 Beobachtungen uber Auskultation der Schwengeren. Zeitschrift fur Geburtskunde VI: 1

Von Winckel F 1893 Lehrbuch der Geburtshilf. Leipzig

Vyas S, Campbell S, Bower S, Nicolaides K H 1990a Maternal abdominal pressure alters fetal cerebral blood flow. British Journal of Obstetrics and Gynaecology 97: 740

Vyas S, Nicolaides K H, Bower S, Campbell S 1990b Middle cerebral artery flow velocity waveforms in fetal hypoxaemia. British Journal of Obstetrics and Gynaecology 97: 797

Walkinshaw S, Cameron H, MacPhail S, Robson S 1992 The prediction of fetal compromise and acidosis by biophysical profile scoring in the small for gestational age fetus. Journal of Perinatal Medicine 20: 227

Watson W J, Katz V L, Bowes W A 1991 Fetal death after normal biophysical profile. American Journal of Perinatology 8: 94

Weiner C P 1990 The relationship between the umbilical artery systolic/diastolic ratio and umbilical blood gas measurements in specimens obtained by cordocentesis. American Journal of Obstetrics and Gynecology 162: 1198

Weingold A B, Yonekura M L, O'Kieffe J 1980 Non-stress testing. American Journal of Obstetrics and Gynecology 138: 195

Wenstrom K D, Weiner C P, Williamson R A 1991 Diverse maternal and fetal pathology associated with absent diastolic flow in the umbilical artery of the high-risk fetus. Obstetrics and Gynecology 77: 374

Weiss E, Ulrich S, Berle P 1992 Condition at birth of infants with previously absent or reverse umbilical artery end-diastolic flow velocities. Archives of Gynaecology and Obstetrics. 252: 37

Wheeler T, Murrills A, Shelley T 1978 Measurements of the fetal heart rate during pregnancy by a new electrocardiographic technique. British Journal of Obstetrics and Gynaecology 85: 12

Wheeler T, Cooke E, Murrills A 1979 Computer analysis of fetal heart rate variation during normal pregnancy. British Journal of Obstetrics and Gynaecology 86: 186

White D N 1982 Johann Christian Doppler and his effect—a brief history. Ultrasound in Medicine and Biology 8: 588

Wilcox A J 1983 Intrauterine growth retardation; beyond birthweight criteria. Editorial. Early Human Development 189

Wilken H P, Hackel B, Wilken H 1980 Klinische Erfahrungn mit den antepartalen CTG-auswerteverfahren nach Fischer, Hammacher, Huch and Kubli. IV Score nach Kubli. Zentralblatt fur Gynaekologie 102: 909

Wladimiroff J W, Tonge H M, Stewart P A 1986 Doppler ultrasound assessment of cerebral blood flow in the human fetus. British Journal of Obstetrics and Gynaecology 93: 471

Wladimiroff J W, van den Wijngaard J A G W, Degani S, Noordam M J, van Eyck J, Tonge H M 1987 Cerebral and umbilical arterial blood-flow velocity waveforms in normal and growth-retarded pregnancies. Obstetrics and Gynecology 69: 705

Wladimiroff J W, Noordam M J, van den Wijngaard J A G W, Hop W C J 1988 Fetal internal carotid and umbilical artery blood flow velocity waveforms as a measure of fetal well-being in intrauterine growth retardation. Pediatric Research 24: 609

Wood C, Walker A, Yardley R 1979 Acceleration of the fetal heart rate. American Journal of Obstetrics and Gynecology 86: 186

Young B K, Katz M, Klein S A 1979 The relationship between heart rate patterns and tissue pH in the human fetus. American Journal of Obstetrics and Gynecology 134: 685

Young B K, Katz M, Wilson S J 1980 Sinusoidal fetal heart rate. I. Clinical significance. American Journal of Obstetrics and Gynecology 136: 587

Zimmer E Z, Divon M Y 1993 Fetal vibroacoustic stimulation. Obstetrics and Gynaecology 81: 451

15. Prenatal diagnosis

Charles H. Rodeck   Pam Johnson

Material in this chapter contains contributions from the first edition and we are grateful to the previous authors for the work done.

INTRODUCTION

Inherited disorders affect a significant number of all populations, although risk factors vary. Some inherited disorders, e.g. colour blindness, permit an affected individual to enjoy a virtually normal life but many are either lethal or result in an individual suffering severe physical or mental handicap. Whilst some aneuploidies are lethal before or soon after birth, others are associated with a life expectancy of three or four decades for an individual impaired both mentally and physically. The ethical problems of termination of pregnancies affected by non-lethal abnormalities will be touched upon later in this chapter, but in terms of reducing the enormous emotional and financial cost associated with the care of these individuals, prenatal diagnosis offers the opportunity to reduce the load on society (Kaback 1984).

A large number of tests are now freely available which can permit prenatal diagnosis of inherited disorders. In the knowledge of a positive diagnosis, obstetrical management, which may include termination of an affected pregnancy, can be focused, immediate relevant postnatal therapy instigated and the overall outcome thus has the potential for improvement. Some of these tests are considered in detail in the chapters of this book. For completeness and to get the overall picture, they are briefly put into context in this chapter.

The aims of prenatal diagnosis are:

1. to reduce the fear of fetal abnormality
2. the prevention of handicap
3. to encourage couples at risk of inherited disease to have healthy children
4. the preparation of the parents for the birth of an abnormal child if an abnormality is detected
5. to provide more rational perinatal management
6. to identify correctly the need for intrauterine treatment.

In order to achieve these aims, certain criteria must be met and these will be dealt with in this chapter. To be amenable to prenatal diagnosis, a condition must be inherited, e.g. chromosomal abnormalities, inborn errors of metabolism and the haemoglobinopathies, or acquired in utero, e.g. fetal infections. The population at risk must be identified and appropriate diagnostic tests performed after counselling. Prenatal screening and diagnosis will be dealt with in Chapter 14 under ultrasound.

Risk factors for many inherited disorders are easily identified. A positive family history, knowledge that one of the parents is a carrier of a recessive or sex-linked disorder or raised maternal age will alert those involved in the care of a woman before and in early pregnancy to the possibility that the index pregnancy might be affected. However, inherited disorders are not confined to the offspring of a couple with obvious risk factors, e.g. chromosomal abnormalities. Confirmation that a particular pregnancy is affected depends on invasive testing which includes amniocentesis, chorion villus sampling and fetal blood or tissue sampling. All these tests carry a risk of miscarriage, fetal death or premature delivery. In addition, the laboratory costs of processing samples so obtained are very high. For these reasons, it is essential to be able clearly to identify the population at risk.

The nature of inheritance of a disorder will determine the ease with which the population at risk can be identified. Autosomal dominant disorders will generally manifest themselves in the affected individual and the family history will be clear, but carrier identification may be of value when there is a positive family history and the disorder has either a variable or late manifestation, e.g.

Huntington's chorea. Disorders of the autosomal recessive or X-linked inheritance pattern may not be apparent until an affected individual is born, e.g. cystic fibrosis, and a positive family history may not be detected. Some inherited disorders occur with a high frequency in particular ethnic groups. These include Tay–Sachs disease in Ashkenazi Jews, sickle cell disease in Afro-Caribbeans and thalassaemia in people of mediterranean origin. In these instances, family history as well as ethnic origin are important when detecting those at risk. However, with the breakdown of the extended family there are many individuals, including those who have been adopted, who do not know their family history. Therefore, while a positive family history is extremely useful in identifying those at risk, a negative history does not exclude risk.

Identification of carrier status before pregnancy occurs permits appropriate genetic counselling and risk evaluation, which will optimize prenatal diagnosis. Screening of ethnic minorities for the haemoglobinopathies is well established both in hospital and primary care (Modell & Modell 1990). Carrier status for the haemoglobinopathies is possible because of easily discernible changes in red blood cell indices and haemoglobin. However, population screening for disorders such as cystic fibrosis has only been possible since the responsible gene has been identified (Rommens et al 1989). There is increasing experience of screening for this gene defect, both in families with a positive history (Super et al 1994) and in the general population (Livingstone et al 1994). Such screening does not appear to cause a great increase in anxiety among the population screened (Thornton et al 1990, Watson et al 1992).

CHROMOSOME ABNORMALITIES

Following the early work of Painter (1923) it was accepted for many years that the normal diploid chromosome number in man was 48. In 1956, Tjio and Levan, studying human fetal lung fibroblasts, found only 46 but were able to describe clearly the pairing of individual chromosomes. They knew that one other group had only been able to find 46 chromosomes, and that this was the correct number was confirmed by Ford and Hamerton in the same year. These studies were made possible by advances in cytogenetics: the use of colchicine as a spindle inhibitor, hypotonic saline to swell the cell, and the technique, borrowed from the botanical cytogeneticists, of squashing the preparation between slide and coverslip to further enhance cell dispersal. These techniques, though refined, are still fundamental in human cytogenetics today. Further advances included the development of a technique for culturing peripheral blood lymphocytes (Nowell & Hungerford 1960), quinacrine banding (Casperson et al 1970) and Giemsa banding (Seabright 1971, Sumner et al 1971). As banding techniques improve further, the

ability to detect chromosome anomalies is increasing (Speleman et al 1992) and fluorescence-in-situ hybridization (FISH) will revolutionize cytogenetics.

Human constitutional chromosomal abnormalities

The first human chromosome abnormality to be discovered was that of Down's syndrome. In 1959, Lejeune et al reported the observation of an extra small acrocentric chromosome in fibroblast cultures of patients with Down's syndrome. At that time, the two pairs of small acrocentrics, 21 and 22, were not readily distinguished and it was decided that the extra chromosome was probably one of the second smallest pairs, number 21. Subsequent studies with meiotic preparations and with banding techniques have shown this conclusion to be wrong and that it is after all the smallest chromosome pair which is affected. However, the term trisomy 21 for the chromosome abnormality in Down's syndrome (Fig. 15.1) had become so well established that we now define the smallest chromosome pair as being number 21 and the second smallest as number 22.

Although trisomy 21 was confirmed as the abnormality in the great bulk of cases, it was found that in about 3% of Down's syndrome children there were 46 chromosomes but that one of these was an abnormal chromosome arising from the centric fusion of a chromosome with another acrocentric chromosome, 13–15 or 21–22, in a Robertsonian translocation (Fig. 15.2; Polani et al 1960). These children are effectively trisomic for 21, having two independent chromosomes 21 and a third 21 fused to another acrocentric chromosome. In about half of these translocation cases, when involving fusion of a 21 with one of the pairs 13–15, usually 14, it is found that one or other parent carries the translocation in a symptomless balanced form (Fig. 15.3; Penrose et al 1960, Penrose & Delhanty 1961, Sergovich et al 1962, Carter et al 1986).

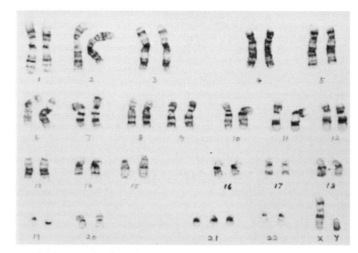

Fig. 15.1 G-banded karyotype of a male Down's syndrome patient with standard trisomy 21.

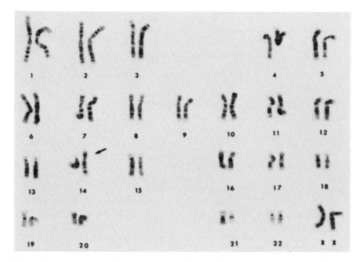

Fig. 15.2   G-banded karyotype of a Down's syndrome patient with a Robertsonian translocation between chromosomes 14 and 21, resulting in effective trisomy for chromosome 21.

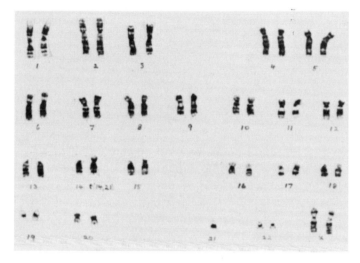

Fig. 15.3   G-banded karyotype of clinically normal female patient with a balanced Robertsonian translocation between chromosomes 14 and 15.

It is important to recognize such cases, both because a parent with a balanced translocation is at increased risk of further Down's syndrome children, and because other relatives may also carry the balanced translocation and should be identified. It should be noted that an individual who carries a 21;21 translocation cannot have a normal child; all will be either monosomic or trisomic for chromosome 21 (Bavin et al 1963).

The well-known association of trisomic Down's syndrome birth and maternal age arises specifically through meiotic errors (non-dysjunction) in the formation of the ovum. There has been speculation for many years as to the likely mechanism for the maternal age effect. One possibility is that the older the mother is the less likely she is to abort a trisomic fetus spontaneously (Stein et al 1986).

Following Lejeune's discovery of trisomy 21 in Down's syndrome there was a spate of discoveries of human syndromes of chromosomal abnormality in 1959 and the early 1960s. These included D trisomy (trisomy 13; Patau et al 1960); E trisomy (trisomy 18; Edwards et al 1960); XXY and variants in Klinefelter's syndrome (Jacobs & Strong 1959) and complete or mosaic 45, X karyotype in Turner's syndrome (Ford et al 1969). Subsequent studies have revealed further sex chromosomal anomalies, including XXX and XYY syndromes and their variants, structural sex chromosome anomalies, the XY sex constitution in testicular feminization and XX males who carry Y chromosomal material translocated to their X (Affara et al 1986). There have also been many new autosomal anomaly syndromes described including further trisomies, such as that for chromosome 8. Many structural deletions or rearrangements such as cri du chat syndrome are found in which there is a deletion of the short arm of chromosome 5, and deletions in several syndromes that are not always chromosomal, at least at a microscopic level, such as bilateral retinoblastoma, Wilm's tumour and Prader–Willi syndrome. In some of the latter conditions the recently described phenomenon, uniparental isodisomy of parentally imprinted genes, is the cause (Malcolm et al 1991). Studies in which tissue from spontaneous abortuses have been karyotyped, especially early abortuses, show a high incidence of chromosomal anomaly—up to 50% or more. Many of the trisomies and other abnormalities found are never seen in term or near-term births, indicating that they are inevitably lethal. Yet other abnormalities, especially most monosomies, which must occur, are not seen even in the earliest abortuses, suggesting an earlier lethality.

Not only is the chromosomal count and configuration important, but advancing techniques have permitted the identification of a fragile site at Xq27.3 or fragile X, the second commonest cause of mental retardation after Down's syndrome. Affected males have moderate to severe intellectual handicap, a long face, large ears and macro-orchidism. Heterozygous females may have lesser degrees of intellectual handicap. Screening is now available for this condition, thus allowing accurate determination of carrier status which permits appropriate selection for prenatal diagnostic techniques (Turner et al 1992).

Screening for chromosomal abnormality

Maternal age

The incidence of chromosomal abnormalities in a fetus increases with advancing maternal age as shown in Table 15.1. As many fetuses with an abnormal karyotype miscarry or die in utero, the incidence of abnormalities *decreases* with advancing gestation, and this has to be considered when screening. In the past, the age of 35 years has been adopted as an arbitrary cut-off point for

Table 15.1 Rates per 1000 of chromosomal abnormality at amniocentesis (amino) and livebirths (LB) by maternal age

Maternal age (years)	47, + 21		47, + 18		47, + 13		47, XXX		47, XXY		Other clinically significant abnormalities‡		All abnormalities§	
	Amnio*	LB**	Amnio	LB	Amnio†	LB††	Amino	LB	Amino	LB	Amino	LB	Amino	LB
33	2.4	1.6	0.6	0.2	0.4	0.2	0.4	0.4	0.4	0.4	1.1	0.8	4.6–5.4	2.9–3.5
34	3.1	2.0	0.8	0.2	0.4	0.2	0.5	0.5	0.5	0.4	1.2	0.8	5.8–6.5	3.7–4.2
35	4.0	2.6	1.0	0.3	0.5	0.3	0.6	0.5	0.6	0.6	1.3	0.9	7.4–8.0	4.7–5.2
36	5.2	3.4	1.3	0.4	0.6	0.3	0.7	0.6	0.8	0.7	1.3	0.9	9.5–9.9	5.9–6.4
37	6.7	4.4	1.6	0.5	0.6	0.4	0.8	0.8	1.0	0.9	1.4	1.0	12.1–12.2	7.6–7.9
38	8.7	5.7	2.1	0.6	0.7	0.4	1.0	0.9	1.2	1.1	1.5	1.0	15.4–15.2	9.7–9.8
39	11.2	7.3	2.6	0.8	0.9	0.5	1.2	1.1	1.5	1.4	1.6	1.1	19.6–19.0	12.3–12.1
40	14.5	9.4	3.3	1.0	1.0	0.5	1.4	1.3	1.9	1.7	1.7	1.2	25.0–23.8	15.7–15.2
41	18.7	12.2	4.2	1.2	1.1	0.6	1.7	1.6	2.4	2.2	1.8	1.2	31.9–29.9	20.1–19.0
42	24.1	15.7	5.2	1.6	1.3	0.7	2.0	1.9	3.0	2.7	1.9	1.3	40.7–37.6	25.6–23.9
43	31.1	20.2	6.6	2.0	1.5	0.8	2.4	2.2	3.8	3.4	2.0	1.4	51.9–47.5	32.6–30.2
44	40.1	26.1	8.4	2.5	1.8	1.0	2.9	2.7	4.7	4.3	2.2	1.5	66.1–60.1	41.6–38.1
45	51.8	33.7	10.6	3.2	2.0	1.1	3.4	3.2	5.9	5.4	2.3	1.6	84.3–76.0	53.0–48.2
46	66.8	43.4	13.3	4.0	2.4	1.3	4.1	3.8	7.4	6.8	2.4	1.7	107.5–96.5	67.6–61.0
47	86.2	56.0	16.9	5.1	2.7	1.5	4.9	4.6	9.3	8.5	2.6	1.8	137.1–122.6	86.2–77.5
48	111.2	72.3	21.3	6.4	3.1	1.8	5.9	5.5	11.7	10.7	2.7	1.9	174.8–155.9	109.9–98.5
49	143.5	93.3	26.9	8.1	3.6	2.0	7.0	6.5	14.6	13.4	2.9	2.0	222.9–198.6	140.1–125.3

*, ** Values of 0.08 and 0.06 respectively should be added to these values to allow for structural rearrangements associated with Down's syndrome.
†, †† Values of 0.06 and 0.03 respectively should be added to these values to allow for structural rearrangements associated with trisomy 13.
‡ Include structural rearrangements associated with trisomies 13 and 21.
§ First value of range given is derived from the regression analysis on all abnormalities; the second by adding the values for all abnormalities.
Reproduced from Tables 1–4 from Hook et al (1983) with permission.

offering prenatal diagnosis. This arose because the assumed risk of invasive testing by amniocentesis was thought to be equal to the risk of a positive result. However, because the majority of babies in the UK are born to women under the age of 35 years, the majority of babies with karyotype anomalies are born to these women. Thus, maternal age alone will only identify a maximum of 30% of pregnancies affected by Down's syndrome, the commonest chromosomal abnormality. Therefore population screening is an area of active research into a screening test which could be applied to the whole population to correctly identify those pregnancies at risk. The ideal test does not yet exist, but maternal serum screening and nuchal translucency studies show promise.

Serum screening for chromosomal anomalies

The observation by Merkatz and colleagues (1984) of a correlation between low maternal serum alphafetoprotein levels (MSAFP) and fetal trisomy raised the possibility of an alternative, or complementary, method of selecting mothers for chromosomal prenatal diagnosis. This observation was rapidly confirmed by several centres (Chard et al 1984, Cuckle et al 1984, Fuhrmann et al 1984, Tabor et al 1984, Baumgarten et al 1985). There is a relatively low MSAFP in fetuses with trisomies even in the presence of a neural tube or abdominal wall defect (Macri et al 1986). Cuckle and colleagues (1984) proposed the use of a scale of cut-off values for MSAFP

and age for selection for amniocentesis. Other workers expressed reservations about using this particular combination on the grounds of a too high false positive rate (7–12%) necessitating too many amniocenteses on woman with an unaffected fetus (Houlsby 1984, Seller 1984, Spencer & Carpenter 1985, Wyatt 1985), with consequent maternal anxiety and some increases in miscarriage. Although in their response, Cuckle and colleagues (1985) accepted that only a 30% detection rate with an 11.5% false-positive rate could be expected, they felt that a pilot study was justified. Murday & Slack (1985) tested this hypothesis, and concluded that the measurement of MSAFP was only useful in women aged 32 years and over.

However, a marked improvement in the antenatal detection of pregnancies at risk of Down's syndrome can be achieved with the additional assay of human chorionic gonadotrophin (hCG) (Bogart et al 1987) and unconjugated oestriol (UE₃) (Wald et al 1988a). With the combination of hCG, UE₃, MSAFP and maternal age, Wald et al (1988b) estimated that 60% of affected pregnancies would be detected at a similar amniocentesis rate to that if screening was based on maternal age alone. Using individual risk estimated from MSAFP and hCG, Lewis et al (1991) concluded that screening was more effective than maternal age and genetic history alone. The success rate in their study was 73%. Other markers have also been investigated, including urea-resistant neutrophil alkaline phosphatase (Cuckle et al 1990) and pregnancy-associated plasma protein A (Wald et al 1992).

The most commonly applied test at present is the so-called *triple test* performed at 16–18 weeks, which measures MSAFP, hCG, UE$_3$ and maternal age in relation to confirmed gestation. The test result is reported as a risk ratio, and described as screen positive if the risk is 1 : 250 or greater. Using this test in over 12 000 women, Wald et al (1992) achieved a detection rate of 48%, with 4.8% false-positives. If the maternal blood result was reported as screen-positive, the risk ratio was 1 : 43. Clearly, while better than a pick-up rate of 30% based on age alone, this method of screening is still far from ideal. Many problems have arisen with serum testing, particularly with regard to maternal anxiety in the case of false-positives and the devastating effect of a false-negative. It has become obvious that many health-care workers in the field of antenatal care are not fully conversant with the implications of triple test screening and results, and further training is required (Statham & Green 1993). It is essential that all implications of a new screening test are fully considered, including the ethical and legal aspects (Edwards & Hall 1992).

Ultrasound screening for chromosomal anomalies

The association between nuchal oedema in the first trimester and structural and karyotype anomalies has become evident with high resolution ultrasound (Ville et al 1992). Clearly, as many pregnancies affected by a karyotypic abnormality miscarry, the earlier the diagnosis is made, the higher the pick-up rate will be. Nicolaides et al (1992) have examined the value of measurement of nuchal translucency by ultrasound at 10–14 weeks' gestation. In this preliminary study of high-risk women, using a cut-off of 3 mm, 18 of 28 (68%) chromosomally abnormal fetuses were detected. The addition of maternal age to nuchal translucency has increased the detection rate, and the study is ongoing. This measurement may pick up many pregnancies destined to miscarry however, as pregnancy loss with chromosomal abnormality is common. Before its introduction into general population screening, a low-risk population must be studied without intervention in order to determine the natural history. In a preliminary low-risk population study, the pick-up of chromosomal anomalies does not appear to be so reliable (Bewley et al 1994).

In addition to early examination of fetal nuchal translucency, there are many structural anomalies detected by ultrasound which may lead to the suspicion that a fetus has aneuploidy. Some anomalies have a very strong association (e.g. 50% of fetuses with an atrioventriculoseptal defect with normal situs have trisomy 21), while others have a much lower incidence (e.g. 1 : 200 fetuses with isolated choroid plexus cysts have abnormal chromosomes). However, if a fetus has more than one structural abnormality, the risk of aneuploidy increases and karyo-

typing may be offered when such anomalies are detected (see Ch. 14).

Counselling

Counselling of patients is an integral part of any screening procedure. As mentioned above, if a new screening test is introduced without adequate assessment and training of relevant health-care workers, many problems will arise. In addition to providing adequate information regarding what a positive result means, and explanation that a negative screening result does not equate with a negative diagnosis, those involved must have a mechanism whereby results of screening tests can be rapidly and sympathetically passed on to the patient, with a set protocol for managing those pregnancies with a positive screen result.

Management of a patient with a screen positive result

A firm diagnosis of chromosomal abnormality can only be made by an invasive test to examine the fetal chromosomes. Women who are screen positive should therefore be offered fetal karyotyping by invasive testing. It is not appropriate to offer a second screening test for reassurance. However, some women, when faced with a screen-positive triple test or nuchal translucency result, do not wish to proceed to invasive testing such as amniocentesis unless there is additional evidence that the fetus may be chromosomally abnormal. They may therefore request a detailed scan looking for ultrasound markers such as choroid plexus cysts. However, they cannot be reassured by a negative scan and must understand that an invasive test to examine the chromosomes is the only way to know definitely if a fetus is chromosomally normal or not.

METABOLIC DISORDERS

The inborn errors of metabolism are single gene defects inherited according to Mendelian patterns. They may be autosomal or X linked. The realization that a pregnancy is at risk will usually come from the recognition that a previous child of the parents was affected. Only in conditions such as Tay–Sachs, where screening of the at-risk population is well established, can a couple be identified as at high risk of having an affected pregnancy before conception occurs. In most circumstances, it is unusual for a carrier couple to be identified prior to an affected pregnancy. Population screening for conditions such as cystic fibrosis may alter this.

Clearly it is preferable for maximum information to be available as soon after an affected child is born, to allow full counselling of the parents and relatives before further pregnancies occur. Whilst confirmation of some metabolic disorders can be difficult, prenatal diagnosis may be relatively easy as investigation often relies upon assessing enzyme activity, which in a homozygous affected individual is usually very low or absent. However, there may be overlap of enzyme activity between a heterozygous (carrier) fetus and homozygous (affected) fetus, and care must be taken. The methods for diagnosing inborn errors of metabolism vary and include biochemical or enzyme assay in amniotic fluid, cultured or uncultured chorionic villi, or fetal fibroblasts (amniocytes). Tests are constantly being developed and refined, and it is important that when a couple at risk is seen for prenatal diagnosis, the obstetrician seeks advice from a genetics centre as to the nature and availability of relevant investigations.

The list of inborn errors of metabolism for which prenatal diagnosis is suitable is long and constantly increasing; Table 15.2 provides a shortened list of some of those conditions amenable to prenatal detection.

Screening for inborn errors of metabolism

The nature and level of sophistication of population screening for metabolic disorders has changed greatly in the recent past. Screening of the population of Ashkenazi Jews, of whom 1 in 30 is a carrier for Tay–Sachs disease, has been possible for over 20 years. This screening initially relied upon measurement of reduced enzyme activity of hexoaminidase A. Screening projects were introduced in the USA in 1970. Couples at risk were offered prenatal diagnosis and termination if the pregnancy was affected, and by 1986 there had been an estimated fall of 70–85% in the incidence of babies being born with the disease

(Chapple 1992). Population screening permits those who are carriers of the disease to adjust to the potential problems *before* embarking on pregnancy, which reduces anxiety and psychological morbidity.

Since the identification of the mutant gene responsible for cystic fibrosis, screening for carrier status has been possible. However, it is not possible to screen for all the numerous cystic fibrosis alleles, and screening would therefore not identify all carriers. If prenatal diagnosis were performed in those identified to be at risk of the commonest mutation (ΔF 508), up to a third of affected fetuses would be missed. Although this may be viewed as insufficient pick up to warrant population screening, many investigators argue that the ability to reduce the birth incidence by two-thirds is a powerful argument for carefully constructed pilot trials.

Cascade screening, where the relatives of an affected individual are screened, offers a much more reliable pickup of cystic fibrosis carriers and is also the method of screening adopted in many of the much less common inborn errors of metabolism. It obviously misses those at risk but without an affected child. The most appropriate method of screening for cystic fibrosis is still not established.

HAEMOGLOBINOPATHIES

Inherited haemoglobin defects are responsible for significant morbidity and mortality worldwide and present a vast public health problem, which is concentrated in

Table 15.2 Disorders for which prenatal diagnosis is currently available

Disorder	Method of prenatal diagnosis
Chromosomal	
Down's syndrome, trisomies 13 and 18, and other autosomal trisomies	Amniocentesis or chorionic villus sampling with chromosome analysis
Klinefelter's syndrome and other sex chromosome aneuploidy in males	Amniocentesis or chorionic villus sampling with chromosome analysis
Turner's syndrome, XXX syndrome, and other sex chromosome aneuploidy in females	Amniocentesis or chorionic villus sampling with chromosome analysis
Chromosome deletions or rearrangements, balanced or aneuploid	Amniocentesis or chorionic villus sampling with chromosome analysis
Fragile (X) syndrome	Fetal blood sample and chromosome analysis
Single gene defects with known gene product	
Sickle cell disease and thalassaemias	Site specific probe and restriction enzymes or DNA deletion
Inborn errors of metabolism	
Mucopolysaccharidoses	Enzyme assay
Aminoacidopathies:	
Phenylketonuria	Restriction fragment length polymorphism
Ornithine carbamoyl transferase deficiency	Enzyme assay on fetal liver biopsy
Citrullinuria	Enzyme assay
Argininosuccinicaciduria	Enzyme assay
Homocystinuria	Enzyme assay
Maple syrup urine disease	Enzyme assay
Carbohydrate disorders:	
Galactosaemia	Enzyme assay with gas chromatography or mass spectroscopy, or both, of amniotic fluid
Galactokinase and galactose 4-epimerase deficiency	Enzyme assay with gas chromatography or mass spectroscopy, or both, of amniotic fluid
Glucose-6-phosphate dehydrogenase deficiency	Enzyme assay
Glycogenoses	Enzyme assay

Table 15.2 (*contd*)

Purine and pyrimidine disorders:	
Lesch–Nyhan syndrome	Enzyme assay with restriction fragment length polymorphism
Adenine phosphoribosyl transferase deficiency	Enzyme assay
Organic acidurias:	
Methylmalonic acidurias	Enzyme assay or gas chromatography and mass spectroscopy
Proprionic acidaemia	Enzyme assay or gas chromatography mass spectroscopy
3-Methylcrotonyl coenzyme A carboxylase deficiency	Enzyme assay
Lipid disorders:	
Anderson–Fabry disease	Enzyme assay with restriction fragment length polymorphism
Farber's disease	Enzyme assay
Fucosidosis	Enzyme assay
Gangliosidoses	Enzyme assay
Gaucher's disease	Enzyme assay
I cell disease	Enzyme assay
Krabbe's disease	Enzyme assay
Mannosidosis	Enzyme assay
Metachromatic leucodystrophy	Enzyme assay
Mucolipidosis III	Enzyme assay
Niemann–Pick disease	Enzyme assay
Sialidosis	Enzyme assay
Wolman's disease	Enzyme assay
Other:	
Acid phosphatasia	Enzyme assay
Adrenal hyperplasia (21-hydroxylase deficiency)	Hormone assay, HLA antigen or HLA DNA linkage, 21-hydroxylase gene restriction fragment length polymorphism
Ccrebrohepatorenal syndrome	Long chain fatty acid assay with enzyme assay
Cystinosis	Uptake of radiolabelled sulphur-35
Hypophosphatasia	Enzyme assay
Placental steroid sulphatase deficiency (X linked ichthyosis)	Hormone assay and enzyme assay
Coagulation defects	
Haemophilia A and B	Factor VIII or factor IX assay with restriction fragment length polymorphism
Factor X deficiency	Restriction fragment length polymorphism
Immune deficiency disorders	
Severe combined immunodeficiency syndrome	Enzyme assay
T cell immunodeficiency	Enzyme assay
Collagen disorders	
Ehlers–Danlos syndrome types II and V (some cases)	DNA delection
Osteogenesis imperfecta types I and II (some cases)	DNA deletion
Single gene defects with unknown gene product	
Cystic fibrosis	Amniotic fluid enzyme assay with restriction fragment length polymorphism
Duchenne and Becker types of muscular dystrophy	Restriction fragment length polymorphism
Huntington's chorea	Restriction fragment length polymorphism
Adult polycystic kidney disease	Restriction fragment length polymorphism
Generalized neurofibromatosis (von Recklinghausen's disease)	Restriction fragment length polymorphism
Tuberous sclerosis	Restriction fragment length polymorphism
Myotonic dystrophy	Restriction fragment length polymorphism
Ataxia telangiectasia	Chromosome breakage
Bloom's syndrome	Increased sister chromatid exchange and increased ultraviolet sensitivity
Fanconi's anaemia	Chromosome breakage
Robert's syndrome	Chromosome puffs
Xeroderma pigmentosum	DNA repair defect
Epidermolysis bullosa syndromes	Fetal skin biopsy and histology
Hypohidrotic ectodermal dysplasia	Restriction fragment length polymorphism
Congenital nephrosis (Finnish type)	Amniotic fluid α fetoprotein
Multiple endocrine neoplasias	Restriction fragment length polymorphism
Fetal infections	
Intrauterine rubella	Viral RNA specific DNA probe
Intrauterine cytomegalovirus	Antibody detection with lymphocyte transformation test
Other	
α_1 Antitrypsin deficiency	Isoelectric focusing, restriction fragment length polymorphism with site-specific probe
Acute intermittent porphyria	Restriction fragment length polymorphism

Reproduced with permission from Crawfurd (1988).
RNA = ribonucleic acid.
* Lower urinary tract obstruction with a greatly enlarged bladder distending the abdomen.

the populations of the eastern Mediterranean, Middle East, parts of India, South-east Asia, Africa and the West Indies. With immigration from these parts of the world to the UK, this group of inherited disorders, rarely seen in the indigenous population, is now more frequently encountered particularly by obstetricians. Prenatal diagnosis is possible for all the haemoglobinopathies, and population screening in communities at risk can identify those with a positive carrier status. In some countries, e.g. Greece and Cyprus, where beta-thalassaemia is a large public health problem, premarital testing is obligatory and this has led to a major reduction in the number of affected children, but this carries enormous emotional and practical problems for couples who find they are both carriers. However, the techniques for screening and prenatal diagnosis are generally restricted to centres in the developed world, the majority of which are in countries such as the UK where the problem is relatively infrequent.

The genetic disorders of haemoglobin structure and synthesis are single gene disorders which consist of two main groups:

1. The structural haemoglobin variants.
2. Inherited abnormalities of the synthesis of the globin chains of haemoglobin, the thalassaemias.

All normal human haemoglobins have a similar structure, consisting of two different pairs of peptide chains (Fig. 15.4), each of which has a haem molecule attached to it. In fetal life the major haemoglobin is haemoglobin F (α_2, γ_2) although small amounts of normal adult haemoglobin A (α_2, β_2) are synthesized from as early as 6 weeks' gestation. Prior to this, there are several embryonic haemoglobins, which disappear after about 6 weeks' gestation (Fig. 15.5). In adult life, the haemoglobin is mainly A, with about 3% being A$_2$ (α_2, δ_2). The major change from fetal to adult haemoglobin production, i.e. gamma to beta chain synthesis, occurs from about 32 weeks' gestation (Fig. 15.5) with gamma chain synthesis declining rapidly after birth.

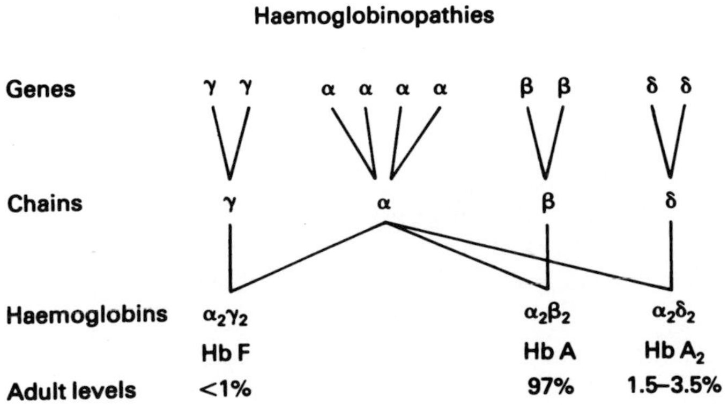

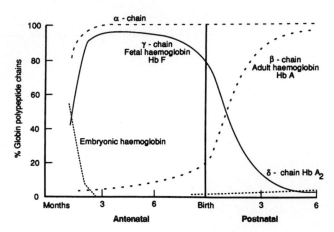

Fig. 15.5 The developmental changes in human haemoglobinopathies. After Huehns et al (1964).

The synthesis and structure of the four globin chains are under separate control. Production of the alpha chain, which is common to all forms of haemoglobin, is under the control of four genes, two inherited from each parent, located on chromosome 16. On the other hand beta chain production is under the control of just two genes, one inherited from each parent, and, together with the genes for gamma and delta chain production, are located on chromosome 11.

From the public health point of view, the most important haemoglobinopathies are the sickling disorders and the thalassaemias, both in the homozygous and heterozygous forms. It must be remembered, of course, that any baby born with homozygous defects of beta chain synthesis or structure will be perfectly healthy at birth and will not develop symptoms and signs of the disorder until 3–6 months of age, when beta chain production usually becomes predominant.

The thalassaemias

This extremely heterogeneous group of genetic disorders of haemoglobin synthesis is characterized by a reduced rate of production of one or more of the globin chains (Weatherall & Clegg 1981). The disorders are classified according to the chain which is inefficiently produced and fall into two main groups: the alpha- and the beta-thalassaemias.

Beta-thalassaemias

The beta-thalassaemias are characterized by an inability to synthesize adult beta chains. Hence these disorders do not present in intrauterine life but only after birth when the effect of the switch from gamma to beta chain synthesis becomes significant. The heterozygous states

Haemoglobinopathies

Genes	γ γ	α α α α	β β	δ δ
Chains	γ	α	β	δ
Haemoglobins	$\alpha_2\gamma_2$		$\alpha_2\beta_2$	$\alpha_2\delta_2$
	Hb F		Hb A	Hb A$_2$
Adult levels	<1%		97%	1.5–3.5%

Fig. 15.4 Genetic control of globin chain synthesis. Adult levels achieved by 6 months of age.

for these conditions are symptomless. However, in the homozygous state for beta-thalassaemia there is marked deficiency of beta chain production and although gamma chain synthesis persists it is usually insufficient to compensate for the deficiency of beta chains and hence there is a severe anaemia. For reasons as yet obscure, the homozygous states for delta-beta thalassaemia are much less severe because compensation by gamma chain synthesis is much more efficient in this disorder.

There are two main forms of beta-thalassaemia, the beta^0-thalassaemia in which no beta chains are produced, and the beta$^+$-thalassaemia in which there is a reduction in the amount of beta chains.

The beta-thalassaemias occur particularly commonly in the Mediterranean island populations, parts of Italy, Greece and the Middle East, in parts of the Indian subcontinent, and throughout South-east Asia. The carrier rates in these populations range from 5% to 20%. The beta^0-thalassaemias are particularly common in Sardinia, the Po valley region of Italy and throughout South-east Asia. The beta$^+$-thalassaemia gene is particularly common in Cyprus, parts of southern Italy and in the Middle East. In many populations, both variants are encountered. Molecular studies have revealed over 91 different mutations (Kazazian 1990).

Thalassaemia major, homozygous thalassaemia resulting from the inheritance of a defective beta globin gene from each parent, was the first identified form of the thalassaemia syndromes. It was described in the 1920s by Cooley, a physician practising in the USA. The first few cases were found in the children of Greek and Italian immigrants. It is a rare inherited abnormality among the indigenous British population. The heterozygote state is found in roughly 1 in 1000 individuals (compared to 1 in 7 in Cyprus) and the birth rate of homozygotes is of the order of 1 in 4 million. Some of the genes involved may be new mutations and some may have been imported from the Mediterranean from as far back as Phoenician times. However, thalassaemia has been brought to the UK in recent years by movements of populations and the arrival of immigrant groups of various ethnic origins.

In the 1950s and 1960s the main source of thalassaemia major cases was from the immigrant Cypriot populations who settled in the Greater London area. From the 1960s there has been a steady increase in the proportion of Asian cases.

Although the majority of the 360 or so patients currently living in the UK are still to be found in and around Greater London, there are increasing numbers of cases in the Midlands, Manchester, Bradford and Leeds. This is not only due to the fact that there has been an influx of Asian immigrants to these areas but that the Cypriot population of Greater London is an homogeneous population which has taken advantage of the availability of prenatal diagnosis and consequently there has been a dramatic reduction in the number of homozygotes born to Cypriot couples at risk.

The Asian immigrant population, unlike the Cypriot, is very heterogeneous, with incidences of thalassaemia varying markedly from group to group. They continue to have a high incidence of first-cousin marriages. Large groups of rural Indians and Pakistanis have settled in the industrial towns of the Midlands. Relatively few of them make use of genetic counselling or fetal diagnosis and the incidence of thalassaemic children in these groups continues to rise.

The modern management of thalassaemia consists of regular blood transfusions, timely splenectomy and iron chelation therapy to avoid iron overload. With these techniques, survival continues to increase and is now well past the third decade. Death can still occur from the effects of iron overload (endocrine, hepatic and myocardial dysfunction). Puberty may be delayed or incomplete, although successful pregnancy in a transfusion-dependent thalassaemic woman can occur (Goldfarb et al 1982). Bone marrow transplantation has been successfully employed, and this suggests that thalassaemia may be amenable to gene therapy in the future (Lancet Editorial 1987).

Alpha-thalassaemias

The alpha-thalassaemias are characterized by an inability to produce the alpha chains which are common to haemoglobins A, A$_2$ and F. In fetal life a deficiency of alpha chains results in the production of excess gamma chains which form γ_4 molecules or haemoglobin Barts (named because it was first identified in a Chinese baby born at St Bartholomew's Hospital, London). In adult life a deficiency of alpha chains leads to excess of beta chains which form β_4 tetramers of haemoglobin (Hb H). Haemoglobin Barts and H are unstable and also useless oxygen carriers. There are many different alpha-thalassaemia determinants which are associated with either a reduced or total absence of alpha chain production. In their heterozygous states these disorders are symptomless but in the homozygous or compound heterozygous states they give rise to a spectrum of disorders ranging from intrauterine death to a haemolytic anaemia of variable severity in adult life.

Normal individuals have four functional alpha genes. Alpha-thalassaemia, unlike beta-thalassaemia, is often but not always a gene deletion. There are two forms of alpha-thalassaemia trait which are the result of inheriting two or three normal alpha genes instead of the usual four. These are called alpha^0- and alpha$^+$-thalassaemia (Fig. 15.6), sometimes known as alpha^1- and alpha^2-thalassaemia respectively. HbH disease is an intermediate form of alpha-thalassaemia in which there is only one functional alpha gene; HbH is the name given to the unstable haemoglobin formed by tetramers of the beta

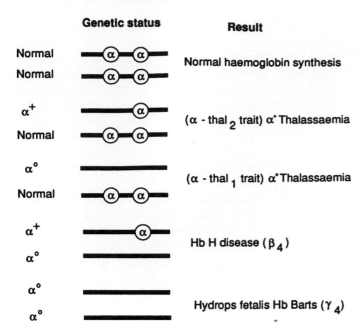

Fig. 15.6 Alpha genes and the various thalassaemias resulting from alpha gene deletion.

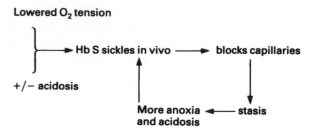

Fig. 15.7 Sequence of events in intravascular sickling.

chains when there is a relative lack of alpha chains. Alpha-thalassaemia major, in which there are no functional alpha genes, is incompatible with life and pregnancy usually ends prematurely in a neonate with hydrops which will only survive a matter of hours if born alive. This is a common condition in South-east Asia.

Pregnancy with an alpha-thalassaemia hydrops is associated with severe, sometimes life-threatening pre-eclampsia. Vaginal deliveries can be associated with obstetric complications due to the increased size of the fetus and placenta. If screening of the parents indicates that there is a risk of alpha-thalassaemia, the couple should be referred for prenatal diagnosis in order to try and avoid such problems. A group highly at risk includes recent refugees from Indo-China.

Sickle cell disease

Over 250 structural variants of the globin chains have been described but the most important by far, both numerically and clinically, is sickle cell haemoglobin (HbS). This is a variant of the beta chain where there is one amino acid substitution at the sixth position, a glutamine replacing a valine residue. HbS has the unique physical property that, despite being a soluble protein in its oxygenated form, in its reduced state the molecules become stacked on one another, forming tactoids, which distort the red cells to the characteristic shape which gives the haemoglobin its name. These sickled cells, because of their rigid structure, tend to block small blood vessels. The sickling phenomenon occurs particularly in conditions of lowered oxygen tension but may also be favoured

by acidosis, dehydration or cooling, causing stasis in small blood vessels (Fig. 15.7).

Sickle cell syndromes

The sickling disorders include the heterozygous state for sickle cell haemoglobin, sickle cell trait (HbAS); homozygous sickle cell disease (HbSS); compound heterozygotes for Hb variants, the most important of which is sickle cell/HbC disease (HbSC), and sickle cell thalassaemia. Although these disorders are more commonly seen in black people of African origin, they can be found in Saudi Arabians, Indians and Mediterraneans.

The characteristic feature of homozygous sickle cell anaemia (HbSS) is the occurrence of periods of health punctuated by periods of crisis. Between 3 and 6 months of age, when normal HbA production usually becomes predominant, a chronic haemolytic anaemia develops with a haemoglobin level between 6 and 9 g/dl. Even if the haemoglobin is in the lower range, symptoms of anaemia are surprisingly few. This is because of the low affinity of HbS for oxygen; oxygen delivery to the tissues is facilitated, and there is little or no cellular anoxia even on exertion.

The acute episodes due to intravascular sickling are of major importance, because they cause vascular occlusion which can lead to tissue infarction. Sickling crises can be precipitated by infection, dehydration and hypoxia. Renal complications are common, due to sickling in the renal medullary circulation. The prognosis depends greatly on the environment; in Africa, probably less than 10% of homozygous children reach adulthood, whereas in the West Indies, where prompt treatment and infection prophylaxis are more easily available, the outlook is better. At present, there is no effective long-term method of reducing the liability of red cells to sickle. Once a crisis is established, adequate fluid replacement and antibiotics are the mainstay of treatment.

Sickle cell haemoglobin C disease (HbSC) is a milder variant of HbSS, with less anaemia. However, these individuals are just as much at risk of sickling crises. Sickle cell trait (HbAS), on the other hand, results in no detectable abnormality under normal circumstances, and sickling crises occur only in situations of extreme anoxia, dehydration and acidosis.

Screening for haemoglobinopathies

In most cases, screening procedures are not instigated until the woman is pregnant or before an anaesthetic. Screening consists of examination of a blood sample for the red cell indices (low MCV), Sickledex, haemoglobin electrophoresis and, if indicated, HbA_2 and HbF quantitation. If a woman is found to be heterozygous for a haemoglobinopathy, it is necessary to check the partner. If he has normal haemoglobin, at worst the offspring will be heterozygotes, like the mother, and prenatal diagnosis is therefore not offered. However, if the male partner is also heterozygous, there is a 1 in 4 risk of a fetus being affected and prenatal diagnosis should then be discussed. All these procedures take time, and therefore, in a first pregnancy, prenatal diagnosis may be delayed considerably. However, in subsequent pregnancies, or where the status of both parents is known before a pregnancy occurs, early prenatal diagnosis by chorion villus sampling can be offered.

FETAL INFECTION

Not all infectious agents are associated with congenital infection but of those that are, some carry the risk of fetal abnormality, organ dysfunction or even death in utero. The approach to the diagnosis of fetal infection includes maternal serology, ultrasound examination of the fetus and assessment of whether the fetus is infected by direct investigation. Confirmation of fetal infection relies on the demonstration of the infectious agent within fetal tissue or the presence of specific IgM within the fetal circulation (IgG crosses the placenta and therefore may be maternal in origin).

There are five main infections where prenatal diagnosis has been employed to assess fetal state.

1. rubella
2. toxoplasmosis
3. cytomegalovirus
4. varicella
5. parvovirus B19.

Rubella

Rubella is a viral illness with mild symptoms which include an erythematous rash. Transmission occurs via direct contact with nasopharyngeal secretions of an infected individual. It generally affects children of school age and it is often subclinical, particularly in adults. However, fetal infection with rubella in the first trimester carries an extremely high morbidity, congenital rubella being a cause of severe and permanent disability. In the UK, there is a national immunization programme and about 2.8–3% of pregnant women fail to demonstrate rubella antibodies, indicating that they are susceptible to the infection (Noah & Fowle 1988). Symptomatic maternal infection is usually mild, occurring 14–21 days after exposure. The fetus may become infected as a result of transplacental passage of the virus during maternal viraemia, and such infection may lead to spontaneous abortion, stillbirth, congenital defects or an apparently normal infant. The majority of congenital rubella follows primary maternal infection, reinfection being rare although it can occur in women with previous naturally acquired rubella or vaccination (Best et al 1989). The risk to the fetus, which is greater in a primary infection, is related to the gestational age at infection, no major defects being found following maternal infection after the 17th week of pregnancy (Munro et al 1987), although deafness can occur.

The abnormalities associated with congenital rubella can be divided into transient, permanent and late. Transient manifestations may persist for up to 6 months and include skin lesions, hepatosplenomegaly, thrombocytopenic purpura and haemolytic anaemia. Permanent sequelae commonly include sensorineural hearing loss, heart defects, cataracts, and encephalopathy which results in severe mental retardation. The structural defects most commonly occur following maternal infection before the 12th week of pregnancy. Endocrinopathies, sensorineural hearing loss and progressive cataracts can be late manifestations. The overall mortality for infants with congenital rubella is 5–35%.

Maternal diagnosis depends upon serology demonstrating rubella-specific IgM within a month of the rash, or a four-fold rise in IgG. However, as the fetus is not invariably infected following proven maternal infection, prenatal investigations are essential. Amniocentesis has been used, but demonstration of the rubella virus in the amniotic fluid is time-consuming and not entirely reliable. Using DNA probes, rubella-specific RNA sequences can be detected in chorionic villi (Terry et al 1986) and thus CVS, which can be performed from the end of the first trimester, has a role in the diagnosis of congenital rubella. Fetal blood sampling, after 20 weeks, can be used to demonstrate IgM in fetal serum (Morgan-Capner et al 1985).

There is no specific treatment for rubella. However, if fetal infection is proven, the option of termination of the pregnancy can be discussed.

Screening for rubella immunity in pregnancy is universal in the UK. If a woman is seronegative, she must be informed, advised to seek medical advice if contact occurs and offered postnatal immunization.

Toxoplasmosis

The domestic cat is the main source of infection with *Toxoplasma gondii*, a zoonotic parasite. The oocytes of the parasite are secreted in cat faeces, from where they can enter intermediate hosts such as birds, rabbits, sheep, cows and humans. Apart from this source of transmission, the eating of undercooked meat places humans at risk of infection.

The clinical manifestations of toxoplasma infection are mild and non-specific, including low-grade fever, headache, malaise and muscular pains. The infection is usually benign, but in some cases can persist and lead to encephalitis, myocarditis, pneumonitis, hepatitis and chorioretinitis. Infection in pregnancy is usually subclinical. The parasite may be transmitted across the placenta in 40–50% of cases, leading to congenital infection which may not be apparent at birth. The risk to the fetus is directly related to the gestational age at which maternal infection occurs, increasing from 10% transmission in the first trimester to 90% at the end of the third trimester (Stray-Pedersen 1993). However, the severity of infection is less the later in the pregnancy it occurs. When maternal infection is acquired before 20 weeks, 25% of infected fetuses will be severely affected, often resulting in spontaneous abortion or intrauterine death. Fifteen percent will be mildly affected and the remainder will be subclinical. Maternal infection in the second half of pregnancy, whilst carrying a higher risk of transmission to the fetus, rarely results in severe fetal infection. Severe fetal infection causes chorioretinitis, hydrocephalus, intracranial calcifications and convulsions, with a 12% mortality and 85% risk of mental retardation in the survivors.

The diagnosis of toxoplasma infection depends on direct identification of the parasite in body fluids or detection of specific antibodies. Serology is the primary method of diagnosis, both in the mother and fetus. IgM appears soon after infection, reaching maximum levels by a month generally decreasing subsequently, although IgM may remain detectable for up to 2 years. IgG appears after a few weeks with peak levels at 2–6 months.

A problem in pregnancy is that accurate timing of infection is very difficult, especially if trying to determine whether infection occurred before or after conception, and repeated measurements of IgM and IgG are necessary.

If maternal infection in pregnancy is diagnosed or suspected, the diagnosis of fetal infection is confirmed if parasites are obtained from amniotic fluid, or if IgM is detected in fetal blood. DNA techniques are now also being used. The high prevalence of toxoplasma infection in France was the main spur behind the development of ultrasound-guided fetal blood sampling (Daffos et al 1983). One difficulty in the interpretation of fetal blood results is that IgM is not produced until the 19th week, and therefore early blood samples may be negative for IgM (Daffos et al 1988). If there is evidence of fetal infection, termination of pregnancy may be considered. The confirmation of intrauterine infection, even with prenatal diagnostic techniques available today, may not be possible and therefore infants of mothers with proven infection during pregnancy should be followed up for 12–18 months.

Screening for toxoplasmosis in pregnancy is commonplace in France, but not in the UK. When screening is employed, repeated blood tests are required in seronegative women to exclude infection. Since half the proven maternal infections do not result in fetal infection, prenatal diagnosis must be offered before any consideration of pregnancy termination.

Toxoplasma infection can be treated, although in the healthy non-pregnant adult it is not necessary. However, in pregnancy treatment reduces the risk of fetal infection and should therefore always be offered. The optimum schedule of treatment is uncertain, but the therapeutic efficiency is known to be dependent upon the gestational age at which infection occurred, early recognition and whether or not the fetus is infected by the time treatment begins. Spiramycin is the drug of choice, capable of killing free and intracellular parasites. It crosses the placenta (Forestier et al 1987) although fetal blood levels are only half maternal levels. However, spiramycin is completely safe to both mother and fetus, with no teratogenic potential. If maternal infection occurs, with no evidence of fetal infection, spiramycin 3 g per day should be given for the remainder of the pregnancy. In definite cases of fetal infection, 3-week courses of spiramycin alternating with 3 weeks of pyrimethamine-sulphadiazine should be given until term.

Cytomegalovirus

Cytomegalovirus (CMV) is the commonest cause of intrauterine infection, with an incidence of 0.2–2.2% of livebirths (Stagno & Whitley 1985). Most CMV infections are subclinical. Maternofetal transmission of CMV can occur during either primary or recurrent infection but is commoner (30–40%) in primary infections. Only 10–14% of the infected fetuses suffer sequelae, usually neurological damage or deafness. The highest risk of transmission is when infection occurs during the first trimester, when the virus can cause a variety of congenital abnormalities. Later infection can lead to growth retardation, hepatosplenomegaly, thrombocytopenia, chorioretinitis, haemolytic anaemia, hydrocephalus and intracranial calcifications. Symptomatic infants have a mortality of 20–30% and most survivors have severe handicap.

Diagnosis of maternal infection is achieved by isolating the active virus from a body fluid such as saliva, or serology where the demonstration of CMV-specific IgM is diagnostic. Amniocentesis is most reliable in fetal diagnosis, for detection of the virus, and fetal blood sampling after 22 weeks may demonstrate IgM (Lange et al 1982). Ultrasound can detect growth retardation, microcephaly and hydrocephalus and aid the diagnosis if maternal and fetal serology are positive.

There is no treatment for CMV infection, but termination may be offered if there is evidence of fetal infection resulting in congenital abnormality.

Varicella-zoster

Varicella-zoster virus may manifest as chickenpox or shingles. Varicella during pregnancy may result in the congenital varicella syndrome (Paryani & Arvin 1986). Maternal infection is usually symptomatic, following an incubation period of 10–20 days. The illness is characterized by fever, malaise and a vesicular rash. In pregnancy, the infection may be complicated by pneumonia with a considerable maternal morbidity and mortality. During maternal infection, transplacental transmission of the virus can occur. The fetal effects of infection depend upon the gestational age at the time of infection. Maternal varicella during the first trimester can result in spontaneous abortion or congenital defects, whereas infection near to term can lead to neonatal infection which, if disseminated, is usually fatal. Congenital defects associated with varicella-zoster infection include skin lesions, limb hypoplasia, muscular atrophy, growth retardation, microcephaly, cortical atrophy, microphthalmia and other neurological sequelae.

Diagnosis in the mother is relatively easy clinically, and can be confirmed by serology or isolation of the virus from the vesicles. Fetal infection can be diagnosed by detection of varicella-zoster-specific IgM in fetal blood or by DNA techniques.

There is no specific treatment for maternal infection, but infants born to women who develop varicella in the peripartum period should receive anti-varicella-zoster immunoglobulin. Treatment with acyclovir is also recommended.

Parvovirus B19

Parvovirus causes the fifth disease or erythema infectiosum. It was first described in 1975 (Cossart et al 1975) and intrauterine infection is known to occur (Knott et al 1984). Transplacental transmission occurs during maternal viraemia, and viral DNA can be isolated in fetal and placental tissues. The virus is fetotropic and fetotoxic, causing myocarditis, bone marrow suppression with resultant anaemia, hydrops fetalis and intrauterine death. No teratogenic effects have been documented in the human fetus.

Human parvovirus infection is frequently subclinical, but diagnosis of maternal infection can be made by the demonstration of specific IgM in blood. Fetal infection should be suspected in cases of non-immune hydrops fetalis (Johnson et al 1993). The diagnosis of fetal infection can be made by demonstration of IgM in fetal blood or the presence of viral DNA in fetal tissues, including chorionic villi.

Whilst no treatment of the viral infection exists, fetal anaemia can be corrected by intrauterine transfusion (Soothill 1990), and myocardial dysfunction treated by direct administration of digoxin to the fetus.

DIAGNOSTIC AND INVASIVE PROCEDURES

The fetus has become a potential patient because of increased accessibility provided by modern high resolution ultrasound. Palpation, auscultation and radiology are no longer the only tools available. Of the non-invasive methods, ultrasound is the most useful although other modalities such as magnetic resonance imaging show promise.

Imaging is only one part of the diagnostic and therapeutic armamentarium. A large variety of samples can now be acquired for analysis by an impressive array of techniques. All should be regarded as ultrasound-guided procedures, as maximal safety and success can only be achieved with the combined use of good ultrasound.

Ultrasound and invasive procedures

The information obtained from ultrasound includes:

1. Fetal viability is confirmed before any procedure.
2. Fetal age is checked by sonographic fetal measurements. This is best done before the procedure so that it can be planned for the optimal gestational age.
3. Multiple pregnancy is diagnosed. If present, it considerably complicates the procedure and its implications, e.g. if twins are discordant for an abnormality.
4. Fetal anatomy is examined to exclude anomalies, and amniotic fluid volume noted.
5. Uterine and adnexal abnormalities can be excluded.
6. The placenta is localized and its margins defined.
7. The target for the procedure is defined.
8. The site of entry of the needle is selected.
9. Simultaneous guidance of the needle during the procedure.
10. Continuous monitoring of the fetal heart rate.
11. Early warning of complications, e.g. fetal bradycardia.
12. The fetal heart rate and signs of bleeding are checked after the procedure.
13. The umbilical artery flow velocity waveform may be examined before and after the procedure.

Most of the items of information above are relevant to all invasive procedures. Initially, lip service was paid to placental localization, some hours or even days before the procedure. It is no surprise that the use of ultrasound in this way showed no benefit to the procedure of amniocentesis (Levine et al 1978) but it was not then appreciated how much the fetal lie and position can change in a few minutes.

It became clear that amniocentesis should be performed in the ultrasound department, initially as quickly as possible after the entry point had been selected sonographically (Harrison et al 1975, Kerenyl & Walker 1977). However, further advances in technique led to the adaptation using real time visualization of the needle throughout the entire procedure, further reducing the risk of dry taps (Jonatha 1974, Jeanty et al 1983). This technique has been adapted for more complex procedures including percutaneous fetal blood sampling, fetal catheterization and fetoscopy (Rodeck 1980), in which the transducer is sterile or held in a sterile polythene bag. Needling techniques can be free hand, where the transducer is held in one hand and the needle in the other, or using a needle guide. The use of a guide limits freedom of movement, especially when considering intrafetal procedures, but is preferred by some. The choice of ultrasound probe lies with the operator, but most find the curvilinear probe most convenient.

In many centres, invasive procedures are done very successfully by a team consisting of operator, assistant and ultrasonographer. This requires extremely close team work and a change in sonographer can be disturbing. The information derived from the scanning is so vital to the decision making that it is more straightforward and in principle better if this is done by the operator. There is then no doubt where the responsibility lies.

Counselling

No patient should have an invasive procedure without previous detailed counselling; in many instances a consent form, if not strictly necessary, is a wise precaution. Counselling may require a geneticist, and may have already been done, but this does not absolve the obstetrician from responsibility for ensuring that the patient is fully informed. She, and her partner, should have the knowledge of:

1. the disease or abnormality being investigated
2. the prognosis
3. the risk of occurrence and recurrence
4. the nature of the procedure, its risks and success rate
5. the possibility of other tests or options, including having nothing done
6. the diagnostic accuracy, and time taken for the result to be available
7. termination of pregnancy, methods and complications
8. what to do in the event of complications.

Ideally most of these points will have been covered before the pregnancy. All too often this is not possible, or the problem may have developed during the pregnancy.

More than one session may be required and couples should have the opportunity to go away to think about and discuss the problem. It is quite unacceptable to burden the patient hastily with new information in a darkened ultrasound room immediately before a procedure.

Amniocentesis

Technique

Regular use of amniocentesis was first advocated by Bevis (1952) in the management of rhesus disease. Many practitioners achieved a high degree of success before ultrasound was available, but few would now wish to perform amniocentesis without it.

After first scanning to confirm the gestation, viability, placental site and liquor volume, the skin is cleansed with antiseptic. Using aseptic technique, the ultrasound transducer is held in one hand while the needle is inserted into a pool of amniotic fluid, avoiding the placenta if possible, under continuous ultrasound visualization (Fig. 15.8). The commonest needle used is a 21 gauge disposable spinal needle with a stylet. Once in place, the stylet is removed, a syringe attached to the hub of the needle and a small quantity of fluid aspirated. The fluid should be clear and a pale straw colour. If blood stained, the initial sample must be discarded and a second syringe attached. 20 ml of fluid is then aspirated, watching for colour change all the time. Once the sample has been collected, the needle is withdrawn and the mother shown the fetal heart movement for reassurance. It is essential that the sample is placed in a sterile container labelled with the mother's name, age and hospital number or address, and that the mother checks the labelling with a member of staff. Anti D gammaglobulin should then be administered if the mother is Rhesus negative. Following the procedure, many women prefer to rest quietly for 20–30 minutes

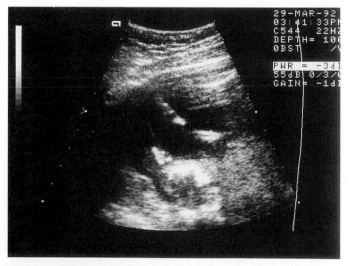

Fig. 15.8   Ultrasound picture of amniocentesis.

Table 15.3 Indications for amniocentesis

Before 20 weeks
1. Chromosome abnormalities (maternal age, translocation carrier, previous affected child)
2. Fetal sexing in X-linked disorders
3. Neural tube defects—raised alpha-fetoprotein or acetylcholinesterase levels
4. Inborn errors of metabolism
5. DNA analysis

After 20 weeks
1. Bilirubin (ΔOD at 450 nm)
2. Phospholipids (for fetal pulmonary maturity)
3. Fetal maturity
4. Amniography or fetography

before going home with the advice to limit activity for 24–48 hours, although this is not of proven value.

Indications

The indications for amniocentesis are shown in Table 15.3. In the past, it has also been used for estimation of fetal maturity, amniography and fetography. In the investigation of inherited disorders, the technique has been performed at 15–16 weeks' gestation. By this time, the uterus is readily accessible abdominally and contains 150–200 ml of liquor, permitting the removal of 15–20 ml with impunity. However, following cell culture and cytogenetic analysis, chromosome results are rarely available before 3 weeks so that the diagnosis cannot be made until 18–20 weeks' gestation, which for many women, and those involved in their care, seems unacceptably late if termination is to be considered. There has therefore been interest in bringing forward the gestation at which amniocentesis is performed.

Early amniocentesis

A number of centres have assessed early amniocentesis, between 10 and 14 weeks' gestation. There are several factors to consider, which include the safety of the procedure, the success of cell culture, accuracy of karyotype and whether the technique is appropriate for investigation of metabolic disorders as well as karyotyping. Culture failure occurs in up to 3% of cases (Stripparo et al 1990, Byrne et al 1991, Fogarty et al 1991), although in some series 100% culture was achieved (Nevin et al 1990, Rebello et al 1990, Hackett et al 1991), but this high level of success is only achieved if amniocentesis is performed when the crown–rump length of the fetus is greater than 37 mm (Byrne et al 1991). DNA has been successfully extracted from amniotic fluid taken between 8 and 14 weeks (Rebello et al 1990), and evaluation of enzyme activity in the investigation of metabolic disease has also been successful (Chadefaux et al 1989).

The technique for early amniocentesis is very similar to that described above, although the volume aspirated is usually 1 ml per week gestation and a slightly smaller, 22 gauge, needle is used (Stripparo et al 1990). One difficulty encountered in this technique is that the amniotic membrane is not yet totally adherent to the uterine wall and at times the extraembryonic coelom is visible and may be entered inadvertently. In order to improve the cell yield of early amniocentesis, amniofiltration has been developed (Sundberg et al 1991) although this is of unproven value and safety.

Risk of procedure

The true risk of any invasive procedure used in prenatal diagnosis is difficult to establish, as there is a background rate of pregnancy loss which is increased with advanced maternal age in pregnancies complicated by fetal anomaly, be it structural, karyotypic or metabolic. Large multicentre trials are complicated by differences in technique used and operator skill. Careful audit of an individual centre's figures is essential to be able to assess the local risk of a procedure. However, with these limitations in mind, there are a number of studies where the risk of pregnancy loss due to amniocentesis performed for prenatal diagnosis has been estimated. The risk of loss in the studies varies from an increase of 0.5% compared with controls (Canadian Medical Research Council 1977, National Institute of Child Health and Development Amniocentesis Register 1978) to 2.1% (MRC study 1978), although when adjusted for age and parity, this UK series gave an increased risk of pregnancy loss of 1%. The best study is that of Tabor et al (1986) who randomized over 4000 women to have ultrasound alone or ultrasound and amniocentesis. There was an increased risk of pregnancy loss of 1% in the amniocentesis group. It would therefore seem appropriate to estimate the risk to be approximately 1%.

As a new technique, early amniocentesis has been subjected to close scrutiny as far as safety of the procedure is concerned. In most series, pregnancy losses have been about 1–1.5% (Nevin et al 1990), although higher if the amniocentesis was performed between 11 and 12 weeks (Stripparo et al 1990). Most of these small studies do not have any control data and there is a need for a large randomized study before early amniocentesis is performed as a routine.

Some studies have suggested that there is an increase in respiratory distress and talipes following amniocentesis (MRC Working Party 1978, Tabor et al 1986). Subclinical but significant inhibition of pulmonary growth may occur as a result of removing a significant amount of liquor at 12–14 weeks' gestation which is the time of maximum sensitivity of lung development. Studies in primates (Hislop et al 1984) have demonstrated this effect, which is a major concern in early amniocentesis.

Chorionic villus sampling

Chorionic villus sampling (CVS) is an example of a technique arriving at the wrong time. The pioneering work in the late 1960s using endoscopes (Hahnemann & Mohr 1968, Kullander & Sandahl 1973) was not taken up, partly because there appeared to be a high complication and failure rate, and partly because it was becoming clear that amniocentesis was safe and reliable for fetal chromosome analysis. Even earlier studies had already been performed on placental biopsy (Alvarez 1964) but within another context.

The report from China (Tietung Hospital 1975) of the successful use of an aspiration cannula, passed blindly in continuing pregnancies, re-awakened interest in the West, although work with ultrasound-guided forceps was also being done in the USSR (Kazy et al 1982). The demonstration that villi could be used for gene analysis (Williamson et al 1981) led to the development of further methods. Blind aspiration was shown to be unreliable (Horwell et al 1983) and endoscopy was too complicated (Gosden et al 1982). Ultrasound-guided transcervical catheters have become the most widely used techniques (Rodeck et al 1983, Ward et al 1983; Fig. 15.9). The similar use of biopsy forceps is also very successful (Goossens et al 1983, Vaughan & Rodeck 1992). Transabdominal CVS has been increasingly used (Smidt-Jensen & Hahnemann 1984; Fig. 15.10) and its main advantage is that it can be used from the first trimester to term (Nicolaides et al 1986a), whereas transcervical CVS has a limit of 10–12 weeks. It is not clear whether one method is better than the other, but many operators are skilled in both approaches and can therefore choose whichever approach seems appropriate.

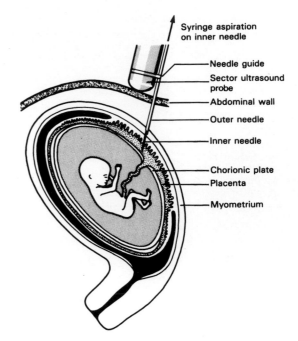

Fig. 15.10   Transabdominal needle aspiration of chorionic villi under ultrasound guidance.

The advantages of CVS are summarized in Table 15.4. Clearly the most important, particularly from the patient's point of view, is the possibility of first-trimester diagnosis.

Indications

The indications for CVS are given in Table 15.5. The advances in molecular genetics have been particularly rapid in the last 15 years and as more genes are cloned and probes developed, more diseases can be diagnosed by this technology.

The enzyme deficiency underlying most inborn errors

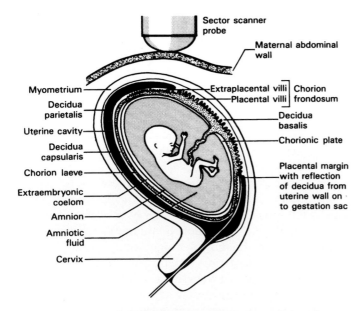

Fig. 15.9   Transcervical passage of an aspiration cannula into the placental site under ultrasound guidance.

Table 15.4   Advantages of chorion villus biopsy

1. Enables first-trimester fetal diagnosis, i.e. early reassurance or early termination; avoidance of long delay and late termination
2. Villi are a good source of DNA
3. Villi are (nearly always) genetically, chromosomally and biochemically identical to the fetus
4. Villi can be sampled without perforating the membranes or fetus

Table 15.5   Indications for chorion villus biopsy

DNA analysis
  Haemoglobinopathies—sickle cell disease, alpha-thalassaemia, most beta-thalassaemias
  Most haemophilias—A and B
  Duchenne muscular dystrophy (not all families)
  Cystic fibrosis (not all families)
  Alpha$_1$-antitrypsin deficiency
Chromosome abnormalities
Inborn errors of metabolism

of metabolism is expressed in villi, and in many cases the villi can be assayed directly, giving a result the next day. However, in some cases, culture of the villi is required.

Techniques

Prior to the procedure of CVS, the patient should be scanned to confirm viability, gestation and placental site. The preferred route can then be chosen. The patient should have received adequate counselling concerning the need for the investigation, time taken for the results to be obtained, the implications of a positive result and the precision of the test. In addition, she must be aware of the risks of the procedure.

All CVS is performed under continuous ultrasound guidance. For the transcervical approach, the patient lies on a couch in a modified lithotomy position (a colposcopy couch is ideal). After cleansing of the vulval area with antiseptic, a sterile bivalve speculum is introduced into the vagina and the cervix visualized. The cervix is then cleansed meticulously with antiseptic. The ultrasonographer or operator will then scan transabdominally to visualize the cervical canal, uterus and placental site. Either an aspiration catheter or biopsy forceps are then gently introduced through the cervix and guided into the placental tissue from where a sample of villi is collected. It is usually unnecessary to steady the cervix with a vulsellum. No more than two passes should be attempted. The material obtained should be examined under a microscope to confirm the presence of villi, to allow removal of decidua if any is present and an assessment of the quantity obtained is made. With biopsy forceps, only villi are obtained, and as these are easily recognized with the naked eye, a microscope is not required.

For transabdominal CVS, the patient lies supine on a couch and the preparation is similar to that for amniocentesis. However, many operators prefer to administer local anaesthetic into the skin and subcutaneous tissues prior to taking the sample. Under continuous ultrasound guidance, the chosen needle is introduced into the placenta. The amniotic cavity should not be entered. A number of techniques exist for transabdominal CVS: single needle, double needle and forceps. For the single needle technique, an 18 gauge needle with stylet is directed into the placenta. The stylet is removed and a syringe containing culture medium or wash is attached to the hub of the needle. With suction applied, the needle is moved vigorously backwards and forwards within the placenta, under continuous ultrasound visualization. With the suction still applied, the needle is withdrawn and the sample thus aspirated into the syringe. One potential problem with this technique is that if the first sample is insufficient, it is necessary to reintroduce the needle. This can be avoided when a double needle technique or biopsy forceps are used. The outer 17 or 18 gauge needle with stylet is inserted as above. The stylet is removed and either a flat-ended 19 gauge needle or a pair of fine biopsy forceps is introduced through the first needle into the placenta. The sample is either aspirated or taken using the forceps, and removed, leaving the outer needle in situ until sufficient tissue has been obtained.

The route chosen depends on gestation, operator preference and site of placenta. Under 12 weeks, many operators choose the transcervical route if the placenta is posterior, and transabdominal for an anterior placenta (Saura et al 1990).

Risks of procedure

From the introduction of the current techniques of CVS, there has been concern that the pregnancy losses after CVS were greater than after amniocentesis. Initially, this was thought to be related to the earlier gestation at which CVS was performed but subsequent studies have shown that the loss rate is indeed greater than after amniocentesis. In the CVS newsletter in 1988, the pregnancy loss rate was quoted as 3.4%. A randomized Canadian study published in 1989 (Canadian Collaborative CVS–Amniocentesis Clinical Trial Group 1989) gave equal loss rates before 28 weeks following amniocentesis and CVS, but more pregnancies were lost after 28 weeks in the group that had CVS performed. The US study (Rhoads et al 1989) also showed no significant difference in fetal loss between CVS and amniocentesis. The Danish study (Smidt-Jensen et al 1991) demonstrated equal pregnancy losses after transabdominal CVS and amniocentesis (6.2% and 6.3% respectively) but 10.1% after transcervical CVS. These loss rates included spontaneous miscarriages, termination and perinatal deaths.

The largest study to address this problem, however, was that supervised by the Medical Research Council and published in 1991. This examined the outcome of 3248 pregnancies, randomly assigned to first-trimester CVS or second-trimester amniocentesis, and measured outcome as a liveborn infant. There was a decrease of 4.6% in the chance of a liveborn baby in the group allocated to CVS which was statistically significant. However, although the centres involved in this study had strict criteria for training for CVS, there was no way of controlling for operator differences and many were inexperienced. Of interest also was that there was no difference in the loss rates after transabdominal or transcervical CVS.

To some extent the question remains unanswered, although most would agree that there is probably a slight increase in the risk of pregnancy loss following first-trimester CVS compared with conventional amniocentesis. Therefore CVS is used here for those women at high risk of an affected pregnancy, i.e. single gene defects, rather than women of advanced maternal age, who have a relatively lower chance of an abnormal fetus. Furthermore, villi is the preferred tissue for DNA analysis or biochemistry.

The question of who should have CVS and whether

it will replace amniocentesis has been addressed many times. The results of the MRC trial (MRC Working Party 1991), together with reports of limb deformities after early CVS (Firth et al 1991), led to doubts over the safety of this procedure. The limb reduction defects reported may be related to the trauma of the technique resulting in fetomaternal haemorrhage, release of vasoactive peptides or emboli (Rodeck 1993, Rodeck et al 1993) and these patients usually had the CVS before 9 weeks' gestation. Although there was a fall in the number of CVS procedures performed in the first 6 months after the publication of these two papers (James et al 1992), that reduction has not persisted and CVS has re-established its role in prenatal diagnosis in all three trimesters of pregnancy (Pijpers et al 1988, Lilford 1991). CVS is clearly of benefit to patients with genetic histories and a 1 : 2 or 1 : 4 chance of recurrence risk, and in this group CVS has replaced amniocentesis and fetal blood sampling.

Fetal blood sampling

When a pure sample can be obtained, fetal blood provides the opportunity for numerous analyses, as do blood samples in postnatal medicine. Not only can lymphocytes be cultured for a rapid karyotype, the result often being available in 48–72 hours, but the full range of haematological, biochemical, pharmacological and immunological investigations can be performed. Initial attempts at fetal blood sampling included placentacentesis where multiple punctures of the chorionic plate were made with a 19 or 20 gauge needle in the hope that a fetal blood vessel would bleed into the amniotic cavity, which was then aspirated (Kan et al 1974). Samples often contained only a very low proportion of fetal cells and 10–15% of patients required a repeat procedure. The fetal loss rate was about 10% (Fairweather et al 1980) and this technique is now obsolete.

Fetoscopy

Early attempts at visualization of the fetus with a rigid endoscope required a maternal laparotomy (Valenti 1972, Scrimgeour 1973). Real-time ultrasound allowed the development of fetoscopy as an ultrasound-guided percutaneous procedure (Hobbins & Mahoney 1974) and initial attempts to obtain fetal blood under fetoscopic guidance involved placentacentesis under direct vision. In order to obtain pure fetal samples, the technique was adapted to permit aspiration of fetal blood from the umbilical cord at the placental insertion with 100% reliability (Rodeck & Campbell 1978, Rodeck & Nicolaides 1986). The technique could be applied from 15 weeks' gestation up to term, and allowed versatile access to the fetus. However, it was not easy to learn and has been superceded by ultrasound-guided fetal blood sampling. There is

currently, however, renewed interest in fetal endoscopic procedures for diagnosis and treatment.

Ultrasound-guided fetal blood sampling

The first large series of ultrasound-guided fetal blood sampling came from France, where the high incidence of toxoplasmosis was the stimulus for the development of a simple method for obtaining pure fetal blood (Daffos et al 1983). The majority of fetal blood sampling procedures performed today take blood from the placental insertion of the umbilical cord, although alternative routes include a free loop of cord, abdominal insertion, intrahepatic vein or fetal heart (Nicolini et al 1988, Westgren et al 1988).

Technique

Fetal blood sampling is easiest to perform between 18 and 28 weeks' gestation. Before 18 weeks, it may be difficult to visualize the cord insertion, and there appears to be a higher risk of pregnancy loss (Orlandi et al 1990). After 28 weeks, as the fetus increases in size, it may obscure the cord insertion and alternative sites may be more appropriate.

Using real-time ultrasound, the cord insertion into the placenta or the intrahepatic umbilical vein is visualized. The choice of transducer obviously depends on what is available, but the curvilinear probe is preferred by most operators (Nicolaides 1988). Under aseptic conditions, the maternal skin is cleansed with antiseptic and local anaesthetic injected into the skin and subcutaneous tissues. Holding the ultrasound transducer in one hand, the operator introduces a 20 or 22 gauge needle with stylet into the target vessel. The stylet is then removed and blood aspirated. The volume required depends upon the investigations being performed and the gestation, but between 0.5 and 2 ml of blood is usually adequate. The blood must be confirmed to be fetal in origin immediately, and this can be effected by passing a sample through a Coulter counter to check the mean corpuscular volume. Subsequently, the Kleihauer–Betke stain will demonstrate the presence or absence of maternal cells. After the procedure, the sampling site should be checked for haemorrhage (which usually settles within 30 seconds) and the fetal heart movement should be shown to the mother. There is generally no indication for any premedication of the mother or fetus, but if the latter is extremely active, it may be necessary to paralyse the fetus with a muscle relaxant administered directly.

Indications

The groups of disorders that can be investigated with fetal blood sampling are shown in Table 15.6.

Table 15.6   Indications for fetal blood sampling

1. Haemoglobinopathies
2. Bleeding disorders
3. Chromosome disorders
4. Immunodeficiencies
5. Viral and other infections
6. Metabolic disorders
7. Unexplained (non-haemolytic) hydrops
8. Fetal blood grouping
9. Assessment of fetal anaemia
10. Assessment of fetal blood gas and acid–base status

The haemoglobinopathies were the classical indication for which the early blood sampling techniques were evolved (Hobbins & Mahoney 1974, Kan et al 1974). The diagnosis was made by studying the biosynthesis of globin chains. More recently, most of these patients have first-trimester CVS and DNA analysis.

Pure fetal blood samples, in which clotting has not been initiated, can be used for bioassay of factor VIIIC and factor IX for diagnosis of fetal haemophilia (Mibashan & Rodeck 1984). Here again, DNA analysis on villi taken at early CVS has superceded fetal blood sampling as the primary method of prenatal diagnosis.

A karyotype can be obtained from cultured fetal lymphocytes within 48–72 hours, far more rapidly than cell culture after amniocentesis. This is particularly useful in the further investigation of fetal abnormalities discovered by mid-trimester ultrasound as these have a much higher incidence of chromosome aberrations than at term (Nicolaides et al 1986b). This is now the largest group of patients having fetal blood sampling. Other indications include fragile X-linked mental retardation, amniotic fluid culture failure and the investigation of mosaicism on amniocyte or villus culture.

Fetal infections can be diagnosed by the demonstration of specific IgM in fetal blood, and on occasion by isolation of the infective agent. Fetal blood also permits the diagnosis of many inborn errors of metabolism, although first-trimester CVS is the method of choice. In the assessment of fetal hydrops, fetal blood sampling is invaluable in the investigation of the underlying cause (Johnson et al 1993). Rhesus disease and alloimmune thrombocytopenia are other areas where fetal blood sampling became an essential part of management.

Blood gas and acid–base measurements may occasionally be valuable in high-risk fetuses (Rodeck & Nicolaides 1986). Doppler blood flow studies may however provide a more useful non-invasive alternative (Nicolini et al 1990b).

Risks of procedure

All invasive procedures carry a risk of pregnancy loss, either by inducing miscarriage, preterm labour or intra-uterine fetal death. The actual risk of any procedure is difficult to define, as the exact causation of pregnancy loss

cannot always be established. Whilst a miscarriage within a few days of a procedure might be said to be a direct result of the procedure, it is much more difficult if the loss occurs 4 or more weeks later. In addition, the underlying reason for the procedure may, in itself, carry a higher risk of pregnancy loss, e.g. investigation of an abnormal or severely growth-retarded fetus. The loss of a pregnancy may be due to bleeding, infection or preterm rupture of the membranes.

Operator technique and experience are obviously important factors that must be taken into account. All operators learning a procedure should receive expert tuition, and ideally have the opportunity to develop their expertise on pregnancies undergoing termination. One problem with many of the multicentre trials that have been carried out to try to assess the true rate of pregnancy loss is that all centres include operators of differing skill, experience and technique. The most reliable estimation of loss rates must be that obtained from careful audit of the figures of the unit in which the procedure is being performed, comparing the operator with others of similar experience.

Careful selection of appropriate cases, impeccable aseptic technique and knowing when to abandon a procedure will all contribute to minimizing the pregnancy losses. The risk of pregnancy loss following ultrasound-guided fetal blood sampling has been estimated at 1–2% (Daffos et al 1985) but there is evidence that this rate is increased with higher risk mothers. There are a large number of individual case reports of complications after fetal blood sampling (Benacerraf et al 1987, Feinkind et al 1990). One retrospective study identified markedly differing loss rates depending on the indication for the procedure, varying from 1% in normal fetuses to 25% losses in the investigation of hydrops (Maxwell et al 1991). However, the advantages of a rapid and reliable result of investigations by fetal blood sampling must be balanced against an increase risk of pregnancy loss if there is a severe abnormality or if the fetus is at risk of intrauterine death as in severe intrauterine growth retardation or hydrops.

Other sampling techniques

Fetal skin biopsies can be taken under fetoscopic or ultrasound control, using cupped biopsy forceps (Rodeck et al 1980). The procedure is indicated in the prenatal diagnosis of the severe genodermatoses such as epidermolysis bullosa letalis and dystrophica, epidermolytic hyperkeratosis, harlequin ichthyosis and oculocutaneous albinism.

Fetal liver biopsy can be performed, using biopsy forceps, under fetoscopic or ultrasound guidance (Rodeck et al 1982, Holzgreve & Golbus 1984). Indications include the diagnosis of some rare inborn errors of metabolism where other tests are not suitable, e.g. defects of the urea cycle such as carbamyl phosphate synthetase deficiency or ornithine carbamyl transferase deficiency.

Fetal tumour biopsies have been obtained and can be used to confirm the diagnosis of teratomas or congenital adenomatoid malformation of the lung.

Aspiration of fluid collections, such as fetal urine from a dilated bladder or a pleural effusion, can be easily performed with ultrasound guidance. Assessment of the biochemistry of fetal urine is of some benefit in the assessment of obstructive uropathy, and the white cell count of pleural fluid may suggest the diagnosis of chylothorax.

Instillation of intraperitoneal saline is also of value in cases of anhydramnios or severe oligohydramnios. This is particularly useful if renal agenesis is suspected as it permits evaluation of the abdominal organs, and renal fossae in particular.

Therapeutic invasive procedures

Ultrasound-guided needling techniques have been adapted to permit the development of a number of fetal therapeutic procedures.

Amniocentesis

The drainage of excess fluid in cases of polyhydramnios has been performed many times to alleviate maternal discomfort, reduce the risk of premature labour and improve fetal oxygenation. Intrauterine manometry can assist in the management of appropriate cases (Nicolini et al 1989).

The instillation of warmed saline into the amniotic cavity in cases of oligohydramnios can aid ultrasound visualization and enhance diagnostic accuracy of ultrasound examination (Fisk et al 1991).

Fetal transfusion

Whilst rhesus immunization is the main indication for intrauterine blood transfusion (Rodeck et al 1981), other causes of fetal anaemia, e.g. parvovirus infection, will respond to blood transfusion. This is usually performed into the umbilical vein, under continuous ultrasound guidance, although the fetal heart and intrahepatic vein have been used. Platelets have also been successfully transfused into the fetal circulation in cases of severe thrombocytopenia (Nicolini et al 1990a).

Intrauterine shunting

Obstructive uropathy. The most common cause of obstructive uropathy is posterior urethral valves, leading to megacystis, megaureter, varying degrees of renal damage, oligohydramnios and resultant pulmonary hypoplasia. With ultrasound alone, it may be difficult to distinguish this from the low-pressure dilatation of the urinary tract seen in prune belly syndrome. An increasing number of

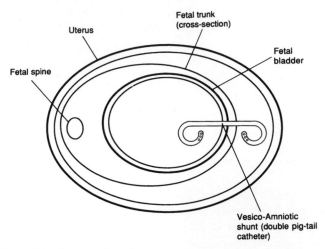

Fig. 15.11   Cross-section of uterus and fetal trunk showing double pigtail catheter (vesico-amniotic shunt) in position.

cases of obstructive uropathy have been managed by the insertion of a vesico-amniotic shunt.

A trochar and cannula are introduced into the fetal bladder under ultrasound guidance and a plastic, double pigtailed catheter is inserted so that one end coils in the bladder and the other in the amniotic cavity (Fig. 15.11). This is not technically difficult to achieve, but the major problem lies with the selection of cases. Obstructive uropathy in utero may be progressive and some cases will have caused irreparable renal damage at the time of diagnosis, whilst some cases will have an excellent prognosis in the absence of any intervention. An attempt must be made, therefore, to assess renal function by a combination of sonography, biochemical analysis of fetal urine and assessment of urine production by measuring the rate of bladder refilling. Where reasonable renal function can be demonstrated, it is hoped that this can be preserved by insertion of a shunt. From data collected by the International Fetal Surgery Registry (Manning et al 1986) this appears to be so, but there is no definite proof that intervention directly benefits these fetuses. It is of vital importance that therapeutic interventions are not considered until other abnormalities, including aneuploidies, have been excluded.

Hydrocephalus. Early attempts to shunt hydrocephalus in utero were extremely disappointing, and this mode of treatment is not used at present.

Hydrothorax. Longstanding fetal pleural effusions are likely to cause pulmonary hypoplasia and, by obstructing venous return to the heart, may cause hydrops. Needle aspiration has been successfully employed (Schmidt et al 1985), but the effusions rapidly reaccumulate. Therefore, in this situation, there is a place for the insertion of a thoraco-amniotic pigtail catheter, which frequently has an excellent outcome (Rodeck et al 1988).

Aspiration of fluid. Large intrafetal collections of fluid, e.g. renal cysts, massive ascites, can be aspirated before delivery, making the delivery less traumatic and often facilitating the resuscitation of the neonate (Bell 1988).

Balloon valvoplasty. Critical aortic stenosis is a progressive condition which, when diagnosed in utero, carries a uniformly poor prognosis. Attempts have therefore been made to relieve the valvular obstruction by the passage of a balloon catheter across the stenotic valve in utero. This has been successful on two occasions out of five (D. Maxwell, personal communication).

Clinically important aspects of laboratory techniques

Cell culture

The mainstay of diagnosis of karyotype abnormalities still relies upon the culture of fetal fibroblasts obtained from liquor taken at amniocentesis. The discovery of mammalian sex chromatin soon led to its demonstration in human amniotic cells and to the suggestion that such cells might be cultured to reveal the fetal karyotype (Fuchs & Riis 1956, Sachs et al 1956, Riis & Fuchs 1960, Austin 1962). In 1966, Steele & Breg demonstrated that human amniotic fluid does contain viable cells, and that they can be cultured and used for the demonstration of sex chromatin or for chromosomal analysis. Their observations were confirmed by Jacobson & Barter (1967) who evaluated 91 amniotic fluid samples taken at varying times from 5 weeks' gestation to term. Their highest success rates were from 12 weeks onwards. Nadler (1968) made similar observations and was one of the first to make a prenatal diagnosis of an abnormal fetus, with an inherited D;G translocation Down's syndrome.

Following these early observations several groups of workers established the optimum period of gestation for amniocentesis for chromosomal analysis at about 16 weeks' gestation and the best methods of cell culture, harvesting, chromosomal preparation and analysis (Lisgar et al 1970, Nadler & Gerbie 1970, Wahlstrom et al 1970, Fuchs 1971, Nadler 1971, Timson et al 1971, Milunsky et al 1972, Warburton & Miller 1972). Chromosomal banding techniques have greatly increased the precision of prenatal as well as postnatal diagnosis of chromosomal disorders. Recent advances in ultrasound have lead to amniocentesis being performed earlier as described above. Cell culture is generally successful in 98% or more of cases.

Several large studies of amniocentesis have reported on the nature and frequency of chromosomal abnormality detected. All manner of abnormalities can be detected by this technique, although some subtle chromosomal rearrangements have only been described using more sophisticated techniques (see below). Mothers aged over 35 years consistently yield chromosomal abnormality on amniocentesis at a frequency of between 1.9% and 2.8%, with an overall frequency of 2.3% (e.g. Squire et al 1982). With changes in screening that are now taking place, the incidence of abnormal karyotype seen in prenatal diagnosis is likely to increase.

Cell culture generally takes about 12 days to harvest in early amniocentesis (12–14 weeks' gestation) and 11 days in standard mid-trimester procedures (Rebello et al 1991). The time taken to report averages 22 days in early and 21 days in standard samples, allowing results to be given to the patient 3 weeks after the procedure. However, if the harvest can take place early (8 days), the result can be ready as quickly as 13 days.

Chorionic villi provide two types of material (trophoblast and mesenchymal core) for examination of the fetal karyotype. Because the trophoblast cells in the villi are dividing rapidly, it is possible to obtain a direct (24–48 hours) karyotype result which does not rely on successful culture and minimizes the risk of contamination. However, direct preparations provide fewer metaphase spreads of poorer quality than those obtained from cultured cells (Brambati et al 1983, Maxwell et al 1985, Czepulkowski et al 1986). This limitation has resulted in some chromosomal rearrangements being undetected in direct analyses. Another limitation of the direct preparation is their higher incidence of mosaicism which is present in trophoblast, but which is not found in either cultures of the villous mesenchyme or in the fetal tissues (Kalousek & Dill 1983, Liu et al 1983). Maternal cells may occasionally contaminate direct preparations and cultures (Simoni et al 1986). Rarely, abnormalities have been detected in cultured villi and in other fetal tissue that have not been detected in direct or short-term cultures (Eichenbaum et al 1986, Martin et al 1986). Whilst the speed of obtaining a result from a direct preparation which will exclude major rearrangements cannot be denied, many laboratories use cultures of the mesenchymal core as their primary technique, even though the results take about 2 weeks.

Direct preparations of chorionic villi permit rapid sexing of the fetus, which is important in the investigation of sex-linked disorders (Lilford et al 1983, Gibbs et al 1984, Gosden et al 1984, Simoni et al 1984). However, disorders such as Fragile X can only be diagnosed after full culture of the villi, which requires a similar time period to amniocentesis culture.

Fetal lymphocytes from blood samples are also cultured. This provides the most rapid and reliable karyotype, with the result frequently being available within 48–72 hours.

Cell culture of all these tissues must be subject to extremely high standards of quality control. Contamination by maternal or foreign tissue must be avoided, as must contamination by infectious agents which usually results in a failed culture. Not only is laboratory quality control necessary, but follow-up on all pregnancies karyotyped is desirable to ensure the accuracy of results. This is most important in cases of mosaicism, common particularly in

CVS direct preparation, but found also in amniocentesis and, rarely, fetal blood. When a mosaic is found, it is necessary to establish whether the abnormality is confined to the placenta or whether it is a true reflection of the fetal karyotype. Expert genetic advice is always necessary for correct interpretation of mosaics.

In addition to the culture of cells from direct sampling of the pregnancy, there has been interest in the possibility of isolation of fetal cells found in the maternal circulation. This approach was first suggested by Walknowska et al more than 20 years ago (Walknowska et al 1969). Whilst culture of the fetal cells found in maternal blood had not been successful, using immunofluorescent techniques and flow cytometry, fetal cells can be identified in maternal blood and modern molecular biology techniques such as DNA amplification and fluorescence in situ hybridization (FISH) permit examination of the fetal karyotype (Lo et al 1989, Elias et al 1992).

Enzyme assay

The methods available for prenatal diagnosis of inborn errors of metabolism vary, but include biochemical assay of enzyme levels. The ideal method is a reliable enzyme assay that can be performed on uncultured and cultured chorionic villus tissue, and also cultured fetal fibroblasts from amniotic fluid. Fujimoto and colleagues (1968) used an autoradiographic method for the detection of hypoxanthine-guanosine ribosyl transferase activity in cultured and uncultured amniotic fluid cells from a female fetus heterozygous for Lesch–Nyhan disease. Quantitative assays can be used, for example in the prenatal diagnosis of Hurler's disease (Stirling et al 1979) and Tay–Sachs disease (Milunsky 1973).

If an enzyme assay is not available for a particular inborn error, it may be possible to measure a specific metabolite in amniotic fluid as in one of the earliest reports of metabolic prenatal diagnosis (Crawfurd et al 1973), but such techniques, which include gas chromatography and mass spectrometry, may not be reliable (Matalon et al 1972). However, the measurement of a metabolite may be a useful check against the possibility of cell contamination of amniotic fluid or chorionic villi if an enzyme assay result is equivocal.

Biochemical assessment of the phenotype was also employed in the detection of abnormal haemoglobin chain synthesis using carboxymethyl cellulose urea chromatography (Huehns et al 1964, Clegg et al 1966), but these methods have been largely superseded by DNA analysis.

Gene identification

The last 20 years have seen major technological advances in molecular biology. Using techniques such as Southern blotting, polymerase chain reaction and fluorescence in situ hybridization, many individual genes or chromosomes can be detected, permitting more sophisticated diagnosis of inherited disorders.

Southern blotting involves the cleavage of chromosomal DNA at specific sites using DNA nucleases of bacterial origin followed by gel electrophoretic separation of fragments. Treatment with sodium hydroxide denatures the DNA. After neutralizing with a suitable buffer, the gel is placed on a filter wick, under a nylon membrane and then compressed. The DNA rises with the high salt solution through to the membrane to which it binds. The Southern blot thus obtained can be hybridized to a radioactive-labelled DNA probe specific to the gene under study. After autoradiography, the location of the bound radioactive probe can be identified, and thus the length of the DNA fragment which contains the gene.

Polymerase chain reaction amplifies specific DNA or RNA fragments, allowing further investigation. Once the sequence of nucleotides is known for a region of DNA strand either side of the area to be studied, complementary oligonucleotides and a polymerase are added to single stranded DNA, which permits replication and therefore doubling of the DNA. This process is repeated up to 30 times until sufficient DNA is available. It requires very high quality control to avoid contamination, as any contaminant will be amplified as well.

This test permits the identification of specific DNA sequences of gene mutations and allows the amplification of DNA from small supplies as diverse as Egyptian mummies and the Guthrie spots from neonates. The need for only a small amount of starting template (e.g. a single cell) is the great advantage of polymerase chain reaction in modern prenatal diagnosis, with the possibility of prenatal diagnosis of inherited disorders being performed on a single cell taken from an embryo prior to transfer after in vitro fertilization (preimplantation diagnosis) (Monk 1992).

Fluorescence in situ hydridization is a technique where a fluorescent probe attached to a known DNA sequence is added to uncultured, non-dividing cells. Under appropriate examination conditions, the presence of the probe in the interphase nuclei of the cells confirms that the DNA sequence is present in the chromosomes. This technique has many potential applications, including the diagnosis of chromosomal anomalies in fetal cells isolated from maternal blood (Elias et al 1992) and the rapid detection (within 6 hours) of aneuploidy in fetal tissue (Pandya et al 1994).

Gene expression can also be studied using modern molecular genetic techniques. This relies on RNA analysis, using similar blot techniques and in situ hybridization (Bennett & Moore 1992). All the modern techniques have applications which are expanding rapidly, and it is difficult to keep up to date with current advances.

However, referral to a genetics centre for advice concerning current diagnostic techniques permits the clinician to optimize the prenatal diagnosis service for every mother at risk.

ETHICAL CONSIDERATIONS

Prenatal diagnosis offers the potential for improvement of the health of future generations, by avoiding handicap and abnormality in the community. However, there are many areas of controversy and ethical difficulty.

Informed consent

Most couples attending for antenatal care do not consider themselves at risk of having a pregnancy affected by an inherited disorder. The approach to the routine ultrasound examination is generally that of confirming normality rather than exclusion of abnormality. Many women, when informed that their baby has an abnormality, will say that they were unaware that abnormalities were looked for. It is essential that all women are allowed to give informed consent to every aspect of prenatal diagnosis, including the routine scan. The introduction of serum screening for chromosomal abnormality has emphasized the fact that many health-care workers do not understand the implications of the tests they are offering, and thus cannot counsel the women appropriately.

Termination of pregnancy

Counselling women for prenatal diagnosis must include non-directive discussion of the options available if an abnormality is confirmed, and this may include termination of an affected pregnancy. Details of the procedure of termination must be given before prenatal testing occurs, as some women faced with a mid-trimester termination would rather not undergo prenatal diagnosis at all.

Improving obstetric management

The diagnosis of an inherited disorder in any pregnancy does not automatically result in termination of that pregnancy. Prenatal diagnosis is an exercise in information gathering, that permits all those involved in an affected pregnancy to give the best management to that couple. The commonest questions, regardless of outcome, asked by the parents of a baby with an inherited disorder are 'Why did it happen, and will it happen again?' Only with appropriate and thorough investigation can these questions be answered.

Appropriate use of prenatal diagnostic techniques will also permit optimal management of subsequent pregnancies, with the potential for early diagnosis.

The organization of prenatal diagnosis services

All obstetricians and midwives involved in antenatal care should have a background knowledge of the conditions which can be diagnosed prenatally, how that diagnosis is made and where the relevant investigations can be performed. However, the sophistication of the techniques involved means that expertise is generally concentrated in regional referral centres for fetal medicine and genetics. Referral across normal administrative boundaries must be smooth and swift, as delays in achieving prenatal diagnosis may deny a couple the opportunity of terminating an affected pregnancy, with the attendant problems. Referral centres must have counsellors trained in prenatal diagnosis and bereavement care. There should ideally be a dedicated perinatal pathology service.

Patient support groups are extremely valuable, and exist for mutual support of families affected by a variety of inherited disorders. In addition, organizations exist for the support of those parents who have lost affected pregnancies (SATFA). Obstetricians should be aware of these groups, and be able to help their patients contact the relevant ones.

REFERENCES

Affara N A, Ferguson-Smith M A, Tolmie J et al 1986 Variable transfer of Y-specific sequences in XX males. Nucleic Acids Research 14: 5375–5387

Alvarez H 1964 Morphology, pathophysiology of the human placenta I. Studies of morphology and development of the chorionic villi by phase-contrast microscopy. Obstetrics and Gynecology 28: 813

Austin C R 1962 Sex chromatin in embryonic and fetal tissue. Acta Cytologica 6: 61–68

Baumgarten A, Schoenfeld M, Mohoney M J, Greenstein R M, Saal H M 1985 Prospective screening for Down syndrome using maternal serum AFP. Lancet i: 1280–1281

Bavin J T R, Marshall R, Delhanty J D A 1963 A mongol with 21 : 22 type chromosomal translocation. Journal of Mental Deficiency Research 7: 84–89

Bell S G 1988 Nonimmune hydrops fetalis. Neonatal Network 7: 15–27

Benacerraf B R, Barss V A, Saltzman D H, Greene M F, Penso C A,

Frigoletto F D 1987 Acute fetal distress associated with percutaneous umbilical blood sampling. American Journal of Obstetrics and Gynecology 156: 1218–1220

Bennett P, Moore G 1992 Studying the expression of genes. In: Molecular biology for obstetricians and gynaecologists. Blackwell Scientific Publications, Oxford, pp 111–117

Best J M, Banatvala J E, Morgan-Capner P, Miller E 1989 Fetal infection after maternal reinfection with rubella: criteria for defining reinfection. British Medical Journal 299: 773–735

Bewley S, Roberts L J, Mackinson A-M, Rodeck C H 1994 First trimester fetal nuchal translucency—problems with screening the general population. British Journal of Obstetrics and Gynaecology (in press).

Bogart M H, Pandian M R, Jones O W 1987 Abnormal maternal serum chorionic gonadotrophin levels in pregnancies with fetal chromosome abnormalities. Prenatal Diagnosis 7: 623–630

Brambati B, Oldrini A, Simoni G et al 1983 First trimester fetal karyotyping in twin pregnancy. Journal of Medical Genetics 20: 58–60

Byrne D, Marks K, Azar G, Nicolaides K 1991 Randomized study of early amniocentesis versus chorionic villus sampling: a technical and cytogenetic comparison of 650 patients. Ultrasound in Obstetrics and Gynaecology 1: 235–240

Canadian Collaborative CVS–Amniocentesis Clinical Trial Group 1989 Multicentre randomized clinical trial of chorion villus sampling and amniocentesis. Lancet i: 1–6

Canadian Medical Research Council 1977 Diagnosis of genetic disease by amniocentesis during the second trimester of pregnancy. A Canadian study. Report No: 5 Supple Services, Ottawa, Canada

Carter C O, Hamerton J L, Polani P E, Gunalp A, Weller S D V 1986 Chromosome translocation as a cause of familial mongolism. Lancet ii: 678–680

Caspersson T, Zech L, Johansson C 1970 Analysis of human metaphase chromosome set by aid of DNA-binding fluorescent agents. Experimental Cell Research 62: 490–492

Chadefaux B, Rabier D, Dumez Y, Oury J F, Kamoun P 1989 Eleventh week amniocentesis for prenatal diagnosis of metabolic diseases. Lancet i: 849

Chapple J C 1992 Genetic screening. In: Brock D J H, Rodeck C H, Ferguson-Smith M A (eds) Prenatal diagnosis and screening. Churchill Livingstone, Edinburgh, pp 579–593

Chard T, Lowings C, Kitau M J 1984 Alphafetoprotein and chorionic gonadotrophin levels in relation to Down's syndrome. Lancet ii: 750

Clegg J B, Naughton M A, Weatherall D J 1966 Abnormal human haemoglobins; separation and characterisation of the γ and β chains by chromatography and the determination of two new variants Hb Chesapeake and Hb J (Bangkok). Journal of Molecular Biology 19: 91–108

Cossart Y E, Field A M, Cant B, Widdows D 1975 Parvovirus-like particles in human sera. Lancet i: 72–73

Crawfurd M d'A 1988 Regular review: prenatal diagnosis of common genetic disorders. British Medical Journal 297: 502–506

Crawfurd M d'A, Dean M F, Hunt D M et al 1973 Early prenatal diagnosis of Hurler's syndrome with termination of pregnancy and confirmatory findings of the fetus. Journal of Medical Genetics 10: 144–153

Cuckle H S, Wald N J, Lindenbaum R H 1984 Maternal serum alpha-fetoprotein measurement: a screening test for Down's syndrome. Lancet i: 926–929

Cuckle H S, Wald N J, Lindenbaum R H 1985 Screening for Down's syndrome using serum alpha-fetoprotein. British Medical Journal 291: 349

Cuckle H S, Wald N J, Goodburn S F, Sneddon J, Amess J A L, Carlson Dunn S 1990 Measurement of activity of urea resistant neutrophil alkaline phosphatase as an antenatal screening test for Down's syndrome. British Medical Journal 301: 1024–1026

Czepulkowski B H, Heaton D E, Kearney L U, Rodeck C H, Coleman D V 1986 Chorionic villus culture for first trimester diagnosis of chromosome defects: evaluation by two London centres. Prenatal Diagnosis 6: 271–282

Daffos F, Capella-Pavlovsky M, Forestier F 1983 Fetal blood sampling via the umbilical cord using a needle guided by ultrasound. Prenatal Diagnosis 3: 271–274

Daffos F, Capella Pavlovsky M, Forestier F 1985 Fetal blood sampling during pregnancy with the use of a needle guided by ultrasound: a study of 606 consecutive cases. American Journal of Obstetrics and Gynecology 153: 655–60

Daffos F, Forestier F, Capella Pavlovsky M et al 1988 Prenatal management of 746 pregnancies at risk for congenital toxoplasmosis. New England Journal of Medicine 318: 271–275

Edwards P J, Hall D M B 1992 Screening, ethics and the law. British Medical Journal 305: 267–268

Eichenbaum S Z, Krumins E J, Fortune D W, Duke J 1986 False negative findings on chorionic villus sampling. Lancet ii: 391

Elias S, Price J, Dockter M et al 1992 First trimester prenatal diagnosis of trisomy 21 in fetal cells from maternal blood. Lancet 340: 1033

Fairweather D V I, Ward R H T, Modell B 1980 Obstetrics aspects of mid-trimester fetal blood sampling by needling or fetoscopy. British Journal of Obstetrics and Gynaecology 87: 87–91

Feinkind L, Nanda D, Delke I, Minkoff H 1990 Abruptio placentae after percutaneous umbilical cord sampling: a case report. American Journal of Obstetrics and Gynecology 162: 1203–1204

Firth H V, Boyd P A, Chamberlain P, MacKenzie I Z, Lindenbaum R H, Huson S M 1991 Severe limb abnormalities after chorion villus sampling at 56–66 days gestation. Lancet 337: 762–763

Fisk N M, Ronderos-Dumit D, Soliani A, Nicolini U, Vaughan J, Rodeck C H 1991 Diagnostic and therapeutic transabdominal amnioinfusion in oligohydramnios. Obstetrics and Gynecology 78: 270–278

Fogarty P, Dornan J C, Magee A, Priest F 1991 Early amniocentesis in Northern Ireland: experience of 561 cases. Abstract: Blair Bell Research Society Meeting, Belfast, September 1991

Ford C E, Hamerton J L 1956 The chromosomes of man. Nature 178: 1020–1023

Ford C E, Jones K W, Polani P E, de Almeida J C, Briggs J H 1969 A sex chromosome anomaly in a case of gonadal dysgenesis (Turner's syndrome). Lancet i: 711–713

Forestier F, Daffos F, Rainaut M et al 1987 Suivi thérapeutique foetomaternel de la spiramycine en cours de grossesse. Archives français de Pédiatrie 44: 539–544

Fuchs F 1971 Amniocentesis and abortion: methods and risks. Birth Defects Original Article Series 7: 18–19

Fuchs F, Riis P 1956 Antenatal sex determination. Nature 177: 330

Fujimoto W Y, Seegmiller J E, Uhlendorf B W, Jacobson C B 1968 Biochemical diagnosis of an X-linked disease in utero. Lancet ii: 511–512

Furhmann W, Wendt P, Weitzel H K 1984 Maternal serum-AFP as screeing test for Down syndrome. Lancet ii: 413

Gibbs D A, McFadyen I R, Crawfurd M d'A et al 1984 First trimester diagnosis of Lesch–Nyhan syndrome. Lancet ii: 1180–1183

Goldfarb A E, Hochner-Celnikier D, Beller U, Menashe M, Dargan I, Palti Z 1982 A successful pregnancy in transfusion dependent homozygous β-thalassaemia: a case report. International Journal of Gynaecology and Obstetrics 20: 319–332

Goossens M N, Dumez Y, Kaplan L et al 1983 Prenatal diagnosis of sickle cell anaemia in the first trimester of pregnancy. New England Journal of Medicine 309: 831–833

Gosden J R, Mitchell A R, Gosden C M, Rodeck C H, Morsman J M 1982 Direct vision chorion biopsy and chromosome specific DNA probes for determination of fetal sex in first trimester prenatal diagnosis. Lancet ii: 1418–1420

Gosden J R, Gosden C M, Christie S, Cooke H J, Morsman J M, Rodeck C H 1984 The use of cloned Y chromosome-specific DNA probes for fetal sex determination in first trimester prenatal diagnosis. Human Genetics 66: 347–351

Hackett G A, Smith J H, Rebello M T et al 1991 Early amniocentesis at 11–14 weeks for diagnosis of fetal chromosomal abnormality—a clinical evaluation. Prenatal Diagnosis 11: 311–315

Hahnemann N, Mohr J 1968 Genetic diagnosis in the embryo by means of biopsy from extra-embryonic membranes. Bulletin of European Society of Human Genetics 2: 23–29

Harrison R, Campbell S, Craft I 1975 Risks of feto-maternal haemorrhage resulting from amniocentesis with and without ultrasound placental localization. Obstetrics and Gynecology 46: 389–391

Hislop A, Fairweather D V I, Blackwell R J, Howard S 1984 The effect of amniocentesis and drainage of amniotic fluid on lung development in Macaca fascicularis. American Journal of Obstetrics and Gynecology 91: 835–842

Hobbins J C, Mahoney M J 1974 In utero diagnosis of hemoglobinopathies. Technic for obtaining fetal blood. New England Journal of Medicine 290: 1065–1067

Holzgreve W, Golbus M S 1984 Prenatal diagnosis of ornithine transcarbamylase deficiency using fetal liver biopsy. American Journal of Human Genetics 36: 320–324

Hook E B, Cross P K, Schreinemachers D M 1983 Chromosomal abnormality rates at amniocentesis and in live-born infants. Journal of the American Medical Association 249: 2034–2038

Horwell D H, Loeffler F E, Coleman D V 1983 Assessment of transcervical aspiration technique for chorionic villus biopsy in the first trimester of pregnancy. British Journal of Obstetrics and Gynecology 90: 196–198

Houlsby W T 1984 Maternal serum AFP as a screening test for Down syndrome. Lancet i: 1127

Huehns E R, Dance N, Beavan G H, Hect F, Motulsky A G 1964 Human embryonic haemoglobin. Cold Spring Harbour Symposium on Quantitative Biology 29: 327–331

Jacobs P A, Strong J A 1959 A case of human intersexuality having a possible XXY sex-determining mechanism. Nature 183: 302–303

Jacobson C B, Barter R H 1967 Intrauterine diagnosis and management of genetic defects. American Journal of Obstetrics and Gynecology 99: 796–807

James D, Bickley D, Davies T, McDermott A 1992 Influence of the Lancet on chorionic villus sampling. Lancet 340: 180–181

Jeanty P, Rodesch F, Romero R, Venus I, Hobbins J C 1983 How to improve your amniocentesis technique. American Journal of Obstetrics and Gynecology 146: 593–596

Johnson P, Allan L D, Maxwell D J 1993 Nonimmune hydrops fetalis. In: Studd J (ed) Progress in Obstetrics and Gynaecology 10. Churchill and Livingstone, London, pp 33–50

Jonatha W D 1974 Amniozentese in der Fruhschwangerschaft unter Sichtkontrolle mit Ultraschall. Elektromedica 3: 94–96

Kaback M M 1984 Utility of prenatal diagnosis. In: Rodeck C H, Nicolaides K H (eds) Prenatal diagnosis (Proceedings of 11th Study Group of Royal College of Obstetricians and Gynaecologists). RCOG, London, pp 1–12

Kalousek D K, Dill F J 1983 Chromosomal mosaicism confined to the placenta in human conceptions. Science 221: 665–667

Kan Y W, Valenti C, Guidotti R, Carnazza V, Rieder R F 1974 Fetal blood sampling in utero. Lancet i: 79–80

Kazazian H H 1990 The thalassaemia syndromes: molecular basis and prenatal diagnosis in 1990. Seminars in Haematology 27: 209–228

Kazy Z, Rozovsky I S, Bakharev V A 1982 Chorion biopsy in early pregnancy: a method of early prenatal diagnosis for inherited disorders. Prenatal Diagnosis 2: 39–45

Kerenyl T D, Walker B 1977 The preventability of 'bloody taps' in second trimester amniocentesis by ultrasound scanning. Obstetrics and Gynecology 50: 61–64

Knott P D, Welply G A C, Anderson M J 1984 Serologically proven intrauterine infection with parvovirus. British Medical Journal 289: 1660

Kullander S, Sandahl B 1973 Fetal chromosome analysis after transcervical placental biopsies during early pregnancy. Acta Obstetrica et Gynecologica Scandinavica 52: 355–359

Lancet Editorial 1987 Marrow transplantation for thalassaemia. Lancet i: 1246

Lange I, Rodeck C H, Morgan-Capner P, Simmons A, Kangro H O 1982 Prenatal serological diagnosis of intrauterine cytomegalovirus infection. British Medical Journal 1: 284–285

Lejeune J, Gautier M, Turpin R 1959 Les chromosomes humains en culture de tissus. Compte Rendus de l'Academie de Science (Paris) 248: 602–603

Levine S C, Filly R A, Golbus M A 1978 Ultrasonography for guidance of amniocentesis in genetic counselling. Clinical Genetics 14: 133

Lewis M, Faed M J W, Howie P 1991 Screening for Down's syndrome based on individual risk. British Medical Journal 303: 551–553

Lilford R, Maxwell D, Coleman D, Czepulkowski B, Heaton D 1983 Diagnosis, 4 hours after chorion biopsy, of female fetus in pregnancy at risk of Duchenne muscular dystrophy. Lancet ii: 1491

Lilford R J 1991 The rise and fall of chorionic villus sampling. British Medical Journal 303: 936–937

Lisgar F, Gertner M, Cherry S, Hau L Y, Hirschorn K 1970 Prenatal chromosome analysis. Nature 225: 280-281

Liu D T Y, Mitchell J, Johnson J, Wass D M 1983 Trophoblast sampling by blind transcervical aspiration. British Journal of Obstetrics and Gynaecology 90: 1119–1123

Livingstone J, Axton R A, Gilfillan A et al 1994 Antenatal screening for cystic fibrosis: a trial of the couple model. British Medical Journal 308: 1459–1462

Lo Y-M, Wainscot J S, Gillmer M D G, Patel P, Sampietro M, Fleming K A 1989 Prenatal sex determination by DNA amplification from maternal peripheral blood. Lancet ii: 1363–1365

Macri J N, Buchanan P D, Gold M P 1986 Low alpha-fetoprotein and trisomy. Lancet ii: 405

Malcolm S, Clayton-Smith J, Nichols M et al 1991 Angelman syndrome can result from uniparental disomy. Lancet 337: 694–697

Manning F A, Harrison M M R, Rodeck C H 1986 Catheter shunts for fetal hydronephrosis and hydrocephalus. Report of the International Fetal Surgery Registry. New England Journal of Medicine 315: 336–340

Martin A O, Elias S, Rosinsky B, Bombard A T, Simpson J L 1986 False-negative finding on chorionic villus sampling Lancet ii: 391

Matalon R, Dorfman A, Nadler H L 1972 A chemical method for the antenatal diagnosis of mucopolysaccharidoses. Lancet i: 798–799

Maxwell D, Czepulkowski B H, Heaton D E, Coleman D V, Lilford R 1985 A practical assessment of ultrasound-guided transcervical aspiration of chorionic villi and subsequent chromosomal analysis. British Journal of Obstetrics and Gynaecology 92: 660–665

Maxwell D J, Johnson P, Hurley P, Neales K, Allan L D, Knott P 1991 Pregnancy loss after fetal blood sampling—an evaluation in relation to indication. British Journal of Obstetrics and Gynaecology 98: 892–897

Medical Research Council 1978 An assessment of the hazards of amniocentesis. British Journal of Obstetrics and Gynaecology 85 (suppl 2)

Merkatz I R, Nitowsky H M, Macri J N, Johnson W E 1984 An association between low maternal serum alpha-fetoprotein and fetal chromosomal abnormalities. American Journal of Obstetrics and Gynecology 148: 886–894

Mibashan R S, Rodeck C H 1984 Haemophilia and other genetic defects of haemostasis. In: Rodeck C H, Nicolaides K H (eds) Prenatal diagnosis. Wiley, Chichester, pp 179–194

Milunsky A 1973 The prenatal diagnosis of hereditary disorders. Thomas, Springfield, Illinois

Milunsky A, Atkins L, Littlefield J W 1972 Amniocentesis for prenatal genetic studies. Obstetrics and Gynecology 40: 104–108

Modell M, Modell B 1990 Genetic screening for ethnic minorities. British Medical Journal 300: 1702–1704

Monk M 1992 Preimplantation diagnosis—a comprehensive review. In: Brock D J H, Rodeck C H, Ferguson-Smith M A (eds) Prenatal diagnosis and screening. Churchill Livingstone, Edinburgh, pp 627–638

Morgan-Capner P, Rodeck C H, Nicolaides K H, Cradock-Watson J E 1985 Prenatal diagnosis of rubella specific IgM in fetal sera. Prenatal Diagnosis 5: 21–26

MRC Working Party 1978 An assessment of the hazards of amniocentesis. British Journal of Obstetrics and Gynaecology 85 (suppl 2): 1–41

MRC Working Party on the Evaluation of Chorionic Villus Sampling 1991 Medical Research Council European trial of chorionic villus sampling. Lancet 337: 1491–1499

Munro N D et al 1987 Temporal relations between maternal rubella and congenital defects. Lancet i: 201

Murday V, Slack J 1985 Screening for Down's syndrome in the north east Thames region. British Medical Journal 291: 1315–1318

Nadler H L 1968 Antenatal detection of hereditary disorders. Pediatrics 42: 912–918

Nadler H L 1971 Indications for amniocentesis in the early prenatal detection of genetic disorders. Birth Defects Original Article Series 7: 5–9

Nadler H L, Gerbie A B 1970 Role of amniocentesis in intrauterine detection of genetic disorders. New England Journal of Medicine 282: 596–599

National Institute of Child Health and Development Amniocentesis Register 1978 The safety and accuracy of mid-trimester amniocentesis. US Department of Health, Education and Welfare, No 78–190

Nevin J, Nevin N C, Dornan J C, Sim D, Armstrong M J 1990 Early amniocentesis: experience of 222 consecutive patients. Prenatal Diagnosis 10: 79–83

Nicolaides K 1988 Cordocentesis. Clinical Obstetrics and Gynaecology 31: 123–135

Nicolaides K H, Rodeck C H, Soothill P W, Warren R C 1986a Why confine chorionic villus (placental) biopsy to the first trimester? Lancet i: 543–544

Nicolaides K H, Rodeck C H, Gosden C M 1986b Rapid karyotyping in non-lethal malformations. Lancet i: 283–286

Nicolaides K H, Azar G, Byrne D, Mansur C, Marks K 1992 Fetal nuchal translucency: ultrasound screening for chromosomal defects in the first trimester of pregnancy. British Medical Journal 304: 867–869

Nicolini U, Santolaya J, Ojo O E et al 1988 The fetal intrahepatic vein as an alternative to cord needling for prenatal diagnosis and therapy. Prenatal Diagnosis 3: 665–671

Nicolini U, Fisk N M, Talbert D G et al 1989 Intrauterine manometry: technique and application to fetal pathology. Prenatal Diagnosis 9: 243–254

Nicolini U, Tannirandom Y, Gonzalez P et al 1990a Continuing controversy in alloimmune thrombocytopenia: fetal hyperimmunoglobulinaemia fails to prevent thrombocytopenia. American Journal of Obstetrics and Gynecology 143: 1144–1146

Nicolini U, Nicolaides P, Fisk N M et al 1990b Limited role of fetal blood sampling in prediction of outcome in intrauterine growth retardation. Lancet 336: 768–772

Noah N D, Fowle S E 1988 Immunity to rubella in women of childbearing age in the United Kingdom. British Medical Journal 297: 1301–1308

Nowell P C, Hungerford D A 1960 Chromosome studies on normal and leukemic human lymphocytes. Journal of the National Cancer Institute 25: 85–109

Orlandi F, Damiani G, Jakil C et al 1990 The risks of early cordocentesis (12–21 weeks): analysis of 500 procedures. Prenatal Diagnosis 10: 425–428

Painter T S 1923 Studies in mammalian spermatogenesis II. The spermatogenesis of man. Journal of Experimental Zoology 37: 291–321

Pandya P P, Kuhn P, Brizot M, Cardy D L, Nicolaides K H 1994 Rapid detection of chromosome aneuploidies in fetal blood and chorionic villi by fluorescence in situ hybridization. British Journal of Obstetrics and Gynaecology 101: 493–497

Paryani S G, Arvin A M 1986 Intrauterine infection with varicella-zoster virus after maternal varicella. New England Journal of Medicine 314: 1542–1546

Patau K, Smith D W, Therman E, Inhorn S L, Wagner H P 1960 Multiple congenital anomaly caused by an extra autosome. Lancet i: 790–793

Penrose L S, Delhanty J D A 1961 Familial Langdon Down anomaly with chromosomal fusion. Annals of Human Genetics 25: 243–252

Penrose L S, Ellis J R, Delhanty J D A 1960 Chromosomal translocations in mongolism and normal relatives. Lancet ii: 409–410

Pijpers L, Jahoda M G J, Reuss A, Wladimiroff J W, Sachs E S 1988 Transabdominal chorionic villus sampling in second and third trimesters of pregnancy to determine fetal karyotype. British Medical Journal 297: 822–823

Polani P E, Briggd J H, Ford C E, Clarke C M, Berg J M 1960 A mongol girl with 46 chromosomes. Lancet i: 721–723

Rebello M T, Hackett G, Smith J et al 1991 Extraction of DNA from amniotic fluid cells for the early prenatal diagnosis of genetic disease. Prenatal Diagnosis 11: 41–46

Rhoads G G, Jackson L G, Schesselman S E et al 1989 The safety and efficacy of chorionic villus sampling for early prenatal diagnosis of cytogenetic abnormalities. New England Journal of Medicine 320: 609–617

Riis P, Fuchs F 1960 Antenatal determination of foetal sex in prevention of hereditary disease. Lancet ii: 180–182

Rodeck C 1980 Fetoscopy guided by real-time ultrasound for pure fetal blood samples, fetal skin samples and examination of the fetus in utero. British Journal of Obstetrics and Gynaecology 87: 449–456

Rodeck C H 1993 Prenatal diagnosis: fetal development after chorionic villus sampling. Lancet 341: 468–469

Rodeck C H, Campbell S 1978 Sampling pure fetal blood by fetoscopy in second trimester of pregnancy. British Medical Journal 2: 728–730

Rodeck C H, Nicolaides K H 1986 Fetoscopy. British Medical Bulletin 42: 296–300

Rodeck C H, Eady R A, Gosden C M 1980 Prenatal diagnosis of epidermolysis bullosa fetalis. Lancet i: 949–952

Rodeck C H, Kemp J R, Holman C A, Whitemore D N, Karnicki J, Austen N A 1981 Direct intravascular fetal blood transfusion by fetoscopy in severe rehesus isoimmunization. Lancet i: 625–627

Rodeck C H, Patrick A D, Pembrey M E, Tzannatos C, Whitfield A E 1982 Fetal liver biopsy for prenatal diagnosis of ornithine carbamyl transferase deficiency. Lancet ii: 297–299

Rodeck C H, Morsman J M, Nicolaides K H, McKenzie C, Gosden C M, Gosden J R 1983 A single operator technique for first trimester chorion biopsy. Lancet ii: 1340–1341

Rodeck C H, Fisk N M, Fraser D I, Nicolini U 1988 Long-term in utero drainage of fetal hydrothorax. New England Journal of Medicine 319: 1135–1138

Rodeck C H, Sheldrake A, Beattie B, Whittle M J 1993 Maternal serum alphafetoprotein after placental damage in chorionic villus sampling. Lancet 341: 500

Rommens J M, Ianuzzi M C, Kerem B-S et al 1989 Identification of the cystic fibrosis gene: chromosome walking and jumping. Science 245: 1059–1065

Sachs L, Serr D M, Danon M 1956 Analysis of amniotic fluid cells for diagnosis of fetal sex. British Medical Journal 2: 795–798

Saura R, Longy M, Horovitz J et al 1990 Risks of transabdominal chorionic villus sampling before the 12th week of amenorrhoea. Prenatal Diagnosis 10: 461–467

Schmidt W, Harms E, Wolf D 1985 Successful treatment of non-immune hydrops fetalis due to congenital chylothorax. British Journal of Obstetrics and Gynaecology 92: 685–687

Scrimgeour J B 1973 Other techniques for antenatal diagnosis. In: Emery A E H (ed) Antenatal diagnosis of genetic disease. Churchill Livingstone, Edinburgh, pp 40–57

Seabright M 1971 A rapid banding technique for human chromosomes. Lancet ii: 971–972

Seller M J 1984 Prenatal screening for Down syndrome. Lancet i: 1359

Sergovich F R, Soltan H C, Carr D H 1962 A 13–15/21 translocation chromosome in carrier father and mongol son. Canadian Medical Association Journal 87: 852–858

Simoni G, Brambati B, Danesino C, Fraccaro M 1984 Antenatal sex determination. Lancet i: 397

Simoni G, Gimelli G, Cuoco C et al 1986 First trimester fetus karyotyping: 1000 diagnoses. Human Genetics 72: 203–209

Smidt-Jensen S, Hahnemann N 1984 Transabdominal fine needle biopsy from chorionic villi in the first trimester. Prenatal Diagnosis 4: 163–169

Smidt-Jensen S, Permin M, Philip J 1991 Sampling success and risk by transabdominal chorionic villus sampling, transcervical chorionic villus sampling, and amniocentesis: a randomised study. Ultrasound in Obstetrics and Gynaecology 1: 86–90

Soothill P 1990 Intrauterine blood transfusion for nonimmune hydrops fetalis due to parvovirus B19 infection. Lancet 336: 121–122

Speleman F, VanRoy N, Wiegant J et al 1992 Detection of subtle reciprocal translocations by fluorescence in situ hybridization. Clinical Genetics 41: 169–174

Spencer K, Carpenter P 1985 Screening for Down's syndrome using serum alpha-fetoprotein: a retrospective study indicating caution. British Medical Journal 290: 1940–1943

Squire J A, Nauth L, Ridler M A C, Sutton S, Timberlake C 1982 Prenatal diagnosis and outcome of pregnancy in 2036 women investigated by amniocentesis. Human Genetics 61: 215–222

Stagno S, Whitley R J 1985 Herpesvirus infections of pregnancy, Part 1. Cytomegalovirus and Epstein Barr virus infections. New England Journal of Medicine 313: 1270–1274

Statham H, Green J 1993 Serum screening for Down's syndrome: some women's experience. British Medical Journal 307: 174–176

Steele M W, Bregg W R 1966 Chromosome analysis of human amniotic fluid cells. Lancet i: 383–385

Stein Z, Stein W, Susser 1986 Hypothesis: attrition of trisomies as a maternal screening device, an explanation of the association of trisomy 21 with maternal age. Lancet i: 944–947

Stirling J L, Robinson D, Fensom A H, Benson P F, Baker J E, Button L R 1979 Prenatal diagnosis of two Hurler fetuses using an improved assay for methylumbelliferyl-alpha-L-iduronidase. Lancet ii: 37

Stray-Pedersen B 1993 Toxoplasmosis in pregnancy. Clinical Obstetrics and Gynaecology 7: 115–137

Stripparo L, Buscaglia M, Longatti L et al 1990 Genetic amniocentesis: 505 cases performed before the sixteenth week of gestation. Prenatal Diagnosis 10: 359–364

Sumner A T, Evans H J, Buckland R A 1971 New technique for distinguishing between human chromosomes. Nature New Biology 232: 31–32

Sundberg K, Smidt-Jensen S, Philip J 1991 Amniocentesis with increased cell yield, obtained by filtration and reinjection of the amniotic fluid. Ultrasound in Obstetrics and Gynaecology 1: 91–94

Super M, Schwarz M J, Malone G, Roberts T, Haworth A, Dermody G 1994 Active cascade testing for carriers of cystic fibrosis gene. British Medical Journal 308: 1462–1468

Tabor A, Norgaard-Pederson B, Jacobsen J C 1984 Low maternal serum AFP and Down syndrome. Lancet ii: 16

Tabor A, Philip J, Marsen M, Bang J, Obel F B, Norgaard-Pederson B 1986 Randomised controlled trial of genetic amniocentesis in 4606 low-risk women. Lancet i: 1287–1293

Terry G M, Ho-Terry L, Warren R C, Rodeck C H, Cohen A, Rees K 1986 First trimester prenatal diagnosis of congenital rubella: a laboratory investigation. British Medical Journal 292: 930–933

Thornton J G, Costain K, Thomas M, Blakeman J M, Hester S A, Lilford R J 1990 Identification of the cystic fibrosis gene. British Medical Journal 300: 1141

Tietung Hospital of Anshan Steelworks, Department of Obstetrics and Gynaecology 1975 Fetal sex prediction by sex chromatin of chorionic villi cells during early pregnancy. Chinese Medical Journal 1: 117–126

Timson J, Harris R, Gadd R L, Ferguson-Smith M E, Ferguson-Smith M A 1971 Down's syndrome due to maternal mosaicism, and the value of antenatal diagnosis. Lancet i: 549–550

Tjio J H, Levan A 1956 The chromosome numbers of man. Hereditas 42: 1–6

Turner G, Robinson H, Laing S et al 1992 Population screening for fragile X. Lancet 339: 1210–1213

Valenti C 1972 Endoamnioscopy and fetal biopsy: a new technique. American Journal of Obstetrics and Gynecology 114: 561–564

Vaughan J I, Rodeck C H 1992 Interventional procedures. In: Meire H, Cosgrove D, Denbury K (eds) Clinical ultrasound—a comprehensive text. Churchill Livingstone, Edinburgh

Ville Y, Lalondrelle C, Doumerc S et al 1992 First-trimester diagnosis of nuchal anomalies: significance and fetal outcome. Ultrasound in Obstetrics and Gynaecology 2: 314–316

Wahlstrom T, Brosset A, Bartsch F 1970 Viability of amniotic cells at different stages of gestation. Lancet ii: 1037

Wald N J, Cuckle H S, Densem J W et al 1988a Maternal unconjugated oestriol as an antenatal screening test for Down's syndrome. British Journal of Obstetrics and Gynaecology 95: 334–341

Wald N J, Cuckle H S, Densem J W et al 1988b Maternal serum screening for Down's syndrome in early pregnancy. British Medical Journal 297: 883–887

Wald N, Stone R, Cuckle H S et al 1992 First trimester concentrations of pregnancy associated plasma protein A and placental protein 14 in Down's syndrome. British Medical Journal 305: 28

Walknowska J, Conte F A, Grumback M M 1969 Practical and theoretical implications of fetal/maternal lymphocyte transfer. Lancet i: 1119

Warburton D, Miller O J 1972 Present status and future trends in prenatal diagnosis of chromosomal disorders. Clinics in Obstetrics and Gynaecology 15: 272–282

Ward R H T, Modell B, Petrou M, Karagozlou F, Douratsos E 1983 Method of sampling chorionic villi in the first trimester of pregnancy under guidance of real-time ultrasound. British Medical Journal 286: 1542–1544

Watson E K, Mayall E S, Lamb J, Chapple J C, Williamson R 1992 Psychological and social consequences of community carrier screening programme for cystic fibrosis. Lancet 340: 217–220

Weatherall D J, Clegg J B 1981 The thalassaemia syndromes, 3rd edn. Blackwell Scientific Publications, Oxford

Westgren M, Selbing A, Stangenberg M 1988 Fetal intracardiac transfusions in patients with severe rhesus isoimmunisation. British Medical Journal 296: 885–886

Williamson R, Eskdale J, Coleman D V, Niazi M, Loeffler F E, Modell B 1981 Direct gene analysis of chorionic villi: a possible technique for the first trimester diagnosis of haemoglobinopathies. Lancet ii: 1125–1127

Wyatt P R 1985 Screening for Down's syndrome using serum alpha-fetoprotein. British Medical Journal 291: 740

Abnormal pregnancy

16. Assisted reproduction

Michael G. Chapman

The birth of Louise Brown following in vitro fertilization (IVF) in 1978 heralded a new era in the management of the infertile couple (Steptoe & Edwards 1978). The ability to deal directly with gametes of both partners has led to the proliferation of techniques aimed at assisting conception.

Many years of failure preceded the final success of Steptoe and Edwards and indeed rates of conception subsequently were poor. In the last 5 years refinements in techniques, a greater understanding of the biological processes which are involved, and advances in technology have led to significantly better outcomes of treatment than in the pioneering years. Indeed, in 1991 in the UK there were more than 1500 babies born by these techniques (Interim Licensing Authority 1991). In the USA more than 5500 babies were born (American Fertility Society Registry 1993).

However, assisted conception is by no means a panacea. At best each treatment cycle may bring success to a third of our patients—two-thirds will fail. Thus failure and its implications—psychological, emotional and physical—must be recognized and dealt with as an integral part of the management of an assisted conception programme. In addition, the subsequent obstetric problems of multiple births, growth retardation and high Caesarean section rates compound the difficulties for these patients.

The infertile couple become desperate for help to achieve their goal of pregnancy and a child. This makes them extremely vulnerable to suggestions that one or other treatment is likely to fulfil their dream. Appropriate selection of patients for specific therapies is therefore a vital aspect of our work. Appropriate counselling to support the couple when the situation is untreatable is also essential. Acceptance of childlessness is almost as important an aim as a successful pregnancy.

INTRODUCTION

The history of assisted conception was limited to the manipulation of sperm until in vitro fertilization (IVF) became a reality in the late 1970s. Intracervical and later intrauterine insemination (IUI) of partner's or donor's sperm has been a routine treatment during most of this century. The techniques to harvest oocytes and fertilize them with prepared sperm in the laboratory have been developed over the last 20 years. Standard IVF remains the mainstay of this approach. However, many variations have been explored and, for individual patients, offer optimum outcomes. Gamete intrafallopian transfer (GIFT) involves the harvesting of oocytes and their transfer to the site of fertilization, i.e. the distal Fallopian tube, with spermatozoa. Fertilization then occurs in vivo. Obviously this requires at least one normal tube. Pronuclear stage transfer (PROST), also known as zygote intrafallopian transfer (ZIFT), uses the normal Fallopian tube as an incubator once fertilization to the pronuclear stage of development has occurred. These latter procedures are generally done laparoscopically but the development of non-traumatic tubal catheters has allowed the gametes as zygotes to be transferred transcervically (Jansen & Anderson 1993).

The most exciting recent development has been the ability to fertilize oocytes with extremely few sperm. Indeed, direct insertion of a single sperm into the ooplasm by microsurgical techniques (ICSI) is now a reality (Van Steirteghem et al 1993). The previously considered infertile male now has a reasonable possibility of producing a child. Other advances have been in the area of cryobiology. The ability to freeze embryos has increased the chances of success from a single treatment from which there is an excess of good quality fresh embryos (Veeck et al 1993) or when immediate transfer of fresh embryos is impossible or contraindicated. Embryo freezing remains relatively inefficient since 50% of the embryos fail to survive the freeze and thawing process. Pregnancy rates with frozen embryos are between 10% and 15% per cycle.

Much effort is now being devoted to perfect the process of oocyte freezing. This technique will benefit women where oophorectomy is due to be undertaken or where chemotherapy may cause premature ovarian failure.

The ethical and moral dilemmas of donation of gametes have always been controversial. After public debate, general guidelines should be agreed (as in the UK by the Human Fertilisation and Embryology Authority (HFEA)); then begins the problems of appropriate counselling for all the parties involved. Detailed consideration of the various implications, e.g. anonymity, legal status of the child, risks of abnormality, is required. No area of medicine has greater interplay of advancing technology and society's acceptance of these improvements.

Assisted conception in its broadest sense encompasses any manipulation of gametes to enhance the possibility of conception. The list of the various techniques is long and increases yearly (Table 16.1).

ARTIFICIAL INSEMINATION

The use of artificial insemination has been documented for over 200 years. At its most elementary, an ejaculated sample of semen is injected into the upper vagina or posterior fornix at the time of ovulation. At its most complex, a selective separation of highly motile spermatozoa is performed and that specimen is injected transcervically into the upper uterus or even directly into the Fallopian tube with fine catheters within hours of ovulation as determined by hormonal and ultrasound tracking of the cycle.

John Hunter, in dealing with an infertile couple in whom the male had hypospadias, advised that the seminal fluid, which had escaped during intercourse, be inserted into the vagina with a warm syringe. This first documented case of artificial insemination by husband was successful (Home 1799). Cases of AIH are reported in the American literature in the nineteenth century. Several

Table 16.1 Abbreviations used for the more common forms of assisted conception

AI	Artificial insemination
AIH	Artificial insemination with husband's sperm
AIH, DI	Artificial insemination with donor sperm
IUI	Intrauterine insemination
IVF	In vitro fertilization
GIFT	Gamete intrafallopian transfer
PROST	Pronuclear stage transfer
ZIFT	Zygote intrafallopian transfer
SUZI	Subzonal insertion of sperm
PZD	Partial zona dissection
ICSI	Intracytoplasmic sperm injection

workers successfully employed AIH in cases of sexual dysfunction in the early twentieth century (Frankel 1909).

Indications

The role of AIH for many of its alleged indications remains controversial. Properly conducted trials of AIH versus natural intercourse are lacking. In unexplained infertility, and even in oligospermia, spontaneous pregnancies do occur. AIH is often credited for the success with little data to support this assumption.

Sexual dysfunction

On the female side, severe vaginismus may be an indication for AIH if penetration is not occurring. After appropriate counselling in relation to the psychosexual aspects and the treatment itself, AIH is commenced. There are concerns that a child resulting from such successful treatment may lead to further psychological problems. Care in selection of cases is obviously vital.

In the male, impotence or premature ejaculation can be considered as indications for AIH. Once again the psychological aspects require full investigation prior to commencing therapy. There is also that group of males with impotence due to medical disorders, e.g. diabetic neuropathy and paraplegics, who may be assisted to fertility with AIH. Electroejaculation in paraplegics is now an established procedure although the semen quality is often poor so that in vitro fertilization is required to achieve a pregnancy (Randolph et al 1990).

Hypospadias and epispadias may result in inadequate deposition of semen at the cervix and such cases may benefit from AIH.

Retrograde ejaculation should be suspected when anejaculation is the complaint. Confirmation can be made by the assessment of a postejaculatory urine specimen for spermatozoa. AIH using sperm recovered from the bladder has been successful (Scammell et al 1989). The urine is neutralized by oral alkalizing agents prior to masturbation and then is centrifuged after ejaculation to collect adequate numbers of sperm for insemination.

Oligospermia

Oligospermia is a debatable indication for AIH. Many publications report successful treatment but none has been properly controlled and all involve small numbers. Thompson (1990) compiled a list of studies which show a 22% pregnancy rate in 550 cases.

Modern semen preparation techniques appear to have defined more clearly those men in whom AIH is worth attempting—a count of >5 million motile sperm after preparation by either swim up or Percoll gradients (see later). This excludes the majority of men with moderate to severe oligospermia on basic semen assessment.

Postcoital tests (PCT) have been used to select couples for AIH. If the semen assessment has been normal but the PCT reveal predominantly or all dead or immotile sperm, some workers regard this as an indication for AIH. The value of the PCT itself is questionable when studies in fertile couples revealed no sperm in 8% of the couples, 12% had less than one sperm per high-powered field (HPF) and 20% had sperm motility which was less than 50% motile (Kovacs et al 1979). In addition, the studies reporting the use of AIH in such cases are poorly documented in that the abnormality on the PCT is undefined and none of the studies is controlled. Certainly the presence of antisperm antibodies is a contraindication to AIH as is poor motility on swim up.

Unexplained infertility

The use of AIH in situations where all investigations have proved negative has gained increasing favour. Data have emerged showing encouraging success rates in association with ovarian stimulation with human menopausal gonadotrophin (hMG) and semen preparation as developed for IVF (Serhal et al 1988, Chaffkin et al 1991). Intrauterine insemination has been used in these studies.

With >5 million motile sperm/ml after preparation, intrauterine insemination at the time of ovulation in women stimulated with hMG will result in rates of pregnancy per cycle of between 15% and 22%. When compared with the complexity of GIFT or IVF, these are very acceptable rates of success.

Cryopreserved semen

Artificial insemination is indicated when cryopreserved semen is to be used. Obviously the major use of such sperm is donor insemination but there are men who have sperm frozen prior to chemotherapy, radiotherapy or surgery for malignant disease. Cumulative pregnancy rates of 45% over six courses of artificial insemination have been reported in this group (Scammell et al 1985). A further group are those men who have stored sperm prior to undergoing vasectomy—an increasingly common procedure.

Insemination techniques

Intravaginal insemination

This merely involves the injection of ejaculated sperm into the upper vagina using a plastic syringe. It is no more successful than natural intercourse. If coitus is not occurring for whatever reason, this technique is simple and straightforward.

Intracervical and pericervical insemination

After revealing the cervix on speculum examination, a small amount (0.2–0.5 ml) of semen is injected into the external cervical canal by means of a syringe. The remainder is placed in the upper vagina. Caps have been developed to place over the cervix to retain sperm at the cervix. There appears no benefit to their use. Once again the evidence that these techniques are any better than natural intercourse is lacking. This is probably because of the difficulty of sperm to pass through the cervical canal (Joyce & Vassilopoulos 1981).

With the use of donor sperm which is provided in small amounts in straws or ampoules, intracervical and pericervical insemination results in reasonable pregnancy rates of 5–10% per cycle when accurate ovulation monitoring is employed.

Intrauterine insemination

In this approach, prepared sperm is placed into the uterine cavity by means of a fine non-toxic plastic catheter. The cervix is exposed with the use of a Cuscoe's speculum. The catheter (external diameter 1–2 mm) is inserted in a sterile manner through the external cervical os and then through the internal os into the uterus. The aim is to place the tip of the catheter as near to the fundus, in as atraumatic manner as possible, so as not to disturb the endometrium. In the majority of cases (>80%) no instrumentation of the cervix is required. In acute uterine retroversion or anteversion, it may be necessary to correct the position by manipulation of the cervix with a tenaculum. Difficulties can also occur with cervix stenosis following surgery, e.g. cone biopsy.

Intrauterine insemination may lead to severe cramping but this is generally related to the volume inseminated (>0.1 ml) and the instrumentation required to achieve the passage of the catheter. With unprepared semen a theoretical risk of infection exists, but is extremely small (Allen et al 1985). The more recent standard semen preparations further decrease the risk by separation of the spermatozoa from the ejaculate.

Intrafallopian insemination

GIFT where prepared spermatozoa are injected into the Fallopian tube together with harvested oocytes via the laparoscope could be considered a form of artificial insemination. However it will be dealt with in more detail below. Techniques to inseminate the Fallopian tube directly using a transcervical route without anaesthesia have been developed but appear to offer no advantage over IUI.

Intraperitoneal insemination

There was an initial enthusiasm when reports appeared suggesting high pregnancy rates following the injection of prepared spermatozoa directly into the pouch of Douglas.

The posterior fornix is visualized by the speculum. A needle is then inserted blindly though the posterior fornix and a small amount of prepared sperm is injected into the pouch of Douglas. This is performed at the time of ovulation. Concerns about the risk of generating anti-sperm antibodies have been expressed, but not proven. Follow-up studies have not borne out the early expectations. Success rates are similar to IUI with hMG stimulation (Turhan et al 1992).

Preparation of semen

The development of IVF has led to new techniques to prepare small concentrated samples of high quality spermatozoa. Centrifugation of the ejaculate was the initial approach but often resulted in decreased motility (Davajan et al 1983). This has been attributed to release of free O_2 radicals during this process.

Various techniques to filter out the dead and abnormal sperm have been tried with initially little increase in pregnancy rates. The two techniques now commonly in use are the swim up technique or the use of a Percoll gradient.

Additives to improve sperm motilities have been tried with AIH. Caffeine (Barkay et al 1977) and kallkrien (Schill 1975) have been reported to enhance conception rates but other studies do not support their use.

Timing of insemination

With natural cycle insemination, tracking can be done relatively crudely with basal body temperature charts (BBT) but is inaccurate for timing in one-third of cycles (Lenton et al 1977). Changes in cervical mucus are a more refined biological method of assessment, but the most accurate method includes the detection of the luteinizing hormone (LH) surge. Ovulation occurs some 20–24 hours after the peak of the LH surge or 40–44 hours after its commencement. Rapid radioimmunoassays can be used to pick up the rise of LH above the baseline. Recently highly sensitive LH monoclonal antibodies have been incorporated into colour-sensitive pads which change colour when the LH in urine applied to them exceeds basal levels. This development allows home testing kits for the LH surge with a high degree of accuracy (>98%). Ovarian follicle tracking with transvaginal ultrasound can be employed to determine when testing for the LH surge should begin.

Pregnancy outcome following artificial insemination with husband's sperm

Despite the possibility that pregnancies following AIH are from men with potentially poorer semen quality, the miscarriage rate and subsequently the incidence of abnormality is no greater than that in the normal fertile population. A slightly higher abortion rate than in the background population has been reported, i.e. 30% versus 15–20%, but review of the literature by Nachtigall et al (1979) showed this was primarily the result of early diagnosis of pregnancy and increased surveillance.

When hMG therapy is used together with AIH, there is a serious risk of high multiple pregnancy, with all its complications, unless appropriate monitoring is undertaken. It is vital not to undertake the insemination if there are many (i.e. >6) mature follicles.

GAMETE DONATION

The use of donated spermatozoa and more recently oocytes provides the opportunity to treat infertile couples in whom the production of gametes is absent or severely restricted. With improvements in IVF supplemented by technological advances in dealing successfully with low spermatozoa numbers, semen donation is no longer the only therapeutic manoeuvre for the male, but still remains the mainstay of treatment.

The ethical and moral issues related to gamete donation continue to be highly debatable. First, there is the acceptance or rejection of the notion that a couple should be able to use another's gametes to produce a child that genetically (at least in part) is not their own. In some societies, e.g. Muslim, the use of donor gametes is banned on religious grounds. In most Western countries, the principle of donation has been accepted, although obviously individual couples will make their own choice. Only a little over half the couples offered donor insemination for severe male factor undertake this step. Once donation programmes are accepted, the next issues relate to their organization, e.g. selection of donors, screening techniques, anonymity, payment to donors, appropriate counselling. Then there are the individual patient issues, e.g. telling the child, telling their family, the rights of the child.

Donor insemination

DI has been practised medically for more than a century. The impregnation by semen from other than the husband has been an accepted, if covert, approach to childlessness in some cultures for generations.

In the latter half of this century it has become an accepted treatment with the advent of clinics primarily set up to provide such a service. This has led to the licensing of such centres and regulation of their programmes, for instance in the UK all donor centres require to be licensed by the Human Fertilisation and Embryology Authority. This regulation extends to control registration of all donors and recipients and restriction of the number of offspring per donor. With regard to payment, travel and expenses are the only allowable recompense to donors.

Semen donors

A successful donor insemination programme is dependent upon a plentiful supply of good quality donor sperm. In the UK, recruitment is primarily from the student population since the recompense is relatively small. Some clinics have been successful in recruiting fertile husbands from their own successfully treated couples. Commercial sperm banks as set up in the USA are of concern where the primary incentive to the donor is financial and so the donors may suppress important clinical history or falsify information which might otherwise make the donor unacceptable. France has centralized donor banks which ensures quality control and monitoring of pregnancy numbers. In the UK the HFEA holds a central register of donors and the use of each donor's sperm together with outcome data.

The criteria for donation include a normal health record, a clear family and genetic history. To minimize the risk of HIV transmission, a sexual history should be taken and those with a homosexual or promiscuous heterosexual history may be considered inappropriate donors. Any history of drug abuse should also exclude a potential donor. A potential donor requires full counselling in regards to his responsibility in relation to such treatment. Confidentiality should be paramount in their participation in the programme.

The investigations for the donor will include a sperm count and culture for bacteriology for *Neisseria gonorrhoeae* and *Chlamydia*. The semen analysis must be >40 million/ml and progressive motility of at least 60%. These are above the normally quoted values for an acceptable analysis as cryopreservation reduces viability and motility by at least 20% and usually more. Today it is unacceptable to use fresh semen for donation with the known risks of HIV transmission (Stewart et al 1985); cryopreservation of 3–6 months quarantine of frozen semen virtually excludes the possibility of this occurrence.

The indications for DI are outlined in Table 16.2. These are not absolute indications particularly with recent advances in technology, e.g. sperm microinjection has been successful with severe oligospermia, preimplantation diagnosis using assisted conception can now be used

to exclude some genetic disorders in the embryos to be replaced. Thus, prior to accepting donor insemination couples should be advised on the options open to them, given their diagnosis. A full and thorough discussion of donor insemination and its implications is then undertaken. All clinics in the UK offer counselling to such couples and in some units it is a mandatory part of the workup prior to commencing treatment.

Investigations of the couple should include blood group, HIV antibodies, venereal disease reference laboratory test (VDRL), Rubella status of the female.

Pamphlets especially prepared for potential recipient couples (e.g. in the UK by the RCOG and by HFEA) enumerate the various procedures involved in the treatment together with the legal and psychological aspects of the outcome. It is good practice to ensure the couple have had time to understand fully DI and its implications prior to signing the consents for the procedure.

Outcome for donor insemination

Pregnancy rates for DI should be as good as for the normal fertile population (i.e. 75% cumulative pregnancy rate over 12 months) provided the female has demonstrable ovulation and tubal patency. Rates/year of between 31.5% (Joyce 1979) and 72% (Chong & Taymer 1975) have been reported. Our own figures at the Bridge Fertility Centre, London over the past 2 years indicate a 60% pregnancy rate after six cycles. The discrepancies between results can be explained in a number of ways; these include the manner in which the data is presented, differing criteria for entry to DI, e.g. partners of azoospermic men have higher success rates than those with oligospermia, and the representation of the groups of ages of the women treated.

Newton (1984) reviewed the outcome of 6587 pregnancies generated by DI over a 7-year period. The early pregnancy loss with miscarriage (12.3%) and ectopics (0.5%) was similar to the normal population. Congenital abnormality rate and perinatal mortality rate is also not changed by DI, despite the careful screening of donors. Data on follow-up of children is obviously difficult as a result of the secrecy surrounding DI. However, in one study Iizuku et al (1968) found the physical and mental development of 54 children to be superior to a control group.

Donor oocytes

Successful ovum donation, fertilization in vitro and embryo transfer were reported in 1984 (Lutjen et al 1984). It is remarkable that the uterus of the recipient can be primed so readily by the use of oral oestrogens followed by the addition of progestagens 2 or 3 days before embryo transfer. Hormonal support is continued for the first trimester

Table 16.2 Indications for donor insemination

Azoospermia
Gross oligospermia
Disorders of sperm motility and morphology
Genetic disease
    Recessive, e.g. cystic fibrosis, Huntingdon's chorea
    X-linked, e.g. muscular dystrophy
Rhesus isoimmunization
Previous vasectomy
Sexual dysfunction
    Paraplegia, impotence, ejaculatory failure

but once placental function becomes established, it can be discontinued.

Ovum donors are difficult to recruit. There are three sources—altruistic anonymous donors, donors related or known to the recipient, and women who are undergoing assisted conception procedures and are prepared to donate excess oocytes.

It is not surprising that women are reluctant to come forward as altruistic donors since it a substantial undertaking to undergo ovarian stimulation and oocyte collection in the same regimen as women for IVF. The accompanying risks of ovarian hyperstimulation and potential pregnancy are also disincentives. With known donors, the possibility of major emotional trauma between recipient and donor, should any problem arise in the offspring, must be raised and some centres do not accept such arrangements. With the advent of cryopreservation of embryos, the desire of a couple to utilize this technique to maximize their chances of success from a single treatment cycle has reduced the occasions when excess oocytes are available for donation. Thus demand for donated oocytes considerably outstrips supply, which has resulted in long waiting lists for treatments. The use of GIFT using donor oocytes and patient's sperm seems to have a better success rate than IVF (Abdalla et al 1990).

The indications for ovum donation include the following groups:

1. Women carrying genetic disorders which have a high transmission rate to the fetus.
2. Women with premature menopause.
3. Women who have repeatedly failed to achieve fertilization in an IVF programme due either to the inability to obtain sufficient numbers of oocytes or to the poor quality of oocytes obtained.
4. Women after a normal aged menopause who still desire a pregnancy.

The ethical and moral issues related to ovum donation have aroused considerable discussion, but it is now accepted in the UK as a licensed form of treatment. In particular the last group has caused extreme controversy with reports of women in their fifties delivering after ovum donation. Most clinics in the UK have an upper age limit of 50 years of age.

Donors are usually restricted to under 35 years of age to reduce the risk of chromosomal abnormalities. They are screened in a similar manner to the semen donors. There is obviously a requirement for detailed counselling with respect to the procedures involved in the treatment and its risks, as well as the legal aspects of their donation.

Outcome for ovum donation

The results from ovum donation are extremely good in comparison with other groups undergoing assisted conception. GIFT results with donor oocytes are in the order of 35%/cycle and IVF results around 30%/cycle. These results are independent of the recipient's age, indicating that the fall in the general fertility of the older age groups is primarily related to oocyte quality not to the uterine environment (Abdalla et al 1993).

The numbers of babies born following ovum donation are still only in the hundreds in the UK and so few data are available on perinatal outcomes or follow-up. No problems have been reported.

On the maternal side, there have been suggestions of an increased risk of pre-eclampsia. This could be related to the unusual situation in that the genotype of the fetus is totally foreign to the mother in comparison to only half the genotype being foreign in normal pregnancy. This intriguing biological experiment demands further study.

SURROGACY

Probably the most controversial area of assisted reproduction for the general public has been the use of IVF technology to allow the carriage of a pregnancy derived from an infertile couple by another woman. The surrogate, having delivered, gives the child to the genetic parents, who then formally adopt the child. Such arrangements are condoned in some countries (e.g. UK, USA) but banned in others (e.g. Germany). Commercialization of the process, particularly in the USA, resulting in substantial payments to surrogates has been a major concern. In addition, the legal basis for transfer of the child from its natural mother to its genetic parents has been challenged when the surrogate refuses to give up the child. Despite these problems, many couples now have their own genetic child in situations where this would previously have been impossible.

Candidates for such an approach are women who have had a hysterectomy (e.g. uterine malignancy, obstetric disasters, uncontrolled uterine haemorrhage) or have congenital absence of the uterus and have not fulfilled their reproductive desires. It has also been used by women with appalling reproductive histories, e.g. recurrent miscarriages or stillbirths or when the medical history indicates that a pregnancy would be severely detrimental to their health or to the pregnancy, e.g. severe systemic lupus erythematosis or congenital heart disease.

A variation of surrogacy involves donor insemination of the surrogate using the husband's sperm. This means the resulting child is genetically half of the adopting parents. This approach is applicable to women who would otherwise be suitable for ovum donation, e.g. premature menopause. It has been suggested that some women will take advantage of surrogacy to avoid the inconvenience of pregnancy and childbirth to their careers; at present this practice is rare.

IN VITRO FERTILIZATION

Indications

When first developed, IVF was designed to solve the problem of bringing sperm and oocytes together when tubal damage had made this process impossible. Tubal disease remains the major reason for undertaking IVF but the list of other indications has grown over the years.

The increasing use of IVF for other causes of infertility is attributable to a number of factors. For instance, the indications previously felt to be better treated by GIFT (outlined below) are now accepted as indications for IVF. This has occurred because the pregnancy rates for IVF have improved to the extent that many clinics have similar rates as for GIFT. The advantage of IVF over GIFT is its ability to be performed in an office situation without general anaesthesia or laparoscopic instrumentation. In addition the clinician can be certain that fertilization has taken place with IVF. Thus, more information is available for the couple should conception fail to occur.

Developments in sperm microinjection techniques have resulted in the ability to attempt treatment in severe male factor infertility where previously conventional IVF was rarely successful. These couples were counselled towards donor insemination as their only hope for a pregnancy. A further advance has been the use of pharmaceutical agents (e.g. pentoxifylline; Yovich 1993) to improve the fertilizing ability of sperm which lack either adequate motility or the capacity to undergo the various changes required to achieve penetration of oocytes, e.g. capacitation, acrosome reaction. Our understanding of these latter processes has increased significantly over recent years and led to success in IVF pregnancies.

The treatment of ovulatory disorders is not a primary indication for IVF. The cumulative pregnancy rates in ovulatory failure are in the order of 80% per year once regular ovulation has been induced using pharmacological treatments. Thus it is poor practice to embark on IVF until there has been a reasonable trial of drug therapy.

Tubal disease

Damage to the Fallopian tubes is generally the result of pelvic inflammatory disease. However, iatrogenic damage is not uncommon, e.g. ovarian cystectomy, appendectomy. Endometriosis is also a factor. Ectopic pregnancies are increasing in frequency and, despite more conservative surgery for their removal, remain a significant indication for IVF; underlying tubal damage may have been the cause of the ectopic in the first place.

Unexplained infertility

While definitions vary as to the minimal requirements to label a couple as suffering from unexplained infertility, it is mandatory to:

1. establish normal tubal anatomy via laparoscopy
2. exclude other pelvic pathology at laparoscopy, e.g. significant endometriosis or paraovarian adhesions
3. demonstrate regular ovulation
4. establish normal semen parameters.

The use of hysteroscopy to establish a normal uterine cavity is now becoming a further requirement for the diagnosis.

Male factor has received increasing interest as it has become clear that a normal sperm assessment does not define any functional aspect of spermatozoa in terms of fertilizing capability nor its ability to traverse the female genital tract. More detailed investigations of the semen are indicated in unexplained infertility, e.g. swim up, 24-hour survival, acrosome reactivity.

The natural history of unexplained infertility is that pregnancies continue to occur with each year of attempted conception. For instance in the second year of trying to conceive, a couple have approximately a 50% chance of success without medical intervention if all investigations are normal. In the third year the spontaneous pregnancy rate is not insignificant—30%. Any intervention must be compared with this background chance of pregnancy. Thus, most clinicians will not recommend IVF until at least 2 years of attempted conception have passed in this group of patients. Obviously other factors may influence this decision, e.g. age older than 35 years, or increasing anxiety of the couple.

Male factor

As suggested above, the only true test of sperm function is fertilization of the oocyte. IVF provides the means to assess this process, although in vitro models, e.g. hamster egg penetration tests (HEPT), do give some indication of the likelihood of success. Semen assessment provides only basic information, but does correlate well with pregnancy rates. However there are some males with a normal semen assessment who do in fact have a fertilizing problem. When these couples with apparently unexplained infertility fail to produce fertilization in vitro further investigation is worthwhile.

The majority of male problems relate to low numbers of sperm produced, poor motility or an excess of abnormal forms. The first stage in their assessment for suitability for IVF is a sperm preparation, e.g. using the swim up technique or Percoll gradient. A prepared sample which contains a minimum of 3 million highly motile sperm is sufficient to undertake standard IVF. Counts below this level will result in poor or nil fertilization rates in the standard systems.

The use of pentoxifylline has increased pregnancy rates

in cases of poor motility (Yovich, 1993). Microinjection techniques where sperm are placed beneath the zona pellucida (SUZI) have achieved pregnancies in cases of low sperm numbers, albeit with relative poor rates of success. Most recently ICSI, where a single sperm is inserted directly into the ooplasm, has produced pregnancies in cases where virtually no spermatozoa have been found on routine semen assessment (Van Steirteghem et al 1993). Success rates approaching standard IVF results have been reported.

Other male factor problems have been tackled with IVF or microinjection techniques. With absence of the vas, blockage of the vas or failed reversal of vasectomy, sperm have been retrieved from the epididymis and achieved conceptions (Jequier et al 1990). Pregnancies have even been reported from immature sperm extracted by testicular biopsy and inseminated using the ICSI technique. Although the pregnancy rates for some of these approaches are low or not fully assessed as yet, it is now clear many males previously labelled infertile may conceive.

Standard in vitro fertilization

Ovarian stimulation

Initial successes with IVF followed oocyte collection during natural cycles. This soon gave way to ovarian stimulation regimens, when it became clear that multiple embryo transfer after several oocytes were collected resulted in better pregnancy rates. There has been a resurgence in interest in natural cycle IVF in the past 5 years (Lenton et al 1992), primarily because of its reduced medical interference and reduced costs. However, at best the oocyte pick-up rate is in the order of 90% and fertilization rates are 80%. Thus, the chances of transferring a single embryo are < 80%. Pregnancy rates of 15% per cycle have been reported (Lenton et al 1992). The other disadvantage is the need for close monitoring to establish timing of oocyte collection which may be at unsociable times at night and weekends.

Human menopausal gonadotrophins. Ovarian stimulation has primarily been with human menopausal gonadotrophins (hMG). The standard protocols developed in the early 1980s involve clomiphene (100 mg for 5 days) in the early follicular phase in conjunction with daily (or alternate daily) injections of hMG (usually 2 or 3 ampoules). When follicular development is felt to be appropriate (see Monitoring below) the final maturation of the oocytes is stimulated by an intramuscular injection of human chorionic gonadotrophin (hCG). During this period the oocyte commences secondary meiosis and the cumulus mass expands. This injection is timed to 34–38 hours prior to planned oocyte collected. With this regimen >90% of women less than 40 years of age will produce more than three mature follicles. In women > 40 years of age 70% will have a reasonable response. Some poor responders will be helped by increased doses of hMG (up to 8 ampoules daily), but for many it is an indication of declining ovarian function which cannot be improved. The problems of natural cycle and stimulated cycle protocols include poor or failed response of the ovaries and premature ovulation (i.e. before oocyte collection can be carried out). The latter problem is minimized by obsessive monitoring by ultrasound and LH measurements. A further difficulty already mentioned is the potential for oocyte collection to be required out of the normal working week. A 7-day a week, 24-hours-a-day service is necessary to obtain the results.

The complications of ovarian stimulation include the patient acceptance of the need for frequent injections, abdomen discomfort from the enlarging ovaries and, most importantly, ovarian overstimulation leading to the ovarian hyperstimulation syndrome (OHSS). In well-controlled programmes where there is close tracking of cycles and a policy to abandon cycles where there is risk (Forman et al 1990), the incidence of clinically significant hyperstimulation is in the order of 1–2%. In these cases pain due to ovarian enlargement and mild ascites is the usual cause for presentation. These problems generally resolve without any intervention other than bed rest and good hydration.

A small percentage have more severe OHSS. In addition to acute pain these patients develop significant abdominal distension, shortness of breath due to pleural effusion and oliguria. They develop substantial biochemical abnormalities primarily related to altered capillary permeability. Albumen moves into the extracellular space producing a colloid pressure which results in intravascular hypovolaemia. The movement of plasma volume from the vasculature accounts for the ascites and effusions, the reduced intravascular perfusion leads to the oliguria. While the condition is generally self-limiting it can be fatal. Death is usually the result of thrombotic episodes, fluid overload or respiratory and circulatory collapse due to effusions, often iatrogenically induced. Therefore, management should be in experienced hands. Central venous pressure monitoring is mandatory to avoid fluid overload while at the same time maintaining circulating volume. Multiple pharmacological approaches have been tried but are of no demonstrable benefit. Tapping the ascites or effusions seems of little value in reducing the severity of the condition.

On the positive side > 50% of patients who have had embryo transfer and subsequently develop OHSS become pregnant but the risks to the mother are significant. Thus, the best approach to OHSS is to avoid it by ceasing hMG and continuing downregulation with gonadotrophin releasing hormone (GnRH) agonists (Forman et al 1990). The hCG injection, which is routinely given to induce the final maturation of the oocytes, should be withheld, as it triggers the OHSS. An alternative approach which has been reported is in fact to give the hCG, harvest the oocytes, then downregulate with GnRH agonists. The fertilized oocytes then generated are not replaced, but cryopreserved since the cycle is basically abandoned. The cryopreserved embryos may be replaced in a subsequent cycle (Amso et al 1989).

A recent epidemiological study (Whittemore et al 1992) and some anecdotal case reports have raised the issue of ovarian cancer in association with hMG therapy. The epidemiological study has been criticized on many counts, primarily in that most cases were treated for infertility prior to the introduction of hMG, but it has focused our attention on this potential risk. Long-term follow-up studies are being mounted to review the situation in the future.

Gonadotrophin releasing hormone analogues. A major advance for IVF has been the development of gonadotrophin releasing hormone agonists (GnRHa). These compounds are structurally similar to GnRH but with one or two amino acids altered. These changes lead to prolongation of their half-life, producing a saturation and downregulation of their receptors in the anterior pituitary. As a result LH and follicle stimulating hormone (FSH) production and release are basically switched off. No endogenous LH surge can then occur. Premature ovulation is therefore prevented. A further advantage is that multiple follicular growth is promoted which results in higher oocyte yields. The major disadvantage is the requirement for twice the amount of hMG to achieve adequate ovarian response, which significantly increases the cost of treatment.

A variety of regimens have evolved for hMG ovarian stimulation in conjunction with GnRH analogues. The most commonly used current regimen is GnRH from either day 1 or day 21 of the cycle preceding the planned oocyte recovery. These are termed the long protocols. Their major advantage is the certainty with which downregulation can be induced and the ability to plan hMG administration to allow oocyte collection on a day of convenience for the laboratory. Other approaches include GnRHa from D1 of the planned cycle for IVF through to the time of oocyte retrieval (short protocol) or the ultrashort protocol which uses GnRHa from day 1 to day 5 only. These latter two approaches take advantage of the initial stimulation of FSH (the flare up) by GnRH agonists to start follicle development. Both regimens and subsequent oocyte retrieval are determined by the day of commencement of the period and are therefore less amenable to organization of the clinic.

Monitoring

It is vital to assess follicular response to hMG to ensure optimal growth, exclude the risk of OHSS and to select the most appropriate day for oocyte retrieval. Such monitoring varies considerably between units. A minimum is follicle tracking with ultrasound alone. A baseline scan is done prior to the commencement of hMG to ensure no follicles remain from the previous cycle. These may be producing progesterone and oestrogen which appears to inhibit optimal follicular growth and in addition their presence can confuse the ultrasound picture later in the cycle. Repeat scans should be done no later than 9 days after hMG has commenced. By this stage the response can be judged as appropriate, excessive or suboptimal. An average woman will have between six and 10 follicles of diameters between 12 and 16 mm on this scan at 9 days of hMG. Dependent upon the response a further scan may be indicated to follow growth. Oocyte collection will generally be on days 12–14 of hMG administration. The addition of oestradiol (E_2) estimations probably improves the accuracy of judging the optimum day of oocyte collection. The IVF units with the high success rates undertake at least one E_2 measurement on day 9 of hMG and will repeat it if levels are low and follicular development retarded.

Some units scan daily after day 7 of hMG and undertake daily E_2 measurements from this time. The value of this rate of increased surveillance is questionable.

Once the optimum stage both on ultrasound and biochemically has been obtained, hCG is administered 34–38 hours prior to planned oocyte recovery. This stimulates the final maturation of the oocytes with the aim being to harvest these just prior to expected ovulation.

Oocyte retrieval

Oocyte collection for IVF was originally performed laparoscopically, although open mini laparotomy was also undertaken. A collection of instruments was developed to optimize the laparoscopic approach. Indeed they are still in use today for GIFT cases and the occasional case where it is felt laparoscopic collection is appropriate, e.g. when IVF is done in conjunction with a diagnostic procedure or when the ovaries are inaccessible to transvaginal ultrasound.

Ultrasound-guided collection began in the early 1980s with a transabdominal transvesical approach (Lenz et al 1985). Subsequently the transurethral method was described by Parsons et al (1985). The development of transvaginal ultrasound probes with their superior images of the pelvic structure have led to their almost universal use for oocyte retrieval (Dellenbach et al 1984).

General anaesthesia is the usual approach for laparoscopic oocyte retrieval. The major advantage of ultrasound-directed oocyte collection, particularly the transvaginal approach, is that analgesia rather than anaesthesia is all that is necessary. A variety of agents have been employed that basically allow oocyte collection to be an outpatient procedure. However, many women having experienced sedation or analgesia, when given the choice elect for general anaesthesia in a subsequent cycle. Epidural anaesthesia has been used to good effect but obviously is more invasive. There is no strong evidence that any of the anaesthetic, analgesic or sedative agents have a deleterious effect on fertilization or embryo development.

The transvaginal procedure involves ultrasonically localizing each ovary in turn and puncturing the vaginal wall with the collection needle. This is usually in the posterior or lateral fornix and preferably with only one puncture (to minimize the risk of introduction of vaginal flora into the pelvis) on each side. The needle is directed into each follicle over 10 mm diameter. Most units employ a double lumen needle which allows initial aspiration of the follicular fluid and the oocyte in 70% of cases. If the oocyte is not in this aspirate, flushing medium is injected into the follicle. The turbulence so created results in the dislodgement of the oocyte from the follicular wall. Repeat flushes are sometimes necessary. It is worthwhile to empty all the follicles > 12 mm to:

1. ensure that maximum number of oocytes are retrieved for fertilization
2. reduce the risk of hyperstimulation syndrome.

The more granulosa cells removed, the lower the levels of circulating E_2 which are subsequently present.

Complications of oocyte retrieval include the general problems associated with anaesthesia and laparoscopy if they are used. For transvaginal ultrasound-directed retrieval the risks are:

1. puncture of major vessels, although these are usually visible on the ultrasound monitor and so avoidable
2. introduction of vaginal organisms into the pelvis with resultant pelvic infection.

Some clinics routinely prescribe antibiotic cover while others do so only in high-risk cases, e.g. endometriosis, recent pelvic infection.

Laboratory procedures

The crucial aspect of a successful IVF programme is high quality embryology. Skill in oocyte handling, sperm preparation and embryo manipulation coupled with meticulous sterile technique appear to be the vital aspects. Quality control in relation to culture medium is obviously critical, although many variations have been developed over the years with good fertilization rates. The major problem is batch to batch variation of in house preparations. Commercial ready-made media with proven high success rates that have little variability in terms of quality control are now available.

The embryological procedures of assisted conception include:

1. *Oocyte recognition*. After each follicular aspirate is given to the embryologist, it is immediately examined microscopically for the oocyte and its accompanying cumulus mass. Once identified, the oocyte is graded in terms of its quality and maturity. It is then placed in culture medium.
2. *Semen preparation*. The aim of this procedure is to produce a small volume of highly motile normal sperm with which to inseminate the oocyte (usually 3–4 hours after aspiration).

    The standard techniques in current use are the swim up technique or the Percoll gradient system.

    The swim up technique involves the semen sample being allowed to liquefy for 30 minutes at 37°C; once it is liquefied, the volume and pH are measured and a rapid assessment of the count and motility of the sperm is carried out. In the multi-tube method 0.2 ml of semen is underlaid under 0.8 ml of medium, sufficient numbers of tubes being used in order to use the whole sample. Alternatively, the entire volume can be underlaid under 2 ml of medium. In each case the preparation is then placed in an incubator at 37°C for 1 hour, after which time the supernatants are carefully removed taking care not to disturb the interface between the semen and the medium, pooled together, diluted with an equal volume of medium, centrifuged at 600 *g* for 10 minutes, the supernatant removed and sufficient medium added to the pellet to give a final concentration of 1 million motile sperm/ml for IVF or 3 million motile sperm/ml for GIFT. The resulting preparation is usually free from debris and dead sperm with > 90% highly motile sperm that have swum up into the overlying medium.

    Percoll gradients allow the separation of motile sperm from immotile sperm and debris by centrifugation through different densities of Percoll.
3. *Incubation*. The oocytes are incubated for 4–16 hours prior to insemination, depending upon their maturity as assessed at the time of oocyte collection. The medium around each oocyte is inseminated with between 50 000 and 100 000 sperm.
4. *Identification of pronuclei*. At 16–20 hours postinsemination, the oocytes are inspected for the presence of the swollen decondensed sperm head or two pronuclei. Oocytes with more than two pronuclei (i.e. where more than one spermatozoa has entered the oocyte) or those with no pronuclei will not be transferred and will be discarded. The demonstration by Angell et all (1983) of numerous chromosome defects in human embryos derived from IVF highlights the importance of checking the pronuclear stage to exclude haploidy or polyploidy.

5. *Embryo transfer.* Further incubation for 30 hours allows the early divisions of the embryo to occur. By this stage or some 48 hours postinsemination, most good quality embryos will be at the 4-cell stage, but some may be at the 2-cell stage or sometimes at the 8-cell stage. The embryos are graded on the basis of simple morphology—the size of the embryo, i.e. the number of cells (blastomeres), whether the blastomeres are all the same size and their granularity. The highest graded embryos will be transferred and at most three embryos will be transferred. There is an increasing trend to transfer two embryos where the implantation rate per embryo is high. This avoids the risk of triplets.

The embryo transfer

The technique of embryo transfer plays an important role in the success of IVF. An easy transfer with no disruption of the endometrium is associated with higher implantation rates. Instrumentation of the cervix to correct malposition or dilatation to aid passage of the catheter, or the presence of blood on the tip of the catheter on withdrawal is associated with poor success rates.

The cervix is identified using a Cuscoe's speculum. The external os is located. The embryologist selects the highest graded embryos and loads them into the tip of a non-toxic, pliable, soft catheter. This is usually stiffened by an outer cannula which is held at the external os. The inner catheter is then threaded gently through the internal cervical os and into the uterine cavity. The tip is introduced halfway to the fundus. The embryos are deposited in 50 µl of culture medium containing 75% albumen. The temptation is to ensure the patient rests for a period following transfer, but the evidence indicates that this is probably irrelevant to the likelihood of conception.

The luteal phase

Following hMG stimulation the luteal phase endometrium is generally supported by either the administration of progestagen, intramuscularly with progesterone in oil or by suppository or pessary with micronized progesterone or natural progesterone. Alternatively, further injections of hCG to stimulate corpus luteal activity have been used. hCG should not be used when E_2 levels are very high and in the presence of large numbers of follicles (> 12) due to the risk of OHSS.

Transport in vitro fertilization

In France and in the UK, programmes of IVF have been successfully developed which involve a central embryological laboratory servicing a number of peripheral units. At the distant site the patient has ovarian stimulation with appropriate monitoring undertaken. The oocyte collection is also performed locally. The oocytes are then transported (usually by the male partner) to the central laboratory where the sperm is produced. The woman then attends the central unit for the embryo transfer 2 days later.

This system allows patients to be treated in their local environment rather than travelling long distances on a frequent basis during their treatment cycle. It also allows the maximum utilization of the highly skilled clinical and laboratory staff at the central clinic. In addition, it provides a single laboratory with a large throughput thereby ensuring better quality control. The major component for the success of such programmes is good communications between the central unit and the peripheral clinics. Reported success rates for transport programmes are similar to standard clinics.

Preimplantation diagnosis

The combination of in vitro fertilization and the technology advances in molecular biology which have allowed genetic sequence identification in single cells, has led to the ability to detect embryos with specific gene defects or at high risk of such abnormalities (e.g. X-linked disorders). From a hypothetical possibility in the 1980s, pregnancies have now been produced following preimplantation diagnosis (Hardy & Handyside 1992).

The woman undergoes standard IVF treatment. Once the cleavage occurs, a single blastomere is extracted from the embryo after dissection of the zona pellucida. The single cell is then probed for the marker gene or group of genes. With in situ hybridization, the blastomere is squashed and the chromosomes exposed to a fluorescent linked marker. If the gene is present, then the fluorescence will be visible. In X-linked genetic disease, the female embryos can be identified and will be replaced.

Probes for more specific genetic defects are now available. The polymerase chain reaction which rapidly amplifies the gene sequence under study is employed to amplify the segment of the chromosome from the single blastomere for which the probe is targeted (Chong et al 1993). Both approaches only take 24–48 hours. Meanwhile the embryo (less the biopsied blastomere) continues to divide. Those embryos of the correct sex or lacking the genetic defect are then replaced into the uterus. The biopsy procedure in skilled hands does not affect the chances of implantation nor alter the normality of the fetus. At this early stage of pregnancy all cells in the embryo are equal in their potential (omnipotent) to grow into a normal child. The loss of one cell appears to make little difference at the 4-cell stage.

Gamete intrafallopian transfer

Gamete intrafallopian transfer (GIFT) was first described

in 1986 (Asch et al 1986). The technique involves the same ovarian stimulation protocols as for IVF. The oocyte collection is usually performed laparoscopically. Transvaginal ultrasound-directed collection is practised by some clinicians, particularly when high multiple follicular development has occurred, to maximize the number of oocytes collected. Up to three of the highest graded oocytes are then loaded into a catheter with 50 000–100 000 motile sperm and introduced under laparoscopic control into the Fallopian tube via the fimbrial end. They are deposited some 2–3 cm from the ostium.

The procedure is relatively more simple than IVF since it excludes the need for culture facilities in its most basic form. However, if its fails, there is no information concerning the presence of fertilization unless excess oocytes are cultured in vitro to check this aspect.

Obviously, GIFT is only possible in the presence of normal tubal architecture. Thus the indications are unexplained infertility or mild male factor problems where the swim up produces a concentrated sample of motile sperm of sufficient numbers, i.e. 50 000–100 000 sperm for insemination.

In the late 1980s GIFT pregnancy rates were significantly better than IVF rates, but recent improvements in IVF success have made the differences marginal. Thus, its frequently of use has diminished since IVF is substantially less traumatic for the patient and does not require inpatient care.

Other laparoscopic tubal cannulation procedures have been described and have been used in particular in ovum donation programmes. Transfer of embryos at the pronuclear stage has been termed PROST or ZIFT, transfer at the embryo stage has been termed TEST. High pregnancy rates have been reported but ectopic pregnancy rates are in the order of 10% or higher. Jansen & Anderson (1993) have described GIFT avoiding laparoscopic oocyte collection and tubal cannulation but the use of transvaginal ultrasound and transvaginal cannulation of the Fallopian tube. This makes the whole procedure possible on an outpatient basis. There is however no clear advantage over IVF in terms of results.

Outcome

Pregnancy rates for IVF even in the 1990s vary from 5% to 35%. By the time IVF had become an established form of treatment in the mid 1980s, results of an 11% pregnancy rate/cycle were reported in a world survey of clinics (Seppala & Edwards 1985). No comparable international data is currently available. However, as governmental control of IVF has increased in most countries, reliable data is now being collected (Ezra & Schenker 1993). It is clear that success rates are rising. Comparison of outcomes from the Reports of the Licensing Authority in the UK over the last seven years shows significant improvement (Statistical Analysis of the United Kingdom IVF and GIFT data 1985–90). Between 1985 and 1992 there has been a 50% increase in pregnancy rates. Despite this increase in success rate, a couple entering an IVF cycle are still faced with a 75% chance of failure to conceive and a less than 1 in 5 chance of a liveborn infant.

EXPRESSION OF RESULTS

Much debate surrounds the appropriate outcome of measures for assisted conception. Table 16.3 demonstrates some aspects. The rates may be expressed as pregnancies, as defined by a positive BhCG estimation or more practically as a gestational sac seen on ultrasound at 5–6 weeks' gestation. From the patient's viewpoint the most important outcome measure is a live birth since this is the goal for which the couple undertook treatment to achieve. As can be seen from Table 16.3, the difference is substantial. Between 20% and 25% of pregnancies are lost between 5 weeks and term, the majority in the first trimester.

The results may be expressed as per embryo transfer. However, a substantial number of patients (10–20%) who commence treatment do not reach transfer. The biggest group fail to achieve sufficient ovarian follicles to undergo oocyte retrieval. In a further small group, aspiration of follicles fails to produce oocytes. Failed fertilization contributes another group who will not achieve transfer. This may be due to poor oocyte quality, poor sperm factor or deficient laboratory standards. Finally, a small number of patients have oocytes which fertilize to the pronuclear stage but which fail to cleave.

From the patient's perspective the most relevant statistic is the chance of a baby once treatment has begun, i.e. live birth rate/cycle started. As yet this is not the accepted performance indicator for a particular unit (Wilcox et al 1993).

Other confounding variables enter into the assessment of success rates. These primarily are the factors which determine the individual woman's chance of conceiving with assisted conception, e.g. age, cause of infertility. A clinic which treats a disproportionately high population of

Table 16.3 IVF data 1985–1991

	No. of cycles	Pregnancy rate/transfer (%)	Live birth/transfer (%)
1985	4308	15.9	12.0
1986	7043	19.9	15.9
1987	8899	17.5	13.6
1988	10489	20.7	14.6
1989	10413	21.7	15.7
1990	11583	24.4	17.6
1991*	15967	24.2	18.1

* Extrapolated data from HFEA 1991 Annual Report.

older women will have a lower success rate. In addition, there is certainly evidence from the UK data that the size of the clinic bears a relationship to success rates, i.e. the larger units with more than 500 cycles per year have better success rates than those with less than 500 cycles per year. This probably reflects better maintenance of quality control in busier units.

It is important to consider the characteristics which are influential in determining the chances of conception in a particular couple when counselling them in relation to IVF. It has long been known that a woman's fertility declines from her 35th year and particularly falls over the age of 40. This is also clearly apparent in IVF results by age. See for example Table 16.4 which is derived from the Interim Licensing Authority figures in 1989 and 1990.

The other aspect to consider is the increasing high pregnancy loss rate with age. In the National Health Service (NHS) with minimal resources to allocate to assisted conception, a number of clinics have opted not to treat women over the age of 40. The figures above are stated per embryo transfer, but, when abandoned cycles due to failed stimulation are added in, the chances of a live birth/treatment cycle over the age of 40 are even smaller. Paternal age has little impact.

Male factor problems will obviously influence outcome. However, this only appears to be important when the swim up of semen produces <1 million highly motile sperm/ml. In these cases there may be an improvement with microinjection techniques.

Previous fertility in the female partner has been thought to be a good prognostic feature, although the data for the Interim Licensing Authority (1989, 1990) does not confirm this aspect. The number of embryos transferred does alter the chances of success, but also changes the risk of multiple pregnancy (Table 16.5).

In part the low success with one embryo may reflect a poor cycle, since virtually no patient would elect to have only one embryo replaced. This probably also applied to two embryo transfers in 1990. However, in 1994 many clinics which have high pregnancy rates (i.e. >30% per cycle) are now recommending only a two embryo transfer

Table 16.4 Pregnancy and live birth rates/embryo transfer stratified by age in 1989 and 1990 (ILA data)

Age (yr)	Cycles	Pregnancy rate/transfer (%)	Live birth/transfer (%)
1989			
<30	1879	22.8	17.8
30–34	4035	22.0	16.6
35–39	3249	19.3	13.4
>40	922	12.6	6.9
1990			
<30	2133	27.0	19.4
30–34	4465	26.2	19.8
35–39	3723	23.0	16.0
>40	1192	11.6	5.7

Table 16.5 Percentage overall pregnancy rate and multiple pregnancy rate stratified by the number of embryos transferred

No. of embryos transferred	Pregnancy rate (%)	Multiple rate (%)
1	6.8	1.2
2	23.9	23.3
3	27.1	28.1
4	21.4	23.7

to avoid an increasing incidence of triplets. As mentioned above, the ease of embryo transfer is an important factor in success in addition to the number of embryos transferred.

The success rate per cycle does not seem to decline with repeated attempts (at least up to five attempts) provided good fertilization rates are achieved on each occasion. Various workers have assessed cumulative pregnancy rates with IVF (Hull 1992). With rates/cycle of 20–25%, the chance of a pregnancy after three attempts is in the order of 50–55%.

Outcome of pregnancies generated by in vitro fertilization

In every respect the pregnancies of successful couples from assisted conception are high risk. Sadly, the problems of assisted conception do not finish with the establishment of a gestation. A number of studies in various countries have produced similar findings.

Miscarriage

As can be seen from Table 16.3, once pregnancy is established, the miscarriage rate may be as high as 25% (or greater in older women). This increase over the accepted normal rate of 15% can in part be explained by the early stage of diagnosis of pregnancy and the obvious high-level reporting of outcome in these carefully monitored patients. However, there is a real increase in mid-trimester abortion which is primarily related to the increased incidence of multiple pregnancy. In an audit of IVF pregnancies in Dundee, 5% of miscarriage occurred between 15 and 24 weeks' gestation (McFaul et al 1993).

Ectopic pregnancy

Ectopic pregnancy occurs more frequently in IVF pregnancies than in the general population. This may seem surprising since the embryos are deposited in the uterine cavity. Rates as high as 10% have been reported, encouraging some clinics to perform elective salpingectomy or proximal tube occlusion. The Dundee study showed a rate of 5%.

In general, the current rates would seem to be in the order of 2–5%—a significant risk for women undertaking

296 TURNBULL'S OBSTETRICS

IVF. Early diagnosis is common, primarily because of the close observation of these cases with ultrasound and BhCG measurements. Heterotopic pregnancy (i.e. a co-incident ectopic and intrauterine gestation) has been reported with increased frequency in assisted conception.

Multiple pregnancy

Multiple pregnancies are a major hazard of assisted conception where multiple oocytes and embryos are generated and replaced. To have achieved conception but to then lose the pregnancy due to premature delivery because of high multiplicity is a devastating event—certainly not a successful outcome.

In the UK in 1990 when four embryos were considered to be the appropriate number to replace, a multiple pregnancy rate of 25% was reported by the ILA. The MRC study (1990) reported a 23% multiple pregnancy rate. Higher birth numbers have received great publicity but generally a poor outcome. These are associated with transfer of large numbers of embryos or oocytes. Thus most countries are limiting the number of embryos to be replaced. In the UK it is illegal to replace more than three embryos. An alternative approach to reduce the high multiple pregnancy rate is to undertake fetal reduction in the first trimester (Boulot et al 1993). The Scottish study (McFaul et al 1993) reported a 27% multiple pregnancy rate with the use of a maximum of three embryos. It is for this reason that some clinics are recommending a two embryo transfer when the embryo quality is good and the patient is under 35 years old.

The impact of assisted conception on the incidence of multiple pregnancy is substantial. For example, in England and Wales the rate has risen from 10/100 000 in 1980 to 30/100 000 in 1989. The problems of early delivery, lower birthweight, higher perinatal mortality and the caring difficulties for parents (particularly of higher order multiples) have significant implications for the proponents of assisted conception.

Prematurity

Not surprisingly the premature delivery rate is high after assisted conception although, interestingly, the rate in singletons is also significantly higher than in the normally conceived population (13% vs 7% in the Scottish Health Service) in 1991. The additional costs to the health care system in provision of neonatal services are substantial.

Low birthweight

A further indication of the high risk of such pregnancies is the higher than expected incidence of small babies, even after correction for multiple pregnancy and gestation.

In the Scottish study 37% of infants were small for gestational age compared to 8% in the normal obstetric population. In the MRC study 32% of babies were of low birthweight compared with 7% in England and Wales.

This effect may be related to the infertility itself or the hMG therapy rather than IVF (Olivennes et al 1993). In their study looking at singleton pregnancies a comparison of natural conception, ovulation induction and IVF conception revealed no difference in the latter two approaches but a worse outcome when compared with the normal population.

Other indices of high-risk pregnancies

In the MRC study (1990) predictors of poor perinatal outcome were present in increased frequency, e.g. maternal age, previous adverse pregnancy outcome, multiple pregnancy, hypertension. Pregnancy-induced hypertension requiring hospital admission occurred in 16% of cases, bleeding during pregnancy requiring admission occurred in 18%.

The perinatal mortality rates were about twice the national average (27.2/1000), mostly accounted for by multiplicity, i.e. singletons 11.7/1000, twins 39.7/1000, triplets or greater 79.3/1000. Other countries, Australia, USA, France, have reported similar outcomes.

Malformations have been carefully studied in many countries. The general conclusion is that the risks are no greater than age-matched populations. Questions have been raised but never proven in relation to central nervous system abnormalities.

Caesarean section

The MRC study which looked at patients in 1983–87 showed Caesarean sections rates of 43% for singletons, 64% for twins and 95% for triplets and higher order births. In the Dundee report which studied women between 1986 and 1989, the Caesarean section rates were 36% for singletons and 50% for twins, respectively, compared with a hospital rate of 15% in the same period. Increased Caesarean rates will always be a factor, to ensure the maximum chances of a non-traumatic delivery of an infant for whom so much effort was expended to achieve conception. The associated maternal morbidity must be considered in this equation.

The future

In the 15 years since the first IVF success our understanding of the processes involved in normal reproduction has expanded immensely. The stimulus to improve pregnancy rates has produced a variety of techniques to help the infertile couple. Virtually any form of infertility can now be treated (albeit with low success rates in some situations). Advances which were theoretical 5 years ago are now reality.

The advances for the next 10 years will be in the areas of oocyte cryopreservation, management of the endometrium to maximize implantation rates and the extension of preimplantation diagnosis to many more genetic diseases. Controversial issues such as the use of fetal ovarian tissue as a source of donor oocytes* and pregnancies in postmenopausal women will continue to push the field of assisted reproduction into the arena of public debate. Technological advances will continue to present ethical and moral dilemmas to clinicians involved in the field.

---

*A change in the law in the UK made this illegal.

REFERENCES

Abdalla H I, Baber R, Kirkland A, Leonard T, Power M, Studd J 1990 A report on 100 cycles of oocyte donation; factors affecting the outcome. Human Reproduction 5: 1018–1022

Abdalla H I, Burton G, Kirkland A et al 1993 Age, pregnancy and miscarriage: uterine versus ovarian factors. Human Reproduction 8: 1512–1517

Allen N C, Herbert C M, Maxon W S, Rogers B J, Diamond M P, Wentz A C 1985 Intrauterine insemination: a critical review. Fertility and Sterility 44: 569–580

American Fertility Society Registry 1991 Assisted reproductive technology in the United States and Canada: 1991 results from the Society for Assisted Reproductive Technology

Amso N N, Ahuja K K, Morris N, Shaw R 1989 Elective preembryo cryopreservation in ovarian hyperstimulation syndrome. Journal of In Vitro Fertilisation and Embryo Transfer 6: 312–314

Angell R R, Aitken R J, Van Look P F A, Lumsden M A, Templeton A A 1983 Chromosome abnormalities in human embryos after in vitro fertilisation. Nature (London) 303: 336–338

Asch R H, Balmaceda J P, Ellsworth L R, Wong P C 1986 Preliminary experiences with gamete intrafallopian transfer (GIFT). Fertility and Sterility 45: 366

Barkay J, Zuckerman H K, Sklan D, Gordon S 1977 Effect of caffeine on increasing the motility of frozen human sperm. Fertility and Sterility 29: 304–308

Boulot P, Hedon B, Pelliccia et al 1993 Multifetal pregnancy reduction: a consecutive series of 61 cases. British Journal of Obstetrics and Gynaecology 100: 63–68

Chaffkin L M, Nulsen J C, Luciano A A, Metzger D A 1991 A comparative analysis of the cycle fecundity rates associated with combined human menopausal gonadotrophin (hMG) and intrauterine insemination (IUI) versus either hMG or IUI alone. Fertility and Sterility 55: 252–257

Chong A P, Taymer M L 1975 Sixteen years of experience with therapeutic donor insemination. Fertility and Sterility 26: 791–798

Chong S S, Kristjansson K, Cota J, Handyside A H, Hughes M R 1993 Preimplantation prevention of X-linked disease: reliable and rapid sex determination of single human cells by restriction analysis of simultaneously amplified ZFX and ZFY sequences. Human Molecular Genetics 2: 1187–1191

Davajan V, Vargyas J M, Kletzky O A et al 1983 Intrauterine insemination with washed sperm to treat infertility. Fertility and Sterility 40: 419–422

Dellenbach P, Nisan I, Moreau L et al 1985 Transvaginal sonographical controlled follicle puncture for oocyte retrieval. Fertility and Sterility 44: 656–662

Ezra Y, Schenker J G 1983 Appraisal of in vitro fertilisation. European Journal of Obstetrics and Gynaecology and Reproductive Biology 48: 127–133

Forman R G, Frydman R, Egan D, Ross C, Barlow D H 1990 Severe ovarian hyperstimulation syndrome using agonists of gonadotrophin-releasing hormone for in vitro fertilisation: a European series and a proposal for prevention. Fertility and Sterility 53: 502–509

Frankel L 1909 Uber kunstliche Befruchtung beim Menschen und ihre gerichtsarztliche Beuerteirling. Arztliche Sachverst Ztg 15: 169

Hardy K, Handyside A H 1992 Biopsy of cleavage stage embryos and diagnosis of single gene defects by DNA amplification. Archives of Pathology and Laboratory Medicine 116: 388–392

Home E 1799 An account of the dissection of a hermaphrodite dog. Philosophical Transactions of the Royal Society, London 89: 157

Hull M G R 1992 Infertility treatment: relative effectiveness of conventional and assisted conception methods. Human Reproduction 7: 785–796

Interim Licensing Authority for Human In Vitro Fertilisation and Embryology 1989 Fifth Report. Summerfield and Day, Eastbourne

Interim Licensing Authority for Human In Vitro Fertilisation and Embryology 1990 Sixth Report. Summerfield and Day, Eastbourne

Interim Licensing Authority for Human In Vitro Fertilisation and Embryology 1991 Statistical Analysis of the United Kingdom IVF and GIFT Data 1985–1990. Summerfield and Day, Eastbourne

Iizuku R, Sawada Y, Nishina N, Ohi M 1968 The physical and mental development of children born following artificial insemination. International Journal of Fertility 13: 24–32

Jansen R P, Anderson J C 1993 Transvaginal versus laparoscopic gamete intrafallopian transfer: a case-controlled retrospective comparison. Fertility and Sterility 59: 836–840

Jequier A M, Cummins J M, Gearon C, Apted S L, Yovich J M, Yovich J 1990 A pregnancy achieved using sperm from the epididymal caput in idiopathic obstructive azoospermia. Fertility and Sterility 53: 1104–1105

Joyce D 1979 The organisation of an NHS Clinic. In: Richardson D, Joyce D, Symonds M (eds) Frozen human semen: proceedings of a workshop upon the cryobiology of human semen and its role in artificial insemination by donor. Royal College of Obstetricians and Gynaecologists, London, pp 234–245

Joyce D, Vassilopoulos D 1981 Sperm–mucus interaction and artificial insemination. Clinics in Obstetrics and Gynaecology 8: 587–610

Kovacs G T, Newman G B, Henson G L 1978 The postcoital test: what is normal? British Medical Journal 1: 818

Lenton E A, Weston G A, Cooke I D 1977 Problems in using basal body temperature recordings in an infertility clinic. British Medical Journal 1: 803–805

Lenton E A, Cooke I D, Hooper M et al 1992 In vitro fertilisation in the natural cycle. Baillières Clinics in Obstetrics and Gynaecology 6: 229–245

Lenz S, Bang J, Lauritsen J G, Lindenberg S 1985 Ultrasonically guided aspiration of oocytes for in vitro fertilisation using a plain needle and syringe under local anaesthesia. Infertility 7: 1–4

Lutjen P J, Trounson A O, Leeton J et al 1984 The establishment and maintenance of pregnancy using in vitro fertilization and embryo donation in a patient with primary ovarian failure. Nature 307: 174–175

McFaul P B, Patel N, Mills J 1993 An audit of the obstetric outcome of 148 consecutive pregnancies from assisted conception: implications for neonatal services. British Journal of Obstetrics and Gynaecology 100: 820–825

MRC Working Party 1990 Births in Great Britain resulting from assisted conception. British Medical Journal 300: 1229–1233

Nachtigall R D, Faure W, Glass R H 1979 Artificial insemination of husband's semen. Fertility and Sterility 32: 141–147

Newton J R 1984 Clinical results of AID. In: Thompson W, Joyce D N, Newton J R (eds) In vitro fertilisation and donor insemination. Royal College of Obstetricians and Gynaecologists, London, pp 307–315

Olivennes F, Rufat P, Andre B, Pourade A, Quiros M C, Frydman R

1993 The increased risk of complication observed in singleton pregnancies resulting from in vitro fertilisation (IVF) does not seem to be related to the IVF method itself. Human Reproduction 8: 1297–1300

Parsons J, Riddle A, Booker M et al 1985 Oocyte retrieval for in vitro fertilisation by ultrasonically guided needle aspiration via the urethra. Lancet i: 1076–1077

Randolph J F, Ohl D A, Bennett C J, Ayers J W, Menge A C 1990 Combined electroejaculation and in vitro fertilisation in the evaluation of anejaculatory infertility. Journal of In Vitro Fertilisation and Embryo Transfer 7: 58–62

Scammell G E, White N, Stedronska J, Hendry W F, Edmonds D K, Jeffcoate S L 1985 Cryopreservation of semen in men with testicular tumours or Hodgkin's disease: results of artificial insemination of their partners. Lancet ii: 31–32

Scammell G E, Stedronska-Clark J, Edmonds D K, Hendry W F 1989 Retrograde ejaculation: successful treatment with artificial insemination. British Journal of Urology 63: 198–201

Schill W B 1975 Caffeine and kallikrein induced stimulation of human sperm motility: a comparative study. Andrologie 7: 229–236

Seppala M, Edwards R G 1985 In vitro fertilisation and embryo transfer. Annals of the New York Academy of Science 442: 1072–1079

Serhal P F, Katz M, Little V, Woronwski H 1988 Unexplained infertility—the value of Pergonal superovulation combined with intrauterine insemination. Fertility and Sterility 49: 602

Steptoe P C, Edwards R G 1978 Birth after the implantation of a human embryo. Lancet ii: 336

Stewart G J, Tyler J P P, Cunningham A L et al 1985 Transmission of human T-cell lymphotrophic virus type III (HTVL-III) by artificial insemination by donor. Lancet ii: 581–585

Thompson W 1990 Artificial insemination. In: Chamberlain G (ed) Turnbull's obstetrics. Churchill Livingstone, London

Turhan N O, Artini P G, D'Ambrogio G, Droghini F, Volpe A, Genazzani A R 1992 Studies on direct intraperitoneal insemination in the management of male factor, cervical factor, unexplained and immunological infertility. Human Reproduction 7: 66–71

Van Steirteghem A C, Nagy Z, Joris H et al 1993 High fertilisation and implantation rates after intracytoplasmic sperm injection. Human Reproduction 8: 1061–1066

Veeck L L, Amudson C H, Brothman L J et al 1993 Significantly enhanced pregnancy rates per cycle through cryopreservation and thaw of pronuclear stage oocytes. Fertility and Sterility 59: 1202–1207

Whittemore A S, Harris R, Intyre J 1992 Characteristics relating to ovarian cancer risk: collaborative analysis of 12 US case-control studies. American Journal of Epidemiology 136: 1212–1220

Wilcox L S, Peterson H B, Haseltine F P, Martin M C 1993 Defining and interpreting pregnancy success rates for in vitro fertilisation. Fertility and Sterility 60: 18–25

Yovich J L 1993 Pentoxifylline: actions and applications in assisted reproduction. Human Reproduction 8: 1786–1791

17. Fetal growth and intrauterine growth retardation

J. Malcolm Pearce   Gillian Robinson

INTRODUCTION

Although birthweight is one of the most widely used parameters to judge the outcome of pregnancy, it is a luxury afforded to paediatricians and epidemiologists and is only of limited value to the obstetrician. By the time the infant is born, the chance to influence fetal growth (and hence birthweight) is lost. Low birthweight is defined by the WHO as a birthweight of less than 2.5 kg and such babies may be premature, growth retarded or both. In absolute terms maturity is probably more important than size (Robertson et al 1992) and this introduces one of the many problems associated with growth, namely the need to assess function rather than size.

The term intrauterine growth retardation (IUGR) may be defined as a process or pathology that impairs the genetic growth potential of the fetus, which, if removed, would allow the resumption of normal growth. This is not a clinically useful definition and as there is no test that can be applied to a baby at birth to determine whether it is pathologically growth retarded, statistical definitions of abnormality are used. From this arises the concept of small for gestational age (SGA), but this assumes knowledge of what constitutes normality at each gestation. This chapter will examine normal fetal growth as defined by birthweight for gestational age charts and ultrasonic charts of fetal parameters. It will then discuss the current methods of screening for and managing both smallness and impaired growth.

FETAL GROWTH

Growth results from an increase in both cell size or number. Fetal growth and eventual birthweight are intrinsically determined by genetic information but are modified by stimuli, which are largely hormonal, and constraints which are largely extrinsic to the fetus (for reviews see von Assche & Robertson 1981, Cockburn 1988). These constraints are poorly understood but some of the more frequently quoted ones are illustrated in Figure 17.1.

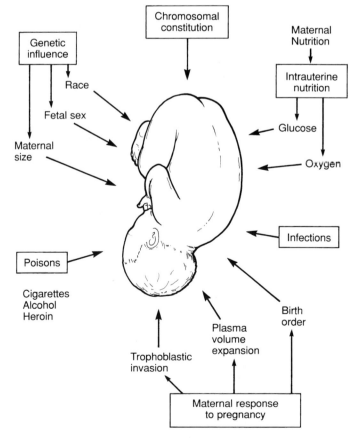

Fig. 17.1   Factors known to constrain fetal growth.

Birthweight charts

These charts are derived by recording the birthweights of a large number of infants with a gestation known accurately and then regressing them against gestational age (Fig. 17.2). These charts have several problems:

1. The statistical cut-off points for normality vary between studies and include less than the 10th, 5th, 3rd, 2/3rd centiles and less than 1, 2 and 3 standard deviations below the mean. Whatever cut-off value is chosen it will, by definition, include a number of normal babies, e.g. 5% of a normal population will give birth to a baby weighing less than the 5th centile for gestational age.
2. Babies born before 37 weeks' gestation cannot be considered normal and are certainly not a representative sample of fetal size at lower gestations.
3. Most charts suggest a sigmoid shape (Fig. 17.2) for growth but this has never been demonstrated by any of the charts of ultrasonically measured growth parameters.
4. The use of different populations affects the mean birthweight as demonstrated in a review of the English literature from 1963 to 1987. Goldenberg was able to demonstrate a difference of up to 500 g for the tenth centile of birthweight at 40 weeks' gestation (Goldenberg et al 1989a). The social and racial composition of the population influenced the results as did the height of the area above sea level. One of the largest sources of variation however was the method used to establish gestational age. Before the introduction of routine ultrasound scanning in early pregnancy, gestational age was uncertain in 20–40% of the population (Hall et al 1985, Warsof et al 1986). This results in a skewing of the birthweight distributions.

Ideally charts should be derived from the local population under study. This is often impractical and other charts are accepted. In the UK the most commonly used are those of Thomson et al (1968), which are age and parity specific and provide corrections for maternal height and weight at mid pregnancy. They are usefully provided in pocket-sized cards (Fig. 17.3).

Using incorrect charts can provide some major anomalies. Table 17.1 is from Kierse (1984) and demonstrates that babies born weighing 600 g at 30 weeks in Baltimore would be considered SGA but would not be so if born in Britain or Portland! In addition babies born with birthweights of 2450 g at 42 weeks in Montreal would be small but would not be considered growth retarded if born 2 weeks later, suggesting that prolonging the pregnancy would be beneficial. Weight for gestational age charts are a simple way of expressing the relationship between gestational age and birthweight and are best termed birthweight for gestational age standards (Altman & Hytten 1989). They should only be used to identify SGA not IUGR, as the charts make the assumption that weight is dependent upon gestational age whereas the very concept of IUGR demonstrates that weight may be independent of gestation.

Fetal growth can only be determined by serial measurements that are compared to longitudinally collected data and this, to all intents and purposes, means the use of ultrasonically measured parameters.

Ultrasonic charts of fetal size and growth

There are many published charts of fetal size but most of the studies are flawed by weakness in design, statistical analysis or both. The charts of fetal measurement are principally used in one of three ways (Altman & Chitty 1993):

1. To compare the size of the fetus (of known gestation) on a single occasion with reference data.
2. To estimate gestational age from fetal size.
3. To compare the growth of the fetus between two occasions with reference data.

Generally studies are either derived from measurements made on a single occasion, i.e. cross-sectional data; or measurements made on a series of occasions, i.e. longitudinal data. Cross-sectional data may be used to assess

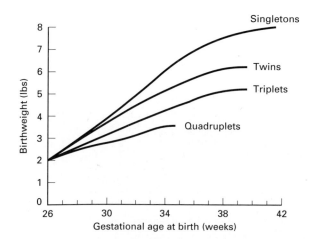

Fig. 17.2 An example of a birthweight for gestational age standards charts (McKeown & Record 1952).

Table 17.1 Birthweight limits (g) for intrauterine growth retardation, defined as a birthweight 2 SD below the mean and calculated from published fetal growth standards for different populations (Keirse 1984)

Gestational age (weeks)	Baltimore	Britain	Montreal	Portland
30	640	300	1023	581
36	1730	1400	1889	1769
40	2380	2450	2560	1769
42	2480	2550	2553	2673
44	2420	2475	2410	2589

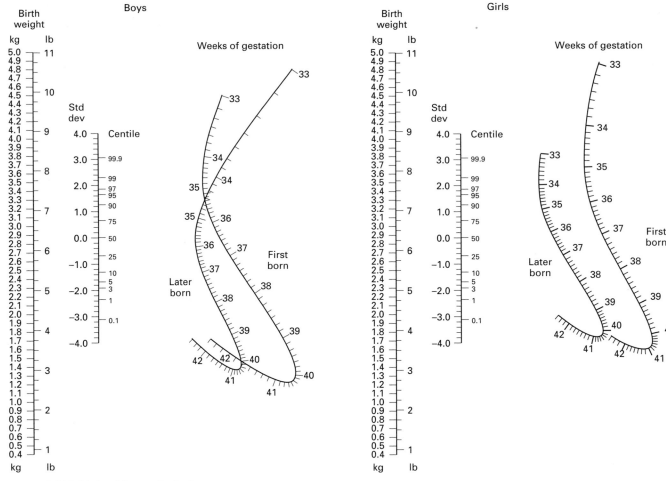

Fig. 17.3 British birthweight standards charts.

size on a single occasion and to estimate gestational age but longitudinal data is required to assess fetal growth. There is much confusion between size and growth and the cross-sectional charts of fetal size are often incorrectly refered to as growth charts.

The published studies of fetal size are subject to major criticisms:

1. The method of sample selection is inappropriate or unclear.
2. The inclusion and exclusion criteria are unclear or unreasonable.
3. Some fetuses are measured on many occasions.
4. The sample size is too small.
5. The method of dating the pregnancy is unclear.
6. It is unclear if the measurements were a single measurement or an average of several.

Sample selection is of crucial importance. The reference data should refer to normal fetuses and not those being scanned for some clinical indication. Ideally the data should be collected specifically for the purposes of the study and each fetus measured only on one occasion. The date of measurement should be allocated at random so that approximately equal numbers are measured at

each gestation. Whilst those measurements from fetuses subsequently found to be chromosomally abnormal or to have a congenital abnormality may be legitimately excluded, as may those from women who have a medical condition such as diabetes which is known to affect fetal growth, all other data should be included in order to collect as representative sample as possible.

The use of serial measurements from the same fetus is utilized in growth charts but not in size charts, since the measurements are highly correlated and so cannot be used to create size centiles.

Reference centiles may be calculated using parametric or non-parametric statistical methods. The latter require several hundred measurements at each week gestation and so are rarely used. Parametric analysis assumes that at each gestational age the data is normally distributed. The mean and standard deviations are calculated for each gestational age and the 5th and 95th centiles calculated as the mean $\pm$ 1.645 SD. The mean itself is calculated from linear or quadratic polynomial regression. The reference centiles should change smoothly with gestation and provide a good fit of the data.

Many studies fail to account for the variability of the measurement with gestation. The variability may increase with gestation and if not accounted for leads to centiles that are too far apart in early pregnancy and too close together in late pregnancy. Inappropriate modelling may not be apparent unless a scatter diagram of the raw data with the centiles superimposed is included (Altman & Chitty 1993).

Attempts to overcome the problems of variability within the populations have resulted in the derivation of individual growth curves. An individual growth standard is an attempt to predict the genetically determined growth potential of a particular fetus. Several measurements of fetal growth are made in early pregnancy and by mathematical modelling (Deter et al 1986) an individual growth curve is constructed. At least two measurements of fetal growth are required with an interval of not less than 6 weeks. Curves are then projected and if serial ultrasound measurements demonstrate growth less than expected the fetus is growth retarded. Deter et al (1990) have combined fetal head, abdominal and thigh circumference with predicted weight to produce a neonatal growth assessment score. The authors claim that the combination of these factors provides a better discriminator of growth retardation than measurement of a single parameter. This is one of the first attempts to study function (i.e. growth) rather than size.

A similar concept is that of customized antenatal growth charts (Gardosi et al 1992). These charts are customized for an individual pregnancy by taking maternal weight at first antenatal attendence, height, ethnic group, birthweight, gestation and sex of previous pregnancies into consideration. Correction factors for these variables are entered into a computer program which adjusts the normal birthweight centiles. The graph has gestation from 28 to 42 weeks on the X axis and birthweight on the Y axis. The tenth, fiftieth and ninetieth centiles curves for boys and girls adjusted according to the variables entered for the individual pregnancy are added and each women has her own growth chart added to her notes. This approach has several merits but has been critized in that the charts were constructed using cross-sectional data on birthweight and thus it is claimed they reflect size rather than growth (Chang et al 1992, Chard et al 1992). Other authorities argue that maternal ethnic group and weight are not known to be physiological variables and could be independent risk factors for growth retardation and thus should not be corrected for in the development of individual charts (Steer 1992). There is not yet data to demonstrate that identification of growth retardation in this manner leads to a reduction in perinatal morbidity or mortality. The construction and use of these charts is labour intensive and demands serial ultrasound examinations. This is not practical because of manpower, time and equipment and because there is little evidence, as yet, that many small fetuses come to any harm.

DETECTION OF SMALL FOR GESTATIONAL AGE

Determination of gestational age

In order to determine whether the size is correct for the gestation the gestational age needs to be accurately known. Apart from a few fertility patients where the date of ovulation, insemination or embryo replacement is known, gestational age is usually determined from the first day of the last menstrual period (LMP). The LMP is usually considered to be reliable if:

1. There is accurate maternal recall of the date of the LMP and that the period occurred at the expected time and was of the usual duration.
2. The menstrual cycle is regular, preferably of 28 days in length.
3. There had been no vaginal bleeding in pregnancy.
4. That the woman had not been using hormonal methods of contraception within the last 3 months of the LMP.

Even if all the above conditions are fulfilled ultrasonic measurements of the crown–rump lenth (CRL) in early pregnancy or biparietal diameter (BPD) up to 20 weeks' gestation will suggest a gestational age that is more than 2 weeks different from the postmenstrual age in at least 25% of women (Bennet et al 1982), with nearly all women being less pregnant than their dates would suggest. There is still much confusion in the literature as to which dates to use and this often leads to both being retained to the confusion of both the mother and her attendents. There is little objective evidence that the ultrasonic dates should be retained (if the discrepancy is greater than 2 weeks), since there have been no randomized controlled trials demonstrating a change in perinatal morbidity or mortality but:

1. There is a reduction in the number of women whose pregnancies are induced for postmaturity (greater than 42 weeks' completed gestation) without apparent harm to the mother or fetus (Bakketeig et al 1984, Eik-Nes et al 1984, Waldenstrom et al 1988, Le Fevre et al 1993).
2. Growth retardation is very rare in the first half of pregnancy.
3. The assessment of future growth in pregnancy will be based upon a change in ultrasound parameters.

Detection of SGA

Abdominal palpation

Many methods (Fig. 17.4) have been used in the detection of the small fetus. The oldest and the most ritualistic is abdominal palpation which is performed at every antenatal visit. However it is a poor indicator of fetal size.

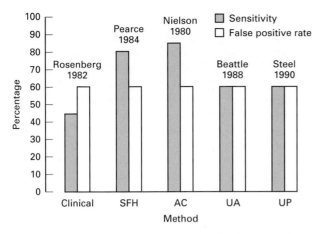

Fig. 17.4 Sensitivity and false-positive rates of various screening methods for detecting babies with birthweights of less than the 10th centile. SFH = symphyseal–fundal height; UA = umbilical artery; UP = uteroplacental waveform; AC = abdominal circumference.

Twenty per cent of assessments made immediately prior to delivery have an error of at least 450 g (Loeffler 1967). In a study of its value in the detection of SGA (less than 10% centile), 50% of those babies affected were not detected. In addition 41% of those that were unsuspected were less than the fifth centile (Rosenberg et al 1982).

Symphyseal–fundal height

The size of the maternal abdomen is a crude measure of both uterine and fetal growth. Measurements of symphysis–fundal height (SFH) and abdominal girth have been studied as screening tests for the detection of small babies, Longitudinal measurements from the same woman might be useful in the assessment of fetal growth but to date no studies have been performed. It has been shown that SFH measurements are a better determinant of fetal size than abdominal girth measurements (Mathai et al 1987).

SFH measurements are made by determining the uterine fundus by abdominal palpation and then measuring the distance from the upper border of the symphysis pubis to the uterine fundus in centimetres. Studies that have evaluated the prediction of SGA by SFH measurement have shown widely differing results, with sensitivities varying between 27% and 86%; specificities between 78% and 93% and positive predictive values between 18% and 79% (Belizan et al 1978, Rosenberg et al 1982, Persson et al 1986). In some of these studies (Belizan et al 1978, Quaranta et al 1981, Wallin et al 1981, Calvert et al 1982) the population studied had a high incidence of SGA babies which increases the sensitivity of the screening procedure. Serial SFH measurements and a single measurement of abdominal circumference by ultrasound in the third trimester were compared in an unselected group of 699 women attending an antenatal clinic (Pearce et al 1987). The sensitivity of SFH measurement was 76% as compared to 83% for abdominal circumference after the specificities of both tests had been set at 79%. The positive predictive values were comparable —36% for SFH measurement and 39% for abdominal circumference. If used alone SFH measurement would identify 28% of the antenatal population as being of risk for SGA and would detect 75% of SGA babies.

The first prospective randomized study of SFH measurement compared abdominal palpation with SFH measurement in 1639 women (Lindhard et al 1990). SFH had a lower detection rate of SGA than abdominal palpation (sensitivities 28% and 48% respectively), but the observers could have been biased by knowledge of the ultrasound scan that was performed on all women at 29 weeks. In addition to those randomized to SFH measurement, 6% did not have any measurements performed and in a further 15% only one or two measurements were taken.

The value of SFH measurement remains unproved and further large prospective studies need to be performed before it can be properly evaluated and either disregarded or incorporated into routine antenatal care. It may prove to be a simple and inexpensive screening tool, particularly in countries where ultrasound is either restricted or unavailable.

Ultrasonic measurement

Ultrasonic assessment of fetal size has a key role to play in the detection of SGA babies and is widely accepted to increase the detection rate above that determined by clinical palpation alone (Fig. 17.4). The ultrasonic measurements that may be used in the assessment of fetal size are illustrated in Table 17.2 (Geirsson & Persson 1984). Accurate ultrasonic confirmation of menstrual dates in the early stages of pregnancy is essential.

The measurement of the biparietal diameter (BPD) was the first method used in the ultrasonic detection of

Table 17.2 Ultrasonic measurements used in the assessment of fetal size (Geirsson & Persson 1984)

One-/two-dimensional growth	
Skeletal	BPD, head area/circumference
	Long bone length
Soft tissue	Trunk diameters/area/circumference
	Thigh thickness
	Subcutaneous fat
Combination	Head/trunk ratio
	CRL and trunk area
Three-dimensional growth	
Weight	Fetal weight assessment
Volume	Fetal volume
	Total intrauterine volume
	Intra-amniotic volume
	Visual assessment of amniotic fluid volume

Table 17.3 Sensitivity and specificity of ultrasonic parameters in the assessment of fetal growth (Neilson et al 1980)

Ultrasonic measurement	Sensitivity (%)	Specificity (%)
BPD	58	90
Head area	59	90
Head circumference	56	92
Trunk area	81	89
Trunk circumference	83	90
Transverse trunk diameter	61	88
CRL	69	88
CRL × trunk area	94	88
Head area/trunk area	44	91

IUGR and a detection rate of 73% was reported from serial scanning in a high-risk population (Campbell & Dewhurst 1971). However the measurement of BPD may be difficult, if not impossible, in late pregnancy due to the lie of the fetus (direct occipito anterior or posterior positions), or because the fetal head is low in the pelvis. Furthermore head measurement may not be the most logical since in some patterns of growth retardation there is a head-sparing effect. Other studies have found BPD measurements to be less useful in screening for SGA than abdominal measurements (Ferrazzie et al 1986, Warsof et al 1986). The results of a study comparing the sensitivities and specificities of different ultrasonic measurements in the prediction of SGA (< 10th centile) babies are illustrated in Table 17.3 (Neilson et al 1980). With real-time ultrasound equipment, measurements of CRL in late pregnancy are not practical so most groups use trunk (abdominal) circumference.

There have been four randomized controlled trials published that compare routine scanning in the third trimester with scanning on indication in the detection of SGA. The sensitivities varied between 62% and 82% in those routinely scanned as compared with 31–45% in those scanned for clinical indication (Wladimiroff et al 1980, Neilson et al 1984, Eik-Nes et al 1984, Secher et al 1986). The predictive values varied between 16% and 70%. Thus many babies considered antenatally to be SGA will be delivered with a birthweight appropriate for gestation. The effect of a routine ultrasound examination in the third trimester had a variable influence on the management of the remainder of the pregnancy. Inconsistant results have been shown in respect of antenatal admission rates (Bakketeig et al 1984, Eik-Nes et al 1984) but a possible increase in the use of antenatal cadiotocography, ultrasound and early induction were found (Cochlin 1984, Hughey 1984). In addition none of the studies has demonstrated any fetal benefit in terms of reduced perinatal morbidity or mortality (Neilson & Graw 1989, Breart & Ringa 1990, Larsen et al 1992).

Doppler ultrasound

The use of umbilical artery Doppler ultrasonography as a screening tool for the detection of SGA babies in low-risk pregnancies has been investigated in five prospective studies. In all but one the clinicians were blinded to the results (Beattie & Doran 1989, Hanretty et al 1989, Sijmons et al 1989, Newnham et al 1990). The predictive values ranged from 11% to 50%; the sensitivity of the test was also low with an overall mean between the studies of 23% (Dornan & Bealtie 1992; Fig. 17.4).

Doppler ultrasound of the uteroplacental circulation (Fig. 17.4) has also been investigated as a screening tool for the detection of SGA. About 50% of SGA (< 10th centile) are thought to be caused by failure of trophoblastic invasion, which is reflected by an increased resistance to flow in the uteroplacental circulation (Sheppard & Bonnar 1976). The fall in the uteroplacental flow velocity waveform resistance indices by 22–24 weeks' gestation is thought to represent the second wave of trophoblastic invasion with the uteroplacental flow velocity waveform reflecting the depth of trophoblastic invasion. Doppler indices in the second trimester might predict problems in the third trimester.

At least seven studies investigating the role of Doppler examination of the uteroplacental circulation have been published demonstrating widely varying results (Campbell et al 1986, Arduini et al 1987, Hanretty et al 1989, Schulman et al 1989, Jacobson et al 1990, Newnham et al 1990). Some of these differences may be explained by the different populations studied, different definitions of pregnancy outcome and different study methodology, however there is little agreement regarding which part of the uteroplacental circulation to study (Bewley et al 1989) and it is not known whether readings obtained from one part of the circulation reflect changes seen in other areas.

It has recently been suggested that the shape of the velocity waveform may prove a better discriminator. The presence of a diastolic notch predicted only 46% of SGA babies in a population sample of 2430 women but there was a trend for these pregnancies so identified to be associated with fetal destress, low Apgar scores at delivery, early delivery and admission to the special care baby unit (Bower et al 1993). This finding requires further study. Doppler examination does not appear to have a role in the screening of a low risk population for SGA.

Conclusion

Currently the best methods of screening for SGA would appear to be ultrasound scanning or SFH measurements where facilities for two ultrasounds scans are not possible.

AETIOLOGY OF SMALL FOR GESTATIONAL AGE

Many factors are associated with SGA (Table 17.4).

Genetic

Weight is multifactorial, being determined both by genes

Table 17.4 Factors associated with SGA

Maternal
  Malnutrition and low body weight
  Pregnancy at age < 16 years or > 35 years
  Low socioeconomic status
  Smoking
  Drug abuse
Fetal
  Chromosome abnormalities
  Structural abnormalities
  Intrauterine infection
Medical conditions
  Pre-eclampsia
  Hypertension
  Antepartum haemorrhage
  Severe chronic disease
  Sickle cell disease
  Anaemia
  Uterine abnormalities
Environmental problems
  High altitude
  Toxic substances
Placental abnormalities
  Impaired trophoblastic invasion
  Placenta circumvallata

on various loci and environmental influences. Studies of twins and siblings have identified the extent of these influences and found that birthweight variation can be accounted for by intrauterine environment (24%), maternal genotype (24%), fetal genotype (18%), environmental influences on the mother (20%) and maternal disease (11%) (Beattie et al 1993).

Chromosome abnormalites are associated with structural deformities, dysmorphic features, mental retardation, intrauterine and postnatal growth retardation. Trisomy 18 results in a much more profound retardation than that seen with either trisomy 13 or 21. Triplody is also associated with severe IUGR and usually early pregnancy loss. The sex chromosome abnormalities do not generally result in IUGR, the exception being Turner's syndrome. The presence of a Y chromosome results in a faster growing fetus which is also heavier. The average male fetus is 150–200 g heavier than its female counterpart at term (Beattie & Whittle 1993, Nicholaides et al 1993).

Infection

Intrauterine infection causes less than 5% of cases of IUGR and the rate is declining. Rubella is the principal infection for which there is good evidence of causation, in that the virus causes a reduction in cell division and hence both the fetus and placenta have fewer cell numbers (Driscoll 1969).

Drugs

Cigarette smoking

Studies of smoking in pregnancy in various populations have consistently shown that the whole distribution of

birthweight is reduced in direct proportion to the number of cigarettes smoked in pregnancy (Murphy 1984). On average babies of smokers are 150–400 g lighter than those of non-smokers (Butler 1972, Murphy et al 1980). The time in pregnancy at which growth is affected is unclear. Ultrasound studies in early pregnancy have demonstrated that fetal growth as assessed by CRL is unaffected up to 14 weeks' gestation (Murphy 1984). However some studies have shown that women who stop smoking in early pregnancy have lighter babies than non-smokers (Herriott et al 1962), whilst others found no difference (Murphy 1984). Placental weight is not affected, although the placenta may be larger and thinner. In addition there may be differences in the ultrastructure of the placental vessels suggesting a faster ageing process (Murphy 1984). Smoking may cause a fetal hypoxia by acute nicotinic activation of adrenergic neurones, resulting in vasoconstriction, reduced uterine perfusion and fetal tachycardia (Kelly et al 1984). It may also have a delayed effect by increasing carboxyhaemoglobin and reducing fetal oxygenation. Nicotine crosses the placenta and depresses cellular metabolism, blocking the active transport of amino acids from the maternal to the fetal circulation.

Alcohol

The effect of moderate and light drinking in pregnancy is controversial. Some studies have shown a reduction in birthweight of 91–160 g in women drinking an average of two drinks a day (Little 1977) and women drinking greater than 10 drinks a week were more than twice as likely to deliver an infant of low birthweight than those drinking less than five drinks a week (Wright et al 1983). In contrast Hingson found no alteration in birthweight in women drinking moderately throughout pregnancy (Hingson et al 1982).

Ethanol has a direct effect on cell growth resulting in a reduction in cell number rather than size. In the fetal brain it interferes with neuronal proliferation and disturbs the migration and integration of neurones. The mechanism is unknown (Beattie 1988).

Maternal weight and nutrition

Pregnant women store nutrients. Healthy women eating a normal diet gain weight at an average of 400–500 g/week during pregnancy. By 30 weeks over 30 kg has been stored as fat in the subcutaneous tissues of the abdomen and thighs. This store is mobilized in later pregnancy when human plasma lactinogen (hPL) influences the lipolysis of the fat stores resulting in a rise in the plasma levels of free fatty acids (Hytten 1982).

The placenta aquires nutrients for the fetus and may transform them into a derivative so they cannot be transfered back to the maternal circulation. The enables the fetus to be supplied with whatever nutrients are required later in the pregnancy. The main exception to this is glucose which is not stored in the placenta. If maternal levels are low the fetus receives little; thus the fetus of a starving mother is well grown but thin due to lack of subcutaneous fat.

The physiology has been well demonstrated in the famines of Holland and Leningrad which occurred in the Second World War. Babies which were conceived prior to the famine but born during it had birthweights between 300 and 550 g less than those born when food was plentiful. However those babies conceived during the famine but born after were of normal weight, demonstrating that compensatory mechanisms can occur.

Women who have a low body weight or who fail to gain much weight in pregnancy are more likely to deliver an infant of low birthweight. In a study of pregnancy outcome in underweight women with spontaneous and induced ovulation, women who had a body mass index less than 19.1 (normal range 20–25) but who ovulated spontaneously had a three times increased risk of a small baby and those who were both underweight and required ovulation induction had a nine times increased risk when compared to women of normal weight who conceived spontaneously (van der Spuy 1988).

Impaired vascularization

The maternal placental bed develops from the original implantation site. At term maternal blood enters the intervillous space through 100–200 spiral arteries. Blood entering the space has a higher pressure than that found within the space, so blood is directed towards the chorionic plate which forms the roof of the space. The blood flows over the fetal villi which allows time for the exchange of gases and nutrients and then drains to the floor of the space where it flows into the endometrial veins. Uteroplacental blood flow increases from approximately 50 ml/minute at 10 weeks' gestation to 600 ml/minute at term. In order to accomodate this huge increase in blood flow the spiral ateries of the non-pregnant uterus are converted into uteroplacental vessels by trophoblastic invasion. The trophoblast disrupts the wall of the spiral artery, destroying the muscle and elastic layers and replacing them with fibrinoid material. This invasion process occurs in two waves; the first occurs at implantation and lasts 10 weeks reaching the decidual layer of the spiral arteries; the second wave starts at 14–16 weeks and lasts for 4–6 weeks. This wave invades as far as the radial artery with a concomitant increase in uteroplacental flow and subsequent resistance to the effects of circulating pressor agents.

Patients with severe pre-eclampsia have a failure of the second wave of trophoblastic invasion. This results in decreased perfusion of the intervillous space, maternal hypertension and persisting responsiveness to circulating pressor agents with subsequent acute necrotizing atherosis

leading to further narrowing of the spiral arteries. In normotensive pregnancies complicated by IUGR similar evidence of incomplete trophoblastic invasion was demonstrated in 50% of placental bed biopsies (Sheppard & Bonnar 1976). This suggests that impaired trophoblastic invasion leading to increased uteroplacental impedence, as demonstrated by Doppler studies, is a significant cause of IUGR.

Pearce (1993) has studied 100 primigravid women who have abnormal uterine artery Doppler waveforms as demonstrated by colour flow, pulsed Doppler ultrasound. Figures 17.5–17.8 demonstrate the way in which the fetus suffers from impaired uteroplacental perfusion. It may be summarized as follows:

1. There is impairment in the growth velocity of the fetal abdominal circumference before any other changes are observed (Fig. 17.5).
2. There is a decrease in the pulsatility index (PI) of the middle cerebral artery (MCA) but the waveforms from the descending aorta and umbilical artery are normal (Fig. 17.6). This may result from a decrease in oxygen transfer and a fetal baroreceptor response.
3. There is further impairment of the growth of the fetal abdomen or it may cease altogether.
4. There is evidence of reduced end-diastolic frequencies in both the umbilical artery and the aorta and in most cases the umbilical artery changes first.

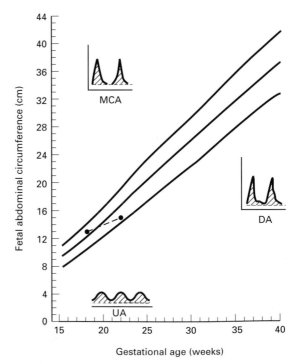

Fig. 17.5 Pattern of growth failure in 100 primigravid women with abnormal uterine artery waveforms. Small figures are the Doppler waveforms from the fetal middle cerebral artery (MCA), descending aorta (DA) and umbilical artery (UA). These are all within normal limits whilst there is biometric evidence of impaired growth.

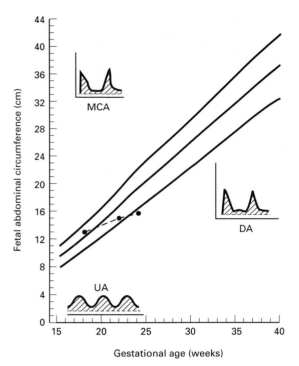

Fig. 17.6 There is now a decrease in the pulsatility of the MCA (see text) in that end-diastolic frequencies are visible in the waveform. Further failure of growth of the abdominal circumference is evident, but the DA and UA waveforms remain within normal limits.

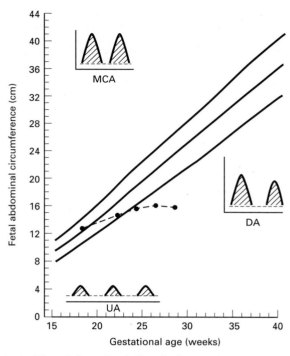

Fig. 17.8 There is loss of end-diastolic frequencies in the MCA, DA and UA. At this stage abnormalities of the cardiotocograph may occur.

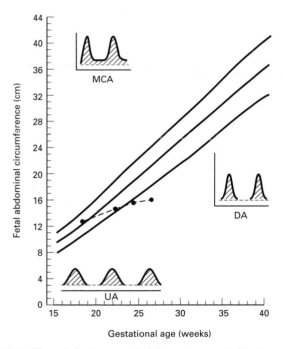

Fig. 17.7 There is further growth failure accompanied by loss of end-diastolic frequencies in the DA and UA. The MCA has increased end-diastolic frequencies.

5. There is loss of end-diastolic frequencies in both the umbilical artery and the descending aorta and the pulsatility index of the middle cerebral artery may be further decreased (Fig. 17.7).

6. There is an increase in the PI from the MCA and at this stage CTG abnormalities may become apparent (Fig. 17.8).
7. There is absence of end-diastolic frequencies in the MCA and then fetal death occurs. Reversed frequencies in end diastole may be observed prior to death.

No pregnancies in which there were bilateral high resistance uterine artery waveforms with bilateral notching went beyond 34 weeks' gestation.

Pearce (1993) matched the primigravidae described above with a control group who had normal waveforms from the uterine artery in the first half of pregnancy. Late onset (after 34 weeks) impairment of growth was observed in 15 women. In these cases uterine artery waveforms were either normal ($n = 8$) or only abnormal on the non-placental side of the uterus ($n = 7$). Impairment of growth of the abdominal circumference (AC) was observed before changes were seen in the fetal circulation and again a decrease in the MCA PI was the first circulatory change observed. Only six women went on to loose end-diastolic frequencies in the umbilical artery and aorta and in all cases this occurred within 2 weeks of the decrease in MCA PI. Abnormal cardiotocographs (CTGs) were observed in four of the six women and these occurred within 7–14 days of loss of end-diastolic flow.

Traditionally IUGR has been divided into two groups: symmetrical which accounts for 20% of cases and asymmetrical which accounts for the remaining 80%. Animal

Table 17.5 Types of intrauterine growth retardation

Fetal tissue	Type 1 (maternal protein restriction)	Type 2 (vascular insufficiency)
Fetal weight	Reduced	Reduced
Organ weight	Symmetrically reduced	Asymmetrical
Brain weight	Reduced	Normal
Brain cell number	Moderately reduced	Normal
Liver cell number	Moderately reduced	Much reduced
Liver glycogen	Slightly depleted	Absent

models suggest two differing causes—maternal starvation and reduced protein supply, and vascular insufficiency. The differing effects on fetal tissues are illustrated below in Table 17.5.

Factors that tend to reduce fetal growth from early in pregnancy produce symmetrically small babies whereas those that take effect from later in pregnancy produce asymmetrical or brain-sparing growth retardation.

MANAGEMENT OF SMALL FOR GESTATIONAL AGE

The management of babies found to be SGA may be thought of in terms of prevention, detection, assessment and delivery.

Prevention

Much of the advice that is given to women either prior to or in the early stages of pregnancy has little if any scientific foundation. Smokers should be advised to stop the habit altogether or if this is not possible to reduce consumption. However much maternal anxiety can be caused by an overzealous approach which results in undue stress, the effects of which are not known. Pregnant women are often advised to stop working and take more rest. Whilst this appears logical it fails to appreciate home circumstances and there is little evidence to show it is beneficial.

Several trials have demonstrated the benefits of low-dose aspirin in the prevention of pre-eclampsia and IUGR. Meta-analysis of these studies has shown that low-dose aspirin in the dose 60–300 mg/day reduces the incidence of pre-eclampsia in selected women at risk of disease based on previous history, increased angiotensin II sensitivity or abnormal vascular patterns on Doppler examination. This effect is thought to be due to a reduction in thromboxane production which prevents vascular vasoconstriction. The effects on growth are less clear. Small studies in women with a history of a previous growth-retarded baby suggest that low-dose aspirin increases birthweight in the current pregnancy (Wallenberg & Rotmans 1987, Elder et al 1988). However results from two larger studies are conflicting. The Italian study failed to demonstrate a benefit from low-dose asprin in terms of prevention of IUGR or pre-eclampsia in 1106 women said to be at immediate risk of the conditions (Italian

Study of Aspirin in Pregnancy 1993). This study had no placebo group and the investigators were not blinded. In addition a larger proportion of the women in the no treatment group were lost to follow up than in the aspirin group. Their findings should be treated with caution. The National Insititutes of Health Multicentre Maternal and Fetal Medicine Network Study in 3135 nulliparous women revealed a 26% reduction in the incidence of pre-eclampsia in the treated group but there was no apparent effect on the incidence of IUGR. More alarming was the sevenfold increase in abruption found in the treated women (Sibai 1993). Currently the role of aspirin in the prevention of IUGR is unclear.

Detection

Table 17.6 illustrates women who are at particular risk of impaired growth. These women should have serial ultrasound examinations performed in the latter half of pregnancy to monitor growth. Where facilites exist it may be more appropriate to use a predictive growth chart (Deter et al 1986) or the customized charts (Gardosi et al 1992). The ultrasonic parameters most frequently used are the head and abdominal circumference together with the H/A ratio (Chudleigh & Pearce 1992).

The best method of detection of SGA in low-risk women is an ultrasound measurement of AC between 30 and 36 weeks. However at least half of those babies suspected of being SGA will be born with an appropriate weight for gestation (Breart & Ringa 1990). Those fetuses with a small AC should then have their head circumference measured and their type of smallness determined. Ultrasound examinations are then repeated every 2 weeks to monitor growth and tests of fetal well-being may in addition be employed.

Management of impaired growth and smallness

Impaired growth

The diagnosis of impaired growth can only be made

Table 17.6 Women at high risk of SGA

Maternal weight less than 10th centile for height (< 45 kg as rough guide)
Previous infant with SGA
Maternal vascular disease
   Essential hypertension
   Pregnancy-induced hypertension
   Diabetes mellitus
   Collagen disorders
Maternal cardiac disease severe enough to cause maternal polycythaemia
Heavy smokers
Alcoholics and drug addicts
Women with sickle cell disease
Women with recurrent APH
Women with raised MSAFP but with structurally normal fetus

by serial ultrasound measurements which are in general only performed in women at high risk. The subsequent management is not universally agreed upon but tests of fetal well-being can be applied in a logical manner based upon knowledge of the pattern and time of detection of IUGR.

Early-onset intrauterine growth retardation (before 34 weeks)

When the diagnosis of IUGR is made prior to 24 weeks, the fetus is often symmetrically small. Indeed the detection of asymetrical growth retardation before twenty weeks suggests a triploid pregnancy (Snijders et al 1993). The subsequent management depends on the Doppler waveforms:

1. *Normal uterine artery waveforms.* In these cases (which are rare) there is an inherent fetal problem which is impairing growth. Detailed ultrasound examination looking for structural abnormalities and markers to suggest a chromosomal abnormality should be performed. A cordocentesis may detect the fetal karyotype and evidence of viral infection. If no abnormality is detected monitoring should continue with serial biometry and Dopplers of the fetal circulation.
2. *Abnormal uterine artery waveforms.* This is the most common clinical situation. Maternal blood should be tested for the presence of Lupus inhibitor and anticardiolipin antibodies which, although rare, indicate a maternal condition which may be improved with steroids. Low-dose aspirin has also been demonstrated to be beneficial (Trudinger et al 1988). Monitoring should continue with Doppler waveforms from the fetal circulation. If the MCA waveform is normal the test may be repeated weekly but once a reduction in the PI is seen then three times weekly examinations are required. If end-diastolic frequencies are lost in the aorta, the oxygen test should be used to predict imminent fetal demise. The mother is given 28% oxygen to breathe via a facemask for 15 minutes and the Doppler examination repeated. If the PI in the MCA increases and end-diastolic frequences reappear in the aorta (reversal of central shunting), that fetus will survive for at least 24 hours (barring acute accidents such as abruption). End-diastolic frequencies do not reappear in the umbilical artery. Should oxygen therapy not reverse the central shunting the fetus will most probably die in the next 48 hours and a clinical judgement based on estimated fetal weight and gestation should be made regarding delivery.

If detailed fetal monitoring is unavailable, umbilical artery waveforms should be measured. As long as end-diastolic frequencies are present the fetus is not in jeapordy, however once they are lost the prediction of fetal demise is difficult. In these circumstances daily monitoring with CTG may be employed.

Late-onset intrauterine growth retardation

After 34 weeks' gestation the detection of impaired growth should lead to Doppler examination of the umbilical artery. If the A/B ratio is within normal limits the test can be repeated weekly and ultrasonic examination repeated every fortnight. In addition low-dose aspirin may be beneficial. The absence of end-diastolic flow is associated with hypoxia and acidosis (Nicolaides et al 1988), an increased perinatal morbidity and mortality (McFarland et al 1991). Routine monitoring in these cases with CTG or biophysical profiles has not improved fetal outcome (Mohide & Keirse 1989) and in our opinion loss of end-diastolic flow in the umbilical artery should be the indication for delivery.

Management of a small fetus

Small babies detected in low-risk women pose a different problem. The type of growth impairment should be identified and all cases should have Doppler examination of the umbilical artery and central vessels if facilities are available.

Symmetrical SGA (Fig. 17.9). Most of these fetuses are normal and simply represent the lower end of the biological spectrum. The fetus should be scanned for structural anomalies and markers of chromosomal abnormality, especially if umbilical end-diastolic frequencies have been lost. Whilst the identification of a maternal factor is of academic interest it is too late to alter the pattern of growth. The reminder of the pregnancy is monitored with weekly Doppler of the umbilical artery and serial ultrasonic measurement. In most cases spontaneous labour occurs but should end-diastolic frequencies be lost delivery should be expedited.

Asymmetrical SGA (Fig. 17.10). We recommend monitoring with weekly Doppler examination of the umbilical and fetal vessels and serial ultrasound examination. In randomized trials CTG and biophysical profiles have not been demonstrated to be of benefit (Mohide et al 1989). Should end-diastolic flow be lost we recommend delivery, measurement of the PI of the MCA will demonstrate a reduction prior to changes in the umbilical artery and may allow time for induction and vaginal delivery.

CONCLUSION

Fetal growth is dependent upon a complex and ill-understood series of factors. Patterns of fetal growth should not be inferred from cross-sectional birthweight for gestational age charts but from correctly constructed charts of ultrasonically determined biometric parameters. Size and growth charts should not be confused.

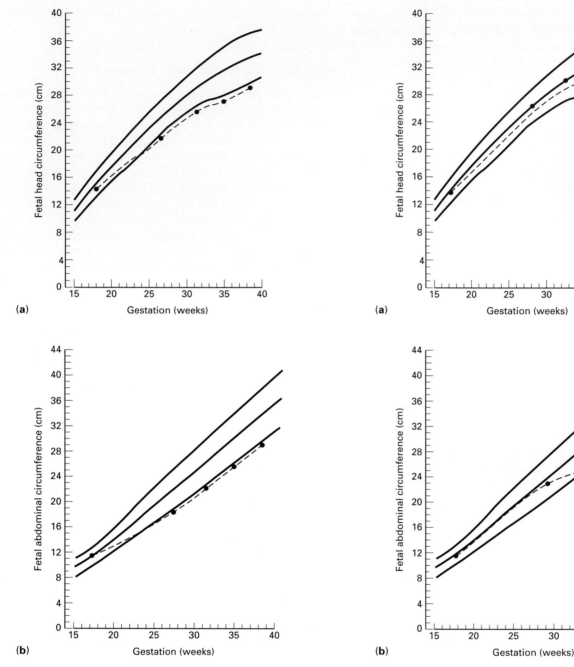

Fig. 17.9 Ultrasonic charts illustrating the growth pattern in symmetrical growth retardation.

Fig. 17.10 Ultrasonic charts illustrating the growth pattern in asymmetrical growth retardation.

Although proof is scarce, gestational age should be determined from ultrasonic parameters (in the absence of more reliable data). Subsequent monitoring of growth should be by serial measurement in high-risk pregnancies but has to be limited to screening for smallness in low-risk pregnancies.

Smallness and growth failure are best evaluated with the aid of Doppler ultrasound examination of both the uterine arteries and the fetal circulation. Symmetrically small fetuses are usually representatives of the lower end of the normal range but rarely may be due to chromo-

somal or viral causes or associated with some maternal problem or habit. In the absence of these, Doppler examinations are usually within normal limits and expectant management is appropriate.

Asymmetry before 34 weeks' gestation is usually associated with abnormal uterine artery waveforms. Subsequent management is dependent upon the state of the fetal circulation. After 34 weeks asymmetry appears to be associated with normal uterine artery Doppler waveforms, suggesting senescence of fetal vessels. Management again depends upon the waveforms from the fetal circulation.

REFERENCES

Altman D G, Chitty L S 1993 Design and analysis of studies to derive charts of fetal size. Ultrasound in Obstetrics and Gynaecology 3: 378–384

Altman G D, Hytten F E 1989 Assessment of fetal size and fetal growth. In: Chalmers I, Enkin M, Keirse M J N C (eds) Effective care in pregnancy and childbirth. Oxford University Press, Oxford, pp 411–418

Anderson G A, Blidner I N, McClemont S, Sinclair J C 1984 Determinants of size at birth in a Canadian population. American Journal of Obstetrics and Gynecology 150: 236

Arduini D, Rizzo G, Romanini C, Mancuso S 1987 Uteroplacental blood flow velocity waveforms as predictors of pregnancy induced hypertension. European Journal of Obstetrics and Gynaecology and Reproductive Biology 26: 335–341

Bakketeig L S, Eik-Nes S H, Jacobsen G et al 1984 Randomized controlled trial of ultrasonographic screening in pregnancy. Lancet ii: 207–211

Beattie J O 1988 Alcohol pregnancy and the fetus. In: Chamberlain G (ed) Contempory obstetrics and gynaecology. Butterworths, London

Beattie R B, Doran J C 1989 Antenatal screening for intrauterine growth retardation using umbilical artery Doppler ultrasound. British Medical Journal 298: 631–635

Beattie R B, Whittle M J 1993 The aetiology of intrauterine growth retardation. Current Obstetrics and Gynaecology 3: 184–189

Belizan J M, Villar J, Nardin J C, Malamud J, Sainz de Vicuna L 1978 Diagnosis of intrauterine growth retardation by a simple clinical method: measurement of the uterine height. American Journal of Obstetrics and Gynecology 131: 643–645

Bennet M J, Little G, Dewhurst J, Chamberlain G 1982 Predictive value of ultrasound measurement in early pregnancy. British Journal of Obstetrics and Gynaecology 89: 338–341

Bewely S, Campbell S, Cooper D 1989 Uteroplacental Doppler flow velocity waveforms in the second trimester. A complex circulation. British Journal of Obstetrics and Gynaecology 96: 1040–1046

Bower S, Schuchter K, Campbell S 1993 Doppler ultrasound screening as part of routine antenatal scanning: prediction of pre-eclampsia and intrauterine growth retardation. British Journal of Obstetrics and Gynaecology 100: 989–994

Breart G, Ringa V 1990 Routine or selective ultrasound. Clinics in Obstetrics and Gynaecology 4: 45–63

Butler N R, Goldstein H, Ross E M 1972 Cigarette smoking and pregnancy. British Medical Journal 2: 127–130

Calvert J P, Crean E E, Newcombe R G, Pearson J F 1982 Antenatal screening by measurement of symphysis fundal height. British Medical Journal 285: 846–849

Campbell S, Dewhurst C J 1971 Diagnosis of small for dates fetus by serial ultrasonic cephalometry. Lancet ii: 1002–1006

Campbell S, Pearce J M F, Hackett G, Cohen-Overbeek T, Hernandez C 1986 Qualitative assessment of uteroplacental blood flow: early screening test for high risk pregnancies. Obstetrics and Gynecology 68: 649–653

Chang T C, Robson S C, Spencer J A D 1992 Customised antenatal growth charts. Lancet 339: 878 (letter)

Chard T, Macintosh M, Yoony A 1992 Customised antenatal growth charts. Lancet 339: 878 (letter)

Chudleigh P, Pearce J M 1992 In: Obstetric ultrasound how why and when, 2nd edn. Churchill Livingstone, London

Cochlin D L 1984 Effects of two ultrasound scanning regiemes on the management of pregnancy. British Journal of Obstetrics and Gynaecology 91: 885–890

Cockburn F (ed) 1988 Fetal and neonatal growth. Perinatal practice, vol 5. Wiley, Chichester

Deter R L, Rossavik I K, Harrist R B, Hadlock F P 1986 Mathematical modeling of fetal growth: development of individual growth curve standards. Obstetrics and Gynecology 68: 156–161

Deter R L, Harris R B, Hill R M 1990 Neonatal growth assessment score: a new approach to the detection of intrauterine growth retardation in the newborn. American Journal of Obstetrics and Gynecology 1990; 162: 1030–1036

Dornan J, Beattie J 1992 Umbilical artery doppler ultrasonography as a screening tool. In: Pearce J M (ed) Doppler ultrasound in perinatal medicine. Oxford University Press, Oxford

Driscoll S G 1969 Histopathology of gestational rubella. American Journal of Diseases of Children 118: 49–53

Edwards L E, Alton I R, Barrada M I, Hakanson E Y 1979 Pregnancy in underweight women. American Journal of Obstetrics and Gynecology 135: 297–301

Eik-Nes S H, Okland O, Aure J C, Ulstein M 1984 Ultrasound screening in pregnancy: a randomised controlled trial. Lancet i: 1347

Elder M G, de Swiet M, Robertson A et al 1988 Low dose aspirin in pregnancy. Lancet ii: 410

Ferrazzie E, Nicoloni U, Kustermann A, Pardi G 1986 Routine obstetric ultrasound; effectiveness of cross sectional screening for fetal growth retardation. Journal of Clinical Ultrasound 1986; 14: 17–22

Gardosi J et al 1992 Customised antenatal growth charts Lancet 339: 283–287

Geirsson R T, Persson P 1984 Diagnosis of IUGR using ultrasound. Clinical Obstetrics and Gynecology 11: 457–480

Goldenberg R L et al 1989a Intrauterine growth retardation: standards for diagnosis. American Journal of Obstetrics and Gynecology 1989; 161: 271–277

Goldenberg R L et al 1989b Prematurity, postdates and growth retardation; the influence of the use of ultrasonography on reported gestational age. American Journal of Obstetrics and Gynecology 160: 462–470

Hall M A 1990 Identification of high risk and low risk. Antenatal care. Clinical Obstetrics and Gynecology 1990; 4: 65–76

Hall M H, Carr-Hill R A 1985 The significance of uncertain gestation on obstetric outcome. British Journal of Obstetrics and Gynaecology 1985; 92: 452–460

Hanretty K P, Primrose M H, Neilson J P, Whittle M J 1989 Pregnancy screening by doppler uteroplacental and umbilical artery waveforms. British Journal of Obstetrics and Gynaecology 1989; 96: 1163–1167

Herriott A, Billewicz W, Hytten F E 1962 Cigarette smoking and pregnancy. Lancet i: 771–773

Hingson R, Alpert J J, Day N et al 1982 Effects of maternal drinking and mari juanna use on fetal growth and development. Paediatrics 70: 539–546

Hughey M J 1984 Routine ultrasound for the detection and management of small for gestational age fetus. Obstetrics and Gynecology 64: 101–107

Hytten F E 1982 Nutritional physiology during pregnancy. In: Campbell D M, Gillmer M D G (eds) Nutrition in pregnancy. Proceedings of the tenth study group of the RCOG. RCOG, London

Italian Study of Aspirin in Pregnancy 1993 Low dose aspirin in the prevention and treatment of intrauterine growth retardation and pregnancy induced hypertension. Lancet 341: 396–400

Jacobson S-L, Imhof R, Manning N et al 1990 The value of doppler assessment of the uteroplacental circulation in predicting pre-eclampsia and intrauterine growth retardation. American Journal of Obstetrics and Gynecology 162: 110–114

Kierse M J N C 1981 Aetiology of intrauterine growth retardation. In: Van Assche F A, Robertson W B (eds) Fetal growth retardation. Churchill Livingstone, London

Kierse M 1984 Epidemiology and aetiology of the growth retarded baby. Clinics in Obstetrics and Gynecology 11: 457–480

Kelly J, Mathews K A, O'Connor M 1984 Smoking in pregnancy: effects on mother and fetus. British Journal of Obstetrics and Gynaecology 91: 111–117

Larsen T, Larsen J F, Peterson S, Greison G 1992 Detection of small for gestational age fetuses by ultrasound screening in a high risk population; a randomised controlled study. British Journal of Obstetrics and Gynaecology 1992; 99: 469–474

Le Fevre M L, Bain R P, Ewigman B G et al 1993 A randomised trial of prenatal ultrasonographic screening: impact on maternal management and outcome. American Journal of Obstetrics and Gynecology 169: 483–489

Lindhard A, Nielsen P V, Mouritsen L A. Zachariassen A, Sorensen H U, Roseno H 1990 The implications of introducing symphsis fundal height measurement. A prospective randomised controlled study. British Journal of Obstetrics and Gynaecology 97: 675–680

Little R 1977 Moderate alcohol intake in pregnancy and decreased infant birthweight. American Journal of Public Health 67: 1154–1156

Loeffler F E 1967 Clinical foetal weight prediction. Journal of Obstetrics and Gynaecology of the British Commonwealth 74: 675–677

Mathai M, Jairaj P, Mulhuratham J 1987 Screening for light for dates gestational infants: a comparison of three simple measurements. British Journal of Obstetrics and Gynaecology 94: 217–221

McFarland P, Steel S A, Pearce J M 1991 The clinical implications of absent or reversed end-diastolic frequencies in the umbilical artery flow velocity waveform. European Journal of Obstetrics and Gynaecology 37: 15–23

McKeown T, Record R G 1952 Observations on foetal growth in multiple pregnancy in man. Journal of Endocrinology 8: 386–401

Mohide P, Keirse M J N C 1989 Biophysical assessment of fetal wellbeing. In: Enkin M, Keirse M J N C, Chalmers I (eds) Effective care in pregnancy and childbirth. Oxford University Press, Oxford

Morrow R, Adamson L, Ritchie K, Pearce M 1992 The pathophysiological basis of abnormal flow velocity waveforms. In: Pearce M J (ed) Doppler ultrasound in perinatal medicine. Oxford University, Oxford

Murphy J F 1984 The effects of maternal smoking on the unborn child. In: Studd J (ed) Progress in obstetrics and gynaecology. Churchill Livingstone, Edinburgh

Murphy J F, Drumm J E, Mulcahy R, Daly L 1980 The effect of maternal smoking on fetal birthweight and on the growth of the fetal biparietal diameter. British Journal of Obstetrics and Gynaecology 1980; 87: 462–466

Neilson J P, Whitfield C R, Aitchison T C 1980 Screening for the small-for-dates fetus: a two stage ultrasound examination schedule. British Medical Journal 1980; 2280: 1203–1206

Neilson J P, Munjanja S P, Whitfield C R 1984 Screening for small for dates fetus: a controlled trial. British Medical Journal 1984; 289: 1179–1182

Neilson J, Grant A 1989 Ultrasound in pregnancy. In: Enkin M, Keirse M J N C, Chalmers I (eds) Effective care in pregnancy and childbirth. Oxford University Press, Oxford

Newnham J P, Lyn L, Patterson R N, James I R, Diepveen D A, Reid S A 1990 An evaluation of the efficacy of doppler flow velocity wave form analysis as a screening test in pregnancy. American Journal of Obstetrics and Gynecology 162: 403–410

Nicolaides K, Bilardo C M, Soothill P W, Campbell S 1988 Absence of end-diastolic frequencies in the umbilical artery a sign of fetal hypoxia and acidosis. British Medical Journal 1988; 297: 1026–1027

Nicolaides K, Shawwa L, Brizot M, Snijders R 1983 Ultrasonographically detectable markers of chromosomal defects. Ultrasound in Obstetrics and Gynaecology 1993; 3: 560–569

Quaranta P, Currell R, Redman C W G, Robinson J S 1981 Prediction of small for dates infants by measurements of symphyseal fundal height. British Journal of Obstetrics and Gynaecology 88: 115–119

Pearce J M 1993 The scientific basis for antenatal fetal monitoring. In: Spencer J A D, Ward R H T (eds) Intrapartum fetal surveillance. RCOG, London, pp 69–76

Pearce J M, Campbell S 1987 A comparison of symphysis fundal height and ultrasound as screening tests for light for gestational age infants. British Journal of Obstetrics and Gynaecology 94: 100–104

Persson B, Stangenberg M, Lunell N O, Broden U, Holmberg N G, Vaclavinkova V 1986 Prediction of size of infants at birth by

measurement of symphysis fundal height. British Journal of Obstetrics and Gynecology 93: 206–211

Robertson P A, Sniderman M D, Laros R K et al 1992 Neonatal morbidity according to gestational age and birthweight from five tertiary care centres in the United States 1983 through 1986. American Journal of Obstetrics and Gynecology 166: 1629–1645

Rosenberg K, Grant J M, Hepburn M 1982 Antenatal detection of growth retardation; actual practice in a large maternity hospital. British Journal of Obstetrics and Gynaecology 98: 12–15

Schulman H, Winter D, Farmakides G et al 1989 Pregnancy surveillance with doppler velocimetry of uterine and umbilical arteries. American Journal of Obstetrics and Gynecology 160: 192–196

Secher N J, Hansen P K, Lenstrup C, Eriksen P S 1986 Controlled trial of ultrasound for light for gestational age infants in late pregnancy. European Journal of Obstetrics and Gynaecology 23: 307–313

Sheppard B L, Bonnard J 1976 The ultrastructure of the human placenta in pregnancy complicated by fetal growth retardation. British Journal of Obstetrics and Gynaecology 83: 948–959

Sijmons E A, Reuwer P J H M, van Beek E, Bruinse H W 1989 The validity of screening for small for gestational age and low birth weight infants by doppler ultrasound. British Journal of Obstetrics and Gynaecology 96: 192–196

Sibai B 1993 American Journal of Obstetrics and Gynecology 168: 286

Snijders R J M, Sherrod C, Gosden C M, Nicolaides K H 1983 Fetal growth retardation: associated malformations and chromosomal abnormalities. American Journal of Obstetrics and Gynecology 168: 547–555

Steel S A, Pearce J M, Chamberlain G V 1988 Doppler ultrasound of the uteroplacental circulation as a screening test for severe pre-eclampsia with intrauterine growth retardation. European Journal of Obstetrics Gynaecology and Reproductive Biology 28: 279–287

Steer P J 1992 Customised antenatal growth charts. Lancet 339: 878

Thompson A M, Billewicz W Z, Hytten F E 1968 The assessment of fetal growth. Journal of Obstetrics and Gynaecology of the British Commonwealth 75: 903–916

Trudinger B J, Cook C M, Thompson R S et al 1988 Low dose aspirin therapy improves fetal weight in umbilical placental insufficiency. American Journal of Obstetrics and Gynecology 159: 681–685

Van Assche F A, Robertson W B (eds) 1981 Fetal growth retardation. Churchill Livingstone, London

Van der Spuy Z M 1988 Outcome of pregnancy in underweight women after spontaneous and induced ovulation. British Medical Journal 296: 962–965

Waldenstrom U, Axelsson O, Nilsson S et al 1988 Effects of routine one stage ultrasound screening in pregnancy: a randomised controlled trial. Lancet ii: 585–588

Wallenberg H C S, Rotmans N 1987 Prevention of recurrent idiopathic fetal growth retardation by low dose aspirin and dipyridamole. American Journal of Obstetrics and Gynecology 157: 1230–1235

Wallin A, Gyllensward A, Westin B 1981 Symphysis–fundus measurement in the prediction of fetal growth disturbances. Acta Obstetricia et Gynecologica Scandinavica 60: 310–323

Warsof S L, Cooper D J, Little D, Campbell S 1986 Routine ultrasound screening for antenatal detection intrauterine growth retardation. Obstetrics and Gynecology 67: 33–39

Wladimiroff J W, Laar J 1980 Ultrasonic measurements of fetal body size; a randomized controlled trial. Acta Obstetrica Gynaecologica Scandinavica 59: 177–179

Wright J, Waterson E J, Barrison I G et al 1983 Alcohol consumption, pregnancy and low birth weight. Lancet i: 663–665

18. Bleeding in pregnancy

S. Leonard Barron

Material in this chapter contains contributions from the first edition and we are grateful to the previous author for the work done.

INTRODUCTION

It has always been the custom to separate the management of bleeding in early pregnancy, associated with the process of miscarriage, from that in late pregnancy where treatment must take account of the interests of the fetus. Over the past decade, our perceptions of the second trimester of pregnancy have been changed by the advances in imaging and by the greatly improved survival of very preterm infants. As a result, the distinction between early and late pregnancy bleeding has become blurred. The diagnosis and management of spontaneous abortion is still considered to a be a gynaecological problem and for an account of that subject, the reader is referred to Chapter 15 in the Companion Volume *Gynaecology* (Edmunds 1992).

A survey of all births in Britain in 1970 found that there was a history of bleeding in one in 10 of all pregnancies (Chamberlain et al 1978). The bleeding varied from a small episode before 28 weeks (4.2%) to placenta praevia (0.5%; Table 18.1). In practice, it is often difficult to allocate cases to simple diagnostic categories, such as premature separation of placenta or placenta praevia, and there is little doubt that small episodes of bleeding often go unreported.

The placenta contains, within the intervillous space, about 700 ml of maternal blood which reaches it via the uterine and ovarian arteries. The open arterioles discharge into the choriodecidual space, which depends for its integrity only on the adherence of the placenta to the maternal decidua. This normally remains intact until after delivery of the fetus, so long as the placenta is inserted into the upper segment of the uterus. Effacement and dilatation of the cervix cause separation from the chorion, from its attachment to the myometrium, sometimes producing a small amount of bleeding (a show). If, however, the placenta is inserted either wholly or partly into the lower segment (placenta praevia) bleeding not only becomes inevitable but may be very heavy.

When bleeding occurs from a normally sited placenta, separation from the decidual bed may lead to a cycle of massive haemorrhage and further separation (placental abruption). The fetus is deprived of placental function and the uterine muscle is suffused with extravasated blood—the Couvelaire uterus (Speert 1957). Such separation is not always catastrophic and the bleeding may be trivial. Nevertheless, the perinatal mortality following even minor episodes of antepartum haemorrhage (APH) is about double that in women without a history of such bleeding (Table 18.1).

Fetal blood in the placenta circulates within the capillaries of the villi and is separated from maternal blood in the intervillous space by the capillary wall and trophoblast. In vasa praevia a placental blood vessel lies in front of the presenting part of the fetus, usually because of anatomical variation such as velamentous insertion of the cord. Rupture of the vessel causes not only vaginal bleeding, but also exsanguination of the fetus.

Table 18.1 Bleeding in pregnancy: frequency and perinatal mortality

Type of bleeding	Incidence (%)	Perinatal mortality rate (per 1000 births)
None	88.7	16.8
Placenta praevia	0.5	81.4
Accidental APH	1.2	143.6
Bleeding < 28 weeks	4.2	61.0
Other specified cause	2.2	39.7
Unspecified	2.4	32.6
No information	0.8	30.3
Total in survey	17005 (100%)	21.4

From Chamberlain et al (1978).
APH = antepartum haemorrhage.

Finally, there are causes of bleeding which are best described as incidental APH because they are unrelated to the placenta. Polyps or carcinoma of the cervix may cause bleeding, especially following coitus, or bleeding can occur from varicosities of the vulva.

Nomenclature

Students of all ages are understandably confused by the term accidental APH, which is sometimes used as a synonym for abruption. The expression dates from the 19th century when obstetricians distinguished unavoidable bleeding due to placental presentation from inadvertent or accidental bleeding (Kerr et al 1954); this had nothing to do with the present-day association of the word accidental with trauma. Abruptio placentae, also called ablatio placentae, indicates that the placenta has separated from its implantation in the uterine wall before delivery of the fetus. In the UK it is usual to use the anglicized version *placental abruption*.

Timing

Until about 15 years ago, APH was defined simply as bleeding from the genital tract after the 28th week of pregnancy and before labour; however, two major advances have changed our understanding and management of bleeding in late pregnancy. The first is the contribution of diagnostic ultrasound which has enabled the placental site to be identified in early pregnancy before the appearance of symptoms. The second advance has been in the paediatric care of very low birthweight infants so that even infants born as early as 24 weeks' gestation now have a good chance of survival. The old legal assumption of 'viability' became outdated and under the Stillbirth (Definition) Act of 1992, stillbirths are now registered in Britain from 24 weeks instead of 28 weeks. The effect of the change is far reaching and pregnancy bleeding is now seen to be a continuum rather than two separate entities split by the perceived date of viability. It therefore seems reasonable that 24 weeks should also form the new boundary between the definition of APH and bleeding of early pregnancy. Britain did not adopt the recommendation of The International Federation of Gynaecology and Obstetrics (FIGO) that perinatal death statistics should include any fetus born after 22 weeks or weighing 500 g or more.

World Health Organization (WHO) rubrics

The International Classification of Diseases (ICD, ninth revision, World Health Organization 1977) recognizes premature separation of placenta (641.2), other APH (641.8) and unspecified APH (641.9). The term acciden-

tal haemorrhage is so well established that it is unlikely to disappear, but it is tolerable only if its meaning is defined. The following nomenclature (with the appropriate ICD code) is therefore suggested as a way of resolving the confusion:

Incidental APH (ICD 641.1)
Placenta praevia
    with haemorrhage (ICD 641.1)
    without haemorrhage (ICD 641.0)
    vasa praevia (ICD 663.5)
Accidental APH
    abruption (ICD 641.2)
    unspecified APH (ICD 641.9)

The radically revised 10th version of ICD (ICD10) (World Health Organization 1992) is due to be introduced in 1995. The nomenclature will change and the term 'accidental haemorrhage' disappears.

(ICD10 O20) Haemorrhage in early pregnancy:
- O44.   Placenta praevia
  - O44.0 Placenta praevia without haemorrhage
  - O44.1 Placenta praevia with haemorrhage
- O45.   Premature separation of placenta (abruptio placentae)
  - O45.0 Premature separation of placenta with coagulation defect
  - O45.8 Other separation of placenta
  - O45.9 Premature separation of placenta, unspecified.
- O46.   Antepartum haemorrhage, not elsewhere classified
  - O46.0 Antepartum haemorrhage with coagulation defect
  - O46.8 Other antepartum haemorrhage
  - O46.9 Antepartum haemorrhage, unspecified.

BLEEDING IN THE SECOND TRIMESTER

As the demarcation between APH and earlier pregnancy bleeding has evaporated, there has been a keener interest in the effect of bleeding in the second trimester. Several authors report that bleeding during early pregnancy is associated with an increased incidence of later abruption. Eriksen et al (1991) found that early bleeding occurred in 10% of patients with abruption, compared with only 3% in controls. Nielson et al (1991) identified 101 patients admitted with bleeding in the second trimester, in Utah, USA, of whom 40 proved later to have had abruption with a fetal loss of 15 (37%). Another 27 had placenta praevia and only two babies were lost (7.4%). There were 11 patients who appeared to have both praevia and abruption (fetal mortality 18.2%) and 23 for whom no cause was identified (17.4% fetal loss). Another study by Lipitz et al (1991) looked at the outcome of women admitted to hospital in Israel with bleeding between 14 and 26 weeks' gestation. Out of the 65 women, 39 went to term and 18 delivered before 26 weeks. The overall fetal loss rate was 31.8%. The factors, identified by discriminant analysis, which were associated with poor outcome were bleeding sufficient to reduce the haemoglobin by 1% or more and the presence of a previous uterine scar.

The findings confirm that second trimester bleeding carries a poor fetal prognosis

PLACENTA PRAEVIA

Definitions

The placenta is partly or wholly inserted in the lower uterine segment and the condition has traditionally been divided into four numbered grades I–IV (Fig. 18.1). With modern management it is more usual to describe only three degrees of severity, lateral, marginal and complete, since there is little point in distinguishing grade III from IV.

Grade I (lateral placenta praevia): the placenta just encroaches on the lower uterine segment.
Grade II (marginal placenta praevia): the placenta reaches the margin of the cervical os.
Grade III (complete placenta praevia): the placenta covers part of the os.
Grade IV (complete placenta praevia): the placenta is centrally placed in the lower uterine segment.

The routine use of ultrasound has revealed that the relationship between the placental site and the lower segment can change as pregnancy progresses, so that the placenta appears to migrate up the uterus. For this reason there is a tendency to overdiagnose grade I placenta praevia. The use of ultrasound also increases the likelihood of diagnosing asymptomatic placenta praevia, before there has been any bleeding (ICD 641.0).

Incidence

Estimates of incidence based on a defined population are hard to find. One source of error is the practice of many

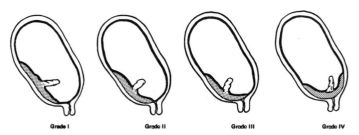

Fig. 18.1 The four grades of placenta praevia (see text for explanations).

Table 18.2 The incidence of placenta praevia in relation to maternal age and parity (rates are per 100 pregnancies)

Reference	Maternal age				
	< 20	20–24	25–29	30–34	35+
Chamberlain et al (1978)	0.1	0.3	0.5	0.6	1.5
Paintin (1962)	0.1	0.2	0.4	⊢—— 0.7 ——⊣	
Clark et al (1985)	0.1	0.2	0.3	0.4	0.9
Naeye (1980)					
Non-smokers	0.2	⊢—— 0.4 ——⊣		⊢—— 0.8 ——⊣	
Smokers	0.3	⊢—— 0.7 ——⊣		⊢—— 1.8 ——⊣	

	Pregnancy number			
	1	2	3–4	5+
Naeye (1980)				
Non-smokers	1.5	1.8	1.7	1.8
Smokers	1.8	1.9	2.2	2.9
Paintin (1962)	0.3	0.3	⊢—— 0.7 ——⊣	
Clark et al (1985)	0.1	0.2	0.4	0.6
Chamberlain et al (1978)	1.1	⊢—— 1.4 ——⊣		1.7

American authors of using 20 weeks as the lower limit of APH and rejecting as irrelevant cases of placenta praevia delivered vaginally. Nevertheless, there is reasonable agreement that placenta praevia occurs in between 0.4% and 0.8% of pregnancies. The incidence of placenta praevia by maternal age and parity is summarized in Table 18.2.

Aetiology

The placenta develops as a discoid condensation of trophoblast on the surface of the chorion at about 8–10 weeks' gestation; the position is determined by the site of implantation (Hamilton & Mossman 1972). Routine ultrasound examination in pregnancy has provided interesting information on the changing anatomical relationship of placental site to the cervix as the uterus enlarges. Low implantation has been observed in 5–28% of pregnancies during the second trimester, but as the uterus grows, the placental site appears to migrate upwards and by term only 3% are praevia. It is possible that the observed migration is due in part to differential development of the placenta, possibly affected by previous scarring or changes in vascularization. There is evidence for this from the observation that the umbilical cord in placenta praevia frequently has a marginal insertion (Hibbard 1986). Adherence to a lower segment scar may also explain the increased incidence of placenta praevia following a previous Caesarean section.

Increased surface area

It is generally accepted that conditions in which the area of the placenta is increased, such as twins, succenturiate lobe and placenta membranacea, have an increased incidence of placenta praevia, but there is little published evidence on the subject apart from the association with placenta extrachorialis (Scott 1960).

Age, parity and previous Caesarean section

The increased incidence of placenta praevia with age and parity is shown in Table 18.2. The relationship between parity and placenta praevia was also found to be true in cases of low implantation diagnosed in the second trimester but which did not prove to be praevia at term (Newton et al 1984). In a study of 147 cases of major placenta praevia, McShane et al (1985) found that 22 (15%) had had a previous Caesarean section. In their study of 97 799 deliveries, Clark et al (1985) found that the incidence of placenta praevia in those who had not had previous Caesarean section was 0.25%; in those with one scar it was 0.65% and with three or more Caesarean section scars it was 2.2% (Table 18.3).

Other gynaecological surgery

It has been suggested that an induced abortion increases the risk of placenta praevia in a subsequent pregnancy, but the studies of Grimes & Techman (1984) and of Newton et al (1984) showed no evidence of such an association. Rose & Chapman (1986) compared the gynaecological history of 80 women with placenta praevia with controls who were matched for age and parity. As well as confirming the association with parity and a history of previous Caesarean section, they also found a significant relation to a history of dilatation and curettage, a less significant relation to evacuation of retained products of conception, but no relation to a previous induced abortion. They concluded that endometrial damage was a factor in the aetiology of placenta praevia.

Cigarette smoking

In a paper based on the large US collaborative study, Naeye (1980) showed that placenta praevia was more frequent in mothers who smoked during pregnancy than those who did not, or who had already stopped smoking. The relationship was not as strong as with placental abruption (Table 18.2) but the finding is difficult to explain.

Association with placenta accreta

Not only does the risk of placenta praevia increase with

Table 18.3 Placenta praevia, placenta accreta and previous Caesarean section

No. of Caesarean sections	Patients (no.)	Placenta praevia		Placenta accreta	
		No.	%	No.	%
0	92 917	238	0.26	12	5
1	3 820	25	0.65	6	24
2	850	15	1.8	7	47
3	183	5	3.0	2	40

From Clark et al (1985).

the number of previous Caesarean sections, but so does the likelihood of placenta accreta (Table 18.3). McShane et al (1985) also reported that of the 22 women in their series with a previous Caesarean section scar, six (27%) of them had placenta accreta.

Clinical aspects

Signs and symptoms

The characteristic feature of placenta praevia is painless bleeding, usually in the third trimester. As pregnancy advances, Braxton Hicks contractions cause the lower segment to thin and in multiparae there is often some dilatation of the cervix. As a result, the abnormally inserted placenta separates from the decidua and bleeding results from the exposed uterine blood vessels. The bleeding is usually unprovoked, although there is sometimes a history of coitus just before. Commonly, the woman wakes because she feels wet and is then alarmed to discover that she has been bleeding. Sometimes there is a history of bleeding in the second trimester, but fortunately, the first episode of bleeding is often minor. Since the lower uterine segment has poor contractility, the bleeding from placenta praevia can be very severe and although it is unusual for it to be so before the 34th week of pregnancy, the exceptions that do occur amply justify hospital admission even for apparently trivial episodes of bleeding. The most catastrophic cases of haemorrhage from placenta praevia occur from ill-advised attempts at vaginal examination.

With routine ultrasound scanning in early pregnancy, most cases of placenta praevia are suspected before there has been any bleeding; indeed, there may be a problem of overdiagnosis and the unnecessary anxiety that it provokes.

Diagnosis

In placenta praevia, the abdomen is soft with no tenderness. The presenting part should be easily felt and the fetal heart unaffected. The low placenta acts as a pelvic tumour, and displaces the presenting part, with a high incidence of malpresentation (Hibbard 1986). In some cases, the condition is suspected because of an unstable lie even before there has been any bleeding. A deeply engaged presenting part is strong evidence that the praevia is of minor degree.

Vaginal examination in a case of placenta praevia may provoke serious bleeding and should therefore only be undertaken in an operating theatre with everything ready for an immediate Caesarean section.

The diagnosis can be particularly difficult when the episode of bleeding occurs with the onset of labour, and there is a grade I praevia. In these circumstances, the presenting part is engaged and the presence of labour contractions obscures the abdominal palpation.

There is some justification for passing a vaginal speculum where there is a suspicion that the bleeding is coming from a local lesion of the vagina or cervix, but this can usually wait until more serious causes have been eliminated. The other reason for inserting a speculum would be to collect a blood sample to test for fetal haemoglobin. Bleeding from vasa praevia is a rare cause of APH but unless it is recognized and the baby delivered by immediate Caesarean section, fetal exsanguination will occur.

Placental localization

Ultrasonography has overtaken other methods of placental localization because of its convenience, safety and accuracy. It is the practice in many British and European obstetric units to offer routine ultrasound scanning at about 16 weeks' gestation. Doubts have been expressed about the wisdom of routine scanning, partly on the grounds that ultrasound has not been proven to be absolutely safe to the fetus, but also (and perhaps more cogently) on the grounds that routine scanning raises false fears which may lead to unnecessary obstetric intervention. This criticism applies particularly to the diagnosis of placenta praevia and the condition should not be diagnosed on the basis of a single observation in the second trimester.

Chapman et al (1979) found a low-lying placenta in 28% of women who were scanned routinely before 24 weeks' gestation; by 24 weeks the incidence had fallen to 18% and by term it was 3%. The apparent change in position is due to formation of the lower segment and the enlargement upwards of the upper uterine segment. There may also be technical errors when the lower margin of the placenta is difficult to define because the bladder is not adequately filled.

Real-time scanners can produce high-quality images (Fig. 18.2) and it is now possible, because of the reduction in size of the equipment, to carry out ultrasound

Table 18.4 Prediction of placenta praevia from early ultrasound scans: results of 632 scans in 503 women

Gestation (weeks)	Praevia at first scan	Significant bleeding or praevia at term	
		No.	%
10–14	65	2	3.1
15–19	157	3	1.9
20–24	125	4	3.2
25–29	97	5	5.2
30–34	46	11	23.9
35–term	13	3	23.1
Total	503	28	5.6

From Comeau et al (1983).

scanning within the delivery room. In early pregnancy, although the placenta can be visualized without difficulty, the diagnosis of placenta praevia cannot be made with confidence, for the reasons given above. The later in pregnancy the scan is performed, the more accurate the prediction (Table 18.4). Of 222 cases of placenta praevia predicted by scan before 20 weeks, only five (2.2%) had significant bleeding or placenta praevia at term (Comeau et al 1983).

Once bleeding has occurred, diagnosis by ultrasound is difficult because of the resemblance of placenta to blood clot and the indistinct appearance of the cervical os. This is particularly true close to term and in such circumstances clinical examination under controlled conditions as described may be necessary.

Radioisotope placentography is an acceptable alternative when sonar is not available or unsatisfactory. The method uses an intravenous injection of ^{99m}Tc bound to red blood cells or radioactive albumin bound to ^{132}I. These substances remain within the vascular compartment and the very vascular placental bed shows up as an area of high radioactivity. By means of a Picker scanner, the area can be pictured as a coloured print-out which delineates the placenta, but of course does not show the site of the fetus or the lower uterine segment (Robertson et al 1968). The isotopes used are considered safe for use in pregnancy because of their short half-life; the procedure itself involves only minimal discomfort to the mother.

Soft-tissue radiography. Although largely eclipsed by ultrasound, X-rays are still used when ultrasound is not available. A lateral film of the lower abdomen is taken with low voltage X-rays. This shows up the lower margin of the placenta by distinguishing it from uterine muscle. If the head presents, then the internal limit of the placenta may also be seen. When the placenta is on the posterior wall, it is more difficult to define because of the overlying bony pelvis and muscle mass, but it may be demonstrated by its ability to displace the presenting part forwards when the patient is X-rayed in a sitting position.

Pelvic angiography involves the injection of a radiopaque medium into the femoral artery after retrograde catheterization with the catheter tip at the bifurcation of the

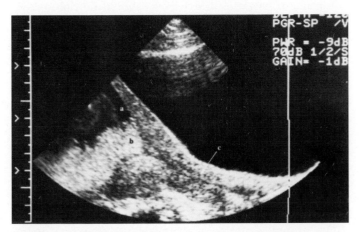

Fig. 18.2 Real-time ultrasonograph showing the edge of placenta overlying the cervical canal. a = liquor; b = edge of placenta; c = cervical canal. Reproduced by kind permission of Dr P. G. Rose.

aorta. It gives a good and reliable picture of the placental site but the procedure is uncomfortable, especially the intra-arterial injection, and carries some risk; it is therefore not used where easier and less invasive methods are available.

Magnetic resonance imaging (MRI). This is a relatively new and expensive method of tissue imaging which is now available in most large centres. When a very powerful magnetic field is passed through the body, the hydrogen atoms become polarized and the H$^+$ ions are aligned. The protons (the hydrogen atom nuclei) are displaced by radio pulses and in returning to their basal state, give out a small radio signal. A series of images can be built up from the proton density maps of a section of the body. The sections may be at any plane of the body and no ionizing radiation is used.

At present, the tissues need to be immobile for some seconds while the imaging is performed; hence clear fetal images are difficult to produce but localization of the placenta is excellent since both the placental edge and the cervical canal can by readily identified (Powell et al 1986). This may become the most precise method of diagnosing placenta praevia in the future.

Clinical management. Most patients with placenta praevia appear with a history of painless APH; there may have been more than one warning show of blood but insufficient to have alarmed the patient. The priority is to assess and deal with the blood loss and arrange for an adequate supply of blood should transfusion become necessary.

Where routine ultrasound is done in early pregnancy, the diagnosis should be easy and further localization of the placenta is not necessary. Only in cases of serious haemorrhage is it necessary to make an immediate diagnosis; the important point is to distinguish placenta praevia from vasa praevia and placental abruption. In such circumstances, ultrasound, if available, may be very helpful.

Expectant management

Unless the bleeding is severe there is much to be gained by expectant management, with the aim of making a correct diagnosis and postponing delivery until about 37 weeks. The benefits of conservative management and the history of its introduction have been well reviewed by Myerscough (1982). The advantage of adequate transfusion is self-evident, but the advantages of avoiding premature delivery to the baby are perhaps less than they used to be, thanks to the improvements in neonatal paediatrics.

Use of tocolytics

When bleeding is complicated by premature labour, it would seem logical to inhibit uterine activity by means of tocolytic agents. Sampson et al (1984) reported the

benefits from an intravenous infusion of terbutaline sulphate, starting with a bolus of 0.25 mg and continuing with 10 µg/min. Silver et al (1984) also advocated aggressive conservatism, which included the use of blood transfusion and tocolytics (type unstated) in all cases of placenta praevia after 21 weeks' gestation. They claimed that by postponing delivery in most cases they achieved a low perinatal mortality rate of 42/1000.

The danger of using tocolytic agents is that they produce tachycardia and palpitations, neither of which are desirable in someone already suffering from hypovolaemia. Furthermore, since they are contraindicated in placental abruption, the diagnosis of placenta praevia must be secure.

Vasa praevia is difficult to diagnose, but must always be borne in mind, particularly where the clinical picture is unusual. The diagnosis is made by testing the vaginal blood for fetal haemoglobin using the alkaline denaturation test or by examining the blood microscopically for the presence of nucleated red cells.

Vaginal delivery

There is no point in postponing delivery beyond 37 weeks' gestation except in women with minor degrees of placenta praevia in whom the placenta is anterior and the head engaged. Such a situation may not be apparent until labour starts or an attempt is made to rupture the membranes. In such circumstances, the bleeding is usually controlled by amniotomy augmented by Syntocinon infusion.

Examination under anaesthesia and amniotomy

The procedure should only be carried out under anaesthesia in an operating theatre, with everything prepared for an immediate transfusion and Caesarean section, should the examination provoke heavy bleeding. The instruments are laid out and the nursing staff scrubbed. The stage of gestation for delivery should be right; there is no point in carrying out an examination when conservative management would be more appropriate. It is a mistake to hurry the examination and it should be performed with the patient in the lithotomy position and using sterile drapes. After catheterizing the bladder, two fingers are introduced into the vagina, avoiding the cervical os. Each vaginal fornix is palpated in turn, the object being to feel whether there is a placenta between the presenting head and the finger. If the four fornices are empty, then a finger can be introduced into the cervical os. If the cervical os is tightly closed and there is significant bleeding it is unwise to use force to dilate the cervix; instead a Caesarean section should be performed.

The presence of clot often makes it difficult to define the edge of the placenta, but if the membranes can be identified then a forewater amniotomy is carried out.

Heavily blood-stained liquor is suspicious of an abruption, but if the bleeding is separate from the liquor and it does not stop within a few minutes, it is best to proceed to Caesarean section.

Examination under anaesthesia is also justified where clinical or ultrasound evidence suggests an anterior grade I placenta praevia. Vaginal delivery is therefore possible and amniotomy may be all that is necessary. Once the membranes are ruptured and the uterus is contracting, the presenting part compresses the lateral edge of the placenta and arrests the bleeding.

Caesarean section

With the exception already mentioned, delivery by Caesarean section is the method of choice for most women with any severe degree of placenta praevia; the operation however can be hazardous. When the placenta is anterior the lower segment can be very vascular with huge veins coursing across the potential site of incision. Once the lower segment has been opened, the placenta must either be incised or separated in order to reach the baby. Each method has its problems. Incising the placenta may be speedy, but dividing fetal vessels can cause fetal exsanguination. On the other hand, separating the placenta may be difficult especially if it is adherent. Once placental separation has been started, the fetus is deprived of maternal oxygen and delivery becomes urgent. Further difficulty can arise if there is a transverse lie and this is one of the few occasions in which it may be prudent to resort to an upper segment incision. An alternative to the classical incision is to convert the transverse lower segment incision into an inverted T, an approach which many obstetricians consider does not heal well, although there is no published evidence on this.

Much will depend on the exact circumstances, but the author's preference is for a lower segment approach, under-running the large vessels with a catgut suture before dividing them. The anterior placenta is then separated with the finger until the edge is reached and the amniotic sac can be opened. If necessary the incision is extended into an inverted T.

Placenta accreta is a serious complication of placenta praevia, leading to uncontrollable bleeding. It is particularly liable to be present in association with anterior placenta praevia in a woman who has had one or more Caesarean sections (Clark et al 1985) and hysterectomy may be necessary. It is one of the reasons why Caesarean section for placenta praevia should always be carried out under the supervision of an experienced obstetrician. It is not an operation for the tyro.

Maternal mortality

The dramatic fall in maternal mortality from APH since

Table 18.5 Maternal and fetal mortality in placenta praevia before and after introduction of conservative management in Belfast

Year	No. of cases	Maternal mortality (%)	Caesarean section(%)	Fetal mortality (%)
1932–1936	76	2.6	—	51
1937–1944	174	0.6	31	24
1945–1952	206	0.0	68	15

From Macafee (1945) and Macafee et al (1962).

the beginning of the century is partly due to the availability of blood transfusion and improved understanding of coagulation failure, but there have also been important changes in management. In placenta praevia, the outlook for mother and child were greatly improved by the introduction of conservative management, pioneered in Belfast and rapidly adopted elsewhere. An expectant regimen was used, with bed rest, blood transfusion and more liberal use of Caesarean section (Macafee et al 1962). The effects of this change in policy on maternal and fetal mortality are shown in Table 18.5.

Perinatal mortality

The fetal outlook following placenta praevia is more favourable than in placental abruption and has continued to improve over the past 50 years (Macafee et al 1962, Crenshaw et al 1973). In 1980, Cotton et al reported a perinatal mortality rate of 126/1000 total births, which is little different from that of Paintin (1962). There have, however, been two reports from the USA that the perinatal mortality rate has been reduced by a more active approach, with rates of 81/1000 (McShane et al 1985) and 42/1000. Scotland, with its system for detailed recording of every pregnancy in the country, provides excellent epidemiological data. During the two years 1984 and 1985, there were 800 cases of placenta praevia with 19 perinatal deaths—a mortality of only 24/1000 (Scottish Health Service, personal communication). Unlike placental abruption, placenta praevia does not cause intrauterine hypoxia and premature delivery is the greatest cause of morbidity and mortality.

PLACENTAL ABRUPTION

Incidence

In the British Births study (Chamberlain et al 1978), placental abruption occurred in about 1% of pregnancies, in close agreement with other reports from the UK. Table 18.6 shows a good deal of variation in the recorded incidence, probably due to differences in definition and accuracy of diagnosis.

There is no agreement if the condition is more common with increasing age and parity. Although Naeye (1980)

Table 18.6 The incidence of placental abruption in relation to maternal age and parity (rates per 100 pregnancies)

Reference	Maternal age				
	< 20	20–24	25–29	30–34	35+
Hibbard & Hibbard (1963)	0.85	0.9	1.1	1.2	1.7
Chamberlain et al (1978)	1.4	1.2	1.0	1.2	1.8
Paintin (1962)	0.9	0.7	0.7	⊢——— 0.8 ———⊣	
Naeye (1980)					
Non-smokers	1.3	⊢——— 1.7 ———⊣		⊢——— 2.3 ———⊣	
Smokers	1.6	⊢——— 2.1 ———⊣		⊢——— 3.3 ———⊣	

	Pregnancy number			
	1	2	3–4	5+
Naeye (1980)				
Non-smokers	1.5	1.8	1.7	1.8
Smokers	1.8	1.9	2.2	2.9
Paintin (1962)	0.7	0.6	0.9	0.9
Hibbard & Hibbard (1963)	0.8	⊢——— 1.0 ———⊣		2.3
Chamberlain et al (1978)	1.1	⊢——— 1.4 ———⊣		1.7

Description of samples

Hibbard & Hibbard (1963)	23 043 consecutive deliveries, Mill Road Hospital, Liverpool, UK
Naeye (1980)	53 518 pregnancies in 12 university hospitals, USA, 1959–66 (collaborative perinatal project)
Chamberlain et al (1978)	17 005 pregnancies born in UK during April 1970 (British births 1970 survey)
Paintin (1962)	30 383 singleton pregnancies to married women resident in Aberdeen, UK, 1949–58

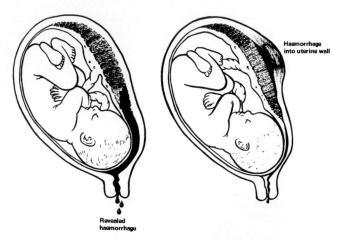

Fig. 18.3 Placental abruption (see text for explanation).

believes that it is, a comparison of the data in Table 18.6 shows that the rise with these parameters is consistent, but not impressive.

Mechanism

The term abruption (Latin: breaking away) describes the process by which the placental attachment to the uterus is disrupted by haemorrhage. According to Egley & Cefalo (1985), the process of abruption begins with uterine vasospasm, followed by relaxation and subsequent venous engorgement and arteriolar rupture into the decidua. The blood then attempts to escape by dissecting under the membranes, sometimes getting into the amniotic sac and producing blood-stained liquor—a common finding in cases of placental abruption. The alternative path is for the blood to dissect under the placenta, causing it to separate from its maternal attachment, and often extending into the uterine muscle itself (Fig. 18.3). The effect on the myometrium is to cause a tonic contraction, which makes the uterus feel woody and hard. The increase of intrauterine pressure embarrasses the placental circulation, adding to the hypoxia already caused by the separation of the placenta.

Examination of the placenta after birth typically shows an area of organizing blood clot with an underlying com-

pression of the maternal surface. Fox (1978) found evidence of retroplacental clot in 4.5% of placentas which he examined routinely. This suggests that small episodes are more common than is realized.

Aetiology

The aetiology remains an enigma. Although the cause is sometimes obvious, as in cases of direct trauma to the uterus, such cases are uncommon and in the majority the cause is obscure. A woman who has suffered from the condition once, has a recurrence rate with subsequent pregnancy of about 6%; this suggests that there may be an underlying abnormality in the uterus or its vasculature.

Egley & Cefalo (1985) found that women who had an unexplained high level of serum alphafetoprotein on routine screening had an increased risk of placental abruption. They suggested that this was evidence of faulty implantation, but it could equally well be due to repeated small episodes of fetomaternal bleeding resulting from decidual necrosis.

Maternal hypertension

There is a wealth of evidence to link maternal hypertension to the occurrence of placental abruption, but there is no agreement on whether the hypertension precedes the abruption or vice versa. Paintin (1962) and Hibbard & Hibbard (1963) looked at the epidemiology of APH in Aberdeen and Liverpool respectively. They concluded that there was no evidence of pre-existing hypertension in most cases of placental abruption and that the hypertension and proteinuria happened as a consequence of the abruption. Naeye et al (1977) came to a similar conclusion from their study of 212 perinatal deaths following placental abruption in the US collaborative study. More recently, Abdella et al (1984) came to the opposite conclusion. They examined 265 consecutive cases of placental abruption in Memphis, USA. The overall incidence in the 24 258 deliveries was 1.2%, but it was 2.3% in those with pre-eclamptic toxaemia, 10% in those with chronic hypertension and 23.6% in those with eclampsia.

Abdominal trauma

A direct blow to the abdomen is a dramatic but infrequent cause of abruption. It can occur from assault or more commonly as a result of injury in a car collision. Crosby & Costiloe (1971), using data from the state of California, found an incidence of 4% of placental abruption in women who survived a car crash whilst wearing a seat belt. Their findings suggest that seat belts, whilst reducing fatal accidents, can also traumatize the pregnant uterus: however, this is not an argument against the use of seat belts.

Abruption was a well-recognized complication of external cephalic version when it was a common practice, especially when performed under anaesthesia. According to Savona-Ventura (1986), who quotes four series of cases, the incidence of abruption following version was between 2% and 9%. The practice of external version is now being revived, with the addition of tocolytic drugs, and the complication rates are reported to be low (Lancet Leader 1984).

Toxins, drugs and nutritional deficiencies

Epidemiological evidence suggests that the incidence of placental abruption is related to social factors. Perinatal mortality rates from APH increase with maternal age and with decreasing social class, suggesting that environmental factors play an important part (Baird & Thomson 1969). Placental abruption was found to be the commonest cause of fetal loss in an African village and was strongly associated with maternal poverty and malnutrition (Naeye et al 1979).

The theory that placental abruption was due to folate or vitamin deficiency was suggested by Hibbard & Hibbard (1963) from their study of APH in Liverpool, but it was not confirmed by others, notably Pritchard (1970). For a time it was fashionable to give folate supplements to reduce the risk of recurrent placental abruption, but the results were disappointing.

Abruption has been reported following snake bite (Zugaib et al 1985) but is not reported as a complication of anticoagulant therapy (Howell et al 1983). It has also been reported in relation to cocaine abuse, possibly related to transient hypertension (Acker et al 1983). One drug, however, is repeatedly implicated—nicotine.

Cigarette smoking. Evidence is accumulating that cigarette smoking increases the risk of placental abruption. Using data from the US collaborative study, Naeye (1980) reported that the incidence of abruption was 1.69% in non-smokers, 2.46% in smokers and 1.87% in smokers who had given up in early pregnancy. These rates were independent of age and parity and the fact that its effect was also found to be dose related suggests that the effect was pharmacological. Naeye found evidence of decidual necrosis at the edge of the placenta and thought that this was ischaemic in origin. Cigarette smoking is known to affect uteroplacental blood flow and to induce uterine contractions (Lehtovirta & Forss 1978).

There is additional evidence from a case-controlled study of 5727 patients in Denmark, which found that cigarette smoking was twice as common in patients who suffered from abruption than among the control cases (Eriksen et al 1991).

Uterine decompression

Sudden decompression of the uterus occurs when the membranes rupture in the presence of polyhydramnios. The reduction of uterine volume causes a corresponding loss of surface area and as a result the placenta sheers off. Nevertheless, according to Pritchard (1970), it is an uncommon cause of abruption.

Abnormalities of the placenta and uterus

In a comprehensive study, Scott (1960) identified a strong association between placenta extrachorialis and all forms of APH, including abruption. This is supported by Wilson & Paalman (1967) who believed that the commonest specific abnormality associated with placental abruption was a circumvallate placenta, in which there is a rim of placental tissue outside the chorial plate. On the other hand, Fox (1978) stated that the commonest findings in placental abruption are necrosis of the decidua and infarcts of the villi, but made no mention of anatomical anomalies.

Vena caval compression syndrome

Although experimental occlusion of the vena cava in animals can produce placental abruption, Pritchard (1970) found no evidence that compression of the inferior vena cava by the uterus (supine hypotension syndrome) was a cause of abruption. In fact, two patients in their series underwent ligation of the inferior vena cava during pregnancy without harm to the fetus.

Lupus anticoagulant

There has been considerable interest in the role of the lupus anticoagulant as a cause of fetal death in the second trimester (Carreras et al 1981, Lubbe et al 1984, Lubbe & Liggins 1985). The factor causes thrombosis of the vessels in the placental bed with severe fetal growth retardation and fetal death. The prognosis can sometimes be improved by the administration of low-dose aspirin and corticosteroids. No evidence has yet been adduced for its role in the genesis of abruption.

Signs and symptoms

The presenting symptoms are bleeding, pain and the onset of premature labour. Hurd et al (1983) reported that 35% of women admitted with abruption were already in labour. About 10% give a history of previous small episodes of vaginal bleeding (Egley & Cefalo 1985). If the separation starts near the placental margin, then vaginal bleeding occurs early and, because there is little concealed haemorrhage, pain is minimal. Here, the diagnosis may be less obvious. Tenderness over the placental site may not be apparent for several hours and since the event may stimulate uterine contractions, the clinical presentation may resemble premature onset of labour with a heavy show.

When bleeding occurs into the uterine muscle there is pain, increased uterine tone and a deceptive absence of vaginal bleeding. When seen at Caesarean section, the Couvelaire uterus is deeply suffused with haematoma, looking like a huge bruise (Speert 1957). The patient looks distressed and unwell, the abdomen is tender and the uterus has a woody consistency. If placental separation is extensive, fetal parts are difficult to identify and the fetal heart beat may be very slow or absent. If the placenta is posterior, tenderness is less marked and the patient complains of backache. The blood pressure is a poor guide to the extent of bleeding. The coexistence of hypertension (whether it is cause or effect) confuses the usual association of haemorrhage with hypotension. Some cases are unsuspected (the silent abruption) and only diagnosed in retrospect (Notelovitz et al 1979).

With such a variation in clinical presentation, the division of placental abruption into three grades (Sher & Statland 1985) has much to commend it as a guide to management:

Grade I — not recognized clinically before delivery and usually diagnosed by the presence of a retroplacental clot.
Grade II — intermediate. The classical signs of abruption are present but the fetus is still alive.
Grade III — severe, the fetus is dead:
   IIIa without coagulopathy, or
   IIIb with coagulopathy.

Differential diagnosis

When vaginal bleeding, a tonically contracted tender uterus and fetal hypoxia occur together, there is little doubt about the diagnosis of placental abruption, but a very similar picture is produced by a ruptured uterus. If the rupture is through a previous Caesarean section scar, the tenderness tends to be localized to the suprapubic area, but real confusion can occur if the scar is from some other operation, such as a myomectomy, or is spontaneous.

In the absence of vaginal bleeding, other conditions causing acute abdominal pain and uterine tenderness in pregnancy which will have to be considered include:

1. haematoma of the rectus sheath
2. retroperitoneal haemorrhage
3. rupture of an appendix abscess
4. acute degeneration or torsion in a uterine fibroid.

A more common problem occurs when there is a small amount of bleeding associated with uterine contractions and a slightly tender uterus. The difficulty is to distinguish a grade I placental abruption from spontaneous preterm labour with a heavy show, especially since a small abruption can itself provoke labour.

Bleeding without pain can also be confusing; it is important to make the distinction from placenta praevia. An ultrasound scan can be very helpful; with a good-quality machine and an experienced operator it is possible to visualize the retroplacental clot or intraperitoneal bleeding. Previous knowledge of the placental site from routine examination in early pregnancy is, of course, very helpful in these circumstances.

Coagulopathy

The first description of a haemophilia-like syndrome associated with a Couvelaire uterus is credited to Dr Lee in 1901, but it was not until 1936 that Dieckman described the presence of hypofibrinogenaemia (see Myerscough 1982). The condition is thought to originate from disseminated intravascular clotting stimulated by the release of thromboplastin from damaged muscle or a dead fetus. The condition is discussed in more detail in Chapter 23.

In a woman already shocked by an abruption, coagulopathy adds considerably to the dangers to the mother and to the problems of management. Successful treatment requires the resources of a competent haematology laboratory and blood transfusion service.

Hypovolaemic shock

The blood loss in cases of placental abruption is nearly always underestimated. This is partly because of the invisible bleeding behind the placenta and into the myometrium, but also because of the association with hypertension which tends to mask the signs of hypovolaemia. Renal necrosis, a serious complication, is the result of undertransfusion rather than anything to do with the hypertension and should be preventable (Pritchard & Brekken 1967).

Management

Initial assessment

Once placental abruption has been suspected, action should be swift and decisive since the prognosis for mother and fetus is worsened by delay. The first step is to set up an intravenous line and to correct blood loss as soon as possible. In severe cases, two lines should be set up in different veins (Department of Health 1991). A central venous catheter is invaluable because it helps to prevent undertransfusion before delivery and over-infusion during the vital hours following delivery. In pre-eclampsia, the circulating blood volume is reduced and there is a risk of pulmonary oedema if too much fluid is infused. The temptation to overinfuse occurs during recovery when there is anxiety about the return of renal function; a good guide is to maintain the central venous pressure at about $+10\,cmH_2O$. Blood is taken for cross-matching and to screen for clotting factors including a platelet count. Urinary output should be monitored by a self-retaining catheter in the bladder, using one of the calibrated collecting systems now available. Secretion of at least 30 ml/h indicates adequate renal perfusion; less raises the possibility of undertransfusion.

There are three practical options for management:

1. Expectant—in the hope that pregnancy will continue.
2. Immediate Caesarean section.
3. Rupture the membranes and aim at vaginal delivery.

Expectant treatment There is a place for conservative treatment when the diagnosis is in doubt or the abruption very minor. Such cases usually present with a small painless vaginal bleed and a localized area of uterine tenderness appears only after several hours or an ultrasound shows a suspicious area of placental separation. In such circumstances, there is something to be gained from allowing the pregnancy to continue, but the decision will depend on the length of gestation, whether there has been a previous episode, the state of the fetus and extent of the placental separation. Abruption occurring in a posteriorly sited placenta can be treacherous because the only symptom may be backache and the site of tenderness is out of reach.

However innocuous the incident of abruption seems to have been, some damage has likely to have been done to the integrity and function of the placenta and the fetus should be carefully monitored. It is a good principle to induce labour in all such patients at or before term.

Caesarean section If the baby is still alive (grade II abruption), electronic fetal monitoring should be started and immediate preparations made for Caesarean section, although the decision to proceed is not always easy. In the first place, the outlook for the fetus is poor, not only in terms of immediate survival but because 15.4% of all liveborn infants did not survive the neonatal period; Abdella et al (1984) reported a 15.4% neonatal mortality. Secondly, the presence of coagulopathy adds considerably to the risks of the operation; it can be difficult to achieve haemostasis when the myometrium is engorged by haematoma without the added problem of hypofibrino-genaemia. If the uterus is already contracting well and delivery appears to be imminent within a few hours, then the membranes should be ruptured and the decision to operate postponed, so long as the fetal heart is satisfactory. In a series reported by Hurd et al (1983), the perinatal mortality following Caesarean section was 3/30 (15%), compared with 6/30 (20%) for those delivered vaginally.

Rupturing the membranes and hastening delivery The main purpose of forewater amniotomy is to hasten the onset of labour and, by encouraging uterine contractions, to reduce uterine bleeding. In most cases it is effective, but also has dangers. If the uterus has become atonic, as happens rarely, the reduction of intrauterine pressure encourages further bleeding which fills the space. Simple observation of the uterine outline gives warning of such continued bleeding. An intravenous infusion of Syntocinon should always be running before starting. The other disadvantage of rupturing the membranes is that a small premature breech baby may slip through a partially dilated cervical os. Rupture of the membranes should therefore be reserved for cases in which the fetus is already dead or labour is already well advanced.

Management of grade III placental abruption

When the baby is dead the only indication for Caesarean section would be uncontrollable bleeding or failure of conservative management. If labour has not already started, the membranes should be ruptured and an infusion of Syntocinon started. The outline of the uterus should be marked with a pen and the girth around the umbilicus measured at hourly intervals to detect bleeding which is not being expelled because the uterus has lost its ability to contract. This is fortunately rare, but if there is no response to Syntocinon and amniotomy and bleeding, visible or concealed, continues, Caesarean section may become needed; even though hazardous, it may be life-saving.

The management of coagulopathy

The sequence of events which lead to coagulopathy involves a cascade of changes affecting both thrombus formation and fibrinolysis and is considered in detail in Chapter 23. The consequences go beyond the loss of fibrinogen from the circulation because the peripheral deposition of fibrin may also affect the blood vessels in other organs such as kidney and liver. In addition there is sometimes a consumptive thrombocytopenia. With the delivery of the placenta and the extrusion of old clot, the whole process reverts to normal and there is a dramatic improvement within a few hours. Rapid delivery is therefore the key to the treatment of coagulopathy.

Adequate blood transfusion is essential, not only to maintain the circulating haemoglobin, but also to replace platelets. If possible the blood should be fresh and supplemented by fresh platelet concentrate if the platelet count falls below 50 000 per ml. Although whole blood is preferable, an alternative will usually be necessary to start with. Packed red cells, with fresh or frozen plasma, can be used together with plasma expanding agents such as degraded gelatin products. Dextrans are nowadays better avoided because they may inhibit blood clotting as well as interfering with cross-matching (see Ch. 23).

Replacement of fibrinogen is of doubtful value, since it is immediately deposited in peripheral veins, but it may be of value in desperate circumstances such as to cover a Caesarean section. An alternative is to use cryoprecipitate. The use of fibrinolytic inhibitors (such as aminocaproic acid or aprotinin) is controversial because it is said that they consolidate the intravascular clot, with serious consequences in the lungs or liver (Sher & Statland 1985). Heparin has also been advocated because of its effect in augmenting antithrombin III, but Sher & Statland do not advocate it and to most obstetricians it seems illogical and dangerous.

Postpartum haemorrhage

The delivery of the placenta represents the end of the acute phase of anxiety, but the battle is not yet over. By this time there are high circulating levels of fibrin degradation products which can have an inhibiting effect on the myometrium (Basu 1969). Postpartum haemorrhage occurs in about 25% of cases and, coupled with the continuing coagulopathy and the heavy blood loss already sustained, severe postpartum haemorrhage can be a *coup de grâce*. This is one of the occasions on which the use of aprotinin is justified.

Renal failure

Ischaemic necrosis of the kidney is a serious complication of placental abruption and the most likely cause is inadequate perfusion during the phase of acute blood loss, but it can also occur from fibrin deposits resulting from disseminated intravascular clotting.

Oliguria during the first 12 hours following an abruption is common and does not necessarily imply permanent renal damage. Even when urinary output falls below the optimum of 30 ml/h, diuretics should be used only with the greatest caution, if at all. They cannot improve renal perfusion and may do harm (Sher & Statland 1985). If the oliguria persists after 12 hours and the central venous pressure indicates a normal circulating blood volume, the most important step is to prevent fluid and electrolyte overload by reducing the volume of the infusion to that of the urinary output. If the serum potassium, blood urea and creatinine start to rise then help is needed from a nephrologist; such experts prefer to be consulted early rather than too late.

Rhesus prophylaxis

Transplacental haemorrhage is likely to occur with any bleeding in pregnancy and can be quite extensive following placental abruption (Pritchard et al 1985). Anti-D immunoglobulin should therefore be given to every rhesus (D)-negative women within 48 hours of placental abruption. The usual dose in the UK is 100 µg, but this is inadequate if the volume of transplacental haemorrhage has exceeded 5 ml fetal blood. A Kleihauer test will give an estimate of the amount of transplacental haemorrhage, but the assessment is complicated by the effect of blood loss and replacement.

Management of a subsequent pregnancy

Abruption is a serious condition, with a high perinatal mortality and a risk of recurrence, estimated at about 7% (Pritchard et al 1985). Although the causes are not known, there is an understandable desire to do something positive in the following pregnancy.

The value of folate supplements during pregnancy has not been proven, but there is little to be lost from their use, preferably before conception. In spite of the uncertainty of the role of hypertension in the causation of abruption, hypertension discovered in such a patient should be investigated after the pregnancy is over and then treated accordingly, with antihypertensive treatment maintained during the next pregnancy. The harmful effects of cigarette smoking are well documented and Naeye (1980) has shown that if smokers give up the habit, even during pregnancy, the risk of abruption is reduced by 23%.

It is important to motivate the patient to take prevention seriously and, above all, to give up smoking. Admission to hospital around the time when the previous episode occurred has no proven value, but it is reassuring to both patient and doctor. It also provides an opportunity to monitor fetal well-being, to treat any existing hypertension, to reinforce the non-smoking advice and to encourage early reporting of pregnancy bleeding.

Table 18.7 Maternal deaths from antepartum haemorrhage in England and Wales (Departments of Health 1994)

	Triennial reports						
	1970–72	1973–75	1976–78	1979–81	1982–84	1985–87*	1988–90*
Placental abruption	6	6	6	2	2	4	6
Placenta praevia	6	2	2	3	2	0	5
Maternal mortality per million maternities	5.2	4.1	4.7	2.7	2.1	2.0	4.7

*Derived from UK figures.

Maternal mortality

Maternal mortality from placental abruption has fallen from 8% in 1917 to under 1% (Egley & Cefalo 1985), and the most recent Report on Confidential Enquiries into Maternal Deaths for 1988–90 (Department of Health 1994) registered five deaths from placenta praevia and six from placenta abruption (Table 18.7). Although maternal mortality from haemorrhage has been falling steadily, the number of cases was double that in the previous report for 1985–87 and the reversal of the downward trend is a sharp reminder of the need to maintain high standards of care. The report contains revised guidelines for the management of massive obstetric haemorrhage. Recommendations include the use of more than one intravenous line, and the use of a central venous catheter, to ensure adequate transfusion.

Perinatal mortality

Perinatal mortality is increased by any kind of bleeding in pregnancy, but is highest following placental abruption. The perinatal mortality of 14.4% reported in the British Births 1970 Study (Chamberlain et al 1978), found that perinatal mortality from placental abruption declined during the 5 years of the study, a comparison with six other reports does not show much evidence of an improvement over the years (Table 18.8).

More than half of the perinatal deaths are stillborn. In a series of 274 admissions with abruption reported by Abdella et al (1984), 57 (23%) babies were stillborn, and of these, 44 (16%) were dead before arrival in hospital. Of the remaining 217 live births, 35 (16%) died

within 28 days, most of them weighing under 2500 g. As would be expected, the chances of survival depended on the gestation and increased from 23% at 28–32 weeks to 87.6% at 37–40 weeks (Paterson 1979). For liveborn babies weighing 2500 g or more the survival rate is reported as 98% (Lunan 1973). According to Abdella et al (1984), the presence of chronic hypertension trebles the fetal mortality from abruption.

There is also concern about the quality of life for the survivors. The Apgar score and the incidence of respiratory distress syndrome are both worse in babies following abruption than would be expected in infants of equivalent birthweight (Niswander et al 1966). The incidence of congenital anomalies was 4.4%, which is about twice that of the population as a whole, and anomalies of the central nervous system are said to be as much as five times as high (Egley & Cefalo 1985).

Placental abruption still makes a significant contribution to perinatal mortality. In the US collaborative study it was the second most frequent cause and accounted for 15% of all perinatal deaths (Naeye et al 1977). More recent population-based statistics from Scotland (Scottish Health Service 1986) reported 72 deaths from placental abruption (12.3% of the total); 81% of these weighed less than 2500 g. There were another 10 deaths among late abortions between 20 and 28 weeks' gestation, but these were not registered as stillbirths.

UNEXPLAINED ANTEPARTUM HAEMORRHAGE

In the British Births 1970 Study (Chamberlain et al 1978), of 1079 cases of APH, 406 (38%) had bleeding of unspecified cause. The fact that perinatal mortality was twice that of those with no history of bleeding (Table 18.1) suggests that placental function is being compromised. Placental anomalies such as circumvallate placenta (Scott 1960) have been implicated and the idea of a ruptured marginal sinus was a popular explanation, but has never been supported by a placental anatomist.

Management

Once other causes of APH have been excluded, the

Table 18.8 Perinatal mortality from placental abruption

Author	Period of study	Perinatal mortality (%)
Paintin (1962)	1949–58	51
Hibbard & Hibbard (1963)	1952–58	25.2
Lunan (1973)	1966–70	38
		(58, 1966; 27.8, 1970)
Chamberlain et al (1978)	1970	14.4
Paterson (1979)	1986–75	34.8
Hurd et al (1983)	1979–81	30.0
Abdella et al (1984)	1970–80	33.5

possibility of a silent abruption must be constantly reviewed. Even when no uterine tenderness develops and there is no ultrasound evidence of retroplacental clot,fetal monitoring with cardiotocography should be performed and the pregnancy should not be allowed to go beyond term.

It is not clear why perinatal mortality is increased in cases of unexplained APH. In some there will have been minor episodes of silent abruption (Notelovitz et al 1979) or there may be anatomical anomalies of the placenta (Scott 1960).

CONCLUSION

Antepartum haemorrhage remains an important cause of fetal loss. Ultrasound has made the diagnosis of placenta praevia possible in early pregnancy and has contributed to the improvement in the outcome of pregnancy for both mother and child. One cause for concern remains: the rising Caesarean section rate, which is happening all over the world, will probably lead to an increase in the incidence of placenta praevia and of placenta accreta in future pregnancies.

The causes and prevention of placental abruption are still not understood and further research is needed. Such evidence as there is suggests that environmental factors play an important part in aetiology and the same factors may be important in the cause of unexplained hypoxic stillbirths. The seed of abruption is probably sown soon after implantation and future improvements in management will depend on a better understanding of the pathology of the placental bed in early pregnancy.

REFERENCES

Abdella T N, Sibai B M, Hays J M, Anderson G D 1984 Relationship of hypertensive disease to abruptio placentae. Obstetrics and Gynecology 63: 365–370

Acker D, Sachs B J, Tracey K J, Wise W E 1983 Abruptio placentae associated with cocaine use. American Journal of Obstetrics and Gynecology 146: 220–221

Baird D, Thomson A M 1969 The effects of obstetric and environmental factors on perinatal mortality. In: Butler N R, Alberman E D (eds) Perinatal problems. Livingstone, Edinburgh, p 223

Basu H K 1969 Fibrinolysis and abruptio placentae. Journal of Obstetrics and Gynaecology of the British Commonwealth 76: 481–495

Carreras L O, Defreyn G, Machin S J et al 1981 Arterial thrombosis, intrauterine death and lupus anticoagulant: detection of immunoglobulin interfering with prostacyclin formation. Lancet i: 244–246

Chamberlain G V P, Philipp E, Howlett B, Masters K 1978 British births, 1970 Heinemann, London, pp 54–79

Chapman M G, Furness E T, Jones W R, Sheat J H 1979 Significance of the ultrasound location of the placental site in early pregnancy. British Journal of Obstetrics and Gynaecology 86: 846–848

Clark S L, Koonings P P, Phelan J P 1985 Placenta previa/accreta and prior cesarean section. Obstetrics and Gynecology 66: 89–92

Comeau J, Shaw L, Marcell C C, Lavery J P 1983 Early placenta previa and delivery outcome. Obstetrics and Gynecology 61: 577–580

Cotton D B, Read J A, Paul R H, Quilligan E J 1980 The conservative aggresive management of placenta previa. American Journal of Obstetrics and Gynecology 137: 687–695

Crenshaw C, Jones D E D, Parker R T 1973 Placenta previa: a survey of 20 years experience with improved perinatal survival by expectant therapy and caesarean delivery. Obstetrical and Gynecological Survey 28: 461–470

Crosby W M, Costiloe J P 1971 Safety of lap-belt restraint for pregnant victims of automobile collisions. New England Journal of Medicine 284: 632–635

Department of Health 1991 Report on Confidential Enquiries into Maternal Deaths in the United Kingdom, 1985–87. HMSO, London, pp 28–44

Edmunds D K 1992 Spontaneous and recurrent abortion. In: Shaw R, Souter P, Stanton S (eds) Gynaecology. Churchill Livingstone, London

Egley C, Cefalo R C 1985 Abruptio placenta. In: Studd J (ed) Progress in obstetrics and gynaecology, vol 5. Churchill Livingstone, London, pp 108–120

Eriksen G, Wohlert M, Ersbak V, Hvidman L, Hedegaard M, Skajaa K 1991 Placental abruption. A case-control investigation. British Journal of Obstetrics and Gynaecology 98: 448–452

Fox H 1978 Pathology of the placenta. Saunders, London, pp 108–112

Grimes D A, Techman T 1984 Legal abortion and placenta previa. American Journal of Obstetrics and Gynecology 149: 501–504

Hamilton W J, Mossman H W 1972 Human embryology, 4th edn. Macmillan, London, p 130

Hibbard L T 1986 Placenta previa. In: Sciarra J J (ed) Gynecology and obstetrics. Harper & Row, Philadelphia

Hibbard B M, Hibbard E D 1963 Aetiological factors in abruptio placentae. British Medical Journal 2: 1430–1436

Howell R, Fidler J, Letsky E, de Swiet M 1983 The risks of antenatal subcutaneous heparin prophylaxis in a controlled trial. British Journal of Obstetrics and Gynaecology 90: 1124–1128

Hurd W W, Miodovnik M, Hertzberg V, Lavin J P 1983 Selective management of abruptio placentae: a prospective study. Obstetrics and Gynecology 61: 467–473

Kerr J M M, Johnstone R W, Phillips M H 1954 Historical review of British obstetrics and gynaecology. Livingstone, Edinburgh, pp 1800–1950

Lancet Leader 1984 External cephalic version. Lancet i: 385

Lehtovirta P, Forss M 1978 The acute effect of smoking on intervillous blood flow in the placenta. British Journal of Obstetrics and Gynaecology 85: 729

Lipitz S, Admon D, Menczer J, Ben-Baruch G, Oelsner G 1991 Mid-trimester bleeding—variables which affect the outcome of pregnancy. Gynecological and Obstetrical Investigation 32: 24–27

Lubbe W F, Liggins C G 1985 Lupus anticoagulant and pregnancy. American Journal of Obstetrics and Gynecology 153: 322–327

Lubbe W F, Butler W S, Palmer S J, Liggins C G 1984 Lupus anticoagulant in pregnancy. British Journal of Obstetrics and Gynaecology 91: 357–363

Lunan C B 1973 The management of abruptio placentae. Journal of Obstetrics and Gynaecology of the British Commonwealth 80: 120–124

Macafee C H G 1945 Placenta praevia — a study of 174 cases. Journal of Obstetrics and Gynaecology of the British Empire 52: 313–324

Macafee C H G, Millar W G, Harley G 1962 Maternal and foetal morbidity resulting from placenta praevia. Obstetrics and Gynecology 65: 176–182

McShane P M, Heyl P S, Epstein M F 1985 Maternal and fetal morbidity resulting from placenta praevia. Obstetrics and Gynecology 65: 176–182

Myerscough P 1982 Munro Kerr's operative obstetrics, 10th edn. Ballière Tindall, London, p 417

Naeye R 1980 Abruptio placentae and placenta previa: frequency, perinatal mortality and cigarette smoking. Obstetrics and Gynecology 55: 701–704

Naeye R L, Harkness W L, Utts J 1977 Abruptio placentae and perinatal death: a prospective study. American Journal of Obstetrics and Gynecology 128: 740–746

Naeye R L, Tafari N, Marboe C C 1979 Perinatal death due to abruptio placentae in an African city. Acta Obstetricia et Gynecologica Scandinavica 58: 37–40

Newton E R, Barss V, Cetrulo C L 1984 The epidemiology and clinical history of asymptomatic midtrimester placenta previa. American Journal of Obstetrics and Gynecology 148: 743–748

Nielson E C, Varner M W, Scott J R 1991 The outcome of pregnancies complicated by bleeding during the second trimester. Surgery, Gynecology and Obstetrics 173: 371–374

Niswander K R, Friedman E A, Hoover D B, Petrowski H, Westphal M C 1966 Fetal morbidity following potentially anoxigenic obstetric conditions. 1. Abruptio placentae. American Journal of Obstetrics and Gynecology 95: 838–845

Notelovitz M, Bottoms S F, Dase D F, Leichter P J 1979 Painless abruptio placentae. Obstetrics and Gynecology 53: 270–272

Paintin D 1962 The epidemiology of ante-partum haemorrhage. Journal of Obstetrics and Gynaecology of the British Commonwealth 69: 614–624

Paterson M E L 1979 The aetiology and outcome of abruptio placentae Acta Obstetricia et Gynecologica Scandinavica 58: 31–35

Powell M C, Buckley J, Price H, Worthington B S, Symonds E M 1986 Magnetic resonance imaging and placenta previa. American Journal of Obstetrics and Gynecology 154: 565–569

Pritchard J A 1970 Genesis of severe placental abruption. American Journal of Obstetrics and Gynecology 108: 22–27

Pritchard J A, Brekken A L 1967 Clinical and laboratory studies on severe abruptio placentae. American Journal of Obstetrics and Gynecology 97: 681–700

Pritchard J A, MacDonald P C, Gant N F 1985 Williams obstetrics, 17th edn. Appleton-Century-Croft, Norwalk, p 399

Robertson E G, Miller D G, Day M J 1968 Placental localization by colorscan using iodine 132 labelled human serum albumin. Journal of Obstetrics and Gynaecology of the British Commonwealth 75: 636–641

Rose G L, Chapman M G 1986 Aetiological factors in placenta praevia. British Journal of Obstetrics and Gynaecology 93: 586–589

Sampson M B, Lastres O, Thomasi A M, Thomason J L, Work B A 1984 Tocolysis with terbutaline sulfate in patients with placenta previa complicated by premature labor. Journal of Reproductive Medicine 29: 248–250

Savona-Ventura C 1986 The role of external cephalic version in modern obstetrics. Obstetrical and Gynecological Survey 41: 393–400

Scott J S 1960 Placenta extrachorialis (placenta marginata and placenta circumvallata). Journal of Obstetrics and Gynaecology of the British Empire 67: 904–918

Scottish Health Service, Information Services Division 1986 Perinatal mortality survey, Scotland 1985. Common Services Agency, Edinburgh

Sher G, Statland B E 1985 Abruptio placentae with coagulopathy: a rational basis for management. Clinical Obstetrics and Gynecology 28: 15–23

Silver R, Depp R, Sabbagha R E, Dooley S L, Socol M L, Tumura R K 1984 Placenta previa: aggressive expectant management. American Journal of Obstetrics and Gynecology 150: 15–22

Speert H 1957 Alexandre Couvelaire and uteroplacental apoplexy. Obstetrics and Gynecology 9: 740–743

Wilson D, Paalman R J 1967 Clinical significance of circumvallate placenta. Obstetrics and Gynecology 29: 774–778

World Health Organization 1977 International classification of diseases, 9th revision. World Health Organization, Geneva

World Health Organization 1992 International statistical classification of diseases and related health problems, 10th revision. World Health Organization, Geneva

Zugaib M, de Barros A C D, Bittar R E, Burdmann E deA, Neme B 1985 Abruptio placentae following snake bite. American Journal of Obstetrics and Gynecology 151: 754–755

19. Multiple pregnancy

William A. W. Walters

Material in this chapter contains contributions from the first edition and we are grateful to the previous author for the work done.

It is distinctly abnormal for the human female to have more than one offspring at a time. It is an atavistic reversion and such reversions are abnormal. (De Lee & Greenhill 1947)

INTRODUCTION

The number of twin births in Western countries has increased dramatically in recent years. For example, in the USA the birth rate of twins has increased at more than twice the rate of singleton births, 35% versus 15%, during the last decade (National Center for Health Statistics 1984, 1991). This increase is due to the increasing use of assisted reproductive technology and a trend in delaying pregnancy and childbirth to a later maternal age. Twins are more than five times as likely to be born before 37 weeks' gestation compared to singletons, and among preterm births, twins are more than twice as likely to be of low birthweight compared to singletons. Twins also have a relative risk of × 6.6 of dying before their first birthday, and among the survivors a relative risk of × 1.4 of handicap compared to singletons (Luke & Keith 1992). More recently, Luke et al (1993) have reported that fetal growth restriction is a major factor in the neonatal morbidity of twins. Furthermore, they found that when fetal growth restriction in twins is accompanied by other neonatal complications such as the respiratory distress syndrome, sepsis or hyperbilirubinaemia, morbidity is increased. Consequently, every attempt should be made to detect fetal growth restriction in twin pregnancies and make appropriate interventions, if adverse outcomes are to be avoided.

Multiple pregnancy provides the obstetrician with the challenge of increased risks to the mother and of both increased fetal morbidity and mortality. Of greatest concern is the fetal loss due largely but not exclusively to preterm delivery. The total loss rate for twin pregnancy, including late abortions (after 20 weeks) and perinatal and infant deaths, is close to 100 per thousand (Neilson & Crowther 1993).

The duration of pregnancy in multiple gestation decreases in proportion to the increase in number of fetuses. The mean duration of pregnancy for twins is 260 days, for triplets 247 days and for quadruplets 196 days compared with 281 days for singleton pregnancies (McKeown & Record 1952, Caspi et al 1976).

As the number of fetuses per pregnancy increases so does the perinatal mortality rate, reaching 416 per 1000 total births for sextuplets (Botting et al 1987). Other causes contributing to the increased fetal wastage include fetal malformations, intrauterine growth retardation and the twin–twin transfusion syndrome.

Apart from their obstetric and paediatric interest, studies of twins have enabled geneticists to differentiate effects of nature (heredity) from those of nurture (environment) in the aetiology of various diseases. Sir Francis

Galton (1911) first drew attention to this concept, when he stated 'twins have a special claim upon our attention; it is, that their history affords means of distinguishing between the effects of tendencies received at birth, and of those that were imposed by the special circumstances of their after lives'. Basically the twin method in studying the aetiology of a particular disease depends upon finding index patients with the disease who were born as one of twins, and then comparing the proportion of monozygotic and same-sex dizygotic co-twins also affected with the disease.

TWINNING

Types of twins

Twins may originate from:

1. two zygotes, when they are called dizygotic, binovular, fraternal or unlike twins, or
2. one zygote when they are called monozygotic, uniovular, identical or like twins.

Dizygotic twins

Dizygotic twins result when two oocytes are simultaneously released from the ovary and fertilized by two separate spermatozoa. In most cases the oocytes are extruded from two separate ovarian follicles but occasionally come from the one follicle (Arnold 1912).

As both zygotes have different genetic constitutions, they give rise to twins that have no more resemblance to each other than do brothers and sisters. They may be of the same or different sexes. To be precise they are littermates rather than twins. Within the uterine cavity the two zygotes implant separately, each developing its own placenta and fetal membranes, although sometimes these may be in such close apposition that the two placentae and the two chorionic membranes fuse.

Monozygotic twins

Monozygotic twins originate by the fertilization of a single ovum by a single sperm and thereafter by division of the zygote into two at a variable stage of early embryonic development. Monozygotic twins most commonly originate at about 1 week of embryonic age by the inner cell mass dividing into two embryonic primordia. Each embryo will have its own amniotic sac but both will develop in a single chorionic sac. The placenta is common to both twins and often there are a number of anastomoses between the two fetal placental circulations, which will be considered later.

The second most common origin of monozygotic twins is a division of cells in the early embryo at 2 or 3 days of age, somewhere between the two-cell and morula stages of embryonic development. Two identical blastocysts then implant, and each embryo develops its own amniotic and chorionic sacs, while the placentae may be separate or fused. In such cases it is impossible to diagnose from the membranes or the placenta alone whether the twins are monozygotic or dizygotic.

The third and least common origin of monozygotic twins is by late division of embryonic cells at 9–15 days of age when the germinal disc has formed, but just before development of the primitive streak (Sadler 1985). The resulting twins share common amniotic and chorionic sacs, thereby allowing their umbilical cords to become entangled. Only 4% of monozygotic twins are of the monoamniotic type (Moore 1982).

Monozygotic twins of opposite sex have been reported in cases where one parent had Turner's syndrome (Edwards et al 1966). Rarely, monozygosity is associated with the occurrence of a numerical chromosome abnormality in one twin. For example, non-disjunction in a 46XY zygote can lead to one twin having a 45X karyotype and the other twin a 46XY karyotype; the former will be a girl with Turner's syndrome and the latter, an apparently normal boy. The very earliest divisions of the embryo sometimes result in one twin with Down's syndrome (trisomy 21) while the other twin has a normal karyotype (Benson 1991).

Zygosity

Twins may be assumed to be dizygotic if they differ in any trait known to be determined by a single genetic locus that exhibits complete penetrance. Thus, if the twins obviously look different physically, extensive zygosity testing is not required (Simpson & Golbus 1992).

Twins of different sex are almost always dizygotic except in rare circumstances when one twin may be 45X with a 46XY co-twin as mentioned above. When twins are of the same sex careful examination of the membranes between the two fetal sacs often helps to establish zygosity. If, after delivery, the dividing membrane between the two sacs is examined macroscopically and microscopically and found to lack chorionic tissue, one can conclude that the twins were separated by two layers of amnion only, with the chorion outermost and encircling the two amniotic sacs. In this case, the twins are monochorionic and therefore monozygotic. On the other hand, if chorionic tissue is present in the middle of the membrane separating the twins, they are dichorionic and hence dizygotic (Fig. 19.1).

Antenatally, some indication of zygosity may be obtained by ultrasonic assessment of the thickness of the membrane dividing the amniotic sacs (Barss et al 1985), the nature of the genitalia and the position of the placental site or sites. A thick membrane between the sacs, fetuses of unlike sex, and widely separated placental sites indicate

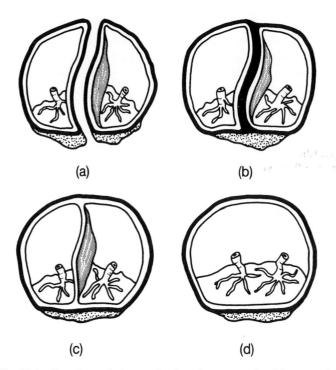

Fig. 19.1 Zygosity and placentation in twin pregnancies. Monozygotic or dizygotic: (**a**) separate diamniotic; (**b**) fused diamniotic. Monozygotic: (**c**) monochorionic diamniotic; (**d**) monochorionic monoamniotic.

dizygosity, whereas the opposite of these findings implies monozygosity. Occasionally, however, it is impossible to diagnose zygosity in twins of the same sex solely by examination of the membranes and placenta. Furthermore, after birth, polymorphic blood groups, enzymes and HLA haplotypes may not be definitive markers as parents may have a similar distribution of antigens to that of the newborn infant.

For a conclusive diagnosis of zygosity DNA fingerprinting is required. This involves the use of DNA probes which are used to identify about 60 dispersed sequences of DNA of variable size. Essentially these are a variable number of tandem repeat (VNTR) markers. The pattern produced is characteristic for an individual and in monozygotic twins the DNA fingerprints are identical. The hypervariability of size of each fragment of DNA is such that the chance of two unrelated individuals having an identical pattern is less than 3×10^{-11} with one probe and less than 5×10^{-9} if two probes are employed (Connor & Fergusson-Smith 1991).

Determination of zygosity of twins is necessary for the following purposes:

1. Legal reasons.
2. If the twins are to be used for genetic studies.
3. To satisfy queries of twins and their relatives concerning their relationship.
4. To assist in diagnosis of the twin–twin transfusion syndrome.
5. Determining feasibility of organ transplantation from one twin to the other.
6. To exclude monozygosity when one twin has a lethal abnormality.
7. Before selective feticide when separate placentae cannot be visualized.

INCIDENCE OF MULTIPLE PREGNANCY

The extensively quoted hypothesis of Hellin (1895), that the natural occurrence of twins is 1 in 80, of triplets 1 in 80^2 and of quadruplets 1 in 80^3, is now known to underestimate the true incidence of multiple pregnancy.

It is difficult to determine the incidence of twins and higher order multiple pregnancies, for serial ultrasound imaging at intervals throughout the same pregnancies has revealed that one or more fetuses often dies in utero during the first trimester. Occasionally this is accompanied by transient blood loss per vaginam, but in some cases there are no clinical signs or symptoms at all. The surviving fetus or fetuses usually develop normally and the pregnancy progresses to term as a normal singleton or lower order multiple pregnancy. The rate of disappearance of a fetus in a multiple pregnancy is at least 21% (Landy et al 1986), but in a recent study using transvaginal ultrasound the spontaneous disappearing twin rate was found to be as high as 48% (Blumenfeld et al 1992). The majority of the spontaneous fetal disappearances occurred during the first trimester. The latter investigators found a multiple pregnancy rate of 2.3% during the first trimester, appreciably higher than the generally accepted twinning rate of 1.89%, which is based upon the number of twins actually delivered. An even higher disappearance rate was reported by Levi (1976) who studied a cohort of 6990 women all of whom had had serial ultrasound scans on 10 occasions throughout pregnancy. Overall, 118 had multiple gestation sacs. In this population, a 71% disappearance rate of twin gestation occurred when the diagnosis was made before 10 weeks' gestation.

During the last two decades, the twin delivery rate has risen in several countries and the delivery rate of triplets has risen more rapidly still. For example, in France between 1972 and 1989 the incidence of twin deliveries of 28 or more weeks' gestation rose from 8.8 to 11.2 per 1000 births and of triplets from 0.9 to 4.4 per 10 000 births. This upward trend was most marked in women between the ages of 30 and 39 years (Tuppin et al 1993). In the USA between 1972–74 and 1985–89, the rate of higher order multiple births increased by 113% among infants of white mothers but by 22% among infants of black mothers (Kiely et al 1992). Similar increases in multiple births have occurred in other industrialized countries including Japan (Imaizumi 1987). These increases have been attributed to the increasing use of ovulation-inducing agents and the development of in vitro fertilization programmes for the treatment of infertility. The mechanisms involved include multiple ovulation, fertilization of more than one ovum, and transfer of more than one embryo to the uterine cavity.

Monozygotic twins

The incidence of spontaneous monozygotic twinning is remarkably constant around the world at an incidence of about 4 per 1000 births. It does not appear to be influenced by race, heredity, age or parity and is largely attributed to chance (MacGillivray 1986). However, recently monozygotic twinning has been reported to be increased after the use of agents to induce ovulation (Derom et al 1987).

Dizygotic twins

The incidence of spontaneous dizygotic twinning in man varies widely from one population to another, as it is probably affected by genetic, nutritional and environmental factors. Among countries which keep good data, it is highest in Nigeria (49 per 1000 maternities) and lowest in Japan (1.3 per 1000 maternities) (MacGillivray 1986) (Table 19.1).

Benirschke & Kaufmann (1990) have suggested that the differences in frequency of dizygotic twinning among various populations is due to genes that regulate follicle stimulating hormone (FSH) and luteinizing hormone (LH) secretions. They point out that both twinning and the FSH/LH ratio in maternal blood increase with age, and that the Japanese, who have a low rate of twinning, have low blood FSH/LH ratios. Support for this suggestion is provided by the finding of higher blood levels of FSH, LH and oestradiol-17β in mothers of dizygotic twins (Martin et al 1984). Such women would be more likely to have multiple ovulation and hence dizygotic twins. Furthermore, it would also account for the fact that mothers of dizygotic twins are more likely to have twins again than women who have not delivered twins before (Nylander 1970).

The twinning rate in the offspring of dizygotic female twins is greatly increased over that observed for the general population, or for spouses of dizygotic and monozygotic male twins (White & Wyshak 1964, Corey et al 1992). Thus it would seem that maternal genetic factors contribute to a predisposition to dizygotic twinning.

The incidence of twinning rises with increasing maternal age (Waterhouse 1950, MacGillivray 1986) and with increasing parity (Petterson et al 1976, Azubuike 1982). With respect to age, the peak incidence occurs in the middle thirties, followed by a decline until 40 years of age, after which it rises again. The influence of age and parity is almost entirely on dizygotic twinning, although age alone has a slight influence on monozygotic twinning (MacGillivray 1986).

Tall women are more likely to produce twins than small women and fat women are more likely to have twins than thin women as the former are generally better nourished. In each instance it is the dizygotic twinning rate that is increased. Fatness increases with maternal age and this explains most of the increased incidence of twins with increasing maternal age (Naeye 1990). Obesity is associated with a higher gonadotrophin production, which would increase multiple ovulation. Thin women have lower gonadotrophin levels and a lower incidence of twinning (MacGillivray 1986). Furthermore, twins occur less often in undernourished women (Campbell et al 1974), who are usually of lesser stature than well-nourished women.

The influence of infertility treatments

The twin and triplet delivery rates have been rising in several countries since the 1970s (Table 19.2). Although the development of ovulation induction and in vitro fertilization have coincided with these observations, it is not yet known to what extent they have been responsible. By comparing over time the incidence of multiple deliveries, the proportion of deliveries resulting from assisted conception, and sales of ovulation-inducing drugs in France, Tuppin et al (1993) found that between 1985 and 1989, 26% of triplet deliveries followed assisted conception and nearly 50% were estimated to be due to ovulation-inducing agents. They concluded that the dramatic

Table 19.1 Twinning rates per 1000 pregnancies in various countries

Country	Monozygotic	Dizygotic	Total
Nigeria	5.0	49.0	54.0
USA			
Black	4.7	11.1	15.8
White	4.2	7.1	11.3
England and Wales	3.5	8.8	12.3
Japan	3.0	1.3	4.3

Adapted from Nylander (1975).

Table 19.2 Multiple births per 1000 pregnancies in various countries

Country	Twins	Triplets	Quadruplets
Nigeria*	66.5	1.78	0.06
USA[†]			
Black	13.4	0.14	0.0018
White	10.0	0.09	0.001
England and Wales[‡]	9.6	0.12	0.009
Japan[§]	6.4	0.056	0.001

*Nylander (1975).
[†]Statistical Bulletin of Metropolitan Life Insurance Company (1960).
[‡]Registrar General (1979).
[§]Imaizumi & Inouye (1984).

increase in triplet deliveries was strongly influenced by infertility treatments, especially ovulation-inducing agents. When clomiphene is used for induction of ovulation the incidence of twin pregnancy is 8% compared with an increased risk of multiple births of 20% after administration of human menopausal gonadotrophin (Martin 1991).

It has been suggested that ultrasound monitoring can help to prevent high-order multiple pregnancies by detecting the presence of more than two ovarian follicles of ovulatory size. Under these circumstances administration of the ovulating dose of human chorionic gonadotrophin could be withheld (O'Herlihy et al 1988). However, despite monitoring ovarian follicular development by measurement of plasma or urinary oestrogen and ovarian ultrasonography, Yu et al (1991) found that prediction of multiple pregnancies in gonadotrophin-stimulated cycles was not accurate. Unfortunately current ovulation induction regimens continue to include an element of uncertainty as far as multiple pregnancy is concerned.

Sex ratios

In the human, as the number of fetuses per pregnancy increases, the percentage of male fetuses diminishes (Strandskov et al 1946). While the cause of this phenomenon is unknown, it is in keeping with the well-known observation of the increased mortality of males in all age groups from infancy to old age. A recent study from the Negev, Israel of 1394 twin deliveries, where each twin weighed 500 g or more, revealed that amongst Jews the proportion of males was significantly lower than in singleton births. By contrast amongst Bedouins, the sex ratio for twins and singletons was similar. This suggests that genetic and lifestyle factors may be responsible for the sex ratio differences between the two ethnic groups comprising the study population (Picard et al 1991).

Superfecundation and superfetation

Superfecundation is rare in women but has been documented on several occasions. It refers to the fertilization of two ova within a short period of time in the same cycle as a result of two separate acts of intercourse. Furthermore, different men may be responsible: the most striking examples of this are the delivery of a mulatto baby and a white baby from dizygotic twins to women who have been inseminated by different partners within a few days of each other (Harris 1982).

Superfetation refers to a second conception that occurs after a period of at least one ovulatory cycle following the first conception. It has never been documented unequivocally in the human. Theoretically, for it to occur the second conception would have to be initiated within the first trimester to allow implantation of the second zygote before obliteration of the uterine cavity by fusion of the decidua capsularis of the first conceptus with the decidua parietalis at about 12 weeks' gestation.

Many alleged cases of superfetation are probably better explained by discordant growth of fetuses of the same gestational age.

ANASTOMOSES BETWEEN TWIN PLACENTAL CIRCULATIONS

Monochorionic twin placentae nearly always have vascular connections between the two fetal circulations. Potentially this could lead to the twin–twin transfusion syndrome. However, this seldom occurs; in one much quoted study it was recognized clinically in only three out of 55 cases (Robertson & Neer 1983). On the other hand dichorionic twin placentae rarely have fetal vascular anastomoses between the two circulations. In Robertson and Neer's study only one of 68 dichorionic placentae showed evidence of transplacental circulation whereas this was seen in 55 of 56 monochorionic placentae. The most common vascular connections were artery-to-artery anastomoses beneath the chorionic plate, with vein-to-vein anastomoses being much less frequent. Arteriovenous anastomoses of variable number and size may also occur. The communication between the fetal artery and vein often develops through the capillary bed of a placental lobule or cotyledon (Benirschke & Kim 1973).

Chimaerism

A chimaera is an individual with two cell lines derived from two separate zygotes. An example of this is blood chimaerism, the finding of discordant blood types in the one individual (Benirschke 1974). The most likely explanation for this is the transfer of haemopoietic stem cells in utero from one of dizygotic twins to the other via transplacental anastomotic vessels connecting their circulations. During early fetal life exposure of one twin to antigens from the other leads to development of immunological tolerance in the recipient fetus.

HYDATIDIFORM MOLE WITH COEXISTENT FETUS

Hydatidiform mole with coexistent fetus occurs in 0.005–0.01% of all pregnancies (McDonald & Ruffolo 1983). It is a variant of twinning, whereby two ova are fertilized, one resulting in a fetus and the other in a hydatidiform mole. In this situation, two placentae are present with one being normal and the other, unrelated to the fetus, being molar tissue. Less commonly a partial mole consisting of hydatidiform hyperplasia in part of the placenta belonging to the fetus develops. Fetal triploidy (69 chromosomes) is often present and responsible for multiple malformations which are not consistent with long-term survival. However, in some cases the fetus has a normal karyotype. In androgenetic (46 XX) and triploid moles, the genetic basis for the abnormal placental morphology appears to be the ratio of male to female chromosomes (Vejerslev 1991). Cytogenetic evidence for dispermic fertilization of an egg with a normal haploid chromosome set was found in all of 24 placental specimens showing both normal villi and vesicles visible to the naked eye, and which contained both maternal and paternal contributions to the genome (Vejerslev et al 1987a).

Prenatal diagnosis of the fetal karyotype is helpful in that a triploid one is virtually incompatible with life and termination of the pregnancy is advisable. On the other hand if the fetal karyotype is normal, attempted continuation of the pregnancy entails a risk of 30% of substantial bleeding or of pre-eclampsia and in about 15% the severity of the condition requires termination on clinical grounds, irrespective of fetal development. No infants survive if delivered before 28 weeks and only about 60% reach this gestation. After 28 weeks, a surviving child may be expected in about 70% of pregnancies, the risk of intrauterine or neonatal death being approximately 30%. Delivery is usually vaginal (85%). In about 9% of continuing pregnancies invasive molar growth or frankly malignant change in the trophoblastic tissue occurs. Unfortunately there is no adequate predictor of this. Furthermore, persistent trophoblastic disease has no correlation with the length of gestation (Vejerslev 1991).

The partial mole is often triploid, the result of two paternal and one maternal halploid complements. This is consistent with animal data in which the paternal haploid is essential for placental development. The most likely explanation is dispermy, the most common chromosome complement being 69 XXY followed by 69 XXX. Parental chromosome analyses have not shown any increase in chromosome anomalies in couples who have had either complete or partial moles (Vejerslev et al 1987b).

Amniocentesis is probably preferable to chorion villus sampling for prenatal diagnosis of the fetal karyotype, given the varying placental morphology and the possibility that trophoblast chromosomal findings may not be representative of the fetus.

Maternal serum human chorionic gonadotrophin levels are usually markedly increased but values within the normal range do not exclude molar change. Alphafetoprotein in maternal serum is also raised significantly above the maximum for non-molar pregnancies in all varieties of complete or partial mole, but again normal values do not necessarily exclude trophoblastic pathology.

Ultrasound imaging is important in the initial examination, for guidance of invasive investigations, and for monitoring of ongoing pregnancies. Magnetic resonance imaging may be especially helpful in detection of invasive growth and metastases (Powell et al 1986).

Azuma et al (1992) examined a spontaneously aborted conceptus comprising two living female fetuses and a molar mass at 19 weeks' gestation, and used DNA fingerprinting to investigate the zygosity of the two fetuses and the pathogenesis of the tumour. The possible explanations were: (i) normal twin pregnancy plus a complete hydatidiform mole, (ii) normal twin pregnancy plus a blighted ovum with diffuse hydropic change and (iii) coexistence of a partial hydatidiform mole with a living fetus plus a normal singleton fetus. Comparison of DNA fingerprints among the fetuses, tumour and parents revealed that this was a triplet pregnancy composed of dizygotic twins and a complete androgenetic hydatidiform mole. The authors pointed out that clinically it is very important to differentiate the multiple pregnancy involving a complete mole from that involving a blighted ovum or partial mole, because the relative risks of choriocarcinoma associated with molar pregnancy have been estimated to be 2000–4000 times higher than those associated with normal or aborted pregnancies (Bracken et al 1984), and because partial hydatidiform mole is probably not associated with an increased risk of choriocarcinoma (Vassilakos et al 1977).

As it is sometimes difficult to distinguish a blighted ovum with severe hydropic change from a complete mole by histological examination only and because karyotyping is time consuming, DNA fingerprinting facilitates an accurate diagnosis.

MATERNAL ADAPTATION TO MULTIPLE PREGNANCY

In multiple pregnancy all of the physiological changes seen in singleton pregnancy occur to a greater degree. Many of these changes are associated with the increased production of steroid and protein hormones by the fetoplacental unit: oestrogens, progesterone, human placental lactogen and pregnancy-specific glycoproteins are all increased beyond levels found in singleton pregnancy. The minor ailments of pregnancy such as nausea and vomiting are similar to but often more severe than those in singleton pregnancy.

Overall women with twin pregnancies gain more weight than women with singleton pregnancies. All of the constituents of weight gain are likely to be increased, including retention of water and deposition of body fat.

Total peripheral resistance declines further in twin than in singleton pregnancy leading to a relatively greater fall in diastolic blood pressure. Cardiac output and blood volume (both plasma volume and red cell mass) are also increased more than in singleton pregnancy. For example, the mean increase in total blood volume in twin pregnancy is about 500 ml greater than in singleton pregnancy (Rovinsky & Jaffin 1965). The increased cardiac output is due mainly to increased heart rate and myocardial contractility rather than to increased blood volume and venous return (Rovinsky & Jaffin 1966, Veille et al 1985).

Although dietary food intake is not increased in women with twin pregnancy over and above that in singleton pregnancies, fetal growth (by weight) is greater in twin pregnancy than when only one fetus is present. This indicates that absorption of nutrients from the diet and use of energy is enhanced to optimal levels in twin pregnancies (Campbell 1986). The concentration of folate in serum falls markedly in twin pregnancies although the total amount of circulating folate and red cell folate is unchanged. In one study in Aberdeen, the incidence of megaloblastic anaemia was the same in both twins and singleton pregnancies (Campbell 1986). Therefore, it is not necessary to give prophylactic iron and folic acid to all women with twin pregnancy, but more frequent examination of peripheral blood should be undertaken during pregnancy to detect anaemia when it occurs. Appropriate treatment can then be started.

Because of the larger uterus in multiple pregnancy, mechanical effects are exaggerated. These include the increased lumbar lordosis when standing causing backache; dyspnoea and dyspepsia due to upward displacement of the diaphragm; partial ureteric obstruction, predisposing to hydroureter, urinary stasis and urinary tract infection; pressure on the abdominal inferior vena cava and aorta in the supine position, leading to the supine hypotensive syndrome; and varicose veins and oedema in the lower limbs due to increased hydrostatic pressure within the veins. Polyhydramnios, especially of the acute type associated with monozygotic twin pregnancies, will cause even greater enlargement of the uterus and further aggravate the various mechanical pressure effects.

MANAGEMENT OF TWIN PREGNANCY

Women with twin pregnancies should be regarded as falling into a high-risk category and therefore should have more intensive antenatal surveillance than women with singleton pregnancies. A good case can be made for 2-weekly antenatal clinic visits until 32 weeks and weekly visits thereafter.

Diagnosis

Management of twin pregnancy begins when the diagnosis has been made. Clinically it may be brought to attention because of a family history of twins, because of hyperemesis in early pregnancy, or unexpected increased uterine size on pelvic or abdominal palpation.

Later in the second trimester, an apparent excess of fetal parts and more than two fetal poles may be palpable abdominally unless hydramnios is present. Auscultation may reveal the presence of two fetal heart rates rarely differing more than a few beats per minute when recorded by two cardiotocographs simultaneously.

The definitive diagnosis is made by ultrasound examination when two embryos or fetuses will be seen. During the second trimester a further ultrasound scan should be performed to determine whether the pregnancy is continuing with triplets, twins or one fetus, to exclude fetal abnormalities, and to attempt diagnosis of zygosity as described earlier. Monozygotic twins have an increased risk of discordant fetal growth, twin–twin transfusion, polyhydramnios and fetal anomalies, leading to a higher perinatal mortality compared with dizygotic twins. Furthermore, when the twins share a single amniotic sac (monoamniotic) they have even greater risk of mortality due to cord entanglement or conjoint development.

Detection of fetal abnormality

It is not unusual to find that a raised maternal serum alphafetoprotein level at 13–15 weeks' gestation can be explained by the presence of a twin pregnancy. Once such a result has been obtained, an ultrasound examination is indicated to assess fetal morphology, which reveals the twin pregnancy.

When a fetal morphological abnormality has been detected in one of twins, expectant management is usually employed to ensure that the normal fetus is not compromised: every effort is made to achieve survival of the normal twin. If a serious fetal abnormality in one twin has been diagnosed during the first trimester or early in the second trimester, selective feticide is an option that should be discussed with the parents. However, counselling should take account of the risks that feticide might impose on continuation of the pregnancy and the well-being of the normal co-twin, especially if the twins are monozygotic, when there are almost always anastomoses between the two fetal circulations within the placenta. Under these circumstances, toxic agents injected into the circulation of the abnormal fetus may cross into the circulation of the normal fetus. In addition, after death of the abnormal fetus, thromboplastins may enter the circulation of the normal fetus to cause disseminated intravascular coagulation and bleeding into various fetal tissues.

Prenatal diagnosis of fetal abnormalities should be offered in twin pregnancies for the same reasons that it is offered in singleton pregnancies. Fetal cells for cytogenetic studies are best obtained by amniocentesis at 15–16 weeks' gestation and alphafetoprotein can be measured in the same amniotic fluid samples. The amniocentesis procedure and interpretation of alphafetoprotein results are discussed below.

Assessment of fetal growth

Clinical assessment of fetal growth in twin pregnancy is unreliable and useless for detecting discordant fetal growth, which is usually regarded as a 25% or more difference in weight between fetuses. Serial ultrasound scans, particularly to measure the head circumference, are required for these purposes, commencing at about 24 weeks' gestation and repeated every 4 weeks or more frequently if clinically indicated.

When discordant fetal growth is diagnosed, Doppler ultrasound studies of the umbilical artery waveforms (Doppler velocimetry) may help to differentiate between the twin–twin transfusion syndrome and idiopathic fetal growth retardation. In the former identical umbilical artery waveforms are seen in the umbilical arteries of both umbilical cords. On the other hand, when one twin is normal and the other growth retarded, the umbilical artery waveforms of only the growth-retarded fetus are abnormal (Giles et al 1985). Twin–twin transfusion syndrome may also be present when polyhydramnios affects one fetal amniotic sac and oligohydramnios affects the other sac (Chescheir & Seeds 1988). Using a 25% or more difference in birthweight between twins as the definition of discordancy, about 10% of twin pregnancies are discordant. Twins in this category have a perinatal mortality rate of 97 per 1000 compared with 37 per 1000 for non-discordant twins (Erkkola et al 1985).

Although claims for the success of Doppler velocimetry for prediction of concordant and discordant fetal growth in twin pregnancies have been reported from some centres (Gerson et al 1987, Gaziano et al 1991, Shah et al 1992), others have found it less helpful (Divon et al 1989). Clearly, the place of Doppler velocimetry in management of twin pregnancy has yet to be clarified.

Antenatal cardiotocography

Several studies of non-stress testing in twin pregnancy have shown antenatal cardiotocography to be a useful investigation for assessing the individual status of twins. High quality simultaneous tracings of both fetal heart rates can be obtained in 85% of cases (Devoe & Azor 1981, Blake et al 1984). When non-stress tests are performed in twin pregnancies during the third trimester, they appear to be prognostically comparable to those performed during the same time period in singleton pregnancies (Devoe & Azor 1981). In a recent Los Angeles study of 665 twin pregnancies, 10 were complicated by fetal death of one or both twins in patients who received prenatal care without non-stress tests, whereas within the group who had received non-stress tests there was only one fetal death. However, this reduction in fetal deaths in the group who had received non-stress tests was not statistically significant ($P = 0.062$) and the authors concluded that a large prospective randomized trial is needed to define the role of non-stress testing in the management of twin pregnancy (Sherman et al 1992).

Nevertheless antenatal cardiotocography may be helpful in diagnosing fetal distress in twin pregnancy, especially when discordant fetal growth or concordant asymmetrical fetal growth have been identified by ultrasound examination. The frequency of cardiotocography recordings should be determined by the clinical circumstances of individual pregnancies, but a recording every 1–2 days is common practice.

COMPLICATIONS OF TWIN PREGNANCY

Spontaneous abortion

The frequency of twins among spontaneous abortuses is approximately three times that among live births. In one study of 2000 abortuses, one set of twin fetuses was found among every 35 abortuses: 88% of the twin fetuses were abnormal and most were of the monozygotic type (Livingston & Poland 1980, Uchida et al 1983).

Pregnancy-induced hypertension

Pregnancy-induced hypertension is two to three times more common in twin pregnancies. It tends to develop earlier and to be more severe than is the case in singleton pregnancies. There is no significant difference in the incidence of proteinuric hypertension between monozygotic and dizygotic twin pregnancies; the incidence is high in both groups, particularly in primigravidae (MacGillivray 1984) (Table 19.3). In an Australian study, Long & Oats (1987) found that 25.9% of 642 women seen consecutively with twin pregnancies developed pre-eclampsia, compared with 9.7% of women with singleton pregnancies. Of the women with twins developing pre-eclampsia, 35.2% were primigravidae and 20.4% multigravidae. The pre-eclampsia was earlier in onset in twin pregnancies than in singleton pregnancies.

The influence of maternal genetic factors

In an epidemiological study of pregnancy complications and outcome in a Norwegian twin population, information on 22 241 pregnancies of 8675 female twins or

Table 19.3 Percentage of women developing pre-eclampsia in monozygotic (MZ) and dizygotic (DZ) twin pregnancies by parity (from MacGillivray 1984)

	Primigravidae (%)		Multigravidae (%)	
	MZ	DZ	MZ	DZ
Proteinuric pre-eclampsia	17.65	18.64	7.18	8.28
Gestational hypertension	26.89	24.15	13.45	17.20
Normotensive	55.46	57.21	79.37	74.52
Total	100	100	100	100
	($n = 119$)	($n = 236$)	($n = 223$)	($n = 628$)

spouses of male twins was obtained by questionnaire. Historical information about pregnancy was provided by both members of 830 monozygotic and 902 dizygotic female twin pairs and by the spouses of both members of 459 monozygotic and 464 dizygotic male twin pairs. It was found that monozygotic female twin pairs were more concordant than dizygotic female twin pairs for the occurrence of nausea and vomiting, miscarriage and hypertension or overt toxaemia. This suggests that maternal genetic factors make an important contribution to the predisposition to risk of miscarriage, nausea, vomiting and pre-eclampsia during pregnancy (Corey et al 1992).

Preterm labour

Idiopathic spontaneous preterm labour occurs in 30% of twin pregnancies, being more common in the monozygotic variety (Hall 1985). Tocolytic drugs such as β-receptor agonists may be helpful in delaying delivery for several hours to allow transfer of the mother with fetuses in utero to a hospital with neonatal intensive care facilities, should these be required. However, most randomized trials of β-receptor agonists in twin pregnancies have not brought about a significant reduction in preterm delivery rates (Marivate et al 1977, O'Connor et al 1979, Gummerus & Halonen 1987, Ashworth et al 1990).

Cervical assessment by digital examination identifies a group of twin pregnancies at especially high risk of preterm labour (Neilson et al 1988). A score, calculated by subtracting cervical dilatation (cm) from cervical length (cm) (Houlton et al 1982), is used for this purpose. Seventy-six per cent of 223 parous women with twin pregnancies who had a cervical score of –2 or less at or before 34 weeks were delivered before 37 completed weeks' gestation.

Bed rest in hospital between 26 and 30 weeks' gestation has long been advocated to prevent preterm delivery but recent controlled trials have shown that it has no significant effect in this regard (Crowther et al 1990,

MacLennan et al 1990). However, Crowther et al (1990) found that although bed rest in hospital from 28 to 30 weeks' gestation until delivery did not increase gestational length in twin pregnancies (Table 19.4), the mean birthweight of twins was greater in the hospitalized group, which included fewer small-for-gestational-age infants than did the control group. Despite this finding, no differences in neonatal morbidity were found between the two groups (Table 19.5). Therefore, little is to be gained by routinely admitting all women with twin pregnancies to hospital at 26–30 weeks' gestation for enforced rest in bed.

Cervical cerclage has also been used prophylactically in twin pregnancies to reduce the preterm delivery rate but has not been found successful (Weekes et al 1977, Dor et al 1982).

Antepartum haemorrhage

It is difficult to assess the true incidence of placental abruption in twin gestation but it is thought to be slightly increased because of the increased incidence of pregnancy-induced hypertension and polyhydramnios. The incidence of placenta praevia may also be increased, probably as a consequence of the larger than usual placental surface area in twin pregnancy. However, at least two studies have shown that antepartum haemorrhage is no more common in twin pregnancies than in singleton pregnancies (Nylander 1975, Scottish Twin Study 1983).

Anaemia

Twin pregnancies are associated with a larger expansion of plasma volume than red cell mass, as in singleton pregnancies, but to a greater degree. Therefore, the haemoglobin concentration is an unreliable indicator of anaemia because of haemodilution. Nylander (1975) suggested that the packed cell volume should be less than 27% before anaemia is diagnosed, and in his study there was

Table 19.4 Pregnancy outcome in a randomized controlled trial of hospitalization for bed rest from 28–30 weeks' gestation until delivery in twin pregnancy. Reproduced from Crowther et al (1990) with permission

	Hospitalized group (n = 58)	Control group (n = 60)		Significance P value
Gestation age at delivery (weeks)	36.1 (2.0)	35.9 (2.1)		NS
Recruitment to delivery interval (days)	49.2 (16.6)	49.3 (20.4)		NS
	n (%)	n (%)	Odds ratio	(95% CI)
Delivery < 37 weeks	36 (62)	40 (67)	0.82	(0.39–1.74)
Delivery < 34 weeks	11 (19)	11 (18)	1.04	(0.41–2.62)
Spontaneous labour	57 (98)	56 (93)	3.35	(0.56–19.92)
Caesarean section	8 (14)	12 (20)	0.65	(0.25–1.68)
Hypertension	3 (5)	9 (15)	0.34	(0.10–1.13)
Prelabour rupture of membranes	7 (12)	5 (8)	1.50	(0.46–4.93)
Other complications	7 (12)	12 (20)	0.56	(0.21–1.49)

NS = Not significant.
Results are means (SD) or n (%) values as appropriate.

Table 19.5 Fetal outcome in a randomized controlled trial of hospitalization for bed rest from 28–30 weeks' gestation until delivery in twin pregnancy. Reproduced from Crowther et al (1990) with permission

	Hospitalized group (n = 116)	Control group (n = 120)	Significance P value
Birthweight (kg)			
Twin I	2.47 (0.49)	2.32 (0.39)	NS
Twin II	2.40 (0.45)	2.28 (0.47)	NS
Both twins	2.43 (0.47)	2.30 (0.43)	0.02
Small-for-gestational age			Odds ratio (95% CI)
Twin I	14 (24)	26 (43)	0.43 (0.20–0.91)
Twin II	20 (35)	25 (42)	0.74 (0.35–1.55)
Both twins	34 (29)	51 (43)	0.57 (0.33–0.96)
Neonatal unit			
Admissions	42 (36)	41 (34)	1.09 (0.64–1.86)
Duration of stay (days)	2.6 (6.1)	3.4 (7.1)	NS
Stillbirths	2	11	0.24 (0.08–0.74)
Early neonatal deaths	2	1	2.03 (0.21–19.69)

Results are mean (SD) or n (%) values as appropriate.

no significant difference in the incidence of anaemia between twin and singleton pregnancies. This has been confirmed by others (Hall et al 1979, Scottish Twin Study 1983), although it is conceded that both iron and folic acid stores may be reduced transiently during twin pregnancy (Hall et al 1979). Results of these studies suggest that routine administration of prophylactic iron and folic acid are not indicated in twin pregnancy and that they should only be prescribed when there is evidence of significant anaemia.

Polyhydramnios

Acute polyhydramnios is an uncommon abnormality occurring in approximately one in 4000 to 12 000 pregnancies. It is defined as an amniotic fluid volume of more than 2000 ml (Queenan et al 1970). Acute polyhydramnios is usually diagnosed before 28 weeks' gestation and is differentiated from the chronic form of the condition by the rapidity of onset over a few days and the increased severity of maternal symptoms. It only occurs in monozygotic monochorionic twin pregnancies.

In a Melbourne study of 774 twin pregnancies delivered after 20 weeks' gestation, the incidence of acute polyhydramnios was 1.7%. The perinatal mortality in this group was 88.5%, largely due to extreme prematurity: there were no fetal abnormalities. The clinical course of the polyhydramnios was fulminating in all cases with a mean duration of 5.5 days (range 1–11 days) between the onset of symptoms and delivery. The average duration of pregnancy reached was 25.5 weeks (range 22–30 weeks) compared to 33 weeks in patients with twins and chronic polyhydramnios (Steinberg et al 1990).

Conservative therapy including bed rest, tocolysis and β-methasone administration is not enough to have any significant impact on the high perinatal wastage associated with acute polyhydramnios. The use of ultrasound-guided serial amniocenteses may help to achieve an increase in the length of gestation (Schneider et al 1985). Alternatively, the maternal administration of the prostaglandin synthetase inhibitor, indomethacin, may reduce amniotic fluid production by suppressing prostaglandin E production in the fetal kidney, thereby reducing the inhibitory action of prostaglandins on vasopressin leading to a reduced fetal urine output (Lange et al 1989).

When acute polyhydramnios develops early in the second trimester selective feticide should be considered to allow the pregnancy to continue long enough to improve fetal outlook for at least one of the two fetuses (Wittmann et al 1986).

Prolonged gestation

It is generally believed that prolongation of twin pregnancy beyond 40 weeks is hazardous because of an increased risk of fetal dysmaturity or placental insufficiency. Indeed the highest mean birthweight of twins has been recorded at 39 weeks compared with 41–42 weeks in singletons, suggesting that twin gestation may be biologically shorter (Greenwald 1970). Furthermore, Keily (1990) reported that twins born in New York city between 1978 and 1984 at and beyond 40 weeks' gestation were lighter in weight than those born at 38–39 weeks, suggesting that intrauterine growth in twins stops after 39 weeks. Luke and colleagues (1993) also found that fetal growth restriction in twins is greatly increased after 38 weeks' gestation. In addition lung maturation in twins occurs earlier than in singletons (Leveno et al 1984) and there is ultrasonographic evidence that the placenta ages more rapidly in twins (Ohel et al 1987). These observations, combined with that of progressively diminishing uterine blood flow in twin pregnancies during the last 2–3 weeks of gestation (Morris et al 1955), has persuaded many obstetricians to recommended delivery of twins between completion of the 37th and 38th weeks. However reasonable this suggestion may seem, we do not have data to allow any dogmatic statement to be made about the risks entailed in prolonged twin gestation.

Fetal death in utero or expulsion of one twin during the second or third trimester

Antepartum death of one twin in the second or third trimester is rare. In a recent British study, the incidence of this complication was 2.3% of twin pregnancies, and in 50% of these the twins were monochorionic (Fusi & Gordon 1990).

The diagnosis should be suspected when fetal movements diminish, when maternal weight gain slows down or when other obstetric complications occur such as antepartum haemorrhage, preterm rupture of membranes or preterm labour. Ultrasound studies will confirm the diagnosis, which may also be established by fetal heart rate monitoring of both fetuses simultaneously, although the latter investigation can be difficult to interpret.

The most important hazard for the surviving twin in monochorionic twin pregnancies is neurological abnormality, which occurs in about 26% of cases (Fusi & Gordon 1990). The cause is unknown but may be due to disseminated intravascular coagulation secondary to thromboplastin from the dead twin entering the circulation of the surviving twin via transplacental anastomoses. Alternatively, sudden changes in fetoplacental haemodynamics at the time of death of one twin may cause disturbances of blood flow in regional circulations of the surviving twin (Benirschke & Kaufmann 1990).

When fetal death occurs in one twin, there is also the risk of disseminated intravascular coagulation occurring in the mother (Romero et al 1984). As in singleton fetal death in utero, it appears that retention of the dead twin for 3–4 weeks is required before maternal disseminated intravascular coagulation occurs. Although Landy & Weingold (1989) estimated the risk of maternal coagulation defects to be 25%, this may be an overestimate (Fusi & Gordon 1990).

Spontaneous preterm delivery is common after death of one twin and not uncommonly elective preterm delivery is indicated for a deterioration of the condition of the mother or the surviving twin. However it has yet to be demonstrated that after fetal death in utero of one twin, delivery of the other twin soon afterwards by elective Caesarean section with a view to improving its chances for survival will lead to any significant improvement in outcome. In some cases brain damage or maldevelopment is likely to have occurred before a decision to deliver can be made, and in those cases where delivery of a very immature fetus occurs, the prognosis is poor.

In the largest reported single study of antepartum loss of a twin with survival of the other twin ($n = 25$),

Sonneveld & Correy (1992) found that there was a higher risk of associated maternal hypertension, antepartum and postpartum haemorrhage and retained placenta compared with the general population of pregnant women. The major risks to the surviving twin were prematurity and low birthweight. Vaginal delivery was achieved in 80% of surviving twins, similar to the method of delivery of all twins during the study period. The authors concluded that the results of their study and those of others reported in the literature support conservative management of this complication during pregnancy.

If fetal death occurs in one of dichorionic twins the conservative approach to management is warranted. In the case of fetal death in one of monochorionic twins, early intervention to deliver may be indicated to avoid the death of the surviving twin, although there is still a significant risk that this fetus will have brain damage. Parents should be given a guarded prognosis.

After preterm rupture of membranes and expulsion of one twin early in pregnancy, the conservative management of the pregnancy including prophylactic antibiotic therapy can be successful in improving the chances of survival of the remaining twin. The time interval between the births of the fetuses has been reported to be as long as 21 days and growth of the fetus retained in utero is often better as a consequence of expulsion of one of the twins (Long et al 1991).

Twin–twin transfusion syndrome

The incidence of the twin–twin transfusion syndrome is 5–15% in twin pregnancies (Naeye 1992). Traditionally it has been attributed to unequal shunting of blood from one twin to the other through placental anastomotic vascular channels (usually artery-to-vein) between the two fetal circulations. This has led to the hypothesis that uteroplacental insufficiency leads to increased peripheral resistance in the placental circulation of the donor twin thereby promoting the shunting of blood to the recipient twin through the fetal vascular anastomoses that are invariably present. The recipient twin reduces the resulting excess fluid by increasing urine production. Consequently polyhydramnios occurs and as the cellular and protein components remain in the fetal circulation, an increase in osmotic pressure causes water to move from the maternal compartment across the placenta into the fetal circulation. Thus a vicious cycle of fetal fluid volume overload and diuresis is established. Polyhydramnios, by increasing intrauterine pressure, would tend to further compromise the placental circulation. Under these circumstances the donor twin becomes anaemic and growth retarded while its amniotic sac shows oligohydramnios due to fetal oliguria. In contrast, the recipient twin becomes plethoric, grows larger and is surrounded by an excess of amniotic fluid, largely because of increased urinary excretion. Ultimately the recipient fetus develops hypertension, congestive cardiac failure and becomes hydropic. A common end-result is the fetal death in utero of one or both twins. When one twin dies before the other, there is some risk of disseminated intravascular coagulation occurring in the surviving fetus (Romero et al 1984). Development of the twin–twin transfusion syndrome in the middle trimester of pregnancy is often associated with preterm labour and delivery and 80% of twins die (Gonsoulin et al 1990).

Recently it has been suggested that velamentous insertion of the umbilical cords, which is more common in monochorionic diamniotic twin gestations, may promote compression of the cord vessels thereby obstructing both umbilical arterial and venous blood flow and leading to a circuit that potentiates twin–twin transfusion (Fries et al 1993).

Classically the twin–twin transfusion syndrome is diagnosed postnatally and is based upon a discordance of more than 15% or 20% in weights of the twin infants and a haemoglobin difference of greater than 5 g/dl, with the smaller twin being anaemic. Obviously this postnatal diagnosis is merely a presumptive one as it does not allow any conclusion to be reached about the antenatal in vivo haemodynamic situation. Nevertheless for clinical purposes, these postnatal characteristics have been extrapolated to the antenatal period: ultrasound examination is used to detect fetal weight discordance and cordocentesis is sometimes used to obtain fetal blood samples to detect haemoglobin and haematocrit differences. However, fetal blood sampling by cordocentesis has recently shown that haemoglobin concentration is not significantly different in the affected twins (Saunders et al 1991). Moreover, when Wenstrom et al (1992) reviewed 97 pathologically proven monochorionic twin pregnancies they found that any combination of fetal weight and haemoglobin/haematocrit discordance can occur. Therefore it was concluded that fetal weight and haemoglobin/haematocrit discordance in themselves are not sufficient to diagnose twin–twin transfusion. Thorough antenatal evaluation with invasive investigations and marker studies to identify anastomotic channels of haemodynamically unbalanced type would be required to make an accurate diagnosis.

The most promising approach to management of this difficult problem is to devise some means of permanently occluding the vascular shunts between the two fetal placental circulations. Recently this has been achieved, with encouraging results, by means of fetoscopy and coagulation of the transplacental shunts in utero with a neodynium–yttrium-aluminium-garnet (Nd : YAG) laser beam (De Lia et al 1990). In the three patients with twins so treated, four of the six fetuses survived. As this technique is still in its early phase of development it requires further assessment before being introduced widely into clinical practice.

In the meantime, a less radical intervention that might be effective is that of repeated amniocenteses to reduce the excessive volume of amniotic fluid in the amniotic sac of the recipient twin. In one study of 19 twin pregnancies, initially seen before 28 weeks' gestation with acute polyhydramnios caused by the twin–twin transfusion syndrome, amniocentesis and removal of amniotic fluid were performed on an average of three times for each patient. Fourteen (37%) of the 28 infants delivered survived the neonatal period (Saunders et al 1992). An even better perinatal survival rate of 79% has been obtained by Elliott et al (1991) using essentially the same method.

Selective feticide has been suggested as an alternative therapy in twin–twin transfusion syndrome when the lives of both twins are threatened (Wittmann et al 1986). However, this is fraught with possible complications in the surviving twin, such as disseminated intravascular coagulation, cerebral ventriculomegaly and unexplained fetal death (Saunders et al 1992).

Cord entanglement

Entanglement of the umbilical cords can only occur in monoamniotic twin pregnancies: a survey of the literature reveals that up to 70% of such twins may develop this complication (Hart & Draw 1991). The umbilical cords may become twisted around each other and even knotted with multiple true knots (Fig. 19.2) or the cord of the second twin may become entangled around the neck, trunk or limbs of the first twin. As cord entanglement can be diagnosed by ultrasound scanning as early as 19 weeks' gestation, twin pregnancies suspected of being monoamniotic should be carefully and repeatedly examined ultrasonically to detect this complication. Failure to recognize cord entanglement may result in one or both fetuses dying in the antenatal or intrapartum periods. Furthermore, it is important to appreciate that continuous fetal heart rate monitoring of both twins does not always reveal abnormalities of the fetal heart rate which would indicate a cord complication.

A strong case can be made for elective Caesarean section for delivery of monoamniotic twins because of the complications with cord entanglement and fetal interlocking that may occur with vaginal delivery (Annan & Hutson 1990).

Genital tract bleeding during early pregnancy may indicate that abortion of the twin conceptus will occur. Alternatively it may, if transient, signify fetal death in utero of one of the twin fetuses with continuation of the pregnancy as a singleton one.

Fetal malformations

The frequency of malformations is nearly twice as great in twins as in singletons, with monozygotic twins being more

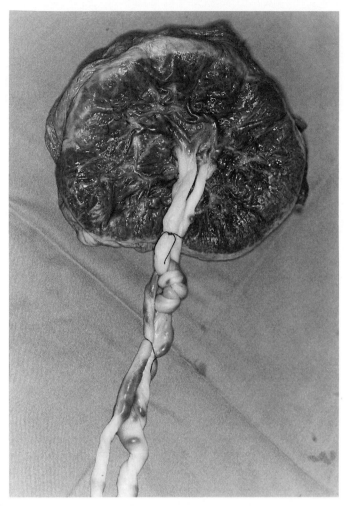

Fig. 19.2 Monoamniotic monochorionic twin placenta showing entanglement of the umbilical cords with knot formation. By courtesy of Dr Andrew Miller.

commonly affected (Kohl & Casey 1975). Onyskowova et al (1970) reported a malformation rate per baby of 1.4% for singletons, 2.7% for twins and 6.1% for triplets: both twins were affected in 14.8% of cases but there were no sets of triplets with all three babies affected. The evidence suggests that an increased incidence of aneuploidy is responsible (Rodis et al 1990).

Some malformations, such as acardia and conjoined twins, appear to be directly related to the twinning process. Furthermore, a group of midline structural birth defects including symmelia, neural tube defects and extrophy of the cloaca may be associated with the same process (Nance 1981). Other malformations, not unique to multiple pregnancy, may also occur in one or both twins.

Fetal malformations unique to multiple pregnancy

Acardia Acardia is a malformation that occurs in one of monozygotic twins or higher order multiple pregnancies with a frequency of about one in 30 000 deliveries

(Benirschke & Kim 1973). Amongst monozygotic twin pairs the incidence of acardia is one in 100. The acardia twin usually has a normally formed co-twin, and is dependent upon a reversed fetal placental circulation, receiving blood flow from the heart of the normal partner. The lower part of the body of the acardia fetus shows varying degrees of development while the cephalad pole fails to develop at all. The heart is absent (holocardia) or rudimentary cardiac tissue (pseudoacardia) only is present. The aetiology of the condition is unknown. It may be the result of a primary failure of cardiac development or atrophy of the heart secondary to passive perfusion and reversal of the circulation.

Conjoined twins When incomplete division of the germinal disc of the embryo occurs in the formation of monozygotic twins various types of conjoined twins result, often referred to as Siamese twins or double monsters. The appellation Siamese refers to a famous pair of conjoined twins, Chang and Eng Bunker, who were born in Siam in 1811 and lived for 63 years. Most of their lives were spent travelling around the world with Barnum's Circus as exhibits. They were xiphopagus twins, that is joined by a band of tissue extending from the umbilicus to the xiphoid cartilage (Harper et al 1980).

While the incidence of conjoined twins varies from one in 2800 to one in 200 000 births, most studies report an incidence of one in 50 000 (Table 19.6). Amongst monozygotic twins one set in 200 are affected (Hanson 1975). With triplets, conjoined pairs occur even more frequently (Schinzel et al 1979). The first report of conjoined twins diagnosed ultrasonographically appeared in 1977 (Fagan 1977). Prior to this the diagnosis was made radiographically during pregnancy or on examination at the time of parturition. Rees et al (1993) reported three sets of conjoined twins over a 10-month period among residents of South Glamorgan in Wales. As this area has approximately 5400 deliveries per year, it represents the highest reported incidence of conjoined twinning described so far.

The cause of conjoined abnormalities is unknown and there are no obvious predisposing factors. Polyhydramnios accompanies half the cases. The site and extent of fusion

Table 19.6 Incidence of conjoined twins (from Hanson 1975 quoted by Rees et al 1993)

Country of report	Incidence	Births (no.)
India	1 : 2800	25 000
Taiwan	1 : 6500	25 814
Rhodesia	1 : 14 000	41 826
Sweden	1 : 20 000	40 000
Atlanta	1 : 20 000	140 000
Chicago	1 : 50 000	100 000
World's literature	1 : 50 000	NA
Los Angeles	1 : 50 000	250 000
New York	1 : 166 000	3 645 622
USA	1 : 200 000	NA

are variable. When each of the conjoined twins is nearly completely separated from its fellow, the attachment is either anterior (thoracopagus), posterior (pyopagus), cephalic (craniopagus) or caudal (ischiopagus). The anterior attachment is the most common (Edmonds & Layde 1982).

The incidence of congenital heart disease is high among thoracopagus twins. Defects include a single ventricle, a common atrium, conotruncal abnormalities, endocardial cushion defects and anomalous pulmonary venous return (Noonan 1978). Nichols and colleagues (1967) found that 90% of thoracopagus twins shared a common pericardium and 75% had conjoined hearts. In addition, about 50% of conjoined twins have malformations not obviously associated with the primary junctional abnormality (Edmonds & Layde 1982).

If considerably immature, and therefore small, conjoined twins may be deliverable vaginally, but usually Caesarean section is necessary.

After delivery the conjoined twins may be separable surgically, depending upon the degree to which they share vital organs. If separation is feasible, two operating teams are required and detailed planning for the surgical procedure is essential.

Fetal malformations not unique to multiple pregnancy

Neural tube defects, particularly anencephaly and encephalocele but not spina bifida, occur more often in twins (Windham et al 1982). Hydrocephaly of the isolated type may also be increased in twins (Layde et al 1980).

A single umbilical artery is found three to four times more often in twins than in singletons (Heifetz 1984). This finding has the same implications for twins as it has for singletons, namely an increased risk (20%) of non-specific malformations.

When polyhydramnios of a persistent or chronic type accompanies twin pregnancies, fetal anomalies of one or both twins are more likely than when the amniotic fluid volume is within normal limits (Hashimoto et al 1986).

Prenatal diagnosis of fetal abnormalities

When an abnormality has been found in one of twins it is important to know the level of risk this entails for the co-twin so that the parents can make an informed decision about further management of the pregnancy. As most abnormalities are discordant, it is likely that the co-twin will be normal and that the parents will be faced with an extremely difficult decision—to opt for uninterrupted continuation of the pregnancy, termination of the entire conceptus or selective feticide.

Maternal serum alphafetoprotein. Maternal serum alphafetoprotein (AFP) screening will identify about half the women with twin pregnancies by detecting levels of AFP greater than 2.5 multiples of the median. In fact levels less than four multiples of the median can be considered as normal for twin pregnancy. When the AFP levels rise above this level more infants of low birthweight are delivered, and preterm delivery and intrauterine fetal growth retardation occur more frequently (Katz et al 1990). If the AFP level is found to be raised more than four multiples of the median in twin pregnancy, both fetuses should have careful ultrasonographic morphological scans at 18–20 weeks' gestation to exclude neural tube and other defects.

Amniocentesis. In twin gestation prenatal diagnosis is usually carried out by amniocentesis in the second trimester to obtain fetal cells from amniotic fluid for cytogenetic studies and measurement of AFP. The problem is to ensure that samples from both amniotic sacs have been obtained. Various procedures have been suggested for this purpose, including injecting a dye such as methylene blue or indigo-carmine into the first sac sampled, single needle insertion sequentially into the separate sacs under ultrasound control, and insertion of separate needles into both sacs with observation of accurate placement by ultrasound. Recent reports of jejunal atresia in fetuses exposed to methylene blue in the second trimester strongly suggest a causal relationship (Van der Pol et al 1992). It is not yet clear how the jejunal atresia is produced but as the amniotic fluid containing the dye is swallowed by the fetus its concentration in the jejunum may exert a local toxic effect, although the clinical features of jejunal atresia suggest that a vascular mechanism may be involved (Louw & Barnard 1955). Therefore the use of all dyes in diagnostic amniocenteses should be avoided, especially now that direct ultrasound guidance suffices.

The safety and reliability of genetic amniocentesis in twin pregnancy has been demonstrated by a study in Rotterdam involving 83 twin pregnancies (Pijpers et al 1988). In 77 (93%) of these both amniotic sacs were successfully sampled: in the other six women the second amniotic sac was not accessible or there was only one amniotic cavity. The total fetal loss within 4 weeks of the amniocentesis was 1.2% and the perinatal mortality rate 55 per 1000 births. This is even lower than in twin pregnancies in which no amniocentesis had been performed.

Amniotic fluid AFP measurement may not be reliable for diagnosis because of the possible difficulties in interpreting the result. Although amniotic fluid can be collected from each amniotic sac without much difficulty, it is important to appreciate that AFP can diffuse between amniotic sacs, particularly in diamniotic monochorionic twin pregnancy thereby leading to possible errors in diagnosis. One fetus may have a neural tube defect while the fetus occupying the adjoining sac may be normal, yet high levels of AFP may be found in both sacs (Duncan et al 1977).

Chorion villus sampling Chorion villus sampling (CVS) in the late first trimester in multiple pregnancies is fraught with technical problems, including that of ensuring that the samples collected are representative of each fetus. Brambati et al (1991) reported on CVS for prenatal diagnosis in 65 women with twins and one with quadruplets. Transabdominal or transcervical CVS under ultrasound guidance was performed in the majority at 9–12 weeks' gestation. Dichorionic pregnancy was predicted ultrasonically when either two distinct placental sites were seen or in cases where the placentae appeared fused, the septal thickness was 2 mm or more. At this stage of gestation ultrasound diagnosis of fetal genital morphology is unreliable. If like-sex dichorionic twins were diagnosed from two different chorionic tissue specimens, cytogenetic DNA polymorphisms were evaluated to prove that separate fetuses had been sampled. When the samples could not be differentiated by this means, later amniocentesis was performed to establish a diagnosis. All monochorionic twin pairs were regarded as monozygotic and therefore a single sample of chorionic tissue was considered sufficient. However, dichorionicity was not helpful in assessing zygosity and each placenta was sampled to avoid missing information. These investigators found that CVS was successful in over 98% of the cases and no failures were reported after a second sampling. In eight of 29 pregnancies with like-sex fetuses the cytogenetic/DNA polymorphism evaluation was not helpful in differentiating between the twin fetuses, and these women underwent amniocentesis at 15 weeks' gestation to confirm the CVS results. The overall resampling rate was 12%.

A prospective study of the relative risks and accuracy of first-trimester CVS and second-trimester amniocentesis in the genetic evaluation of twin pregnancies was carried out in Philadelphia between 1984 and 1990. Of 81 women who had amniocentesis, nine also had previous CVS and 152 women had CVS alone. All fetuses in both groups were sampled and karyotyped successfully. From the time of sampling until the 28th week of pregnancy loss of the entire pregnancy followed amniocentesis in 2.9% of cases and CVS in 3.2%. The total fetal loss rate of 9.3% following amniocentesis was not significantly different from that (4.9%) following CVS. Both of these studies have shown that in the hands of the skilled operator CVS is at least as safe and effective as amniocentesis for prenatal diagnosis investigation of twin pregnancy (Wapner et al 1993).

Cordocentesis to collect fetal blood samples for genetic studies carries a greater risk of fetal complications than does amniocentesis. Furthermore, it may be difficult to differentiate one umbilical cord from the other even with ultrasound visualization, especially in cases of monochorionic monoamniotic twin pregnancies when cord entanglement may be present.

INTRAPARTUM MANAGEMENT OF TWIN PREGNANCY

Because of the high-risk nature of multiple pregnancy and delivery, all such pregnancies should be managed in a tertiary level hospital with neonatal intensive care facilities. An operating theatre should be available for immediate Caesarean section if required and a skilled anaesthetist should be available at all times during labour and delivery in case urgent operative intervention is necessary.

Fetal presentations

In a serial ultrasonographic study of 119 twin pregnancies (of mean duration of 37 weeks and mean birthweight 2640 g) the rate of spontaneous version was found to decrease significantly as gestational age increased, but remained relatively high (25–30%) even at term. This spontaneous version rate is considerably higher than the 5% cephalic version reported in singleton breech presentations at term (Westgren et al 1985). Of patients who have both twins presenting cephalically, very few will experience any changes in fetal position and presentation. All other fetal presentations are relatively unstable and spontaneous versions are likely at any time up to term. However, the presenting twin is less likely than the second twin to undergo spontaneous version. Because of the high rate of spontaneous version during the third trimester in twin pregnancies, the final decision regarding mode of delivery should be decided at the onset of labour (Divon et al 1993).

The changes in fetal presentation throughout pregnancy were studied in 332 sets of twins by serial ultrasound examinations (Santolaya et al 1992). The incidence of non-vertex presentations for the first twin decreased from 41% at 15–20 weeks to 19% at 35–38 weeks. When the first twin was a vertex presentation, the incidence of a non-vertex second twin decreased from 50.8% at 15–20 weeks to 40.4% at 35–38 weeks. The total number of pregnancies in which either twin was non-vertex also decreased from 90.3% to 59.55 at term. The most common presentations near term were vertex–vertex (40%) which were much less frequent earlier in gestation (8% at 15–20 weeks). If the first twin presented by the vertex, the chances of vertex–vertex presentations increased from 26 weeks onwards. There was a steady decrease in the incidence of transverse lie of the first twin with advancing gestational age. Thus it is now possible to predict the chance of Caesarean section for malpresentation(s) alone at different gestational ages in twin pregnancies.

Labour at term

When both twins are presenting cephalically and are appropriate in size for gestation and there are no other maternal or fetal complications, vaginal delivery can be anticipated. Labour may occur spontaneously or may be induced; the reasons for the latter usually being term (40 weeks) or fetal growth retardation in one or both twins. Prolongation of twin pregnancy beyond 40 weeks may be a fetal hazard because of the risk of fetal hypoxia, although as mentioned earlier there are no adequate data to support this hypothesis. Nevertheless, many obstetricians advocate induction of labour in twin pregnancies between 37 and 40 weeks.

During labour, both fetal heart rates should be continuously and simultaneously monitored by means of a scalp electrode applied to the first twin and an external maternal abdominal wall ultrasound transducer for the second twin. Should fetal heart rate abnormalities appear in the cardiotocographic tracing of the first twin, collection of a fetal scalp blood sample for pH measurement may be helpful. Fetal acidosis would indicate immediate delivery by Caesarean section. Otherwise the labour could be allowed to progress normally. If fetal heart rate abnormalities occur in the second twin before the cervix has reached full dilatation, delivery of both twins by Caesarean section is indicated. When uterine inertia is responsible for slow progress of labour, augmentation of uterine contractility with Syntocinon is warranted.

Pain relief in labour is best achieved by epidural anaesthesia, which also has the advantage of permitting manipulative procedures, if required, for delivery of the second twin (Jarvis & Whitfield 1981).

After delivery of the first twin, the umbilical cord is ligated and divided. The lie and presentation of the second twin should be determined by ultrasound imaging but if this is not immediately available, by abdominal palpation and vaginal examination. During the latter, care should be taken not to rupture the membranes until the presenting part has descended well into the pelvis, otherwise cord prolapse or a malpresentation of the fetus may result.

Usually after delivery of the first twin there is a transient reduction in uterine contractility. Occasionally stimulation of uterine activity with Syntocinon is required at this time to facilitate engagement of the presenting part and delivery of the second twin. If the second twin is lying obliquely or transversely an attempt at external cephalic version may be successful in bringing about a longitudinal lie so that the fetal head or breech presents.

After return of uterine contractility and descent of the fetal head or breech into the pelvis, the membranes can be ruptured artificially and the fetus delivered vaginally. In the case of the fetus presenting cephalically, spontaneous delivery can be awaited unless fetal distress develops when immediate forceps delivery is indicated.

The time interval between delivery of the first and second twins is variable and as long as continuous fetal heart rate monitoring of the second twin shows no abnormality, interference to expedite delivery is not required (Cetrulo et al 1980, Rayburn et al 1984). In the study of Rayburn and colleagues (1984) the mean interval between delivery of twins was 21 minutes although it ranged from 1 to 134 minutes. In those babies delivered after the 21-minute period, there was no evidence of depression of fetal vital centres nor was excessive trauma evident.

If external cephalic version is unsuccessful in achieving a longitudinal lie of the second twin, internal podalic version and breech extraction should be carried out unless the operator is inexperienced with this procedure, when early recourse to Caesarean section is the alternative. Several studies have now confirmed that for infants weighing more than 1500 g at delivery, vaginal delivery of the non-vertex second twin is a safe intrapartum management option. No statistically significant difference in perinatal mortality or morbidity has been found when comparing non-vertex second twins delivered vaginally with those delivered by Caesarean section (Adam et al 1991, Davison et al 1992, Fishman et al 1993). Rabinovici et al (1988) have drawn attention to the advantages of performing internal podalic version and breech extraction of the second twin through unruptured membranes. Under epidural or general anaesthesia in the operating theatre set up for Caesarean section, the fetal feet are palpated through the intact membranes and grasped. Gentle continuous traction is applied to the fetal feet while the operator gently manipulates the fetal head towards the uterine fundus with the other hand externally placed on the maternal abdominal wall. The membranes are kept intact for as long as possible after the fetal lie has been corrected to a longitudinal one, and the traction is continued until delivery is achieved.

When the cervix closes and partially reconstitutes itself after delivery of the first twin, Caesarean section may be the most appropriate mode of delivery.

Amnioinfusion of normal saline into the amniotic sacs of three labouring women with twin gestations complicated by oligohydramnios was described by Strong et al (1993). All the twins were delivered safely per vaginam.

Elective Caesarean section

When the first (leading) twin presents other than by the vertex, Caesarean section appears to be the method of choice for delivery (Chervenak 1986). External cephalic version would be difficult and there would also be a risk of interlocking of the heads of the twins should labour occur.

Previous Caesarean section

Multiple pregnancy occurring in a woman who has previously had a Caesarean section is an uncommon complication. In a recent Sheffield study, 25 cases of multiple pregnancy occurred in women with a lower uterine segment scar during the 11-year period 1975–85. The Caesarean section rate in this group of women increased from 20% in the first 6 years to 70% in the latter years for no obvious reason. This change in management did not improve fetal outcome. Analysis of the individual cases and a review of the literature suggested that multiple pregnancy is not in itself an indication for elective repeat Caesarean section (Gilbert et al 1988).

Preterm labour

Particularly during preterm labour twins are exposed to an increased risk of placental abruption, cord prolapse, dystocia, hypoxia and problems related to malpresentation. These factors are all associated with an increased rate of perinatal mortality. Consequently, Caesarean section has been advocated for delivery of twins when both twins fail to present by the vertex, for preterm breech presentations, and for twins of very low birthweight (< 1500 g). Some clinicians have expressed the view that Caesarean section is indicated for all twin deliveries in the interests of the second twin (Ware 1971). However, a major Swedish study on 9368 low birthweight twins (< 2500 g) revealed that despite a dramatic increase in the Caesarean section rate between 1973 and 1985 from 7–10% to 45–50% with a concomitant sharp decrease in perinatal mortality, no correlation was found between these two variables. Factors other than the mode of delivery had a greater impact on fetal outcome (Rydhström et al 1990).

Spontaneous preterm labour occurs in 30% of twin pregnancies, and is most common in association with monozygotic twins (Hall 1985). The administration of tocolytic agents has some benefit in delaying labour long enough to allow the patient to be transferred to a centre with neonatal intensive care facilities, should these be required (King et al 1985).

At one Australian high-risk perinatal centre over a 9-year period, 103% of 124 sets of liveborn twins with gestational ages less than 33 weeks were delivered vaginally. In this cohort, in-hospital mortality and morbidity were statistically independent of the mode of delivery (Doyle et al 1988).

Recent trends suggest that elective Caesarean section for delivery of all women with twin pregnancies of less than 36 weeks' gestation is being abandoned in favour of vaginal delivery.

Occasionally, uterine contractility ceases after delivery of the first twin, especially in very premature labours. Under these circumstances a policy of non-intervention may achieve a gestational age for the remaining fetus(es) such that neonatal survival and outlook are improved. Management entails ligation and division of the umbilical cord of the delivered fetus as high as possible under aseptic conditions, antibiotic therapy if indicated by culture of high vaginal swabs, prophylactic tocolysis, and maternal administration of corticosteroids. Cervical cerclage does not appear to improve the duration of pregnancy. Interestingly, the retained placenta does not seem to have adverse effects on blood clotting. If this conservative regimen is implemented, the patient should remain in bed in hospital, and be very carefully watched for evidence of intrauterine infection and vaginal blood loss (Poeschmann et al 1992).

Locked twins

Fortunately locked twins are rare. In this complication, the aftercoming head of the first twin, presenting by the breech, is prevented from entering the pelvis by the presenting head of the second twin. Usually the diagnosis is not made until the second stage of labour. In these circumstances it may be possible under general anaesthesia to manually push the head of the second twin out of the maternal pelvis, thereby allowing the aftercoming head of the first twin to enter the pelvis and be delivered manually by the Mauriceau–Smellie–Veit procedure or by forceps extraction. Thereafter, the second twin can be delivered normally or with the assistance of forceps. Alternatively, under general anaesthesia, the head of the second twin may be extracted past the first with Kjelland's forceps, followed by delivery of the first twin using the customary methods. If the first twin dies of asphyxia, decapitation of this fetus would allow its body to be delivered vaginally, followed by delivery of the living second twin and lastly retrieval of the head of the first twin. However, many obstetricians have no experience of decapitation and it might be safer for the mother under these circumstances if Caesarean section was performed.

If locked twins are diagnosed early in labour and both are alive, Caesarean section is the best method of delivery.

The third stage of labour

The third stage of labour is more likely to be complicated by haemorrhage from the extensive placental site. Often uterine atony is a predisposing factor. Therefore a prophylactic intramuscular injection of 10 international units of oxytocin is indicated immediately after delivery of the second twin.

POSTPARTUM MANAGEMENT OF MULTIPLE PREGNANCY

During the puerperium the parturient is at risk of complications similar to those experienced by mothers of singleton infants. However fatigue and emotional depression may be prominent features, probably due to the psychological and physical stresses associated with looking after more than one infant. Hence there is much to be said for mothers of twins and higher order multiple infants remaining in hospital for a longer period of time in the puerperium to allow adequate rest and to increase their confidence in mothercraft.

When one twin is lost at some stage during the pregnancy the birth of the surviving twin is usually accompanied by a mixed emotional response; elation with the advent of a new member of the family and grief for the twin that died. In fact the parental response to antenatal loss of a twin is similar to that experienced after loss of a singleton pregnancy (Sonneveld & Correy 1992). Skilled psychological counselling and emotional support for affected parents is often required in the puerperium.

PERINATAL MORTALITY AND MORBIDITY AND BIRTHWEIGHT

Perinatal mortality and morbidity

Although twins represent only 2% of live births, they account for approximately 10% of perinatal deaths. In addition, infant death rates among twins are estimated to be 4–10 times those of singleton births. During 1983–84, birth cohorts from the National Center for Health Statistics in the United States were used to identify maternal and infant characteristics related to twin infant mortality: 41 554 white and 10 062 black liveborn matched twin pairs were evaluated. Approximately two-thirds of the twin pairs were of like-sex in both racial groups. Half the white twins and two-thirds of the black twins were of low birthweight (< 2500 g) whereas 9% of white and 16% of black twins were of very low birthweight (< 1500 g). These data were in sharp contrast to national data regarding singleton births in which only about 5% of white and 11% of black singleton babies were in the low birthweight category and only 1% of white and 2% of black singleton babies were of very low birthweight. Among both white and black twins, there were more low and very low birthweight babies among the second-born twins. Overall infant mortality rates for white and black twins were 47.1 and 79.3 per 1000 live births, respectively. These rates are approximately five times those for white and black singletons. Three-quarters of infant twin deaths in both races occurred in the very low birthweight category. Four-fifths of white and three-quarters of black twins died in the neonatal period (0–27 days). White like-sex twins had about twice the risk of both twins dying compared with unlike-sex twins. Similarly, white twin pairs with > 25% birthweight disparity had a 40–80% increased risk of both twins dying compared with twins whose weights were within 10% of each other. Twins born to high-risk women, on the basis of demographic factors, were twice as likely to die as twins born to low-risk women. Clearly much of the high infant mortality among twins is associated with consequences of very low birthweight. Thus the challenge is to develop strategies that will reduce the number of preterm and growth-retarded twins, particularly in high-risk mothers (Fowler et al 1991).

Birthweight

As the duration of multiple pregnancy decreases so does the birthweight. About 50% of all twins weigh less than 2500 g at birth (Powers 1973). Retarded fetal growth and prematurity are both important causes of low birthweight in multiple pregnancies. After 24 weeks' gestation, the growth of fetuses in multiple pregnancies is often found to be impaired on serial ultrasound scans compared with the growth of the fetus in a singleton pregnancy.

Data from the Oxford Twin Survey (Corney et al 1972) and the Louisville Twin Study (Wilson 1976) show that among dizygotic twins the birthweight correlations for like-sex twins are higher than for those of unlike sex. Moreover, the lowest correlations occur in monozygotic twins. When data from the Oxford study are analysed to reveal the effect of placentation it is then apparent that the lower birthweight correlation for monozygotic twins is associated with monochorionic placentation and is presumably the consequence of shared placental circulation. Dichorionic monozygotic twins have a higher birthweight correlation than dizygotic twins but the difference is small. A comparison of birthweights of dichorionic monozygotic twins with those of like-sex dizygotic twins suggests that the variation in birthweight attributable to fetal genotype is about 8%. In the case of monozygotic co-twins, the maternal and fetal genotypes, parity, maternal age, past environmental influences on the mother and present environmental influences on mother and fetus should be identical. Therefore, any variation in birthweight of the co-twins must be the result of differences in the local intrauterine environment. The birthweight correlation for dichorionic monozygotic twins is 0.76, indicating that local intrauterine factors account for some 24% of birthweight variation (Robson 1978).

In the USA the proportion of multiple births has risen rapidly during the last decade, yet as a proportion of total births it is relatively small. The majority of infants born of multiple pregnancies have low (< 2500 g) or very low birthweights (< 1500 g) which increase their risks of developing short- and long-term complications. The relative risks of low birthweight are 10.3-fold and 18.8-fold, of very low birthweight 9.6-fold and 32.7-fold and infant mortality 6.6-fold and 19.4-fold higher in twins and triplets respectively compared with singletons. Furthermore, among postneonatal survivors the relative risks of severe handicap are 1.7-fold and 2.9-fold and for overall handicap 1.4-fold and 2.0-fold higher among twins and triplets, respectively, than among singletons (Luke & Keith 1992). Consideration of weight and gestational age-specific morbidity and mortality, however, reveals that twins of very low birthweight do not suffer greater morbidity or mortality than do singletons of comparable birthweight and gestational age, and actually develop less bronchopulmonary dysplasia (Wolf et al 1992).

Maternal weight gains during twin pregnancies of 18–20 kg (40–45 lb) are associated with highest birthweights among infants (Brown & Schloesser 1990). A higher birthweight of twins has an immediate and long-term benefit for the child, the family and society. Hence antenatal interventions aimed at improving fetal growth are advocated. Such interventions include early and comprehensive antenatal care, reduction of physical effort to decrease the likelihood of preterm delivery and increased dietary awareness to ensure adequate weight gain. However, Lawrence et al (1991) found in their study of urban Scottish housewives that women who gained more fat during pregnancy did not give birth to heavier babies. Therefore, increasing energy intake may do nothing more than increase maternal fat deposition. In this regard a recent study indicates that despite large weight gains during pregnancy, mothers of twins return to their pregravid weight within the first few years after delivery (Luke et al 1991).

GENETIC STUDIES

Twins share a common environment in utero, and although monozygotic twins are genetically identical, dizygotic twins are no more alike than any other pair of siblings. This provides the basis for studying twins to determine the genetic contribution in various disorders, by comparing the rates of concordance or discordance for a particular trait between pairs of monozygotic and dizygotic twins. The rate of concordance in monozygotic twins is high for disorders in which genetic predisposition plays a major role in the aetiology of the disease. The phenotypic variability of genetic traits can be studied in monozygotic twins and the effects of a shared environment can be studied in dizygotic twins (Kingston 1990).

Concordance is said to exist if both members of a twin pair either have or do not have the trait in question. Discordance is present when only one of the twins has the trait. Investigations usually involve comparisons of concordance versus discordance in monozygotic twins, concordance rates in monozygotic versus dizygotic twins, monozygotic twins in specific environments, and monozygotic twins reared apart versus those reared together.

SUBSEQUENT DEVELOPMENT OF TWINS

Each fetus delivered from a multifetal pregnancy is at some disadvantage compared with the fetus of a singleton pregnancy. Quite apart from the hazards of the newborn period, those twins who survive, especially the smaller of the two, have a greater risk of physical, intellectual or psychological handicap. The smaller twin at birth usually remains smaller throughout life. When there is a large difference in size of fetuses at birth these differences become less later in childhood (Wilson 1979).

In a Norwegian study, 56 male twins born in 1962–63 were followed up at 18 years of age at drafting for military service. Of this group of twins, 14.4% were unfit for military service compared with 6.2% of the total population of Norwegian conscripts in the same year. This finding was attributed to preterm delivery rather than to twinning per se. There was a higher incidence of impaired vision in the preterm twins than in the total group of conscripts, and again this was related to preterm birth. The general intelligence of the twins, measured by standardized tests, did not differ significantly from the control group (Nilsen et al 1984).

TRIPLET, QUADRUPLET AND HIGHER ORDER MULTIPLE PREGNANCY

In higher order multiple pregnancies, the number of ova fertilized and twinning of one or more of these with possible loss of one or more embryos will explain the ultimate number of fetuses carried throughout pregnancy and delivered. Multiple ovulation stimulated by maternal administration of gonadotrophin or clomiphene has resulted in as many as seven fetuses in the one pregnancy (Hamilton et al 1976).

Pregnancies with three or more fetuses are characterized by problems similar to those of twin pregnancies, albeit usually intensified. While vaginal delivery of the first fetus often occurs normally when the spontaneous onset of labour is awaited, malpresentations of subsequent fetuses are common, especially as labour often commences well before term. To avoid difficult manipulative obstetric procedures with the risk of inflicting trauma on the fetuses and to diminish the risk of fetal asphyxia caused by cord complications or early placental separation, Caesarean section is the recommended mode of delivery. Vaginal delivery should be reserved for those women with complications that would render operative delivery hazardous or when very small immature fetuses have to be delivered.

In the USA, a recent population-based study of high-order multiple births (triplets and higher orders) born during the years 1983–85 showed that their mortality rate was about 15 times that of singletons. This was largely due to the lower birthweight distribution of infants of high-order multiple births. Their weight-specific mortality compared favourably with that of singletons (Kiely et al 1992).

Ron-El et al (1992) reported on the management

and outcome of 37 triplet, seven quadruplet and two quintuplet pregnancies delivered in Tel Aviv during the years 1970–84. Management included bed rest, administration of beta-mimetic agents for tocolysis, selective cervical cerclage, and maternal administration of dexamethasone to improve fetal lung maturity. Fifty-four per cent of the deliveries were by Caesarean section, the remainder being vaginal deliveries. The mean weight of the neonates was 1809 g for the triplets, 1837 g for the quadruplets and 1284 g for the quintuplets. Seventy-eight per cent of the babies were delivered prematurely. The total perinatal mortality rate was 14.8% but for babies delivered after 28 weeks' gestation it was 9.4%. There was no statistically significant difference in the outcome for triplets born vaginally or by Caesarean section. The rates of small-for-dates (below 10th percentile) babies were 15.2% for triplets, 12.6% for quadruplets and 17.3% for quintuplets. Pre-eclampsia developed in 15% of patients, while 21.7% had haemoglobin levels less than 10 g/dl. Preterm rupture of the membranes occurred in 13% of patients with latent periods between 8 and 12 days before delivery. Subsequent to the introduction of a neonatal intensive care unit in 1976, the total perinatal mortality fell to 10.3% between 1976 and 1984. For the same period, the perinatal mortality in the group delivered after 28 weeks' gestation fell to 4.4%. The improvement observed was largely due to a reduction in neonatal deaths from hyaline membrane disease and cerebral haemorrhage (Ron-El et al 1992).

In a series of 10 quadruplet pregnancies reported from Phoenix, Arizona, pregnancy-induced hypertension developed in nine and was the indication for delivery in seven. Although the mean gestational age at delivery was 32.5 weeks, there were no perinatal deaths or long-term morbidity. In discussing their management regimen, the authors emphasized the importance they placed on prophylactic administration of low-dose aspirin, home monitoring of uterine contractility, use of terbutaline pump tocolysis, and bed rest at home commencing at 16 weeks' gestation (Elliott & Radin 1992).

SELECTIVE FETICIDE

High-order multiple pregnancies are fraught with maternal and fetal hazards including hyperemesis gravidarum, anaemia, pregnancy-induced hypertension, polyhydramnios, malpresentations, cord accidents, operative delivery, postpartum haemorrhage, thrombophlebitis, increased perinatal morbidity and mortality associated with extreme prematurity, handicapped infants and the social, financial and emotional stresses consequent upon rearing an unexpectedly large number of children.

Selective feticide, by reducing the number of fetuses, theoretically allows continuation of the pregnancy with less risks. Boulot and colleagues (1993) in France per-

formed selective feticide in 61 multiple pregnancies (37 triplets, 18 quadruplets, five quintuplets and one heptuplets) before 13 weeks' gestation with the aim of reducing most to twins. Two methods were used: the first was transcervical perforation of the gestation sac followed by crushing of the embryo contained therein, and the second involved percutaneous maternal abdominal wall puncture of the uterus, gestation sac and embryo followed by intracardiac or pericardiac injection of potassium chloride or hypertonic sodium chloride. The choice of fetuses for termination was based upon technical accessibility. Antibiotic prophylaxis was used in most cases. After the procedure, 54 twins, four singletons and three triplets resulted. The rate of unplanned fetal loss was 13% and was related to the number of suppressed fetuses. The preterm labour rate was 56.6% and the mean gestation at delivery 35.6 weeks. A comparison with published data indicated that selective feticide reduced the rate of preterm labour in high-order multiple pregnancies. The perinatal mortality rate of surviving fetuses was 10.8%. The authors concluded that selective feticide reduces the risk of, but does not entirely prevent, preterm labour and that it is of value in pregnancies with more than three fetuses and should also be considered for triplet pregnancies.

Selective feticide carries small risks, not yet quantified, of complete termination of the entire pregnancy and of unintentional permanent damage to one or more of the surviving fetuses. When successful it avoids both, which is most important for those parents who have planned and wanted the pregnancy and who would have opted for complete termination of the pregnancy had selective feticide not been available. Because the procedure enables parents to achieve the goal of having their own child, and reduces the risks to mothers and surviving fetuses of serious complications during pregnancy and delivery, a good ethical argument can be made for it.

Selective feticide is, however, a new technique. Its place in obstetric practice has yet to be determined. In spite of encouraging reports of its success (Berkowitz et al 1988, Wapner et al 1990, Boulot et al 1993, Evans et al 1993, Tabsh 1993) with a low incidence of complications to mothers and the remaining fetuses in the uterus, it is still too early to be confident about its safety. However, a recent multicentre report on the safety and efficacy of transabdominal multifetal pregnancy reduction in the management of iatrogenic and spontaneous multifetal pregnancies has confirmed that it is an efficient and safe method for improving the outcome of quadruplet and higher order multiple pregnancies and probably that of triplets (Evans et al 1993). Nevertheless, in multiple pregnancies resulting from treatment of infertility, where all fetuses appear normal on ultrasonography, it is still difficult to decide which particular fetuses should have their existence terminated. For example it might only be discovered later in pregnancy or at birth that one or more of the fetuses not selected for termination had some unexpected abnormality. Another possible hazard is the monozygotic twin pregnancy in which there is an anastomosis between the two fetal circulations in the placenta. Under these circumstances, the injection of a substance into the circulation of one fetus may gain access to that of the other. While naturally conceived monozygotic twins are much less common than dizygotic twins and rare as the result of treatment for infertility, this hazard must be considered before selective feticide is carried out.

Obviously, it would be better to prevent multifetal pregnancies in infertility programmes by improved methods of induction of ovulation and a reduction in the number of embryos transferred to the uterus after in vitro fertilization, rather than having to rely on selective feticide to solve such problems.

The ethical issues associated with selective feticide are many and complex but well discussed by Evans et al (1988). Legally, selective feticide may be viewed differently from abortion as the intention is for the pregnancy to continue. Therefore, it is unlikely that existing abortion laws would be applicable to selective feticide. Practitioners would be well advised to seek a legal opinion before using the procedure in their own jurisdictions.

REFERENCES

Adam C, Allen A C, Baskett T F 1991 Twin delivery: influence of the presentation and method of delivery on the second twin. American Journal of Obstetrics and Gynecology 165: 23–27

Annan B, Hutson R C 1990 Double survival despite cord entwinement in monoamniotic twins. Case report. British Journal of Obstetrics and Gynaecology 97: 950–951

Arnold L 1912 Adult human ovaries with follicles containing several oocytes. Anatomical Records 6: 413–422

Ashworth M F, Spooner S F, Verkuyl D A, Waterman R, Ashurst H M 1990 Failure to prevent preterm labour and delivery in twin pregnancy using prophylactic oral salbutamol. British Journal of Obstetrics and Gynaecology 97: 878–882

Azubuike J C 1982 Multiple births in Igbo women. British Journal of Obstetrics and Gynaecology 89: 77–79

Azuma C, Saji F, Takemura M et al 1992 Triplet pregnancy involving complete hydatidiform mole and two fetuses: genetic analysis by deoxyribonucleic acid fingerprint. American Journal of Obstetrics and Gynecology 166: 664–667

Barss V A, Benacerraf B R, Frigoletto F D 1985 Ultrasonographic determination of chorion type in twin gestation. Obstetrics and Gynecology 66: 779–783

Benirschke K 1974 Chimerism and mosaicism—two different entities. In: Wynn R M (ed) Obstetrics and gynecology annual. Appleton, New York, p 33

Benirschke K, Kim C K 1973 Multiple pregnancy. New England Journal of Medicine 288: 1329–1336

Benirschke K, Kaufmann P 1990 Pathology of the human placenta. Springer Verlag, New York, pp 636–732

Benson R C 1991 Multiple pregnancy. In: Pernoll M L (ed) Current obstetric and gynecologic diagnosis and treatment, 7th edn. Appleton and Lange, Prentice Hall, New Jersey, ch 16, pp 352–363

Berkowitz R L, Lynch L, Chitkara U, Wilkins I A, Mehalek K E, Alvarez E 1988 Selective reduction of multifetal pregnancies in the first trimester. New England Journal of Medicine 318: 1043–1047

Blake G D, Knuppel R A, Ingardia C J, Lake M, Aumann G, Hanson M 1984 Evaluation of nonstress testing in multiple gestations. Obstetrics and Gynecology 63: 528–532

Blumenfeld Z, Dirnfeld M, Abramovici H, Amit A, Bronshtein M, Brandes J M 1992 Spontaneous fetal reduction in multiple gestations assessed by transvaginal ultrasound. British Journal of Obstetrics and Gynaecology 99: 333–337

Botting B H, McDonald-Davies I, McFarlane A J 1987 Recent trends in the incidence of multiple births and associated mortality. Archives of Diseases of Childhood 62: 941–950

Boulot P, Hedon B, Pelliccia G et al 1993 Multifetal pregnancy reduction: a consecutive series of 61 cases. British Journal of Obstetrics and Gynaecology 100: 63–68

Bracken M B, Brighton L A, Hayashi K 1984 Epidemiology of hydatidiform mole and choriocarcinoma. Epidemiological Reviews 6: 52–75

Brambati B, Tului L, Lanzani A, Simoni G, Travi M 1991 First-trimester genetic diagnosis in multiple pregnancy: principles and potential pitfalls. Prenatal Diagnosis 11: 767–774

Brown J E, Schloesser P T 1990 Pre-pregnancy weight status, prenatal weight gain and the outcome of term twin gestations. American Journal of Obstetrics and Gynecology 162: 182–186

Campbell D M 1986 In: Creasy R K and Warshaw J B (eds) Maternal adaptation in twin pregnancy. Seminars in Perinatology 10: 14–18

Campbell D M, Campbell A, MacGillivray I 1974 Maternal characteristics of women having twin pregnancies. Journal of Biosocial Science 6: 463–470

Caspi E, Ronen J, Schreyer P, Goldberg M D 1976 The outcome of pregnancy after gonadotrophin therapy. British Journal of Obstetrics and Gynaecology 83: 967–973

Cetrulo C L, Ingardia C J, Sbarra A J 1980 Management of multiple gestations. Clinical Obstetrics and Gynecology 23: 533–548

Chervenak F A 1986 In: Creasy R K and Warshaw J B (eds) The controversy of mode of delivery in twins: the intrapartum management of twin gestation (Part II). Seminars in Perinatology 10: 44–49

Chescheir N C, Seeds J W 1988 Polyhydramnios and oligohydramnios in twin gestations. Obstetrics and Gynecology 71: 882–884

Connor J M, Ferguson-Smith M A 1991 Essential medical genetics. DNA fingerprinting, 3rd edn. Blackwell Scientific Publications, Oxford, p 130

Corey L A, Berg K, Solaas M H, Nance W E 1992 The epidemiology of pregnancy complications and outcome in a Norwegian twin population. Obstetrics and Gynecology 80: 989–994

Corney G, Robson E B, Strong S J 1972 The effect of zygosity on the birth weight of twins. Annals of Human Genetics 36: 45–59

Crowther C A, Neilson J P, Ashurst H M, Verkuyl D A, Bannerman C 1990 The effects of hospitalization for rest on fetal growth, neonatal morbidity and length of gestation in twin pregnancy. British Journal of Obstetrics and Gynaecology 97: 872–877

Davison L, Easterling T R, Jackson J C, Benedetti T J 1992 Breech extraction of low-birth-weight second twins: can Caesarean section be justified? American Journal of Obstetrics and Gynecology 166: 497–502

De Lee J B, Greenhill J P 1947 Multiple pregnancy. In: Principles and practice of obstetrics, 9th edn. WB Saunders, Philadelphia, ch XXXII, p 417

De Lia J E, Cruikshank D P, Keye W R 1990 Fetoscopic neodynium : YAG laser occlusion of placental vessels in severe twin–twin transfusion syndrome. Obstetrics and Gynecology 75: 1046–1053

Derom C, Derom R, Vlietinck R, Van den Berghe H, Thiery M 1987 Increased monozygotic twinning rate after ovulation induction. Lancet i: 1236–1238

Devoe L D, Azor H 1981 Simultaneous nonstress fetal heart rate testing in twin pregnancy. Obstetrics and Gynecology 58: 450–455

Divon M Y, Marin M J, Pollack R N et al 1993 Twin gestation: fetal presentation as a function of gestational age. American Journal of Obstetrics and Gynecology 168: 1500–1502

Divon M Y, Girz B A, Sklar A, Guidetti D A, Langer O 1989 Discordant twins—a prospective study of the diagnostic value of real time ultrasonography combined with umbilical artery velocimetry. American Journal of Obstetrics and Gynecology 161: 757–760

Dor J, Shalev J, Masiarch J, Blankstein J, Serr D M 1982 Elective cervical suture of twin pregnancies diagnosed ultrasonically in the first trimester following induced ovulation. Gynecologic and Obstetric Investigation 13: 55–60

Doyle L W, Hughes C D, Guaran R L, Quinn M A, Kitchen W H 1988 Mode of delivery of preterm twins. Australian and New Zealand Journal of Obstetrics and Gynecology 28: 25–28

Duncan S L B, Ginz B, Milford-Ward A, Hingley S M 1977 Letter: amniotic fluid AFP in multiple pregnancy. British Medical Journal 1: 1354

Edmonds L D, Layde P M 1982 Conjoined twins in the United States 1970–1977. Teratology 25: 301–308

Edwards J H, Dent T, Kahn J 1966 Monozygotic twins of different sex. Journal of Medical Genetics 3: 117–123

Elliott J P, Radin T G 1992 Quadruplet pregnancy: contemporary management and outcome. Obstetrics and Gynecology 80: 421–424

Elliott J P, Urig M A, Clewell W H 1991 Aggressive therapeutic amniocentesis for treatment of twin–twin transfusion syndrome. Obstetrics and Gynecology 77: 537–544

Erkkola R, Ala-Mello S, Piiroinen O, Kero P, Sillanpää M 1985 Growth discordancy in twin pregnancies: a risk factor not detected by measurements of biparietal diameter. Obstetrics and Gynecology 66: 203–206

Evans M I, Fletcher J C, Zador I E, Newton B W, Quigg M H, Struyk C D 1988 Selective first-trimester termination in octuplet and quadruplet pregnancies: clinical and ethical issues. Obstetrics and Gynecology 71: 289–296

Evans M I, Dommergues M, Wapner R J et al 1993 Efficacy of transabdominal multifetal pregnancy reduction: collaborative experience among the world's largest centers. Obstetrics and Gynecology 82: 61–66

Fagan C J 1977 Antepartum diagnosis of conjoined twins by ultrasonography. American Journal of Roentgenology 129: 921–922

Fishman A, Grubb D K, Kovacs B W 1993 Vaginal delivery of the non-vertex second twin. American Journal of Obstetrics and Gynecology 168: 861–864

Fowler M G, Kleinman J C, Keily J L, Kessel S S 1991 Double jeopardy: twin infant mortality in the United States, 1983 and 1984. American Journal of Obstetrics and Gynecology 165: 15–22

Fries M H, Goldstein R B, Kilpatrick S J, Golbus M S, Callen P W, Filly R A 1993 The role of velamentous cord insertion in the etiology of twin–twin transfusion syndrome. Obstetrics and Gynecology 81: 569–574

Fusi L, Gordon H 1990 Twin pregnancy complicated by single intrauterine death. Problems and outcome with conservative management. British Journal of Obstetrics and Gynaecology 97: 511–516

Galton F 1991 Inquiries into human faculty and its development, 2nd edn. J M Dent & Sons, London, p 155

Gaziano E P, Knox E, Bendel R P, Calvin S, Brandt D 1991 Is pulsed Doppler velocimetry useful in the management of multiple-gestation pregnancies? American Journal of Obstetrics and Gynecology 163: 1426–1433

Gerson A G, Wallace D M, Brigens N K, Ashmead G G, Weiner S, Bolognese R J 1987 Duplex Doppler ultrasound in the evaluation of growth in twin pregnancies. Obstetrics and Gynecology 70: 419–423

Gilbert L, Saunders N, Sharp F 1988 The management of multiple pregnancy in women with a lower-segment Caesarean scar. Is a repeat Caesarean section really the 'safe' option? British Journal of Obstetrics and Gynaecology 95: 1312–1316

Giles W B, Trudinger B J, Cook C M 1985 Fetal umbilical artery flow velocity waveforms in twin pregnancies. British Journal of Obstetrics and Gynaecology 92: 490–497

Gonsoulin W, Moise K J Jr, Kirshon B, Cotton D B, Wheeler J M, Carpenter R J Jr 1990 Outcome of twin–twin transfusion diagnosed before 28 weeks' gestation. Obstetrics and Gynecology 75: 214–216

Greenwald P 1970 Environmental influences on twins apparent at birth. Biology of the Neonate 15: 79–93

Gummerus M, Halonen O 1987 Prophylactic long-term oral tocolysis of multiple pregnancies. British Journal of Obstetrics and Gynaecology 94: 249–251

Hall M H 1985 Preterm labour and its consequences. Proceedings of the Thirteenth Study Group of the Royal College of Obstetricians and Gynaecologists, p 11

Hall M H, Campbell D M, Davidson R J L 1979 Anaemia in twin pregnancy. Acta Geneticae Medicae et Gemellologiae 28: 279–284

Hamilton W J, Boyd J D, Mossman H W 1972 Determination, differentiation, the organiser mechanism, abnormal development and twinning. In: Hamilton W J, Boyd J D (eds) Human embryology, 4th edn. W Heffer & Sons, Cambridge, pp 216–222

Hanson J W 1975 Letter: incidence of conjoined twinning. Lancet ii: 1257

Harper R G, Kenigsberg K, Sia C G 1980 Xiphopagus conjoined twins: a 300-year review of the obstetric, morphopathologic, neonatal and surgical parameters. American Journal of Obstetrics and Gynecology 137: 617–629

Harris D W 1982 Letter to the editors. Journal of Reproductive Medicine 27: 39

Hart I, Daw E 1991 Mono-amniotic twin pregnancy with entanglement of the umbilical cords, but no fetal heart rate abnormality. Journal of Obstetrics and Gynaecology 11: 347–348

Hashimoto B, Callen P W, Filly R A, Laros R K 1986 Ultrasound evaluation of polyhydramnios and twin pregnancy. American Journal of Obstetrics and Gynecology 154: 1069–1072

Heifetz S A 1984 Single umbilical artery, a statistical analysis of 237 autopsy cases and review of the literature. Perspectives in Paediatric Pathology 8: 345–378

Hellin D 1895 Die Ursache der Multiparität der uniparen Tiere überhaupt und der Zwillingsschwangerschaft beim Menschen insbesonderer. Seitz und Schauer, München

Houlton M C C, Marivate M, Philpott R H 1982 Factors associated with preterm labour and changes in the cervix before labour in twin pregnancy. British Journal of Obstetrics and Gynaecology 89: 190–194

Imaizumi Y 1987 The recent trends in multiple births and stillbirth rates in Japan. Acta Geneticae Medicae et Gemellologiae 36: 325–334

Imaizumi Y, Inouye E 1984 Multiple birthrates in Japan. Further analysis. Acta Geneticae Medicae et Gemollologiae 33: 107–114

Jarvis G T, Whitfield M F 1981 Epidural analgesia and the delivery of twins. Journal of Obstetrics and Gynaecology 2: 90–92

Katz V L, Chescheir N C, Cefalo R C 1990 Unexplained elevations of maternal serum alpha-fetoprotein. Obstetrical and Gynecological Survey 45: 719–726

Kiely J L 1990 The epidemiology of perinatal mortality in multiple births. Bulletin of the New York Academy of Medicine 66: 618–637

Kiely J L, Kleinman J C, Kiely M 1992 Triplets and higher-order multiple births. Time trends and infant mortality. American Journal of Diseases of Childhood 146: 862–868

King J F, Keirse M J N C, Grant A, Chalmers I 1985 Preterm labour and its consequences. Proceedings of the Thirteenth Study Group of the Royal College of Obstetricians and Gynaecologists, p 206

Kingston H M 1990 ABC of clinical genetics. British Medical Journal, London, p 16

Kohl S G, Casey G 1975 Twin gestation. Mount Sinai Journal of Medicine 42: 523–539

Landy H J, Weingold A B 1989 Management of a multiple gestation complicated by an antepartum fetal demise. Obstetrical and Gynecological Survey 44: 171–176

Landy H J, Weiner S, Corson S L, Batzer F R, Bolognese R J 1986 The 'vanishing twin': ultrasonographic assessment of fetal disappearance in the first trimester. American Journal of Obstetrics and Gynecology 155: 14–19

Lange I R, Harman C R, Ash K M, Manning F A, Menticoglou S 1989 Twins with hydramnios: treating premature labour at source. American Journal of Obstetrics and Gynecology 160: 552–557

Lawrence M, McKillop F M, Durnin J V G A 1991 Women who gain more fat during pregnancy may not have bigger babies: implications for recommended weight gain during pregnancy. British Journal of Obstetrics and Gynaecology 98: 254–259

Layde P M, Erickson J D, Falek A et al 1980 Congenital malformations in twins. American Journal of Human Genetics 32: 69–78

Levi S 1976 Ultrasonic assessment of the high rate of human multiple pregnancy in the first trimester. Journal of Clinical Ultrasound 4: 3–5

Leveno K J, Quirk J G, Whalley P J, Herbert W N P, Trubey R 1984

Fetal lung maturation in twin gestation. American Journal of Obstetrics and Gynecology 148: 405–411

Livingston J E, Poland B J 1980 A study of spontaneously aborted twins. Teratology 21: 139–148

Long M G, Gibb D M F, Kempley S, Cardozo L D, Nicolaides K, Gamsu H 1991 Retention of the second twin: a viable option? Case reports. British Journal of Obstetrics and Gynaecology 98: 1295–1299

Long P A, Oats J N 1987 Pre-eclampsia in twin pregnancy—severity and pathogenesis. Australian and New Zealand Journal of Obstetrics and Gynaecology 27: 1–5

Louw J H, Barnard C N 1955 Congenital intestinal atresia: observations on its origin. Lancet ii: 1065–1067

Luke B, Keith L G 1992 The contribution of singletons, twins and triplets to low birth weight, infant mortality and handicap in the United States. Journal of Reproductive Medicine 37: 661–666

Luke B, Keith L, Johnson T R, Keith D 1991 Pregravid weight, gestational weight gain and current weight of women delivered of twins. Journal of Perinatal Medicine 19: 333–340

Luke B, Minogue J, Witter F R 1993 The role of fetal growth restriction and gestational age on length of hospital stay in twin infants. Obstetrics and Gynecology 81: 949–953

McDonald T W, Ruffolo E H 1983 Modern management of gestational trophoblastic disease. Obstetrical and Gynecological Survey 38: 67–83

MacGillivray I 1984 The Aberdeen contribution to twinning. Acta Geneticae Medicae et Gemellologiae 33: 5–12

MacGillivray I 1986 In: Creasy R K and Warshaw J B (eds) Epidemiology of twin pregnancy. Seminars in Perinatology 10: 4–8

McKeown T, Record R G 1952 Observations on foetal growth in multiple pregnancy in man. Journal of Endocrinology 8: 386–401

MacLennan A H, Green R C, O'Shea R, Brookes C, Mooris D 1990 Routine hospital admission in twin pregnancies between 26 and 36 weeks' gestation. Lancet 335: 267–269

Marivate M, De Villiers K O, Fairbrother P 1977 Effect of prophylactic outpatient administration of fenoterol on the time of onset of spontaneous labour and fetal growth rate in twin pregnancy. American Journal of Obstetrics and Gynecology 128: 707–708

Martin M C 1991 Infertility. In: Pernoll M L (ed) Current obstetric and gynaecologic diagnosis and treatment, 7th edn. Appleton & Lange, New York, pp 1025–1036

Martin N G, Olsen M E, Theile H, El Beaini J L, Handelsman D, Bhatnagar A S 1984 Pituitary-ovarian function in mothers who have had two sets of dizygotic twins. Fertility and Sterility 41: 878–880

Moore K L 1982 The developing human, 3rd edn. WB Saunders, Philadelphia, pp 130–139

Morris N, Osborn S B, Wright N P 1955 Effective circulation of the uterine wall in late pregnancy measured with ^{24}NaCl. Lancet i: 323–325

Naeye R L 1990 Maternal body weight and pregnancy outcome. American Journal of Clinical Nutrition 52: 273–279

Naeye R L 1992 Disorders of the placenta, fetus and neonate. Diagnosis and clinical significance. Mosby Year Book, St Louis, pp 284–288

Nance W E 1981 Malformations unique to the twinning process. Progress in Clinical Biological Research 69A: 123–133

National Cancer for Health Statistics 1984 Vital statistics of the United States, 1979. Vol I, Natality. Public Health Service, Hyattsville, Maryland

National Center for Health Statistics 1991 Advance report of final natality statistics, 1989. Monthly vital statistics report, vol 40, No 8, Supplement. Public Health Service, Hyattsville, Maryland

Neilson J P, Crowther C A 1993 Preterm labour in multiple pregnancies. Fetal and Maternal Medicine Reviews 5: 105–119

Neilson J P, Verkuyl D A A, Crowther C A, Bannerman C 1988 Preterm labour in twin pregnancies: prediction by cervical assessment. Obstetrics and Gynecology 72: 719–723

Nichols B L, Blattner R S, Rudolf A J 1967 General clinical management of thoracopagus twins. Birth Defects 3: 38–51

Nilsen S T, Bergsjø P, Nome S 1984 Male twins at birth and 18 years later. British Journal of Obstetrics and Gynaecology 91: 122–127

Noonan J A 1978 Twins, conjoined twins and cardiac defects. American Journal of Diseases of Childhood 132: 17–18

Nylander P P S 1970 The inheritance of dizygotic twinning. A study of 18 737 maternities. Acta Geneticae Medicae et Gemellologiae 19: 36–39

Nylander P P S 1975 In: MacGillivray I, Corney G, Nylander P P S (eds) Human multiple reproduction. Saunders, London, p 142

O'Connor M C, Murphy H, Dalrymple I J 1979 Double blind trial of ritodrine and placebo in twin pregnancy. British Journal of Obstetrics and Gynaecology 86: 706–709

Ohel G, Granat M, Zeevi D et al 1987 Advanced ultrasonic placental maturation in twin pregnancies. American Journal of Obstetrics and Gynecology 156: 76–78

O'Herlihy C, de Crespigny L J, Robinson H P 1988 Ultrasound monitoring of ovulation. In: Progress in infertility, 3rd edn. Boston, Little Brown and Company, pp 479–497

Onyskowová Z, Doležal A, Jedlička V 1970 The frequency and character of malformations in multiple births. Acta Universitatis Carolinae; Medica (Praha) 16: 333–376

Petersson F, Smedby B, Lindmark G 1976 Outcome of twin birth. Review of 1636 children born in twin birth. Acta Paediatrica Scandinavica 64: 473–479

Picard R, Fraser D, Picard E 1991 Ethnicity and sex ratio in twin births. Acta Geneticae Medicae et Gemellologiae 40: 311–317

Pijpers L, Jahoda M G J, Vosters R P L, Niermeijer M F, Sachs E S 1988 Genetic amniocentesis in twin pregnancies. British Journal of Obstetrics and Gynaecology 95: 323–326

Poeschmann P P, Van Oppen C A, Bruinse H W 1992 Delayed interval delivery in multiple pregnancies: report of three cases and review of the literature. Obstetrical and Gynaecological Survey 47: 139–147

Powell M C, Buckley J, Worthington B S, Symonds E M 1986 Magnetic resonance imaging and hydatidiform mole. British Journal of Radiology 59: 561–564

Powers W F 1973 Twin pregnancy: complications and treatment. Obstetrics and Gynecology 42: 795–808

Queenan J T, Gadow E C 1970 Polyhydramnios: chronic versus acute. American Journal of Obstetrics and Gynecology 108: 349–355

Rabinovici J, Barhai G, Reichman B, Serr D M, Mashiach S 1988 Internal podalic version with unruptured membranes for the second twin in transverse lie. Obstetrics and Gynecology 71: 428–430

Rayburn W F, Lavin J P Jr, Miodovnik M, Varner M W 1984 Multiple gestation: time interval between delivery of the first and second twins. Obstetrics and Gynecology 63: 502–506

Rees A E J, Vujanic G M, Williams W M 1993 Epidemic of conjoined twins in Cardiff. British Journal of Obstetrics and Gynaecology 100: 388–391

Robertson E G, Neer K J 1983 Placental injection studies in twin gestation. American Journal of Obstetrics and Gynecology 147: 170–174

Robson E B 1978 In: Falkner F, Tanner J M (eds) The genetics of birth weight. Human growth, vol 1: principles and prenatal growth. Plenum, New York, pp 285–287

Rodis J F, Egan J F, Craffey A, Ciarleglio L, Greenstein R M, Scorza W E 1990 Calculated risk of chromosomal abnormalities in twin gestations. Obstetrics and Gynecology 76: 1037–1041

Romero R, Duffy T P, Berkowitz R L, Chang E, Hobbins J C 1984 Prolongation of a preterm pregnancy complicated by death of a single twin in utero and disseminated intravascular coagulation. New England Journal of Medicine 310: 772–774

Ron-El R, Mor Z, Weinraub P, Schreyer P et al 1992 Triplet, quadruplet and quintuplet pregnancies: management and outcome. Acta Obstetrica Gynecologica Scandinavica 71: 347–350

Rovinsky J J, Jaffin H 1965 Cardiovascular haemodynamics in pregnancy. I. Blood and plasma volumes in multiple pregnancy. American Journal of Obstetrics and Gynecology 93: 1–15

Rovinsky J J, Jaffin H 1966 Cardiovascular haemodynamics in pregnancy. II. Cardiac output and left ventricular work in multiple pregnancy. American Journal of Obstetrics and Gynecology 95: 781–786

Rydhström H, Ingermarsson I, Ohrlander S 1990 Lack of correlation between a high Caesarean section rate and improved prognosis for low-birthweight twins (< 2500 g). British Journal of Obstetrics and Gynaecology 97: 229–233

Sadler T W 1985 Langman's medical embryology, 5th edn. Williams and Wilkins, Baltimore, pp 102–108

Santolaya J, Sampson M, Abramowicz J S, Warsof S L 1992 Twin pregnancy: ultrasonographically observed changes in fetal presentation. Journal of Reproductive Medicine 37: 328–330

Saunders N J, Snijders R J M, Nicolaides K H 1991 Twin–twin transfusion syndrome in the second trimester is associated with small inter-twin haemoglobin differences. Fetal Diagnosis and Therapy 6: 34–36

Saunders N J, Snijders R J M, Nicolaides K H 1992 Therapeutic amniocentesis in twin–twin transfusion syndrome appearing in the second trimester of pregnancy. American Journal of Obstetrics and Gynecology 166: 820–824

Schneider K T M, Vetter K, Huch R, Huch A 1985 Acute polyhydramnios complicating twin pregnancies. Acta Geneticae Medicae et Gemellologiae 34: 179–184

Schinzel A A G L, Smith D W, Miller J R 1979 Monozygotic twinning and structural defects. Journal of Pediatrics 95: 921–930

Scottish Twin Study 1983 Preliminary Report. Social Paediatric and Obstetric Research Unit, University of Glasgow and Greater Glasgow Health Board, Glasgow

Shah Y G, Gragg L A, Moodley S, Williams G W 1992 Doppler velocimetry in concordant and discordant twin gestations. Obstetrics and Gynecology 80: 272–276

Sherman S J, Kovacs B W, Medearis A L, Bear M B, Paul R H 1992 Nonstress test assessment of twins. Journal of Reproductive Medicine 37: 804–808

Simpson J L, Golbus M S 1992 Twinning. In: Genetics in obstetrics & gynecology. WB Saunders, Philadelphia, ch 13, pp 173–179

Sonneveld S W, Correy J F 1992 Antenatal loss of one of twins. Australian and New Zealand Journal of Obstetrics and Gynaecology 32: 10–13

Steinberg L H, Hurley V A, Desmedt E, Beischer N A 1990 Acute polyhydramnios in twin pregnancies. Australian and New Zealand Journal of Obstetrics and Gynaecology 30: 196–200

Strandskov H H, Edelen E W, Siemens G J 1946 Analysis of the sex ratios among single and plural births in the total 'white' and 'colored' US populations. American Journal of Physical Anthropology 4: 491–501

Strong T H, Howard M W, Wade B K, Miura C S, Elliott J P 1993 Intrapartum amnioinfusion in twin gestation. A preliminary report of three cases. Journal of Reproductive Medicine 38: 397–399

Tabsh K M A 1993 A report of 131 cases of multifetal pregnancy reduction. Obstetrics and Gynecology 82: 57–60

Tuppin P, Blondel B, Kaminski M 1993 Trends in multiple deliveries and infertility treatments in France. British Journal of Obstetrics and Gynaecology 100: 383–385

Uchida I A, Freeman V C P, Gedeon M, Goldmaker J 1983 Twinning rate in spontaneous abortions. American Journal of Human Genetics 35: 987–993

Van der Pol J G, Wolf H, Boer K et al 1992 Jejunal atresia related to the use of methylene blue in genetic amniocentesis in twins. British Journal of Obstetrics and Gynaecology 99: 141–143

Vassilakos P, Ritton G, Kajii T 1977 Hydatidiform moles: two entities. A morphologic and cytogenetic study with some clinical considerations 127: 167–170

Veille J C, Morton M J, Burry K J 1985 Maternal cardiovascular adaptations to twin pregnancy. American Journal of Obstetrics and Gynecology 153: 261–263

Vejerslev L O 1991 Clinical management and diagnostic possibilities in hydatidiform mole with co-existent fetus. Obstetrical and Gynecological Survey 46: 577–588

Vejerslev L O, Dissing J, Hansen H E, Poulsen H 1987a Hydatidiform mole: genetic origin in polyploid conceptuses. Human Genetics 76: 11–19

Vejerslev L O, Fisher R A, Surti V, Wake N 1987b Hydatidiform mole: parental chromosome aberrations in partial and complete moles. Journal of Medical Genetics 24: 613–615

Wapner R J, Davis G H, Johnson A et al 1990 Selective reduction of multifetal pregnancies. Lancet i: 90–93

Wapner R J, Johnson A, Davis G, Urban A, Morgan P, Jackson L 1993 Prenatal diagnosis in twin gestations: a comparison between second-trimester amniocentesis and first-trimester chorionic villus sampling. Obstetrics and Gynecology 82: 49–56

Ware H H 1971 The second twin. American Journal of Obstetrics and Gynecology 110: 865–869

Waterhouse J A H 1950 Twinning in twin pedigrees. British Journal of Social Medicine 4: 197–216

Weekes A R L, Menzies D N, De Boer C H 1977 The relative efficacy of bed rest, cervical suture and no treatment in the management of twin pregnancy. British Journal of Obstetrics and Gynaecology 84: 161–164

Wenstrom K D, Tessen J A, Zlatnik F J, Sipes S L 1992 Frequency, distribution, and theoretical mechanisms of hematologic and weight discordance in monochorionic twins. Obstetrics and Gynecology 80: 257–261

Westgren M, Edvall H, Nordstrom L, Svanelius E, Ranstam J 1985 Spontaneous cephalic version of breech presentation in the last trimester. British Journal of Obstetrics and Gynaecology 92: 19–22

White C, Wyshak G 1964 Inheritance of human dizygotic twinning. New England Journal of Medicine 271: 1003–1112

Wilson R S 1976 Concordance in physical growth for monozygotic and dizygotic twins. Annals of Human Biology 3: 1–10

Wilson R A 1979 Twin growth: initial deficit, recovery, and trends in concordance from birth to nine years. Annals of Human Biology 6: 205–220

Windham G C, Bjerkedal T, Sever L E 1982 The association of twinning and neural tube defects: studies in Los Angeles, California and Norway. Acta Geneticae Medicae et Gemellologiae 31: 165–172

Wittmann B K, Farquharson D F, Thomas W D S, Baldwin V J, Wadsworth L D 1986 The role of feticide in the management of severe twin transfusion syndrome. American Journal of Obstetrics and Gynecology 155: 1023–1026

Wolf E J, Vintzileos A M, Rosenkrantz T S, Rodis J F, Lettieri L, Mallozzi A 1992 A comparison of pre-discharge survival and morbidity in singleton and twin very low birth weight infants. Obstetrics and Gynecology 80: 436–439

Yu S L, Pepperell R J, Evans J H 1991 Can ultrasonography reliably predict the occurrence of multiple pregnancies in gonadotrophin ovulation induction? Australian and New Zealand Journal of Obstetrics and Gynaecology 31: 58–62

20. Rhesus and other red cell isoimmunization in pregnancy

C. R. Whitfield

Material in this chapter contains contributions from the first edition and we are grateful to the previous author for the work done.

Effective management of any disease must be based on understanding its aetiology, its perhaps variable course and the pathological effects it may have. The story of how rhesus (Rh) disease became usually manageable and then mostly preventable, within less than three decades of its aetiology becoming understood, is an example of effective clinical application of successful research. In the process the fetus at last became, in a real sense, a patient amenable to direct diagnosis and treatment, rather than only indirectly and less certainly via the mother. It marked the birth of fetal medicine as a subspecialty; it is therefore of interest, and also very instructive, to take note of the milestones of the Rh story, firstly how our understanding of the clinical process and its aetiology was achieved.

Historical background

The first description of the birth of a hydropic fetus has been variously attributed to Hippocrates in the year 400 BC, to Plater (1641) and to several reports in the German literature of the mid-nineteenth century in which its usual association with congenital syphilis was noted. It was Jakesch (1878) in Prague who, in describing the delivery of a stillborn fetus, first reported the association of fetal and massive placental oedema, yellow amniotic fluid, marked splenomegaly, and on microscopy 'a leukaemic diathesis and corresponding findings in the spleen and liver', which Rautman (1912) later recognized as an excess of nucleated primitive red cells, due to extramedullary haemopiesis, which he named erythroblastosis. Ballantyne (1892), a pathologist by initial training, described the same findings in more detail, differentiating the condition from congenital syphilis and reporting a familial incidence;

he added an association with maternal hypertension and oedema—was this the so-called *maternal syndrome*?

Buchan & Comrie (1909) first reported that in icterus gravis neonatorum there is an excess of nucleated erythrocytes in the peripheral blood, and 20 years later Diamond et al (1932) in Boston linked together the triad of hydrops fetalis, icterus gravis and neonatal anaemia (without jaundice at the time of birth) as manifestations of the single process of erythroblastosis fetalis. It is interesting, in view of what we now know about the protective effect of ABO blood group incompatibility (below), that Diamond and his colleagues reported no examples of fetomaternal ABO incompatibility between the mothers and babies they reported. Having reviewed the literature on erythroblastosis fetalis, Darrow (1938) made the correct deduction that its most likely explanation was a fetomaternal antigen–antibody reaction, but the wrong speculation in suggesting that this must be due to maternal sensitivity to the fetal type of haemoglobin. In the same year Hellman & Hertig (1938) confirmed the familial occurrence that Ballantyne had noted, and reported the rarity of erythroblastosis fetalis in first-born babies.

The basic aetiology was unravelled during the next 3 years. First, Levine & Stetson (1939) reported a severe transfusion reaction in a woman following stillbirth and leading to the development of antibodies in her blood, which agglutinated red blood cells from her husband and also from the majority of a large number of Group O subjects. They suggested that the mother became immunized to a fetal antigen from her husband which she lacked. Then, at the Rockefeller Institute, Landsteiner & Wiener (1940) identified the Rh antibody in rabbits following injection of blood from rhesus monkeys, and the serum so produced agglutinated about 80% of human bloods (i.e. the Rh-positive ones). Finally, in the same year, Wiener & Peters (1940) put together the human and animal evidence by demonstrating these Rh antibodies in three further examples of human blood transfusion reactions. It had now become clear that almost all transfusion reactions, which could not be explained on the basis of Group A or B incompatibility, had occurred either in men or women who had recently been transfused or in women who had recently carried a pregnancy that aborted or ended in stillbirth; in the latter case they concluded that the maternal antibodies arose as a reaction to leakage of erythrocytes from the placental circulation of a Rh-positive fetus into the circulation of a Rh-negative mother, a suggestion already made 2 years before by Levine & Stetson (1939) and which Dienst (1905) had been inspired to suggest more than 30 years before. Levine et al (1941) provided the final serological proof that the erythroblastosis of neonatal haemolytic disease is due to Rh immunization, in the process going back to the father of the stillborn baby reported in 1939 to confirm that he was in fact Rh-positive.

It remained to be proved that fetal red cells could cross the placental barrier into the mother's circulation.

THE Rh SYSTEM

Whether three allelic genes each with two major variables (C or c, D or d, E or e) or a group of regulatory genes produce the two triple-antigen complexes making up a person's Rh genotype, inheritance follows Mendelian principles and the individual is either homozygous or heterozygous for each antigen represented in the genotype. Of the two systems designating the different Rh antigens, that of Fisher & Race (1946) is preferred to the alternative nomenclature (Wiener 1944). The former system is generally neater, its more distinctive symbols D and d, C and c, and E and e, are logically and easily recognizable as indicating pairs of alleles (compared with the corresponding two-letter symbols Rh_o and rr_o, rh′ and hr′, and rh″ and hr″), the same symbols are used to describe genotypes, e.g. CDe/cde (rather than introducing yet more symbols for each complex in the genotype, e.g. R′ and r) and the symbol D, for the most powerful and important of the Rh antigens, is now universally used in some contexts, e.g. anti-D immunoglobulin. Certain antigen combinations are more common than others, showing considerable ethnic variation, e.g. in Caucasians CDe, cde and cDE are the commonest in that order of frequency, whereas cDe, which is unusual in Caucasians, is common in Africa, and genotypes that include d are uncommon in most African and Asian races. For completeness both systems are included in Table 20.1, but for clarity that of Fisher & Race will be used in the remainder of this text.

So much more important is D than the other antigens, that its presence or absence is generally used to classify a person as Rh-positive or Rh-negative. Antibodies are made to the other Rh antigens, sometimes together with anti-D antibody, and they can cause erythroblastosis fetalis and haemolytic disease, occasionally even fatally particularly with anti-c. Indeed, although isoimmunization to D remains the most common cause of severe

Table 20.1 Terminology and frequency of the most common Rh genotypes in Caucasian populations

Fisher & Race (1946)	Wiener (1944)	Frequency (%)
CDe/cde	R^1r	33
CDe/CDe	R^1R^1	18
cde/cde	r r	15
CDe/cDE	R^1R^2	12
cDE/cde	R^2r	11

erythroblastosis fetalis, successful prophylaxis with anti-D immunoglobulin has resulted in an increasing proportion of haemolytic disease being caused by Rh antibodies other than anti-D, and two-thirds of antenatal patients found to have irregular red blood cell antibodies are themselves Rh(D)-positive (Bowell et al 1986). It is also unfortunate that donor blood for the transfusion of Rh(D)-negative women in their reproductive years is often not matched for the other Rh factors.

Fetomaternal haemorrhage

The train of events leading to and resulting from red cell isoimmunization is the same whichever antigen/antibody is involved, and is initiated by entry into the maternal circulation of erythrocytes carrying an antigen which the mother lacks. It is now extremely rare for this to follow a Rh(D)-incompatible blood transfusion, there being only one example of this (transfusion and tonsillectomy during childhood overseas) in more than 300 consecutive pregnancies with anti-D antibodies at The Queen Mother's Hospital in Glasgow, but it still occasionally occurs from transfusion of blood containing one of the other Rh antigens, or more frequently a non-Rh (e.g. Kell) antigen. Almost always, therefore, immunization of a Rh(D)-negative women results from transplacental bleeding from a Rh(D)-positive fetus.

Chown (1954) and Gunson (1957) made the first reports of fetomaternal haemorrhage. In each case more than 100 ml of fetal blood, estimated by differential agglutination, was demonstrated in the mother's circulation, and both these mothers subsequently became Rh(D)-immunized. The frequency of fetomaternal haemorrhage, exceptionally of such magnitude, became well recognized when the much simpler Kleihauer–Bettke test (Kleihauer et al 1957) or modifications of it came into general use. By acid or alkali denaturation these tests distinguish between the fetal red cells which maintain their colour (due to uneluted fetal haemoglobin) from the ghosted maternal cells (from which adult haemoglobin has been eluted).

In their work to establish prophylaxis with anti-D immunoglobulin, investigators in Liverpool (Woodrow & Finn 1966, Woodrow & Donohoe 1968) carried out extensive studies of fetomaternal haemorrhage, using the Kleihauer technique to make fetal red cell counts in maternal blood samples, and their findings have been amply confirmed by others. They found the following:

1. Fetal erythrocytes were present in the blood of about 3% of women during the third trimester, in half of them in sufficient amount (corresponding to at least 0.2–0.25 ml of fetal blood in the maternal circulation) to possibly cause isoimmunization, and an estimated fetomaternal haemorrhage of 7 ml was reported.
2. After delivery more than 50% of mothers had fetal erythrocytes in their blood, equivalent to more than 0.2 ml of fetomaternal haemorrhage in 18% when there was ABO compatibility between mother and baby, compared with 1.9% when there was ABO incompatibility, and a fetomaternal haemorrhage of 170 ml was reported. However, using the Kleihauer staining technique but a different method for cell counting, Zipursky & Israels (1967) reported that Rh immunization could follow postpartum fetomaternal haemorrhage of as little as 60 μl (i.e. about one-third of the critical volume suggested from Liverpool). It seems likely that the difference lies simply in the counting methods used.

Two techniques of more accuracy than the Kleihauer test have been introduced. An immunofluorescence technique differentiates Rh(D)-positive and Rh(D)-negative cells and is obviously also more specific, but a more practical alternative is the widely available assay of maternal serum alphafetoprotein (used for the prenatal diagnosis of fetal neural tube defects) which has received less attention than it merits as a measure of fetomaternal haemorrhage (Lachman et al 1977).

It is during labour, presumably in the third stage when placental separation occurs, that transplacental bleeding is most likely to occur, especially of a large amount of fetal blood. The incidence and volume of fetomaternal haemorrhage is increased following manual removal of the placenta, multiple births or Caesarean section, in the last mentioned when some (perhaps most) of the fetal blood is absorbed from the mother's peritoneal cavity. Antepartum fetomaternal haemorrhage may be silent, occurring in the absence of any obvious clinical complication, but it is much more likely to occur in association with certain complications and procedures. Thus, fulminant pre-eclampsia or antepartum haemorrhage, especially when due to placental abruption, is associated with a high rate of fetomaternal haemorrhage, including sometimes very large bleeds. Fetomaternal haemorrhage has also been reported following abdominal trauma, external cephalic version, chorion villus sampling and early or late amniocentesis. Incidences as high as 30% or 40% following amniocentesis in late pregnancy were observed before ultrasound was used to guide the needle, but this has been virtually eliminated with good ultrasound imaging.

Fetomaternal haemorrhage has been described following abortion, whether spontaneous or therapeutic and at different stages of gestation, and there has been some controversy over the need for anti-D immunoprophylaxis after early losses (see below). In early spontaneous abortion, the amount of fetomaternal haemorrhage is probably insufficient to cause isoimmunization up to 10 or 12 weeks, but the risk increases through the second trimester to reach 3% or 4% (Freda et al 1970, Queenan et al 1971a). Significant fetomaternal haemorrhage is even more likely to occur during therapeutic termination of pregnancy, which was shown to carry a 5.5% risk of immunization in the absence of anti-D prophylaxis (Queenan et al 1971b). It may well be that the risk is reduced by use of the newer aspiration or medical techniques for termination.

Development of Rh antibodies

Whether or not transplacental bleeding from a Rh-positive fetus to a Rh-negative mother leads to immunization, and how strong that immunization may be, depends on several factors. Firstly, it depends on her inborn responsiveness which varies considerably from woman to woman, about one-third of whom are unresponsive. Secondly, there is variation in the strength of the antigenic stimulus, D being the most potent Rh antigen, especially when CDe/cde is the fetal genotype. Thirdly, the volume of fetomaternal haemorrhage is important, with placental abruption, severe pre-eclampsia, multiple birth, Caesarean section and manual removal of the placenta being examples of complications which, by causing large fetomaternal haemorrhages, may lead to such severe Rh-immunization that the next Rh-positive fetus is critically or fatally affected (Whitfield 1976). The fourth factor determining the response to a Rh-incompatible fetomaternal haemorrhage is the relationship between the ABO blood groups of the mother and fetus. ABO incompatibility between them (e.g. a Group O mother bearing a Group A or B fetus) provides substantial protection against Rh-immunization, reducing its incidence to about one-tenth of that when there is ABO compatibility. Levine (1958), who had first drawn attention to this phenomenon, later outlined its mechanism.

Thus, when ABO-incompatible fetal red cells enter the mother's bloodstream, they combine with her naturally occurring anti-A and/or anti-B agglutinins and are neutralized by sequestration in her liver, unless the fetomaternal haemorrhage has been so large that enough fetal erythrocytes remain free to stimulate sufficient immunologically competent maternal lymphocytes to mount an antibody response. In contrast, ABO-compatible fetal cells will persist for their normal lifespans, before being scavenged and releasing their antigens, but, because of the time involved, no more than 1% of Rh(D)-negative mothers will have detectable antibodies before delivery of their first Rh(D)-positive baby. When antibodies become detectable then or soon after a first Rh(D)-positive pregnancy, it probably indicates that the mother is a strong responder, in whom the fetus or the next Rh(D)-positive one can become so severely affected that it is at risk of being stillborn. Presumably, primary immunization will occur antepartum in the same proportion (1%) during each subsequent Rh(D)-positive pregnancy. Because most fetomaternal haemorrhages occur during labour, immunization is more likely to occur during the ensuing weeks, and antibodies can be detected in about 8% of at-risk mothers 6 months after delivery. In other immunized mothers the level of circulating antibody is too small to be detected, sometimes even by very sensitive enzyme techniques, or they may have been detectable transiently before declining to undetectable levels in the absence of any further antigenic stimulus.

Once a woman has developed Rh(D) antibodies, even if they have declined below the sensitivity of laboratory tests, they will almost always become detectable from an early stage in a further pregnancy, especially when the pregnancy is again Rh(D)-positive, but sometimes even if it is Rh(D)-negative (the anamnestic response). By the end of the second Rh(D)-positive pregnancy, 17% of Rh(D)-negative mothers will have detectable antibodies, most of which will have resulted from primary immunization by the first of these pregnancies but 1% will be from primary immunization by the second one. After each further Rh(D)-positive pregnancy there will be the same immunological possibilities, namely:

1. Failure to respond.
2. A slow response that may or may not be detectable by 6 months' postpartum.
3. Fetomaternal haemorrhage may have occurred in sufficient volume and early enough in the pregnancy to have brought about antepartum immunization which may be first detected then or in the routine postpartum blood sample.

IgM antibody develops first, followed by IgG antibody which persists at a higher concentration in the mother's serum long after IgM is no longer detectable. The next Rh-positive pregnancy will stimulate a very rapid rise in IgM and a more sustained increase in IgG. Thus, it is IgM antibody that provides the first evidence that immunization has occurred, but it is IgG that is small enough to cross the placenta to cause haemolysis and erythroblastosis in a Rh-positive fetus.

Fetal and neonatal effects

Having crossed the placenta, anti-Rh IgG attaches to antigen sites on the surface of the fetal red cells and causes their destruction with release of bilirubin. The rate of haemolysis, and thus the severity of fetal anaemia, depends not only on the amount of anti-Rh IgG entering the fetal circulation and the ability of the reticuloendothelial system to remove antibody-coated cells, but also on the ability of the fetus to compensate by increased production of new erythrocytes. There is increased erythropoiesis in the bone marrow, and other sites of red cell production, especially the spleen and liver, are activated. Immature nucleated erythroblasts enter the circulation and, as a result of the extramedullary erythropoiesis, the liver and spleen enlarge. In the most severely affected fetuses their lower edges may reach the iliac crests. Before birth the excess of bilirubin is cleared mainly through the placenta into the mother's circulation and thence to her liver, but some reaches the amniotic fluid where it provides a useful marker of the severity of the disorder.

In the more severely affected fetuses, increased haemopoiesis can no longer make up for the excessive destruction of red cells so that significant, perhaps severe, anaemia develops. This induces a compensatory placental hyperplasia to increase oxygen transfer. Following birth, because excess bilirubin and free IgG antibody are no longer being cleared into the mother's circulation, jaundice develops rapidly and the anaemia increases.

In a critically affected fetus, anaemia is so severe that there is tissue hypoxia and acidosis, circulatory failure with generalized oedema including scalp oedema, ascites and often pleural and pericardial effusions. Frank hydrops to this degree, to which a contributory factor is hypoproteinaemia from protein loss into the fluid collections, may sometimes be reversed by immediate direct fetal therapy, but other such fetuses often die in utero. Some of these babies, and others less critically affected during fetal life, require prolonged assisted ventilation, parenteral nutrition and other intensive neonatal support, and they are liable to such serious complications as disseminated intravascular coagulation, severe thrombocytopenia, necrotizing enterocolitis and later also bronchopulmonary dysplasia. If hyperbilirubinaemia is not controlled and a critical level of about 310–345 µm/l of unconjugated bilirubin is reached, it will cross the blood–brain barrier to stain and damage the basal nuclei in the brain, causing the permanently crippling disorder of kernicterus described first by Orth (1875) almost 80 years before its causation by indirect bilirubin was revealed (Claireaux et al 1953). To the dangers of haemolytic disease itself, may be added the hazards to the newborn of preterm birth, occurring either spontaneously or electively as part of management, and of invasive treatment.

MANAGEMENT

Antibody screening

The first step is to identify all pregnancies at risk. As well as blood grouping and Rh typing, at first attendance in pregnancy every woman's blood should be screened for irregular red cell antibodies, using a non-specific test with red cells carrying a full representation of those antibodies that, by crossing the placenta, have the potential to cause haemolytic disease. When the screening test is positive the specific antibody, or each such antibody if more than one is present, is identified and quantified by titration using the Coombs indirect anti-human-globulin test in both saline (for IgM) and in albumen (for IgG). If necessary ultrasensitive enzyme tests are available. Even when antibodies are not found initially, screening should be repeated because they may develop later, even in a first pregnancy, and mothers already very weakly immunized may not have detectable antibody in the early months. Rh(D)-negative women, in whom immunization has not already been detected, should be screened again at 20–24 weeks and then several more times up to delivery, but for Rh(D)-positive women a second screening test at 28–30 weeks will suffice.

Management following detection of Rh antibodies

Referral centres

Well before the effect of immunoprophylaxis became apparent, the best results were achieved by concentrating Rh disease in regional centres, where obstetric/paediatric teams and their supporting diagnostic and transfusion services had become well experienced in all aspects of its management. Now that the incidence is greatly reduced, referral to such centres, and in Britain perhaps sometimes to supraregional teams, is even more necessary to maintain specialized expertise in invasive intrauterine procedures and in managing the severely affected newborn. It also makes use of accumulated experience of the different courses that Rh disease may follow to plan a provisional management strategy for each patient, which should be kept under review and revised if necessary. This applies even when at first it seems unlikely that the fetus may be more than mildly affected because, presumably as a result of further fetomaternal haemorrhages, antibody production may be boosted and an acute haemolytic crisis in the fetus can occur. However, with careful liaison, and especially if the mother lives far away, a shared care schedule can be arranged with her local obstetrician, but overall responsibility for further management must lie with the central Rh team. These rules apply when Rh antibodies other than anti-D are present or there are non-Rh irregular antibodies which may affect the fetus.

Serological surveillance

When Rh antibodies or important non-Rh antibodies have been detected they should be quantified and the father's probable Rh genotype determined. For anti-D quantitation automated immunoassay is available, it is accurate and reproducible and so will reveal any significant change between separate measurements. It should now be relied on in preference to indirect Coombs titres which, because of poor reproducibility, may be misleading in this respect. Although automated immunoassay can be set up for other antibodies this is not generally available, so that these less potent antibodies must still be quantified by titration.

The level of maternal antibody and its trend, in conjunction with the previous history, provide the guide to the timing of amniocentesis or fetal blood sampling to predict severity. Thus, when no previous baby has been affected by Rh disease (as indicated by the direct Coombs testing of cord blood samples), a maternal anti-D concentration persistently at or below 2.5 iu/ml on continued 4-weekly testing indicates that term delivery without amniocentesis is a safe policy, while concentrations exceeding 20 iu/ml raise the possibility of very severe erythroblastosis fetalis, especially in a first affected pregnancy. A sharp increase over 4 weeks, e.g. from below 5 to 20 iu/ml or from less than 15 to 40 iu/ml, should always suggest that a dangerously acute haemolytic crisis may be occurring or is threatening, and this is an indication for immediate amniocentesis or fetal blood sampling or for delivery if already near term.

Knowing the partner's probable Rh genotype may be helpful. It may confirm the half-chance that the fetus is negative for Rh(D) or for whichever Rh or other antigen the mother has developed antibodies to, and this may be helpful when there are favourable amniotic fluid bilirubin estimations despite previous severely affected babies.

Biophysical surveillance

Ultrasound   The first role of ultrasound is to make accurate fetal measurements in early pregnancy in order to confirm or adjust dating from the menstrual history. This becomes important later when interpreting amniotic fluid bilirubin values and timing invasive tests and delivery, all of which must be related to gestational age. The performance of amniocentesis without ultrasound guidance is indefensible, and fetal blood sampling or intrauterine transfusion by the intravascular route cannot be performed without good quality imaging. Although intraperitoneal transfusion was first carried out under radiological control, this technique too is made less difficult and safer when navigated by ultrasound.

Fetal oedema, ascites and pleural or pericardial effusions are revealed by ultrasound scanning, and the appearance of any of these features may be the first warning that the fetus is more severely affected than had been expected. Whenever serum antibody, amniotic fluid bilirubin measurements or the history suggest the fetus may be more than mildly affected, regular imaging should become part of surveillance, usually monthly but more often if the measurements are increasing, and at once if they suggest that an acute haemolytic crisis may be occurring or threatened. Dilatation of the inferior vena cava is another sign that should suggest that the fetus is already severely affected, and it had been hoped that changes in Doppler flow velocity waveforms might also be helpful in this respect, but in practice this has yet to be established on a sound basis (Copel et al 1989).

External cardiotocography   When regular ultrasound scanning has become advisable (see above), weekly external cardiotocography should also be initiated. Occasionally it can be a useful arbiter for or against immediate intervention. Thus, a reactive fetal heart rate tracing may suggest that intrauterine transfusion or delivery can be delayed, while a smooth trace due to sustained loss of baseline variability suggests otherwise, and a sinusoidal rhythm that is not very transient or is repetitive almost certainly shows that there is already extreme fetal anaemia.

Amniocentesis and amniotic fluid analysis

Management of pregnancies complicated by isoimmunization is based on determining the optimal timing for intervention by intrauterine transfusion or delivery. From the history, the level and trend of the mother's serum antibody and other factors including accurate dating of the pregnancy, the first major decision to make is usually when to perform the initial amniocentesis, unless anti-D concentration of no higher than 2.5 iu/ml by repeated automated assay or a weak titre (less than 1 in 8) of some other significant antibody excludes the need for amniocentesis, or, at the other extreme, the risk of intrauterine death is judged to require fetal blood sampling before the amniotic fluid could give a clinically useful guide (below).

It was Bevis (1952, 1956) who first pointed to the potential use of amniocentesis, when he showed that there was a correlation between the severity of erythroblastosis fetalis and the amount of certain haemoglobin breakdown products, including bilirubin, in the amniotic fluid. For several years, however, no way was devised to use this information clinically.

Liley (1961) made the first of his breakthroughs when he showed the following points which are still important to understand:

1. Amniotic fluid bilirubin is more accurately estimated by spectrophotometry than by standard biochemical tests, and he devised his now very widely used measurement of the optical density deviation at the peak wavelength of 450 nm for bilirubin ($\Delta OD450$).
2. The concentration of bilirubin usually present in the amniotic fluid normally declines towards zero during the last trimester, and therefore in attempting to evaluate any excess of bilirubin present as a result of abnormal haemolysis, an allowance must be made for this physiological reduction by relating values to gestational age.

3. These $\Delta OD450$ measurements, and especially the trend between separate estimations in the third trimester, could be plotted against gestational age (on a logarithmic vertical scale) in his three prediction zones to give useful separation between pregnancies proceeding to stillbirth, the birth of babies with different degrees of anaemia, and unaffected infants.
4. In most cases (about two-thirds) the $\Delta OD450$ trend was roughly parallel to the decline observed in normal pregnancies, but in the remainder it moved towards or entered a different prediction zone.
5. These methods might be less reliable before the last trimester.
6. A third measurement of $\Delta OD450$ usually maintains the trend between the first two values in the third trimester.

Finally, he reported that adoption of these methods and principles throughout New Zealand had improved the management of Rh disease, particularly a reduction in stillbirths and in identifying most unaffected babies and some of those only mildly affected.

Liley's methods or modifications of them, including various transfusion zones superimposed on his charts, were soon successfully adopted very widely, in Britain almost exclusively. Queenan & Goetschel (1968) held that it was sufficient to distinguish ominous rising or horizontal $\Delta OD450$ trends from favourable falling trends, without needing prediction zones, although there is an area of overlap between survivors and fatally affected babies if only single $\Delta OD450$ values are plotted. With any of these methods there remains the problem of somehow converting predictions of severity into decisions on when to intervene. Freda (1965) achieved this by grading the $\Delta OD450$ in terms of how long the pregnancy might be left to continue without risk of fetal death before further sampling, but, because his grading makes no allowance for the normal fall in amniotic fluid in the third trimester, it underestimates severity progressively towards term so that some unexpected fetal deaths then occur. Also, his method usually requires very frequently repeated amniocenteses.

An alternative approach was to devise, instead of prediction zones, a single action line (Whitfield 1970) to which the trend between (usually) two $\Delta OD450$ measurements is extrapolated to indicate when continued non-intervention will become less safe than delivery, intrauterine transfusion or fetal blood sampling (Fig. 20.1). Based initially on retrospective experience in more than 100 pregnancies, the line runs close to the first part of Liley's upper dividing line and most proposed transfusion zones, but from 33 weeks it curves down through the middle zone to select almost all of the unaffected babies and many of those only mildly affected for delivery at or near term. It proved an effective, readily used and easily taught method when used as the mainstay of managing almost 1400 consecutive

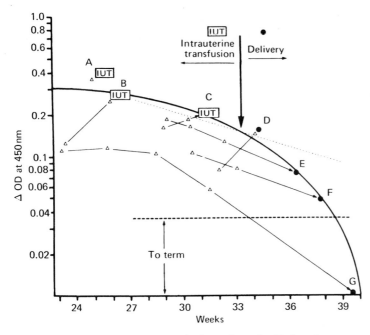

Fig. 20.1 The curved action line is shown from the 23rd week to term; before 27 weeks it would run below an extension of the lower limit of Liley's upper prediction zone (marked by the sloping dotted line) which almost coincides with the action line between 27 and 33 weeks; after 33 weeks the action line curves downwards through Liley's middle zone to reach its lower limit in the 40th week. The horizontal broken line represents an ΔOD450 value of 0.035, below which amniocentesis is not repeated and the pregnancy is allowed to proceed to term. In the case examples, amniocenteses are depicted by triangles, FT indicates fetal tranfusions, and solid dots depict delivery. The original policy of electing intrauterine transfusion when action is required before 33 weeks, but delivery after that time, is shown.

In Case A transfusion was indicated by the ΔOD450 already beyond the action line, and in Case B when the ΔOD450 trend extrapolated to the line at 26 weeks; in Cases C and E, because the initial ΔOD450 was close to the action line, amniocentesis was repeated soon, the unfavourable trend in C indicating transfusion at 31 weeks, but the more favourable trend in E being confirmed by a third amniotic fluid analysis and indicating delivery could be safely postponed to the 37th week; in Case D a steeply rising ΔOD450 trend suggested that acute haemolysis might be occurring and a severely affected baby was delivered at 34 weeks; like Case E, Case F shows the usually expected decline in ΔOD450 and a moderately affected baby was delivered at 38 weeks; two early amniocenteses were performed in Case G because of the history of two stillbirths due to erythroblastosis, but these showed a more favourable trend than was expected, so the trend was re-set by further tests in the second trimester and an unaffected baby was born at term. From Whitfield (1970) with permission.

isoimmunized pregnancies in a combined Rh service at two Belfast hospitals during 6 years. With experience, it was applicable from as early as 22 weeks in mothers with previous losses from Rh disease, as are both Freda's and Queenan's systems. However, if ΔOD450 measurements have not already called for intervention before 27 weeks, when physiological levels of amniotic fluid bilirubin are beginning to decline, the trend should not be extrapolated into the third trimester. Instead, further amniotic fluid samples are needed to reset the bilirubin trend. This is an essential but often misunderstood point.

The timing of the first amniocentesis is important. As

a general rule it should be performed at 28–30 weeks, and usually repeated 3 or 4 weeks later, but earlier if the first value was already close to the action line. With a bad history, the first sample is required 10 weeks before the gestational age at which the earliest previous fetal death, intrauterine transfusion or birth of a critically or fatally affected baby took place, but not before 22 weeks. Additional samples are sometimes obtained to confirm a bilirubin trend that is quite unexpected from the history, e.g. a favourable trend when previous babies were severely affected and the supposed father is homozygous for whichever antigen(s) the maternal antibodies are related.

Fetal blood sampling

Fetal blood sampling was introduced as a procedure in Paris in 1985 by Daffos and his team who went on to describe its use in 606 samplings for various prenatal diagnoses, reporting a 1.9% fetal loss rate in completed pregnancies, including one certainly attributable to the procedure itself (Daffos et al 1983, 1985). Members of his team reported haematological values for normal fetuses, including haemoglobin concentration rising from 11.5 to 13.5 g/dl between 20 and 30 weeks and haematocrit from 37% to 42% over the same period (Forestier et al 1986).

Fetal blood sampling has two roles in managing iso-immunized pregnancies. First, in early pregnancy it may be useful to determine the fetal Rh genotype (or e.g. Kell type) and carry out a direct Coombs test when there have been previous losses or very severely affected survivors and the supposed father is heterozygous for the Rh or other antigen(s) to which the mother is immunized. If the fetus is negative for these, no further intervention need be planned, but it is wise to repeat serological screening of the mother later because additional antibodies, for which the father is antigenic, may appear. If the father has the relevant antigen(s) and the previous history is very bad, the couple may consider the pregnancy being terminated. Fetal blood sampling should perhaps be used more often to determine the fetal Kell-type in the minority (8%) of Kell-immunized mothers who have Kell-positive partners, the great majority of whom are heterozygotes. Almost half of these mothers will be carrying Kell-negative fetuses and do not need amniocentesis or any other special care on account of their antibodies.

Fetal blood sampling and amniocentesis as complementary tests

Secondly, fetal blood sampling is an alternative to amnio-centesis in the prediction of severity, and the question 'Have Liley charts outlived their usefulness'? has been asked (Nicolaides et al 1986a) but this related only to the second trimester when, as Liley (1961) had warned, his system might in any case not be applicable. If a lower critical ΔOD450 value is used in the second trimester, e.g. the action line at this stage, and attention is directed to trends between measurements rather than single values, the great majority of already significantly anaemic fetuses are identified and a guide is provided to the appropriate time for fetal blood sampling. The undoubted value of a precise measurement of haemoglobin or haematocrit, assuming there is no contamination of the fetal blood sample with either maternal blood or amniotic fluid, should be balanced against the greater simplicity of amniocentesis, its lesser direct risk to the fetus, and much smaller risk of fetomaternal haemorrhage. With fetal blood sampling there is a significant risk of, perhaps substantial, fetomaternal haemorrhage, especially when the sample is obtained by transplacental needling which is the usual route when the placenta lies anteriorly. The consequence may be boosted antibody levels with, in turn, an incremental effect on fetal anaemia in the current pregnancy, and probably to an even greater extent in a subsequent incompatible fetus.

In taking these factors into account and regarding fetal blood sampling and amniocentesis as complementary procedures, a practical general rule is as follows. Fetal blood sampling should be used up to 22 weeks in the few cases when the history suggests that fetal death may occur as early as that stage, and it is simply the first step of an emergency intravascular intrauterine transfusion when either generalized hydrops has been shown by ultrasound or a sustained or recurrent sinusoidal heart rhythm has been recorded. If there is fetal ascites (without oedema) suggesting that hydrops may soon develop, or if there is very obvious polyhydramnios with its diluting effect on bilirubin concentration, the fetal haematocrit or haemoglobin concentration is probably a more reliable guide than the ΔOD450 in the amniotic fluid at any stage of gestation. Otherwise, between 22 and 27 weeks amniocentesis, repeated if necessary, can be relied on as the primary method to decide the need for fetal blood sampling and its timing. In the third trimester until the fetus is judged viable for delivery the ΔOD450 and a reliable prediction method (e.g. Liley's or the action line) suffice.

There is as yet no agreement on the haematological criteria for intrauterine transfusion. At King's College Hospital during 6 years (1985–90), fetal blood sampling was performed 1017 times on 272 fetuses in red cell isoimmunized pregnancies, leading to 716 intravascular transfusions. The indication for the initial intrauterine transfusion was a fetal haemoglobin concentration below the fifth centile of the normal range for the gestational age (Nicolaides et al 1993). In most other centres a defined haematocrit value is taken as the indication, and it is generally between 25% (Reece et al 1988) and 30% (Weiner et al 1991) and no account is taken of the normal increase in fetal haematocrit as gestation proceeds. The lower of these values (25%) leaves a clear margin of safety from the 15% haematocrit above which hydrops does not occur (Grannum et al 1988). The higher value (30%) represents a deficit below the normal mean values (Forestier et al 1986) which increases from −7% at 20 weeks to −12% at 30 weeks. Altering the indication for the first intrauterine transfusion to rise from a haematocrit of 25% at 20 weeks to 30% at 30 weeks would adjust the indicative haematocrit deficit to 12% at any time during this range of gestation.

Intrauterine transfusion

Liley's second great breakthrough was in first performing intrauterine transfusion of a severely affected fetus through an epidural catheter threaded via a needle inserted into its peritoneal cavity, with the aid of X-rays, radiopaque contrast injected into the amniotic cavity and swallowed by the fetus to outline its gut in the target area, and paper clips as markers on the mother's abdomen (Liley 1963). His basic technique was soon adopted widely and refinements introduced, in particular the substitution of fluoroscopy with image intensification instead of several X-ray exposures, giving continuous imaging with less radiation. Before the full impact of prophylaxis with anti-D immunoglobulin on case numbers, several large series of intraperitoneal intrauterine transfusions were described from referral centres in New Zealand (Liley 1970), North America (Bowman 1978, Frigoletto et al 1981), Britain (Karnicki 1968, Whitfield, 1976) and elsewhere. In these series survival rates around 40% were reported, rising as high as 70% during the last 8 years of Bowman's 14-year review of 611 transfusions on 257 fetuses in Winnipeg. A collaborative survey of 1074 intrauterine transfusions on 591 fetuses at 15 centres in the USA showed an overall survival rate of 34%, operative deaths within 4 days of 4.8% of the transfusions, and premature labour by 35 weeks in 30% of the pregnancies (Queenan 1969).

The indications for intrauterine transfusion, while based on the history and amniotic fluid spectrophotometry, were not the same in each of these and other series, this variation and increasing experience being the main reasons for different survival rates. A few survivals were reported in hydropic fetuses, but without an agreed definition of radiologically obvious hydrops. Thus, at some centres fetal ascites without any oedema qualified as hydrops, and among such fetuses survival rates sometimes approached the rates in fetuses without oedema, ascites or any other effusion; however, when only fetuses with generalized oedema (anasarca) were regarded as hydropic very few, if any at all, survived.

Once correct catheter placement was confirmed, by injection of radiopaque contrast, a fairly uniform technique resembling Liley's was followed in most centres. Donor blood, compatible with the mother and packed to a haematocrit of about 70%, was infused, usually slowly, the volume given increasing with gestational age, and transfusion was usually repeated about every 2 weeks until the fetus was considered viable for delivery.

Guidance of intrauterine transfusion was improved considerably when real-time ultrasound came into use for this purpose (Hobbins et al 1976). At first, this was sometimes used in conjunction with X-rays or fluoroscopy, but with growing experience and improving equipment radiology was dispensed with. Today, high-resolution real-time ultrasound remains the standard method for:

1. Preliminary inspection of the fetus, including occasionally enabling it to be manipulated into a favourable lie and position.
2. To provide imaging during intrauterine transfusion.
3. To help assess the response of the fetus to the transfusion, by its biophysical profile, the rate of absorption of the transfused blood and sometimes the resolution of ascites and perhaps hydrops.

The continued experience of the Winnipeg intrauterine transfusion team, the great majority of whose referrals come from outside the province of Manitoba, underlines the importance of concentrating today's reduced case numbers on a limited number of specialist centres. Real-time ultrasound was used by this team from 1980 and, despite a short period of increased mortality attributed to catheter-induced haemolysis of the donor blood due to too narrow side-holes on the epidural catheters used (Bowman & Manning 1983), a survival rate of 74% was achieved in 75 fetuses receiving 202 intraperitoneal intrauterine transfusions during the 6 years to 1988 (Harman & Bowman 1993). Although since 1986 intravascular intrauterine transfusion has become the method of choice, as in other centres, the Winnipeg team has the view that their 'experience with intravascular transfusion has demonstrated a clear, although limited, need to continue familiarity with the intraperitoneal approach'. They recommend that when there is non-hydropic disease and a posterior placenta, indications for the intraperitoneal method are a cord insertion that is inaccessible or abnormal (e.g. velamentous), a cord haematoma or thrombus following an unsuccessful intravascular procedure, or an abnormally narrow umbilical vein (< 4 mm), to which may be added its occasional use to top-up an incomplete intravenous intrauterine transfusion following displacement of the needle. The latest report from Winnipeg contains an excellent and very detailed description of the pathophysiology of peritoneal absorption, the now limited but essential role and the achievable results of intraperitoneal intrauterine transfusion, its technical minutiae and complications (Harman and Bowman 1993) to which the reader seeking specialized information may wish to refer.

At four centres in the American cooperative study (Queenan 1969), 23 hysterotomy-type procedures were carried out; 13 fetuses received multiple transfusions through an indwelling intraperitoneal catheter but none survived, and 10 were transfused through the femoral or jugular vein or the umbilical artery and three survived. There have also been single case reports of hysterotomy exchange transfusion by cannulation of the fetal femoral artery (Freda & Adamsons 1964), of a vein on the fetal aspect of the placenta (Seelen et al 1966) and of the jugular vein of an exteriorized fetus (Asensio et al, 1968). One of these fetuses died 2 days later, premature labour followed shortly in both the other cases and one of these babies succumbed. Not surprisingly, hysterotomy to facilitate transfusion, either exchange or straight, has failed to become an established option.

The fetal blood sampling technique was first adapted for intravascular intrauterine transfusion by Rodeck et al (1981) using an umbilical vessel viewed at ultrasound-guided fetoscopy. Subsequently, with this technique, the survival of 29 of 34 severely affected fetuses (84%) including 13 of 15 with hydrops first transfused before 25 weeks (87%) was reported (Nicolaides & Rodeck 1985). The survival of these hydropic fetuses receiving early transfusions represented a breakthrough in the attempted treatment of generalized hydrops fetalis.

With its establishment as a much less cumbersome diagnostic technique, ultrasound-directed percutaneous umbilical blood sampling (cordocentesis) replaced the fetoscopic method for intravascular transfusion (Berkowitz et al 1986, Nicolaides et al 1986b). Exchange transfusion is usually feasible by this approach and was initially the preferred option in a few centres, including Yale/New Haven (Grannum et al 1988) where the policy has since been revised to limit this to fetuses that are already hydropic or are considered to be in serious danger of volume overload (Grannum 1993) and where 28 of 37 hydropic fetuses (76%) have survived a combination of exchange and simple transfusions. The largest series of intravascular exchange transfusions, reported from Paris (Poissonnier et al 1989), was of 200 exchanges to 107 fetuses with reversal of hydrops in utero in 33 of them, and an eventual overall survival rate of 77%, including 27 of 47 initially hydropic fetuses (57%). The technique of fetal exchange transfusion by cordocentesis is well described in these reports.

At most centres intravascular fetal exchange transfusions are not carried out. Several referral teams have achieved better results by straight transfusions, e.g. survival rates of 96% in Iowa in 48 fetuses having 142 transfusions (3.0 per fetus) with the loss of two from 13 with anasarca and fluid collections in at least two cavities (Weiner et al 1991), and of 91% in Winnipeg in 44 fetuses having 174 transfusions (3.9 per fetus) with the loss of three of the 13 fetuses which fulfil the Iowa criterion (above; shared by this author) for frank hydrops (Harman et al 1990). By far the largest experience of ultrasound-guided straight intravascular transfusion is at King's College Hospital, where during 6 years fetal blood sampling by cordo-centesis showed that 221 of 272 fetuses from red cell isoimmunized pregnancies were Coombs-positive, and in these 716 intravascular intrauterine transfusions were performed (Nicolaides et al 1993). It is not stated how many of the Coombs-positive fetuses had transfusions or how many were hydropic, but simply that there were eventually 24 intrauterine, neonatal and infant deaths among the 221 Coombs-positive fetuses (11%), leaving an overall survival rate of 88% in all 272 fetuses including the 51 (19%) which were Coombs-negative. This makes the report difficult to evaluate with regard to the role and results of intravascular transfusion, but it contains a useful description of the technique, as do the other reports cited here.

Shortly after Rodeck's first fetoscopic intravascular transfusions, Bang et al (1982) demonstrated the feasibility of ultrasound-guided transfusion into the intra-hepatic part of the umbilical vein which is a stable target and in severe haemolytic disease is usually dilated. This has become the preferred route of some operators (de Crespigny et al 1985, Nicolini et al 1988). Cardiac puncture, used for genetic diagnosis (Bang 1985), is another alternative when access to a cord vessel has been impossible, although this is a less safe procedure (Westgren et al 1988).

In summary, it is clear that intrauterine transfusion in the management of the fetus severely affected by Rh or other red cell isoimmunization, should be restricted to specialized tertiary referral teams. Ideally perhaps each should serve a population of at least five million. One is left to share the Winnipeg group's view that intravascular transfusion is usually the method of choice, and that it can save the majority of frankly hydropic fetuses, but there remains a small but important place for the intra-peritoneal route for various forms of fetal therapy in which teams should therefore maintain their expertise. It would also seem that the capacitance of the fetoplacental circulation protects against cardiac overload so that the more complex procedure of exchange transfusion is not necessary. It is also to be hoped that the potential complications of intrauterine transfusion by whatever method will be kept in mind, especially the risk of fetomaternal haemorrhage and consequent exacerbation of isoimmunization during the current or any further incompatible pregnancy. The temptation to proceed to a prepared-for transfusion should not be yielded to if the fetal blood sampling shows a haematocrit or haemoglobin value that does not quite meet the agreed criterion.

Early rescue

The continued improvements in specialized neonatal care should also be kept in mind, and integration with an expert paediatric team is essential. Early rescue to intensive neonatal care may be the preferred option when intervention is required as early as 28 or 30 weeks. However, for the severely anaemic fetus, especially if hydropic, an emergency intrauterine transfusion to restore haemoglobin and oxygen-carrying capacity, and to correct acidosis, prior to elective Caesarean section may be the surest way to effect delivery in the best possible condition and circumstances. If, instead, labour is to be induced or allowed to proceed if occurring spontaneously, there must be close and continuous monitoring of the fetal condition and prompt rescue by Caesarean section if necessary, because these fetuses are at particular risk from intra-partum hypoxia and acidosis.

Other managements

Medical treatment A number of medical treatments have been tried but found wanting, even as supplementary measures. They include intensively repeated plasma exchange from early pregnancy in a usually unsuccessful attempt to achieve and maintain low maternal antibody levels (Robinson 1984), attempted immunosuppression with promezathine (Gusdon 1981), corticosteroids alone (Navot et al 1982) or combined with azothioprine (Odendaal et al 1986) and attempted maternal desensitization by the injection of gastric acid-resistant capsules containing material from Rh(D)-positive erythrocyte membrane (Bierme et al 1979). These methods have not been shown to affect the incidence of severe erythroblastosis fetalis, and when there is very serious disease, they are no substitute for giving the fetus stable blood and/or rescuing it at the optimal time from its dangerously incompatible environment.

Selective termination and artificial insemination When there is a very bad previous history, especially if there have been early intrauterine deaths from Rh disease despite adequate management, and when the partner is probably heterozygous for Rh(D) or whichever other antigens have immunized the mother, fetal blood sampling or chorion villus sampling in early pregnancy enables the fetus to be typed (Kanhai et al 1987) and for therapeutic abortion if it proves to have the responsible antigen(s) or, if not, for the pregnancy to continue. When the partner is probably homozygous, the couple can be offered artificial insemination with sperm from an antigenically compatible donor.

Counselling and contraception

Counselling, backed by appropriate contraceptive advice, is an essential part of supporting couples with the problem of red cell isoimmunization. Even when there has already been haemolytic disease, and perhaps unsuccessful pregnancies as a result, a fully informed and frank but sympathetically conducted discussion will be welcomed by the couple. There is not only considerable individual variation in the course of Rh isoimmunizations in successive pregnancies, but because of the impact of immunoprophylaxis and the new methods of treatment, prognostic guidelines can no longer be based on the experience derived from large series. However, each referral centre should have available updated prognostic information based on its own results.

RHESUS MORTALITY

Since 1977 Clarke and his associates have performed a valuable service in auditing registered stillbirths and deaths certified as due, or partly due, to haemolytic disease in England and Wales. They have been provided with the hospital records for scrutiny and have described their findings in a series of reports. However, because in Britain stillbirth was not registered when a dead fetus is born before the end of the 28th week, the survey necessarily underestimates the full wastage due or partly due to Rh incompatibility or to its treatment. This is usefully designated as 'total Rh mortality', a comprehensive category including all attributable abortions, stillbirths, early and late neonatal deaths, and also a few later infant deaths from complications of the disease or its treatment. A proportion of the deaths notified to the survey each year, usually between 20% and 26%, have been wrongly certified as due to haemolytic disease (Clarke & Whitfield 1979). This raises the opposite question of how many deaths from the disease are not registered as so; some of these are found by the Office of Population Censuses and Surveys from multiple coding of a sample of the certificates, but almost certainly there are others in which haemolytic disease is not coded at all.

A 15-year survey of 339 Rh(D)-immunized pregnancies in women referred to The Queen Mother's Hospital confirms that restricting reproductive mortality statistics to only perinatal deaths as presently defined in Britain (7.5% in this series) seriously underestimates the total Rh(D) mortality (14%). Of 45 attributable abortions, stillbirths and deaths of liveborns during this period, 20 were late abortions and two were deaths after the first week of life so that 49% would be excluded from perinatal mortality statistics. In the last 7 years of the Glasgow series this effect has been even more striking, with only two stillbirths and three first week neonatal deaths, a rate of only 3.2% representing little more than one-fifth of the total wastage of 22 (or 13.5%).

Nevertheless, the annual statistics provided by Clarke's uninterrupted survey give useful information on mortality trends and on changes in the relative importance of the different causes of Rh immunization. There was a steady fall in these deaths from 106 (at 18.4 per 100 000 live births) in 1977, to 44 (at 7.0 per 100 000 live births) in 1977, to 44 (at 7.0 per 100 000 live births) in 1982,

reflecting the growing impact of anti-D prophylaxis. This was followed by a steady loss of about 30 each year (at roughly 4.0 per 100 000 live births) up to 1987 which closed the first decade of the survey (Clarke & Mollison 1989). A parallel reduction in Rh-isoimmunized pregnancies, followed by a plateau of little change, was observed in several parts of Britain during the same period. The most recent report, covering the next 3 years, shows a resumed reduction in deaths due to Rh(D) disease to only 10 (at 1.6 per 100 000 live births) during 1990 (Hussey & Clarke 1992). This may at last reflect a response to increasing awareness that the national prophylaxis programme has not been implemented thoroughly, but also better salvage by improvements in both intensive neonatal care and intrauterine transfusion techniques. In Scotland, where an annual perinatal mortality survey is conducted, two or three Rh deaths are now usually identified each year (about four per 100 000 live births).

Regarding deaths attributed to haemolytic disease caused by other antibodies, mostly anti-c and anti-Kell, the survey in England and Wales shows three or four of these in most years since 1977. Interestingly, Clarke has raised the point that the persistence of deaths due to anti-c, despite improved treatment, could be because the antigens C and D usually coexist in a genotype, and therefore a woman liable to anti-c immunization will usually test as D-positive and may be wrongly thought not to be at risk (C Clarke, 1993, personal communication). This emphasizes the importance of screening every D-positive pregnant woman for all atypical red cell antibodies, as was made very clear by the results of a screening survey of 70 000 antenatal patients in Oxford, which showed that about 1% of these women had irregular antibodies, that almost half of the antibodies were not against Rh antigens, and that two-thirds of all the antibody-producers were Rh(D) positive (Bowell et al 1986).

PROPHYLAXIS

The protective mechanism whereby ABO fetomaternal incompatibility gives Rh(D)-negative mothers considerable protection against immunization by Rh(D)-positive red cells has been noted already. It was this that led Finn (1960) to reason that nature might be mimicked effectively by injecting anti-D antibodies, to give a temporary passive immunity to mothers that would neutralize the D-positive red cells entering her circulation before they could induce a lasting active immunization. Following a series of investigations in Liverpool and New York, experimental studies of Rh(D) immunoprophylaxis in male volunteers (Finn et al 1961) led to the demonstration that anti-D IgG could prevent immunization of D-negative women after delivery. This observation was then confirmed by a combined clinical trial in several English cities and Baltimore, in which anti-D immunoglobulin gave almost complete protection to high-risk D-negative primiparas with at least 0.2 ml of circulating fetal blood after being delivered of ABO-compatible D-positive babies (Combined Study from Centres in England and Baltimore 1966); at the end of a further D-positive pregnancy, which is the crucial test, only two of 86 of these mothers had anti-D antibodies, compared with 20 out of 65 controls (Combined Study from Centres in England and Baltimore 1971). Since then there has been ample evidence that when anti-D immunoglobulin is given by intramuscular injection within 72 hours after delivery, it will prevent immunization if the mother has not already been sensitized and if enough anti-D is given to neutralize the volume of fetomaternal haemorrhage she has received, even when as much as 170 ml of fetal blood has entered her circulation (Woodrow et al 1968).

In North America a relatively large standard dose of RhoGAM (Ortho Diagnostics), equivalent to 1500 iu, is used and this can neutralize 15 ml of D-positive blood. In Britain, when a Medical Research Council Working Party (1974) reported that the very small failure rate was similar with doses equivalent to 1000, 500 and 250 iu, but higher with only 100 iu, the standard national dose was reduced from 200 to 100 µg (equivalent to 500 iu). Since this is given for every 4 ml of fetal blood, and for every further 4 ml or fraction thereof, there is a safety margin with the lower British dose. Using a commercial product, the American programme was introduced rapidly for routine postpartum prophylaxis, regardless of parity or ABO grouping. The same occurred in most other developed countries where a significant proportion of the population is Rh(D)-negative. In Britain, using a nationally produced non-commercial product, there was a gradual step-by-step introduction of postpartum prophylaxis beginning with primiparas giving birth to ABO-compatible babies, and extending over a number of years until all as yet unimmunized Rh(D)-negative mothers giving birth to Rh(D)-positive babies qualified, as well as limited antepartum prophylaxis to cover potentially immunizing events, e.g. abortion, external version, antepartum haemorrhage or intrauterine procedures. As a further economy, a half-standard dose is given for any of these events occurring before 20 weeks. This will neutralize a 2.0 ml transplacental bleed of D-positive blood, which is not often exceeded before 20 weeks, although if a greater fetomaternal haemorrhage is demonstrated by Kleihauer testing the dose administered should be increased appropriately. Detailed recommendations for the use of anti-D prophylaxis were updated recently by the National Blood Transfusion Service Immunoglobulin Working Party (1991). To maximize implementation of the programme a fail-safe system of clinical documentation is essential, and a Kleihauer or alternative test must be carried out to estimate the volume of any fetal blood in the circulation of

every as yet unimmunized D-negative mother following delivery or a potentially immunizing event so that additional anti-D is given if required. Immediately before giving anti-D immunoglobulin in any of these circumstances, a sample of the mother's blood should be drawn for antibody testing to detect when any apparent failure of prophylaxis in reality results from the woman already having been immunized. This information may be of clinical interest, and possibly also of medicolegal importance.

Prophylaxis following abortion

The need for anti-D immunoglobulin after early abortion remains in dispute, in particular whether or not the family doctor should order it for a Rh(D)-negative woman threatening to miscarry or following spontaneous abortion in the early weeks. Evidence that fetomaternal haemorrhage can result from spontaneous or therapeutic abortion has been noted earlier in this chapter, but there is little or no evidence suggesting that isoimmunization is a risk following spontaneous abortion before 12 weeks. One of the problems is that the gestational age may not be known with any certainty, and ultrasonic dating is of course not possible if products of conception have already been lost. Since the risk of significant fetomaternal bleeding and isoimmunization increases as the pregnancy grows, the prudent course is to assume and act on the longest possible gestational age.

The National Blood Transfusion Service's Working Party has made the following proposals for the administration of anti-D immunoglobulin to as yet unimmunized D-negative women in relation to abortion. It should be given at any gestational age following (i) therapeutic abortion or (ii) instrumentation for removal of products of conception, and after 12 weeks for any (iii) threatened or (iv) completed spontaneous abortion; (v) if the pregnancy and vaginal bleeding persist it should be repeated every 6 weeks until fresh bleeding stops. Up to 20 weeks the dose is 250 iu, but thereafter the standard 500 iu dose should be given and any transplacental bleeding should be quantified in case any additional anti-D is required. All too frequently it is not realized that a late abortion, especially if associated with abdominal pain and heavy vaginal bleeding, may be due to placental abruption in which case a large fetomaternal haemorrhage may have occurred with the real risk that the next pregnancy, if D-positive, may be compromised by severe Rh disease.

Prophylaxis following large fetomaternal haemorrhages

The problem of large fetomaternal haemorrhage has been referred to several times, and attention was drawn to several circumstances in which these are most likely to occur and may cause such severe immunization that the next Rh-positive baby is critically or fatally affected. This was documented in 81 cases in Belfast, in which the immunizing pregnancy had been otherwise uncomplicated in only one-fifth of them, the remainder having one or more of the following complications: fulminant pre-eclampsia, placental abruption, twin births, Caesarean section, and manual removal of the placenta. The increased risk of a large fetomaternal haemorrhage in these circumstances, and its possible implications, must be borne in mind if a mother is D-negative and the fetus D-positive, and special attention paid to the need to quantify the fetomaternal haemorrhage to give anti-D immunoglobulin in adequate dosage. It is also useful to test again for antibodies several months after the pregnancy. At Caesarean section, as an additional practical contribution towards prevention, a rushed manual removal of the placenta should not be undertaken, and spillage of blood (which will inevitably include some fetal blood) into the peritoneal cavity (from whence it will be absorbed) should be reduced to a minimum by careful packing and swabbing out.

Failed prophylaxis and the case for antepartum prophylaxis

At the McMaster Conference on Rh Prevention in 1977 (Davey & Zipursky 1979) attention was directed to the importance of thorough documentation to audit the causes of Rh(D) isoimmunization to highlight gaps in the prophylactic programme. Evidence from that conference and from surveys in Yorkshire (Tovey et al 1978) and Glasgow (Whitfield 1984) at about the same time showed that, while incompatible blood transfusion still caused very occasional Rh(D) isoimmunization, one-third of pregnant women with Rh(D) antibodies had been immunized before anti-D prophylaxis became available (in 1969 in Britain), in a similar number there had been a failure to provide prophylaxis in the previous pregnancy, in 10% immunization had occurred despite prophylaxis correctly given, and in the remaining 20% immunization had occurred during a pregnancy. Evidence was also presented at the McMaster Conference to show that when antepartum immunization occurred, it was after 28 weeks in about 90% of cases, and that this could be prevented by administration of anti-D immunoglobulin then and at 34 weeks. Alternatively, a single injection of the larger North American dose at 28 weeks proved effective in Manitoba (Bowman & Pollock 1978).

The pattern of causes of Rh(D) disease has changed, mainly as a result of immunoprophylaxis and also because, when there is already a history of affected babies, couples now seem less likely to embark on further pregnancies.

In the referral service at The Queen Mother's Hospital during the 15 years from 1977 to 1991, the causes of the initial anti-D immunization were classified by thorough documentation in the hospital, supplemented by obtaining as much relevant information as possible from referring hospitals and transfusion services, including from overseas. Mothers who had developed their anti-D antibodies before immunoprophylaxis became available accounted for almost 15% of the whole series, but for none of those managed during the last 3 years (1989–91). One woman had been immunized by an incompatible blood transfusion. So-called administrative failures of prophylaxis, signifying that anti-D immunoglobulin was indicated by the national criteria in effect at the time but had not been given, accounted for 10%, slightly reduced to 8% in the last 3 years. There was virtually no difference in the incidence of correctly given but unsuccessful prophylaxis (14%), termed therapeutic failure, between the whole series and the last 3 years.

There was clear documentary evidence that in 53% of all the pregnancies the initial immunization had occurred antepartum, either in the index pregnancy or a previous one. This proportion had reached 71% in the last 3 years, and it was even more significant that antepartum immunization now accounted for 91% of the total Rh mortality. The contribution of antepartum immunization to the series as a whole and to the wastage is probably even greater, because it was the commonest possible cause in the 8% of cases in which classification could not be made with certainty.

This experience reinforces the view that, while not slackening efforts to achieve full implementation of post-partum prophylaxis and full protection after abortion or a large fetomaternal haemorrhage, there is a very strong case that Britain should follow other developed countries in instituting routine antepartum prophylaxis, and indeed this would be to follow the example of some British centres which have already adopted such a policy.

Antepartum prevention, using the standard British dose of anti-D immunoglobulin (500 iu) at 28 and 34 weeks, proved effective in a trial in primigravidas in Yorkshire (Tovey at al 1983), with only two cases of mild haemolytic disease in 1238 Rh(D)-positive newborns, compared with 16 examples of haemolytic disease (two needing exchange transfusions) in 2000 Rh(D)-positive babies born to untreated historical control mothers. Three hundred and twenty-five of the antepartum-treated mothers and 528 of the controls were documented through further Rh(D)-positive pregnancies, in respectively two and 11 of which anti-D antibodies were detected for the first time. About 600 of each group have now been followed through at least one further Rh(D)-positive pregnancy (Thornton et al 1989) with only one further example of active anti-D immunization (in a fourth pregnancy) in the originally treated group (without further antepartum prophylaxis) compared with four more examples among the controls. This suggests that the beneficial effect of antepartum prophylaxis in one pregnancy may persist through one or several further Rh(D)-positive pregnancies. There was also no evidence of any subsequent detrimental effect, maternal or fetal, of antepartum immunoprophylaxis.

In the hope that, for reasons of logistics and cost-effectiveness, the available national half-dose (250 iu) of anti-D immunoglobulin, given at 28 and 34 weeks, would prove adequate, a multicentre low-dose trial was started in Britain. Unfortunately, the trial had to be abandoned before reaching a statistically valid result. However, because there were examples of antepartum immunization in the group of treated patients, it does seem that the 250 iu dose cannot be relied on for routine antepartum prophylaxis. A single standard dose (500 iu) at 28 weeks might be more effective, while increased harvesting of anti-D immunoglobulin from hyperimmunized volunteer donors, the purchase of commercially available supplies, and eventually the production of monoclonal anti-D IgG are other possibilities.

Although no cost–benefit analysis of antepartum anti-D prophylaxis has been undertaken in Britain, or in the USA, two such assessments have been made in Canada. In Ontario, Torrance & Zipursky (1984) found that, while treating primigravidas was twice as cost-effective as treating multiparas, comprehensive prophylaxis (regardless of parity) was cost-effective by current standards in comparison with other accepted health care expenditures. More recently in Nova Scotia, Baskett & Parsons (1990) showed that the cost per case of Rh(D) isoimmunization

prevented was 2.7 times less than the cost per case treated.

NON-Rh ANTIBODIES

For some time a steadily increased detection of non-Rh antibodies has been the general experience of obstetric units and their supporting haematology and transfusion services (Hardy & Napier 1981), and the observation that now two-thirds of pregnant women with red cell antibodies are Rh(D)-positive (Bowell et al 1986) was mentioned earlier in considering serological screening. The commonest of the non-Rh antibodies are anti-Kell, present in about one pregnancy in each thousand and occasionally causing lethal haemolytic disease (Caine et al 1986). In most cases they have been induced by an incompatible (Kell-positive) blood transfusion, and it is for this reason that the Australian Red Cross avoids providing Kell-positive donor blood for premenopausal women requiring transfusion (Beal 1979).

The management of pregnancies with non-Rh antibodies that can cross the placenta is similar to that of Rh immunization, although with anti-Kell the amniotic fluid $\Delta OD450$ values have been said to underpredict the severity of erythroblastosis fetalis and haemolytic disease (Caine et al 1986), although that has not always been the experience elsewhere. It certainly makes for efficiency to manage such pregnancies in the same way as for those with Rh antibodies, and at or in conjunction with a referral centre. More frequent recourse to early fetal blood sampling to determine the fetal Kell-type (Reece et al 1988) should be considered, as noted earlier.

REFERENCES

Asensio S H, Figueroa-Longo J G, Pelegrina I V 1968 Intrauterine exchange transfusion. Obstetrics and Gynaecology 32: 350–355

Ballantyne J W 1892 General dropsy of the foetus. In: The diseases and deformities of the foetus, vol 1. Oliver and Boyd, Edinburgh

Bang J 1985 Intrauterine needle diagnosis. In: Bang J (ed) International ultrasound. Munksgaard, Copenhagen, pp 122–128

Bang J, Bock J E, Trolle D 1982 Ultrasound-guided fetal transfusion for severe rhesus haemolytic disease. British Medical Journal 284: 373–374

Baskett T F, Parsons M L 1990 Prevention of Rh(D) alloimmunisation: a cost-benefit analysis. Canadian Medical Association Journal 142: 337–339

Beal R W 1979 Non-rhesus (D) blood group isoimmunisation in obstetrics. Clinical Obstetrics and Gynecology 6: 493–508

Berkowitz R L, Chitkara U, Goldberg J D, Wilkins I, Chervenak F A, Lynch L 1986 Intrauterine intravascular transfusions for severe red blood cell isoimmunisation: ultrasound-guided percutaneous approach. American Journal of Obstetrics and Gynecology 155: 574–581

Bevis D C A 1952 The antenatal prediction of haemolytic disease of the newborn. Lancet i: 395–398

Bevis D C A 1956 Blood pigments in haemolytic disease of the newborn. Journal of Obstetrics and Gynaecology of the British Commonwealth 63: 68–75

Bierme S J, Blanc M, Abbal M, Fournie A 1979 Oral Rh treatment for severely immunised mothers. Lancet i: 604–605

Bowell P J, Allen D L, Enwistle C C 1986 Blood group antibody screening tests during pregnancy. British Journal of Obstetrics and Gynaecology 93: 1038–1043

Bowman J M 1978 The management of Rh-isoimmunisation. Obstetrics and Gynecology 52: 1–16

Bowman J M, Manning F A 1983 Intrauterine fetal transfusions: Winnipeg, 1982. Obstetrics and Gynecology 61: 203–209

Bowman J M, Pollock J M 1978 Antenatal prophylaxis of Rh isoimmunization: 28-weeks-gestation service program. Canadian Medical Association Journal 118: 627–630

Buchan A H, Comrie J D 1909 Four cases of congenital anaemia with jaundice and enlargement of the spleen. Journal of Pathology and Bacteriology 13: 398–413

Caine M E, Mueller-Heubach E 1986 Kell sensitization in pregnancy. American Journal of Obstetrics and Gynecology 154: 85–90

Chown B 1954 Anaemia from bleeding of the fetus into mother's circulation. Lancet i: 1213–1215

Claireaux A E, Cole P G, Lathe G H 1953 Icterus of the brain in the newborn. Lancet ii: 1226–1230

Clarke C, Whitfield A G W 1979 Deaths from rhesus haemolytic disease in England and Wales in 1977: accuracy of records and assessment of anti-D prophylaxis. British Medical Journal 1: 1665–1669

Clarke C A, Mollison P L 1989 Deaths from Rh haemolytic disease of the fetus and newborn, 1977–87. Journal of the Royal College of Physicians of London 23: 181–184

Combined Study from Centres in England and Baltimore 1966 Prevention of Rh haemolytic disease: results of the clinical trial. British Medical Journal 2: 907–914

Combined Study from Centres in England and Baltimore 1971 Prevention of Rh haemolytic disease: final results of the 'high-risk' clinical trial. British Medical Journal 1: 607–609

Copel J A, Grannum P A, Green J J, Belanger K, Hobbins J C 1989 Pulsed Doppler flow velocity waveforms in the production of fetal haematocrit of the severely isoimmunised pregnancy. American Journal of Obstetrics and Gynecology 161: 341–344

Daffos F, Capella-Pavlovsky M, Forestier F 1983 Fetal blood sampling via the umbilical cord using a needle guided by ultrasound: report of 66 cases. Prenatal Diagnosis 3: 211–217

Daffos F, Capella-Pavlovsky M, Forestier F 1985 Fetal blood sampling during pregnancy with use of a needle guided by ultrasound: a study of 606 cases. American Journal of Obstetrics and Gynecology 153: 655–660

Darrow R R 1938 Icterus gravis (erythroblastosis) neonatorum: examination of aetiologic considerations. Archives of Pathology 25: 378–417

Davey M G, Zipursky A M 1979 McMaster Conference on prevention of Rh immunization. Vox Sanguinis 36: 50–64

de Crespigny L Ch, Robinson H P, Quinn M, Doyle L, Ross A, Cauchi M 1985 Ultrasound guided fetal blood transfusion for severe Rhesus isoimmunisation. Obstetrics and Gynaecology 66: 529–532

Diamond L K, Blackfan K D, Baty J M 1932 Erythroblastosis fetalis and its association with universal oedema of the fetus, icterus gravis neonatorum and anaemia of the newborn. Journal of Pediatrics 1: 269–309

Dienst A 1905 Eclampsia: further studies. Zentralblatt fur Gynakologie 20: 353–364

Finn R 1960 Erythroblastosis. Lancet i: 526–527

Finn R, Clarke C A, Donohoe W T A et al 1961 Experimental studies on the prevention of Rh haemolytic disease. British Medical Journal 1: 1486–1490

Fisher R A, Race R R 1946 Rh gene frequencies in Britain. Nature 157: 48–49

Forrestier F, Galacteros F, Bardakjian J, Rainaut M, Beuzard Y 1986 Haematological values in 163 normal fetuses between 18 and 30 weeks of gestation. Pediatric Research 20: 342–346

Freda V J 1965 The Rh problem in obstetrics and a concept of its management using amniocentesis and spectrophotometric scanning of amniotic fluid. American Journal of Obstetrics and Gynecology 92: 341–374

Freda V J, Adamsons K 1964 Exchange transfusion in utero. American Journal of Obstetrics and Gynecology 89: 817–821

Freda V J, Gorman J G, Galen R S, Treacy N 1970 The threat of Rh isoimmunisation from abortion. Lancet ii: 147–148

Frigoletto F D, Umansky I, Birnholz J et al 1981 Intrauterine fetal transfusion in 365 fetuses during 15 years. American Journal of Obstetrics and Gynecology 139: 781–787

Grannum P A T 1993 In utero intravascular exchange transfusion for severe erythroblastosis fetalis. In: Chervenak F A (ed) Ultrasound in obstetrics and gynecology, vol 2. Little, Brown and Company, Boston, pp 1321–1326

Grannum P A T, Copel J A, Moya F R et al 1988 The reversal of hydrops fetalis by intravascular intrauterine transfusions in severe isoimmune fetal anaemia. American Journal of Obstetrics and Gynecology 158: 914–919

Gunson H H 1957 Neonatal anaemia due to fetal haemorrhage into the maternal circulation. American Journal of Clinical Pathology 20: 3–8

Gusdon J P 1981 In discussion of Gall S A and Miller J M Rh isoimmunization. American Journal of Obstetrics and Gynecology 140: 906–907

Hardy J, Napier J A F 1981 Red cell antibodies detected in antenatal tests in Rhesus positive women in South and Mid Wales 1948–1978. British Journal of Obstetrics and Gynaecology 88: 91–100

Harman C R, Bowman J M 1993 Intraperitoneal fetal transfusion. In: Chervenak F A (ed) Ultrasound in obstetrics and gynecology, vol 2. Little, Brown and Company, Boston, pp 1295–1313

Harman C R, Bowman J M, Manning F A, Mentiglou S M 1990 Intrauterine transfusion—intraperitoneal versus intravascular

approach: a case-control comparison. American Journal of Obstetrics and Gynecology 162: 1053–1059

Hellman L M, Hertig A T 1938 Pathological changes in the placenta associated with erythroblastosis of the fetus. American Journal of Pathology 14: 111–120

Hobbins J C, Davis C D, Webster J 1976 A new technique utilising ultrasound to aid intrauterine transfusion. Journal of Clinical Ultrasound 4: 135–137

Hussey R, Clarke C 1992 Deaths from haemolytic disease of the newborn in 1990. British Medical Journal 304: 444

Jakesch W 1878 A case of hydrops universalis of the foetus and hydrops placentae. Centralblatt fur Gynakologie 26: 619–624

Kanhai H H, Gravenhorst J B, Gemke R J, Overbeeke M A, Bernini L F, Beverstock G C 1987 Fetal blood group determination in first trimester pregnancy for the management of severe immunization. American Journal of Obstetrics and Gynecology 156: 120–123

Karnicki J 1968 Results and hazards of prenatal transfusion. Journal of Obstetrics and Gynaecology of the British Commonwealth 75: 1209–1213

Kleihauer E, Braun H, Betke K 1957 Demonstration of fetal haemoglobin in the circulating erythrocytes. Klinische Wochenschrift 35: 637–642

Lachman E, Hingley S M, Ward A M, Stewart C R, Duncan S L B 1977 Detection and measurement of fetomaternal haemorrhage: serum alphafetoprotein and Kleihauer techniques. British Medical Journal 1: 1377–1379

Landsteiner K, Wiener A S 1940 An agglutinable factor in human blood recognised by immune sera for rhesus blood. Proceedings of the Society for Experimental Biology and Medicine 43: 223

Levine P 1958 The influence of the ABO system on Rh haemolytic disease. Human Biology 30: 14–28

Levine P, Stetson R E 1939 Unusual cases of intra group agglutination. Journal of the American Medical Association 113: 126–127

Levine P, Katzin E M, Burnham L 1941 Isoimmunisation in pregnancy: its bearing on the aetiology of erythroblastosis fetalis. Journal of the American Medical Association 116: 825–817

Liley A W 1961 Liquor amnii analysis in the management of the pregnancy complicated by rhesus sensitisation. American Journal of Obstetrics and Gynecology 82: 1359–1370

Liley A W 1963 Intrauterine transfusion of foetus in haemolytic disease. British Medical Journal 2: 1107–1109

Liley A W 1970 Intrauterine transfusion. In: Robertson J G, Dambrosio F (eds) The Rh problem. Annali Obstetrica Ginecologica Special Number, Milan, pp 130–133

Medical Research Council Anti-D Working Party 1974 Controlled trial of various anti-D dosages in suppression of Rh sensitization following pregnancy. British Medical Journal 2: 175–180

National Blood Transfusion Service Immunoglobulin Working Party 1991 Recommendations for the use of anti-D immunoglobulin. Prescribers' Journal 31: 137–145

Navot D, Rozen E, Sodovsky E 1982 Effect of dexamethasone on amniotic fluid absorbance in Rh-sensitised pregnancy. British Journal of Obstetrics and Gynaecology 89: 456–458

Nicolaides K H, Rodeck C H 1985 Fetal therapy. In: Studd J (ed) Progress in obstetrics and gynaecology, vol 5. Churchill Livingstone, Edinburgh, pp 48–51

Nicolaides K H, Rodeck C H, Mibashan R S, Kemp J R 1986a Have Liley charts outlived their usefulness? American Journal of Obstetrics and Gynecology 155: 90–94

Nicolaides K H, Soothill P W, Clewell W, Rodeck C H, Campbell S 1986b Rh disease: intravascular fetal blood transfusion by cordocentesis. Fetal Therapy 1: 185–192

Nicolaides K H, Thorpe-Beeston J G, Salvesen D R, Snijders R J N 1993 Fetal blood transfusion by cordocentesis. In: Chervenak F A (ed) Ultrasound in obstetrics and gynecology, vol 2. Little Brown and Company, Boston pp 1315–1320

Nicolini U, Santolaya J, Ojo O E 1988 The fetal intrahepatic vein as an alternative to cord needling for prenatal diagnosis and treatment. Prenatal Diagnosis 8: 655–671

Odendaal H J, King J B, Oosthuizen O J 1986 Severe rhesus immunization successfully treated with apheresis and azothioprine. South African Medical Journal 69: 122–124

Orth J 1875 Uber das Vorkommen von bilirubinkrystallen

beinengeborenen kindern. Virchow's Archives of Pathology and Anatomy 63: 647

Plater F 1641 Observationum: Basie p. 748

Poissonnier M-H, Brossard Y, Demedeiros N et al 1989 Two hundred intrauterine exchange transfusions in severe blood incompatibilities. American Journal of Obstetrics and Gynecology 161: 709–713

Queenan J T 1969 Intrauterine transfusion: a cooperative survey. American Journal of Obstetrics and Gynecology 104: 397–405

Queenan J T, Goetschel E 1968 Amniotic fluid analysis for erythroblastosis fetalis. Obstetrics and Gynecology 32: 120–133

Queenan J T, Gadow E C, Lopes A C 1971a Role of spontaneous abortion in Rh-immunization. American Journal of Obstetrics and Gynecology 110: 128–130

Queenan J T, Shah S, Kubarych S F, Holland B 1971b Role of induced abortion in rhesus immunization Lancet i: 815–817

Rautman H 1912 Uber blutbildung bei totales allgeneiner wasserucht. Beitrage Anatomie Pathologie 54: 332–349

Reece E A, Copel J A, Scioscia A L, Grannum P A T, DeGennaro N, Hobbins J C 1988 Diagnostic fetal umbilical sampling in the management of isoimmunization. American Journal of Obstetrics and Gynecology 159: 1057–1062

Robinson E A E 1984 Principles and practice of plasma exchange in the management of Rh haemolytic disease of the newborn. Plasma Therapy and Transfusion Technology 5: 7–14

Rodeck C H, Holman C A, Karnicki J, Kemp J R, Whitmore D N, Austin M A 1981 Direct intravascular fetal blood transfusion by fetoscopy in severe rhesus isoimmunisation. Lancet i: 625–627

Seelen J, Van Kessel H, Eskes T et al 1966 A new method of exchange transfusion in utero. American Journal of Obstetrics and Gynecology 95: 812–816

Thornton J G, Page C, Foote G, Arthur G R, Tovey L A D, Scott J S 1989 Efficacy and long-term effects of antenatal prophylaxis with anti-D immunoglobulin. British Medical Journal 298: 1671–1673

Torrance G W, Zipursky A 1984 Cost-effectiveness of antepartum prevention of Rh immunization. Clinics in Perinatology 11: 267–281

Tovey L A D, Murray J, Stevenson B J, Taverner J M 1978 Prevention of Rh haemolytic disease. British Medical Journal 2: 106–108

Tovey L A D, Townley A, Stevenson B J, Taverner J M 1983 The Yorkshire antenatal anti-D immunoglobulin trial in primigravidae. Lancet ii: 244–246

Weiner C P, Williamson R A, Wenstrom K D et al 1991 Management of fetal ahemolytic disease by cordocentesis II: outcome of treatment. American Journal of Obstetrics and Gynecology 165: 1302–1308

Westgren M, Selberg A, Strangenberg M 1988 Fetal intracardiac transfusion in patients with severe Rhesus isoimmunisation. British Medical Journal 296: 885–886

Whitfield C R 1970 A three-year assessment of an Action Line method of timing intervention in rhesus isoimmunization. American Journal of Obstetrics and Gynecology 108: 1239–1244

Whitfield C R 1976 Rhesus haemolytic disease. Journal of Clinical Pathology 29, Suppl (Royal College of Pathologists) 103: 54–62

Whitfield C R 1984 An obstetric overview of trends in the management of Rh haemolytic disease. Plasma Therapy and Transfusion Technology 5: 47–55

Wiener A S 1944 Nomenclature of Rh blood types. Science 99: 532–533

Wiener A S, Peters H R 1940 Haemolytic reactions following transfusions of blood of the husband's group with three cases in which the same agglutinogen was responsible. Annals of Internal Medicine 13: 2306–2322

Woodrow J C, Finn R 1966 Transplacental haemorrhage. British Journal of Haematology 12: 297–309

Woodrow J C, Donohoe W T A 1968 Rh-immunization by pregnancy: results of a survey and their relevance to prophylactic therapy. British Medical Journal 2: 139–144

Zipursky A, Israels L G 1967 The pathogenesis and prevention of Rh immunisation. Canadian Medical Association Journal 97: 1245–1257

21. Cardiovascular problems in pregnancy

Michael de Swiet

Material in this chapter contains contributions from the first edition and we are grateful to the previous author for the work done.

Cardiovascular disease in pregnancy is a worrying condition for the obstetrician. Even excluding hypertensive disease (considered in Chapter 24), cardiovascular disease and specifically heart disease has an appreciable maternal mortality (10 per 100 000 in the most recent Report on Confidential Enquiries into Maternal Deaths Series (Department of Health and Social Security 1994). If the presence of a heart murmur is considered indicative of heart disease, the majority of women are at risk, for as many as 90% have systolic murmurs in pregnancy. Yet the prevalance of heart disease in pregnancy in the West is probably no more than 1%.

In this chapter we will consider, as they refer to pregnancy, the physiology of the cardiovascular system, the epidemiology of heart disease, the general management of patients with heart disease and certain specific conditions. For further reviews see de Swiet (1995), Elkayam & Gleicher (1982) and Sullivan & Ramanathan (1985).

THE PHYSIOLOGY OF THE CARDIOVASCULAR SYSTEM IN PREGNANCY

During pregnancy, oxygen consumption at rest increases by about 50 ml/min, i.e. from 300 to 350 ml/min. The oxygen is used by the fetus and other contents of the developing uterus, and to support the increased metabolic rate of the mother. Arterial blood is fully saturated. The only ways in which the mother can increase the supply of oxygen to peripheral tissues are either to increase the quantity of oxygen removed from the blood (increased arteriovenous oxygen difference) or to increase the delivery of oxygenated blood to the tissues (increased cardiac output). The pregnant woman chooses the latter course and, as in so many other physiological adaptations to pregnancy, overcompensates for the increased load, so that cardiac output increases to such an extent that arteriovenous oxygen difference decreases from 100 ml/l in the non-pregnant state to 80 ml/l in pregnancy.

The 40% increase in cardiac output from 3.5 to 6.0 l/min occurs early in pregnancy; at least two-thirds of the increase has occurred by the end of the first trimester. Although some studies have suggested that cardiac output falls at the end of pregnancy, even in patients in the left lateral position where the uterus does not obstruct venous return (Rubler et al 1977, James et al 1985, Davies et al 1986), measurements made with pulsed Doppler have shown no fall (Robson et al 1989b) and this must be considered the most reliable technique (Easterling et al 1990).

It is not clear to what extent myocardial contractility increases in pregnancy independently of the increase in preload and decrease in afterload. However, echocardiographic studies show an increase in the speed of circumferential shortening (Rubler et al 1977), which would suggest some increase in contractility.

Most studies have been performed at rest. Cardiac output rises still further on exertion and in labour. Each uterine contraction will increase cardiac output by about 20% (Ueland & Hansen 1969) by increasing preload (increased venous return). The pain of contractions is another important contributing factor. Cardiac output does increase on exercise in pregnancy, but as pregnancy progresses, the increase gets smaller. Limitation of venous return is a probable reason (Morton et al 1985). Although heart rate increases by about 10% in pregnancy, this is not sufficient to account for the 40% increase in cardiac output and so there is also an increase in stroke volume.

In normal pregnancy, blood pressure does not rise and, indeed, usually falls in the second trimester. The increased cardiac output is therefore accommodated by a decrease in peripheral resistance. Although some of these effects are probably caused by increased oestrogen levels, other mechanisms must be implicated since maximal oestrogen stimulation does not cause such large changes as are seen in pregnancy (Slater et al 1986). It is very likely that prostanoids and locally acting agents such as NO also contribute. Further support for active vasodilatation in pregnancy comes from the refractoriness to angiotensin infusion, as measured by a relative lack of pressor response to angiotensin infusion in normal pregnancy compared to the non-pregnant state (Gant et al 1973). This effect of pregnancy has also been associated with prostanoids and, in particular, prostacyclin.

Cardiac output also increases in pregnancy because of the increased preload caused by increased circulating blood volume. Blood volume rises very early in pregnancy; the total increase is about 40%, and this rise is maintained until delivery (Hytten & Paintin 1963).

The cardiac output has nearly returned to normal by 2 weeks after delivery (Robson et al 1987), but it may take up to 3 months for the blood pressure to return to normal.

The rise in cardiac output and associated vasodilatation in pregnancy cause changes in the circulation which may mimic heart disease. Heart rate increases and it is likely that arrhythmias are more common in pregnancy. Pulse volume is increased. Jugular venous pressure waves are more prominent, though the height of the venous pressure is not increased in pregnancy. Heart size increases and displacement of the apex beat by up to 1 cm from the mid-clavicular line should not be considered abnormal. The first heart sound is loud; there is often a very prominent third heart sound and an ejection systolic murmur up to grade 3/6 in intensity is heard over the whole praecordium in up to 90% of pregnant women. Venous hums—continuous murmurs usually audible in the neck which can be modified by stethoscope pressure—may also be heard in pregnancy.

In addition, peripheral oedema is very common in pregnancy, and usually does not indicate heart disease.

NATURAL HISTORY

Prevalance of heart disease

The prevalence and incidence of all heart disease in pregnancy varies between 0.3% (MacNab & MacAfee 1985) and 3.5% (Mendelson 1956). The figures vary because of differences in the prevalence of heart disease in different communities at different times. Thus rheumatic heart disease is becoming less common and congenital heart disease is proportionately more important. In addition, diagnostic criteria change, so that, for example, most cases of mitral valve abnormality are now thought to be congenital rather than rheumatic. It is also likely that we will see a change in the pattern of congenital heart disease in pregnancy following the increase in paediatric cardiac surgery which occurred between 1965 and 1975.

In all series, the dominant lesion in rheumatic heart disease has been mitral stenosis. In 1048 patients with rheumatic heart disease reported from Newcastle, Szekely et al (1973) found dominant mitral stenosis in 90%, mitral regurgitation in 6.6%, aortic regurgitation in 2.5% and aortic stenosis in 10%.

At present, the experience of congenital heart disease in pregnancy is limited to relatively simple defects. Five representative series are shown in Table 21.1. Although the total numbers in each series are very different, the overall pattern is similar. The most common lesions are atrial septal defect and patent ductus arteriosus, which account for about 50% of cases, followed by ventricular septal defect, pulmonary stenosis and Fallot's tetralogy which together contribute another 20%. In the more modern series from Dublin and Connecticut, we see the effect of surgery, as more women with patent ductus arteriosus and atrial septal defect have had these corrected in earlier life and are now childbearing.

Maternal mortality

Although sporadic fatalities will be seen in all forms of

Table 21.1 The prevalence (percentage) of various forms of congenital heart disease in pregnancy

	Ohio[1] (n = 125)	Queensland[2] (n = 93)	Dublin[3] (n = 74)	Connecticut[4] (n = 482)	Leicester[5] (n = 73)
Patent ductus arteriosus	24	27	9	22	11
Atrial septal defect	29	26	38	14	22
Pulmonary stenosis	4	12	6	10*	11
Ventricular septal defect	22	14	13	20	16
Tetralogy of Fallot	4	4	13	8†	8
Coarctation of the aorta	10	6	6 }	12	7
Aortic valve disease	3	4	6 }		7
Mitral valve disease				7	14
Other	2	2		7	4
Unclassified	5	5			

[1]Copeland et al (1963); [2]Neilson et al (1970); [3]Sugrue et al (1981); [4]Whittemore et al (1982); [5]MacNab and MacAfee (1985).
*Includes all pregnancies where mother had obstruction to right ventricular outflow.
†Expressed as percentage of all 233 mothers who became pregnant (some had more than one pregnancy).

heart disease in pregnancy, maternal mortality is most likely in those conditions where pulmonary blood flow cannot be increased (Jewett 1979). This occurs because of obstruction, either within the pulmonary blood vessels or at the mitral valve. The situation is documented clearly in Eisenmenger's syndrome, where up to now there has been no effective treatment, and where the maternal mortality is between 30 and 50% (Morgan Jones & Howitt 1965, Gleicher et al 1979.) An elevation in pulmonary vascular resistance is also seen in primary pulmonary hypertension in which the reported maternal mortality is 40–50% (Morgan Jones & Howitt 1965, McCaffrey & Dunn 1974, Tsou et al 1984).

In contrast, in women with Fallot's tetralogy in which pulmonary vascular resistance is normal, the reported maternal mortality varies between 4 and 20% (Jacoby 1964, Morgan Jones & Howitt 1965). Furthermore, the figure of 20% is only based on one maternal death in five pregnancies reported by Jacoby. The Connecticut series (Whittemore et al 1982) shows how good the results can be with obsessional care, since in 482 pregnancies from 233 women, including 8 mothers with Eisenmenger's syndrome, there were no maternal deaths.

In Ehlers–Danlos syndrome, the arterial and classical forms have also been associated with a high mortality due to arterial dissection and bleeding (Barabas 1967, Pearl & Spicer 1981, Rudd et al 1983).

In rheumatic heart disease, maternal mortality can now be very low. Szekely et al (1973) report 26 mortalities (about 1%) in 2856 pregnancies complicated by rheumatic heart disease between 1942 and 1969. Half of the deaths were due to pulmonary oedema, which became much less common once mitral valvotomy was freely available. These authors reported no maternal deaths in about 1000 pregnancies occurring after 1960. Rush et al (1979) also reported a maternal mortality of 0.7% in 450 mothers with rheumatic heart disease in South Africa.

There is no evidence that a well managed pregnancy is detrimental to the long term health of the woman with heart disease, providing she survives pregnancy itself. Chesley (1980) has reported a group of 38 patients with 51 pregnancies occurring after they were diagnosed as having severe heart disease. These were compared with a group of 96 women with equally severe rheumatic heart disease who did not have any pregnancies after diagnosis. The mean survival time (14 years) was no less and, in fact, was greater in the group that did have further pregnancies, compared to the group that did not (12 years).

Fetal outcome

The fetal outcome among those whose mothers have rheumatic heart disease in pregnancy is usually good and little different from that in those who do not have heart disease (Rush et al 1979, Sugrue et al 1981). How-ever, the babies are likely to be lighter at birth (Ueland et al 1972) by about 200 g, as reported in the study of Ho et al (1980).

In the five series of patients with congenital heart disease in pregnancy cited in Table 21.1, there was no excess fetal mortality, except in the group with cyanotic congenital heart disease. Here the babies are generally growth-retarded (Batson 1974, Whittemore et al 1982), and the fetal loss including abortion may be as high as 45% (Copeland et al 1963, Batson 1974, Gleicher et al 1979, Whittemore et al 1982). This is hardly surprising, in view of the inefficient mechanisms of placental exchange which cannot compensate for maternal systemic hypoxaemia. It is likely that the fetus dies because of inadequate oxygen supply or because of immaturity (Gleicher et al 1979) which may be iatrogenic.

Of great importance is the prevalence of congenital heart disease in the infants of mothers who themselves have congenital heart disease; this prevalence varies according to series from 3 to 14% (Nora 1978, Whittemore et al 1982). This compares with a prevalence of 1% in the general population (Nora 1978). The highest prevalence was in infants whose mothers had outflow obstruction, particularly left-sided. Most congenital abnormalities were represented in the infants; in about one-half, the child had the same abnormality as the mother.

MANAGEMENT

If possible, all women with heart disease attending one maternity hospital should be managed in a combined obstetric/cardiac clinic by one obstetrician and one cardiologist. In this way, the number of visits the patient makes to the hospital is kept to a minimum, and the obstetrician and cardiologist obtain the maximum experience in the management of relatively rare conditions.

History

As in all forms of medicine, the history is the most important single factor in the assessment of a patient who may have heart disease. In developed countries, most patients know whether they have heart disease. Even in developing countries it is very unusual though not unknown to have haemodynamically significant heart disease with no symptoms.

The most frequent symptom of heart disease in pregnancy is breathlessness. This can be difficult to assess because it is a variable feature of all pregnancies (Milne et al 1978); it is therefore important to consider whether the woman was breathless before she became pregnant. Syncope occurs in severe aortic stenosis, hypertrophic cardiomyopathy or subaortic stenosis, Fallot's tetralogy and Eisenmenger's syndrome; it is also a feature of normal pregnancy. Syncope, like chest pain, may occur because of dysrhythmias. The pregnant woman may also be aware of the dysrhythmia as a feeling of palpitations. Chest pain is usually a feature of ischaemic disease which is uncommon in pregnancy; chest pain may also occur in severe aortic stenosis, or, more commonly in pregnancy, in hypertrophic cardiomyopathy.

Physical signs

As noted above, the hyperdynamic circulation of pregnancy causes alterations in the cardiovascular system which mimic heart disease. Thus 20% of patients originally thought to have rheumatic heart disease may have none at all, following a reassessment performed up to 30 years later (Gleicher et al 1979). The changes which occur in the cardiovascular system associated with normal pregnancy have already been considered. Any other murmurs or additional heart sounds should be considered to be significant. Particular difficulty occurs with systolic murmurs, since they are so common in pregnancy. Those that are significant are:

1. Pansystolic murmurs of ventricular septal defect, mitral regurgitation or tricuspid regurgitation.
2. Late systolic murmurs of mitral regurgitation, mitral valve prolapse or hypertrophic cardiomyopathy.
3. Ejection systolic murmurs louder than grade 3/6 of aortic stenosis.
4. Ejection systolic murmurs which vary with respiration in pulmonary stenosis.
5. Ejection systolic murmurs associated with other abnormalities, e.g. ejection clicks—valvar pulmonary and aortic stenosis.

In addition, an assessment of the patient's cardiac status should also include the signs of heart failure: whether the patient is cyanosed or has finger-clubbing, the presence of pulse deficits and other peripheral signs of endocarditis such as splinter haemorrhages.

Investigations

Chest radiography

The chest radiograph is unhelpful in the diagnosis of minor degrees of heart disease but will, of course, show typical changes in those who have haemodynamically significant heart pathology. In pregnancy patients with normal hearts show slight cardiomegaly, increased pulmonary vascular markings and distension of the pulmonary veins.

Electrocardiography

In pregnancy, T wave inversion in lead III, S-T segment changes and Q waves, which would usually be considered pathological, occur frequently. In pregnancy, therefore, the electrocardiograph is more helpful in the diagnosis of dysrhythmias than in the demonstration of a structural abnormality of the heart.

Echocardiography

Recent studies have shown that the majority of structural cardiac abnormalities can be detected by echocardiography. This is the investigation of choice in pregnancy, since there is no radiation hazard, and because of the detailed information available in skilled hands. However most murmurs can be evaluated by clinical criteria alone and echocardiography is only necessary when there is doubt about their significance (Mishra et al 1992).

Clinical management

The nature and severity of the heart lesion should first be assessed in the combined clinic. In practice, many patients will have no evidence of any lesion at all and no further follow-up will be required. Some may only have a mild lesion with no haemodynamic problems, such as congenital mitral prolapse which has such an excellent prognosis (Rayburn & Fontana 1981) that again, no further follow-up is necessary. The remainder will have a condition with real or potential haemodynamic implications. These women must first be assessed as to the need for termination, if seen early enough in pregnancy, and secondly, as to the need for surgery. In patients with well managed heart disease, these assessments would have been made before the patient became pregnant.

Because of the mortality statistics indicated above, Eisenmenger's syndrome and primary pulmonary hypertension are absolute indications for termination of pregnancy. Very rarely, termination may also be indicated in patients with such severe pulmonary disease that they have pulmonary hypertension. In all other cases, the decision whether the pregnancy should continue depends on an individual assessment of the risk of pregnancy compared to the patient's desire to have children.

In general, the indications for surgery in pregnancy are similar to those in the non-pregnant state: failure of medical treatment with either intractable heart failure or intolerable symptoms. However, because of the bad reputation of severe mitral stenosis in pregnancy, mitral valvotomy (Pavankumar et al 1988) or valvuloplasty (Mangione et al 1989) is performed relatively commonly in patients with suitable heart valves, whereas open heart surgery is only performed with reluctance because of worries about the fetus (Zitnik et al 1969). More recent studies suggest that these worries about fetal survival are not justifiable, at least in the short term (Eilen et al 1981, Becker 1983). Possible long-term effects on the development of the child are unknown.

Antenatal care

After the initial assessment of the pregnant woman, the remainder of medical management during pregnancy is associated with avoiding, if possible, those factors which increase the risk of heart failure, and the vigorous treatment of any heart failure if it occurs. Risk factors for heart failure in pregnancy include infections (particularly urinary tract infection), hypertension (both pregnancy-associated and pregnancy-induced), obesity, multiple pregnancy, anaemia, the development of arrhythmias and, very rarely, hyperthyroidism. The increase in cardiac output in twin pregnancy, which is about 30% greater than in singleton pregnancy, is achieved by increasing heart rate and contractility rather than by increasing venous return. This suggests that cardiac reserve is particularly compromised in multiple pregnancy (Veille et al 1985).

Treatment of heart failure

The principles of treatment of heart failure in pregnancy are the same as in the non-pregnant state.

Digoxin The indications for the use of digoxin are to control the heart rate in atrial fibrillation and some other supraventricular tachycardias, and, when given acutely in heart failure, to increase the force of contraction. Dosage requirements of digoxin are the same in pregnancy as in the non-pregnant state. Both digoxin (Rogers et al 1972) and digitoxin (Okita et al 1956) cross the placenta, producing similar drug levels in the fetus to those seen in the mother (Rogers et al 1972, Saarikosi 1976). Digoxin enters the umbilical circulation within 5 minutes of intravenous administration to the mother (Saarikosi 1976). In general, there is no evidence that therapeutic levels of digoxin in the mother affect the neonatal electrocardiograph (Rogers et al 1972) or cause any harm to the fetus. However, although therapeutic drug levels in the mother do not harm the fetus, toxic levels do.

There may be a place for prophylactic digoxin therapy in selected women who are not in heart failure. This is most likely to be of value in those at risk from developing atrial fibrillation, i.e. those with rheumatic mitral valve disease with an enlarged left atrium, and possibly those who have paroxysmal atrial fibrillation or frequent atrial ectopic beats. However, this form of treatment has not been subjected to formal clinical trial, and there is certainly no case for digitalization of all women with heart disease in pregnancy. Digoxin is also secreted in breast milk, but since the total daily excretion in the mother with therapeutic blood levels should not exceed 2 µg (Levy et al 1977), this too is unlikely to cause any harm to the neonate, unless it suffers from some other disorder predisposing to digitalis toxicity, such as hypokalaemia.

Diuretic therapy Frusemide is the most commonly used and rapidly acting loop diuretic for the treatment of pulmonary oedema. In congestive cardiac failure where speed of action is not so important, oral thiazides are normally used in the first instance, although the extra potency of the loop diuretics may be necessary in a minority of cases. The use of thiazide in late pregnancy is not associated with any significant salt or water depletion in the neonate (Andersen 1970).

There are no risks with the use of diuretics for the treatment of heart failure specific to pregnancy, but, as in the non-pregnant state, hypokalaemia is an important complication in the woman who may also be taking digoxin. Treatment of pulmonary oedema should also include opiates such as morphine, which reduces anxiety and decreases venous return by causing venodilatation, and also aminophylline if there is associated bronchospasm. Angiotensin converting enzyme inhibitors should not be used in general in pregnancy because they may cause lethal renal failure in the neonate. But they may also be life saving in heart failure and in these circumstances should not be withheld. Life-threatening pulmonary oedema that does not respond to drug therapy may be helped by mechanical ventilation. If this is successful, and in other cases which do not respond to medical treatment, cardiac surgery should be considered if the patient has a potentially operable lesion.

Dysrhythmias

Most dysrhythmias that require treatment are due to ischaemic heart disease, which usually presents in women after their childbearing years and is rare in pregnancy. Therefore, there is limited experience in the treatment of dysrhythmias during pregnancy. Nevertheless, the problem does exist, particularly in patients who have non-ischaemic abnormalities of cardiac-conducting tissue, such as are believed to occur in the Wolff–Parkinson–White, Lown–Ganong–Levine (Carpenter & Decuir 1984) and Long Q-T syndromes (Bruner et al 1984). Furthermore, paroxysmal atrial tachycardia is said to occur more frequently in pregnancy than in the non-pregnant state (Szekely & Snaith 1953).

The antidysrhythmic drugs used most frequently in pregnancy are digoxin, quinidine and beta-adrenergic blocking agents, in particular propranolol, oxprenolol and atenolol. The indications for the use of these drugs are unaltered by pregnancy. Although there are isolated case reports of intrauterine growth retardation, acute fetal distress in labour and hypoglycaemia in the newborn in patients taking beta-adrenergic blocking agents, these have not been confirmed in clinical trials of oxprenolol used for treating hypertension in pregnancy. It would seem reasonable, therefore, to use propranolol or oxprenolol in both the acute and long-term treatment of supraventricular and ventricular tachycardia in pregnancy.

Atenolol is associated with growth retardation if given in the first half of pregnancy and probably is best avoided at this time.

Quinidine is used to maintain or induce sinus rhythm in patients either after DC conversion or when taking digoxin. It is well tolerated in pregnancy and has only minimal oxytocic effect. There is much less experience with other antidysrhythmic drugs such as verapamil, diltiazem, amiodarone or disopyramide. The use of disopyramide has been associated with hypertonic uterine activity on one occasion (Leonard et al 1978). Therefore disopyramide should be used in pregnancy with caution. The long-term risks of phenytoin are well known. However, this drug is only likely to be used in the acute treatment of dysrhythmias, particularly those induced by digitalis intoxication. Procainamide has also been used successfully to abolish atrial fibrillation in pregnancy (Szekely & Snaith 1974). Amiodarone has been used in several cases in pregnancy (Pilcher et al 1983). The drug contains substantial quantities of iodine and may cause transient abnormalities in fetal thyroid function and temporary goitre in the fetus, but no long-term problems have been reported. On the basis of this one report, it would seem reasonable to use amiodarone for resistant arrhythmias in late pregnancy that cannot be treated in any other way. Amiodarone and verapamil have been successfully used for the intrauterine treatment of fetal supraventricular tachycardia (Rey et al 1985); flecainamide is being used with increasing frequency for this indication.

DC conversion for tachyarrhythmias is safe in pregnancy and does not harm the fetus (Finlay & Edmunds 1979). Intravenous adenosine is so effective in terminating supraventricular tachycardias that it is now the treatment of choice (Garratt et al 1992). It has been used safely in pregnancy and is most unlikely to affect the fetus since its half-life is less than 2 seconds.

The difficulty arises in considering long-term prophylactic treatment with antidysrhythmic drugs which have not been extensively used in pregnancy. Here each case must be considered on its own merits, paying particular attention to the frequency and severity of the attacks of dysrhythmia. A single short episode of supraventricular tachycardia associated with no other symptoms does not require prophylactic treatment. Frequent attacks of ventricular tachycardia associated with syncope would require prophylaxis whatever the outcome in the fetus.

Anticoagulant therapy is a major problem in the management of patients with heart disease in pregnancy and is considered in the section on artificial heart valves, below.

Labour

Heart disease per se is not an indication for induction of labour; indeed, the risks of failed induction and of possible sepsis are relative contraindications. Nevertheless, these risks are slight, and induction should not be withheld if it is necessary for obstetric reasons. Furthermore, in complicated cases requiring optimal medical support, induction near term may be justified to plan delivery in daylight hours.

Fluid balance necessitates careful and expert attention during labour in women with significant heart disease. Many women in labour are given copious quantities of intravenous fluid and if they have normal hearts, can cope with the resultant increase in circulating blood volume. Patients with heart disease cannot, however, and may easily develop pulmonary oedema. This effect is exacerbated by the tendency to use crystalloid intravenous fluids which decrease the colloid osmotic pressure of plasma by about 5 mmHg over the course of labour (Gonik et al 1985).

Some centres are gaining increasing experience in the use of elective central catheterization (Swan–Ganz technique) to measure right atrial pressure, wedge pressure (indirect left atrial pressure) and cardiac output in labour in patients with heart disease. There is no doubt that this technique facilitates a more rational use of fluid therapy, diuretics and inotropes. Preliminary results also suggest that measurement of central venous pressure alone is so misleading as an index of left ventricular filling pressure that it should not be used for this purpose (although it is still invaluable in managing patients with bleeding problems). The technique of Swan–Ganz catheterization is quite difficult, however, and has a significant morbidity. Therefore, it should only be used in centres where there is sufficient experience.

Women with heart disease are also particularly sensitive to the effects of aortocaval compression by the gravid uterus when lying in the supine position. Marked hypotension can develop, causing maternal and fetal distress. The risk of this complication developing is even greater after epidural anaesthesia (Ueland et al 1968).

Most patients with heart disease do have quite rapid, uncomplicated labours, particularly if they are taking digoxin (Weaver & Pearson 1973). In the majority, analgesia is best given by epidural anaesthesia since it is an effective analgesic which also decreases cardiac output, by causing peripheral vasodilation and decreasing venous return, and reduces heart rate. However, epidural anaesthesia is inadvisable in Eisenmenger's syndrome and contraindicated in hypertrophic cardiomyopathy.

Most obstetric emergencies arising in labour, including the need for Caesarean section, can be managed using epidural anaesthesia and in general is commonly believed to be safer than general anaesthesia (Department of Health and Social Security 1994) though not necessarily in cardiac patients. Epidural block causes less haemodynamic changes than spinal (Robson et al 1991) and in normal patients did not affect haemodynamics (Robson

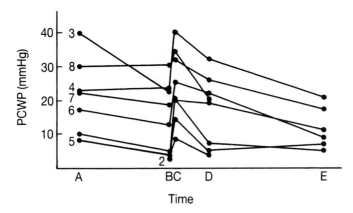

Fig. 21.1 Intrapartum alterations in pulmonary capillary wedge pressure (PCWP) in eight patients with mitral stenosis. A = First-stage labour; B = second-stage labour, 15–30 min before delivery; C = 5–15 min postpartum; D = 4–6 h postpartum; E = 18–20 h postpartum. From Clark et al (1985) with permission.

et al 1989a). There are few adequate comparisons of these forms of anaesthesia in comparable patients, and much depends on the skill and preference of the anaesthetist.

In women with heart disease, it seems sensible to keep the second stage of labour short in order to decrease maternal effort, but there is obviously no advantage in performing forceps delivery in a woman who would deliver easily by herself.

The use of oxytocic drugs in the third stage of labour is much debated. The theoretical disadvantage is that ergometrine and Syntocinon will cause a tonic contraction of the uterus, expressing about 500 ml of blood into a circulation whose capacitance has also been reduced by associated venoconstriction. The consequent rise in left atrial pressure (Fig. 21.1), which averages 10 mmHg in patients with mitral stenosis, may be quite sufficient to precipitate pulmonary oedema. However, the management of postpartum haemorrhage in a patient with heart disease is not easy. Syntocinon should be used in all patients in the third stage, unless they are in failure, since it has less effect on blood vessels than ergometrine and can be given by intravenous infusion, which can be accompanied by intravenous frusemide.

Endocarditis and its prevention in pregnancy

The Report on Confidential Enquiries into Maternal Deaths in England and Wales (Department of Health and Social Security 1994) shows that there were 10 such deaths from endocarditis in England and Wales between 1970 and 1975. There were another three deaths from endocarditis in the most recent report (Department of Health and Social Security 1994). However, the case for antibiotic prophylaxis in labour has not been proven. There are several large series of women with heart disease in pregnancy in whom no antibiotics were given and in whom no endocarditis was observed (Fleming 1977,

Sugrue et al 1981). Yet, the data in the Confidential Enquiries into Maternal Deaths series suggests that women are at increased risk from endocarditis in pregnancy. What is not clear from these reports is whether the endocarditis was contracted during labour and therefore potentially preventable by antibiotics, or whether it arose at some other time. Until more details are available, the author continues to use antibiotic prophylaxis. For patients not allergic to penicillin and who have not had a penicillin more than once in the preceding month, amoxycillin 1 g i.v. plus gentamicin 120 mg i.v. at the onset of labour or induction followed by amoxycillin 500 mg i.v. 6 hours later. For patients who are allergic to penicillin or who have had a penicillin more than once in the preceding month, teicoplanin 400 mg i.v. and gentamicin 120 mg i.v. at the onset of labour or induction. (Teicoplanin is easier to give and has less side-effects than vancomycin which was previously recommended; Recommendations from the Endocarditis Working Party 1990, Simmons et 1992.)

SPECIFIC CONDITIONS OCCURRING DURING PREGNANCY

Acquired heart disease

Chronic rheumatic heart disease

As already indicated, this form of heart disease has been commonest in pregnancy in the UK and still is in many parts of the world. By far the most important lesion is mitral stenosis, which may be the only lesion or the dominant abnormality amongst several others. Women with mitral stenosis are particularly likely to develop pulmonary oedema in pregnancy because of the increase in cardiac output, the increase in heart rate preventing ventricular filling and the increase in pulmonary blood volume. Mitral stenosis is the lesion that is most likely to require treatment for pulmonary oedema or heart failure and also to require surgery during pregnancy. The haemodynamic changes associated with labour in patients with mitral stenosis have been documented by Swan–Ganz catheterization. Women entering labour with a wedge pressure (indirect left atrial pressure) less than 14 mmHg are unlikely to develop pulmonary oedema (Clark et al 1985).

Mitral regurgitation puts a volume load on the left atrium and left ventricle, but it does not cause pulmonary hypertension until late in the condition, and heart failure is rare in pregnancy; it occurs usually in older women.

Rheumatic aortic valve disease is much less common in women than in men, and much less common that mitral valve disease in pregnancy. Severe aortic regurgitation causes pulmonary oedema; aortic stenosis may be associated with chest pain, syncope and sudden death, but aortic valve disease is usually not severe enough to be a problem in pregnancy. Severe aortic stenosis has a 17% maternal mortality (Arias & Pineda 1978).

Disease of the tricuspid valve almost never occurs in isolation. Also, tricuspid valve disease rarely requires specific treatment; the patient improves when the rheumatic disease of the other valves is treated, either medically or surgically.

Pregnancy in women with artificial heart valves

Anticoagulation is the major problem in this group. Those who have successful isolated aortic or mitral valve replacements usually have near normal cardiac function and do not incur haemodynamic problems in pregnancy (Oakley 1983). Even those with multiple valve replacements usually have sufficient cardiac reserve for a successful pregnancy (Andrinopoulos & Arias 1980).

The problem of anticoagulation is shown in Table 21.2. The combined fetal morbidity and mortality rates varied between 31 and 50% in women who were anticoagulated with warfarin compared with 4–9% in those were not anticoagulated.

For conditions such as pulmonary embolism, subcutaneous heparin is safer than warfarin (see Ch. 44). There appears to be less maternal bleeding and less fetal risk of congenital abnormalities such as chrondrodysplasia punctata or optic atrophy. However, where there is a risk of systemic thromboembolism as with artificial heart valves, subcutaneous heparin treatment does not seem to be adequate; indeed there are reports of Starr Edwards aortic and Björk–Shiley mitral valves that have thrombosed during pregnancy when the mothers were either managed with subcutaneous heparin (Bennett & Oakley 1968, McLeod et al 1978) or were not anticoagulated (Chen et al 1982). There is no ideal solution to this problem. Even though the risk of fetal malformations may persist after 16 weeks' gestation (Shaul & Hall 1977), warfarin should be used from before conception until about 37 weeks' gestation, because subcutaneous heparin does not give adequate protection (subcutaneous heparin therapy also has the risk of maternal bone demineraliza-

tion (de Swiet et al 1983), while the risks of warfarin therapy have probably been overestimated (Chong et al 1984)). The optimal INR with warfarin appears to be three times control. Any further prolongation does not decrease the thromboembolism risk but does increase the risk of bleeding. Alternative approaches to management in early pregnancy are to use intravenous heparin given by a Hickman catheter (Nelson et al 1984), or through a heparin lock (Pearson 1984) or to use high-dose continuous subcutaneous infusion of heparin (Rabinovici et al 1987), in all cases aiming to achieve a heparin level (protamine sulphate neutralization test; Dacie 1975) of 0.4–0.6 u/ml. Such treatment, which ideally should be given from before conception, must be considered experimental at present and is unlikely to suit all patients.

At 37 weeks, when the risk of fetal bleeding associated with labour in patients treated with warfarin seems to be too great, the patient should be admitted to hospital and given continuous intravenous heparin to produce a heparin level of 0.4–0.6 u/ml, as assayed by protamine sulphate neutralization (Dacie 1975). Heparin does not cross the placenta and therefore will not cause bleeding in the fetus. It is believed that the clotting system of the fetus will return to normal after warfarin has been withheld for 1 week. At that time maternal heparin therapy should be reduced to give a heparin level of less than 0.2 u/ml and a normal thrombin time. Under these circumstances the woman is not at risk of bleeding and labour should be induced. If the woman inadvertently goes into labour while taking warfarin, she should be given vitamin K to reverse the action of warfarin in the fetus and started on heparin therapy as above. In extreme cases vitamin K has been given intramuscularly to the fetus in utero by transamniotic injection (Larsen et al 1978).

After delivery, because of the risk of maternal postpartum haemorrhage, the patient should continue to receive heparin for 7 days, when warfarin may be recommenced. This is not a contraindication to breastfeeding, since insignificant quantities of warfarin are secreted in breast milk (Orme et al 1977). However, Dindevan is

Table 21.2 Fetal outcome of oral anticoagulation in pregnancy in mothers with artificial heart valves

	Hammersmith[1]	Dublin[2]	Hong Kong[3]	Barcelona[4]
Number of pregnancies	39	18	41	46
Number anticoagulated (fetal mortality and morbidity % of those anticoagulated)	15 (53)	18 (50)	30 (40)	42 (31–38)*
Cause of fetal mortality and morbidity (% of those anticoagulated)				
Abortion	3 (20)	8 (44)	10 (33)	12 (21–29)*
Perinatal deaths	4 (27)	0 (0)	0 (0)	2 (0–5)*
Fetal malformation	1 (7)	1 (5)	2 (7)	2 (0–5)*
Number not anticoagulated (fetal mortality and morbidity % of those not anticoagulated)	24 (4)	0	11 (9)	3 (?–?)*

[1]Oakley & Doherty (1976); [2]O'Neill et al (1982); [3]Chen et al (1982); [4]Javares et al (1984).
*Not stated which of the fetal losses etc. were in the anticoagulated group so possible range is given.

excreted in breast milk (Eckstein & Jack 1970); women taking it should not breastfeed.

Myocardial infarction

Myocardial infarction is rare in pregnancy (1 in 10 000 gravidas or less) and in young women in general. Most cases occur in women aged 30–40 years. About 40% of women die in pregnancy or within 1 week of delivery. However, infarction occurring in the first two trimesters has a lower mortality (23%) than that occurring in the last trimester (45%; Hawkins et al 1985). Successful outcomes have been reported following cardiac arrest (Stokes et al 1984) and the development of left ventricular aneurysm in pregnancy (Roberts et al 1983). In contrast to myocardial infarction during pregnancy, infarction in the puerperium occurs in younger, often primigravid women. Their pregnancies have frequently been complicated by pre-eclampsia (Beary et al 1979). The precise mechanism of myocardial infarction is open to speculation in all patients. Women have a particularly high incidence of coronary spasm, and atypical mechanisms seem to be common in pregnancy. Patients with myocardial infarction occurring in the puerperium are most likely to have spasm or coronary artery thrombosis unassociated with atherosclerotic narrowing. Another possible cause is primary dissection of the coronary arteries.

The diagnosis of myocardial infarction in pregnancy is made on the basis of chest pain, with possible pericardial friction rub and fever supported by the typical changes in the electrocardiogram. Moderate elevations of the white cell count and erythrocyte sedimentation rate are seen in normal pregnancy, when the level of lactic acid dehydrogenase may also be raised (Stone et al 1960). The serum glutamine acid transaminase level may also be elevated due to contraction of the uterus and is certainly elevated in the puerperium when the uterus is involuting. However the creatine kinase MB isoenzyme is specific to heart muscle and is the test of choice for the diagnosis of myocardial infarction in pregnancy (Donnelly et al 1993).

It is difficult to be dogmatic about management, for there is little experience and the pathology may be diverse. It would be sensible to treat the initial episode in a coronary care unit, with conventional opiate analgesics and medication for complications such as dysrhythmias. Because of the possibility of coronary spasm, nitroglycerine or other vasodilators should be used early in women with continuing pain. Once delivery has occurred, there is a good case for coronary arteriography. The angiographic demonstration of coronary embolus would be an indication for anticoagulation, but otherwise the benefits of anticoagulation in myocardial infarction unassociated with pregnancy do not seem great enough to justify the considerable extra risks imposed on the pregnancy (Borchgrevnik et al 1968). Streptokinase and other thrombolytic drugs are contraindicated because of the risk of bleeding. Spontaneous vaginal delivery should be allowed unless there are good obstetric reasons for interfering. Epidural anaesthesia should be used because of its efficacy as an analgesic and in reducing cardiac output by reducing preload. As in other cases of heart disease, the second stage should be limited by forceps delivery. Syntocinon infusion should be used rather than ergometrine in the third stage, since ergometrine is more likely to cause coronary artery spasm.

There is no evidence that pregnancy specifically predisposes women to myocardial infarction. Unless it is thought that the woman has had a coronary embolus, pregnancy should not be discouraged in patients who have had myocardial infarction in the past.

Cardiomyopathy in pregnancy

Cardiomyopathy may arise de novo during pregnancy, and there is probably at least one form of cardiomyopathy (peripartum cardiomyopathy) that is specific to pregnancy. Alternatively, any form of cardiomyopathy due to other causes may complicate pregnancy.

Hypertrophic obstructive cardiomyopathy

The most common of these other causes is hypertrophic obstructive cardiomyopathy or subaortic stenosis. The cause is not known but the pathological features are hypertrophy and disorganization of cardiac muscle, particularly that of the left ventricular outflow tract. Women present with chest pain, syncope, arrhythmias or the symptoms of heart failure. They should not be allowed to become hypovolaemic, since this too increases the risk of obstruction of the left ventricular outflow tract. Particular care should be taken to give adequate fluid replacement if there is antepartum haemorrhage and also in avoiding postpartum haemorrhage. During labour, those with hypertrophic obstructive cardiomyopathy should not have epidural anaesthesia, since this causes relative hypovolaemia by increasing venous capacitance in the lower limbs. Beta-blocking drugs are often used in women with symptoms (Oakley et al 1979) and should be considered safe in pregnancy (see Ch. 24), apart from the risk of intrauterine growth retardation best described with atenolol taken in the first half of pregnancy.

Peripartum cardiomyopathy

For reviews of this important condition see Stuart (1968), Homans (1985) and Julian & Szekely (1985). The woman usually presents with heart failure, which is usually right-sided, either at the end of pregnancy or more commonly in the puerperium (Fig. 21.2). There is no predisposing cause for the heart failure and the heart is grossly dilated.

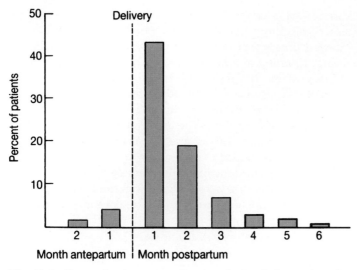

Fig. 21.2 Onset of peripartum cardiomyopathy in relation to time of delivery. From Homans (1985) with permission.

The diagnosis is made by excluding all other causes of right and left ventricular dysfunction. Patients tend to be multiparous, black, relatively elderly and socially deprived. Pregnancy has often been complicated by hypertension. Pulmonary, peripheral and particularly cerebral embolization are major causes of morbidity and mortality. Apart from conventional antifailure treatment, these women should also receive anticoagulant therapy until heart size has returned to normal, and until they have no further dysrhythmias. Immunosuppressive therapy with prednisone and azathioprine has been used to improve left ventricular function (Midei et al 1990). If they recover from the initial episode, the long-term prognosis is good, but the condition may recur in future pregnancies, particularly if there is evidence of even subclinical left ventricular dysfunction.

The pathogenesis is unknown; immunological (Rand et al 1975), nutritional and infective (Melvin et al 1982) aetiologies have been proposed.

A specific form of peripartum cardiac failure occurs in the Hausa tribe in northern Nigeria (Davidson & Parry 1978). The peak incidence is 4 weeks postpartum. During this period, for up to 40 days after delivery, the Hausa woman spends 18 h/day lying on a mud bed, heated so that the ambient temperature reaches 40°C. She also increases her sodium intake to 450 mmol/day by eating *kanwa* salt from Lake Chad. Many are hypertensive, but the condition regresses rapidly with diuretic and digoxin therapy. The contribution of hypertension to the heart failure is debated (Sanderson 1977), but this would seem an extreme example of the instability of the cardiovascular system in the first few weeks of the puerperium interacting with the particular susceptibility of West Africans to dilated cardiomyopathy (Lancet Editorial 1985).

Congenital heart disease

Eisenmenger's syndrome

Eisenmenger's syndrome has a very high maternal mortality, particularly if there is superimposed pre-eclampsia. Only recently has there been any form of surgical treatment—heart and lung transplantation—and that must be considered experimental.

Most of those with Eisenmenger's syndrome who die do so in the puerperium. Although death may be occasionally sudden, due to thromboembolism, this is unusual. More frequently, these women die due to a slowly falling systemic Po_2 with associated decrease in cardiac output. It is likely that this is due to a change in the shunt ratio whereby pulmonary blood flow decreases at the expense of systemic flow (Fig. 21.3).

What can be offered to the pregnant woman with Eisenmenger's syndrome? Unfortunately, abortion would appear to be the answer. The maternal mortality associated with abortion is only 7% in comparison to 30% for continuing pregnancy (Gleicher et al 1979). However, if she decides to continue with pregnancy, prophylactic anticoagulation, probably with subcutaneous heparin, should be offered, because of the risk of systemic and pulmonary thromboembolism. Labour should not be induced unless there are good obstetric reasons. Induced labour carries a higher risk of Caesarean section, which is associated with a particularly high maternal mortality in Eisenmenger's syndrome (Gleicher et al 1979).

There is controversy concerning the place of epidural anaesthesia for the management of labour. Although

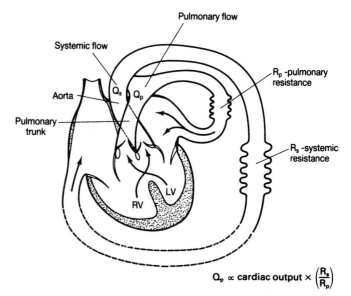

$$Q_p \propto \text{cardiac output} \times \left(\frac{R_s}{R_p}\right)$$

Fig. 21.3 Pulmonary (Q_p) and systemic (Q_s) blood flows and resistances (R_p, R_s) in Eisenmenger's syndrome associated with ventricular septal defect. From de Swiet & Fidler (1981) with permission.

epidural anaesthesia could decrease the shunt ratio by decreasing systemic vascular resistance, this is not invariable (Midwall et al 1978). On balance, an elective epidural anaesthetic carefully administered at the beginning of labour is probably preferable to emergency epidural or general anaesthesia needed if a sudden decision is made to perform instrumental delivery (Gleicher 1979).

If the woman does become hypotensive with increasing cyanosis and decreasing cardiac output, high inspired oxygen concentrations will decrease pulmonary vascular resistance, increasing the pulmonary blood flow and increasing peripheral oxygen saturation (Midwall et al 1978). In addition, alpha-sympathomimetic agents, such as phenylephrine, methoxamine and noradrenaline, will increase systemic resistance and thus divert blood to the lungs (Devitt & Noble 1980). However, drugs such as tolazoline, phentolamine, nitroprusside and isoprenaline, which have been used to decrease pulmonary vascular resistance in other clinical situations, probably should not be given since they will also decrease the systemic vascular resistance. The same problem may occur with dopamine and beta-sympathomimetic drugs which have been given to increase cardiac output.

Inhaled nitric oxide has been used successfully to reduce pulmonary vascular resistance in both neonates (Roberts et al 1992) and adults (Pepke-Zaba et al 1991) with other conditions and might be helpful in Eisenmenger's syndrome.

Coarctation of the aorta and Marfan's syndrome

In both these conditions, the maternal risk is of dissection of the aorta associated with the hyperdynamic circulation of pregnancy and possibly with an increased risk of medial degeneration due to the hormonal environment of pregnancy (Konishi et al 1980). Although earlier studies of coarctation had indicated a high maternal mortality, they date from the period before surgery was available for correction of severe cases. There were no maternal deaths among 83 patients studied from 1960 (Deal & Wooley 1973). Only those who already have evidence of dissection should have the coarctation repaired in pregnancy. Any upper limb hypertension should be treated aggressively with anti-hypertensive drugs. If there is gross widening of the ascending aorta, suggesting intrinsic disease, the woman should be delivered by elective Caesarean section to reduce the risk of dissection associated with labour.

In Marfan's syndrome there is also a risk of dissection of the aorta. Dilatation of the aorta to more than 40 mm (determined echocardiographically) is the limit at which pregnancy is contraindicated (Pyeritz 1981). As in coarctation of the aorta, any associated hypertension should be treated aggressively and delivery should be by Caesarean section if there is evidence of aortic disease.

Congenital heart block

This usually presents no problem in pregnancy. Although part of the normal response to pregnancy includes an increase in heart rate to increase the cardiac output, this is not obligatory. There are many records of successful pregnancy among those with heart block (Ginns & Holinrake 1970, Szekely & Snaith 1974). Presumably, they are able to increase stroke volume sufficiently to cope with the increased demands of pregnancy. A few are unable to increase cardiac output sufficiently at the end of pregnancy or during labour (Bowman & Millar-Craig 1980). Therefore, women with heart block who are not paced, or those in whom there is any possibility of pacemaker failure, should be managed in obstetric units where there is access to pacing facilities.

CONCLUSIONS

Heart disease in pregnancy remains a worrying problem for the obstetrician because of those women (very much in the minority) who are at risk. Future advances will help us to define this minority with more precision and optimize management strategies for these patients.

REFERENCES

Andersen J B 1970 The effect of diuretics in late pregnancy on the new born infant. Acta Paediatrica Scandinavica 59: 659–663
Andrinopoulos G C, Arias F 1980 Triple heart valve prosthesis and pregnancy. Obstetrics and Gynecology 55: 762–764
Ardias F, Pineda J 1978 Aortic stenosis and pregnancy. Journal of Reproductive Medicine 20: 229–232
Barabas A P 1967 Heterogeneity of the Ehlers–Danlos syndrome: description of three clinical types and a hypothesis to explain the basic defect(s). British Medical Journal 2: 612–613
Batson G A 1974 Cyanotic congenital heart disease and pregnancy. British Journal of Obstetrics and Gynaecology 81: 549–553
Beary J F, Sumner W R, Bulkley B H 1978 Postpartum acute myocardial infarction: a rare occurrence of uncertain etiology. American Journal of Cardiology 43: 158–160
Becker R M 1983 Intracardiac surgery in pregnant women. Annals of Thoracic Surgery 36: 453–458
Bennett G G, Oakley C M 1968 Pregnancy in a patient with a mitral valve prosthesis. Lancet i: 616–619
Borchgrevink C F, Bjerkelund C, Abrahamsen A M et al 1968 Long-term anticoagulant therapy after myocardial infarction in women. British Medical Journal 2: 571–574
Bowman P R, Millar-Craig M W 1980 Congenital heart block and pregnancy: a further case report. Journal of Obstetrics and Gynaecology 1: 98–99
Bruner J P, Barry M J, Elliott J P 1984 Pregnancy in a patient with idiopathic long QT syndrome. American Journal of Obstetrics and Gynecology 149: 690–691
Carpenter R J, Decuir P 1984 Cardiovascular collapse associated with oral terbutaline tocolytic therapy. American Journal of Obstetrics and Gynecology 148: 821–823

380   TURNBULL'S OBSTETRICS

Chen W W C, Chan C S, Lee P K, Wang R Y C, Wong V C W 1982 Pregnancy in patients with prosthetic heart valves: an experience with 45 pregnancies. Quarterly Journal of Medicine 51: 358–365

Chesley L C 1980 Severe rheumatic cardiac disease and pregnancy: the ultimate prognosis. American Journal of Obstetrics and Gynecology 136: 552–558

Chong M K B, Harvey D, de Swiet M 1984 Follow-up study of children whose mothers were treated with warfarin during pregnancy. British Journal of Obstetrics and Gynaecology 91: 1070–1073

Clark S L, Phelan J P, Greenspoon J, Aldahl D, Horenstein J 1985 Labor and delivery in the presence of mitral stenosis: central hemodynamic observations. American Journal of Obstetrics and Gynecology 152: 984–1088

Copeland W E, Wooley C F, Ryan J M, Runco V, Levin H S 1963 Pregnancy and congenital heart disease. American Journal of Obstetrics and Gynecology 86: 107–110

Dacie J 1975 Practical haematology. Churchill Livingstone, Edinburgh, pp 413–414

Davidson N McD, Parry E H O 1978 Peri-partum cardiac failure. Quarterly Journal of Medicine 47: 431–461

Davies P, Francis R I, Docker M F, Watt J M, Selwyn Crawford J 1986 Analysis of impedance cardiography longitudinally applied in pregnancy. British Journal of Obstetrics and Gynaecology 93: 717–720

Deal K, Wooley C F 1973 Coarctation of the aorta and pregnancy. Annals of Internal Medicine 78: 706–710

Department of Health and Social Security 1994 Report on Confidential Enquiries into Maternal Deaths in England and Wales 1987–1990. HMSO, London

de Swiet M 1995 Heart disease in pregnancy. In: de Swiet M (ed) Medical disorders in obstetric practice, 3rd edn. Blackwell Science, Oxford, pp 143–181

de Swiet M, Fidler J 1981 Heart disease in pregnancy: some controversies. Journal of the Royal College of Physicians 15: 183–186

de Swiet M, Dorrington Ward P, Fidler J et al 1983 Prolonged heparin therapy in pregnancy causes bone demineralisation (heparin-induced osteopenia). British Journal of Obstetrics and Gynaecology 90: 1129–1134

Devitt J H, Noble W H 1980 Eisenmenger's syndrome and pregnancy. New England Journal of Medicine 302: 751

Donnelly S, McKenna P, McGing P, Sugrue D 1993 Myocardial infarction during pregnancy. British Journal of Obstetrics and Gynaecology 100: 781–782

Easterling T R, Carlson K L, Schmucker B C et al 1990 Measurement of cardiac output in pregnancy by Doppler technique. American Journal of Perinatology 7: 220–222

Eckstein H, Jack B 1970 Breast feeding and anticoagulant therapy. Lancet i: 672–673

Eilen B, Kaiser I H, Becker R M, Cohen M N 1981 Aortic valve replacement in the third trimester of pregnancy: case report and review of the literature. Obstetrics and Gynecology 57: 119–121

Elkayam U, Gleicher N 1982 Cardiac problems in pregnancy. Diagnosis and management of maternal and fetal disease. Alan R Liss, New York

Finlay A Y, Edmunds V 1979 DC cardioversion in pregnancy. British Journal of Clinical Practice 33: 88–94

Fleming H A 1977 Antibiotic prophylaxis against infective endocarditis after delivery. Lancet i: 144–145

Gant N F, Daley G L, Chand S, Whalley P J, MacDonald P C 1973 A study of angiotensin II pressor response throughout primigravid pregnancy. Journal of Clinical Investigation 52: 2682–2689

Garratt C J, Malcolm A D, Camm A J 1992 Adenosine and cardiac arrhythmias. British Medical Journal 305: 3–4

Ginns H M, Holinrake K 1970 Complete heart block in pregnancy treated with an internal cardiac pacemaker. Journal of Obstetrics and Gynaecology of the British Commonwealth 77: 710

Gleicher N, Midwall J, Hochberger D, Jaffin H 1979 Eisenmenger's syndrome and pregnancy. Obstetrical and Gynecological Survey 34: 721–741

Gonik B, Cotton D, Spillman T, Abouleish E, Zavisca F 1985 Peripartum colloid osmotic pressure changes: effects of controlled fluid management. American Journal of Obstetrics and Gynecology 151: 812–815

Hawkins G D V, Wendel G D, Leveno K J, Stoneham J 1985 Myocardial infarction during pregnancy: a review. Obstetrics and Gynecology 65: 139–147

Ho P C, Chen T Y, Wong V 1980 The effect of maternal cardiac disease and digoxin administration on labour, fetal weight and maturity at birth. Australian and New Zealand Journal of Obstetrics and Gynaecology 20: 24–27

Homans D C 1985 Peripartum cardiomyopathy. New England Journal of Medicine 312: 1432–1436

Hytten F E, Paintin D B 1963 Increase in plasma volume during normal pregnancy. Journal of Obstetrics and Gynaecology of the British Commonwealth 70: 402–407

Jacoby W J 1964 Pregnancy with tetralogy and pentalogy of Fallot. American Journal of Cardiology 14: 866–873

James C F, Banner T, Levelle P, Caton D 1985 Noninvasive determination of cardiac output throughout pregnancy. Anesthesiology 63: A434

Javares T, Coto E C, Maiques V, Rincon A, Such M, Caffarena J M 1984 Pregnancy after heart valve replacement. International Journal of Cardiology 5: 731–739

Jewett J F 1979 Pulmonary hypertension and pre-eclampsia. New England Journal of Medicine 301: 1063–1064

Julian D G, Szekely P 1985 Peripartum cardiomyopathy. Progress in Cardiovascular Disease 27: 223–240

Konishi Y, Tatsuta N, Kumada K et al 1980 Dissecting aneurysm during pregnancy and the puerperium. Japanese Circulation Journal 44: 726–732

Lancet Editorial 1985 Dilated cardiomyopathy in Africa. Lancet i: 557–558

Larsen J F, Jacobsen B, Holm H H, Pedersen J F, Mantoni M 1978 Intrauterine injection of vitamin K before the delivery during anticoagulant treatment of the mother. Acta Obstetricia et Gynecologica Scandinavica 57: 227–230

Leonard R F, Braun T E, Levy A M 1978 Initiation of uterine contractions by disopyramide during pregnancy. New England Journal of Medicine 299: 84

Levy M, Grait L, Laufer N 1977 Excretion of drugs in human milk. New England Journal of Medicine 297: 789

MacNab G, MacAfee C A J 1985 A changing pattern of heart disease associated with pregnancy. Journal of Obstetrics and Gynaecology 5: 139–142

McCaffrey R M, Dunn L J 1974 Primary pulmonary hypertension in pregnancy. Obstetrical and Gynecological Survey 19: 567

McLeod A A, Jennings K P, Townsend E R 1978 Near fatal puerperal thrombosis on Björk-Shiley mitral valve prosthesis. British Heart Journal 40: 934–937

Mangione J A, Zuliani M F, Del Castillo J M et al 1989 Percutaneous double balloon mitral valvuloplasty in pregnant women. American Journal of Cardiology 1989; 64: 99–102

Melvin K R, Richardson P J, Olsen E G J, Daly K, Jackson G 1982 Peripartum cardiomyopathy due to myocarditis. New England Journal of Medicine 307: 731–734

Mendelson C L 1956 Disorders of the heart beat during pregnancy. American Journal of Obstetrics and Gynecology 72: 1268–1301

Midei M G, DeMent S H, Feldman A M et al 1990 Peripartum myocarditis and cardiomyopathy. Circulation 81: 922–928

Midwall J, Jaffin H, Herman M V, Kuper Smith J 1978 Shunt flow and pulmonary haemodynamics during labor and delivery in the Eisenmenger syndrome. American Journal of Cardiology 42: 299–303

Milne J A, Howie A D, Pack A I 1978 Dyspnoea during normal pregnancy. British Journal of Obstetrics and Gynaecology 85: 260–263

Mishra M, Chambers J B, Jackson G 1992 Murmurs in pregnancy: an audit of echocardiography. British Medical Journal 304: 1413–1414

Morgan Jones A, Howitt G 1965 Eisenmenger syndrome in pregnancy. British Medical Journal 1: 1627–1631

Morton M J, Paul M S, Campos G R, Hart M V, Metcalfe J 1985 Exercise dynamics in late gestation: effects of physical training. American Journal of Obstetrics and Gynecology 152: 91–97

Neilson G, Galea E G, Blunt A 1970 Congenital heart disease and pregnancy. Medical Journal of Australia 1: 1086–1088

Nelson D M, Stempel L E, Fabri P J, Talbert M 1984 Hickman

catheter use in a pregnant patient requiring therapeutic heparin anticoagulation. 149: 461–462

Nora J J 1978 The evolution of specific genetic and environmental counselling in congenital heart disease. Circulation 57: 205–213

Oakley C M 1983 Pregnancy in patients with prosthetic heart valves. British Medical Journal 286: 1680–1682

Oakley C M, Doherty P 1976 Pregnancy in patients after valve replacement. British Heart Journal 38: 1140–1148

Oakley G D G, McGarry K, Limb D G, Oakley C M 1979 Management of pregnancy in patients with hypertrophic cardiomyopathy. British Medical Journal 1: 1749–1750

Okita G T, Plotz E J, Davis M E 1956 Placental transfer of radioactive digitoxin in pregnant woman and its fetal distribution. Circulation Research 4: 376–380

O'Neill H, Blake S, Sugrue D, MacDonald D 1982 Problems in the management of patients with artificial heart valves during pregnancy. British Journal of Obstetrics and Gynaecology 89: 940–943

Orme M l'E, Lewis P J, de Swiet M et al 1977 May mothers given warfarin breast-feed their infants? British Medical Journal 1: 1564–1565

Pavankumar P, Venugopal P, Kaul U et al 198 Closed mitral valvotomy during pregnancy. Scandinavian Journal of Thoracic and Cardiovascular Surgery 22: 11–15

Pearl W, Spicer M 1981 Ehlers–Danlos syndrome. Southern Medical Journal 74: 80–81

Pearson J N 1984 Outpatient intravenous heparin. American Journal of Obstetrics and Gynecology 149: 108

Pepke-Zaba J, Higenbottam T W, Dinh-Xuan A T et al 1991 Inhaled nitric oxide as a cause of selective pulmonary vasodilatation in pulmonary hypertension. Lancet 338: 1173–1174

Pilcher D, Leather H M, Storey G C A, Holt D W 1983 Amiodarone in pregnancy. Lancet ii: 597–598

Pyeritz R E 1981 Maternal and fetal complications of pregnancy in the Marfan syndrome. American Journal of Medicine 71: 784–790

Rabinovici J, Mani A, Barkai G, Hod H, Frenkel Y, Mashiach S 1987 Long-term ambulatory anticoagulation by constant subcutaneous heparin infusion in pregnancy. British Journal of Obstetrics and Gynaecology 94: 89–91

Rand R J, Jenkins D M, Scott D G 1975 Maternal cardiomyopathy of pregnancy causing stillbirth. British Journal of Obstetrics and Gynaecology 82: 172–175

Rayburn W F, Fontana M E 1981 Mitral valve prolapse and pregnancy. American Journal of Obstetrics and Gynecology 14: 9–11

Recommendations from the Endocarditis Working Party of the British Society for Antimicrobial Chemotherapy 1990 Antibiotic prophylaxis of infective endocarditis. Lancet 335: 88–89

Rey E, Duperron L, Gauthier R, Lemay M, Grignon A, LeLorier J 1985 Transplacental treatment of tachycardia-induced fetal heart failure with verapamil and amiodarone: a case report. American Journal of Obstetrics and Gynecology 153: 311–312

Roberts A D G, Low R A L, Rae A P, Hillis W S 1983 Left ventricular aneurysm complicating myocardial infarction occurring during pregnancy. Case report. British Journal of Obstetrics and Gynaecology 90: 969–970

Robert J D, Polaner D M, Lang D, Zapol W M 1992 Inhaled nitric oxide in persistent pulmonary hypertension of the newborn. Lancet 340: 818–819

Robson S C, Boys R, Rodeck C, Morgan B 1991 Haemodynamic changes during epidural and spinal anaesthesia for elective caesarean section: correlation with umbilical artery pH. Clinical Science 11: 301

Robson S C, Hunter S, Moore M, Dunlop W 1987 Haemodynamic changes during the puerperium; a Doppler and M-mode echocardiographic study. British Journal of Obstetrics and Gynaecology 94: 1028–1039

Robson S C, Dunlop W, Hunter S et al 1989a Haemodynamic changes associated with caesarean section under epidural anaesthesia. British Journal of Obstetrics and Gynaecology 96: 642–647

Robson S C, Hunter S, Boys R J, Dunlop W 1989b Serial study of factors influencing changes in cardiac output during human pregnancy. American Journal of Physiology 256: H1060–H1065

Rogers M E, Willerson J T, Goldblatt A, Smith T W 1972 Serum digoxin concentrations in the human fetus, neonate and infant. New England Journal of Medicine 287: 1010–1013

Rubler S, Prabod Kumar M D, Pinto E R 1977 Cardiac size and performance during pregnancy estimated with echocardiography. American Journal of Cardiology 40: 534–540

Rudd N L, Nimrod C, Holbrook K A, Byers P H 1983 Pregnancy complications in type IV Ehlers–Danlos syndrome. Lancet i: 50–53

Rush R W, Verjans M, Spracklen F H N 1979 Incidence of heart disease in pregnancy. A study done at Peninsular Maternity Services Hospital. South African Medical Journal 55: 808–810

Saarikoski S 1976 Placental transfer and fetal uptake of ^{3}H-digoxin in humans. British Journal of Obstetrics and Gynaecology 83: 879–884

Sanderson J E 1977 Oedema and heart failure in the tropics. Lancet ii: 1159–1161

Shaul W L, Hall J G 1977 Multiple congenital anomalies associated with oral anticoagulants. American Journal of Obstetrics and Gynecology 127: 191–198

Simmons N A, Ball A P, Cawson R A et al 1992 Antibiotic prophylaxis and infective endocarditis. Lancet 339: 1292–1293

Slater A J, Gude N, Clarke I J, Walters W A W 1986 Haemodynamic changes in left ventricular performance during high-dose oestrogen administration in transsexuals. British Journal of Obstetrics and Gynaecology 93: 532–538

Stokes I M, Evans J, Stone M 1984 Myocardial infarction and cardiac output in the second trimester followed by assisted vaginal delivery under epidural anaesthesia at 38 weeks gestation. Case report. British Journal of Obstetrics and Gynaecology 91: 197–198

Stone M L, Lending M, Slobody L B, Mestern J 1960 Glutamine oxalacetic transaminase and lactic acid dehydrogenase in pregnancy. American Journal of Obstetrics and Gynecology 80: 104

Stuart K L 1968 Cardiomyopathy of pregnancy and the puerperium. Quarterly Journal of Medicine 37: 463–478

Sugrue D, Blake S, MacDonald D 1981 Pregnancy complicated by maternal heart disease at the National Maternity Hospital, Dublin, Ireland, 1969 to 1978. American Journal of Obstetrics and Gynecology 139: 1–6

Sullivan J M, Ramanathan K B 1985 Management of medical problems in pregnancy—severe cardiac disease. New England Journal of Medicine 313: 304–309

Szekely P, Snaith L 1953 Paroxysmal tachycardia in pregnancy. British Heart Journal 15: 195

Szekely P, Snaith L 1974 Heart disease and pregnancy. Churchill Livingstone, Edinburgh

Szekely P, Turner R, Snaith L 1973 Pregnancy and the changing pattern of rheumatic heart disease. British Heart Journal 35: 1293–1303

Tsou E, Waldhorn R E, Kerwin D M, Katz S, Patterson J A 1984 Pulmonary venoocclusive disease in pregnancy. Obstetrics and Gynecology 64: 281–284

Ueland K, Hansen J M 1969 Maternal cardiovascular dynamics. II. Posture and uterine contractions. American Journal of Obstetrics and Gynecology 103: 1–7

Ueland K, Gills R, Hansen J M 1968 Maternal cardiovascular dynamics. I. Caesarean section under subarachnoid block anesthesia. American Journal of Obstetrics and Gynecology 100: 42–53

Ueland K, Novy M J, Metcalfe S 1972 Hemodynamic responses of patients with heart disease to pregnancy and exercise. American Journal of Obstetrics and Gynecology 113: 47–59

Veille J C, Morton M J, Burry K J 1985 Maternal cardiovascular adaptations to twin pregnancy. American Journal of Obstetrics and Gynecology 153: 261–263

Weaver J B, Pearson J F 1973 Influence on time of onset and duration of labour in women with cardiac disease. British Medical Journal 2: 519–520

Whittemore R, Hobbins J C, Engle M A 1982 Pregnancy and its outcome in women with and without surgical treatment of congenital heart disease. American Journal of Cardiology 50: 641–651

Zitnik R S, Brandenburg R O, Sheldon R, Wallace R B 1969 Pregnancy and open heart surgery. Circulation 39 (suppl): 257

22. Medical disorders in pregnancy: diabetes, thyroid disease, epilepsy

Michael de Swiet

INTRODUCTION

Medical disorders in pregnancy cover a wide field and for further details the reader is referred to other texts (e.g. de Swiet 1985, Barron & Lindheimer 1991). In this chapter we consider diabetes, thyroid disease and epilepsy. Thromboembolism is considered in Chapter 23, cardiovascular disease in Chapter 21 and hypertension in Chapter 24.

DIABETES

Banting & Best published their first paper on the discovery of insulin in 1922 and revolutionized the management of insulin-dependent diabetes, a condition which up to that time had been invariably fatal. Diabetic pregnancy pre-insulin had a very high maternal and fetal mortality. There were 10 pregnancies among 650 diabetic women attending the Joselin Clinic between 1898 and 1917: of these two were terminated, two babies were stillborn, two women died undelivered and only four women were delivered of a liveborn child. Even as late as 1922 Joselin could only describe 108 cases of diabetic pregnancy with a perinatal mortality rate of 440 per 1000 births. Once insulin was available maternal mortality in diabetic pregnancy fell sharply but perinatal mortality remained high and was still in the region of 400 per 1000 by the 1940s. Since that time, however, perinatal mortality has fallen steadily with increasingly good control of maternal diabetes and a better understanding of the problems of the fetus.

Carbohydrate metabolism in pregnancy

Hormonal changes occur in pregnancy which profoundly affect carbohydrate metabolism. The levels of oestrogen and progesterone, human placental lactogen, cortisol and prolactin rise progressively as pregnancy advances. Of these a number, notably human placental lactogen and cortisol, are insulin antagonists and so insulin resistance develops in the mother as the pregnancy advances, and is most marked in the last trimester. In response to this change the normal woman produces an increased amount of insulin to keep carbohydrate metabolism stable. In normal pregnancy the increased insulin production counters the rise in insulin resistance and blood glucose levels are kept within a very narrow range of between 4 and 6 mmol/l during much of every 24 hours.

As a result of the hormonal changes carbohydrate metabolism in pregnancy undergoes characteristic changes. The fasting level of glucose is significantly lower than normal from the 10th week until the 16th week when there is a slow but significant rise up to 32 weeks. Thereafter the fasting level falls again slowly so that at term it is not significantly different from the non-pregnant level (Baird 1986). The peak levels of glucose after a carbohydrate load are higher than normal, especially after the 20th week. In response to an intravenous injection of glucose the rate of disappearance of glucose is increased in early pregnancy and returns to a normal level in late pregnancy. The insulin response to oral or intravenous glucose is substantially increased during the third trimester of pregnancy. In the second half of pregnancy, especially during the third trimester, there is an increase in insulin resistance with a slight deterioration in glucose tolerance and the hypoglycaemic effect of intravenous insulin is less. Pregnancy-onset gestational diabetes is most commonly seen at this time.

Animal experimental work suggests that the increased insulin action on carbohydrate metabolism in early human pregnancy is reduced in later pregnancy so as to provide ample glucose to the fetus at a time when its growth is maximal and its preferential utilization of this substance reaches a peak. The extent to which blood glucose levels are kept within a relatively narrow range cannot be matched when the mother is diabetic, no matter how good the diabetic control may be.

Fetomaternal blood glucose relationships

Glucose crosses the placenta by a process of facilitated diffusion and the fetal blood glucose level follows closely the maternal level. The glucose transport mechanism protects the fetus from excessively high levels becoming saturated by maternal blood glucose levels of 10 mmol/l or more so that the fetal blood glucose level peaks at 8–9 mmol/l. This ensures that in normal pregnancy the fetus is not overstimulated by postprandial peaks in the maternal blood glucose levels. In diabetic pregnancy although the protective action of the placental barrier persists, higher levels of glucose in the fetus will occur in response to maternal hyperglycaemia.

Glycosuria

Glycosuria is common in pregnancy, starting within 6 weeks of the last menstrual period. The mean excretion rate of glucose per 24 hours is 76 mg in the pregnant woman and a minority of women secrete significantly larger amounts of glucose, up to 1 g or more in 24 hours, in the last 4 weeks of pregnancy. There is a tendency for glycosuria to increase as pregnancy advances but there is a great deal of diurnal and day-to-day variation in excretion rate. There is no constant relationship between urinary and blood glucose levels.

Lipid metabolism

Every aspect of lipid metabolism is affected by pregnancy, particularly free fatty acids, triglycerides, phospholipids and cholesterol. The plasma level of free fatty acids falls from early to mid-pregnancy and thereafter shows a significant rise. The same is true of the plasma level of glycerol. This is in keeping with the accumulation of body fat that occurs during the anabolic phase of pregnancy (first two trimesters). In the catabolic phase of pregnancy (last trimester) raised free fatty acid and glycerol level are available as fuel to the maternal tissues to offset the increasing diversion to the rapidly growing fetus of glucose and amino acids. Free fatty acids and glycerol levels fall postpartum, followed by a rise during breastfeeding, presumably to allow similar diversion of the ingested maternal nutrients for the synthesis of breast milk.

As with free fatty acids, glycerol and triglycerides, plasma levels of cholesterol and phospholipid are increased in pregnancy. The increase in the latter two substances accounts for the predisposition of the pregnant woman to gall stones, especially as there is a relative reduction in the excretion of bile acids (O'Sullivan et al 1975). The significance of changes of lipid metabolism in pregnancy

is not clear, but they are mediated by hormonal changes and fit into the general pattern of an increase in storage of glycogen and fat in most maternal tissues during the anabolic first two trimesters of pregnancy followed by the mobilization of fuel for the benefit of both mother and fetus in the catabolic third trimester (Kalkhoff et al 1979).

Diabetes mellitus defined

Diabetes mellitus is a clinical syndrome characterized by hyperglycaemia due to a deficiency or diminished effectiveness of insulin. The metabolic disturbances affect the metabolism of carbohydrate, protein, fat, water and electrolytes. The deranged metabolism depends on the loss of insulin activity in the body, in many cases eventually leading to cellular damage, especially to vascular endothelial cells in the eye, kidney and nervous system. Diabetes mellitus is not a single disease but a group of diseases.

The classification of diabetes mellitus suggested by the National Diabetes Data Group in 1979 is generally accepted. The three main clinical types of interest to the obstetrician are insulin-dependent diabetes (IDD or type 1), non-insulin-dependent diabetes (NIDD or type 2) and gestational diabetes though the existance of gestation diabetes as a significant entity is becoming increasingly doubtful (see below).

Insulin-dependent diabetes rarely needs a glucose tolerance test (GTT) for diagnosis in pregnancy. Because the maximum age of incidence is 11–14 years, most women have been diagnosed and are taking insulin before they become pregnant. A few women develop IDD in pregnancy; indeed it is more common to develop IDD in pregnancy than in the non-pregnant state in women of childbearing age. The diagnosis is rarely in doubt for such women since they are usually symptomatic at presentation, with very high blood sugars and often keto-acidosis (Buschard et al 1990).

NIDD does require a GTT for diagnosis; as we will see it is important since it carries risks for the fetus almost as great as those of IDD. Since the patients are not symptomatic, a GTT is necessary for diagnosis and the possibility of diagnosing NIDD is probably the only valid justification for a glycaemic screen in all patients. In Caucasians the prevalence of NIDD is so low that such a universal screen is not justified. In Asians (Matther & Keen 1985) and Afro-Carribeans (Dooley et al 1991) the prevalence is higher and such patients should probably be screened in pregnancy but this policy should be formally evaluated.

In general, the WHO classification was of great value since it separated patients with diabetes who needed to be treated from those with impaired glucose tolerance whose only risk was the long-term one of vascular disease. However the study was not performed with pregnancy in mind. Erring on the side of caution the authors stated that in pregnancy all patients with impaired glucose tolerance should be treated as if they were diabetic. In this respect the WHO classification did more harm than good since it put a relatively low cut-off point for the diagnosis of diabetes in pregnancy and increased the potential number of patients suffering from gestational diabetes, a condition which may well not be of clincal significance at least in the index pregnancy.

Gestational diabetes

The concept of gestational diabetes is that some women cannot increase insulin production sufficiently to remain euglycaemic in pregnancy and that as a consequence the fetus is put at risk. The first statement may well be true; the second is unproven. Originally glucose tolerance was required to return to normal after delivery for the definition. More pragmatically gestational diabetes has been redefined to include all patients who are shown to be diabetic for the first time in pregnancy, though this is confusing epidemiologically since the group will include a few patients with IDD (see above) and a varying proportion with NIDD depending on the population.

The original criteria for the diagnosis of gestational diabetes were the GTT data of O'Sullivan & Mahan (1964) in Boston which were based on the likelihood of developing a very mild form of diabetes 6 years later (Jarrett 1993). This form of diabetes would be impaired glucose tolerance rather than diabetes by WHO criteria (Jarrett 1993).

Even O'Sullivan was not able to show a statistically significant increase in perinatal mortality in the Boston group and all of the increase in perinatal mortality could be accounted for by increased maternal age and weight. Subsequent data from Belfast have shown no increased risk of perinatal mortality (Hadden 1980).

What of perinatal morbidity? Certainly women with gestational diabetes however defined tend to have bigger babies who are more likely to be delivered by Caesarean section; there is some evidence that aggressive treatment with diet and insulin will lower the birth weight (O'Sullivan et al 1971, 1975). However, the increase in fetal size can again be largely though not entirely (Maresh 1993) accounted for by maternal age and weight and the current studies of Barker's group (1992) would suggest that a reduction in birthweight leads to the long-term development of chronic illness in adults, particularly hypertension.

Furthermore once a patient has been labelled as diabetic in pregnancy, she is made to feel abnormal and the treatment is time consuming, invasive and painful, i.e. diet, home glucose monitoring and insulin.

At present there does not seem to be sufficient evidence that gestational diabetes causes harm to the fetus to justify treating the condition. It also does not meet the criteria for screening since it is not a condition in which intervention makes any difference. In addition there is no uniformity about the definition of gestational diabetes, if indeed it exists at all (Ales & Santini 1989). Unselected screening of Caucasian populations should cease (Hunter & Kierse 1989).

The condition for which we should screen is NIDD and we would suggest using the WHO criteria for diabetes to define this in pregnancy, i.e. fasting blood glucose > 7.0 mmol/l or 2 hour blood glucose > 10.0 mmol/l, venous whole blood.

Who should have a GTT in pregnancy? What is needed is a controlled clinical trial of the value of screening and treatment compared to no screening. Until the results of such a trial are available a selective screen is suggested for patients who may be at risk because of racial characteristics (Dooley et al 1991) plus those who have had serious fetal morbidity or mortality in the past that might be due to NIDD, i.e. stillbirth or birth trauma of a macrosomic baby. The most widely accepted screen is O'Sullivan's using a 50-g load of glucose without fasting and checking the blood glucose 1 hour later. This could be performed at any time in the second trimester since it is only NIDD that is being sought for. Those with venous plasma glucose greater than 8.3 screen positive and should have a GTT. Only those who then meet the WHO criteria for diabetes in pregnancy (see above) should be considered to have NIDD and only those should have any further intervention.

Insulin-dependent diabetes

Insulin-dependent diabetes (IDD) occurs most often in young adults; the prevalence rate is about 0.2% in whites under the age of 30. It is unusual in newborn children but the incidence increases with increasing age to reach a peak at 11–14 years. Thereafter, the incidence declines slowly to a plateau of about eight per 100 000 (Lernmark 1985). Shortly after the diagnosis of IDD has been made, inflammatory cells are found infiltrating and surrounding the islets of Langerhans. There is a marked decrease in the number of beta cells.

A number of factors are involved in the aetiology of IDD: genetic determinants involve certain human leucocyte antigens (HLA) on chromosome 6 (Cudworth & Woodrow 1976), especially HLA-DR3 and DR4 which are associated with an increased incidence of IDD. Given that these genetic markers indicate an increased susceptibility to diabetes for the individuals concerned, there are a number of possible initiators of the disease, including environmental factors and viruses such as the coxsackie B4 and rubella and chemicals such as streptozocin and certain rodenticides. IDD patients have a cellular and humoral autoimmunity to pancreatic β cells. The current hypothesis as to the cause of the IDD is that a combination of specific antigen molecules with an invading antigen, virus, bacteria or chemical triggers the formation of effector cells which cross-react with the islet beta cells. When sufficient of these are destroyed IDD is precipitated (Lernmark 1985).

Non-insulin-dependent diabetes

The majority of all diabetics are non-insulin-dependent but non-insulin-dependent diabetes (NIDD) is less common in the childbearing age group than among older women. There is an association between obesity and NIDD which is more common in fat than thin women. Obesity is associated with insulin insensitivity and glucose tolerance improves with weight loss. However, most obese women are not diabetic and many NIDD women are not obese, so the exact role of obesity in the pathogenesis of NIDD is uncertain.

There is a heriditary element in NIDD; 25% of NIDD patients have a first-degree family history of the disease and nearly all identical twins with NIDD have a similarly affected co-twin. Certain racial groups have a tendency to NIDD, especially those of Indian origin. The NIDD woman has few symptoms and is not prone to ketosis but in pregnancy the management needs to be just as careful as for IDD if perinatal losses are to be avoided. (Johnstone et al 1990, Nasrat et al 1990).

The diagnosis of diabetes mellitus (non-pregnant patients)

In a patient with symptoms, the diagnosis of diabetes mellitus is established by a raised fasting blood glucose level of 7 mmol/l or more or 10 mmol/l or more after food (venous whole blood). A fasting level of less than 6 mmol/l usually excludes the diagnosis of diabetes. When the fasting level is between 6 and 7 mmol/l a glucose tolerance test (GTT) should be performed. Although there are variations of oral GTTs and an extensive literature on intravenous GTTs, the 75 g oral GTT, as advocated by the World Health Organization (WHO 1980) is likely to become the most widely used in the future and has the virtue of simplicity in interpretation. A standard load of 75 g of glucose in 250 ml of water is given after an overnight fast following 3 days of adequate carbohydrate intake (greater than 250 g/day). Blood samples are taken before and at 1 and 2 hours after the load. The test distinguishes between normal, diabetes mellitus and impaired glucose tolerance (IGT) (Table 22.1).

Potential abnormality of glucose tolerance

Certain groups of women are more likely to develop diabetes mellitus at some time during their life than normal

Table 22.1 Diagnostic glucose concentrations (from World Health Organization 1980)

Diagnosis	Venous blood (mmol/l)	Capillary whole blood (mmol/l)	Venous plasma (mmol/l)
Diabetes mellitus*			
Fasting	≥ 7.0	≥ 7.0	≥ 8.0
2-h blood glucose	≥ 10.0	≥ 11.0	≥ 11.0
Impaired glucose tolerance			
Fasting	< 7.0	< 7.0	< 8.0
2-h blood glucose	≥ 7.0 – < 10.0	≥ 8.0 – < 11.0	≥ 8.0 – < 11.0

*In the absence of diabetic symptoms an abnormal 1-h level is required in addition to the 2-h figure to confirm the diagnosis of diabetes mellitus.

and are labelled potential diabetics. From the obstetrician's point of view the risk that these individuals will develop NIDD in pregnancy is low but the risk factors remain useful criteria where routine screening of the whole antenatal population is not carried out. The risk factors that are important to the obstetrician are given below.

Family history

Genetic factors play a part in the development of diabetes although the exact mode of inheritance is not established. Approximately 1% of all offspring of IDD parents may be expected to develop the disease themselves—an incidence of between 5 and 10 times greater than that of a child with non-diabetic parents. A history of IDD in the father is of greater predictive value than in the mother and even greater when a sibling is diabetic. A family history in grandparents is less significant. If both parents are diabetic the incidence of diabetes in the offspring rises, depending upon the age at which the parents became diabetic. The greatest risk of the offspring developing diabetes occurs when one or both parents developed the disease before the age of 40. Even so, not more than 25% of their children will become diabetic and the figure is lower in children of parents with diabetes of late onset. The extent to which a positive family history makes an individual a potential diabetic will therefore vary with circumstances (Pyke 1968).

Previous heavy babies

The incidence of babies weighing 4.5 kg or more is about 1.5% of all births. Among the children of women who later develop diabetes the rate is much higher, varying in different reports from 4% to 31% (Pyke 1962). A tendency to bear heavy babies may precede the development of clinical diabetes by many years. There is no clearcut evidence to support the idea that the proportion of heavy babies increases as the time of diagnosis draws near, suggesting that genetic factors are more important than environmental factors, particularly maternal hyperglycaemia.

Obesity

Women who are obese (weight exceeding 90 kg) have a greater tendency to become diabetic in later life than non-obese women.

Classification of severity of diabetes in pregnancy

In general terms the more severe the diabetes the greater the risk of maternal complications in pregnancy and perinatal mortality and morbidity. Severity in this context is measured by the presence of diabetic vascular complications and by the duration of the diabetes. Traditionally the classification used is that of White (1965) but this now seems unnecessarily complicated. In practice a classification based on the severity of vascular complications is used instead of White's classification. There are three groups:

Group 1 Diabetes diagnosed during pregnancy (synonymous with gestational diabetes in most modern publications).
Group 2 Established diabetes without retinopathy (i.e. less than six microaneurysms seen on ophthalmoscopy).
Group 3 Established diabetes with retinopathy and/or nephropathy.

This simple classification indicates the distribution of diabetic pregnancies by severity of maternal disease in a given population and the effect which severity has on clinical outcome, particularly perinatal mortality. The distribution of diabetic mothers, insulin-dependent and non-insulin-dependent, at King's College Hospital in 1981–1985 is shown in Table 22.2.

The effect of diabetic complications on pregnancy outcome

Diabetes is associated with an increased incidence of

Table 22.2 Classification of diabetic mothers (1981–85). Proportions of groups (%) and perinatal mortality rates (per thousand) are given in parentheses

	Group	IDD	NID	Total	Neonatal deaths
Gestational	1	1	29	30 (16%)	0 (0)
Established	2	116	17	133 (70%)	0 (0)
Established with complications	3	27	0	27 (14%)	2 (74)
Total		144 (75%)	46 (25%)	190 (100%)	2 (10)

vascular disease. Diabetic vasculopathy develops to a variable extent and over a variable period of time in many diabetics. Diabetic retinopathy, diabetic vascular disease and neuropathy are common in diabetics but tend to develop late and are not adversely affected by pregnancy so long as the diabetes is well controlled. However diabetic symptoms increase the risk of perinatal mortality and morbidity when they are present (Table 22.2).

Diabetic retinopathy is the most easily documented diabetic vascular lesion. Background retinopathy follows a benign course during pregnancy and does not require treatment but proliferative retinopathy may require treatment with an argon laser. Diabetic nephropathy is commonly associated with hypertension and the pregnancy may be complicated by intrauterine growth retardation. The series reported by Kitzmiller et al (1981) and Jovanovic & Jovanovic (1984) indicate that the outlook for the fetus in diabetic pregnancy with nephropathy is good as long as hypertension and significant renal impairment are absent at the outset of the pregnancy. Most patients show an increase in proteinuria during pregnancy and have a stable or falling creatinine clearance. These changes return to prepregnancy levels after delivery and pregnancy has no long-term adverse effects on the course of the disease (Reece et al 1988).

Several cases of diabetic pregnancy following renal transplantation have been reported (Penn et al 1980, Grenfell et al 1986). It should be borne in mind that the long-term prospects for patients with diabetic renal disease are not generally good and many will require renal transplantation or long-term dialysis when the disease has progressed. Ischaemic heart disease is occasionally seen. One case has been reported of an IDD woman who had a pregnancy following a coronary artery bypass operation for coronary artery disease (Reece et al 1986).

Glycosylated haemoglobin

Haemoglobin A (HbA) constitutes about 90% of the haemoglobin of adults and infants above the age of 6 months (Gabbay et al 1977). Glycosylation of haemoglobin occurs as a two-stage process. The first is a rapid and reversible non-enzymatic attachment between the glucose molecule and the N-terminal amino group of the chains of the beta haemoglobin molecule (Schiff base linkage) and to a lesser extent the N-terminal groups in the alpha chains and the N group in epsilon lysine (Gabbay et al 1979). The second is the Amadori rearrangement leading to the formation of a stable ketoamine linkage HbA_1. This comprises HbA_{1a}, HbA_{1b} and HbA_{1c}, and these together with HbA_2 and HbF make up the remaining 10%. Of the total haemoglobin, HbA_{1c} may comprise up to 4%. The level of HbA_1 is raised in diabetes, reflecting diabetic control over the previous 2 or 3 months. During rapid changes of diabetic control, the

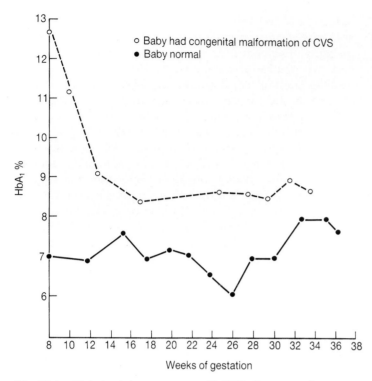

Fig. 22.1 HbA$_1$ levels in two women with IDD. One was well controlled throughout pregnancy and had a normal baby. The other had a high level of HbA$_1$ initially and the baby had a congenital cardiac lesion (truncus arteriosus).

Table 22.3 HbA$_1$ in first trimester and major congenital malformations: King's College Hospital 1981–85

HbA$_1$ (%)	Congenital malformations
8.9	Microcephaly
11.0	Absent radius, deformed thumbs
	Hemivertebrae
11.6	Caudal regression
12.3	Truncus arteriosus
12.4	Microcephaly
13.8	Multiple (including exomphalos)

HbA$_1$ levels of six severely congenital malformed babies born to diabetic mothers at King's College Hospital.

labile fraction, which is thought to be the Schiff base, reflects transient rather than long-term changes which occur throughout the lifespan of the red cell.

Since glycosylated haemoglobin measurement in the first trimester will give retrospective assessment of diabetic control at this critical time in development, various studies have examined HbA$_1$ at this stage (Fig. 22.1).

It was observed (Leslie et al 1978) that three out of five women with high glycosylated haemoglobin measurements at presentation had babies with congenital malformations including hemivertebrae, neural tube defects and congenital heart disease. This led to a multicentre study in the UK. Out of 168 women with an HbA$_1$ < 12%, three had babies with major malformations (1.8%). In 62 women with HbA$_1$ > 12%, there were four babies with major malformations (6.8%; Stubbs et al 1987). The study also showed that the two groups had similar miscarriage rates: 20/168 had an HbA$_1$ < 12% (12%) and 7/62 had an HbA$_1$ > 12% (11%). Two other studies have reported a high incidence of miscarriage—26% (Wright et al 1983) and 30% (Miodovnik et al 1984). In the former series HbA$_1$ was found to be significantly higher in those who aborted spontaneously. Ylinen et al (1984) in Finland looked at 142 pregnancies and found that the incidence of major malformation rose progressively with increasing levels of HbA$_1$ (between the 6th and 15th weeks) rising to

an incidence of 23.5% in 17 pregnancies with an initial HbA$_1$ > 10%.

Table 22.3 shows the congenital abnormalities seen in diabetic pregnant patients at King's College Hospital between 1981 and 1985 and indicates that most were associated with raised levels of HbA$_1$.

Figure 22.1 shows HbA$_1$ levels in two women with IDD. One was well controlled throughout pregnancy and had a normal delivery of a normal-sized baby. The other had a high level of HbA$_1$ at the start of the pregnancy; her diabetes was quickly brought under control and the HbA$_1$ was lowered and remained lowered for the rest of the pregnancy. Sadly, however, the baby had a truncus arteriosus which was not detected at the 18-week fetal anomaly scan.

HbA$_1$ has been found to increase in anaemia (Brooks et al 1980) and to be decreased in chronic renal failure (Dandona et al 1979). The latter is probably related to the shortened lifespan of erythrocytes, with the result that those in circulation have a relatively short time to glycosylate haemoglobin. The same applies to haemolytic disease.

Maternal HbA$_1$ correlation with birthweight
Birthweight ratio (birthweight divided by the 50th centile birthweight for gestational age) did not correlate with cord or maternal HbA$_1$ at delivery in one series (Worth et al 1983) and was explained by relatively tight control of maternal diabetes towards the end of pregnancy. There have been conflicting reports about the correlation of maternal HbA$_1$ with birthweight or birthweight ratio. Stubbs et al (1981), Fadel et al (1981), Miller et al (1981), O'Shaughnessy et al (1979), Poon et al (1981) and Sosenko et al (1982) did not find such a correlation but others have found a link between third-trimester HbA$_1$ and relative birthweight (Widness et al 1978, Ylinen et al 1981). Russell et al (1984) and Knight (1983) found near normal HbA$_1$ levels in macrosomic pregnancy.

HbA$_1$ estimation has proved a valuable additional aid to good control and when elevated in early pregnancy serves as a warning to the obstetrician to be on the look-out for major congenital abnormality.

Fructosamine

Fructosamine is glycosylated albumin. It reflects the mean blood glucose over a period of 2 weeks rather than 3 months as in the case of glycosylated haemoglobin. The normal level varies between laboratories but the mean in non-diabetics is about 2.2 mmol/l with the 95th centile 2.5 mmol/l (Roberts et al 1990). Fructosamine levels are insensitive as a predictor of abnormal glucose tolerance in pregnancy (Comtois et al 1989, Roberts et al 1990) or of fetal hyperinsulinaemia (Hofmann 1990) but may be of use in the management of diabetes to confirm home blood glucose monitoring (Roberts et al 1988), particularly when short-term changes in mean blood glucose are anticipated.

Lung function in the infants of diabetic mothers

Fetal hyperinsulinaemia consequent upon maternal hyperglycaemia inhibits the production of surfactant by the fetal lung cells. The occurrence of respiratory distress in the infants of diabetic mothers has fallen sharply since the introduction of strict control of maternal diabetes. In strictly controlled diabetic pregnancy fetal lung maturation at 37 weeks and thereafter is no different from in a non-diabetic pregnancy (Tyden et al 1984). When delivery occurs between 32 and 37 weeks respiratory complications are more likely to occur but if maternal diabetic control has been good severe respiratory distress is uncommon. When control has been poor, delivery before 37 weeks, but especially before 34 weeks, is likely to be complicated by respiratory distress and all cases of surfactant-deficient respiratory distress syndrome will be identified by standard estimates of fetal lung maturity, i.e. lecithin sphingomyelin (L : S) ratio > 2, phosphatidyl glycerol > 72% and optical density at 650 nm > 0.150 (Kjos et al 1990). Unfortunately all these tests have a high false-positive rate so that in gestational diabetics 21% may be phosphatidyl glycerol negative as late as 38 weeks' gestation (Ojomo & Coustan 1990). Therefore since surfactant-deficient respiratory distress is now very rare in well-controlled diabetics delivering after 34 weeks (Kjos et al 1990), there does not seem to be any place for routine amniocentesis for lung maturity testing in patients delivering near term.

Congenital abnormality in diabetic pregnancy

Congenital abnormality is now the most important contributor to perinatal mortality and morbidity in diabetic pregnancy (Centers for Disease Control 1990). It is now accepted that the diabetic woman is three to four times more likely to have a congenitally malformed baby than her non-diabetic counterpart (Malins 1979, Fuhrmann et al 1983). This is in accord with experience at King's College Hospital (see Table 22.4, which also lists the range of abnormalities). Table 22.5 illustrates the contribution which fatal congenital malformations have made to perinatal mortality during the years 1951–85. To the clinician, the interest lies in two aspects: what causes the abnormalities, and can good diabetic control decrease the incidence of abnormality?

The cause of congenital abnormality in diabetic pregnancy

The most important time for organogenesis is the first 7 weeks of intrauterine life and it is during this period that abnormal carbohydrate metabolism might cause abnormality (Mills et al 1979). In the female rat with streptozocin-induced diabetes, pregnancy results in a high incidence of congenital abnormality, especially visceral eversion and incomplete ossification of the sacrum (Deuchar 1979). The latter anomaly is particularly significant in diabetes (See 'Caudal regression syndrome' below).

So far it has not been possible to identify the exact cause of the abnormalities. Experimental ketoacidosis in mice causes chromosomal abnormalities with and without

Table 22.4 Major congenital abnormalities in diabetic pregnancies at King's College Hospital 1971–85

System/abnormality	Number
Central nervous system	11
Skeletal	10
Cardiac	9
Alimentary	3
Caudal regression	2
Multiple abnormalities	2
Hypoplastic lungs	1
Potter's syndrome	1
Total	39

Prevalence = 39/545 = 7.2%.

Table 22.5 Diabetic pregnancies at King's College Hospital 1951–85

	No.	Perinatal deaths	Fatal congenital malformations	% of perinatal deaths contributed by malformation	TOP for congenital malformations
1951–60	318	72	6	8	—
1961–70	389	39	5	13	—
1971–80	352	13	6	46	5
1981–85	193	2	2	100	3

TOP = termination of pregnancy.

manifest deformities (Enricho & Ingalls 1968) so the effect of maternal diabetes may be on the chromosomes of the oocyte or the pre- or postimplantation embryo. Once the embryo is implanted and starts to develop, a direct effect on the process of organogenesis is possible. Since most pregnant diabetic women do not become ketoacidotic in early pregnancy, hyperglycaemia seems the most likely culprit.

Goldman et al (1985) proposed that hyperglycaemia causes a functional deficiency of arachidonic acid at a critical stage of organogenesis and have shown experimentally that supplementation of the diet of rats and mice exerts a protective effect against the teratogenic action of hyperglycaemia in vivo (rat) and in vitro (mouse animal models).

The effect of good diabetic control on the incidence of abnormality

There is good evidence that abnormality occurs less frequently in well controlled diabetics (Pedersen 1979, Fuhrmann et al 1983) and it has long been recognized that diabetic mothers with vascular complications, i.e. severe diabetics, are more prone to have abnormal babies (Baker et al 1981).

The emergence of HbA_1 estimation as a means of judging diabetic control retrospectively has shed further light on the question of the effect of hyperglycaemia on fetal development in the first trimester. Since HbA_1 levels reflect the blood glucose concentrations during the preceding 4–8 weeks it is not surprising that those patients with a low HbA_1 level at 12 weeks' gestation have a lower risk of having an abnormal baby than those with a high level. For example increase in the glycosylated haemoglobin level from about 10% to 14% (more than 2 standard deviations) was associated with a five-fold risk in minor malformation rate, i.e. a rate of about 30% (Rosen et al 1990).

Preventing congenital abnormality in diabetic pregnancy

All diabetic women should be made aware of the need for prepregnancy counselling so as to ensure that their diabetes is well controlled from the very start of the pregnancy. Diabetic clinics, general practitioners and obstetricians seeing non-pregnant women should take the opportunity to press this point (Watkins 1982). Tight control of diabetes before pregnancy has been shown to reduce both the glycosylated haemoglobin level and the malformation rate (Steel et al 1990, Kitzmiller et al 1991, Willhoite et al 1993). In dealing with those women who report to the clinic when already pregnant, those who are most at risk should be recognized; they include the badly controlled, the long-standing IDD with vascular complications and those women who have previously had

an abnormal baby. A high HbA_1 level ($> 12\%$) during the first 12 weeks or at the 12th week should alert the obstetrician since it is highly likely that such high levels are associated with an increased risk of abnormality. The risks are relative however, and as indicated above, the majority of women with badly controlled diabetes and high HbA_1 levels in early pregnancy will have normal babies—the incidence in both cases is, however, increased.

Detecting congenital abnormalities

Ultrasound scanning has made possible early detection of congenital abnormality and the opportunity to offer the mother a termination if the abnormality is severe. It has been suggested that delayed fetal growth in very early pregnancy (between 7 and 14 weeks) may indicate fetal abnormality (Pedersen & Mølsted-Pedersen 1981). All diabetic women should have a full fetal anomaly scan done at 18–20 weeks with the possibility of increased fetal abnormality borne in mind, especially where earlier HbA_1 levels have been high.

Caudal regression syndrome (caudal dysplasia syndrome)

This congenital abnormality, described by Hohl in 1852, is rare and consists of absence of vertebrae from any level below T10 and the consequent deformities. If the sacrum is missing (sacral agenesis) the transverse diameter of the pelvis is reduced, the buttocks are flattened and there is muscular atrophy in the legs. There may be dislocation of the hips, talipes, spina bifida, renal anomalies and urinary and faecal incontinence. Lesser degrees of abnormality of the lower limbs not amounting to true caudal regression are also seen. The caudal regression syndrome is akin to rumplessness in chickens. This abnormality occurs as a hereditary condition or spontaneously. More interestingly it can be produced experimentally in white leghorn chickens by injecting insulin into the incubating eggs. This suggests that either insulin itself or the hypoglycaemia produced by it may be teratogenic. This observation does not fit in with clinical experience which, as noted above, does not implicate either insulin or hypoglycaemia in the aetiology of congenital abnormality in women with IDD. Nevertheless, it is of some interest because although the caudal regression syndrome does not only occur in IDD, its incidence in diabetic pregnancy does seem to be considerably higher.

The estimates of incidence of caudal regression syndrome in diabetic pregnancy vary widely but it is probably of the order of one in 1000 (Leny & Maier 1964). This level accords with the experience of King's College Hospital in recent years. Any woman who is not diagnosed as being diabetic giving birth to a baby showing caudal regression syndrome should have a GTT.

The combined approach of prevention and early detection of congenital abnormality and selected termination in diabetic pregnancy should ensure a decrease in congenital abnormality as a cause of perinatal mortality and morbidity.

Perinatal mortality in diabetic pregnancy

The high perinatal mortality seen in diabetic pregnancy 30 years ago has diminished sharply to the present time, as shown in Table 22.5. This table also illustrates the changing pattern of perinatal mortality. Deaths from obstetric causes (Table 22.6), mainly birth trauma, pre-eclampsia, antepartum haemorrhage and acute hydramnios, were relatively common in the early years but have completely disappeared latterly with better obstetric care. Fetal death as a result of diabetic ketoacidosis in the mother has shown a similar decline, as has perinatal death from respiratory distress. Unexplained late intrauterine death, the classic problem of diabetic pregnancy, has also fallen sharply and no deaths from this cause occurred at King's College Hospital in the 1981–1985 quinquennium. It seems likely that these unexplained late intrauterine deaths in late diabetic pregnancy are due to fetal anoxia. Although the delivery of blood to the intervillous space is normal in uncomplicated diabetic pregnancy, blood flow through the intervillous space is slowed and transfer of oxygen to the fetal circulation is impaired. HbA_{1c}, often raised in badly controlled diabetes, has an increased affinity for oxygen so when levels of HbA_1 in the maternal blood are high the release of oxygen to the fetal circulation is further reduced. The placenta and especially the fetal consumption of oxygen are increased in the presence of hyperinsulinaemia. This combination of factors leads occasionally to a fatal degree of fetal hypoxia. Proof that the diabetic fetus may be hypoxic is suggested by some preliminary studies of Po_2 levels on samples of fetal blood obtained by cordocentesis but further work needs to be done before hypoxia can be finally identified as the cause of this type of fetal loss.

Only congenital abnormalities continue to pose problems. Indeed the only two deaths that occurred in this latter quinquennium were from serious congenital abnormalities which had not been diagnosed antenatally.

Table 22.6 Obstetric causes of perinatal death (King's College Hospital)

	1951–1970	1971–1985
Birth trauma	9	0
Pre-eclampsia	9	0
Antepartum haemorrhage	4	2
Acute hydramnios	4	0
Intrauterine growth retardation	3	0
Intrapartum asphyxia	3	0
Rhesus incompatibility	2	0
Unexplained	8	0

Maternal mortality in diabetic pregnancy

A general fall in maternal mortality for all pregnancies is reflected in the fall in maternal mortality for diabetic pregnancy, so that it is now extremely rare for a diabetic woman to die as a result of pregnancy. This contrasts sharply with the maternal mortality figures in the pre-insulin era; these were as high as 45% in the 66 diabetic pregnancies reported by Williams in 1909. There was only one maternal death in diabetic pregnancy at King's College Hospital from 1971 to 1986 and this occurred in a patient with advanced diabetic nephropathy who died from renal failure 11 months after successful delivery. Of the seven maternal deaths in diabetic pregnancy reported in the Reports on Confidential Enquiries into Maternal Deaths in England and Wales (1976–81), three resulted from infection, one from myocardial infarction, one from severe hypoglycaemia, one from pulmonary embolus and one from cardiac arrest of unknown origin during induction of anaesthesia prior to Caesarean section. In all seven cases diabetic control was less than optimal—an important practical point in the management of diabetic pregnancy.

Medical management of diabetic pregnancy

Prepregnancy care

Diabetic women who plan to become pregnant should ensure that their diabetes is as well controlled as it can be in order to reduce the risk of congenital abnormality. Diabetic women with vascular complications should also discuss fully the implications of pregnancy with the diabetic physician and, in the case of retinopathy, may need to have appropriate local treatment.

Patients attending for prepregnancy advice should have a complete physical examination to confirm their fitness for pregnancy and their routine blood glucose and urine tests (to detect albuminuria), as well as an HbA_1 estimation. Based on the results of these investigations appropriate adjustments may need to be made to diet and insulin to ensure tight control of the maternal diabetes. For women with NIDD the importance of sticking closely to diet in order to keep blood glucose levels as near normal as possible may need to be emphasized.

Women who are not doing home monitoring of blood glucose levels should be encouraged to do so using either a glucose oxidase stick alone or a glucose meter. The results of these tests should be recorded and kept, so that at the next diabetic clinic visit the diabetic physician can confirm that control is good. Patients are advised to maintain fasting blood glucose less than 6 mmol/l and postprandial blood glucose less than 7.5 mmol/l as far as possible and an HbA_1 preferably below 10% and not above 12%. A simple prepregnancy advice sheet to diabetic women who are planning to become pregnant, which is also relevant when they do achieve a pregnancy, is helpful.

The obstetrician's contribution to prepregnancy care

The obstetrician should also see diabetic women planning to become pregnant in order to deal with any anxieties they may have about the pregnancy. The importance of keeping a menstrual calendar should be emphasized so that pregnancy can be accurately dated. When infertility is a problem, suitable investigations can be undertaken. Rubella status, blood pressure and weight need to be checked and the patient who smokes should be discouraged from doing so.

Prepregnancy care is the most important aspect of the management of diabetic pregnancy and holds out the best hope for reducing the number of congenital abnormalities (see above). Taking folic acid is not a substitute for good diabetic control.

Pregnancy

Medical management of diabetic pregnancy is based on diet alone or diet and insulin, depending on the type of the maternal diabetes. Oral hypoglycaemic agents are not recommended for the patient who is planning a pregnancy unless she is unable to control her diabetes adequately with diet alone or to use insulin where diet is not adequate. In developing countries oral hypoglycaemics may have an important role to play but in developed countries insulin is preferable when diet alone is not sufficient.

Diet

Proper diet is an essential part of the management of all pregnant diabetic women. It is important that pregnant women do not become hungry and an increased allowance of carbohydrate to meet the extra energy requirements of pregnancy may be needed. An increase in dietary fibre is helpful since it exerts a flattening effect on the postprandial rise of blood glucose concentration (Eastwood & Kay 1979). An experienced dietitian should supervise the patient's diet and it will be necessary to take note of the patient's ethnic requirements. In Asian communities it has been shown that in many groups diet consists of a low carbohydrate and high fat content and appropriate adjustments will have to be made although it is not always an easy task to restructure eating habits in these patients.

Insulin

There are no advantages in any particular type of insulin. All are now purified at a single strength of 100 u/ml. Nearly all are monocomponent or human insulin preparations but there are no special advantages to the patient and there is no indication for changing patients from an established insulin regime using one species of insulin to another species. Instances of insulin allergy or resistance are extremely rare. Increasingly, patients are using pen systems for insulin administration because of increased convenience, whether they are pregnant or not.

The majority of women with IDD require insulin injections at least twice daily. The best regime uses a mixture of short-acting (soluble) and medium-acting (isophane or insulin zinc suspensions) insulin and given 20–30 minutes before the main morning and evening meals. The proportions and amounts of each type of insulin are determined by trial and error, by examining blood glucose profiles measured by the patients themselves and when they attend hospital. Self-monitoring of blood glucose levels by patients is an important aspect of diabetic care during pregnancy and all patients should now undertake some form of blood glucose measurement. When unacceptable swings of blood glucose occur they do so more frequently during the middle of the night or at noon, when hypoglycaemia may be a problem, and during the 2 hours after breakfast when hyperglycaemia is often seen. The splitting of the twice-daily double-mix regime, giving the soluble insulin alone before the main evening meal and the medium-acting insulin before the bedtime snack, may improve matters (Peacock et al 1979). Many patients take an additional injection of soluble insulin before the midday meal.

Continuous subcutaneous insulin has become less popular since it has been realized that it does not achieve better control than with the same amount of care given to intermittent insulin therapy. Also some patients have had very severe rebound hypergylcaemia if there is pump failure.

When IDD develops acutely during pregnancy—a comparatively rare occurrence—soluble insulin is used two or three times daily initially, with the medium-acting insulin being added as the diabetes comes under control. Women with NIDD whose diet alone has failed to give adequate control will also need insulin during pregnancy. In these patients it is often sufficient to use a single dose of medium-acting insulin starting with approximately 10 u/day or small doses of soluble insulin (6 units) given before each meal. Decisions about therapy should of course be made on the basis of home blood glucose monitoring.

First trimester

Although the insulin requirement increases later in pregnancy it does not do so in the first trimester. Hypoglycaemia at this stage is common especially if the insulin dose is inappropriately increased and may result in part from anorexia and vomiting or due to normal pregnancy.

Second and third trimesters

The degree of cooperation on the part of the pregnant women and the enthusiasm of her diabetic physician and the rest of the team (diabetic nurse, dietician and midwife) are key factors in achieving the necessary tight control of diabetes during the second and third trimesters of pregnancy. The insulin dose increases steadily, especially after the 28th week. Most patients learn how to make their own adjustments to the insulin dose to maintain control between visits to hospital but it is important that they are able to contact the hospital (ideally the diabetic nurse) in any case of doubt. The increase in insulin requirement varies considerably from a negligible amount to two or three times normal requirements. Sometimes there is a small decrease in the last weeks of pregnancy; this is not in itself an ominous feature. The need for high insulin dosage ceases abruptly at the time of delivery, when it is important to reduce the dose to its prepregnancy level immediately, otherwise profound hypoglycaemia will develop. The aim of control is to keep preprandial blood glucose levels between 5 and 6 mmol/l, postprandial less than 7.5 mmol/l and the HbA_1 below 8%. Both postprandial and preprandial blood glucose levels are important determinants of fetal weight (Jovanovic-Peterson et al 1991).

Labour

Labour, and any acute situation arising during pregnancy, e.g. severe infection, call for a change to intravenous insulin and glucose to ensure close control at these critical times. The intravenous insulin infusion should be started as soon as labour is established or whenever food is to be withheld if labour is to be induced electively. An infusion pump enables fine adjustments to be made and is the best method of administration. Soluble insulin is diluted in normal saline—1 unit of insulin per 1 ml of saline—and is delivered initially at 1 u/h. Blood glucose is checked every hour and kept within the range 3–8 mmol/l; in general, small variations of insulin rate in the range of 0.5–2 u/h are sufficient to achieve this. Along with the intravenous insulin an intravenous infusion of 10% glucose is maintained at 1 litre every 8 hours; oral feeding is discontinued during the whole of the labour. The same regimen is employed when delivery is by elective Caesarean section; insulin and glucose infusions are commenced 2 hours prior to the time of the operation.

Obstetric management of diabetic pregnancy

Early pregnancy

There is an increased risk of miscarriage in early pregnancy as well as the increased risk of congenital fetal abnormality; both these risks are reduced sharply by good diabetic control, especially if this has been achieved prior to conception. Indeed with good control there may be no increased risk compared to non-diabetics (Mills et al 1988). Early attendance at the combined diabetic–antenatal clinic should ensure that diabetic control is optimal and also give the obstetrician an opportunity to confirm that the pregnancy is proceeding normally. Early ultrasound scan establishes the maturity of the pregnancy and the size of the embryo as well as detecting early failure of embryonic development or growth abnormality.

Combined diabetic–antenatal clinic

Essential to good management of diabetic pregnancy is the combined diabetic–antenatal clinic where both diabetic physician and obstetrician work together in the same clinic seeing the pregnant woman together. Equally important are the other members of the team—diabetic nurse, dietician and a midwife that understands diabetic pregnancy who the patient can relate to and with whom she can discuss her usually considerable anxieties. Free communication between the doctors involved and the patient herself greatly increases understanding and ensures the best possible patient cooperation. Specialized diabetic–antenatal clinics in hospitals with intensive special care baby units are a feature of many regions of the UK and the results obtained in such units are usually better than those in isolated units where the numbers of cases seen do not give enough experience to either obstetrician or diabetic physician to be confident in the handling of the complex problems that may arise during the course of the pregnancy and labour.

Routine antenatal care

The routine obstetric antenatal care of the patient does not differ greatly from that of the non-diabetic patient. Diagnostic ultrasound is important but routine clinical observation remains very important.

The use of ultrasound in diabetic pregnancy

Diagnostic ultrasound plays an important part in the management of diabetic pregnancy. Before 12 weeks the object of the early pregnancy scan is to establish maturity and the well-being of the embryo as well as detecting gross abnormality. The diagnosis of maturity of the pregnancy is based on crown–rump length. Pedersen (1979) found that crown–rump lengths were, on average, 5.4 days smaller than those in non-diabetics of the same age. More recent studies suggest that this is due to delayed ovulation. A number of factors affect fetal growth in early pregnancy and it is always wise to confirm maturity at a later stage by biparietal diameter and femur length measurements. Early fetal growth delay may result from poor diabetic control or may be associated with a congenital abnormality.

At 18–20 weeks detailed anomaly scans are essential and are particularly important in those women whose diabetic control in the first trimester, as indicated by blood glucose levels and/or HbA_1 estimations at 12 weeks, has been bad. From 24 weeks onwards the task of the ultrasonographer in a diabetic pregnancy is to detect the development of fetal macrosomia and polyhydramnios (see later) which may occur even though maternal diabetes is impeccably controlled. Evidence of fetal macrosomia can be obtained by serial measurements of the fetal abdominal and head circumference starting at 24 weeks and continuing at 2-weekly intervals until delivery. Developing macrosomia is evident by 32–34 weeks and is an indication that the maternal diabetes may be affecting fetal growth. Macrosomia may, of course, occur in the absence of maternal diabetes but it is wise to assume that macrosomia developing in a pregnant diabetic woman is due to the maternal diabetes and check that diabetic control is satisfactory. If the maternal diabetes is not well controlled then urgent steps must be taken to correct it. Where diabetic control is satisfactory the obstetrician can only observe and plot the developing macrosomia by the evidence of serial ultrasound scan but can time the planning and mode of delivery from this point of view.

Ultrasound is also helpful in late pregnancy in observing fetal movements and can form part of the biophysical profile used to evaluate fetal well-being. Ultrasound can also be used to study blood flow on the fetal and maternal sides of the placenta, using a duplex pulse Doppler system. This is particularly of value where diabetic pregnancy is complicated by uterine growth retardation but does not seem to be of any particular help in normal diabetic pregnancy or diabetic pregnancy complicated by developing fetal macrosomia.

Maternal obstetric complications in pregnancy

There are three important obstetric complications in diabetic pregnancy: pre-eclampsia, polyhydramnios and preterm labour.

Pre-eclampsia

Pre-eclampsia, often severe, was a common occurrence in diabetic pregnancy and a cause of perinatal mortality in the past. More recently it has become much less common and there have been no perinatal deaths due to pre-eclampsia at King's College Hospital from 1971 to 1985. Broughton Pipkin et al (1982) showed that in diabetic pregnancy the plasma renin and aldosterone concentrations were higher than in non-diabetic pregnancy and the plasma renin substrate was lower. Plasma angiotensin too showed a strong inverse relationship to serum sodium

and was directly proportional to blood glucose concentrations. These differences from normal may contribute to the raised incidence of hypertension in diabetic pregnancy and explain why good control leads to a lower incidence.

In the UK Diabetic Pregnancy Survey (Brudenell 1982) the overall incidence of pre-eclampsia in established diabetics was 14.4% but there was no increase in perinatal mortality in these patients, so that although pre-eclampsia remains a more common occurrence in diabetic than in non-diabetic pregnancy, it does not present a particular problem in antenatal care, since it is detected and managed as in non-diabetic pregnancy. In Canada, Garner (1990) found that pre-eclampsia was twice as common in diabetics (9.9%) as in non-diabetics but the incidence did not relate to glycaemic control. Siddiqi (1991) found that pregnancy-induced hypertension was three times as common (15%) but by contrast was related to diabetic control.

Polyhydramnios

Polyhydramnios complicates 25% of pregnancies in established diabetics included in the UK Diabetic Pregnancy Survey (Brudenell 1982). Severe acute polyhydramnios which was responsible for perinatal deaths in the past is not now seen but the development of any degree of polyhydramnios during the course of diabetic pregnancy is an indication to look closely at the level of diabetic control, since there is a definite clinical relationship between mean glucose levels and polyhydramnios. It is likely that fetal hyperglycaemia resulting from maternal hyperglycaemia leads to fetal polyuria and hence polyhydramnios. Patients who seem to be developing polyhydramnios quickly should be admitted to hospital for closer supervision. This will often halt the progress of developing polyhydramnios and postpone the onset of preterm labour, which may otherwise complicate it.

Preterm labour

Preterm labour, i.e. labour starting prior to the completion of the 37th week of pregnancy, is more common in diabetic than in non-diabetic pregnancy. It occurred in 17% of diabetic patients at King's College Hospital in recent times. When it occurs it is usually associated with urinary infection or more often with polyhydramnios; hence the chances that it will occur are reduced if maternal diabetes is well controlled. The management of preterm labour calls for fine judgement on the part of the obstetrician.

Management of preterm labour In general if pregnancy has reached 32 weeks no attempt should be make to stop the labour. If, however, preterm labour begins with spontaneous rupture of membranes unaccompanied by uterine contractions, a sample of liquor should be obtained either by vaginal collection or ultrasound-directed amniocentesis to assess the maturity of the fetal lungs. If the fetal lungs are immature, as judged by the L : S ratio and the presence or absence of phosphatidyl-glycerol, a course of dexamethasone 4 mg 8-hourly for 48 hours should be given to accelerate lung function. This will cause a marked rise in blood glucose which needs to be anticipated (see below). In all cases of preterm labour with ruptured membranes a sample of liquor obtained by amniocentesis or vaginal swab should be sent for bacteriological examination and the patient meanwhile started on amoxycillin to counter the risk of intrauterine infection, especially by beta-haemolytic streptococci.

Preterm labour with intact or ruptured membranes before 32 weeks should generally be stopped unless it is clear that the labour is fully established, as evident by the strength and frequency of the contractions and by cervical dilatation. Beta-agonists such as salbutamol or ritodrine to inhibit uterine contractions and corticosteroids to accelerate lung function cause hyperglycaemia and keto-acidosis so that, if they are used, they should be given in conjunction with an intravenous infusion of soluble insulin to keep blood glucose levels within the normal range of 3–5 mmol/l. A glucose level should be estimated every hour and the plasma potassium every 2 hours. An intravenous 5% glucose drip may be needed to counteract transient hypoglycaemia and intravenous potassium supplements up to 100 mmol/24 h should be given, if necessary, to maintain normal potassium levels. The maternal pulse rate and blood pressure are taken hourly and a continuous cardiotocographic trace taken of the fetal heart. This regimen is continued for 48 hours.

Thereafter, if the membranes are ruptured, no further attempts should be made to inhibit labour and delivery should be allowed to occur vaginally or by Caesarean section. If the membranes are intact and the contractions have been successfully inhibited, the beta-agonist infusion is slowly reduced over the succeeding 48 hours. The insulin infusion should be continued at the appropriate rate until the beta-agonist is discontinued, the dose being adjusted according to blood glucose levels. Preterm labour often recurs after successful inhibition and the regime may have to be reinstated.

If preterm labour has been successfully inhibited in those cases with intact membranes an amniocentesis should be performed to obtain a liquor sample to assess further fetal lung maturity. A mature fetal lung should encourage the obstetrician to abandon attempts to inhibit preterm labour if it threatens again. If the pregnancy proceeds, a repeat course of corticosteroids should be given at weekly intervals after the first until 36 weeks. With regard to delivery, Caesarean section should be considered unless labour and vaginal delivery seem likely to be straightforward. In the presence of added complications such as severe pre-eclampsia, unstable presentation or malpresentation or an increased risk of intrauterine infection, a Caesarean section should generally be performed but each case needs to be considered individually.

Late pregnancy admission to hospital

In well controlled uncomplicated diabetic pregnancy antenatal care can follow a normal pattern up to full term. Where complications arise during the last several weeks, e.g. difficulty in diabetic control or developing poly-hydramnios or pre-eclampsia, admission to hospital is advisable so that diabetic control can be kept closely supervised and fetal well-being monitored. Patients whose serial ultrasound scans show developing fetal macrosomia should also be admitted. Diabetic control may be better at home than in hospital (Stubbs et al 1980), but this is only true with well motivated patients who make regular checks of their own blood glucose levels. Less intelligent or less well motivated patients are likely to be better controlled in hospital.

Monitoring of fetal well-being in late pregnancy

When the patient is admitted to hospital because of complications, biophysical tests are employed to assess fetal well-being. Biochemical tests, e.g. estimations of oestriol and placental lactogen levels in maternal serum, were employed formerly but have been replaced now by biophysical testing which relies on the recording of fetal movements by the patient and observations by regular ultrasound scan and on antenatal fetal cardiotocography. Any abnormality in the cardiotocograph calls for a full fetal biophysical profile, and if there is any doubt about fetal well-being immediate delivery is called for by induction of labour or by Caesarean section. A normal biophysical profile is helpful in providing reassurance to the clinician and to the patient that a conservative policy with regard to delivery can be continued.

Delivering the infant of a diabetic mother

Apart from preterm labour and unless complications occur indicating earlier delivery, diabetic patients are not nowadays delivered before 37 weeks and in well controlled uncomplicated diabetes with normal fetal growth pregnancy is allowed to proceed to 40 weeks. Once the patient has reached full term it is our present policy to induce labour or, if indicated, deliver the patient by Caesarean section. It is not felt desirable at present to allow a diabetic pregnancy to continue beyond full term since experience of the management of diabetic pregnancy beyond established ultrasound-confirmed full term is extremely limited and the risk of unexplained intrauterine death may still exist in these patients.

Planned Caesarean section

Every effort should be made to avoid complicated, difficult or prolonged labour in diabetic woman. Planned Caesarean section will therefore be appropriate in a number of cases and will usually be performed between 38 and 40 weeks. Of the indications shown in Table 22.7, disproportion is probably the most important in modern practice since the prevalence of macrosomia means that the risk of disproportion and difficult vaginal delivery is always present in diabetic pregnancy. Birth trauma has often featured in diabetic deliveries in earlier series (Stallone & Ziel 1974) and was a major cause of perinatal mortality at King's College Hospital in 1951–1970. If macrosomia has been detected by serial ultrasound scanning it is likely that shoulder dystocia will result. Serious consideration must then be given to a planned Caesarean section.

The management of planned Caesarean section

The obstetric management is no different from that in non-diabetic pregnancy. Either general anaesthesia or epidural analgesia is appropriate. The use of the latter facilitates control of maternal diabetes pre- and immediately postoperatively since the patient is able to take carbohydrate by mouth. Intravenous insulin and glucose will often be preferred by the diabetic physician if general anaesthesia is used and in any complicated case this is the best way of ensuring good control throughout the perioperative period.

Induction of labour

The indications for the induction of labour are shown in Table 22.8. The indications for the induction of labour in diabetic pregnancy have changed during the past decade, reflecting the growing confidence obstetricians have in managing the well controlled patient and the diminishing risk of unexplained intrauterine death up to full term. Uncomplicated diabetes per se therefore does not normally constitute an indication to induce labour before term.

Table 22.7   Indications for planned Caesarean section

Previous Caesarean section
Malpresentation
Disproportion
Severe pre-eclampsia
Age 35 or over
Long history of infertility
Diabetic complications

Table 22.8   Indications for induction of labour

Uncomplicated diabetes at 40 weeks
Developing fetal macrosomia
Pre-eclampsia and hypertension
Diabetic complications

Full-term uncomplicated diabetes   Once the diabetic woman reaches full term labour should be induced. Cordocentesis studies at King's College Hospital indicate that the diabetic fetus is often hypoxic in utero. Postmaturity is likely to make this worse and may lead occasionally to intrauterine death. There is, however, no substantial clinical evidence to support this view but, for the present, it seems a reasonable compromise and the result of its application to diabetic pregnancy is satisfactory in terms of perinatal mortality and morbidity.

Developing fetal macrosomia   A baby that is growing excessively as judged by serial ultrasound scans is clearly being affected by the maternal diabetes and becoming hyperinsulinaemic. Induction of labour at 38 weeks seems reasonable then since a considerable increase in body size and weight may occur in the last 2 weeks. By inducing the patient at 38 weeks the possible risk of late unexplained intrauterine death in the remaining 2 weeks of the pregnancy is also avoided.

Pre-eclampsia and hypertension   The indications for induction for pre-eclampsia and hypertension in diabetic women are the same as for non-diabetic women. In hypertension in diabetic pregnancy there may be a degree of intrauterine growth retardation which can be, to some extent, masked by the macrosomia-inducing effect of the mother's diabetes. The timing of induction for hypertension will depend on the progress of the condition and on the fetus. As long as the blood pressure does not rise significantly above the early pregnancy readings, there is no proteinuria and the fetal parameters of growth and well-being are satisfactory, induction is not indicated but a rise in blood pressure, especially if proteinuria develops or if there is a definite falling off in the fetal growth pattern, indicates the need for induction or, in some cases, the need for elective Caesarean section.

Diabetic microvasculopathy   Diabetic retinopathy or nephropathy are not thought generally to be made worse by pregnancy or by labour but in the case of nephropathy pre-eclampsia is more likely to be superimposed on pregnancy and induction, therefore, may be indicated for this reason.

Obstetric management of induced labour

Induction of labour can be achieved by the use of a single prostaglandin pessary (PGE_2 3 mg) inserted into the posterior fornix; when contractions are established and the cervix starts to dilate, this is followed by a simple forewater rupture. If necessary, labour contractions are augmented by the cautious use of intravenous oxytocin, taking great care to avoid hyperstimulation. Continuous fetal heart monitoring using an external ultrasound sensor or a fetal scalp electrode and, if indicated, fetal scalp blood sampling are an essential part of the management of diabetic labour because of an increased risk of fetal distress (Brudenell 1978). Epidural analgesia has much to commend it but there is no objection to any of the alternative forms of analgesia commonly used in labour.

Spontaneous labour

When labour starts spontaneously it is managed in the same way as induced labour, expect that the need for augmentation is less likely.

Delivery

When labour progresses normally and the baby is not macrosomic, spontaneous vaginal delivery can be confidently expected. However, the obstetrician will often be called upon to decide whether or not to terminate a labour by operative delivery. Delay in progress in the first or second stages, fetal distress or difficulty in controlling the maternal diabetes—a rare occurrence nowadays—all indicate the need to expedite delivery. Caesarean section will often be the method of choice but, when the patient is fully dilated, if an easy forceps delivery can be carried out this is preferable. A difficult forceps delivery, bearing in mind that the baby may be big if not actually macrosomic, should be avoided because of the risk of shoulder dystocia and birth trauma. A very careful assessment of the patient in the operating theatre with preparations made for immediate Caesarean section is often helpful. In this circumstance a tentative attempt at forceps delivery can be made and if easy vaginal delivery is effected this is clearly desirable; otherwise immediate recourse should be made to Caesarean section. A neonatal paediatrician should always be present when a diabetic patient is delivered so that paediatric care of the baby can be started immediately after birth.

Mode of delivery

The actual mode of delivery at King's College Hospital in the years 1970–1985 is shown in Table 22.9. The overall Caesarean section rate remains higher than in non-diabetic pregnancy and this is true for both primigravidae and multigravidae, although the rate for primigravidae is less than the overall rate because of the influence which repeat Caesarean section has on the multigravidae rate.

Table 22.9 Mode of delivery of diabetic mothers at King's College Hospital

	1971–80	1981–85
Spontaneous onset followed by vaginal delivery	41 (12%)	33 (17%)
Induction followed by vaginal delivery	132 (38%)	60 (31%)
Induction followed by Caesarean section	45 (13%)	30 (16%)
Spontaneous onset followed by Caesarean section	11 (3%)	23 (12%)
Planned Caesarean section	123 (34%)	47 (24%)

Given the problems of diabetic pregnancy and labour a delivery by Caesarean section is a small price to pay by those women whose diabetic and obstetric complications make labour more hazardous for the fetus.

The anticipation of problems in labour is an essential part of all antenatal care but this is especially true of diabetic pregnancy when a decision to perform a planned rather than an emergency Caesarean section will relieve the patient as well as the obstetric and diabetic team of a great deal of anxiety. The same readiness to perform an emergency Caesarean section when labour is not progressing satisfactorily is an equally important part of the management of the pregnant diabetic.

Judgement

With careful monitoring in both pregnancy and labour the overall rate of Caesarean section should fall, and especially in primigravidae.

The infant of the diabetic mother

The characteristic appearance of the infant of the diabetic mother as described by Farquhar (1959) is well known. The tomato baby is most often associated with a diabetic pregnancy where maternal control has been bad, but may occur where maternal care has been good. The management of all infants of diabetic mothers, whether presenting characteristic appearance or not, calls for expert neonatal care.

Neonatal morbidity

The neonatal morbidity in these infants has changed considerably over the past 20 years and many now have a normal and uncomplicated neonatal course. Most will not require to be admitted to a special care baby unit.

Asphyxia

Asphyxia is more common in the infant of the diabetic mother. About one-third of all cases require intubation, although this figure includes a number of preterm and other compromised infants. Acidosis (pH < 7.20) is seen in about 10% and may require intravenous sodium bicarbonate.

Respiratory distress syndrome

The importance of respiratory distress syndrome (RDS) as a cause of perinatal mortality and morbidity has diminished sharply in recent times, although it remains a hazard for the preterm infant of the diabetic mother. The infant of a well controlled diabetic mother delivered

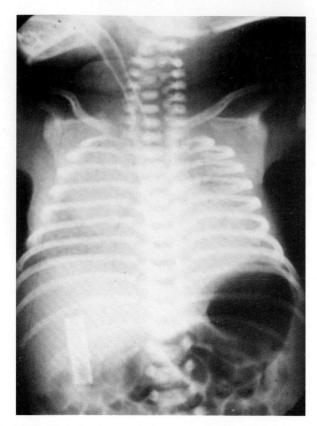

Fig. 22.2 RDS showing a typical air bronchogram.

after 37 weeks is unlikely to develop RDS (Fig. 22.2). Diagnosis is made by the typical air bronchogram appearance on chest X-ray. Prompt raising of the ambient oxygen concentration is called for. Only the very premature infant of a diabetic mother is likely to succumb to this cause given good modern neonatal paediatric care.

Hypoglycaemia

Blood glucose levels of < 1.1 mmol/l occur more frequently in the infant of a diabetic mother. The lowest levels are seen in the first hour of life, after which the concentration begins to rise. Hypoglycaemia is more commonly seen in macrosomic babies or after birth asphyxia. Hypoglycaemia is usually asymptomatic in these infants, but apnoea attacks, hypertonia, extreme excitability and frank convulsions may occur. The condition results from hyperinsulinaemia which is in turn a reflection of maternal hyperglycaemia. Whether hyperinsulinaemia is the sole cause of neonatal hypoglycaemia in such babies is debated, but it is probably the major factor. Hypoglycaemia is best prevented by early breastfeeding. The blood glucose levels should be measured at 2 and 4 hours after birth. If the level is < 2.5 mmol/l on both occasions intravenous glucose is commenced and continued until a sustained rise in glucose levels is obtained.

Hypocalcaemia and hypomagnesaemia

Neonatal hypocalcaemia (serum < 1.65 mmol/l) and hypomagnesaemia (serum magnesium < 0.62 mmol/l) are more common in these babies. Hypocalcaemia may lead to increased neuromuscular excitability, causing apnoeic spells and fits. If the levels are low, intravenous calcium gluconate 5% (50–100 mg/kg) is given.

Polycythaemia

Polycythaemia is more common in infants of diabetic mothers. It seems likely to be a response to intrauterine fetal anoxia. The increased maternal levels of HbA_1 may cause a degree of fetal anoxia and account for some decrease in the transfer of oxygen across the placenta. It seems unlikely that this is the sole explanation however. Polycythaemia is less of a problem in those pregnancies where maternal diabetic control has been good. If the haematocrit is more than 65% (20 g% of Hb) during the first 8 hours after birth venesection is recommended, with 10% of the infant's blood volume being removed. The red cells are centrifuged off and the plasma replaced.

Jaundice

Hyperbilirubinaemia may result from neonatal polycythaemia. Like polycythaemia it is much less common nowadays. Other contributors to hyperbilirubinaemia are bruising, including cephalhaematoma following a traumatic delivery and sepsis. Jaundice is of course more likely to occur in premature babies and in those who have had respiratory distress. A careful check on the level of bilirubin in these newborn babies is necessary and phototherapy or, rarely, exchange transfusion is carried out as required.

Cardiomyopathy

Some babies from women with diabetes are born with a form of cardiomyopathy which is similar to hypertrophic obstructive cardiomyopathy both on ultrasound examination and on histology (Reiler & Kaplan 1988). The abnormalities have been demonstrated from 34 weeks and are not eliminated by good diabetic control (Weber et al 1991). The impaired cardiac function may be the cause of some cases of respiratory distress (Kjos et al 1990). Although some babies die, most make a complete recovery.

Birth trauma

Birth trauma results from a difficult vaginal delivery often because of fetal macrosomia. In general, difficult vaginal delivery has no place in the modern management of diabetic pregnancy. Macrosomia should be diagnosed by routine antenatal ultrasound scanning and, where disproportion exists, the baby delivered by planned Caesarean section. Birth trauma should be rare in modern obstetric practice.

The long-term outlook for infants of diabetic mothers

The infants of diabetic mothers have a greater than average chance of developing diabetes in later life, but the actual risk is of the order of 1% as against 0.1% in infants of mothers who are not diabetic. A study by Persson (1986) found that 2 (3%) of 73 such children had developed diabetes in the first 10 years of life. Macrosomic babies tend to become obese and obesity may then be associated with abnormal glucose tolerance, but the majority of these babies, macrosomic or otherwise, usually exhibit normal physical development. Mental development is also usually normal, although there is a risk of neurological abnormality where prolonged neonatal hypoglycaemia occurs (Gamsu 1978).

Breastfeeding for the diabetic mother

Breastfeeding should be encouraged in diabetic women, as in non-diabetic women. In a survey by Whichelow & Doddridge (1983) it was found that three-quarters of the diabetic mothers at King's College Hospital were breastfeeding at 6 weeks. Those babies who were encouraged to suckle within 12 hours of delivery were more likely to be weaned later than those put to the breast after that time. An increase in the dietary allowance of carbohydrate by 50 g as a contribution for the extra 600 calories per day needed for lactation is essential. Insulin requirements are about 25% less than prepregnancy in women who are breastfeeding (Alban Davies et al 1989). In particular most mothers need less long-acting insulin at night to prevent nocturnal hypoglycaemia if they have to get up to feed their baby.

Family planning and the diabetic woman

For the average diabetic woman who wishes to have children a small family should be the aim. The problem of managing her diabetes and the possibility that long-term vascular complications will at some stage further impair her health make pregnancy and the addition of children to her life much more of a burden than for the non-diabetic woman. Family planning for the diabetic woman should result in a planned family and in the timing of conception in order to ensure that it occurs at a time when diabetic control is optimal. Diabetic women should aim to have their children as early as possible in their reproductive lives since the vascular complications of diabetes are more likely to arise after some years.

The traditional methods of contraception—sheath and contraceptive diaphragm—are appropriate for a woman who is well motivated toward family planning and has a caring partner. They offer a reasonable degree of safety from unplanned pregnancy with no risk of complications.

The intrauterine contraceptive device is a safer option and although it has certain disadvantages it has the important advantage that once placed in position the woman and her partner need take no further contraceptive measures. It is not suitable as a method of contraception for a nulliparous woman unless no alternative method can be used. The risk of intrauterine infection does not seem to be greater in well controlled diabetic women and a reported higher failure rate among diabetic intrauterine contraceptive device users (Steel & Duncan 1980) has not been borne out by experience or by subsequent papers (Thiery 1982).

The combined oral contraceptive pill is the most effective contraceptive method available, but has a slight but definite risk of causing venous thromboembolism; it is this complication rather than its minor effects on carbohydrate lipid metabolism which gives the greatest cause for concern in diabetic women, particularly amongst those known to have vascular disease or hypertension. Adjustment of insulin dosage may be required but the majority of diabetic women suffer no disturbance of diabetic control when taking the pill. Diabetic women who wish to use the pill should be examined carefully for evidence of microvasculopathy and hypertension and should be encouraged to lose weight if they are obese. They should also be strongly discouraged from smoking.

When diabetic women do opt for oral contraception the low-dose triphasic pill or the progesterone-only pill should be advised. The progesterone-only pill is not associated with increased risk of venous thromboembolism and from this point of view is suitable for the diabetic woman. It does sometimes cause irregular menstrual periods with intermenstrual spotting and has a higher failure rate than the combined pill. The failure rate can be kept to acceptably low levels if the patient takes the pill without fail every day, starting immediately after delivery; it is useful if the patient is breastfeeding. If it proves successful, it can be continued thereafter.

To the average non-pregnant diabetic woman who wishes to use oral contraception a low-dose triphasic preparation with its regularity of menstrual periods and very low failure rate is probably the pill of choice but the progesterone-only pill is a valuable alternative.

Laparoscopic sterilization is an easily performed gynaecological procedure with a low failure rate (one in 500 cases). It offers the diabetic woman who has completed her family the most satisfactory long-term solution to family planning problems and should be freely available. It is best performed 6 weeks postpartum and the patient can usually be dealt with on a day-case basis. Sterilization at the time of Caesarean section is an option which should be discussed with diabetic patients during the antenatal period and generally will only be applicable to those women having planned repeat Caesarean sections. Vasectomy may be an appropriate alternative to female sterilization in some cases, but only if the male partner is certain he will not want to bear more children under any circumstances.

THYROID DISEASE

Physiology

The clearance of iodine by the kidneys is increased because of the increase in renal blood flow in pregnancy. Therefore the thyroid responds by an increase in metabolic activity to trap iodine and convert it to iodinated tyrosines including thyroxine (T_4) and triiodothyronine (T_3). This is the cause of the increase in size of the thyroid gland observed in many communities in pregnancy, called the physiological goitre. However it is not physiological but pathological since it does not occur in populations that are iodine replete either because of a very high dietary intake, e.g. the Icelandic people who eat a lot of fish (Crooks et al 1964) or Americans whose salt is artificially iodised (Long et al 1985).

In pregnancy thyroid binding globulin levels are increased by the high oestrogen activity. This therefore increases the total thyroxine, but it is the free thyroxine that is metabolically active and this declines slightly in the latter part of pregnancy. Normal ranges are non-pregnant 9–23 pmol/l, first trimester 10–24 pmol/l, second trimester 9–19 pmol/l, third trimester 7–17 pmol/ (Parker 1985).

It is generally believed that TSH levels are not affected by pregnancy and this is important since a high TSH level is taken to indicate hypothyroidism and a low TSH level indicates hyperthyroidism. However hCG shares some immunological and physiological features with TSH and hCG levels are markedly elevated in early pregnancy. In some assays for TSH there may be cross-reaction with hCG giving apparently elevated TSH levels; by contrast the activity of hCG in stimulating the thyroid and thyroxine production may depress TSH levels by negative feedback. So minor changes in TSH levels should be interpreted with caution in pregnancy.

Pathologically elevated hCG levels in choriocarcinoma can cause frank hyperthyroidism but this resolves as the choriocarcinoma is treated. Commoner and more perplexing is the relation between hyperemesis gravidarum and elevated thyroxine levels. It is more likely that both conditions are also caused by elevated hCG but some authors have reported success in the management of hyperemesis treating concomitant hyperthyroidism with antithyroid drugs.

Thyroid disease

Four common methods of presentation need to be considered:

1. Hyperthyroidism—treated or arising de novo.
2. Hypothyroidism—treated or arising de novo.
3. Postpartum thyroiditis.
4. Thyroid nodules.

Hyperthyroidism

It is uncommon for women to present with hyperthyroidism in pregnancy because untreated the condition causes menstrual irregularity and failure of ovulation. Also Graves' disease tends to improve in pregnancy, possibly due to a direct effect of pregnancy inhibiting thyroid stimulating antibodies (TSA). However some women are found to be hyperthyroid for the first time in pregnancy or have only partially treated Graves' disease. It is important therefore to be able to assess thyroid status accurately. This is not easy since pregnancy itself mimics hyperthyroidism. Patients are often anxious, sweaty and complain of increased frequency of bowel movement. On examination they may have a tremor, tachycardia and goitre all due to pregnancy. Eye signs such as exophthalmos and lid retraction do not correlate with thyroid activity since they are caused by autoantibodies that are different from TSA, but eye signs are a marker for thyroid disease, either current or in the past. Loss of weight does not occur in normal pregnancy and would indicate hyperthyroidism unless some other abnormality were present. For the above reasons, a clinical diagnosis of hyperthyroidism should be supported by elevated free T_4 or free T_3 levels with suppression of the TSH.

Treatments available for hyperthyroidism in general are radioiodine, surgery and antithyroid drugs. Radioiodine is given with reluctance to young people and should be avoided altogether in pregnancy because it will cross the placenta and ablate the fetal thyroid. In the UK, surgery is reserved for failed medical therapy or where the patient is unable to take medical treatment for personal or social reasons. Medical therapy is therefore the treatment of choice. The two groups of drugs used are propylthiouracil (PTU) and carbimazole. In the UK there is more experience in general with carbimazole but PTU is probably the agent of choice in pregnancy: it is less likely to cause congenital malformations (aplasia cutis), although this scalp defect has been reported with PTU as well as with carbimazole. This drug has an additional effect in inhibiting TSA, independent of its antithyroid action, and is secreted less in breast milk. Antithyroid drugs are one of the few classes of drugs that are secreted in breast milk in amounts sufficient to harm the infant (Williams et al 1944).

The aim of antithyroid therapy is to use the minimum quantity of pharmacological agents to alleviate the patient's symptoms and to suppress the free thyroxine into the normal range. Under these circumstances the fetus should not be affected although excessive maternal drug treatment can certainly render the fetus hypothyroid (Mamotani et al 1986). Therefore there is no place for the previous management option of giving the mother high-dose antithyroid drug therapy to render her euthyroid as quickly as possible while at the same time giving her thyroxine to ensure that she and the fetus do not become hypothyroid, particularly since very little maternally administered thyroxine crosses to the fetus.

Antithyroid drug therapy needs to be given for a total of 1 year to minimize the chance of recurrence. In practice most patients have treatment initiated either before pregnancy or in the first trimester. The dose of antithyroid drugs is reduced to a maintance dose equal or equivalent to 15 mg of carbimazole by the third trimester and this can be continued or discontinued at the time of delivery. This level of treatment is unlikely to affect the infant if the mother is breastfeeding (Lamberg et al 1984) but the infant should have regular paediatic assessment and thyroid function tests.

The other way in which the fetus can be affected is by maternal TSA which can cross the placenta since they are IgG antibodies. They bind to the TSH receptor in the fetal thyroid and the fetus may therefore develop hyperthyroidism in utero (Pekonen et al 1984). This can lead to growth retardation and the development of fetal goitre which in turn can obstruct delivery, but these are very rare complications. More common, occurring in perhaps 10% of babies delivered to women who have Graves' disease in pregnancy, is hyperthyroidism developing up to 2 weeks after delivery (Zakarija et al 1983, 1986). It usually presents with failure to thrive and irritability but the baby can have all the clinical features of adult Graves' disease. The late presentation of neonatal hyperthyroidism suggests that there may be blocking substances analogous to alphafetoprotein in myasthenia gravis which inhibit the action of TSA in utero. It may also be the reason why neonatal hyperthyroidism has a bad prognosis and significant mortality. The babies present after they have left hospital and when they are no longer under routine paediatric care. Providing that paediatricians are involved, the condition responds quickly to medical therapy (either antithyroid drugs or simple sedatives) and is unlikely to reoccur since the autoantibodies are not produced in the infant, only transferred from its mother.

Hypothyroidism

Patients with extreme degrees of hypothyroidism do not become pregnant because they do not ovulate. Lesser degrees of hypothyroidism have been associated with a variety of causes of pregnancy failure such as preterm labour and accidental haemorrhage but these are old reports (Niswander & Gordon 1972) and such risks have not been confirmed recently. In general if patients with hypothyroidism conceive, their pregnancies are no more complicated than those of euthyroid patients. There is always concern that fetuses carried by women who are hypothyroid will themselves be hypothyroid and will suffer long-term brain damage. This concern is unfounded (Montoro et al 1981) since the fetus is autonomous for its thyroid function from very early in pregnancy. It is only iodine deficiency that relates to permanent brain damage (neurological cretinism) for then the fetus cannot synthesize thyroid homones.

Most women with hypothyroidism are already taking thyroxine before pregnancy. It is disputed whether the dose of thyroxine needs to be increased in pregnancy. Mandel et al (1990) studied 12 patients and found that nine needed to increase thyroxine from a mean of 100 µg per day at the beginning of pregnancy to 150 µg by the end of pregnancy. The need for increasing the dose was based on free T_4 and TSH measurements and was thought to be due to the increase in body weight. We studied 25 patients and found that if they were taking the correct dose of thyroxine in early pregnancy, this did not need to be increased as pregnancy continued, also as judged by TSH measurements (Girling & de Swiet 1992).

Postpartum thyroiditis

This condition occurs surprisingly frequently, in 5–9% of populations as diverse as the Welsh and the Japanese (Lazarus & Othman 1991). The patients usually have underlying autoimmune thyroid disease as shown by the presence of autoantibodies to thyroid tissue during pregnancy (Rasmussen et al 1990), but at that time they are often asymptomatic and have normal thyroid function. About 3 months after delivery, possibly due to a decline in blocking antibody, the titre of cytotoxic thyroid autoantibodies becomes raised. Thyroid cells are destroyed and excessive thyroxine is liberated so that the patients are temporarily hyperthyroid and they may have symptoms of this. However subsequently due to the decreased number of functioning thyroid cells, they become hypothyroid and this is much more likely to cause symptoms. Unfortunately the symptoms of tiredness, weakness and depression (Pop et al 1991) are those which women are expected to have in the first few months of motherhood; the patients typically develop symptoms at 3 months postdelivery when they are no longer in hospital care but in the care of the community where this condition is insufficiently known. They are reassured that they will get better and nothing more is done. The condition does remit spontaneously but may take 6 months to do so, a period of time when they could be made much happier by a short course of thyroxine treatment.

Thyroid nodules

Any asymptomatic enlargement of the thyroid gland is a cause for concern that the condition may be due to cancer. If there is a long history, this is unlikely to be the case but it is impossible to exclude cancer clinically. Such patients should be managed with a surgeon experienced in thyroid disease. Again radioactive iodine cannot be used to show whether the nodule is inactive (cold) or active (hot) (cold nodules are more likely to be cancerous than hot nodules). All patients should have an ultrasound examination of the nodule. Cystic lesions are unlikely to be cancerous (Miller et al 1974). The decision as to whether to perform fine needle biospy in solid nodules before or after delivery needs to be discussed with the surgical colleague.

If there is any suspicion of trachael compression, an X-ray should be taken of the thoracic inlet (notwithstanding the pregnancy) and the patient should be discussed with the anaesthetic team; intubation problems if the patients requires a general anaesthetic are much better anticipated than encountered for the first time in an emergency.

EPILEPSY

Up to 1% of the population have epilepsy (O'Brien & Gilmour White 1993), though not all are taking treatment, so it is a common complication of pregnancy. In general, pregnancy does not affect the frequency of epileptic attacks except for its effects on the metabolism of anticonvulsant drugs and the effects of stress and fatigue. Most patients with epilepsy are aware that these factors will make them more prone to seizures and pregnancy can be a time of considerable stress.

Apart from the question of teratogenicity, there is little evidence that epilepsy affects the outcome of pregnancy once adjustments have been made for other factors such as social class. There is no evidence that fetal outcome relates to the number of fits, which is reassuring for women who do have epileptic attacks in pregnancy. It is however difficult to believe that the fetus would not be affected if the women was having a succession of major seizures as in status epilepticus, particularly in view of the degree of hypoxia that can occur.

All series of epileptic patients have shown an increased malformation risk of the order of twice background. A slight increase can be shown in the children of women with epilepsy who are taking no drugs (Friis et al 1986); also in the children of fathers with epilepsy. However the risk is certainly increased with anticonvulsant therapy

and all anticonvulsant drugs should be considered teratogenic. All seem capable of inducing dysmophic facies, a funny-shaped face with a long philltrum and slanting epicanthic folds, but most children grow out of this (Meadow 1987). Abnormalities of neuromotor development including impaired intelligence have also been described, particularly for carbamazepine (Lyons Jones et al 1989), but in general such studies have not included appropriate controls of the children of women with epilepsy who are not taking anticonvulsant drugs. There is no doubt of the risks of facial clefts and congenital heart disease and these have best been described with phenytoin therapy. Valproate (Bailey et al 1983) and more recently carbamazepine (Rosa et al 1991) are associated with increased risk of neural tube defect; for valproate this risk is about 1%.

The management of women with epilepsy in pregnancy should start with prepregnancy counselling. Because of the teratogenic risk women should consider stopping anticonvulsant drugs before conception and either restarting after the first trimester or not restarting at all. This is a very difficult decision to make and only a small proportion of patients should consider it, mostly those who have had no seizures for at least 1 year. These however are the very women who are likely to loose their driving licences if they did have a fit at a time when they are most likely to want to be able to drive for they often have a young family. There is no easy solution to this personal and social dilemma.

In the majority of cases the women will continue to take anticonvulsants but anticonvulsant therapy should be reduced to the minimum dose of the minimum number of anticonvulsants. Although the teratogenic risk increases markedly with multiple anticonvulsant drug therapy (Nakane et al 1980), such patients are also more likely to have more severe epilepsy and to be taking higher doses; so multiple drug therapy does not necessarily per se increase the teratogenic risk.

Folic acid supplementation (5 mg rather than 400 μg per day) should be taken by those taking anticonvulsants in view of its protective effects against neural tube defect and malformations in general. It will not impair anticonvulsant control.

Once pregnant, the patient should be screened for neural tube defect and receive additional detailed scanning for congenital malformations in general, particularly for facial clefts and heart disease.

During pregnancy there are a number of factors that affect anticonvulsant drug effects. The metabolism and excretion of anticonvulsant drugs is increased, leading to lower drug levels and absorption is decreased. However these effects are partially offset by decreased protein binding. Nevertheless the net effect is a decrease in drug efficacy. There are undoubtedly some patients who have very brittle epilepsy and who require to maintain precise drug levels for anticonvulsant control. They will deteriorate unless frequent blood levels (preferably of the free drug) are obtained with appropriate dose adjustment. However the majority of patients do not have such severe epilepsy. Our practice is to check the blood level at the beginning of pregnancy to know what level controls their fits, and then only increase therapy if the patient has an increase in fit frequency.

Because of the risk of megaloblastic anaemia, folic acid supplementation should be continued with 5 mg daily. Once the patient becomes pregnant. There is also a risk of haemorrhage in the fetus and the mother due to a deficiency of vitamin K-dependent clotting factors induced by anticonvulsant drugs (Deblay et al 1984, Davies et al 1985). This risk is greatest at the time of delivery so we give supplemental oral vitamin K 10 mg daily from 36 weeks' gestation. Folic acid stores will be replete by this stage so folic acid can be discontinued.

Epileptic patients require particular care in the puerperium when they are very likely to have seizures partly because of stress, tiredness and major changes in their physiology and partly because they may have omitted or not absorbed anticonvulsant drugs in labour. They seem specially prone to have fits while having a bath, perhaps induced by vasovagal syncope. These fits have been associated with fatal drowning. Therefore after delivery women with epilepsy should either only take baths when supervised (Department of Health and Social Security 1989) or preferably take showers.

If the dose of anticonvulsant therapy has been increased in pregnancy then it will need to be decreased after delivery or else the woman will become intoxicated. The time-course over which the patient loses pregnancy effects seems quite variable after delivery. Usually the dose can be reduced in stages aided by blood levels over a 4-week period.

Although anticonvulsant drugs are secreted in breast milk, the amount secreted is so small that it will not harm the baby. Indeed the fetus will have become habituated to the drugs in utero and breast feeding is a very good way for the mother to gently withdraw anticonvulsants from her baby.

REFERENCES

Alban Davies H, Clark J D A, Dalton K J, Edwards O M 1989 Insulin requirements of diabetic women who breast feed. British Medical Journal 298: 1357–1358

Ales K L, Santini D L 1989 Should all pregnant women be screened for gestational glucose intolerance? Lancet i: 1187–1191

Bailey C J, Pool R W, Foskitt E M E, Harris F 1983 Valproic acid and fetal abnormality. British Medical Journal 286: 190

Baird J D 1986 Some aspects of metabolism and hormonal adaptation to pregnancy. Acta Endocrinologica (suppl) 277: 11–18

Baker L, Egler J M, Klein S H, Goldman A S 1981 Meticulous control of diabetes during organogenesis prevents congenital lumbo-sacral defects in rats. Diabetes 30: 955–959

Banting F G, Best C H 1922 The internal secretion of the pancreas. Journal of Laboratory and Clinical Medicine 7: 1–5

Barker D J P, Martyn C N 1992 The maternal and fetal enquiry of cardiovascular disease. Journal of Epidemiology 46: 8–11

Barron W M, Lindheimer M D (eds) 1991 Medical disorders during pregnancy. Mosby Year Book, St Louis

Brooks A P, Metcalfe J, Day J L, Edwards M S 1980 Iron deficiency and glycosylated haemoglobin A1. Lancet ii: 141

Broughton Pipkin F, Hunter J C, Oats J J N, O'Brien P M S 1982 The renin angiotensin system in normal and diabetic pregnancy. In: Sammour M B, Symonds E M, Zuspan F P, El Tomi N (eds) Pregnant hypertension. Ain Sham University Press, Cairo, pp 185–192

Brudenell M 1978 Delivering the baby of a diabetic mother. Proceedings of the Royal Society of Medicine 71: 207–211

Brudenell M 1982 Obstetric complications in the antenatal period in diabetic pregnancy. Results of UK Diabetic Pregnancy Survey (Beard R W & Lowy C (eds)) presented at RCOG scientific meeting 1982

Buschard K, Hougaard P, Molsted-Pedersen L, Kuhl C 1990 Type 1 (insulin-dependent) diabetes mellitus diagnosed during pregnancy: a clinical and prognostic study. Obstetrical and Gynecological Survey 607–608

Centers for Disease Control 1990 Leads from the morbidity and mortality weekly report. Perinatal mortality and congenital malformations in infants born to women with insulin-dependent diabetes mellitus—United States, Canada, and Europe, 1940–1988. Journal of the American Medical Association 39: 363–365

Comtois R, Desjarlais F, Nguyen M, Beauregard H 1989 Clinical usefulness of estimation of serum fructosamine concentration as screening test for gestational diabetes. American Journal of Obstetrics and Gynecology 160: 651–654

Crooks J, Aboul-Khair S A, Turnbull A C, Hytten F E 1964 The incidence of goitre during pregnancy. Lancet ii: 334–336

Cudworth A G, Woodrow J C 1976 Genetic susceptibility in diabetes mellitus: analysis of the HLA association. British Medical Journal 2: 1333–1336

Damm P, Molsted-Pedersen L 1989 Significant decrease in congenital malformations in newborn infants of an unselected population of diabetic women. Obstetrical and Gynecological Survey 161: 1163

Dandona P, Freedman D, Moorhead F J 1979 Glycosylated haemoglobin in chronic renal failure. British Medical Journal i: 1183–1184

Davies V A, Argent A C, Staub H et al 1985 Precursor prothrombin status in patients receiving anticonvulsant drugs. Lancet i: 126–128

de Swiet M (ed) 1995 Medical disorders in obstetric practice, 3rd edn. Blackwell Science, Oxford

Deblay M F, Vert P, Andre M, Marchal F 1982 Transplacental vitamin K prevents haemorrhagic disease of infant of epileptic mother. Lancet i: 1247

Department of Health and Social Security 1989 Report on Confidential Equiries on Maternal Deaths in England and Wales 1982–1984. HMSO, London

Deuchar E M 1979 Experimental evidence relating fetal abnormalities to diabetes. In: Sutherland H W, Stowers J M (eds) Carbohydrate metabolism in pregnancy and the newborn. Springer Verlag, Berlin, pp 519–522

Dooley S L, Metzger B E, Cho N, Liu K 1991 The influence of demographic and phenotypic heterogeneity on the prevalence of gestational diabetes mellitus. International Journal of Gynaecology and Obstetrics 35: 13–18

Eastwood M A, Kay R M 1979 An hypothesis for the action of dietary fibre along the gastrointestinal tract. American Journal of Clinical Nutrition 32: 364–367

Enricho A, Ingalls T M 1968 Chromosomal anomalies in the embryos of diabetic mice. Archives of Environmental Health 16: 316–325

Essex N, Pyke D A 1978 Management of maternal diabetes in pregnancy. In: Sutherland H W, Stowers J M (eds) Carbohydrate metabolism in pregnancy and the newborn. Springer Verlag, Berlin, pp 357–368

Fadel H E, Reynolds A, Stallings M, Abraham E C 1981 Minor (glycosylated) hemoglobins in cord blood of infants of normal and diabetic mothers. Journal of Obstetrics and Gynaecology 139: 397–402

Farquhar J W 1959 The child of the diabetic woman. Archives of Disease in Childhood 34: 76–96

Friis M L, Holm N V, Sindrup E H et al 1986 Facial clefts in sibs and children of epileptic patients. Neurology 36: 346–350

Fuhrmann K, Reiher H, Semmler K, Fischer F, Fischer M, Glockner E 1983 Prevention of congenital malformations in infants of insulin-dependent diabetic mothers. Diabetes Care 6: 219–223

Gabbay K H, Hasty K, Breslow J L, Ellison R C, Bunn H F, Fallop P M 1977 Long term blood glucose control in diabetes mellitus. Journal of Clinical Endocrinology and Metabolism 44: 859–864

Gabbay K H, Sosenko J M, Banuchi C A, Mininsohn M J, Fluckiger R 1979 Glycosylated hemoglobins: increased glycosylation of hemoglobin A in diabetic patients. Diabetes 28: 337–340

Gamsu H R 1978 Neonatal morbidity in infants of diabetic mothers. Proceedings of the Royal Society of Medicine 71: 211–221

Garner P R, D'Alton M E, Dudley D K et al 1990 Preeclampsia in diabetic pregnancies. American Journal of Obstetrics and Gynecology 163: 505–508

Gillmer M D G, Oakley N W, Beard R W et al 1980 Antenatal screening for diabetes mellitus by random blood glucose sampling. British Journal of Obstetrics and Gynaecology 87: 377–382

Girling J C, de Swiet M 1992 Thyroxine dosage during pregnancy in women with primary hypothyroidism. British Journal of Obstetrics and Gynaecology 99: 368–370

Goldman A S, Baker L, Piddington R, Marx B, Harold R, Egler J 1985 Hyperglycaemia induced teratogenesis is mediated by a functional deficiency of arachidonic acid. Proceedings of the National Academy of Sciences (USA) 82: 8227–8231

Grenfell A, Bewick M, Brudenell M et al 1986 Diabetic pregnancy following renal transplantation. Diabetic Medicine 3: 177–179

Hadden D R 1980 Screening for abnormalities of carbohydrate metabolism in pregnancy 1966–1977: the Belfast experience. Diabetes Care 3: 440–446

Hofmann H M H 1990 Fructosamine in relation to maternofetal glucose and insulin homeostasis in gestational diabetes. Archives of Gynecology and Obstetrics 247: 173–185

Hunter D J S, Keirse M J N C 1989 Gestational diabetes. In: Chalmers I, Enkin M, Keirse M J N C (eds) Effective care in pregnancy and childbirth, vol 1. Oxford University Press, Oxford, pp 403–409

Jarrett R J 1993 Gestational diabetes: a non-entity? British Medical Journal 306: 37–38

Johnstone F D, Nasrat A A, Prescott R J 1990 The effect of established and gestational diabetes on pregnancy outcome. British Journal of Obstetrics and Gynaecology 97: 1009–1015

Jovanovic R, Jovanovic L 1984 Obstetric management when normoglycaemia is maintained in diabetic pregnant women with vascular compromise. American Journal of Obstetrics and Gynecology 149: 617–623

Jovanovic-Peterson L, Peterson C H, Reed G F et al 1991 Maternal postprandial glucose levels and infant birth weight: the diabetes in early pregnancy study. American Journal of Obstetrics and Gynecology 164: 103–111

Kalkhoff R, Kissebah A H, Hak Joong K 1979 Lipid metabolism during normal pregnancy. In: Merkatz K R, Adam P A J (eds) The diabetic pregnancy; a perinatal perspective. Grune & Stratton, New York, pp 10–17

Kitzmiller J L, Brown E R, Phillipe M 1981 Diabetic nephropathy and perinatal outcome. American Journal of Obstetrics and Gynecology 141: 741–751

Kitzmiller J L, Gavin L A, Gin G D et al 1991 Preconception care of diabetes. Glycemic control prevents congenital anomalies. Journal of the American Medical Association 265: 731–736

Kjos S L, Walther F J, Montoro M et al 1990 Prevalence and etiology of respiratory distress in infants of diabetic mothers: predictive value of fetal lung maturation tests. American Journal of Obstetrics and Gynecology 163: 898–903

Knight A 1983 Concerning macrosomy in diabetic pregnancy. Lancet ii: 1431

Lamberg B A, Ikonen E, Osterlund K et al 1984 Antithyroid treatment of maternal hyperthyroidism during lactation. Clinical Endocrinology 21: 81–87

Lazarus J H, Othman S 1991 Thyroid disease in relation to pregnancy. Clinical Endocrinology 34: 91–98

Leny W, Maier W 1964 Congenital malformations and maternal diabetes. Lancet ii: 1124

Lernmark A 1985 Causes of insulin dependent diabetes. Medicine International 13: 535–538

Leslie R D G, Pyke D A, John P N, White J M 1978 Haemoglobin A$_1$ in diabetic pregnancy. Lancet ii: 958–959

Lind T, McDougall A N 1972 Antenatal screening for diabetes mellitus by random blood glucose sampling. British Journal of Obstetrics and Gynaecology 112: 213–220

Long T J, Felice M E, Hollingsworth D R 1985 Goiter in pregnant teenagers. American Journal of Obstetrics and Gynecology 152: 670–674

Lyons Jones K, Lacro R V, Johnson K A, Adams J 1989 Pattern of malformations in the children of women treated with Carbamazepine during pregnancy. New England Journal of Medicine 320: 1661–1666

Mandel S J, Larsen P R, Seely E W, Brent G A 1990 Increased need for thyroxine during pregnancy in women with primary hyperthyroidism. New England Journal of Medicine 323: 91–96

Malins J 1979 Fetal anomalies related to carbohydrate metabolism: the epidemiological approach. In: Sutherland H W, Stowers J M (eds) Carbohydrate metabolism in pregnancy and the newborn. Springer Verlag, Berlin, pp 229–246

Mamotani N, Noh J, Oyanagi H et al 1986 Antithyroid drug therapy for Graves' disease in pregnancy. New England Journal of Medicine 1986; 315: 24–28

Maresh M 1993 Gestational diabetes mellitus. British Medical Journal 306: 581

Mather H M, Keen H 1985 The Southall Diabetes Survey: prevalence of diabetes in Asians and Europeans. British Medical Journal 291: 1081–1084

Meadow S R 1987 The teratogenic associations of epilepsy and anticonvulsant drugs. In: Hopkins A (ed) Epilepsy. Chapman and Hall, London

Miller E, Hare J W, Cloherty J P et al 1981 Elevated maternal haemoglobin A$_{1c}$ in early pregnancy and major congenital anomalies in infants of diabetic mothers. New England Journal of Medicine 304: 1331–1334

Miller J M, Zafar S U, Karo J J 1974 The cystic thyroid nodule: recognition and management. Radiology 110: 257–261

Mills J L, Baker L, Goldman A S 1979 Malformations in infants of diabetic mothers occur before the 7th gestational week. Implications for treatment. Diabetes 28: 292–293

Mills J L, Leigh Simpson J, Driscoll S G et al 1988 Incidence of spontaneous abortion among normal women and insulin-dependent diabetic women whose pregnancies were identified within 21 days of conception. New England Journal of Medicine 1988; 319: 1617–1623

Miodovnik M, Lavin J P, Knowles H C et al 1984 Spontaneous abortion among insulin-dependent diabetic women. American Journal of Obstetrics and Gynecology 150: 372–376

Montoro M, Collea J V, Frasier S D et al 1981 Succesful outcome of pregnancy in women with hypothyroidism. Annals of Internal Medicine 94: 31–34

Nakane Y, Okuma T, Takahashi R et al 1980 Multi-institutional study on the teratogenicity and fetal toxicity of antiepileptic drugs: a report of a collaborative study group in Japan. Epilepsia 21: 663–680

Nasrat H, Warda M, Ardawi H et al 1990 Pregnancy in Saudi Arabian non-insulin dependent diabetics. Journal of Obstetrics and Gynaecology 10: 357–362

National Diabetes Data Group 1979 Classification and diagnosis of diabetes mellitus and other categories of glucose tolerance. Diabetes 28: 1039–1057

Niuswander K R, Gordon M 1972 The women and their pregnancies. W B Saunders, Philadelphia, p 264

O'Brien M D, Gilmour-White S 1993 Epilepsy and pregnancy. British Medical Journal 307: 492–495

Ojomo E O, Coustan D R 1990 Absence of evidence of pulmonary maturity at amniocentesis in term infants of diabetic mothers. American Journal of Obstetrics and Gynecology 1990; 163: 954–957

O'Shaughnessy R, Cuss J, Zuspan F P 1979 Glycosylated hemoglobins and diabetes mellitus in pregnancy. American Journal of Obstetrics and Gynecology 135: 783–790

O'Sullivan G C, Walker K, Bondar G F 1975 Effects of pregnancy on bile acid metabolism. Surgical Forum 26: 442–444

O'Sullivan J B 1975 Prospective study of gestational diabetes and its treatment. In: Stowers J M, Sutherland H W (eds) Carbohydrate metabolism in pregnancy and the newborn. Churchill Livingstone, Edinburgh, pp 195–204

O'Sullivan J B, Clark D, Dandrour R V 1971 Treatment of verified pre-diabetes in pregnancy. Journal of Reproductive Medicine 1971; 7: 21–24

O'Sullivan J M, Mahan D H 1964 Criteria for the oral glucose tolerance test in pregnancy. Diabetes 13: 278

Paker J H 1985 Amerlex free triiodothyronine and free thyroxine levels in normal pregnancy. British Journal of Obstetrics and Gynaecology 1985; 92: 1234–1238

Peacock I, Hunter J C, Walford S et al 1979 Self-monitoring of blood glucose in diabetic pregnancy. British Medical Journal 2: 1333–1336

Pedersen J 1979 Congenital malformations in newborns of diabetic mothers. In: Sutherland H W, Stowers J M (eds) Carbohydrate metabolism in pregnancy and the newborn. Springer Verlag, Berlin, pp 264–276

Pedersen J F, Mølsted-Pedersen L 1981 Early fetal growth delay detected by ultrasound marks increased risk of congenital malformation in diabetic pregnancy. British Medical Journal 283: 269–271

Pekonen F, Teramo K, Makinen T et al 1984 Prenatal diagnosis and treatment of fetal thyrotoxicosis. American Journal of Obstetrics and Gynecology 150: 893–894

Penn K, Makowski E L, Harris P 1980 Parenthood following renal transplantation. Kidney International 18: 221–233

Persson B 1986 Long term morbidity in the offspring of diabetic mothers. Acta Endocrinologica (Copenhagen) (suppl) 277: 150–155

Poon P, Turner R C, Gillmer M D G 1981 Glycosylated fetal haemoglobin. British Medical Journal 283: 469

Pop V J M, De Rooy H A M, Vader H L et al 1991 Postpartum thyroid dysfunction and depression in an unselected population. New England Journal of Medicine 324: 1815–1816

Pyke D A 1962 Pre-diabetes. In: Pyke D A (ed) Disorders of carbohydrate metabolism. Pitman, London

Pyke D A 1968 Aetiology of diabetes mellitus. In: Oakley W G, Pyke D A, Taylor K W (eds) Clinical diabetes. Blackwell, Oxford, pp 220–221

Rasmussen N G, Hornnes P J, Hoier-Madsen M et al 1990 Thyroid size and function in healthy pregnant women with thyroid autoantibodies. Relation to development of postpartum thyroiditis. Acta Endocrinologica (Copenhagen) 123: 395–401

Reece E A, Eagan J F X, Constan D R et al 1986 Coronary artery disease in diabetic pregnancies. American Journal of Obstetrics and Gynecology 154: 150–151

Reece E A, Coustan D R, Hayslett J P et al 1988 Diabetic nephropathy: pregnancy performance and fetomaternal outcome. American Journal of Obstetrics and Gynecology 159: 56–66

Reller M D, Kaplan S 1988 Hypertrophic cardiomyopathy in infants of diabetic mothers: an update. American Journal of Perinatology 1988; 5: 353–358

Report on Confidential Enquiries into Maternal Deaths in England and Wales 1979–1981 (1986) HMSO, London

Roberts A B, Baker J R, James A G, Henley P 1988 Fructosamine in the management of gestational diabetes. American Journal of Obstetrics and Gynecology 159: 66–71

Roberts A B, Baker J R, Metcalf P, Mullard C 1990 Fructosamine compared with a glucose load as a screening test for gestational diabetes. Obstetrics and Gynecology 76: 773–775

Rosa F W 1991 Spina bifida in infants of women treated with Carbamazepine during pregnancy. New England Journal of Medicine 324: 674–677

Rosen B, Miodovnik M, St John Dignan P et al 1990 Minor congenital malformations in infants of insulin-dependent diabetic women: association with poor glycemic control. Obstetrics and Gynecology 76: 745–749

Russell G, Farmer G, Lloyd D et al 1984 Macrosomia despite well-controlled diabetic pregnancy. Lancet i: 283–284

Siddiqi T, Rosenn B, Mimouni F et al 1991 Hypertension during pregnancy in insulin-dependent diabetic women. Obstetrics and Gynecology 77: 514

Sosenko J M, Kitsmiller J L, Fluckiger R et al 1982 Umbilical cord glycosylated hemoglobin in infants of diabetic mothers: relationships to neonatal hypoglycaemia macrosomia and cord serum C-peptide. Diabetes Care 5: 566–570

Stallone L A, Ziel H K 1974 Management of gestational diabetes. American Journal of Obstetrics and Gynecology 119: 1191–1194

Steel J, Duncan L J P 1980 Contraception for insulin dependent diabetics. Diabetes Care 3: 557

Steel J M 1985 The prepregnancy clinic. Practical Diabetes 2(6): 8–10

Steel J M, Thomson P, Johnstone F et al 1981 Glycosylated haemoglobin concentrations in mothers of large babies. British Medical Journal 282: 1357–1358

Steel J M, Johnstone F D, Hepburn D A, Smith A F 1990 Can prepregnancy care of diabetic women reduce the risk of abnormal babies? British Medical Journal 301: 1070–1074

Stubbs S M, Brudenell J M, Pyke D A, Watkins P J, Stubbs W A, Alberti K G M M 1980 Management of the pregnancy diabetic: home or hospital, with or without glucose meters. Lancet i: 1122

Stubbs S M, Leslie R D G, John P N 1981 Fetal macrosomia and maternal diabetic control in pregnancy. British Medical Journal 282: 439–440

Stubbs S M, Doddridge M, John P N, Steel J M, Wright A D 1987 Haemoglobin A$_1$ and congenital malformations. Diabetic Medicine 4: 156–159

Thiery M 1982 Intra-uterine contraceptive devices for diabetics. Lancet ii: 883

Tyden O, Berne C, Eriksson U J et al 1984 Fetal maturation in strictly controlled diabetic pregnancy. Diabetes Research 1: 131–134

Watkins P J 1982 Congenital malformations and blood glucose control in diabetic pregnancy. British Medical Journal 284: 1357–1358

Weber H S, Copel J A, Reece E A et al 1991 Cardiac growth in fetuses of diabetic mothers with good metabolic control. Journal of Pediatrics 118: 103–107

Whichelow M J, Doddridge M C 1983 Lactation in diabetic women. British Medical Journal 287: 649–650

White P 1965 Pregnancy and diabetes, medical aspects. Medical Clinics of North America 49: 1015

Widness J A, Schartz H C, Thompson D et al 1978 Haemoglobin A$_{1c}$ (glycohaemoglobin) in diabetic pregnancy: an indicator of glucose control and fetal size. British Journal of Obstetrics and Gynaecology 85: 812–817

Willhoite M B, Bennett H W, Palomaki G E et al 1993 The impact of preconception counselling on pregnancy outcomes. Diabetes Care 16: 450–455

Williams R H, Kay G A, Jandorf B J 1944 Its absorption, distribution and excretion. Journal of Clinical Investigation 1944; 23: 613–627

World Health Organization Expert Committee on Diabetes 1980 Second report. WHO Technical Report Series 646, Geneva

Worth R, Ashworth L, Home P et al 1983 Glycosylated haemoglobin in cord blood following normal and diabetic pregnancies. Diabetologia 25: 482–485

Wright A D, Nicholson H O, Pollock A, Taylor K G, Betts S 1983 Spontaneous abortion and diabetes mellitus. Postgraduate Medical Journal 59: 295–298

Ylinen K, Hekali R, Teramo K 1981 Haemoglobin A$_{1c}$ during pregnancy of insulin dependent diabetics and healthy controls. Journal of Obstetrics and Gynaecology 1: 223–228

Ylinen K, Aula P, Stenman U-H et al 1984 Risk of minor and major fetal malformations in diabetics with high haemoglobin A$_{1c}$ values in early pregnancy. British Medical Journal 289: 345–346

Zakarija M, McKenzie J M, Munro D S 1983 Immunoglobulin G inhibitor of thyroid-stimulating antibody is a cause of delay in the onset of neonatal Graves' disease. Journal of Clinical Investigations 1983; 72: 1352–1356

Zakarija M, McKenzie J M, Hoffman W H 1986 Prediction and therapy of intrauterine and late-onset neonatal hyperthyroidism. Journal of Clinical Endocrinology and Metabolism 62: 368–371

23. Coagulation defects in pregnancy

Elizabeth A. Letsky

HAEMOSTASIS AND PREGNANCY

Healthy haemostasis depends on normal vasculature, platelets, coagulation factors and fibrinolysis. These act together to confine the circulating blood to the vascular bed and arrest bleeding after trauma. Normal pregnancy is accompanied by dramatic changes in the coagulation and fibrinolytic systems (Letsky 1991a). There is a marked increase in some of the coagulation factors, particularly fibrinogen. Fibrin is laid down in the uteroplacental vessel walls and fibrinolysis is suppressed. These changes, together with the increased blood volume, help to combat the hazard of haemorrhage at placental separation, but play only a secondary role to the unique process of myometrial contraction which reduces the blood flow to the placental site. They also produce a vulnerable state for intravascular clotting, and a whole spectrum of disorders involving coagulation occur in complications of pregnancy, falling into two main groups—thromboembolism (see Ch. 44) and bleeding due to disseminated intravascular coagulation (DIC). To make more understandable the measures taken to deal with these obstetric emergencies,

a short account follows of haemostasis during pregnancy and how it differs from that in the non-pregnant state.

VASCULAR INTEGRITY

It is not known how vascular integrity is normally maintained but it is clear that the platelets have a key role to play because conditions in which their number is depleted or their function is abnormal are characterized by widespread spontaneous capillary haemorrhages. It is thought that the platelets in health are constantly sealing microdefects of the vasculature, with mini fibrin clots being formed and the unwanted fibrin being removed by a process of fibrinolysis. Generation of prostacyclin appears to be the physiological mechanism which protects the vessel wall from excess deposition of platelet aggregates, and explains the fact that contact of platelets with healthy vascular endothelium is not a stimulus for thrombus formation (Moncada & Vane 1979).

Prostacyclin is an unstable prostaglandin first discovered in 1976. It is the principal prostanoid synthesized by blood vessels, a powerful vasodilator and potent inhibitor of platelet aggregation. Moncada & Vane (1979) have proposed that there is a balance between the production of prostacyclin by the vessel wall, and the production of the vasoconstrictor and powerful aggregating agent thromboxane by the platelet. Prostacyclin prevents aggregation at much lower concentrations than are needed to prevent adhesion, therefore vascular damage leads to platelet adhesion but not necessarily to aggregation and thrombus formation.

When injury is minor, small platelet thrombi form and are washed away by the circulation as described above, but the extent of the injury is an important determinant of the size of the thrombus—and of whether or not platelet aggregation is stimulated. Prostacyclin synthetase is abundant in the intima and progressively decreases in concentration from the intima to the adventitia, whereas the proaggregating elements increase in concentration from the subendothelium to the adventitia. It follows that severe vessel damage or physical detachment of the endothelium will lead to the development of a large thrombus as opposed to simple platelet adherence.

There are several conditions in which the production of prostacyclin could be impaired, thereby upsetting the normal balance. Deficiency of prostacyclin production has been suggested in platelet consumption syndromes such as haemolytic uraemic syndrome and thrombotic thrombocytopenic purpura (Lewis 1982). Prostacyclin production has been shown to be reduced in fetal and placental tissue from pre-eclamptic pregnancies, and the current role of prostacyclin in pathogenesis of this disease and potential for treatment in hypertension of pregnancy is undergoing active investigation. However, endothelial cell injury leads to platelet activation and triggering of the coagulation system; it is possible that the changes in haemostatic components are purely a secondary response to underlying vascular disease.

Some studies have shown an increased oxygen free radical production in pre-eclampsia which will in turn decrease vascular prostacyclin and endothelial dependent relaxing factor (EDRF) release and increase thromboxane A_2 and endothelin release. The whole subject of endothelial function in normal and pre-eclamptic pregnancy has been well reviewed recently (Zeeman et al 1992).

Platelets are produced in the bone marrow by the megakaryocytes and have a lifespan of 9–12 days. At the end of their normal lifespan the effete cells are engulfed by cells of the reticuloendothelial system and most damaged platelets are sequestered in the spleen.

There have been conflicting reports concerning the platelet count during normal pregnancy. A review of publications over the past 25 years (Sill et al 1985) revealed a majority consensus (of six) suggesting a small fall in the platelet count towards term during normal pregnancy; two publications suggested that there is no change and one early, probably inaccurate, study documented a rise. However, few of these studies obtained data on a longitudinal basis and in none of them was a within-patient analysis performed.

Recent studies surveying large populations with the use of automated counting equipment suggest that if mean values for platelet concentration are analysed throughout pregnancy there is a downward trend (Fay et al 1983) even though most values fall within the accepted non-pregnant ranges (Fentan et al 1977, Fay et al 1983, Beal & de Masi 1985, Sill et al 1985).

There appears to be more evidence suggesting that there is an increased platelet turnover and low-grade platelet activation as pregnancy advances, with a larger proportion of younger platelets with a greater mean platelet volume (Fay et al 1983, Sill et al 1985). However, other studies have shown no significant difference in platelet lifespan between non-pregnant and healthy pregnant women (Wallenberg & Van Kessel 1978, Rakoczi et al 1979).

Most investigators agree that low-grade chronic intravascular coagulation within the uteroplacental circulation is a part of the physiological response of all women to pregnancy. This is partially compensated and it is not surprising that the platelets should be involved at some level, even in healthy pregnancy.

A recent prospective study of 2263 healthy women delivering during one year at a Canadian obstetric centre (Burrows & Kelton 1988) showed that 112 (8.3%) had mild thrombocytopenia at term (platelet counts 97–150 $\times 10^9$/l). The frequency of thrombocytopenia in their offspring was no greater than that of babies born to women with platelet counts in the normal accepted range and no infant had a platelet count $< 100 \times 10^9$/l. An extension of this study to include 6715 deliveries substantiates these original findings (Burrows & Kelton 1990a).

One study (Lewis et al 1980) demonstrated significantly more aggregated platelets in a small number of women during late pregnancy and the puerperium compared with non-pregnant controls. In another more recent study, patients with a normal pregnancy were compared with non-pregnant controls (O'Brien et al 1986). They were shown to have a significantly lower platelet count and an increase in circulating platelet aggregates. In vitro the platelets were shown to be hypoaggregable. This was interpreted as suggesting platelet activation during pregnancy causing platelet aggregation and followed by exhaustion of platelets (O'Brien et al 1986).

Earlier publications suggesting that there was no evidence of changes in platelet function (Shaper et al 1968) or differences in platelet lifespan (Rakoczi et al 1979, Romero & Duffy 1980) between healthy non-pregnant and pregnant women must be re-evaluated in the face of more recent investigations, but it is clear that normal pregnancy has little significant effect on the screening parameter usually measured, namely the platelet count.

The problem remains in defining completely normal pregnancy. Certain disease states specific to pregnancy have profound effects on platelet consumption lifespan and function. For example, a decrease in platelet count (Redman et al 1978) and changes in platelet function (Ahmed et al 1991) have been observed in pregnancies with fetal growth retardation and the lifespan of platelets is shortened significantly even in mild pre-eclampsia (Lin et al 1991, Ballegeer et al 1992).

Arrest of bleeding after trauma

An essential function of the haemostatic system is a rapid reaction to injury which remains confined to the area of damage. This requires control mechanisms which will stimulate coagulation after trauma, and limit the extent of the response. The substances involved in the formation of the haemostatic plug normally circulate in an inert form until activated at the site of injury, or by some other factor released into the circulation which will trigger intravascular coagulation.

Local response

Platelets adhere to collagen on the injured basement membrane, which triggers a series of changes in the platelets themselves, including shape change and release of adenosine diphosphate and other substances. Adenosine diphosphate release stimulates further aggregation of platelets, which triggers the coagulation cascade, and the action of thrombin leads to the formation of fibrin which converts the lone platelet plug into a firm, stable wound seal. The role of platelets is of less importance in injury involving large vessels, because platelet aggregates are of insufficient size and strength to breach the defect. The coagulation mechanism is of major importance here, together with vascular contraction.

COAGULATION SYSTEM

The end-result of blood coagulation is the formation of an insoluble fibrin clot from the soluble precursor fibrinogen in the plasma. This involves a complex interaction of clotting factors, and a sequential activation of a series of proenzymes which has been termed the coagulation cascade (Fig. 23.1).

When a blood vessel is injured, blood coagulation is initiated by activation of factor XII by collagen (intrinsic mechanism) and activation of factor VII by thromboplastin release (extrinsic mechanism) from the damaged tissues. Both the intrinsic and extrinsic mechanisms are activated by components of the vessel wall and both are required for normal haemostasis. Strict divisions between

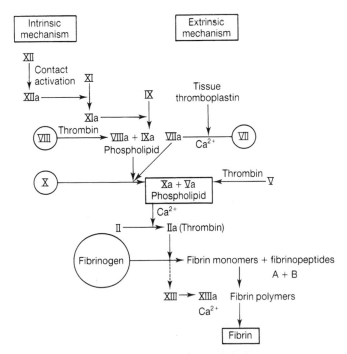

Fig. 23.1 The factors involved in blood coagulation and their interactions. The circled factors show significant increases in pregnancy.

the two pathways do not exist and interactions between activated factors in both pathways have been shown. They share a common pathway following the activation of factor X.

The intrinsic pathway (or contact system) proceeds spontaneously and is relatively slow, requiring 5–20 minutes for visible fibrin formation. All tissues contain a specific lipoprotein, thromboplastin (particularly concentrated in lung and brain), which markedly increases the rate at which blood clots. The placenta is also very rich in tissue factor; tissue factor produces fibrin formation within 12 seconds. The acceleration of coagulation is brought about by bypassing the reactions involving the contact (intrinsic) system (see Fig. 23.1).

Normal pregnancy is accompanied by major changes in the coagulation system, with increases in levels of factors VII, VIII and X, and a particularly marked increase in the level of plasma fibrinogen (Bonnar 1987; Fig. 23.1), which is probably the chief cause of the accelerated erythrocyte sedimentation rate observed in pregnancy. The effect of pregnancy on the coagulation factors can be detected from about the third month of gestation, and the amount of fibrinogen in late pregnancy is at least double that of the non-pregnant state (Bonnar 1987, Forbes & Greer 1992).

Blood coagulation is strictly confined to the site of tissue injury in normal circumstances. Powerful control mechanisms must be at work to prevent dissemination of coagulation beyond the site of trauma.

THE NATURALLY OCCURRING ANTICOAGULANTS

Mechanisms that limit and localize the clotting process at sites of trauma are critically important to protect against generalized thrombosis, and also to prevent spontaneous activation of those powerful procoagulant factors which circulate in normal plasma.

In recent years, in the investigation of healthy haemostasis, emphasis has been switching from the factors which promote clotting to those that prevent generalized and spontaneous activation of these factors. It is not appropriate to give an account of the complex interactions and biochemistry of all of these factors here. Only those of major importance in haemostasis and relevance to pregnancy will be mentioned. The balance of procoagulant and inhibitory factors is discussed in a review by Lammle & Griffin (1985).

Antithrombin III (ATIII)

Antithrombin III (ATIII) is considered to be the main physiological inhibitor of thrombin and factor Xa. It is well known that heparin greatly enhances the reaction rate of enzyme ATIII interaction and this is the rationale for the use of small-dose heparin as prophylaxis in patients at risk of thromboembolic phenomena postoperatively, in pregnancy and the puerperium. An inherited deficiency of ATIII is one of the few conditions in which a familial tendency to thrombosis has been described.

ATIII is synthesized in the liver. Its activity is low in cirrhosis and other chronic diseases of the liver, as well as in protein-losing renal disease. DIC and hypercoagulable states. The commonest cause of a small reduction in ATIII is use of oral contraceptives and this has been shown to be related to the oestrogen content.

During pregnancy there appears to be little change in ATIII levels but some decrease at parturition and an increase in the puerperium (Hellgren & Blomback 1981), but there must be increased synthesis in the antenatal period to maintain normal mean levels in the face of an increasing plasma volume.

Protein C, activated Protein C cofactor (APC)

Protein C inactivates factors V and VIII in conjunction with its cofactors thrombomodulin and protein S. Protein C is a vitamin K-dependent anticoagulant synthesized in the liver. To exert its effect it has to be activated by an endothelial cell cofactor termed thrombomodulin. The importance of the protein C thrombomodulin protein S system is exemplified by the absence of thrombomodulin in the brain where the priority for haemostasis is higher than for anticoagulation.

Many kindreds with a deficiency or a functional deficit of protein C with associated recurrent thromboembolism have been described (Bertina et al 1988). Purpura fulminans neonatalis is the homozygous expression of protein C deficiency with severe thrombosis and neonatal death (Seligsohn et al 1984).

Protein S, also a vitamin K-dependent glycoprotein, acts as a cofactor for activated protein C by promoting its binding to lipid and platelet surface, thus localizing the reaction. Several families have been described with protein S deficiency and thromboembolic disease.

Data on protein C and protein S levels in healthy pregnancy are sparse. One study showed a significant reduction in functional protein S levels during pregnancy and the puerperium (Comp et al 1986). More recently, 14 patients followed longitudinally throughout gestation and postpartum showed a rise of protein C within the normal non-pregnant range during the second trimester. In contrast, free protein S fell from the second trimester onwards but remained within the confines of the normal range (Warwick et al 1989). Another study supported these findings and extended the study to women using oral contraceptives in whom similar changes were found (Malm et al 1988).

The investigation of natural anticoagulants has revealed a system of growing complexity (Alving & Comp 1992). The recent identification of a new protein C co-factor and

its inherited abnormality, activated protein C resistance (APCR), has been shown to be associated with venous thromboembolism in pregnant women in approximately 50% of cases (Hellgren et al, 1995). An understanding of the delicate balance between procoagulant and anticoagulant factors controlling healthy haemostasis (Salem 1986) will enable us to manage the complex hypercoagulable states in pregnancy successfully (Walker 1991).

Fibrinolysis

Fibrinolytic activity is an essential part of the dynamic interacting haemostatic mechanism, and is dependent on plasminogen activator in the blood (Fig. 23.2). Fibrin and fibrinogen are digested by plasmin, a proenzyme derived from an inactive plasma precursor plasminogen.

Increased amounts of activator are found in the plasma after strenuous exercise, emotional stress, surgical operations and other trauma. Tissue activator can be extracted from most human organs, with the exception of the placenta. Tissues especially rich in activator include the uterus, ovaries, prostate, heart, lungs, thyroid, adrenals and lymph nodes. Activity in tissues is concentrated mainly around blood vessels; veins show greater activity than arteries. Venous occlusion of the limbs will stimulate fibrinolytic activity, a fact which should be remembered if tourniquets are applied for any length of time before blood is drawn for measurement of fibrin degradation products.

The inhibitors of fibrinolytic activity are of two types— antiactivators (antiplasminogens) and the antiplasmins. Inhibitors of plasminogen include epsilon amino caproic acid (EACA) and tranexamic acid. Aprotinin (Trasylol) is another antiplasminogen which is commercially prepared from bovine lung.

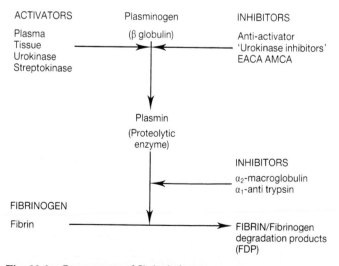

Fig. 23.2 Components of fibrinolytic system.

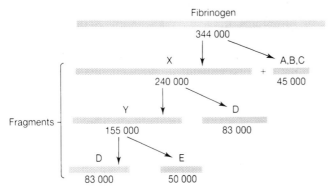

Fig. 23.3 Fibrin degradation products produced by degradation of fibrinogen by plasmin. Molecular weights are shown.

Platelets, plasma and serum exert a strong inhibitory action on plasmin. Normally plasma antiplasmin levels exceed levels of plasminogen and hence the levels of potential plasmin; otherwise we would dissolve away our connecting cement! When fibrinogen or fibrin is broken down by plasmin, fibrin degradation products are formed: these comprise the high molecular weight slip products X and Y, and smaller fragments A, B, C, D and E (Fig. 23.3). When a fibrin clot is formed 70% of fragment X is retained in the clot; Y, D and E are retained to a somewhat lesser extent. Therefore serum, even under normal circumstances, may contain small amounts of fragment X and larger amounts of Y, D and E. All of these components have antigenic determinants in common with fibrinogen and will be recognized by antifibrinogen antisera. It is important to be aware of this when examining blood for the presence of fibrin degradation products as confirmation of excess fibrinolytic activity (e.g. in DIC). Blood should be taken by clean venepuncture and the tourniquet should not be left on too long. The blood should be allowed to clot in the presence of an antifibrinolytic agent such as EACA to stop the process of fibrinolysis which would otherwise continue in vitro.

Plasma fibrinolytic activity is decreased during pregnancy, remains low during labour and delivery and returns to normal within 1 hour of delivery of the placenta (Bonnar et al 1970). This is thought to be due to the effect of plasminogen activator inhibitor type II (PA1-2) derived from the placenta which is present in abundance during pregnancy (Booth et al 1988). In addition the activity in the fibrinolytic system in response to stimulation has been found to be significantly reduced in pregnancy (Ballegeer et al 1987).

SUMMARY OF CHANGES IN HAEMOSTASIS IN PREGNANCY (LETSKY 1992)

The changes in the coagulation system in normal pregnancy are consistent with a continuing low-grade process of coagulant activity. Using electron microscopy, fibrin

deposition can be demonstrated in the intervillous space of the placenta and in the walls of the spiral arteries supplying the placenta (Sheppard & Bonnar 1974). As pregnancy advances, the elastic lamina and smooth muscle of these spiral arteries are replaced by a matrix containing fibrin. This allows expansion of the lumen to accommodate an increasing blood flow and reduces the vascular resistance of the placenta. At placental separation during normal childbirth, a blood flow of 500–800 ml/min has to be staunched within seconds, or serious haemorrhage will occur. Myometrial contraction plays a vital role in securing haemostasis by reducing the blood flow to the placental site. Rapid closure of the terminal part of the spiral artery will be further facilitated by the structural changes within the walls. The placental site is rapidly covered by a fibrin mesh following delivery. The increased levels of fibrinogen and other coagulation factors will be advantageous to meet the sudden demand of haemostasis components.

The changes also produce a vulnerable state for intravascular clotting (Letsky 1991a) and a whole spectrum of disorders involving coagulation occur in complications of pregnancy (Letsky 1985).

DISSEMINATED INTRAVASCULAR COAGULATION

The changes in the haemostatic system and the local activation of the clotting system during parturition carry with them a risk not only of thromboembolism (see Ch. 44) but also of DIC. This results in consumption of clotting factors and platelets, leading in some cases to severe, particularly uterine and sometimes generalized, bleeding Letsky (1987).

The first problem with DIC is in its definition. It is never primary, but always secondary to some general stimulation of coagulation activity by release of procoagulant substances into the blood (Fig. 23.4). Hypothetical triggers of this process in pregnancy include the leaking of placental tissue fragments, amniotic fluid, incompatible red cells or bacterial products into the maternal circulation. There is a great spectrum of manifestations of the process of DIC (Table 23.1), ranging from a compensated state with no clinical manifestation but evidence of increased production and breakdown of coagulation factors, to the condition we all fear of massive uncontrollable haemorrhage with very low concentrations of plasma fibrinogen, pathological raised levels of fibrin degradation products and variable degrees of thrombocytopenia.

Another confusing entity is that there appears to be a transitory state of intravascular coagulation during the whole of normal labour, maximal at the time of birth (Gilabert et al 1978, Stirling et al 1984, Wallmo et al 1984).

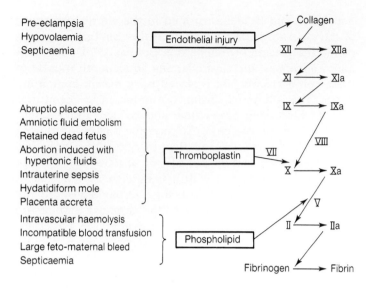

Fig. 23.4 Trigger mechanisms of disseminated intravascular coagulation during pregnancy. Interactions occur in many of these obstetric complications.

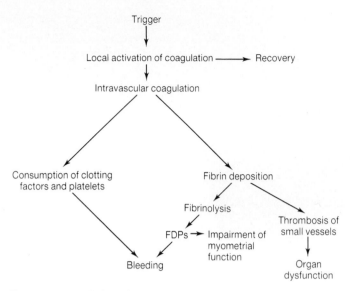

Fig. 23.5 Stimulation of coagulation activity and its possible consequences. FDPs = fibrin degradation products.

Fibrinolysis is stimulated by DIC, and the fibrin degradation products resulting from the process interfere with the formation of firm fibrin clots. Thus a vicious circle is established, resulting in further disastrous bleeding (Fig. 23.5). Fibrin degradation products also interfere with myometrial function and possibly cardiac function and therefore in themselves aggravate both haemorrhage and shock.

Obstetric conditions classically associated with DIC include abruptio placentae, amniotic fluid embolism, septic abortion and intrauterine infection, retained dead fetus, hydatidiform mole, placenta accreta, pre-eclampsia and eclampsia and prolonged shock from any cause (see Fig. 23.4).

Despite the advances in obstetric care and highly developed blood transfusion services, haemorrhage still constitutes a major factor in maternal mortality and morbidity.

The most recent Confidential Enquiries into Maternal Mortality (Department of Health 1994) reports that deaths due to haemorrhage have doubled, making this one of the three leading causes of maternal deaths for the first time during recent years. No one person or unit is likely to see enough cases to randomize patients into groups in which the numbers would achieve statistical significance to assess therapeutic measures. Also the complex and variable nature of the conditions associated with DIC, which are often self-correcting and treated with a variety of strategies, make it impossible to make an objective assessment of the published reports.

HAEMATOLOGICAL MANAGEMENT OF THE BLEEDING OBSTETRIC PATIENT

The management of the bleeding obstetric patient is an acute and frightening problem. There is little time to think

Table 23.1   Spectrum of severity of DIC: its relationship to specific complications in obstetrics

	Severity of DIC	In vitro findings	Obstetric condition commonly associated
Stage 1	Low-grade compensated	FDPs ↑ Increased soluble fibrin complexes Increased ratio $\dfrac{vWF^\star}{factor\ VIIIC}$	Pre-eclampsia Retained dead fetus
Stage 2	Uncompensated but no haemostatic failure	As above, plus fibrinogen ↓ platelets ↓ factors V and VIII ↓	 Small abruptio Severe pre-eclampsia
Stage 3	Rampant with haemostatic failure	Platelets ↓↓ Gross depletion of coagulation factors, particularly fibrinogen FDPs ↑	Abruption placentae Amniotic fluid embolism Eclampsia

Rapid progression from stage 1 to stage 3 is possible unless appropriate action is taken.
★ von Willebrand factor.

and there must be in every unit a planned practice decided on by haematologist, physician, anaesthetist, obstetrician and nursing staff to deal with this situation whenever it arises. This should be read by all junior staff and attention should be drawn to it frequently, for when the emergency occurs there is little time for leisurely perusal. Good reliable communication between the various clinicians, nursing, paramedical and laboratory staff is essential.

It is imperative that the source of bleeding, often an unsuspected uterine or genital laceration, should be located and dealt with. Prolonged hypovolaemic shock, or indeed shock from any cause, may also trigger off DIC and this may lead to haemostatic failure and further prolonged haemorrhage.

The management of haemorrhage is virtually the same whether the bleeding is caused or augmented by coagulation failure or not (Letsky 1992). The clinical condition usually demands urgent treatment and there is no time to wait for results of coagulation factor assays or sophisticated tests of the fibrinolytic system activity for precise definition of the extent of haemostatic failure, although blood can be taken for this purpose and analysed at leisure once the emergency is over.

Simple rapid tests, recommended below, will establish the competence or otherwise of the haemostatic system. In the vast majority of obstetric patients, coagulation failure results from a sudden transitory episode of DIC triggered by a variety of conditions (Fig. 23.4).

As soon as there is any concern about a patient bleeding from any cause, venous blood should be taken and delivered into a set of bottles kept in an emergency pack with a set of laboratory request forms previously made out which only require the patient's name and identification number added to them.

In order to avoid testing artefacts it is essential that the blood is obtained by a quick, efficient non-traumatic technique. Thromboplastin release from damaged tissues may contaminate the specimen and alter the results. This is likely to occur if difficulty is encountered in finding the vein, if the vein is only partly canalized and the flow is slow, or if there is excessive squeezing of tissues and repeated attempts to obtain a specimen with the same needle. In such circumstances the specimen may clot in the tube in spite of the presence of anticoagulant, or the coagulation times of the various tests will be altered and not reflect the true situation in vivo. The platelets may aggregate in clumps and give a falsely low count, be it automated or manual.

Heparin characteristically prolongs the partial thromboplastin time and thrombin time out of proportion to the prothrombin time. As little as 0.05 units of heparin per ml will prolong the coagulation test times. It is customary, though not desirable, to take blood for coagulation tests from lines which have been washed through with fluids containing heparin to keep them patent. It is almost impossible to overcome the effect on the blood passing through such a line, however much blood is taken and discarded before obtaining a sample for investigation. It is strongly recommended that blood is taken from another site not previously contaminated with heparin.

Any blood taken into a glass tube without anticoagulant will clot within a few minutes and natural fibrinolysis will continue in vitro. Unless the blood is taken into a fibrinolytic inhibitor such as EACA, a falsely high level of fibrin in degradation products will be found which bears no relationship to fibrinolysis in vivo. Similarly, leaving a tourniquet on too long before taking the specimen will stimulate local fibrinolytic activity in vivo.

Useful rapid screening tests for haemostatic failure include the platelet count, partial thromboplastin time or accelerated whole-blood clotting time (which tests intrinsic coagulation), prothrombin time (which tests extrinsic coagulation), thrombin time and estimation of fibrinogen (Fig. 23.6).

The measurement of the products of plasmin digestion of fibrinogen or fibrin provides an indirect test for fibrinolysis. Fibrin degradation products can be detected in several ways. They interfere with the production of fibrinogen by thrombin and will prolong the thrombin time. The most sensitive methods are immunological.

In practice the most rapid assessment of fibrin degradation products in the circulation is to add particles coated with fibrinogen antibody (raised in rabbits) to dilutions of the patient's serum taken into EACA to prevent in vitro fibrinolysis. In obstetric practice the measurement of fibrin degradation products is usually part of the investigation of suspected acute or chronic DIC. In the

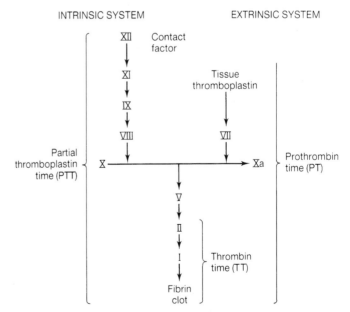

Fig. 23.6 In vitro screening tests of coagulation competence and their relationship to the systems involved.

acute situation raised fibrin degradation products only confirm the presence of DIC, but are not diagnostic and once the specimen is taken the laboratory measurement should be delayed until after the emergency is over, so that skilled laboratory workers can be performing a much more valuable service in providing results of coagulation screening tests and blood and blood products suitable for transfusion. Of the tests of coagulation, probably the thrombin time, an estimation of the thrombin clottable fibrinogen in a citrated sample of plasma, is the most valuable overall rapid screen of haemostatic competence of coagulation factors. The thrombin time of normal plasma is adjusted in the laboratory to 10–15 seconds, and the fibrin clot formed is firm and stable. In the most severe forms of DIC there is no clottable fibrinogen in the sample, and no fibrin clot appears even after 2–3 minutes. Indication of severe DIC is obtained usually by a prolonged thrombin time with a friable clot which may dissolve on standing owing to fibrinolytic substances present in the plasma.

Prolongation of the thrombin time is observed not only with depleted fibrinogen but in conditions where fibrin degradation products are increased, and even traces of heparin will significantly prolong the time it takes for a clot to be formed.

There is no point whatsoever in the obstetrician, anaesthetist or nursing staff wasting time trying to perform bedside whole-blood clotting tests. Whole-blood clotting normally takes up to 7 minutes and should be performed in clean tubes in a 37°C water bath with suitable controls. It furnishes little information of practical value and only creates more panic. The valuable hands at the bedside are of more use doing the things they are trained to do in this emergency situation rather than wasting time performing a test which is time-consuming, of little value or significance unless performed under strict control conditions, and which will not contribute anything to management. The alerted laboratory worker will be able to provide significant results within half an hour at the most of receiving the specimen in the laboratory.

The tests referred to above are straightforward and should be available from any routine haematology laboratory. It is not necessary to have a high-powered coagulation laboratory to perform these simple screening tests to confirm or refute a diagnosis of DIC.

Treatment of severe haemorrhage must include prompt and adequate fluid replacement in order to avoid renal shut-down. If effective circulation is restored without too much delay, fibrin degradation products will be cleared from the blood mainly by the liver, which will further aid restoration of normal haemostasis. This is an aspect of management which is often not appropriately emphasized.

Plasma substitutes

There is much controversy about which plasma substitute to give to any bleeding patient. The remarks which follow are very much slanted towards the supportive laboratory management of acute haemorrhage from the placental site and should not be taken to apply to those situations in which hypovolaemia may be associated with severe hypoproteinaemia, such as occurs in septic peritonitis, burns and bowel infarction. The choice lies between simple crystalloids, such as Hartmann's solution or Ringer's lactate, and artificial colloids, such as dextran, hydroxyethyl starch and gelatin solution or the very expensive preparations of human albumin (albuminoids). If crystalloids are used, two or three times the volume of estimated blood loss should be administered because the crystalloid remains in the vascular compartment for a shorter time than colloids if renal function is maintained.

The infusion of plasma substitutes, i.e. plasma protein, dextran, gelatin and starch solutions, may result in adverse reactions. Although the incidence of severe reactions is rare, they are diverse in nature, varying from allergic urticarial manifestations and mild fever to life-threatening anaphylactic reactions due to spasm of smooth muscle, with cardiac and respiratory arrest (Doenicke et al 1977).

Dextrans adversely affect platelet function, may cause pseudoagglutination and interfere with interpretation of subsequent blood grouping and cross-matching tests. They are, therefore, contraindicated in the woman who is bleeding due to a complication associated with pregnancy where there is a high chance of there being a serious haemostatic defect already. Dextrans are also associated with allergic anaphylactoid reactions. The anaphylactoid reactions accompanying infusion of dextrans are probably related to IgG and IgM antidextran antibodies (Richter & Hedin 1982) which are found in high concentrations in all patients with severe reactions.

Albuminoids are thought to be associated less with anaphylactoid reactions but they may be particularly harmful when transfused in the shocked patient by contributing to renal and pulmonary failure, adversely affecting cardiac function and further impairing haemostasis (Cash 1987).

Many studies have suggested that the best way to deal with hypovolaemic shock initially is by transfusing simple balanced salt solutions (crystalloid) followed by red cells and fresh frozen plasma (Carey et al 1970, Moss 1972, Virgilio et al 1979). More recent work (Hauser et al 1980) has challenged this approach and suggests that albumin-containing solutions are superior to crystalloids for volume replacement in postoperative shocked patients with respiratory insufficiency. This aspect of management of shocked patients with blood loss will remain controversial pending the results of further clinical trials.

In many hospitals nowadays, the derivatives of gelatin (Haemaccel or Gelofusine) are the first-line fluids in resuscitation. They have a shelf-life of 8 years and can be stored at room temperature. They are iso-oncotic and do not interfere with platelet function or subsequent blood grouping or cross-matching. Renal function is improved when they are administered in hypovolaemic shock. They are generally considered to be non-immunogenic and do not trigger the production of antibodies in man, even on repeated challenge. The reactions which occur related to Haemaccel infusion are thought to be due to histamine release (Lorenz et al 1976), the incidence and severity of reactions being proportional to the extent of histamine release. There have been a few rare reports of severe reactions with bronchospasm and circulatory collapse and there has been one report of a fatality (Freeman 1979). Nevertheless, whatever substitute is used it is only a stopgap until suitable blood component therapy can be administered.

The use of whole blood and component therapy

Whole blood may be the treatment of choice in coagulation failure associated with obstetric disorders (Phillips 1984), but whole fresh blood is not generally available in the UK nowadays, because there is insufficient time to complete hepatitis surface antigen, human immunodeficiency virus antibody and blood grouping tests before it is released from the transfusion centre. To release it earlier than the usual 18–24 hours would increase the risk of transmitting viral B hepatitis, human immunodeficiency virus (HIV) and acquired immune deficiency syndrome (AIDS). Serologically incompatible transfusions, syphilis, cytomegalovirus and Epstein–Barr virus are examples of other infections which may be transmitted in fresh blood. Their viability diminishes rapidly on storage at 4°C. These infections, particularly in immunosuppressed or pregnant patients, can be particularly hazardous. Apart from the hazards of giving whole blood which is less than say 6–24 hours old, its use in the UK today represents a serious waste of vitally needed components required for patients with specific isolated deficiencies (Letsky 1992). The use of fresh frozen plasma followed by bank red cells provides all the components, apart from platelets, which are present in whole fresh blood and allows the plasma from the freshly donated unit to be used to make the much needed blood components.

Plasma component therapy

Fresh frozen plasma (FFP) contains all the coagulation factors present in plasma obtained from whole blood within 6 hours of donation. Frozen rapidly and stored at −30°C, the factors are well preserved for at least 1 year. Plasma stored at −20°C does degenerate and should be used within 6 months of preparation.

Plasma Protein fraction (albumin) does not contain coagulation factors but does not carry the risk of transmitting infection. It can be of value in providing colloid in the management of haemorrhage. Concentrated fibrinogen which does not contain the labile clotting factors

V and VIII is no longer available and carried the hazard of transmitting infection. Moreover its use in the past was noted to result in a sharp fall of AT III—suggesting that the concentrate may aggravate intravascular coagulation by adding fuel to the fire.

Although cryoprecipitate is richer in fibrinogen than FFP it lacks AT III which is rapidly consumed in obstetric bleeding associated with DIC. The use of cryoprecipitate also exposes the recipient to more donors and the potential associated hazards.

Platelets, an essential haemostatic component, are not present in FFP and their functional activity rapidly deteriorates in stored blood. The platelet count reflects both the degree of intravascular coagulation and the amount of bank blood transfused. A patient with persistent bleeding and a very low platelet count (less than 20×10^9/l) may be given concentrated platelets, although they are seldom required in addition to FFP to achieve haemostasis. Indeed it has been suggested that platelet transfusions are more likely to do harm than good in this situation since most concentrates contain some damaged platelets which might in themselves provide a fresh trigger or mediator of DIC in the existing state (Sharp 1977). A spontaneous recovery from the coagulation defect is to be expected once the uterus is empty and well contracted, provided that blood volume is maintained by adequate replacement monitored by central venous pressure and urinary output.

Problems arise when bleeding is difficult to control and the woman has a low haemoglobin before blood loss, but this is unusual at term in a well managed obstetric patient.

Red cell transfusion

Cross-matched blood should be available within 40 minutes of the maternal specimen reaching the laboratory. If the woman has had normal antenatal care and carries her cooperation card her blood group will be known. There is a good case for giving uncross-matched blood of her group should the situation warrant it, provided that blood has been properly processed at the transfusion centre. If the blood group is unknown, uncross-matched group O rhesus-negative blood may be given if necessary. By this time laboratory screening tests of haemostatic function should be available. If these prove to be normal, but vaginal bleeding continues, the cause is nearly always trauma or bleeding from the placental site due to failure of the myometrium to contract. It is imperative that the source of bleeding, often an unsuspected uterine or genital laceration, should be located and dealt with. Prolonged hypovolaemic shock or indeed shock from any cause may also trigger DIC and this may lead to haemostatic failure and further prolonged haemorrhage.

Stored whole blood, even under optimal conditions, undergoes certain deleterious changes. The oxygen affinity of red cells increases. Plasma ionic concentrations of potassium and hydrogen increase but these changes are not significant until after 4 days of shelf-life. Platelets deteriorate rapidly within the first 24 hours and after 72 hours they have lost all haemostatic function.

The activity of the labile coagulation factors V and particularly factor VIII decrease within the first 24 hours of donation. After 6 days' storage microaggregates of platelets, white cells and fibrin form.

If the blood loss is replaced only by stored bank blood which is deficient in the labile clotting factors V and VIII and platelets, then the circulation will rapidly become depleted in these essential components of haemostasis even if there is no DIC initially as the cause of haemorrhage. It is advisable to transfuse 1 unit of fresh frozen plasma for every 4–6 units of bank red cells administered.

SAG-M blood

The concept of removing all the plasma from a unit of blood and replacing it with a crystalloid solution has now become routine procedure in the UK in many regional blood transfusion centres so that maximum use of a donated unit can be made.

The process involves centrifuging the anticoagulated unit of whole blood, removing all the plasma and resuspending the packed red cells in 100 ml of sodium chloride, adenine, glucose and mannitol—so-called SAG-M. The resulting unit of packed red cells has better flow properties than plasma-reduced blood and is very suitable for top-up transfusion, but contains practically no protein and no coagulation factors whatsoever. It is not ideal to transfuse in an obstetric emergency or any situations of massive rapid blood loss, but if this is all that is available on site at the time, then the following guidelines should be followed.

The regional transfusion centres do not recommend the use of any more than 4 units of SAG-M blood, but in an emergency after the first 4 units of SAG-M red cells, 1 unit of albumin should be given for every 2 units of SAG-M blood in order to maintain plasma oncotic pressure. FFP should be considered after 8 units of SAG-M red cells have been transfused. In an obstetric emergency FFP should have been administered long before this. Most hospital blood banks are now provided almost exclusively with red cells suspended in SAG-M. Whole blood or plasma-reduced red cells are always available on request to the regional transfusion centre.

It seems sensible in any event, whatever the cause of bleeding, to change the initial plasma substitute and transfuse 2 units of FFP once it has thawed, while waiting for compatible blood to be available.

A spontaneous recovery from the coagulation defect is to be expected once the uterus is empty and well contracted, provided that blood volume is maintained by adequate replacement monitored by central venous pressure and urinary output.

Clinicians may be helped in the decision of which replacement fluid to give in an obstetric emergency with the knowledge that very few bleeding patients die from lack of circulating red cells, the oxygen-carrying moiety of the blood. Death in the majority of cases results from hypovolaemia leading to poor tissue perfusion. Every effort should be made to maintain a normal blood volume and restoration of red cell mass can be delayed until suitable compatibility tests have been performed and bleeding is at least partially controlled (Marshall & Bird 1983).

The single most important component of haemostasis at delivery in normal circumstances is contraction of the myometrium stemming the flow from the placental site. All the clotting factors and platelets in the world will not stop haemorrhage if the uterus remains flabby. Vaginal delivery will make less severe demand on the haemostatic mechanism than delivery by Caesarean section which requires the same haemostatic competence as any other major surgical procedure. Should DIC be established with the fetus in utero, rather than to embark on heroic surgical delivery, it is better to wait for spontaneous delivery if possible, or to stimulate vaginal delivery, avoiding soft-tissue damage.

DISSEMINATED INTRAVASCULAR COAGULATION IN CLINICAL CONDITIONS

In vitro detection of low-grade disseminated intravascular coagulation

Rampant uncompensated DIC results in severe haemorrhage with characteristic findings in vitro dealt with above. However, low-grade DIC does not usually give rise to any clinical manifestations although the condition is potentially hazardous for both mother and fetus.

Many in vitro tests have been claimed to detect low-grade compensated DIC and space does not allow an account of all of these.

Fibrin degradation products

Estimation of fibrin degradation products will give some indication of low-grade DIC if these are significantly raised when fibrinogen, platelets and screening tests of haemostatic function appear to be within the normal range.

Soluble fibrin complexes

The action of thrombin on fibrinogen is crucial in DIC. Thrombin splits two molecules of fibrinopeptide A and two molecules of fibrinopeptide B from fibrinogen. The remaining molecule is called a fibrin monomer and polymerizes rapidly to fibrin (Fig. 23.3). Free fibrinopeptides

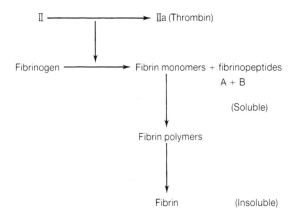

Fig. 23.7   Generation of soluble complexes during the conversion of fibrinogen to insoluble fibrin.

in the blood are a specific measure of thrombin activity and high levels of fibrinopeptide A have been shown to be associated with compensated DIC in pregnancy (Wallmo et al 1984).

Soluble fibrin complexes made up of fibrin–fibrinogen dimers are increased in conditions of low-grade DIC (Aznar et al 1982). These complexes are generated during the process of thrombin generation and the conversion of soluble fibrinogen to insoluble fibrin (Fig. 23.7). Levels of soluble fibrin complexes are increased in patients with severe pre-eclampsia and with a retained dead fetus (Hafter & Graeff 1975).

Factor VIII

During normal pregnancy the levels of both von Willebrand Factor (vWF) and factor VIII coagulation activity (VIII:C) rise in parallel (Whigham et al 1979, Fournie et al 1981). An increase in the ratio of vWF to factor VIII:C has been observed in conditions accompanied by low-grade DIC whether associated with pregnancy or not. An increase in the ratio has been observed in pregnancy with a retained dead fetus and with pre-eclampsia (Caires et al 1984) without any alteration in the simple screening tests of haemostatic function previously described.

The stages in the spectrum of severity of DIC (see Table 23.1) are not strictly delineated and there may be rapid progression from low-grade compensated DIC as diagnosed by paracoagulation tests described above, to the rampant form with haemostatic failure.

There now follows an account of the obstetric conditions most commonly associated with DIC, the past rationale for specific measures as well as those being used at present to manage haemostatic failure optimally.

Abruptio placentae

Premature separation of the placenta or abruptio placentae is a well-known cause of coagulation failure in most obstetric units. Many of the problems which confront the attendant in this situation are common to other conditions associated with DIC in pregnancy, therefore this will be used as the central focus of discussion of some of the controversial methods of management.

Abruptio placentae may occur in apparently healthy women with no clinical warning or may be in association with established pre-eclampsia. It is possible that clinically silent placental infarcts may predispose to placental separation by causing low-grade abnormalities of the haemostatic system such as increased factor VIII consumption and raised fibrin degradation products (Redman 1979).

There is a great spectrum in the severity of the haemostatic failure in this condition (Gilabert et al 1985) which appears to be related to the degree of placental separation. Only 10% of patients overall with abruptio placentae show significant coagulation abnormalities (Naumann & Weinstein 1985). In some cases of a small abruptio, there is a minor degree of failure of haemostatic processes and the fetus does not succumb (Table 23.1). When the uterus is tense and tender and no fetal heart can be heard, the separation and retroplacental bleeding are extensive. No guide to the severity of the haemorrhage or coagulation failure will be given by the amount of vaginal bleeding. Often there is no external vaginal blood loss, even when the placenta is completely separated, the fetus is dead, the circulating blood is incoagulable and there is up to 5 litres of concealed blood loss resulting in hypovolaemic shock.

Haemostatic failure may be suspected if there is persistent oozing at the site of venepuncture or bleeding from the mucous membranes of the mouth or nose. Simple rapid screening tests will confirm the presence of DIC. There will be a low platelet count, greatly prolonged thrombin time, low fibrinogen and raised fibrin degradation products, due to secondary fibrinolysis stimulated by the intravascular deposition of fibrin (Estelles et al 1980). The mainstay of treatment is to maintain the circulating blood volume. This not only prevents renal shutdown and further haemostatic failure caused by hypovolaemic shock, but helps clearance of fibrin degradation products which in themselves act as potent anticoagulants. It has also been suggested that fibrin degradation products inhibit myometrial activity; serious postpartum haemorrhage in women with abruptio placentae was found to be associated with high levels of fibrin degradation products (Basu 1969, Sher 1977). High levels of fibrin degradation products may also have a cardiotoxic effect.

If the fetus is dead the aim should be prompt vaginal delivery avoiding soft-tissue damage. Once correction of hypovolaemia is underway, measures to speed up delivery should be instituted. Amniotomy, or if this fails, prostaglandin or oxytocin stimulation can be used. There is no evidence that the use of oxytocic agents aggravates thromboplastin release from the uterus (Bonnar 1978).

Following emptying of the uterus, myometrial contraction will greatly reduce bleeding from the placental site and spontaneous correction of the haemostatic defect usually occurs shortly after delivery if the measures recommended above have been taken. However, postpartum haemorrhage is a frequent complication and is the commonest cause of death in abruptio placentae (Department of Health 1991).

In cases where the abruptio is small and the fetus is still alive, prompt Caesarean section may save the baby if vaginal delivery is not imminent. FFP, bank red cells and platelet concentrates should be available to correct the potentially severe coagulation defect in the maternal circulation.

In rare situations where vaginal delivery cannot be stimulated and haemorrhage continues. Caesarean section may be indicated even in the presence of a dead fetus.

Despite extravasation of blood throughout the uterine muscle its function is not impaired and good contraction will follow removal of fetus, placenta and retroperitoneal clot. Hysterectomy should be avoided as delayed internal bleeding may occur. Regional anaesthesia or analgesia is contraindicated. Expansion of the lower limb vascular bed resulting from regional block can add to the problem of uncorrected hypovolaemia, plus in the presence of haemostatic failure there is the additional hazard of bleeding into the epidural space (Bonnar 1981).

In recent years, heparin has been used to treat all kinds of DIC, whatever their cause. There is, however, no objective evidence to demonstrate that its use in abruptio placentae has decreased morbidity and mortality, although anecdotal reports continue to suggest this (Thragarajah et al 1981). Very good results have been achieved without the use of heparin (Pritchard 1973). Its use, with an intact circulation, would be sensible and logical to break the vicious circle of DIC, but in the presence of already defective haemostasis with a large bleeding placental site, it may prolong massive local and generalized haemorrhage (Feinstein 1982).

Treatment with an antifibrinolytic agent such as tranexamic acid (Cyclokapron) or Trasylol can result in blockage with fibrin of small vessels in vital organs such as the kidney or brain. It is therefore contraindicated, although Bonnar (1981) suggests that delayed severe and prolonged haemorrhage from the placental site several hours post-delivery may respond to antifibrinolytic therapy if all other measures fail.

It has been suggested (Sher 1977, Sher & Statland 1985) that aprotinin (Trasylol) may be helpful in the management of abruptio placentae, particularly in those cases with uterine inertia associated with high levels of fibrin degradation products. There is a high incidence (1.5%) of abruptio placentae in the obstetric admissions (18 000 per annum) at the Groote Scheur Obstetric Unit, Cape Town, South Africa, where the first study was carried out.

There has been a resurgence of usage of Trasylol recently, particularly in cardiac surgery (Bidstrup et al 1989) where significant reduction in blood loss has been shown following cardiac bypass operations. This is thought to be due predominantly to platelet sparing. It is doubtful whether Trasylol would have any advantage in management of obstetric DIC. In recent years, obstetricians appear unconvinced of the benefits of Trasylol in the treatment of DIC and abruptio placentae, judging by many published reports.

Prompt supportive measures alone, maintaining central venous pressure and replacing blood loss together with essential coagulation factors, will of course result in reduction in fibrin degradation products. This will improve myometrial function and contribute to the return of healthy haemostasis.

One patient with recurrent abruptio placentae successfully treated with the fibrinolytic inhibitor tranexamic acid has been reported (Astedt & Nilsson 1978). Investigations in this woman suggested abnormally increased fibrinolytic activity in the 26th week of her third pregnancy. The previous two pregnancies had been complicated by abruptio placentae associated with a neonatal death and a stillbirth respectively. The intravenous administration of tranexamic acid following a small vaginal bleed resulted in restoration of normal coagulation status and the bleeding stopped; oral administration was continued. Another small bleed occurred at 33 weeks' gestation, treated again with intravenous tranexamic acid. The eventual successful outcome of this pregnancy was attributed by the authors to the use of this agent but many other variables may have been involved. A recent report on reducing the frequency of severe abruptio placentae from Dallas, Texas (Pritchard et al 1991) noted that the reduction in *fetal* death associated with abruptio by 50% over a period covering more than 30 years (1958–90) could be accounted for by the decrease in women of very high parity and an increase in the proportion of Latin-American as opposed to black women in the population served. Abruptio placentae in the latter part of the study recurred in 12% of subsequent pregnancies and proved fatal to the fetus in 7%, which was unchanged from earlier experience. With modern supportive measures, maternal death due directly to abruptio placentae is now extremely rare.

Amniotic fluid embolism

Amniotic fluid embolism is very rare but one of the most dangerous and untreatable conditions in obstetrics. The incidence has been estimated as between one in 8000 and one in 80 000 in various reports (Morgan 1979) but the latter figure is probably nearer the true incidence.

During the triennium 1979–81 in England and Wales, 18 histologically confirmed and six suspected fatal cases occurred associated with 1 942 859 maternities. This gives an incidence of fatal amniotic fluid embolism of approximately one in 81 000 (Department of Health and Social Security 1986). The maternal mortality is very high—over 80% in most reports. An excellent review of 272 cases in the English literature reported that only 39 survived, giving a mortality rate of 86% (Morgan 1979). Amniotic fluid embolism is the most common cause of death in the immediate postpartum period (Herbert 1982).

Amniotic fluid embolism is said to occur most frequently in elderly multiparous patients with large babies at or near term following a short tumultuous labour associated with the use of uterine stimulants. However, the review quoted (Morgan 1979) did not substantiate this statement. Reports on Confidential Enquiries into Maternal Deaths (Department of Health 1991) confirmed that there were higher rates of mortality at older ages and higher parity but the relationship between violent contractions and rapid labour was less apparent.

There have been some reports of this complication of pregnancy occurring in different situations: in young primiparous women (Morgan 1979), during the second trimester (Meier & Bowes 1983), in women undergoing legally induced terminations (Guidotti et al 1981), after evacuation of a missed abortion (Stromme & Fromke 1979) and even after deliberate termination of pregnancy (Cates et al 1981).

The passage of amniotic fluid into the maternal circulation is thought to occur through the endocervical veins, the normal placental site, through uterine trauma at Caesarean section or if the uterus ruptures. Torn fetal membranes is a prerequisite of amniotic fluid embolism. Lethal amniotic fluid embolism is most commonly associated with small tears in the uterus, cervix or vagina which have not totally disrupted the wall (Rushton & Dawson 1982). This is not surprising since a complete tear would allow amniotic fluid to escape into the peritoneal cavity or the vagina.

The clinical features associated with amniotic fluid embolism are respiratory distress, cyanosis, cardiovascular collapse, haemorrhage and coma. Although coagulation failure occurs rapidly the presenting clinical feature is sudden extreme shock with cyanosis due to an almost complete shut-down of the pulmonary circulation, followed by the onset of intractable uterine bleeding. The coagulation abnormalities are ascribed to the thromboplastic activity of amniotic fluid (Courtney & Allington 1972, Yaffe et al 1977). Massive intravascular coagulation occurs and consumption of the clotting factors can be almost total (Bonnar 1981). Platelet fibrin thrombi are formed and trapped within the pulmonary blood vessels.

Profound shock follows, accompanied by respiratory distress and cyanosis. There is a high mortality at this stage from a combination of respiratory and cardiac failure; if the mother survives long enough the effect of massive intravascular coagulation will invariably follow with bleeding from venepuncture sites and severe haemorrhage from the placental site after delivery (Gregory & Clayton 1973).

Confirmation of diagnosis in the past could only be made at autopsy by finding histological evidence of amniotic fluid and fetal tissue within the substance of the maternal lungs, with or without identification of the portal of entry in the placenta or uterine wall (Rushton & Dawson 1982). It is therefore difficult to assess the value of therapeutic measures suggested in the few reports which have appeared of successful management of a clinical syndrome diagnosed clinically as amniotic fluid embolism (Skjodt 1965, Bonnar 1973, Chung & Merkatz 1973, Resnik et al 1976).

More recent techniques of diagnosis include detection of squamous cells and lanugo hair on cytological examination of blood aspirated through a Swan–Ganz catheter and detection of squamous cells in maternal sputum (Herbert 1982). Dolyniuk & colleagues (1983) describe a case in which the diagnosis of amniotic fluid embolism was made using these techniques and the patient survived. In a 19-year-old primigravida acute respiratory failure developed following Caesarean section; fragments of vernix caseosa were identified in a pulmonary artery blood sample obtained through a Swan–Ganz catheter. The patient received intensive supportive care and recovered completely. However, fetal tissue has been found in pulmonary arterial blood in some women who had not suffered amniotic fluid embolism (Clark et al 1986). Therefore this finding should not be considered pathognomonic for amniotic fluid embolism.

The management of cardiorespiratory failure associated with amniotic fluid embolism must be carefully planned. This condition is similar to pulmonary embolism but there is also profound haemorrhage; too rigorous attempts at maintenance of the circulation, as recommended above for other conditions associated with DIC, may result in cardiac failure. There should be careful monitoring of the central venous pressure to avoid cardiac overload; the object is to sustain the circulation while the intravascular thrombin in the lungs is cleared by the naturally stimulated intense fibrinolytic response of the endothelium of the pulmonary vessels.

Measures to stimulate uterine contraction to reduce blood loss from the placental site are important in maintaining the blood volume. If bleeding from the placental site can be controlled by stimulation of uterine contraction then the logical treatment is carefully monitored transfusion of FFP and packed red cells, with heparin administration and, if indicated, positive pressure ventilation (Bonnar 1981). It is obviously essential that a competent intensive care unit should be immediately available for any obstetric service to deal promptly with this rare but often lethal complication of pregnancy.

Retention of dead fetus

The question of intrauterine fetal death and haemostatic failure has been reviewed by Romero et al (1985). There is a gradual depletion of maternal coagulation factors following intrauterine fetal death and the changes are not usually detectable in vitro until after 3–4 weeks (Hodgkinson et al 1964). Thromboplastic substances released from the dead tissues in the uterus into the maternal circulation are thought to be the trigger of DIC in this situation, which occurs in about one-third of patients who retain the dead fetus for more than 4–5 weeks (Pritchard 1959). There is depletion of fibrinogen, factor VIII and platelets, together with elevation of fibrin degradation products. Gross increase of soluble fibrin–fibrinogen complexes amounting to 25% of the total fibrinogen in association with a dead fetus has been described (Hafter & Graeff 1975). Around 80% of pregnant women will go into spontaneous labour within 3 weeks of intrauterine fetal death. Problems arising from defective haemostasis are much less common with this situation in modern obstetric practice because labour is induced promptly following diagnosis of fetal death before clinically significant coagulation changes have developed.

Rupture of the membranes is recommended once induced labour is established in such patients, as there is a risk of precipitate labour and amniotic fluid embolism has been known to occur (Bonnar 1978).

If the screening tests previously described indicate that there is defective haemostasis the coagulation factors should be restored to normal before delivery is attempted. Where the circulation is intact heparin is the logical treatment to interrupt the activation of the coagulation systems. Intravenous infusion of 1000 iu heparin hourly for up to 48 hours is usually sufficient to restore the number of platelets and the levels of fibrinogen and factors V and VIII to normal (Bonnar 1978). The heparin should then be discontinued and onset of labour stimulated. There should be a plentiful supply of compatible red cells and FFP prepared to treat any haemorrhage at placental separation promptly. If the patient goes into spontaneous labour while heparin is being administered the infusion should be stopped. It is not necessary to neutralize the heparin with protamine sulphate unless the patient is bleeding. There is no rational basis for the use of fibrinolytic inhibitors in the management of the patient with coagulation failure associated with a retained dead fetus. The increased fibrinolytic activity is secondary to DIC and the defective haemostasis will be corrected by the powerful anticoagulant effect of heparin in the presence of an intact circulation before the onset of labour.

Retained dead fetus and living twin

The occurrence of single fetal death in a preterm multiple pregnancy poses unique therapeutic dilemmas. Prolongation of the pregnancy could result in life-threatening maternal haemostatic failure. Termination of the pregnancy for maternal indications would result in the birth of an immature infant. The incidence of this problem is unknown but is likely to be observed more frequently with the advent of widespread use of ultrasound in obstetrics. In addition, on occasion selective termination of the life of the affected twin is being offered in situations where only one fetus has been shown to be affected with a genetic disorder.

A report of the successful prolongation of pregnancy with the spontaneous death in utero of one of the twins at 26 weeks' gestation has been published by Romero et al (1986). The patient was treated with intravenous heparin and the reversal of the consumption coagulopathy resulted in the uneventful prolongation of pregnancy for 8 weeks, by which time the fetus had achieved lung maturity.

Abortion

Changes in haemostatic components consistent with DIC have been demonstrated in patients undergoing abortion induced with hypertonic solutions of saline and urea (Stander et al 1971, Spivak et al 1972, Van Royen 1974, MacKenzie et al 1975, Grundy & Craven 1976).

The stimulus appears to be the release of tissue factor into the maternal circulation from the placenta which is damaged by the hypertonic solutions. DIC has been described in association with late dilatation and evacuation procedures (Davis 1972), and also in association with prostaglandin and oxytocin methods (Savage 1982).

The risk of DIC was increased five times in women receiving oxytocin while undergoing induced saline abortions (Cohen & Ballard 1974), but in another study the risk of DIC in women given urea plus prostaglandin or oxytocin was only one-quarter of that for women receiving saline alone (Burkman et al 1977). The resulting haemorrhage may be massive and has resulted in maternal deaths. Prompt restoration of blood volume and transfusions with red cells and FFP as described above should resolve the situation which, once the uterus is empty, is self-limiting.

A unique case of DIC associated with chronic ectopic pregnancy has been reported (Collier & Birrell 1983).

Intrauterine infection

The interactions of sepsis and coagulation in obstetrics have been reviewed by Beller (1985).

Endotoxic shock associated with septic abortion, antepartum or postpartum intrauterine infection can trigger DIC in pregnancy and the puerperium (Steichele & Herschlein 1968, Graeff et al 1978). Infections with Gram-negative micro-organisms is the usual finding. Fibrin is deposited in the microvasculature owing to endothelial damage by the endotoxin, and secondary red cell intravascular haemolysis with characteristic fragmentation, so-called microangiopathic haemolysis, is characteristic of the condition.

The patient is usually alert and flushed with a rapid pulse and low blood pressure. Transfusion, unlike in other obstetric emergencies complicated by DIC, has little or no effect on the hypotension. Some few centres in Europe have used heparinization in the management of septic abortion and have claimed a decrease in mortality (Bonnar 1978). In the situation where the uterus is empty and contracted and there is no undue risk of severe bleeding from the placental site with evidence of a consumptive coagulopathy, heparin may be useful as part of the management of this hazardous emergency (Clarkson et al 1969).

Elimination of the uterine infection remains the most important aspect of management; claims that therapy with heparin has significantly decreased maternal mortality in septic abortions are in doubt (Beller & Uszynski 1974) and use of heparin remains controversial (Beller 1985).

Purpura fulminans

This rare complication of infection sometimes occurs in the puerperium, precipitated by Gram-negative septicaemia.

Extensive haemorrhage occurs into the skin in association with DIC. The underlying mechanism is unknown but there appears to be an acute activation of the clotting system resulting in the deposition of fibrin thrombi within blood vessels of the skin and other organs (McGibbon 1982). The extremities and face are usually involved first; the purpuric patches have a jagged and erythematous border, which can be shown histologically to be the site of a leukocytoclastic vasculitis. Rapid enlargement of the lesions, which become necrotic and gangrenous, is associated with shock tachycardia and fever. Without treatment the mortality rate is high and among those who survive digit or limb amputation may be necessary. The laboratory findings are those of DIC with leukocytosis. In this situation treatment with heparin should be started as soon as the diagnosis is apparent, to prevent further consumption of platelets and coagulation factors. It should always be remembered, however, that bleeding from any site in the presence of the defective coagulation factors will be aggravated by the use of heparin.

Survival in purpura fulminans is currently much improved because of better supportive treatment for the shocked patient and effective control of the triggering infection, together with heparin therapy.

Acute fatty liver of pregnancy

This is a rare complication of pregnancy and it is included in this section because it is often, if not always, associated with variable degrees of DIC, which contributes significantly to its morbidity and mortality (Feinstein 1982, Laursen et al 1983). First identified by Sheehan (1940) as a separate entity, there are now about 90 patients documented in the English literature (Burroughs et al 1982) and probably less than 150 cases in the world literature (Hague et al 1983). The salient histological factors on which the diagnosis is ultimately based are the presence of fat in small vacuoles in centrilobular hepatocytes while a ring of normal hepatocytes remains around the portal systems without any evidence of cellular necrosis (Davies et al 1980). Renal failure with tubular necrosis is a common association (Rushton & Dawson 1982). The aetiology of this rare condition remains unknown.

Clinical presentation is typically during the last trimester with sudden onset of malaise, nausea, repeated vomiting and abdominal pain followed by jaundice. Haematemesis often occurs (Burroughs et al 1982) and is part of a bleeding diathesis due to thrombocytopenia, consumption coagulopathy and defects of coagulation factor synthesis (Lancet Editorial 1983).

The fetus is usually stillborn and, following delivery, the mother lapses into deeper coma associated with progressive hepatic and renal failure. The maternal mortality is between 75 and 85% and the fetal mortality is around 85% (Burroughs et al 1982). There are some few reports of this condition presenting in the puerperium (Lancet Editorial 1983).

Diagnosis during life has usually been made in the past on clinical grounds alone because the severe coagulation defect precludes liver biopsy. Even at post-mortem the acute fatty liver may well go undiagnosed unless the liver is carefully examined histologically using specific stains. An apparently normal liver to naked-eye inspection may show severe fatty infiltration on microscopic examination (Lancet Editorial 1983).

Proteinuria, hypertension and oedema are frequent accompanying features (Burroughs et al 1982) but pre-eclampsia is a much more common complication of pregnancy than acute fatty liver of pregnancy. Thus, with the possibility of the missed histological diagnosis, the validity of statistics concerning the incidence of acute fatty liver of pregnancy must be questioned. Confidential Enquiries into Maternal Deaths in England and Wales (Department of Health and Social Security 1986) attributed 36 deaths to hypertensive diseases of pregnancy of which 16 were associated with cerebral haemorrhage, cerebral oedema, DIC and hepatorenal failure, all of which are well recognized features of acute fatty liver of pregnancy. In the same period only six deaths were attributed to liver disorders. The distinction between eclampsia and acute fatty liver of pregnancy may not be as clear as has been previously assumed (De Swiet 1985): they may represent different clinical expressions of the same underlying disorders, and deaths due to acute fatty liver of pregnancy may have been underestimated.

Most observers agree that prompt delivery of the fetus offers the best chance of survival for both mother and child. Both Caesarean section and induction of labour led to a lower than expected maternal and fetal mortality in a series of 13 patients reported from the Royal Free Hospital (Burroughs et al 1982). This being so, early accurate diagnosis would seem to be a prerequisite for improving survival of both mother and child.

There should be a high order of suspicion when nausea and vomiting occur late in pregnancy, particularly if accompanied by abdominal pain and heartburn and associated with twins. This combination warrants immediate admission to hospital for investigation and observation. Further studies are required to establish the value of liver function tests, uric acid levels, amino acid profiles and examination of the blood film to achieve an early diagnosis of acute fatty liver of pregnancy. Biopsy of the liver obtained before delivery would be valuable in establishing the diagnosis but is often precluded because of the severe haemostatic defect.

At present the clinical problem of acute fatty liver of pregnancy remains that of early diagnosis since prompt delivery seems to be the specific management which limits progression of the disease and decreases both maternal and fetal mortality.

Summary on disseminated intravascular coagulation

As emphasized, DIC is always a secondary phenomenon and the mainstay of management is therefore to remove the initiating stimulus if possible.

With rampant DIC and haemorrhage, recovery will usually follow delivery of the patient provided the blood volume is maintained and shock due to hypovolaemia is prevented. An efficiently acting myometrium post-delivery will stem haemorrhage from the placental site. Measures taken to achieve a firm contracted uterus will obviously contribute one of the most important factors in preventing continuing massive blood loss from the placental site.

It is of interest that the maternal mortality of DIC associated with placental abruption is less than 1% (Pritchard & Brekken 1967), whereas that associated with infection and shock is 50–80% (Mant & King 1979). The mortality rate reported in series of patients with DIC due to various aetiologies is 50–85% and the wide variation probably reflects the mortality rate of the underlying disorder, not of DIC per se (Feinstein 1982). There is no doubt that the major determinant of survival is our ability to identify the underlying trigger and manage it successfully.

ACQUIRED PRIMARY DEFECTS OF HAEMOSTASIS

Thrombocytopenia

The commonest platelet abnormality encountered in clinical practice is thrombocytopenia. During the hundred years since platelets were first described, an increasing understanding of their role in haemostasis and thrombosis has taken place. At the same time there have been dramatic reductions in maternal and fetal mortality, but maternal thrombocytopenia remains a difficult management problem during pregnancy and can have profound effects on fetal and neonatal well-being. The causes and management of maternal and fetal thrombocytopenia have been reviewed (Colvin 1985, Pillai 1993). Emphasis here will be laid on those conditions which cause particular diagnostic and management problems in obstetric practice.

A low platelet count is seen most frequently in association with DIC, as already described. Sometimes severe megaloblastic anaemia of pregnancy is accompanied by thrombocytopenia, but the platelet count rapidly returns to normal after therapy with folic acid (Bonnar 1981). Toxic depression of bone marrow megakaryocytes in pregnancy can occur in association with infection, certain drugs and alcoholism. Neoplastic infiltration may also result in thrombocytopenia. Probably the single most important cause of isolated thrombocytopenia is autoimmune thrombocytopenic purpura (AITP), which is a disease primarily of young women in their reproductive years (McMillan 1981).

Autoimmune thrombocytopenic purpura

Autoimmune thrombocytopenic purpura (AITP) is common in women of childbearing age with an incidence of one to two per 10 000 pregnancies (Kessler et al 1982). Cases may present with skin bruising, and platelet counts between 30 and 80 × 10^9/l, but it is rare to see severe bleeding associated with low platelet counts in the chronic form.

With the screening of pregnant women, very mild thrombocytopenia may be discovered as an incidental finding and is not associated with risk to the mother or infant (Hart et al 1986, Burrows & Kelton 1988). It may be that incidental thrombocytopenia represents a very mild AITP but as it is not associated with adverse effects it must be distinguished from cases of AITP resulting in infants affected with severe thrombocytopenia and intracranial haemorrhage (Kelton 1983, Kaplan et al 1990, Samuels et al 1990). There are no serological tests or clinical guidelines which reliably predict the hazard of thrombocytopenia in an individual fetus and correlation between maternal and neonatal counts is poor (Samuels et al 1990, Kaplan et al 1990). It has been assumed that

Caesarean section delivery is less traumatic to the fetus than vaginal delivery and whilst that premise could be debated, recognizing and investigating the minority of pregnancies at risk of significant fetal thrombocytopenia would avoid many unnecessary fetal blood samples and Caesarean sections.

Diagnosis of autoimmune thrombocytopenic purpura

There have been a number of analyses of outcome of cases of maternal AITP from the 1950s onwards. The findings may not be entirely applicable to current management because some of the documented poor fetal outcomes may have been associated with unrecognized maternal lupus, pre-eclampsia or alloimmune thrombocytopenia. Only symptomatic women and neonates were investigated because there was no general screening of the platelet count in healthy women. This resulted in an exaggerated incidence of both neonatal thrombocytopenia and the rates of morbidity and mortality arising from it.

AITP is a diagnosis of exclusion with peripheral thrombocytopenia and normal or increased megakaryocytes in the bone marrow and the documented absence of other diseases. The red and white cells are essentially normal unless there is secondary anaemia. AITP requires the exclusion of systemic lupus erythematosis (SLE), lupus anticoagulant and anticardiolipin antibody as they may co-exist with thrombocytopenia.

The majority of thrombocytopenic patients are asymptomatic and tests to estimate the bleeding risk in these patients would obviously be helpful.

In chronic platelet consumption disorders, a population of younger larger platelets is established which have enhanced function. Measurement of the mean platelet volume (MPV) or, if not available, examination of the stained blood film will detect the presence of these large platelets. The risk of bleeding at any given platelet count is less in those patients with younger large platelets. The bleeding time, which has recently been severely criticized (Channing et al 1990, Lind 1991) as a predictor of bleeding at surgery, still has a place in this context according to some respected workers (Burrows & Kelton 1992). A bleeding time of greater than 15 minutes indicates a greater risk than in those with a normal bleeding time.

The mechanism of immune destruction of platelets has been shown to be due to autoantibodies directed against platelet surface antigens. This has special relevance in pregnancy because the placenta has receptors for the constant fragment (Fc) of the IgG immunoglobulin molecule facilitating active transport of immunoglobulin across the placenta to the fetal circulation. The immunoglobulin passage increases with advancing pregnancy (Tchernia et al 1984, Nicolini et al 1990) and may result in fetal thrombocytopenia.

The role of circulating globulin in the pathogenesis of immune thrombocytopenia was first documented in the 1950's (Evans et al 1951, Harrington et al 1953). However antibody on the platelet membrane and in the plasma, demonstrated by tests analogous to the direct and indirect Coombs tests on red cells, have been slow to enter the repertoire of routine haematological laboratories because they have been fraught with technological difficulties such as the intrinsic reactivity of platelets and the presence of some platelet-associated immunoglobulin in normal individuals.

Antibody from some cases of AITP demonstrates a specificity for the platelet glycoprotein IIb/IIIa (Van Leeuwen et al 1982, Woods et al 1984a) or for glycoprotein Ib (Woods et al 1984b). In one study, the minority of cases of AITP demonstrating this specificity fared less well in their responses to splenectomy (Woods & McMillan 1984).

Whilst some cases of AITP have normal or increased amounts of immunoglobulin on the platelets or in the plasma (Cines & Schreiber 1979, Mueller-Ekhardt et al 1980, von dem Borne et al 1980), 10–35% of patients have no demonstrable platelet-associated IgG (PAIgG). The presence of IgG rather than IgM antibodies (Hegde et al 1985) has relevance to the pregnant patient because only IgG antibodies can be transported across the placenta and cause thrombocytopenia in the fetus.

In a study of 162 consecutive pregnant patients with platelet counts $< 150 \times 10^9/l$ gathered over 11 years, the absence of circulating IgG antiplatelet antibody at term, despite a history of thrombocytopenic purpura, was associated with minimal risk of thrombocytopenia in the fetus (Samuels et al 1990). However no currently available serological test can be used to predict reliably thrombocytopenia in the fetus (Harrington 1987).

The absence of a history of AITP prior to the index pregnancy is a low risk indicator for neonatal thrombocytopenia (Samuels et al 1990). In contrast, 18 neonates who were born with platelet counts of less than $50 \times 10^9/l$, out of a total of 178, were all born to mothers with a history of AITP prior to pregnancy. In addition, 40% of mothers with a preceding history delivered infants with platelet counts below $100 \times 10^9/l$. Of 162 infants delivered in the index pregnancy, 10 had bleeding complications of which five were serious. Intracranial haemorrhage in infants born to women with a prior history of AITP and delivered vaginally numbered two out of 17, whilst there were no cases of intracranial haemorrhage in women with similar histories who were delivered by Caesarean section (Samuels et al 1990). A more recent review of the literature of AITP in pregnancy (Burrows & Kelton 1992) shows a neonatal mortality rate of six per 1000 AITP patients, about the same or better than the overall perinatal mortality rate. All the deaths in this survey occurred in babies delivered by Caesarean section, unlike other reports, and all events appeared more than 24–48 hours after delivery, the time of the platelet count nadir in the neonate.

Management of autoimmune thrombocytopenic purpura in pregnancy

Management of pregnancy in AITP is directed at three aspects: antenatal care of the mother, management of the mother and fetus during delivery and, lastly, the management of the neonate from the time of delivery.

The most important decision to make is whether the mother requires treatment at all. Many patients have significant thrombocytopenia (platelet count $< 100 \times 10^9/l$) but no evidence of an in vivo haemostatic disorder. In general the platelet count must be $< 50 \times 10^9/l$ for capillary bleeding and purpura to occur.

There is no need to treat asymptomatic women with mild to moderate thrombocytopenia (count above $50 \times 10^9/l$) and a normal bleeding time. However, the maternal platelet count should be monitored at every clinic visit and signs of haemostatic impairment looked for. The platelet count will show a downward trend during pregnancy with a nadir in the third trimester and active treatment may have to be instituted to achieve a safe haemostatic concentration of platelets for delivery at term. The incidence of antepartum haemorrhage is not increased in maternal AITP but there is a small increased risk of postpartum haemorrhagic complications not from the placental bed but from surgical incisions such as episiotomy and from soft tissue lacerations.

Intervention in the antenatal period is based on clinical manifestations of thrombocytopenia. The woman with bruising or petechiae requires measures to raise the platelet count but the woman with mucous membrane bleeding which may be life threatening requires urgent treatment with platelet transfusions and i.v. IgG (see below) and occasionally emergency splenectomy.

The real dilemma in the pregnant woman with AITP is that nearly all patients have chronic disease. The long-term effects of treatment, which is happily embarked on outside pregnancy, have to be considered in the light of the possible complications on the progress of pregnancy in the mother and of any effects on the fetus. The hazard for the mother who is monitored carefully and where appropriate measures have been taken is negligible, but most of her management is orientated towards what are thought to be optimal conditions for the delivery of the fetus who in turn may or may not be thrombocytopenic (see later).

Corticosteroids are a satisfactory short-term therapy but are unacceptable as long-term support unless the maintenance dose is very small (Carloss et al 1980, McMillan 1981). Side-effects for the mother include weight gain, subcutaneous fat redistribution, acne, and hypertension, which are undesirable during pregnancy. In addition, the prevalence of pre-eclampsia, gestational diabetes, post-partum psychosis and osteoporosis are all increased with the use of corticosteroids. Nevertheless, they are often used but should be reserved as short-term therapy for patients with obvious risk of bleeding or to raise the platelet count of an asymptomatic woman at term, allowing her to have epidural or spinal analgesia for delivery if desired or indicated.

A suggestion in the older literature of an association between steroid administration and cleft lip or palate has been refuted by more recent studies. Suppression of fetal adrenal glands is a theoretical hazard but approximately 90% of a dose of prednisolone or hydrocortisone is metabolized in the placenta and never reaches the fetus (Smith & Torday 1982). This is in contrast to dexamethosone and betamethosone which cross the placenta freely. It has been suggested (Hegde 1985) that high doses of corticosteroids given to elevate platelet counts at or near term should be avoided since they may increase the transplacental passage of IgG antibody and thus expose the fetus to greater risk of severe thrombocytopenia. In my experience this is a theoretical hazard not seen in practice.

Intravenous IgG The recent introduction of a highly successful treatment for AITP has altered the management options dramatically. It is known that intravenous administration of monomeric polyvalent human IgG in doses greater than those produced endogenously prolongs the clearance time of immune complexes by the reticuloendothelial system. It is thought that such a prolongation of clearance of IgG-coated platelets in AITP results in an increase in the number of circulating platelets but the mechanism is as yet unknown (Dwyer 1992). Used in the original recommended doses of 0.4 g/kg for 5 days by i.v. infusion, a persistent and predictable response was obtained in more than 80% of reported cases. More recently, alternative dosage regimens of this very expensive treatment have been suggested which are just as effective, but easier to manage and uses less total immunoglobulin (Burrows & Kelton 1992). A typical dose is 1 g/kg over 8 hours on one day. This dose will raise the platelet count to normal or safe levels in approximately half of the patients. In those in whom the platelet count does not rise, a similar dose can be repeated 2 days later. The advantages of this treatment are that it is safe, has very few side-effects and the response to therapy is more rapid than with corticosteroids. The response usually occurs within 48 hours and is maintained for 2–3 weeks. The main disadvantage is that it is very expensive and seldom produces a long-term cure of the AITP.

It has been suggested that IgG given intravenously can cross the placenta and should provoke an identical response in the fetus at risk but this has never been proved (Morgenstern et al 1983). Indeed, analysis of more recent literature indicates that the postulated transplacental effect is unreliable (Tchernia et al 1984, Nicolini et al 1990) and that exogenous IgG may not cross the placenta (Pappas 1986). The use of IgG has been recommended (Hegde 1985, 1987) in all pregnant patients with platelet counts of less than $75 \times 10^9/l$ regardless of history or symptoms. There is no doubt about the value of IgG in selected cases of severe symptomatic thrombocytopenia where a rapid response is required but its indiscriminate use in all cases with significant thrombocytopenia would have to be shown to dramatically improve both maternal and fetal outcome to justify the high cost.

Splenectomy will produce a cure or long-term drug-free remission in 60–80% of all patients with AITP. This is because the main site of antibody production is often the spleen and because many of the IgG-coated platelets are sequestered there. All patients should receive pneumovax before splenectomy and twice daily oral penicillin for life following surgery to protect against pneumococcal infection. Reviews of management of AITP have associated splenectomy during pregnancy with high fetal loss rates (Carloss et al 1980) and even an approximate 10% maternal mortality rate in the past (Bell 1977) but modern supportive measures and improved surgical practices have reduced the fetal loss rate considerably and the risk of maternal mortality is negligible (Martin et al 1984). In current practice, splenectomy is hardly ever indicated in the pregnant patient and should be avoided given the success of medical management. However, removal of the spleen remains an option if all other attempts to increase the platelet count fail. Splenectomy should be performed in the second trimester because surgery is best tolerated then and the size of the uterus will not make the operation technically difficult. The platelet count should be raised to safe levels for surgery if possible by i.v. IgG. Although transfused platelets will have a short life in the maternal circulation, they may help to achieve haemostasis at surgery. Platelet concentrates should be available but given only if abnormal bleeding occurs.

Other therapy   There are a number of other medications which have been used in AITP but most of them are contraindicated in pregnancy and only have moderate success rates. Danazol, an attenuated anabolic steroid, has been used with moderate success in a few patients. Vincristine has a transient beneficial effect in many patients but it is not recommended in pregnancy and long-term associated neurotoxicity limits its usefulness.

Very occasionally immunosuppressives such as azathioprine and cyclophosphamide have to be used in severe intractable thrombocytopenia which does not respond to any other measures. Cyclophosphamide should be avoided in pregnancy. However, experience with relatively low doses of azathioprine in the increasing numbers of transplant patients who have now negotiated a subsequent pregnancy suggests that this drug is not associated with increased fetal or maternal morbidity. The most contentious issue in the management of AITP in pregnancy is the mode of delivery given that the fetus may also be thrombocytopenic and may bleed from trauma during the birth process.

Assessment of the fetal platelet count   Hegde (1985) analysed the reported cases in the literature from 1950 to 1983 which suggested an overall incidence of neonatal thrombocytopenia of 52% with significant morbidity in 12% of births. The incidence increases to 70% of deliveries if maternal platelet counts were less than $100 \times 10^9/l$ at term. The probability of fetal thrombocytopenia increased with the severity of maternal thrombocytopenia. As a result of this and other analyses many strategies were developed to predict the fetal platelet count and to determine the optimal mode of delivery, since it was believed that elective Caesarean section was the best option for an affected fetus at risk from trauma during a vaginal delivery.

We know now that the incidence in these retrospective analyses was distorted because only symptomatic women were likely to have been investigated and reported (see above). A recent report (Samuels et al 1990) studied the outcome of 162 consecutive pregnancies in women with presumed AITP presenting in the decade 1979–89. The overall incidence of thrombocytopenia (11.0%) in the offspring of these women was much lower than the earlier reported analyses but two factors emerged of importance in predicting neonatal thrombocytopenia. In the absence of a history of AITP before pregnancy or in the absence of circulating platelet IgG antibodies in the index pregnancy in those with a history, the risk of severe thrombocytopenia in the fetus at term was negligible.

These findings are supported by another recent report (Burrows & Kelton 1990) of 61 infants born to 50 mothers with confirmed AITP. Only three (4.9%) had a cord platelet count $< 50 \times 10^9/l$. None of the infants had morbidity or mortality as a result of the thrombocytopenia. Two-thirds of the infants had a further fall in platelet count in the first 2 or 3 days after birth but in all the thrombocytopenia could easily be corrected. Some investigators have suggested that maternal splenectomy increases the probability of neonatal thrombocytopenia (Carloss et al 1980, Van Leeuwen et al 1981). Closer scrutiny of published reports (Burrows & Kelton 1992) shows that it is only in those women with splenectomy and persistent thrombocytopenia (less than $100 \times 10^9/l$) that the risk of neonatal thrombocytopenia is increased. What has become clear over the years is that analysis of the older literature gave an exaggerated incidence of neonatal thrombocytopenia and of the morbidity and mortality arising from it. However, even with the benefit of accurate automated, easily repeated platelet counts, estimation of IgG platelet antibodies and taking into consideration splenectomy status, it is still impossible to predict the fetal platelet count in any individual case (Kaplan et al 1990) and to plan the mode of delivery based on these maternal parameters is not logical or sensible.

Fetal blood sampling A method for direct measurement of the fetal platelet count in scalp blood obtained transcervically prior to or early in labour has been described (Ayromlooi 1978, Scott et al 1980, Tchernia 1988). The authors recommend that Caesarean section be performed in all cases where the fetal platelet count is less than $50 \times 10^9/l$. This approach is more logical than a decision about the mode of delivery made on the basis of maternal platelet count, concentration of IgG or splenectomy status, but it is not without risk of significant haemorrhage in the truly thrombocytopenic fetus, often gives false positive results (Burrows & Kelton 1992) and demands urgent action to be taken on the results. Also the cervix must be sufficiently dilated to allow the fetal scalp to be sampled and the uterine contraction to achieve this may have caused the fetus to descend so far in the birth canal that Caesarean section is technically difficult and also traumatic for the fetus.

The only way a reliable fetal platelet count can be obtained so that a decision concerning the optimal mode of delivery can be taken is by a percutaneous fetal cord blood sample taken before term (Daffos et al 1988, Moise et al 1988, Scioscia et al 1988). This gives time for discussion with obstetrician, paediatrician, haematologist, anaesthetist and anyone else involved concerning delivery. It should be performed at 37–38 weeks' gestation under ultrasound guidance as the transfer of IgG increases in the last weeks of pregnancy and an earlier sample may give a higher fetal platelet count than one taken nearer term. There is no need for sampling earlier in gestation because the fetus is not at risk from spontaneous intracranial haemorrhage in utero (cf. fetus with alloimmune thrombocytopenia).

There is a risk associated with the sampling but in skilled hands this is no more than 1% (Nicolini et al 1990). A Caesarean section may be precipitated because of fetal distress during the procedure even if the platelet count proves to be normal. This is another good reason for performing a fetal blood sample as late as possible in gestation if it is thought to be necessary. There is no point in performing serial fetal platelet counts from earlier in gestation because the fetus is not at risk from spontaneous haemorrhage before labour unlike the fetus in alloimmune thrombocytopenia. Given the low risk of identifying a problem and the risk of associated complications in utero, fetal blood sampling cannot be justified in all AITP pregnancies.

Neonatal platelet count After birth the platelet count will continue to fall for 2–5 days. If the cord platelet count shows severe thrombocytopenia and especially if there is evidence of skin or mucous membrane bleeding, measures can be taken to prevent this predicted fall. Intravenous hydrocortisone and platelet transfusion have been used with success but the recommended therapy nowadays should be intravenous IgG because of its relative safety and the rapidity with which a response is observed.

Mode of delivery in autoimmune thrombocytopenic purpura There is little risk to the mother whatever the mode of delivery. In most cases the maternal platelet count can be raised to haemostatic levels to cover the event. Even if the mother has to deliver in the face of a low platelet count, she is unlikely to bleed from the placental site once the uterus is empty but she is at risk of bleeding from any surgical incisions, soft tissue injuries or tears. Platelets should be available but not given prophylactically. It should be remembered that the unnecessary transfusion of platelet concentrates in the absence of haemostatic failure may stimulate more autoantibody formation synthesis and thus increase maternal thrombocytopenia. Most anaesthetists require that the platelet count is at least $80 \times 10^9/l$ and preferably over $100 \times 10^9/l$ before they will administer an epidural anaesthetic, but there is no good evidence that counts above $50 \times 10^9/l$ are not sufficient to achieve haemostasis in AITP (Letsky 1991b).

The major risk at delivery is to the fetus with thrombocytopenia who as the result of birth trauma may suffer intracranial haemorrhage. If there is any question that a vaginal delivery will be difficult because of cephalopelvic disproportion, premature labour, previous history etc., then elective Caesarean section should be carried out.

For many centres the availability of planned or emergency transabdominal fetal blood sampling is severely limited or non-existent and so decisions concerning the mode of delivery will have to be taken without knowing the fetal platelet count.

As discussed earlier, maternal platelet count, maternal platelet-associated IgG, history and splenectomy status show trends regarding the incidence of fetal and neonatal thrombocytopenia but can never be used to predict fetal thrombocytopenia with absolute confidence in an individual case. It does appear however that it is very unlikely for the fetus to have severe thrombocytopenia if the mother has no previous history of AITP before the index pregnancy and if she has no detectable free IgG platelet antibody (Samuels et al 1990).

Many of the options proposed in the literature presuppose that Caesarean section is less traumatic than an uncomplicated vaginal delivery. There is no objective evidence to support this contention and there are undesirable associated complications of Caesarean section per se for both mother and fetus. The only advantage is that there is more overall control of the delivery if it is by elective Caesarean section and there are usually no unpredictable complications.

Based on an estimate of a 12.7–21% perinatal mortality associated with AITP, it was proposed (Murray & Harris 1976) that all patients should be delivered by Caesarean section. The mortality rate quoted is a gross overestimate, probably for reasons previously stated of selection of severe symptomatic cases for the analysis. A recent review of the literature of AITP in pregnancy shows a neonatal mortality rate of six per 1000 AITP patients (Burrows & Kelton 1992), about the same as or better than the overall perinatal mortality rate. All these deaths occurred in babies delivered by Caesarean section and all events appeared more than 24–48 hours after delivery, the time of the platelet count nadir in the neonate.

The incidence of severe thrombocytopenia in the fetus of a woman with proven AITP is not more than 10%. Even if Caesarean section is the optimum mode of delivery for the thrombocytopenic fetus, this does not justify this mode of delivery for the nine out of ten fetuses without thrombocytopenia.

It is not now thought to be optimum management to deliver all fetuses with potential or identified thrombocytopenia by Caesarean section. If delivery by Caesarean section is indicated for obstetric reasons there is no point in fetal blood sampling to obtain the platelet count and elective Caesarean section should be performed.

In our hospital there is considerable expertise in intrauterine fetal blood sampling but we only recommend this procedure:

1. where the women enters pregnancy with a history of AITP together with currently identifiable platelet-associated IgG antibodies, or
2. in those women who have to be treated for AITP during the index pregnancy.

Our obstetricians, like many others, prefer to deliver a fetus with significant thrombocytopenia (platelet count $< 50 \times 10^9/l$) by Caesarean section. However, individual units may need different policies depending on local expertise and practice.

The management of the neonate

An immediate cord platelet count should be performed following delivery in all neonates of mothers with AITP whenever or however diagnosed. The vast majority of babies will have platelet counts well above $50 \times 10^9/l$ and will be symptom free. For those with low platelet counts, petechiae and purpura, steroids or preferably i.v. IgG should be administered. If there is mucous membrane bleeding, platelet concentrates should be administered also.

It should be borne in mind that the neonatal platelet count will fall further in the first few days of life and it is at the nadir that most complications occur, rather than at delivery. Measures should be taken to prevent the fall

if the cord blood platelet count warrants this. The platelet count should be repeated daily for the first week in those neonates with thrombocytopenia at delivery.

The development of techniques to obtain fetal blood with relative safety to perform a fetal platelet count and the widely held concept that Caesarean section is less traumatic for the fetus than a normal vaginal delivery has led to often unnecessary intervention with risks to both mother and fetus.

At the time of writing the emphasis of management is to return to a non-interventional policy (Aster 1990) of sensible monitoring, supportive therapy, and a mode of delivery determined mainly by obstetric indications and not primarily on either the maternal or fetal platelet count.

Autoimmune thrombocytopenic purpura associated with HIV infection

Thrombocytopenia is a well-recognized complication of HIV infection and may be due to drugs and severe infection. The subject has been reviewed (Walsh et al 1984, Costello 1988). However, patients with the immune deficiency syndromes may have thrombocytopenia otherwise indistinguishable from AITP. This may be due to immune platelet destruction resulting from cross-reaction between the Human Immunodeficiency Virus and the platelet glycoproteins IIb/IIIa (Bettaieb et al 1992) which may explain AIDS-free, HIV-associated AITP. It has also been suggested that disturbances in the B-cell subset, CD5, in HIV-infected patients may cause immunological changes correlating with the platelet count (Kouri et al 1992). In addition it has been suggested that non-specific deposition of complement and immune complexes on platelets leads to their removal from the circulation (Hughes 1987).

Whilst most HIV patients have so far been young men, it is possible that this complication will become commoner in young pregnant women although the degree of heterosexual spread of HIV is uncertain. Certainly, young pregnant women in a high risk group for HIV with thrombocytopenia should be considered for HIV testing.

Thrombocytopenia and systemic lupus erythematosus

Systemic lupus erythematosus (SLE) is frequently complicated by thrombocytopenia but this is seldom severe: less than 5% of cases have platelet counts below $30 \times 10^9/l$ during the course of the disease (Hughes 1979). Thrombocytopenia is often the first presenting feature and may outdate any other manifestations by months or even years. Such patients are often labelled as suffering from AITP, unless appropriate additional tests are carried out. Platelet-associated IgG is often found on testing but it is not clear whether this is due to antiplatelet antibody, immune complexes or both. The management of isolated thrombocytopenia associated with SLE in pregnancy does not differ substantially from that of AITP but immuno-suppressive therapy should not be reduced or discontinued during pregnancy (Varner et al 1983). However, the main management problem of systemic lupus erythematosus and pregnancy is the complication of the variably present in vitro lupus anticoagulant and its paradoxical association with in vivo thromboembolism and recurrent mid-trimester abortion.

Alloimmune thrombocytopenia (Levine & Berkowitz 1991)

Fetal alloimmune thrombocytopenia (AIT) is a syndrome that develops as a result of maternal sensitisation to fetal platelet antigens. The antibody, usually Hpa[1] (formerly known as Pla[1]), is directed specifically against a paternally derived antigen which the mother lacks (cf. Rh(D) haemolytic disease).

The mother is not thrombocytopenic herself but the fetal platelets in utero have altered function. The platelet-specific antibody attaches to the membrane of the Hpa[1] binding site and interferes with the function of the glycoprotein IIb–IIIa ligand binding sites thus impairing platelet aggregation. The affected thrombocytopenic fetus is at risk of spontaneous intracranial haemorrhage from early in gestation, unlike the fetus affected by maternal ITP.

It is obvious that the fetus at risk must be identified early in gestation if measures are to be taken to prevent intrauterine intracranial haemorrhage occurring but this is not easy. In the vast majority of cases, a fetus at risk is identified because of a previously affected sibling. Hpa[1] (previously Pla[1]) is the most common antigen associated with AIT. The antigen is present in 97–98% of the population. Two alleles are present, Hpa[1] and Hpa[2], and 69% of the population are homozygous for Hpa[1], the stronger sensitising antigen. The immune response of the Hpa[1]-negative mother seems to be determined in part by genes of the histocompatibility complex and antibody formation appears to be confined to those with HLA-B8 and HLA DR3 antigens. First pregnancies may be affected (unlike Rh disease). Subsequent affected pregnancies will be of similar or increased severity and the recurrence rate is estimated to be between 75% and 90%.

The monitoring of severity of the disease process also differs greatly from Rh haemolytic disease. The absence of antibodies does not guarantee a normal fetal platelet count although women with identifiable antibodies are at risk of producing a fetus with thrombocytopenia. Rises in titre and concentration of antibody do not correlate with severity.

To identify all women at risk of developing platelet alloantibodies by platelet (Hpa[1]) grouping and HLA typing of all pregnant women is not cost-effective or feasible at the moment but the appropriate investigations should be carried out on all female relatives of women known to have had a baby affected by this disorder.

The incidence of neonatal AIT has been estimated to be one per 5000 births, although more recent studies give a higher frequency of one in 2–3000 births. Not all cases necessarily have severe manifestation. We have identified at least one symptomless case on routine screening of neonatal cord blood of an Rh(D)-negative woman at delivery.

Management of alloimmune thrombocytopenia

All management protocols currently involve fetal blood sampling early in gestation but preferably after 22 weeks' gestation when the risk of the procedure is reduced. In the identified affected fetus, subsequent management is controversial. Weekly maternal IgG infusion 1 g/kg with or without prednisone has been used in the successful management of pregnancies at risk of AIT (Lynch et al, 1992). This has not been the universal experience however. Others recommend weekly HPa[1] negative platelet infusions until fetal lung maturity is achieved. All protocols involve frequent ultrasound examinations to check that no intracranial bleeds have occurred. The mode of delivery will be determined by maturity, fetal platelet count and obstetric indications.

The use of maternal platelet infusions to the fetus or neonate should be discouraged. Unless they are repeatedly washed the infused anti HPA[1] antibody has a much longer half-life than the platelets themselves. Repeated washing of platelets also reduces their function (Pillai 1993). Moreover, suitably prepared platelets from accredited donors provided by the regional Blood Transfusion Service are more effective and probably much safer. Post delivery, the disease is usually self-limiting within a few weeks. If therapy is required, Hpa-compatible platelets are the treatment of choice. The aim of all controversial antenatal management is to deliver a relatively mature infant who has not suffered intracranial haemorrhage antenatally or during delivery.

Alloimmune thrombocytopenia can be a devastating fetal disease and it should be excluded in all cases of fetal intracranial haemorrhage, unexplained porencephaly and neonatal thrombocytopenia.

Unlike ITP, because of the risk of spontaneous intrauterine fetal haemorrhage, early fetal blood sampling is indicated and a mother with this potential problem should be referred early in pregnancy to an expert fetal medicine unit for investigation and management although delivery of a treated infant may still take place at the centre of referral.

At Queen Charlotte's Maternity Hospital we have successfully managed this condition with serial weekly fetal platelet transfusions starting as early as 22 weeks' gestation.

Management of a previous similar case with platelet transfusions starting at 34 weeks resulted in delivery of a baby who had no thrombocytopenia or bleeding but had intracranial cysts, presumably due to bleeds sustained before treatment was started in utero. This infant is now severely handicapped (De Vries et al 1988).

Preliminary encouraging reports of successful management with maternally administered i.v. IgG (Bussel et al 1988) have not been borne out in other centres (Kaplan et al 1988, Nicolini et al 1990). This may have something to do with the different preparations of immunoglobulin available for use and the effects of variable content of contaminating CD4 and CD8 molecules (Blasczyk et al 1993). In contrast to AITP, fetal blood sampling is both justified and indicated. Management of all cases should involve a fetal medicine unit skilled in intrauterine investigation and procedures.

Pre-eclampsia and platelets

There have been many reports showing that the circulating platelet count is reduced in pre-eclampsia and these have been recently reviewed (Romero et al 1989). It has also been shown that the platelet count can be used to monitor severity of the disease process and as an initial screening test if there is concern about significant coagulation abnormalities (Redman et al 1978, Spencer et al 1983, Leduc et al 1992). A fall in the platelet count precedes any detectable rise in serum fibrin(ogen) degradation products in women subsequently developing pre-eclampsia (Redman et al 1978).

The combination of a reduced platelet lifespan and a fall in the platelet count without platelet-associated antibodies (see below) indicates a low-grade coagulopathy. Platelets may either be consumed in thrombus formation or may suffer membrane damage from contact with abnormal surfaces and be prematurely removed from the circulation.

Rarely, in very severe pre-eclampsia the patient develops microangiopathic haemolytic anaemia. These patients have profound thrombocytopenia and this leads to confusion in the differential diagnosis between pre-eclampsia, TTP and HELLP syndrome.

The activation of the haemostatic mechanisms in normal pregnancy has led to the view that the haematological manifestations of pre-eclampsia merely represent augmentation of the hypercoagulable state which accompanies normal pregnancy.

Many studies have been carried out on levels of individual coagulation factors. No clear pattern emerges but there appear to be some significant correlations of severity of the disease process with both the factor VIII complex (Redman et al 1977) and antithrombin III (Weiner et al 1985).

A readily available and sensitive indicator of activation of the coagulation system is assay of fibrinopeptide A concentration in the plasma. Although in mild pre-eclampsia patients may have a normal or only slight increase in fibrinopeptide A levels, marked increases occur in patients with severe pre-eclampsia (Borok et al 1984, Wallmo et al 1984).

Most studies in pre-eclampsia have shown increased levels of fibrinogen/fibrin degradation products in serum and urine. Plasma levels of soluble fibrinogen/fibrin complexes are also raised in pre-eclampsia compared with normal pregnancies (Edgar et al 1977, Estelles et al 1987). Borok and colleagues (1984) found that fibrinolytic activity is more pronounced than fibrin formation in patients with severe pre-eclampsia.

A recent study (Thornton et al 1989) estimated kaolin cephalin clotting time, prothrombin time, thrombin time, fibrinogen, englobulin clot lysis time, FDPs, platelet count, β thromboglobulin and platelet factor 4, and fibrinopeptide A in 400 women at 28 weeks' gestation. None of these tests proved predictive but once the disease process is established the most relevant coagulation abnormalities appear to be the platelet count, factor VIII and FDP. Those women with the most marked abnormalities in these parameters suffer the greatest perinatal loss.

Thrombotic thrombocytopenic purpura and haemolytic-uraemic syndrome

These conditions share so many features that they should probably be considered as one disease with pathological effects confined largely to the kidney in haemolytic-uraemic syndrome (HUS) and being more generalized in thrombotic thrombocytopenic purpura (TTP). These conditions are extremely rare and fewer than 100 cases have been reported in pregnancy (Pinette et al 1989). HUS usually presents in the postpartum period with renal failure.

These conditions are both due to the presence of platelet thrombin in the microcirculation which causes ischaemic dysfunction and microangiopathic haemolysis. In HUS, the brunt of the disease process is taken by the kidney and has rarely been associated with pregnancy, particularly in the postnatal period. It has also been seen during pregnancy and in association with ectopic pregnancy (Creasy & Morgan 1987). It has been postulated that endothelial damage is mediated through neutrophil adhesion in association with infection and leads to the formation of platelet thrombin (Forsyth et al 1989).

In TTP, the focus shifts to multisystem disease, often with neurological involvement and fever. It has been associated with pregnancy and the post-partum period (Weiner 1987) and with the platelet anti-aggregating agent, ticlopidine (Page et al 1991). It is associated with abnormal patterns of von Willebrand factor (vWF) multimers in the plasma (Moake et al 1982). Immunohistochemistry has shown the presence of vWF but not fibrinogen in the platelet aggregates in TTP (Asada et al 1985). It has been suggested that a calcium-dependent cysteine protease present in patient's plasma may interact with vWF to render it highly reactive with platelets and thus contributing to the formation of platelet aggregates (Moore et al 1990). The underlying aetiology of TTP in pregnancy remains unknown and the various abnormalities which have been described may only be epiphenomenon. It is feasible that there is a deficiency of prostacyclin activator or synthesis. The aetiology has been reviewed (Machin 1984, Aster 1985).

The pentad of fever, normal coagulation tests with low platelets, haemolytic anaemia, neurological disorders and renal dysfunction are virtually pathognomonic of TTP. The thrombocytopenia may range from 5 to $100 \times 10^9/l$. The clinical picture is severe with a high maternal mortality.

A crucial problem when dealing with TTP is to establish a correct diagnosis, because this condition can be confused with severe pre-eclampsia and placental abruption, especially if DIC is triggered (although DIC is uncommon in TTP).

Unlike fatty liver of pregnancy there is no evidence that prompt delivery affects the course of HUS or TTP favourably. Most clinicians would recommend delivery if these conditions are present in late pregnancy so that the mother can be treated vigorously without fear of harming the fetus.

Empirical therapeutic strategies hinge on intensive plasma exchange or replacement. In a random allocation study of 102 non-pregnant patients with TTP, plasma exchange was found to be more effective than plasma infusion, with more than seven exchanges over 9 days (Rock et al 1991). It has been suggested that plasma supplies a factor lacking in patients with TTP that stimulates the release of prostacyclin. Regimens may be supplemented with antiplatelet drugs to prevent relapse (Machin 1984), although their use has been contested by some authors (Bell et al 1991). Platelet infusions are contraindicated. Cryosupernatant has been shown to control the metabolism of unusually large vWF multimers (Moake et al 1985) in vivo.

In one large series of 108 patients with HUS/TTP, of whom 9% were pregnant, steroids alone were judged to be effective in mild cases, whilst there were eight deaths and 67 relapses in a group of 78 patients with complicated disease. They were treated with steroids and plasma exchange infusions. The overall survival was 91%.

Relapses occurred in 22 of 36 patients given maintenance plasma infusions.

Of the nine pregnant patients, all were in the third trimester and all were delivered of normal infants. Five women went on to further normal pregnancies and deliveries (Bell et al 1991).

In summary, it seems reasonable to treat all TTP patients with steroids. Severe cases will benefit from intensive plasma exchange but where that is difficult, intensive plasma infusion is indicated. Unresponsive cases may benefit from cryosupernatant infusions. The use of antiplatelet drugs seems non-contributory (Moake 1991). Plasma infusion should be tapered but continued until all objective signs have been reversed, in order to prevent recurrence.

Factor VIII antibody

An inhibitor of antihaemophilic factor is a rare cause of haemorrhage in previously healthy postpartum women (O'Brien 1954, Marengo Rowe et al 1972, Voke & Letsky 1977, Coller et al 1981, Reece et al 1982). There are fewer than 50 documented cases in the literature (Voke & Letsky 1977, Reece et al 1982). Women who may have had this type of haemorrhagic disorder were first reported in the late 1930s and the nature of the defect was first reported in 1946, when the plasma of two such patients was shown not only to resemble haemophilic plasma but to have an inhibitory effect on normal clotting. In the late 1960s it was demonstrated that these inhibitors of factor VIII were immunoglobulins, as are the factor VIII antibodies found in treated haemophiliacs (for references see Voke & Letsky 1977). Of the postpartum coagulation defects of this type reported, nearly all were found on in vitro testing to be directed against factor VIII. Only two were found to be anti-factor IX antibodies.

Aetiology

The aetiology of antibodies to factor VIII is complex. The appearance of anti-VIIIC in non-haemophilic individuals is usually attributed to an autoimmune process, or in postpartum women to isoimmunization. However, no difference between maternal and fetal factor VIII has been demonstrated and neutralization of both maternal and fetal factor VIII by the antibody is similar.

There is at present no definite experimental evidence that factor VIII antigen allotypes exist. If the bleeding tendency is to be explained, the antibody formed by stimulation of the maternal immune system by fetal factor VIII has to cross-react with maternal factor VIII. One would expect such an antibody to reappear after some of the subsequent pregnancies (by analogy with rhesus sensitization), but relapses have not been reported. Assuming that these inhibitors are IgG antibodies, they are likely to cross the placenta and persist for several weeks in the neonate, as do anti-rhesus or antiviral antibodies. However, although factor VIII antibody and low levels of factor VIIIC have been found in neonates born to mothers with antibody, there have been no case reports of haemorrhagic problems in their offspring.

The variable nature of this disorder argues in favour of a more complex pathogenesis. There is an association between factor VIII antibodies and autoimmune disorders such as rheumatoid arthritis and systemic lupus erythematosus. There is also a well known alteration of immune reactivity in normal pregnancy. These observations suggest that a likely explanation of postpartum factor VIII antibodies is that of a temporary breakdown in the mother's tolerance to her own factor VIII (or factor IX). This rare disorder resembles other autoimmune states in its variable onset and is still a mystery (Voke & Letsky 1977).

Clinical manifestations

The patient usually presents within 3 months of delivery with severe bleeding, extensive painful bruising, bleeding from the gastrointestinal or genitourinary tract and occasional haemarthroses. The reported confirmed cases presented in a period of 3 days to 17 months postpartum. The factor VIII antibody is associated with life-threatening haemorrhage at various sites, not necessarily related to parturition.

Diagnosis of factor VIII antibody

The diagnosis is established on the basis of characteristic laboratory findings. The prothrombin time and thrombin time are normal but the partial thromboplastin time is very long. The partial thromboplastin time is not corrected by the addition of normal plasma or factor VIII.

The potency of the antibody is determined by an assay in which the ability of concentrations of the patient's plasma to destroy factor VIIIC is observed, the result being expressed in units per millilitre. The unit is defined as that quantity of antibody contained in undiluted patient's plasma which will destroy 0.5 iu VIIIC in 4 hours at 37°C.

Management

Any woman who develops such an antibody should be under the care of an expert coagulation unit. Treatment of the acute bleeding episode is difficult because conventional amounts of factor VIII may merely enhance antibody formation and fail to control the bleeding. Immunosuppressive agents in combination with corticosteroid have been suggested to reduce the antibody production and there are reports of a decrease or disappearance of the antibody in response to treatment (Coller et al 1981).

In one reported case (Reece et al 1982) after failure of factor VIII concentrate and fresh plasma, improvement in the clinical status was achieved by administration of an anti-inhibitor coagulation complex (Autoplex), a preparation of pooled fresh plasma containing precursors and activated clotting factors. The mechanism of action of Autoplex is unknown. It does not suppress or destroy the inhibitor but seems to control the acute haemorrhage diathesis (Reece et al 1982).

The natural history is for the antibody to disappear gradually, usually within 2 years. Women should be advised to avoid further pregnancy until coagulation is back to normal, although in the one documented case where conception occurred in the presence of clinically active antibody, the antibody disappeared during the course of the pregnancy (Voke & Letsky 1977).

GENETIC DISORDERS OF HAEMOSTASIS

It is important to recognize these uncommon conditions not only because the morbidity and mortality they cause in the sufferer is almost completely preventable by correct diagnosis and treatment, but also because carriers of the most devastating of these conditions, particularly the X-linked haemophilias, can be identified and prenatal diagnosis offered if couples at risk so desire.

However, because of the profound changes in haemostasis during normal pregnancy it is desirable to establish a correct diagnosis with appropriate family studies and DNA analysis where relevant, before conception, so that appropriate management, and in conditions where DNA prenatal diagnosis is feasible, chorionic villus sampling can be planned in advance.

Severe congenital disorders of haemostasis are nearly always apparent early in life so that they will have been diagnosed before the obstetrician has to deal with the patient. Milder forms may go unrecognized until adult life and are more of a diagnostic challenge.

Patients with thrombocytopenia or platelet function abnormalities suffer primarily from mucosal bleeding with epistaxes, gingival and gastrointestinal bleeding and menorrhagia. Bleeding occurs immediately after surgery or trauma and may not occur at all if primary haemostasis can be achieved with suturing.

In contrast patients with coagulation disorders typically suffer deep muscle haematomata and haemarthroses. Bleeding after trauma or surgery may be immediate or delayed. A history of previous vaginal deliveries without undue bleeding does not exclude a significant coagulopathy because of the increase in coagulation factors, particularly factor VIII, which occurs during normal pregnancy and the fact that powerful uterine contractility is the most important haemostatic factor at parturition.

Complete laboratory evaluation of a patient giving a

history of easy bleeding or bruising is time-consuming and expensive and a history of significant previous haemostatic challenges should be obtained. For example, a patient who has undergone tonsillectomy without transfusion or special treatment and lived to tell the tale cannot possibly have an inherited haemostatic disorder.

Of more relevance perhaps is any history of dental extractions where haemorrhage can occur with both platelet disorders and coagulopathies. If prolonged bleeding has occurred and particularly if blood transfusion has been required, then a high index of suspicion of a congenital haemorrhagic disorder is justified. In such cases, even if initial laboratory screening tests—partial thromboplastin time, prothrombin time, platelet count and bleeding time—are normal, the diagnosis should be vigorously pursued in consultation with an expert haematologist.

The most common congenital coagulation disorders are von Willebrand's disease, factor VIII deficiency (haemophilia A) and factor IX deficiency (haemophilia B). Less common disorders include factor XI deficiency, abnormal or deficient fibrinogen and deficiency of factor XIII (fibrin-stabilizing factor). All other coagulation factor disorders are extremely rare. The most frequent disorders of platelet function are von Willebrand's disease and storage pool disease (How et al 1991).

INHERITED PLATELET DEFECTS

Qualitative platelet abnormalities

Serious bleeding disorders due to genetic abnormalities of platelet function are rare, the inheritance being autosomal recessive. Clinically, the signs and symptoms are similar to those of von Willebrand's disease, with skin and mucosal haemorrhages. Spontaneous bruises are common but hemiarthroses are not. Although these disorders can lead to life-threatening haemorrhage, particularly after surgery or trauma, the bleeding tendency is usually mild. The essential defect is intrinsic to the platelet. Bleeding time is prolonged and platelet function tests are abnormal, showing reduced aggregation and/or adhesion. In thrombasthenia (Glanzmann's disease), the platelets appear morphologically normal but they fail to aggregate with collagen adenosine diphosphate (ADP) or ristocetin. There is a risk of intracranial haemorrhage in utero in the affected fetus (cf. all-immune thrombocytopenia). In the very rare Bernard–Soulier syndrome, the aggregation defect is similar but the platelets have a characteristically abnormal giant appearance. Serious bleeding episodes in pregnancy have been treated with plasmapheresis and fresh platelet concentrate infusions (Peaceman et al 1989).

Thrombocytopenia

Genetically determined thrombocytopenia may be associated with aplastic anaemia or isolated megakaryocytic aplasia. The thrombocytopenia-absent radius (TAR) syndrome is thought to be an autosomal recessive defect and has been successfully diagnosed prenatally by examination of fetal blood sample (Daffos et al 1988, Nicolaides et al 1985). Patients with May–Heggelin anomaly, an autosomal dominant condition with variable thrombocytopenia and giant platelets, may receive platelet concentrates to achieve haemostasis at delivery and should be offered prenatal diagnosis (Colvin 1985).

Von Willebrand's disease

Von Willebrand's disease (Holmberg et al 1985) is the most frequent of all inherited haemostatic disorders with an overt disease incidence of more than 1 in 10 000, similar to that of haemophilia A. Because subclinical forms of the disorder are common, the total incidence of von Willebrand's disease is actually greater than that of haemophilia. In contrast to haemophilia (an X-linked condition), von Willebrand's disease has an autosomal inheritance and equal incidence in males and females and therefore is the most frequent genetic haemostatic disorder encountered in obstetric practice.

Nature of the defect

Von Willebrand's disease is a disorder of the von Willebrand factor portion of the human factor VIII complex. Factor VIII circulates as a complex of two proteins of unequal size. There is a low molecular weight portion (VIIIC), which promotes coagulation, linked to a large multimer known as von Willebrand factor (vWF). The larger vWF, under autosomal control, serves as a carrier for VIIIC, coded for on the X-chromosome. The complex is found in the circulation as polymers of varying size. vWF is the major protein in plasma which promotes platelet adhesion by forming a bridge between the subendothelial collagen and a specific receptor on the platelet membrane. Reduction in vWF usually leads to comparable decrease in VIIIC activity.

There are subgroups of von Willebrand's disease based on qualitative and quantitative changes in the multimers of the factor VIII complex (see Caldwell et al 1985).

Clinical features

Clinical manifestations of the disease are primarily those of a platelet defect, namely spontaneous mucous membrane or skin bleeding and prolonged bleeding following trauma or surgery. There are also manifestations of a coagulation defect due to VIIIC activity reduction. The most frequent problem encountered in the non-pregnant female is menorrhagia which may be quite severe. Patients with mild abnormalities may be asymptomatic and the diagnosis made only after excessive haemorrhage has followed trauma or related to surgery. The severity of the disorder does not run true within families and fluctuates from time to time in the same individual.

Treatment

Several treatments in von Willebrand's disease are in current use, the choice depending on the severity and type of the disease and on the clinical setting. The aim is to correct the platelet and coagulation disorder by achieving normal levels of factor VIII coagulant activity and a bleeding time within the normal range. The key feature in treatment is substitution with plasma concentrates containing functional von Willebrand's factor and VIIIC. In less severe cases the vasopressin analogue I-desamino-8-arginine-vasopressin (DDAVP) has been used with success. Contraceptive hormones have been used with success in the treatment of menorrhagia in von Willebrand's disease (Holmberg & Nilsson 1985). Aspirin and related anti-inflammatory drugs should not be used in von Willebrand's disease as they will further compromise platelet function.

The main treatment in von Willebrand's disease was replacement therapy with cryoprecipitate or FFP. The latter is efficient, but large volumes may be required to secure haemostasis. In obstetric practice, however, this does not usually cause any problems when covering delivery. Cryoprecipitate was the product of choice to cover cold surgery. Factor VIII concentrates were not used in the management of von Willebrand's disease because, in commercial preparations, the factor promoting platelet adhesion may be lost and because of the increased risk of transmitting infection. Newer preparations of factor VIII concentrate now retain some platelet promoting activity and have the added advantage of being heat-treated and therefore sterile. They now no longer carry the hazard of transmitting HIV and other viral infections. The use of cryoprecipitate and FFP is now contraindicated and cannot be recommended.

DDAVP has been shown to cause release of von Willebrand's factor from endothelial cells where it is synthesized and stored. It is particularly effective in mildly affected patients and may in some cases replace the use or need for blood products in patients undergoing surgery. Toxicity associated with use of this product has been trivial. Occasional patients experience flushing and dizziness (Holmberg & Nilsson 1985, Davison et al 1993). The theoretical risk of water intoxication and hyponatraemia due to a vasopressive effect has not been observed using the current dosage schedules. The recommended dose is an intravenous infusion of 0.3 µg/kg DDAVP given over 30 minutes up to a total dose of 15–25 µg. This may be repeated every 12–24 hours (Linkler 1986). In patients with severe von Willebrand's disease, DDAVP has no effect and replacement therapy must be used.

Von Willebrand's disease and pregnancy

A rise in both factor VIIIC and von Willebrand's factor is observed in normal pregnancy. Patients with all but the severest forms of von Willebrand's disease show a similar but variable rise in both these factors, although there may not be a reduction in the bleeding time (Caldwell et al 1985, Chediak et al 1986, Conti et al 1986, How et al 1991).

After delivery, normal women maintain an elevated factor VIIIC level for at least 5 days. This is followed by a slow fall to baseline levels over 4–6 weeks. The duration of factor VIII activity postpartum in women with von Willebrand's disease seems to be related to the severity of the disorder. Women with more severe forms of the condition may have a rapid fall in factor VIII procoagulant and platelet haemostatic activity. They are then at risk of quite severe secondary postpartum haemorrhage.

Published reports of 33 pregnancies in 22 women showed abnormal bleeding in 27% at the time of abortion, delivery or postpartum (Conti et al 1986). The general consensus is that the most important determinant for abnormal haemorrhage at delivery is a low factor VIIIC plasma level. The vast majority of women will have increased their factor VIIIC production to within the normal range (50–150%) by late gestation and although factor VIII concentrate should be standing by at delivery it will probably not be needed to achieve haemostasis (Milaskiewicz et al 1990).

While there is virtually no place for DDAVP in obstetric practice it is valuable in the management of women with von Willebrand's disease undergoing gynaecological surgery.

The haemophilias

The haemophilias are inherited disorders associated with reduced or absent coagulation factors VIII or IX with an incidence of around 1 in 10 000 in developed countries (Jones 1977). The most common is haemophilia A which is associated with deficiency of factor VIII; about one-sixth of the 3000–4000 cases in Britain today have a condition known as Christmas disease due to a lack of coagulation factor IX (haemophilia B). Clinical manifestations of the two conditions are indistinguishable; symptoms and signs are variable and depend on the degree of the lack of the coagulation factors concerned. Severe disease with frequent spontaneous bleeding (particularly haemarthroses) is associated with clotting factor levels of 0–1%. Less severe disease is found in subjects with clotting factors of 1–4%. Spontaneous bleeding and severe bleeding after minor trauma are rare even in cases with coagulation factor levels between 5% and 30%; the danger is that the condition may be clinically silent but during the course of major surgery or following trauma, such subjects behave as if with the severest forms of haemophilia. Unless the defect is recognized and replacement of the lacking coagulation factor replaced, such patients will continue to bleed. The inheritance of both haemophilias is X-linked—recessive—being expressed in the male and carried by the female.

The risks in pregnancy for a female carrier of haemophilia are twofold:

1. She may, by process of Lyonization, have a very low factor VIII or IX level which puts her at risk of excessive bleeding, particularly following a traumatic or surgical delivery.
2. Fifty per cent of her sons will inherit haemophilia and 50% of her daughters will be carriers like herself.

This has important implications now that prenatal diagnosis of these conditions is possible.

Management of haemophilia in pregnancy

On average female carriers of haemophilia do not have clinical manifestations but in rare individuals in whom the factor VIIIC or IX levels are unusually low (10–30% of normal), abnormal bleeding may occur after trauma or surgery (Luscher & McMillan 1978). It is important to identify carriers prior to pregnancy, not only to provide genetic counselling (Peake et al 1993) but so that appropriate provision can be made for those cases with pathologically low coagulation factor activity. Fortunately the level of the deficient factor tends to increase during the course of pregnancy, as in normal women. There have been anecdotal reports of female homozygotes for haemophilia A who have negotiated pregnancy successfully (Luscher & McMillan 1978). Haemorrhage postpartum does not appear to be a consistent feature, particularly if delivery is by the vaginal route at term with little or no soft-tissue damage. The effect of pregnancy on factor VIIIC levels in these rare cases has not been studied.

If the factor VIII level remains low in carriers of haemophilia, heat-treated factor VIII concentrates should be given to cover delivery.

DDAVP has been shown to be of benefit in patients with mild haemophilia, as with von Willebrand's disease (see above). However, the storage pools of factor VIII released during treatment may become exhausted and tachyphylaxis does occur (Linkler 1986). There are no controlled studies concerning the use of DDAVP during pregnancy and its safety and efficacy in obstetric practice remain to be determined.

The effects of DDAVP on uterine contractability could limit its use, although it has been employed in the management of diabetes insipidus in pregnancy with no harm to the fetus (Caldwell et al 1985). However, as pointed out previously, if the stimulus of pregnancy has not raised the level of factor VIII as expected in mild haemophilia, it is unlikely that DDAVP will do so.

A clinical problem is more likely in carriers of factor IX deficiency (Christmas disease) than in women with factor VIII deficiency (Luscher & McMillan 1978, Levin 1982). In the exceptionally rare situations where factor IX level is very low and remains low during pregnancy, the patient should be managed with high purity factor IX concentrates to cover delivery and for 3–4 days postpartum. Low purity factor IX concentrates (prothrombin concentrate) contain factors II, VII and X, as well as factor IX, and therefore carry a much greater thrombogenic hazard adding to the innate risk of thromboembolism in pregnancy. Fresh frozen plasma will carry the remote hazard (in the UK) of transmitting HIV infection (Acheson 1987). The produce of choice is therefore high purity factor IX concentrate. These patients should be managed in a unit with access to expert advice, 24-hour laboratory coagulation service and immediate access to the appropriate plasma components required for replacement therapy.

Factor XI deficiency (plasma thromboplastin antecedent (PTA) deficiency)   This is a rare coagulation disorder which is less common than the haemophilias but more common than the very rare inherited deficiencies of the remaining coagulation factors. It is inherited as an autosomal recessive, predominantly in Ashkenazi Jews and both men and women may be affected. Usually only the homozygotes have clinical evidence of a coagulation disorder, though occasionally carriers may have a bleeding tendency. It is a mild condition in which spontaneous haemorrhages and haemarthroses are rare but the danger lies in the fact that profuse bleeding may follow major trauma or surgery if no prophylactic factor XI concentrate is given. Indeed it is often diagnosed late in life following surgery in an individual who was unaware of a serious haemostatic defect. The diagnosis is made by finding a prolonged partial thromboplastin time, with a low factor XI level in a coagulation assay system but in which all other coagulation tests are normal. Management consists of replacement with factor XI concentrates as prophylaxis for surgery or to treat bleeding and to cover operative delivery.

The effective haemostatic level of factor XI has a half-life of around 2 days. To cover surgery or delivery women can be treated with one infusion of factor XI concentrate to raise the level to 80–100% and until primary healing is established.

Fortunately the condition rarely causes problems either during pregnancy and labour or in the child; in particular, prolonged bleeding at ritual circumcision is not usual. There is therefore, no justification in screening routinely for this condition in the mother, fetus or neonate.

Genetic disorders of fibrinogen (factor I) Fibrinogen is synthesized in the liver, has a molecular weight of 340 000 and circulates in plasma at a concentration of 300 mg/dl. Both quantitative and qualitative genetic abnormalities are described.

Afibrinogenaemia or hypofibrinogenaemia These are rare autosomal recessive disorders resulting from reduced fibrinogen synthesis. Most patients with hypofibrinogenaemia are heterozygous.

Congenital hypofibrinogenaemia has been associated with recurrent early miscarriages and with recurrent placental abruption (Ness et al 1983).

Afibrinogenaemia is characterized by a lifelong bleeding tendency of variable severity. Prolonged bleeding after minor injury and easy bruising are frequent symptoms. Menorrhagia can be very severe. Spontaneous deep tissue bleeding and haemarthroses are rare, but severe bleeding can occur after trauma or surgery and several patients have suffered intracerebral haemorrhages. In afibrinogenaemia all screening tests of coagulation are prolonged, but corrected by addition of normal plasma or fibrinogen. A prolonged bleeding time may be present. The final diagnosis is made by quantitating the concentration of circulating fibrinogen.

There are no fibrinogen concentrates available and plasma or cryoprecipitate have to be used as replacement therapy to treat bleeding, cover surgery or delivery. The in vivo half-life of fibrinogen is between 3 and 5 days. Initial replacement should be achieved with 25 ml plasma/kg and daily maintenance with 5–10 ml/kg for 7 days.

Dysfibrinogenaemia Congenital dysfibrinogenaemia is an autosomal dominant disorder. In contrast to patients with afibrinogenaemia, patients with this disorder are often symptom-free. Some have a bleeding tendency; others have been shown to have thromboembolic disease. The diagnosis is made by demonstrating a prolonged thrombin time with a normal immunological fibrinogen level.

Affected women like those with hypofibrinogenaemia may have recurrent spontaneous abortion or repeated placental abruption (Ness et al 1983).

Factor XIII deficiency (fibrin-stabilizing factor deficiency)

This is an autosomal recessive disorder classically characterized by bleeding from the umbilical cord during the first few days of life and later by ecchymoses, prolonged post-traumatic haemorrhage and poor wound healing. Bleeding is usually delayed and characteristically of a slow oozing nature. Cases of intracranial haemorrhage have been described in a significant proportion of reported cases. Spontaneous recurrent abortion with excessive bleeding occurs in association with factor XIII deficiency (Kitchens & Newcomb 1979). All standard coagulation tests are normal. Diagnosis of severe factor XIII deficiency is made by the clot solubility test. Normal fibrin clots will not dissolve when incubated overnight in 5 mol/l urea solutions, whereas the unstable clots formed in the absence of factor XIII will be dissolved.

Since factor XIII has a half-life of 6 days to 2 weeks and only 5% of normal factor XIII levels is needed for effective haemostasis, patients can be treated with FFP in doses of 5 ml/kg repeated every 3 weeks. Using this therapy, pregnancy has progressed safely to term in a woman who had previously suffered repeated abortions. Because of the high incidence of intracranial haemorrhage, replacement therapy is recommended for all individuals known to have factor XIII deficiency (Kitchens & Newcomb 1979).

Other plasma factor disorders Congenital deficiencies of factors II, V, VII and X are extremely rare and the reader is referred to Caldwell et al's review of hereditary coagulopathies in pregnancy for an account of their diagnosis and special management problems (Caldwell et al 1985).

REFERENCES

Acheson D 1987 Department of Health and Social Security press release 87/5

Ahmed Y, Sullivan M H, Pearce J M et al 1991 Changes in platelet function in pregnancies complicated by fetal growth retardation. European Journal of Obstetrics, Gynecology and Reproductive Biology 42: 171–175

Alving B M, Comp P C 1992 Recent advances in understanding clotting and evaluating patients with recurrent thrombosis. American Journal of Obstetrics and Gynecology 167(4 Pt 2): 1184–1191

Asada Y, Sumiyoshi A, Hayashi T et al 1985 Immunohistochemistry of vascular lesion in TTP with special reference to factor VIII related antigen. Thrombosis Research 38: 469–479

Astedt B, Nilsson I M 1978 Recurrent abruptio placentae treated with the fibrinolytic inhibitor tranexamic acid. British Medical Journal 1: 756–757

Aster R H 1985 Plasma therapy for thrombotic thrombocytopenic purpura. New England Journal of Medicine 312: 985–987

Aster R H 1990 'Gestational' thrombocytopenia: a plea for conservative management. New England Journal of Medicine 323: 264–266

Ayromlooi J 1978 A new approach to the management of immunologic thrombocytopenic purpura in pregnancy. American Journal of Obstetrics and Gynecology 130: 235–236

Aznar J, Gilabert J, Estelles A, Fernandez M A, Villa P, Aznar J A 1982 Evaluation of the soluble fibrin monomer complexes and other coagulation parameters in obstetric patients. Thrombosis Research 27: 691–701

Ballegeer V C, Mombaerts P, Declerck P J et al 1987 Fibrinolytic response to venous occlusion and fibrin fragment D-dimer levels in normal and complicated pregnancy. Thrombosis and Haemostasis 58: 1030–1032

Ballegeer V C, Spitz B, De Baene L A et al 1992 Platelet activation and vascular damage in gestational hypertension. American Journal of Obstetrics and Gynecology 166: 629–633

Basu H K 1969 Fibrinolysis and abruptio placentae. Journal of Obstetrics and Gynaecology of the British Commonwealth 76: 481–496

Beal D W, de Masi A D 1985 Role of the platelet count in the management of the high-risk obstetric patient. Journal of the American Osteopathic Association 85: 252–255

Bell W R 1977 Hematologic abnormalities in pregnancy. Medical Clinics of North America 61: 1–165

Bell W R, Braine H G, Ness P M et al 1991 Improved survival in thrombotic thrombocytopenic purpura-hemolytic uremic syndrome. New England Journal of Medicine 325: 398–403

Beller F K 1985 Sepsis and coagulation. Clinical Obstetrics and Gynecology 28: 46–52

Beller F K, Uszynski M 1974 Disseminated intravascular coagulation in pregnancy. Clinical Obstetrics and Gynecology 17: 264–278

Bertina R M, Briet E, Engesser L et al 1988 Protein C deficiency and the risk of venous thrombosis. New England Journal of Medicine 318: 930–931

Bettaieb A, Fromont P, Louache F et al 1992 Presence of cross-reactive antibody between human immunodeficiency virus (HIV) and platelet glycoproteins in HIV-related immune thrombocytopenic purpura. Blood 80: 162–169

Bidstrup B P, Royston D, Sapsford R N et al 1989 Reduction in blood loss and blood use after cardiopulmonary bypass with high dose aprotinin (Trasylol). Journal of Thoracic and Cardiovascular Surgery 97: 364–372

Blasczyk R, Westhoff U, Grosse-Wilde H 1993 Soluble CD4, CD8, and HLA molecules in commercial immunoglobulin preparations. Lancet 341: 789–790

Bonnar J 1973 Blood coagulation and fibrinolysis in obstetrics. Clinics in Haematology 2: 213–233

Bonnar J 1978 Haemorrhagic disorders during pregnancy in perinatal coagulation. In: Hathaway W E, Bonnar J (eds) Monographs in neonatology. Grune & Stratton, New York

Bonnar J 1987 Haemostasis and coagulation disorders in pregnancy. In: Bloom A L, Thomas D P (eds) Haemostasis and thrombosis, 2nd edn. Churchill Livingstone, Edinburgh, pp 570–584

Bonnar J, Prentice C R M, McNicol G P, Douglas A S 1970 Haemostatic mechanism in uterine circulation during placental separation. British Medical Journal 2: 564–567

Booth N A, Reith A, Bennett B 1988 A plasminogen activator inhibitor (PA1–2) circulates in two molecular forms during pregnancy. Thrombosis and Haemostasis 59: 77–79

Borok Z, Weitz J, Owen J et al 1984 Fibrinogen proteolysis and platelet α-granule release in pre-eclampsia/eclampsia. Blood 63: 525–531

Burkman R T, Bell W R, Atizenza M F, King T M 1977 Coagulopathy with midtrimester induced abortion. Association with hyperosmolar urea administration. American Journal of Obstetrics and Gynecology 127: 533–536

Burroughs A K, Seong N G, Dojcinoov D M, Scheuer P J, Sherlock S V P 1982 Idiopathic acute fatty liver of pregnancy in 12 patients. Quarterly Journal of Medicine 51: 481–497

Burrows R F, Kelton J G 1988 Incidentally detected thrombocytopenia in healthy mothers and their infants. New England Journal of Medicine 319: 142

Burrows R F, Kelton J G 1990a Thrombocytopenia at delivery: a prospective survey of 6715 deliveries. American Journal of Obstetrics and Gynaecology 162: 731–734

Burrows R F, Kelton J G 1990b Low fetal risks in pregnancies associated with idiopathic thrombocytopenic purpura. American Journal of Obstetrics and Gynecology 163: 1147–1150

Burrows R F, Kelton J G 1992 Thrombocytopenia during pregnancy. In: Greer I A, Turpie A G, Forbes C D (eds) Obstetrics and gynaecology. Chapman and Hall, London, pp 407–429

Bussel J B, Berkowitz R L, McFarland J G, Lynch L, Chitkara U 1988 Antenatal treatment of neonatal alloimmune thrombocytopenia. New England Journal of Medicine 319: 1374–1378

Caires D, Arocha-Pinango C L, Rodriguez S, Linares J 1984 Factor VIII R : Ag/Factor VIII : C and their ratio in obstetrical cases. Acta Obstetricia et Gynecologica Scandinavica 63: 411–416

Caldwell D C, Williamson R A, Goldsmith J C 1985 Hereditary coagulopathies in pregnancy. Clinical Obstetrics and Gynecology 28: 53–72

Carey L C, Cloutier C T, Lowery B D 1970 The use of balanced electrolyte solution for resuscitation. In: Fox Nahas (ed) Body fluid replacement in the surgical patient. Grune & Stratton, New York

Carloss H W, McMillan R, Crosby W H 1980 Management of pregnancy in women with immune thrombocytopenia purpura. Journal of the American Medical Association 244: 2756–2758

Cates W Jr, Boyd C, Halvorson-Boyd G I, Holck S, Gilchrist T F 1981 Death from amniotic fluid embolism and disseminated intravascular coagulation after a curettage abortion. American Journal of Obstetrics and Gynecology 141: 346–348

Channing Rodgers R P, Levin J 1990 A critical reappraisal of the bleeding time. Seminars in Thrombosis and Hemostasis 16: 1–19

Chediak J R, Alban G M, Maxey B 1986 Von Willebrand's disease and pregnancy: management during delivery and outcome of offspring. American Journal of Obstetrics and Gynecology 155: 618–624

Chung A F, Merkatz I R 1973 Survival following amniotic fluid embolism with early heparinization. Obstetrics and Gynecology 42: 809–814

Cines D B, Schreiber A D 1979 Immune thrombocytopenia: use of a Coombs' antiglobulin test to detect IgG and C3 on platelets. New England Journal of Medicine 300: 106–111

Clark S L, Pavlova Z, Greenspoon J, Hortenstein J, Phelan J P 1986 Squamous cells in the maternal pulmonary circulation. American Journal of Obstetrics and Gynecology 154: 104–106

Clarkson A R, Sage R E, Lawrence J R 1969 Consumption coagulopathy and acute renal failure due to Gram negative septicaemia after abortion. Complete recovery with heparin therapy. Annals of Internal Medicine 70: 1191–1199

Cohen E, Ballard C A 1974 Consumptive coagulopathy associated with intra-amniotic saline instillation and the effect of intravenous oxytocin. Obstetrics and Gynecology 43: 300–303

Coller B S, Hultin M B, Homer L W et al 1981 Normal pregnancy in a patient with a prior post-partum factor VIII inhibitor: with observations on pathogenesis and prognosis. Blood 58: 619–624

Collier C B, Birrell W R S 1983 Chronic ectopic pregnancy complicated by shock and disseminated intravascular coagulation. Anaesthesia in Intensive Care II: 246–248

Colvin B T 1985 Thrombocytopenia. Clinics in Haematology 14: 661–681

Comp P C, Thurnau G R, Welsh J, Esmon C T 1986 Functional and immunologic protein S levels are decreased during pregnancy. Blood 68: 881–885

Conti M, Mari D, Conti E, Muggiasca M L, Mannuci P M 1986 Pregnancy in women with different types of von Willebrand disease. Obstetrics and Gynecology 68: 282–285

Costello C 1988 Haematological abnormalities in human immunodeficiency virus (HIV) disease. Journal of Clinical Pathology 41: 711–715

Courtney L D, Allington M 1972 Effect of amniotic fluid on blood coagulation. British Journal of Haematology 29: 353–356

Creasy G W, Morgan J 1987 Haemolytic uremic syndrome after ectopic pregnancy: post ectopic nephrosclerosis. Obstetrics and Gynecology 60: 448–449

Daffos F, Forestier F, Kaplan C et al 1988 Prenatal diagnosis and management of bleeding disorders with fetal blood sampling. American Journal of Obstetrics and Gynecology 158: 939–946

Davies M H et al 1980 Acute liver disease with encephalopathy and renal failure in late pregnancy and the early puerperium. A study of 14 patients. British Journal of Obstetrics and Gynaecology 87: 1003–1014

Davis G 1972 Midtrimester abortion. Late dilation and evacuation and DIC. Lancet ii: 1026

Department of Health 1991 Report on Confidential Enquiries into Maternal Deaths in the United Kingdom 1985–1987. HMSO, London, pp 37–45

Department of Health 1994 Report on Confidential Enquiries into Maternal Deaths in the United Kingdom 1988–1990. HMSO, London

Department of Health and Social Security 1986 Report on Confidential Enquiries into Maternal Deaths in England and Wales 1979–81. Report on Health and Social Services no. 29. HMSO

de Swiet M 1985 Some rare medical complications of pregnancy. British Medical Journal 290: 2–4

De Vries L S, Connell J, Bydder G M et al 1988 Recurrent intracranial haemorrhages in utero in an infant with allo-immune thrombocytopenia. British Journal of Obstetrics and Gynaecology 95: 299–302

Doenicke A, Grote B, Lorenz W 1977 Blood and blood substitutes in management of the injured patient. British Journal of Anaesthesia 49: 681–688

Dwyer J M 1992 Manipulating the immune system with immune globulin. New England Journal of Medicine 326: 107–116

Edgar W, McKillop C, Howie P W 1977 Composition of soluble fibrin complexes in pre-eclampsia. Thrombosis Research 10: 567–574

Estelles A, Aznar J, Gilabert J 1980 A quantitative study of soluble fibrin monomer complexes in normal labour and abruptio placentae. Thrombosis Research 18: 513–519

Estelles A, Gilabert J, Espana F et al 1987 Fibrinolysis in pre-eclampsia. Fibrinolysis 1: 209–214

Evans R S, Takahashi K, Duane R T et al 1951 Primary thrombocytopenic purpura and acquired hemolytic anemia: evidence for a common etiology. Archives of Internal Medicine 87: 48–65

Fay R A, Hughes A D, Farron N T 1983 Platelets in pregnancy: hyperdestruction in pregnancy. Obstetrics and Gynecology 61: 238–240

Feinstein D I 1982 Diagnosis and management of disseminated intravascular coagulation: the role of heparin therapy. Blood 60: 284–287

Fenton V, Saunders K, Cavill I 1977 The platelet count in pregnancy. Journal of Clinical Pathology 30: 68–69

Forbes C D, Greer I A 1992 Physiology of haemostasis and the effect of pregnancy. In: Greer I A, Turpie A G G, Forbes C D (eds) Haemostasis and thrombosis in obstetrics and gynaecology. Chapman and Hall, London, pp 1–25

Forsyth K D, Simpson A C, Fitzpatrick M M et al 1989 Neutrophil mediated endothelial injury in HUS. Lancet ii: 411–414

Fournie A, Monrozies M, Pontonnier G, Boneu B, Bierne R 1981 Factor VIII complex in normal pregnancy, pre-eclampsia and fetal growth retardation. British Journal of Obstetrics and Gynaecology 88: 250–254

Freeman M 1979 Fatal reaction of Haemaccel. Anaesthesia 34: 341–343

Gilabert J, Aznar J, Parilla J, Reganon E, Vila V, Estelles A 1978 Alteration in the coagulation and fibrinolysis system in pregnancy, labour and puerperium, with special reference to a possible transitory state of intravascular coagulation during labour. Thrombosis and Haemostasis 40: 387–396

Gilabert J, Estelles A, Aznar J, Galbis M 1985 Abruptio placentae and disseminated intravascular coagulation. Acta Obstetricia et Gynecologica Scandinavica 64: 35–39

Goodlin R C 1984 Acute fatty liver of pregnancy. Acta Obstetricia et Gynecologica Scandinavica 63: 379–380

Graeff H, Ernst E, Bocaz J A 1978 Evaluation of hypercoagulability in septic abortion. Haemostasis 5: 285–294

Gregory M G, Clayton E M J 1973 Amniotic fluid embolism. Obstetrics and Gynecology 42: 236–244

Grundy M F B, Graven E R 1976 Consumption coagulopathy after intra-amniotic urea. British Medical Journal 2: 677–678

Guidotti R J, Grimes D A, Cates W Jr 1981 Fatal amniotic fluid embolism during legally induced abortion. United States, 1972–1978. American Journal of Obstetrics and Gynecology 141: 257–261

Hafter R, Graeff H 1975 Molecular aspects of defibrination in a reptilase treated case of 'dead fetus syndrome'. Thrombosis Research 7: 391–399

Hague W M, Fenton D W, Duncan S L B, Slater D N 1983 Acute fatty liver of pregnancy. Journal of the Royal Society of Medicine 76: 652–661

Harrington W J 1987 Are platelet-antibody tests worthwhile? New England Journal of Medicine 316: 211–212

Harrington W J, Sprague C C, Minnich V et al 1952 Immunologic mechanisms in idopathic and neonatal thrombocytopenic purpura. Annals of Internal Medicine 38: 433–469

Hart D, Dunetz C, Nardi M et al 1986 An epidemic of maternal thrombocytopenia associated with elevated antiplatelet antibody: platelet count and antiplatelet antibody in 116 consecutive pregnancies: relationship to neonatal platelet count. American Journal of Obstetrics and Gynecology 154: 878–883

Hauser C J, Shoemaker W C, Turpin I, Goldberg S J 1980 Oxygen transport responses to colloids and crystalloids in critically ill surgical patients. Surgica Gynecologica Obstetrica 159: 181–186

Hegde U M 1985 Immune thrombocytopenia in pregnancy and the newborn. British Journal of Obstetrics and Gynaecology 92: 657–659

Hegde U M 1987 Immune thrombocytopenia in pregnancy and the newborn: a review. Journal of Infection 15: 55–58

Hegde U M, Gordon-Smith E C, Worrlledge S M 1977 Platelet antibodies in thrombocytopenic patients. British Journal of Haematology 56: 191–197

Hegde U M, Ball S, Zuiable A et al 1985 Platelet associated immunoglobulins (PAIgG and PAIgM) in autoimmune thrombocytopenia. British Journal of Haematology 59: 221–226

Hellgren M, Blomback M 1981 Blood coagulation and fibrinolysis in pregnancy, during delivery and in the puerperium. Gynecologic Obstetric Investigation 12: 141–154

Hellgren M, Svensson P J, Dahlbäck B 1995 Resistance to activated protein C as a basis for venous thromboembolism associated with pregnancy and oral contraceptives. American Journal of Obstetrics and Gynecology (in press)

Herbert W N P 1982 Complications of the immediate puerperium. Clinical Obstetrics and Gynecology 25: 219–232

Hodgkinson C R, Thompson R J, Hodari A A 1964 Dead fetus syndrome. Clinics in Obstetrics and Gynaecology 7: 349–35

Holmberg L, Nilsson I M. 1985 Von Willebrand disease. In: Ruggeri A M (ed) Coagulation disorders. Clinics in Haematology 14: 461–488

How H Y, Bergmann F, Koshy M et al 1991 Quantitative and qualitative platelet abnormalities during pregnancy. American Journal of Obstetrics and Gynecology 164(1 Pt 1): 92–98

Hughes G R V 1979 Systemic lupus erythematosus in connective tissue diseases. Blackwell Scientific Publications, Oxford

Hughes G R V 1987 Systemic lupus erythematosus. In: Hughes G R V (ed) Connective tissue diseases, 3rd edn. Blackwell Scientific Publications, Oxford, pp 3–71

Jones P 1977 Developments and problems in the management of haemophilia. Seminars in Haematology 14: 375–390

Kaplan C et al 1988 Management of alloimmune thrombocytopenia: antenatal diagnosis and in utero transfusion of maternal platelets. Blood 72: 340–343

Kaplan C, Daffos F, Forestier F et al 1990 Fetal platelet counts in thrombocytopenic pregnancy. Lancet 336: 979–982

Kelton J G 1983 Management of the pregnant patient with idiopathic thrombocytopenic purpura. Annals of Internal Medicine 99: 796–800

Kessler I, Lancet M, Borenstein R et al 1982 The obstetrical management of patients with immunologic thrombocytopenic purpura. International Journal of Gynaecology and Obstetrics 20: 23–28

Kitchens C S, Newcomb T F 1979 Factor XIII. Medicine 58: 413–429

Kouri Y H, Basch R S, Karpatkin S 1992 B-cell subsets and platelet counts in HIV-1 seropositive subjects. Lancet 339: 1445–1446

Lammle B, Griffin J H 1985 Formation of the fibrin clot: the balance of procoagulant and inhibitory factors. In: Ruggeri Z M (ed) Coagulation disorders. WB Saunders, London, pp 281–342

Lancet Editorial 1983 Acute fatty liver of pregnancy. Lancet i: 339

Laursen B, Mortensen J Z, Frost L, Hansen K B 1981 Disseminated intravascular coagulation in hepatic failure treated with antithrombin III. Thrombosis Research 22: 701–704

Laursen B, Frost L, Mortensen J Z, Hansen K B, Paulsen S M 1983 Acute fatty liver of pregnancy with complicating disseminated intravascular coagulation. Acta Obstetricia et Gynecologica Scandinavica 62: 403–407

Lavery J P, Koontz W L, Liu Y K, Howell R 1985 Immunologic thrombocytopenia in pregnancy: use of antenatal immunoglobulin therapy: case report and review. Obstetrics and Gynecology 66: 41S–43S

Leduc L, Wheeler J M, Kirshon B et al 1992 Coagulation profile in severe pre-eclampsia. Obstetrics and Gynecology 79: 14–18

Letsky E A 1985 Coagulation problems during pregnancy. Current Reviews in Obstetrics and Gynaecology, vol 10. Churchill Livingstone, Edinburgh, pp 1–133

Letsky E A 1987 Disseminated intravascular coagulation. In: Morgan B (ed) Problems in obstetric anaesthesia. Wiley, Chichester, pp 69–87

Letsky E A 1991a Mechanisms of coagulation and the changes induced by pregnancy. Current Obstetrics and Gynaecology 1: 203–209

Letsky E A 1991b Haemostasis and epidural anaesthesia. International Journal of Obstetrics and Anesthesia 1: 51–54

Letsky E A 1992 Management of massive haemorrhage—the haematologists role. In: Patel N (ed) Maternal mortality—the way forward. Royal College of Obstetricians and Gynaecologists, London, pp 63–71

Levin J 1982 Disorders of blood coagulation and platelets. In: Barrow G N, Ferris T F (eds) Medical complications during pregnancy, 2nd edn. WB Saunders, London, pp 70–73

Levine A B, Berkowitz R L 1991 Neonatal alloimmune thrombocytopenia, Seminars in Perinatology 15(3,2): 35–40

Lewis P J 1982 The role of prostacyclin in pre-eclampsia. British Journal of Hospital Medicine 62: 1048–1052

Lewis P J, Boylan P, Friedman L A, Hensman C N, Downing I 1980 Prostacyclin in pregnancy. British Medical Journal 280: 1581–1582

Lin K C, Chou T C, Yin C S et al 1991 The role of aggregation of platelets in pregnancy-induced hypertension: a comprehensive and longitudinal study. International Journal of Cardiology 33: 125–131

Lind S E 1991 The bleeding time does not predict surgical bleeding. Blood 77: 2547–2552

Linkler C A 1986 Congenital disorders of haemostasis. In: Laros R K (ed) Blood disorders in pregnancy. Lea & Febiger, Philadelphia, p 160

Lorenz W, Doenicke A, Messmer K et al 1976 Histamine release in human subjects by modified gelatin (Haemaccel) and dextran: an explanation for anaphylactoid reactions observed under clinical conditions. British Journal of Anaesthesia 48: 151–165

Lucher J M, McMillan C W 1978 Severe factor VIII and IX deficiency in females. American Journal of Medicine 65: 637–648

Lynch L, Bussel J B, McFarland J G, Chitkara V, Berkowitz R L 1992 Antenatal treatment of alloimmune thrombocytopenia. Obstetrics and Gynecology 80: 67–71

Machin S J 1984 Thrombotic thrombocytopenic purpura. British Journal of Haematology 56: 191–197

Machin S J, Defrey N G, Vermylen J, Willoughby M L N 1981 Prostacyclin deficiency in thrombotic thrombocytopenic purpura (TTP) and the haemolytic uraemic syndrome (HUS). British Journal of Haematology 49: 141–142

MacKenzie I Z, Sayers L, Bonnar J et al 1975 Coagulation changes during second trimester abortion induced by intra-amniotic prostaglandin E_{2+} and hypertonic solutions. Lancet ii: 1066–1069

Malm J, Laurell M, Dahlback B 1988 Changes in the plasma levels of vitamin K-dependent proteins C and S and of C4b-binding proteins during pregnancy and oral contraception. British Journal of Haematology 68: 437–443

Marengo Rowe A J, Murff G, Leveson J E, Cook J 1972 Haemophilia-like disease associated with pregnancy. Obstetrics and Gynecology 40: 56–64

Marshall M, Bird T 1983 Blood loss and replacement. Edward Arnold, London

Martin J N, Morrison J C, Files J C 1984 Autoimmune thrombocytopenia purpura: current concepts and recommended practices. American Journal of Obstetrics and Gynecology 150: 86–96

McGibbon D H 1982 Dermatological purpura. In: Ingram G I C, Brozovic M, Slater N G P (eds) Bleeding disorders—investigation and management. Blackwell Scientific Publications, Oxford

McMillan R 1981 Chronic idiopathic thrombocytopenic purpura. New England Journal of Medicine 304: 1135–1147

Meier P R, Bowes W A 1983 Amniotic fluid embolus-like syndrome presenting in the second trimester of pregnancy. Obstetrics and Gynecology 61(suppl 3): 31S–34S

Milaskiewicz R M, Holdcroft A, Letsky E A 1990 Epidural anaesthesia and von Willebrand's disease. Anaesthesia 45: 462–464

Moake J L 1991 TTP—desperation, empiricism, progress. New England Journal of Medicine 325: 426–428

Moake J L, Byrnes J J, Troll J H et al 1985 Effects of fresh-frozen plasma and its cryosupernatant fraction on von Willebrand factor multimeric forms in chronic relapsing thrombotic thrombocytopenic purpura. Blood 65: 1232–1236

Moake J L, Rudy C K, Troll J H et al 1982 Unusually large plasma factor VIII: vWF multimers in chronic relapsing TTP. New England Journal of Medicine 307: 1432–1435

Moise K J, Carpenter R J, Cotton D B et al 1988 Percutaneous umbilical cord sampling in the evaluation of fetal platelet counts in pregnant patients with autoimmune thrombocytopenia purpura. Obstetrics and Gynecology 72: 346–350

Moncada M D, Vane J R 1979 Arachidonic acid metabolites and the interactions between platelets and blood-vessel walls. New England Journal of Medicine 300: 1142–1147

Moore J C, Murphy W G, Kelton J G 1990 Calpain proteolysis of vWF enhances its binding to platelet membrane glycoprotein IIbIIIa: an explanation for platelet aggregation in TTP. British Journal of Haematology 74: 457–464

Morgan M 1979 Amniotic fluid embolism. Anaesthesia 34: 20–32

Morgenstern G R, Measday B, Hegde U M 1983 Auto-immune thrombocytopenia in pregnancy. New approach to management. British Medical Journal 287: 584

Moss G 1972 An argument in favour of electrolyte solutions for early resuscitation. Surgical Clinics of North America 52: 3–17

Mueller-Ekhardt C, Kayser W, Mersh-Baument K et al 1980 The clinical significance of platelet-associated IgG: a study on 298 patients with various disorders. British Journal of Haematology 46: 123–131

Murray J M, Harris R E 1976 The management of the pregnant patient with idiopathic thrombocytopenic purpura. American Journal of Obstetrics and Gynecology 126: 449–451

Naumann R O, Weinstein L 1985 Disseminated intravascular coagulation—the clinician's dilemma. Obstetrical and Gynecological Survey 40: 487–492

Ness P M, Budzynski A Z, Olexa S A et al 1983 Congenital hypofibrinogenemia and recurrent placental abruption. Obstetrics and Gynecology 61: 519–523

Nicolaides K H, Rodeck C H, Mibasham R S 1985 Obstetric management and diagnosis of haematological disease in the fetus. In: Letsky E A (ed) Haematological disorders in pregnancy. Clinical Haematology 14: 775–804

Nicolini U, Tannirandorn Y, Gonzales P et al 1990 Continuing controversy in alloimmune thrombocytopenia; fetal hypergammaglobulinemia fails to prevent thrombocytopenia. American Journal of Obstetrics and Gynecology 163: 1144–1146

O'Brien J R 1954 An acquired coagulation defect in a woman. Journal of Clinical Pathology 7: 22–25

O'Brien W F, Saba H I, Knuppel R A, Scerbo J C, Cohen G R 1986 Alterations in platelet concentration and aggregation in normal pregnancy and pre-eclampsia. American Journal of Obstetrics and Gynecology 155: 486–490

Page Y, Tardy B, Zeni F et al 1991 Thrombotic thrombocytopenic purpura related to ticlopidine. Lancet 337: 774–776

Pappas C 1986 Placental transfer of immunoglobulins in immune thrombocytopenic purpura. Lancet i: 389

Peaceman A M, Katz A R, Laville M 1989 Bernard–Soulier syndrome complicating pregnancy. A case report. Obstetrics and Gynecology 73: 457–459

Peake I R, Lilleycrap D P, Boulyjenkov V et al 1993 Report of a joint WHO/WFH meeting on the control of haemophilia: carrier detection and prenatal diagnosis. Blood Coagulation and Fibrinolysis 4: 313–344

Phillips L P 1984 Transfusion support in acquired coagulation disorders. Clinics in Haematology 13: 137–150

Pillai M 1993 Platelets and pregnancy. British Journal of Obstetrics and Gynaecology 100: 201–204

Pinette M G, Vintzileos A M, Ingardia C J 1989 Thrombotic thrombocytopenia purpura as a cause of thrombocytopenia in pregnancy: literature review. American Journal of Perinatology 6: 55–57

Pritchard J A 1959 Fetal death in utero. Obstetrics and Gynecology 14: 573–580

Pritchard J A 1973 Haematological problems associated with delivery, placenta abruption, retained dead fetus and amniotic fluid embolism. Clinics in Haematology 2: 563–580

Pritchard J A, Brekken A L 1967 Clinical and laboratory studies on severe abruptio placentae. American Journal of Obstetrics and Gynecology 57: 681–695

Pritchard J A, Cunningham F G, Pritchard S A et al 1991 On reducing the frequency of severe abruptio placentae. American Journal of Obstetrics and Gynecology 165(5 Pt 1): 1345–1351

Rakoczi I, Tallian F, Bagdan Y S, Gati I 1979 Platelet lifespan in normal pregnancy and pre-eclampsia as determined by a non-radioisotope technique. Thrombosis Research 15: 553–556

Redman C W G 1979 Coagulation problems in human pregnancy. Postgraduate Medical Journal 55: 367–371

Redman C W, Denson K W, Beilin L J et al 1977 Factor VIII consumption in pre-eclampsia. Lancet ii: 1249–1259

Redman C W G, Bonnar J, Bellin C 1978 Early platelet consumption in pre-eclampsia. British Medical Journal 1: 467–469

Reece A, Fox H E, Rapoport F 1982 Factor VIII inhibitor: a cause of severe postpartum haemorrhage. American Journal of Obstetrics and Gynecology 144: 985–987

Resnik R, Swartz W H, Plumer M H I, Bernirske K, Stratthaus M E 1976 Amniotic fluid embolism with survival. Obstetrics and Gynecology 47: 395–398

Richter A W, Hedin H I 1982 Dextran hypersensitivity. Immunology Today 3: 132–138

Rock G A, Shumack K H, Buskard N A et al 1991 Canadian Apheresis Study Group. Comparison of plasma exchange with plasma infusion in the treatment of thrombotic thrombocytopenic purpura. New England Journal of Medicine 325: 393–397

Romero R, Duffy T P 1980 Platelet disorders in pregnancy. Clinics in Perinatology 7: 327–348

Romero R, Copel J A, Hobbins J C 1985 Intrauterine fetal demise and hemostatic failure: the fetal death syndrome. Clinical Obstetrics and Gynecology 28: 24–31

Romero R, Duffy T, Berkowitz R L, Change E, Hobbins J C 1986 Prolongation of a preterm pregnancy complicated by death of a single twin in utero and disseminated intravascular coagulation. New England Journal of Medicine 310: 772–774

Romero R, Mazor M, Lockwood C J et al 1989 Clinical significance, prevalence and natural history of thrombocytopenia in pregnancy-induced hypertension. American Journal of Perinatology 6: 32–38

Rushton D I, Dawson I M P 1982 The maternal autopsy. Journal of Clinical Pathology 350: 909–921

Salem H H 1986 The natural anticoagulants: In: Chesterman C N (ed) Thrombosis and the vessel wall. Clinics in Haematology 15: 371–391

Samuels P, Bussel J B, Braitman L E et al 1990 Estimation of the risk of thrombocytopenia in the offspring of pregnant women with presumed immune thrombocytopenic purpura. New England Journal of Medicine 323: 229–235

Savage W 1982 Abortion: methods and sequelae. British Journal of Hospital Medicine 27: 364–384

Schultz J, Adamson J, Workman W, Norman T 1983 Fatal liver disease after intravenous administration of tetracycline in a high dose. New England Journal of Medicine 269: 999–1004

Scioscia A L, Grannum P A T, Copel J A et al 1988 The use of percutaneous umbilical blood sampling in immune thrombocytopenia purpura. American Journal of Obstetrics and Gynecology 159: 1066–1068

Scott J R, Cruickshank D P, Kochenou R M D, Pitkin R M, Warenski J C 1980 Fetal platelet counts in the obstetric management of immunologic thrombocytopenia purpura. American Journal of Obstetrics Gynecology 136: 495–499

Seligsohn U, Berger A, Abend M et al 1984 Homozygous protein C deficiency manifested by massive venous thrombosis in the newborn. New England Journal of Medicine 310: 559–562

Shaper A G, Kear J, MacIntosh D M, Kyobe J, Njama D 1968 The platelet count, platelet adhesiveness and aggregation and the mechanism of fibrinolytic inhibition in pregnancy and the puerperium. Journal of Obstetrics and Gynaecology of the British Commonwealth 75: 433–441

Sharp A A 1977 Diagnosis and management of disseminated intravascular coagulation. British Medical Bulletin 33: 265–272

Sheehan H 1940 The pathology of acute yellow atrophy and delayed chloroform poisoning. Journal of Obstetrics and Gynaecology of the British Empire 47: 49–62

Sheppard B L, Bonnar J 1974 The ultrastructure of the arterial supply of the human placenta in early and late pregnancy. Journal of Obstetrics and Gynaecology of the British Commonwealth 81: 497–511

Sher G 1977 Pathogenesis and management of uterine inertia complicating abruptio placentae with consumption coagulopathy. American Journal of Obstetrics and Gynecology 129: 164–170

Sher G, Statland B E 1985 Abruptio placentae with coagulopathy: a rational basis for management. Clinical Obstetrics and Gynecology 28: 15–23

Sill P R, Lind T, Walker W 1985 Platelet values during normal pregnancy. British Journal of Obstetrics and Gynaecology 92: 480–483

Skjodt P 1965 Amniotic fluid embolism—a case investigated by coagulation and fibrinolysis studies. Acta Obstetricia et Gynecologica Scandinavica 44: 437–457

Smith B T, Torday J S 1982 Steroid administration in pregnant women with autoimmune thrombocytopenia. New England Journal of Medicine 306: 744–745

Spencer J A, Smith M J, Cederholm-Williams S A et al 1983 Influence of pre-eclampsia on concentrations of haemostatic factors in mothers and infants. Archives of Disease in Childhood 58: 739–741

Spivak J L, Sprangler D B, Bell W R 1972 Defibrination after intra-amniotic injection of hypertonic saline. New England Journal of Medicine 287: 321–323

Stander R W, Flessa H C, Glueck H C et al 1971 Changes in maternal coagulation factors after intraamniotic injection of hypertonic saline. Obstetrics and Gynecology 37: 321–323

Steichele D F, Herschlein H J 1968 Intravascular coagulation in bacterial shock. Consumption coagulopathy and fibrinolysis after febrile abortion. Medizinische Welt 1: 24–30

Stirling Y, Woolf L, North W R S, Seghatchian M J, Meade T W 1984 Haemostasis and normal pregnancy. Thrombosis in Haematology 52: 176

Stromme W B, Fromke V L 1979 Amniotic fluid embolism and disseminated intravascular coagulation after evacuation of missed abortion. Obstetrics and Gynecology 52: 76S–80S

Tchernia G 1988 Immune thrombocytopenic purpura and pregnancy. Current Studies in Haematology and Blood Transfusion 55: 81–89

Tchernia G, Dreyfus M, Laurian Y, Derycke M, Merica C, Kerbrat G 1984 Management of immune thrombocytopenia in pregnancy: response of infusions of immunoglobulins. American Journal of Obstetrics and Gynecology 14: 225–226

Thornton J G, Molloy B J, Vinall P S et al 1989 A prospective study of haemostatic tests at 28 weeks gestation as predictors of pre-eclampsia and growth retardation. Thrombosis and Haemostasis 61: 243–245

Thragarajah S, Wheby M S, Jarn R, May H V, Bourgeois J, Kitchin J D 1981 Disseminated intravascular coagulation in pregnancy. The role of heparin therapy. Journal of Reproductive Medicine 26: 17–24

Van Leeuwen E F, Helmerhorst F M, Engelfriet C P, Von Dem Borne A E G Kr 1981 Maternal autoimmune thrombocytopenia and the newborn. British Medical Journal 283: 104

Van Leeuwen E F, Van der Ven J T M, Englefreit C P et al 1982 Specificity of autoantibodies in autoimmune thrombocytopenia. Blood 59: 23–26

Van Royen E A 1974 Haemostasis in human pregnancy and delivery. MD thesis, University of Amsterdam

Varner M W, Meehan R T, Syrop C H, Strottmann M P, Goplerud C P 1983 Pregnancy in patients with systemic lupus erythematosus. American Journal of Obstetrics and Gynecology 145: 1025–1037

Virgilio R W K, Rice C L, Smith D E et al 1979 Crystalloid versus colloid resuscitation: is one better? Surgery 85: 129–139

Voke J, Letsky E 1977 Pregnancy and antibody to factor VIII. Journal of Clinical Pathology 30: 928–932

von dem Borne A E G Kr, Helmerhorst F M, von Leeuwen E F et al 1980 Autoimmune thrombocytopenia: detection of platelet autoantibodies with the suspension immunofluorescence test. British Journal of Haematology 45: 319–327

Walker I D 1991 Management of thrombophilia in pregnancy. Blood Reviews 5: 227–233

Wallenberg H C S, Van Kessel P H 1978 Platelet lifespan in normal pregnancy as determined by a non-radioisotopic technique. British Journal of Obstetrics and Gynaecology 85: 33–36

Wallmo L, Karlsson K, Teger-Nilsson A C 1984 Fibrinopeptide A and intravascular coagulation in normotensive and hypertensive pregnancy and parturition. Acta Obstetrica et Gynecologica Scandinavica 63: 636–640

Walsh C M, Nardi M A, Karpatkin S 1984 On the mechanism of thrombocytopenic purpura in sexually active homosexual men. New England Journal of Medicine 311: 635–639

Warwick R, Hutton R A, Goff L, Letsky E, Heard M 1989 Changes in protein C and free protein S during pregnancy and following hysterectomy. Journal of the Royal Society of Medicine 82: 591–594

Weiner C P 1987 Thrombotic microangiopathy in pregnancy and the postpartum period. Seminars in Haematology 2: 119–129

Weiner C P, Kwaan H C, Xu C et al 1985 Antithrombin III activity in women with hypertension during pregnancy. Obstetrics and Gynecology 65: 301–306

Whigham K A E, Howie P W, Shaf M M, Prentice C R M 1979 Factor VIII related antigen and coagulant activity in intrauterine growth retardation. Thrombosis Research 16: 629–638

Woods V L Jr, Kurata Y, Montgomery R R et al 1984a Autoantibodies against platelet glycoprotein 1b in patients with chronic Immune Thrombocytopenia Purpura. Blood 64: 156–160

Woods V L Jr, Oh E H, Mason D et al 1984b Autoantibodies against the platelet glycoprotein IIb/IIIa complex in patients with chronic ITP. Blood 63: 368–375

Woods V L Jr, McMillan R 1984 Platelet autoantigens in chronic ITP. British Journal of Haematology 57: 1–4

Yaffe H, Eldor A, Hornshtein E, Sadovsky E 1977 Thromboplastin activity in amniotic fluid during pregnancy. Obstetrics and Gynecology 50: 454–456

Zeeman G G et al 1992 Endothelial function in normal and preeclamptic pregnancy: a hypothesis. European Journal of Obstetrics, Gynecology and Reproductive Biology 43: 113–122

24. Hypertension in pregnancy

Christopher W. G. Redman

INTRODUCTION

The arterial pressure of pregnant women would be of little or no interest to obstetricians were it not for the conditions of pre-eclampsia and eclampsia. These specific disorders of pregnancy are common, dangerous and poorly understood. Hypertension is one of the signs by which they are recognized and for that reason has become a focus of obstetric interest and research. In this chapter, pre-eclampsia and its sequelae will be described. Other hypertensive conditions will also be mentioned. They can predispose to, or mimic, pre-eclampsia but otherwise, conceptually, should be considered a completely separate topic.

TERMINOLOGY

The concept of hypertension is imprecise and usually invested with a spurious significance. An arbitrary threshold is used to divide normotensive from hypertensive individuals, although there is no intrinsic difference between people whose pressures are just below or just above a cut-off reading. To label some as hypertensive, is to say no more than that their blood pressures are in an upper centile range—they may be unusual but they are not necessarily abnormal.

Even if a blood pressure is high enough to be abnormal, hypertension is a sign, not a disease (Pickering 1968). In clinical terms, a discussion of hypertension is as useful as a discussion of pyrexia. The sign may reveal the disease, but not its origin, significance or all of its dangers. After all, individuals with pulmonary tuberculosis may die, but not of the pyrexia by which their condition may be first recognized. In this chapter the term hypertension is used loosely to mean a blood pressure that is higher than average.

Pregnancy-induced hypertension (PIH), transient hypertension of pregnancy, or gestational hypertension are terms used to describe new hypertension which appears after mid-term (20 weeks) and resolves after delivery.

The terms given above describe *one* of the signs of pre-eclampsia. However pre-eclampsia is more than just PIH. It is a syndrome, that is, a combination of abnormal signs that occur together. For reasons that are historical, not logical and, to some extent arbitrary, PIH is deemed to be a mandatory part of the pre-eclampsia syndrome. Thus PIH on its own (a common clinical presentation) is not pre-eclampsia; at least one more sign is required; by convention the second sign is proteinuria (Davey et al 1988). Because fluid retention is a common (but not invariable) symptom, easily detected, it has also featured in some of the older definitions (reviewed by Redman 1987). It is to be regretted that many clinicians and investigators use the terms PIH and pre-eclampsia interchangeably, so muddling an already muddled subject.

The cluster of features that comprise a syndrome are chosen for convenience, describe outward appearances and embody no special truth about the underlying disease or diseases. When a syndrome such as pre-eclampsia is defined, rules are set that bring consistency to what is being discussed. The rules may be sensible or not but their validity cannot be tested because there is no standard to which to refer. All the definitions of pre-eclampsia suffer from these limitations; nor will there be progress until the disease or diseases that contribute to the syndrome are defined. Later different features of pre-eclampsia will be described; most of them could be used legitimately as part of a definition of the syndrome. PIH and proteinuria are not more specific components, merely the conventional ones.

In this chapter, the single term pre-eclampsia is used to label a pregnancy-specific syndrome which may terminate in eclampsia (convulsions), and is characterized by a group of signs of which hypertension is one. The use of one word to describe the syndrome does not exclude the possibility that it may have several causes. Toxaemia is an obsolete expression previously used to describe any hypertension or proteinuria in pregnancy, whether pregnancy induced or not.

THE THREE LEVELS OF PRE-ECLAMPTIC PATHOLOGY

There are three levels of the pathology of pre-eclampsia. The primary pathology must be placental or of the placental bed (Redman 1991) because the condition is pregnancy specific, always resolves after delivery, but does not require the presence of the fetus as it can develop with hydatidiform mole (Chun et al 1964). The secondary pathology comprises the subcritical signs of the placental problem, both maternal and fetal, which can be detected but fall short of overt illness. These disturbances can progress to decompensation of one system or another; the ensuing crises comprise the tertiary pathology.

The primary placental pathology

The underlying problem appears to be uteroplacental arterial insufficiency causing placental ischaemia and hypoxia. There are two lesions involving the spiral arteries which are the end-arteries supplying the intervillous space. The first is a relative lack of the trophoblast infiltration of the arterial walls during placentation (Brosens et al 1972). This occurs between weeks 8 and 18, and is thought to be essential to dilate the arteries for the expanded uteroplacental blood flow of the second half of the pregnancy (Fig. 24.1). The second is acute atherosis—aggregates of fibrin, platelets and lipid-loaded macrophages (lipophages) which partially or completely block the arteries (Robertson et al 1967). Neither change is specific to pre-eclampsia but can also occur with intrauterine growth retardation without a maternal syndrome (de Wolf et al 1980).

Once pre-eclampsia is established functional and structural changes in the placenta are consistent with poor perfusion. Uteroplacental (Johnson & Clayton 1957) and intervillous (Kaar et al 1980) blood flow are reduced, intervillous blood becomes desaturated (Howard et al 1961), and there are functional changes ascribable to poor placental perfusion (Gant et al 1976). Placental infarcts occur more commonly (Little 1960) as structural evidence for ischaemia, although they are not specific to pre-eclampsia.

The concept of placental ischaemia as the cause of pre-eclampsia is also supported by animal experiments. Although other mammals do not seem to get pre-eclampsia, a similar illness can be induced by surgical restriction of the uteroplacental blood supply in several mammalian species including the baboon (Cavanagh et al 1977).

It is important to recognize the implications of the concept that pre-eclampsia is a placental, not a hypertensive,

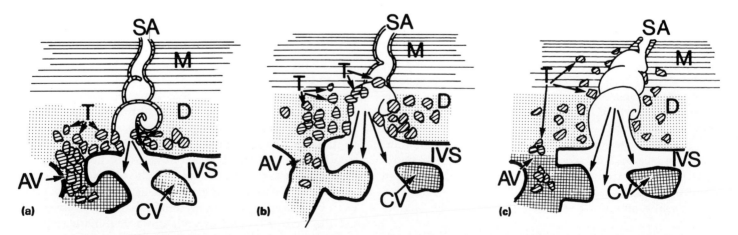

Fig. 24.1 Placentation and pre-eclampsia. Trophoblast (T) from an anchoring villus (AV) invades the decidua (D) and the distal end of a spiral artery (SA) — a process well established by 6 weeks after the last menstrual period ((**a**) left). At this stage the spiral artery is thick walled but the action of the trophoblast breaks down the arterial structure so that the vessel becomes thin walled and dilated, at first in its decidual segment (**b**), extending, by 18 weeks, into the myometrial (M) segment ((**c**), right). The effect is to allow the blood flow into the intervillous space (IVS) to increase. A chorionic villus (CV) is also shown. In pre-eclampsia this process fails to extend beyond the normal stage for 12 weeks so that the ability of the spiral artery to deliver an adequate flow of blood is impaired.

condition (Roberts et al 1993). One implication is that the fetus whose well-being is inevitably linked to the state of the placenta must be involved so there is also a pre-eclamptic fetal syndrome, principally of intrauterine growth retardation and respiratory insufficiency. Secondly, the concept provides a reason why the syndrome is so variable not only with respect to the maternal signs but in the balance of the maternal and fetal syndromes: some may have severe maternal involvement with a relatively normal fetus, others the converse. Thirdly, it becomes sensible to consider that pre-eclampsia could be just one manifestation of a broader group of clinical disorders secondary to similar, or identical, placental problems including cases of fetal growth retardation without maternal hypertension, and even some cases of early miscarriage.

The secondary and tertiary pathology

The secondary pathology of pre-eclampsia results from the maternal adaptation to the ischaemic placenta and includes the defining signs of pre-eclampsia (hypertension and proteinuria) as well as other changes (Table 24.1).

Under certain circumstances the secondary disturbances of pre-eclampsia can become so severe that they initiate new or tertiary pathology—when the regulation of the affected maternal systems is pushed beyond its limits. The tertiary pathology of pre-eclampsia is what makes it so dangerous for the mother. It comprises a number of crises of which eclampsia is one.

Secondary involvement of maternal systems

The maternal cardiovascular, renal, clotting, liver and central nervous systems may all be involved in the highly variable presentations of pre-eclampsia.

Involvement of the cardiovascular system Hypertension is usually the first sign of pre-eclampsia but the exact time-course is largely undefined. In most instances

Table 24.1 Secondary pathology of pre-eclampsia

Cardiovascular system
  Increased arterial sensitivity to angiotensin II
  Increased peripheral resistance
  Raised blood pressure
  Reduced circulating blood volume
Renal system
  Reduced uric acid clearance
  Reduced glomerular function
  Reduced renal blood flow
  Proteinuria
  Glomerular endotheliosis
Coagulation system
  Increased fibrinogen–fibrin turnover
  Reduced platelet count
Hepatic system
  Raised liver enzymes
  Jaundice
Miscellaneous
  Abnormal fluid retention

what is detected is what is sought, that is, confined to the screening of arterial pressure and urine; many other features of the disorder are not noted because their detection involves laboratory investigation. Usually hypertension precedes proteinuria (Redman et al 1976b), although the converse is sometimes encountered.

The hypertension of pre-eclampsia is caused by an increased peripheral resistance (Assali et al 1964) but there is no consistent haemodynamic pattern. Measurements or estimates of the cardiac output have been variable, with values which are normal (Assali et al 1964), increased (Benedetti et al 1980) or decreased (Groenendijk et al 1984). Some of the differences between studies may reflect drug use rather than the characteristics of the disease itself. For example, treatment with vasodilators stimulates cardiac output in pre-eclamptic women by reducing afterload (Groenendijk et al 1984).

However in a serial study, with Doppler ultrasound measurements, those who developed pre-eclampsia had higher estimates of cardiac output before, during and after the episode of pre-eclampsia unrelated to treatment (Easterling et al 1990). Clearly other undefined factors are also involved to account for this heterogeneity.

Many have sought a circulating vasoactive substance to explain pre-eclamptic hypertension. Increased circulating concentrations of catecholamines or angiotension II have not been consistently found. Plasma serotonin, presumably released from platelets, is increased (Middelkoop et al 1993) as is its urinary metabolite 5-hydroxyindole acetic acid (Filshie et al 1992).

Until recently the best explanation for the vasospasm of pre-eclampsia was the hypothesis that it resulted from an imbalance in the production of prostanoids: prostacyclin (a vasodilator and inhibitor of platelet aggregation) and thromboxane (a vasoconstrictor and stimulant of platelet aggregation) (Ylikorkala et al 1992). There is reasonable evidence that pre-eclampsia involves a relative deficiency of prostacyclin and a relative excess of thromboxane at least in terms of intravascular production. Circulating prostacyclin is probably mainly derived from the vessel wall whereas the principal sources of circulating thromboxane are platelets (Fitzgerald et al 1987).

Nevertheless there are other possible factors involved including two intrinsic to the vessel wall—endothelin 1 and endothelium-derived relaxing factor or nitric oxide—both synthesized by the endothelium. The former is a potent vasoconstrictor which probably acts locally; nevertheless circulating levels are increased in pre-eclampsia (many reports, e.g. Sudo et al 1993). Indeed pre-eclampsia is the only form of hypertension so far identified to which increased production of endothelin may contribute (Vanhoutte 1993). Nitric oxide, synthesized from l-arginine, causes endothelium-dependent vascular relaxation. Direct studies of maternal vessels taken at Caesarean section show a reduced activity in pre-eclampsia (McCarthy et al 1993).

Thus pre-eclampsia seems to be associated more with a generalized disturbance of local control of vascular tone (excessive endothelin-1 production, deficient prostacyclin and nitric oxide production) rather than an excess of a single circulating vasoconstrictor substance.

These changes are associated with a much studied increase in arterial reactivity to angiotensin II (Gant et al 1973), whereas in normal pregnancy arterial reactivity to exogenous angiotensin II (AII) is reduced relative to the non-pregnant state (Abdul-Karim et al 1961). Sensitivity to AII is thought to reflect the number of receptors on vascular smooth muscle. These cannot be measured directly; but AII receptors on platelets appear to be a good surrogate marker in that they follow the expected pattern, being down-regulated early in normal pregnancy as the pressor responses to AII diminish (Baker et al 1990), but significantly increased in the third trimester in pre-eclampsia (Baker et al 1991). It is not clear whether increase AII sensitivity contributes to the increase arterial pressure because, as mentioned above, circulating angiotensin II concentrations are reduced in pre-eclampsia (many reports, for example (Graves et al 1992)).

Plasma volume, colloid osmotic pressure and oedema   Maternal plasma volume increases during the second and third trimesters of pregnancy (Pirani et al 1973). The extent of the increase depends on the size of the conceptus, being higher in women with multiple pregnancy (Rovinsky et al 1965), and least in those with fetuses which are small for gestational age (Duffus et al 1971, Pirani et al 1973). Maternal plasma volume is reduced in pre-eclampsia in relation to normal pregnancy (Gallery et al 1979). Pre-eclampsia is frequently associated with intrauterine growth retardation, which accounts for some of the observed change in plasma volume. Whether the plasma volume is further decreased, even given fetal size, has not been determined. Hypertension itself may be a factor, because it is associated with reduced plasma volumes in non-pregnant subjects (Bing et al 1981). Another factor is the hypoalbuminaemia characteristic of the disorder (Studd et al 1970) which causes a lower colloid osmotic pressure (Zinaman et al 1985). This alters the Starling forces governing fluid transport across the capillaries, so that the vascular system in pre-eclampsia becomes leaky, with a maldistribution of fluid: too much in the interstitial spaces (oedema) and too little in the vascular compartment (hypovolaemia).

Atrial natriuretic peptide (ANP), secreted in response to atrial stretch following blood volume expansion, is a vasodilator that opposes the vasopressor actions of noradrenaline and angiotensin II (summarized by Sagnella et al 1984). In normal pregnancy circulating ANP is increased (Thomsen et al 1987), as might be expected given the physiological expansion of blood volume. In pre-eclampsia associated with plasma volume depletion and vasoconstriction, plasma ANP is increased yet further (Thomsen et al 1987), whereas in pregnancies complicated by chronic hypertension alone there is no change (Sumioki et al 1989). Renal impairment is associated with high plasma ANP concentrations and is also a feature of pre-eclampsia (Anderson 1987). However in pre-eclampsia, higher circulating concentrations can be detected before the overt disorder is apparent, and well before there is any renal impairment (Malee et al 1992). There is, as yet, no explanation for this paradoxical response in pre-eclampsia.

Involvement of the renal system   The involvement of the kidneys in pre-eclampsia is one of its more consistent features. Proteinuria reflects advanced disease, associated with a poorer prognosis (Naeye & Friedman 1979) than if it is absent. It has no specific features, is moderately selective (Simanowitz et al 1973), increases until delivery and not uncommonly exceeds 10 g/24 hours—pre-eclampsia being the commonest cause of heavy proteinuria in pregnancy (Fisher et al 1977). A nephrotic syndrome may ensue: apart from generalized oedema, there is hypoproteinaemia (Horne et al 1970), a reduced plasma oncotic pressure (Jouppila et al 1980) and hypovolaemia as discussed above. Serous effusions, particularly ascites, are not uncommon. The oedema may cause tertiary pathology such as laryngeal oedema (Jouppila et al 1980), pulmonary oedema (Benedetti et al 1979); cerebral oedema (Kirby & Jaindl 1984) is a feature, and possibly contributes to at least some cases of eclampsia.

Renal involvement in pre-eclampsia has other well-documented features, including characteristic glomerular histology and changes in function. The glomerular lesion is glomerular endotheliosis (Fig. 24.2); the endothelial cells of the glomeruli swell and block the capillary lumina so that the glomeruli appear enlarged and bloodless (Spargo et al 1959). Renal biopsy is never indicated to resolve the differential diagnosis of pre-eclampsia, however atypical or difficult the presentation. The investigation is reserved for those who continue to have significant proteinuria and renal impairment at a remote time after delivery.

The urinary sediment contains hyaline, granular, red cell and tubular casts indicating both glomerular and tubular damage (Leduc et al 1991). The glomerular pathology correlates with the degree of hyperuricaemia (Pollak et al 1960), the latter being a well-documented component of the condition. It is usually an early feature (Redman et al 1976b), preceding the onset of proteinuria and useful for diagnosis at that stage. The hyperuricaemia results from a reduced renal urate clearance (Chesley & Williams 1945), also observed in pre-eclampsia superimposed on chronic hypertension (Hayashi 1956). The reduction in the renal clearance of urate is proportionally more than that of inulin (Chesley & Williams 1945). As

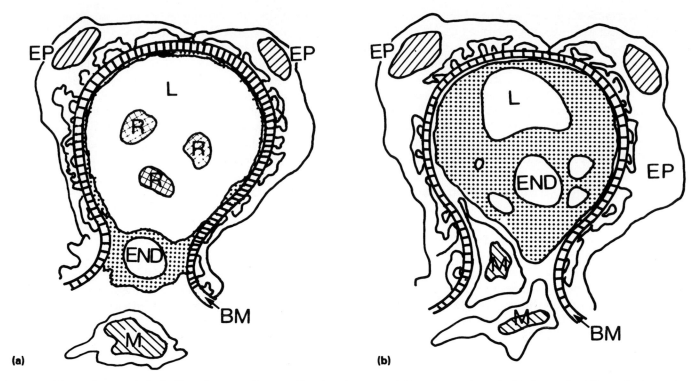

Fig. 24.2 Glomerular endotheliosis. Two diagrams of one capillary loop in a normal (**a**) and pre-eclamptic (**b**) glomerulus. The main change is gross swelling of the endothelial cell's (END) cytoplasm with partial obliteration of the capillary lumen (L). The basement membrane (BM) is intact as are the foot processes of the epithelial cells (EP). There is a slight increase in the numbers of the mesangial cells (M). Red blood cells (R) are squeezed out of the glomerulus, which on light microscopy appears swollen and bloodless.

the plasma urate rises, the plasma concentrations of urea and creatinine at first remain steady, tending to increase slowly after proteinuria has become established.

Hypocalciuria (Taufield et al 1987) is also characteristic of pre-eclampsia but not of other forms of hypertension in pregnancy. Although it is a relatively early event it is not consistent enough to be useful for clinical prediction (Raniolo & Phillipou 1993).

The mechanisms underlying these changes are not understood.

The tertiary pathology of renal involvement in pre-eclampsia is acute renal failure arising from either tubular or cortical necrosis.

Involvement of the clotting system In normal pregnancy the concentrations of several circulating clotting factors increase (fibrinogen, factors VII, VIII, X and XI—Bonnar 1975) and the activity of the fibrinolytic system appears to be inhibited (Bonnar & McNicol 1969). The platelet counts are unchanged (Tygart et al 1986) or slightly reduced (Bonnar & McNicol 1969). There is greater platelet reactivity (Morrison et al 1985) with higher concentrations of the platelet-specific protein beta thromboglobulin in peripheral plasma (Douglas et al 1982).

These trends are exaggerated in some, but not all, cases of pre-eclampsia with a progressive fall in the platelet count (Redman et al 1978), a reduced platelet lifespan (Boneu et al 1980) and circulating plasma concentrations of beta thromboglobulin which are increased (Douglas et al 1982). The platelets tend to become progressively larger (Ahmed et al 1993), which is thought to reflect an influx of younger platelets (Giles et al 1981), even in the absence of thrombocytopenia (Stubbs et al 1986). Their reactivity to various standard stimuli is reduced which is interpreted as platelet exhaustion (Norris et al 1993).

Platelet abnormalities are, however, an inconsistent part of the syndrome, for example only 29% of one series of eclamptic women showed thrombocytopenia, that is, platelets less than $150 \times 10^9/l$ (Pritchard et al 1976). Nevertheless a fall in the platelet count may be an early sign (Redman et al 1978).

Many components of the clotting or fibrinolytic systems or their inhibitors have been studied and found to be altered in pre-eclampsia. A detailed review is impossible. In brief, excess intravascular thrombin formation is reflected in increased formation of circulating complexes with antithrombin III (TAT complexes—Reinthaller et al 1990); the action of thrombin on fibrinogen generates the fragment—fibrinopeptide A—whose circulating concentrations may also be increased (Douglas et al 1982, Saleh et al 1992); lysis of the fibrin that is formed by thrombin—

fibrinogen interaction releases various fragments, including d-dimer, a specific fibrin degradation product, also increased in pre-eclampsia (Trofatter et al 1989). In addition concentrations of circulating factors released by the endothelium—von Willebrand factor (Caron et al 1991), fibronectin (Lockwood & Peters 1990), type 1 plasminogen activator inhibitor (Caron et al 1991)—tend to be greater, as a reflection of generalized endothelial disturbances.

The coagulation disturbances may decompensate to give the tertiary pathology of overt disseminated intravascular coagulation (DIC). Before then, other signs of coagulation disturbances are hard to elicit, although there may be increased plasma concentrations of markers of endothelial activation.

DIC is a rare and dangerous end stage of the clotting abnormalities for which the original evidence was obtained post-mortem (McKay et al 1953). When it develops clotting factors and platelets are consumed and although there are widespread microthromboses the blood becomes incoagulable with problems of severe intractable bleeding. A further complication is microangiopathic haemolysis (Vardi & Fields 1974), which may cause a sudden drop in haemoglobin associated with haemoglobinuria, and fragmented or distorted red cells (schistocytes) on the peripheral blood film. Free haemoglobin forms complexes with haptoglobin which are promptly cleared from the circulation. In consequence low plasma haptoglobin concentrations are a sensitive index of haemolysis in pre-eclampsia (Schrocksnadel et al 1992).

The severe clotting abnormalities of the disorder are particularly associated with liver pathology, now recognized as an important and dangerous component of the disorder.

Involvement of the liver Liver dysfunction occurs in pre-eclampsia and can be detected by elevations of circulating hepatic enzymes (Shukla et al 1978); it may progress to jaundice and severe hepatic impairment (Davies et al 1980). Unless evidence for hepatic derangement is sought in all cases of proteinuric pre-eclampsia, dangerous presentations will be missed.

About two-thirds of women dying from eclampsia have specific lesions in the liver (Sheehan & Lynch 1973b) including periportal lake haemorrhages and various grades of ischaemic damage, including complete infarction (Sheehan & Lynch 1973c). The haemorrhages arise from the arteries and arterioles of the portal tract, which show diffuse mural damage (Sheehan & Lynch 1973a). In addition there are thromboses in the portal tract vessels which may extend into the tributaries of the portal vein. Most of this pathology has been defined post-mortem. Clearly the origins of these problems are in the circulation; whether they are due directly to endothelial damage in the relevant vessels has not been determined.

The HELLP syndrome Liver damage is particularly associated with DIC in pre-eclampsia. If there is also microangiopathic haemolysis the acronym HELLP syndrome has been used to label the concurrence of *H*aemolysis, *E*levated *L*iver enzymes and *L*ow *P*latelet counts (Weinstein 1982, Sibai 1990a). This brings into focus a presentation—which has been documented, albeit incompletely, for many years (Pritchard et al 1954).

The problem may be preceded by clear signs of pre-eclampsia but also can be unheralded (as can eclampsia) by either hypertension or proteinuria. Even more difficult is the fact that, at first presentation, there still may be none of the classical signs of pre-eclampsia (Sibai 1990a, Sibai et al 1993b).

The typical presenting complaint is of right-sided *epigastric pain* (Table 24.2) associated with malaise. Less often there are headaches and vomiting. On examination there is hepatic tenderness. Because there may be no other symptoms or signs the HELLP syndrome can be easily confused with non-specific or viral gastroenteritis or heartburn. For this reason it is important that such complaints are not disregarded. The epigastric pain of the HELLP syndrome is not burning in quality, does not spread upwards towards the throat, is associated with hepatic tenderness, may radiate through to the back and is not relieved by antacid. It is often very severe—described by sufferers as the worst pain that they have ever experienced. Affected women are not uncommonly referred to general surgeons as suffering from an acute abdomen, for example, acute cholecystitis.

The fulminant condition presents very suddenly, often in the immediate postpartum period. It can be associated with eclampsia and acute renal failure. Recovery from the primary problem may take up to 11 days (Martin et al 1990) and may be complicated by rebound hypercoagulability which can cause fatal thrombosis (Katz et al 1989).

In certain severe cases, typically of multiparae rather than primiparae, there may be bleeding under the liver capsule. Subsequently this may rupture to cause massive haemoperitoneum, shock and usually maternal death (Bis et al 1976), although successful treatment with liver transplantation (Erhard et al 1993) or arterial embolization (Terasaki et al 1990) has been reported.

Table 24.2 Presenting symptoms of 442 women with HELLP syndrome (adapted from Sibai et al 1993b)

Symptom	%
Right-sided epigastric pain	65
Nausea/vomiting	36
Headache	31
Visual disturbances	10
Bleeding	9
Jaundice	5
Diarrhoea	5
Shoulder or neck pain	5

Involvement of the nervous system

The incidence of eclampsia For many years in New Zealand, eclampsia was a notifiable condition. Its incidence dropped from 32 to 8 per 10 000 maternities between 1928 and 1958 (Corkill 1961). In more recent years, the incidences have been 6–9 per 10 000 in the Grampian region (Templeton & Campbell 1979), 4–10 per 10 000 in South Wales (Wightman et al 1978) and 8.8 per 10 000 in the National Birthday Trust Survey of 1958 (Butler et al 1963). In 1992 a survey of all the cases in the UK revealed 4.9 cases per 10 000 (Douglas & Redman 1994). This is similar to that in the USA (4.3/10 000 in 1983–86) (Saftlas et al 1990) but higher than that in Sweden (2.7/10 000 in 1976–80 (Moller & Lindmark 1986).

The survey of all the cases of eclampsia in the UK in 1992 (Douglas & Redman 1994) showed that teenagers and women with multiple pregnancy were particularly susceptible. Postnatal eclampsia was the commonest (nearly half the cases). However antepartum eclampsia was associated with significantly more maternal complications than intrapartum or postpartum eclampsia and was more likely to occur in relation to preterm delivery. The maternal case fatality rate was 1.8% and the extended perinatal case fatality rate was 7.8%. Thirty-five per cent of all women had at least one major complication.

Eclampsia and hypertensive encephalopathy Eclampsia resembles hypertensive encephalopathy in non-pregnant individuals. Headaches, nausea, vomiting and convulsions are typical symptoms (Chester et al 1978). It frequently occurs in the context of acute nephritis, and, like eclampsia, is not normally associated with papilloedema or retinopathy (Jellinek et al 1964). Average blood pressures in eclampsia are high (170–195/110–120—Sibai et al 1981), but cases with much lower blood pressures are not rare, which is also true of hypertensive encephalopathy. Another similarity is that both can be complicated by cortical blindness (Jellinek et al 1964, Grimes et al 1980).

The cerebral pathologies of the two conditions both comprise thrombosis, fibrinoid necrosis of the cerebral arterioles, diffuse microinfarcts and petechial haemorrhages (Sheehan & Lynch 1973c, Chester et al 1978). In women with eclampsia, computerized tomography has shown diffuse (Kirby & Jaindl 1984) and focal oedema (Beeson & Duda 1982) as well as haemorrhages (Beck & Menezes 1981) and infarcts (Gaitz & Bamford 1982); radiological evidence of diffuse oedema appears to be relatively unusual (Milliez et al 1990). Reversible foci of cerebral ischaemia or oedema have also been identified on magnetic resonance imaging (Vandenplas et al 1990), usually in the posterior cerebral circulation (Sanders et al 1991). The appearances with eclampsia and hypertensive encephalopathy are similar (Schwartz et al 1992).

The medical condition can be reversed by control of the blood pressure, although it is not clear from the anecdotal reports how much of the recovery may arise from sponta-neous resolution (e.g. of an underlying acute nephritis). The obstetric condition is resolved by delivery so it would not be sensible or ethical to test stringently the effect of antihypertensive medication on the encephalopathy.

What causes the cerebral dysfunction of eclampsia? The cause of eclampsia is not known. However the available evidence is consistent with the concept that it results from changes in the cerebral circulation, which can, in part, be ameliorated by administration of magnesium sulphate, a cerebral vasodilator. This is supported by autopsy evidence that the problem is of ischaemia secondary to intense vasoconstriction (Sheehan & Lynch 1973c). Vasoconstriction is an appropriate, indeed essential, local protective reflex in response to extremes of arterial pressure (Johansson et al 1974). Otherwise there would be an uncontrolled increase in tissue perfusion and rupture of the microcirculation distally. In normal individuals arterial constriction ensures that cerebral perfusion remains constant, when the mean arterial pressure varies from 60 to 150 mmHg (Strandgaard et al 1973).

Beyond the limit of its strength, at very high arterial pressures, the vascular smooth muscle begins to yield, at first in short segments which progressively extend until the whole length of the small artery or arteriole is blown-out (Goldby & Beilin 1972). At the same time cerebral blood flow increases out of control, these events demarcating the upper limit of autoregulation of cerebral blood flow.

Eclampsia may occur at such low arterial pressures to make it unlikely that this mechanism of hypertensive injury is involved. However in those cases with extreme hypertension this type of arterial damage would be expected to aggravate the other problems of the cerebral circulation. This concept provides the rationale for antihypertensive treatment in such women. In previously normotensive pregnant women the upper limit of cerebral autoregulation is probably around 150 mmHg (an actual reading of about 200/130 mmHg), but it has never been measured directly. Thus the extreme hypertension of pre-eclampsia can damage the cerebral circulation and must be presumed to be a key factor underlying cerebral haemorrhages which are a prime cause of maternal death in this condition.

Since it is more likely that eclampsia itself results from inappropriate vasoconstriction secondary to endothelial damage, good control of the arterial pressure could not be expected to prevent eclampsia. The apparently beneficial effects of magnesium sulphate in the same context are also explained.

Involvement of the fetus
Impairment of the uteroplacental circulation affects the placental functions that sustain the fetus. Pre-eclampsia is conventionally considered to be a maternal disorder in which the fetus is an incidental participant, but from the fetus's point of view, it could be seen as a fetal disorder in which the mother is an incidental participant. In fact it is a placental disorder

so that it is predictable that it can cause both maternal and fetal syndromes (Redman 1991).

The fetal syndrome comprises the consequences of respiratory and fetal deprivation.

Pre-eclampsia is an important cause of intrauterine growth retardation in congenitally normal singletons (Gruenwald 1966). Fetal growth failure is more a feature of early-onset disease (Moller & Lindmark 1986, Douglas et al 1994). Ninety per cent of a series presenting with proteinuria before 34 weeks delivered infants weighing less than the 25th centile (Moore & Redman 1983).

Perinatal mortality increases once proteinuria is established. About three-quarters of the excess mortality can be explained by overt placental pathology (Naeye & Friedman 1979), consistent with the view that pre-eclampsia is a primary placental disease. Intrauterine deaths were previously the most significant (Nelson 1955b), sometimes comprising as many as 8.5% of all perinatal deaths from pre-eclampsia (Fitzgerald & Clift 1958). It is one of the achievements of modern antenatal care that this is no longer the case. However, the perinatal mortality remains high in eclampsia, ranging in the past from 13% in Memphis in 1977–80 (Sibai et al 1981) to 64% in Cardiff in 1965–74 (Wightman et al 1978). In the 1992 eclampsia survey of the UK, 7.8% of the babies did not survive including losses after 20 weeks (Douglas & Redman 1994).

Not surprisingly the perinatal death rate is also very high if the mother dies (Department of Health 1994). As a certified cause of perinatal death pre-eclampsia ranks seventh in importance (Edouard & Alberman 1980). This may not be an accurate estimate because complications caused by the pre-eclampsia (prematurity, abruption, placental insufficiency) may be given precedence on the death certificate. A well-timed elective delivery should pre-empt the fetal and maternal complications, but may expose the neonate to the hazards of prematurity—pre-eclampsia being the commonest reason for elective preterm delivery (Rush et al 1976).

Tertiary pathology and maternal mortality

The systemic upsets of pre-eclampsia eventually can progress to decompensation which presents as one of a number of possible crises. It is tertiary pathology (summarized in Table 24.3) that kills women suffering from pre-eclampsia. Pre-eclampsia and eclampsia are the most important causes of maternal death in the USA (Kaunitz et al 1985) and the five Nordic countries comprising Scandinavia, Iceland and Finland (Augensen & Bergsjo 1984). In the UK it remains the foremost direct cause of maternal death (Department of Health 1994). In the third world only infection and haemorrhage are more dangerous (Duley 1992). The pattern of pathology varies but in the UK cerebral pathology is the most significant, particularly cerebral haemorrhage (Table 24.4).

Table 24.3 Tertiary pathology of pre-eclampsia

Eclampsia
Cerebral haemorrhage
Cerebral oedema
Retinal detachment
Pulmonary oedema
Adult respiratory distress syndrome
Laryngeal oedema
Disseminated intravascular coagulation
HELLP syndrome
Renal cortical necrosis
Hepatic rupture

Table 24.4 Maternal deaths from hypertensive disease England and Wales 1973–84; UK 1985–87

Cause of death	1976–78	1979–81	1982–84	1985–87	1988–90
Cerebral haemorrhage	17 (59%)	9 (25%)	13 (52%)	11 (41%)	12 (44%)
Hepatic pathology	1	8	1	1	1
Pulmonary pathology	1	2	3	12	10

Figures derived from: Department of Health (1991); Department of Health (1989); Department of Health and Social Security (1986); Department of Health and Social Security (1982)

In that cerebral haemorrhage is a known complication of severe hypertension in other contexts, it must be assumed, although it has not been proved, that it is a major predisposing factor in this situation. For this reason, pre-eclamptic hypertension is extremely important, as well as being an early, defining sign of the disorder.

The other causes of maternal death include hepatic pathology to the extent that liver involvement must be regarded as the second, most dangerous presentation of the disorder after eclampsia itself.

Role of maternal endothelium

The maternal syndrome is surprisingly variable in the time of onset, speed of progression and the extent to which it involves different systems. Until recently it was impossible to explain a condition that could present not only with hypertension but also other symptoms such as convulsions, jaundice, abdominal pain or normotensive proteinuria by a single underlying pathological process; certainly hypertension could not account for all these features.

The concept that the maternal endothelium is the target organ for the pre-eclampsia process has resolved this difficulty (Roberts et al 1989). In short the maternal syndrome can be explained if it is seen not as a hypertensive problem, but as the sum of the consequences of diffuse endothelial dysfunction and the generalized circulatory disturbances that ensue.

There is both structural and functional evidence for endothelial dysfunction in pre-eclampsia. One example is the renal lesion of glomerular endotheliosis (see above).

Endothelial swelling is also seen in uterine venules (Shanklin & Sibai 1990) and myocardial vessels (Barton et al 1991a). In pre-eclamptic women there are circulating factors that damage endothelium (Rodgers et al 1988, Tsukimori et al 1992) or that alter their lipid metabolism and ability to release prostacyclin (Lorentzen et al 1991). It has been proposed that these factors might include products of free radical activity (lipid peroxides) perhaps derived from hypoxic placental tissue (Hubel et al 1989) or aberrantly released components of the syncytiotrophoblast apical membrane (Smarason et al 1993).

Endothelial dysfunction can explain the increased plasma concentrations of such factors as cellular fibronectin, the von Willebrand factor and type 1 plasminogen activator inhibitor that, as previously mentioned, are increased in pre-eclampsia. It also becomes possible to explain the hypertension of pre-eclampsia as a disturbance of endothelial control of vascular tone as described earlier in this chapter.

Pre-eclampsia: organization of antenatal care

The principles of management are early diagnosis, early admission to hospital, well-timed delivery to pre-empt complications and postpartum follow-up to define underlying medical problems and the outlook for another pregnancy. Although this sounds simple in theory, it is difficult in practice. Only if the clinician can keep one step ahead of events at all stages will dangerous situations be avoided.

There is a particular problem with unheralded crises of eclampsia (Douglas & Redman 1994) or HELLP syndrome (Sibai et al 1993b) for which, it would seem, that these principles of care have nothing to offer. But such crises do not negate the value of what is outlined here, that is their occurrence does not indicate that routine antenatal care does not work. Rather, it is to be expected that the successful application of screening and pre-emptive delivery would leave only these rare cases as outstanding problems.

For convenience, the progression of pre-eclampsia can be divided into three stages, which lead to eclampsia or other crises (Table 24.5). This grossly oversimplifies the problem: every clinician will regularly see cases that do not conform to this pattern. However the staging dovetails with the requirements of management and provides a convenient framework for dealing with the problem in everyday practice. Ideally, cases should be diagnosed in stage 1, admitted to hospital as soon as stage 2 is detected, and delivered before the onset of stage 3. Stage 3 is an obstetric emergency which in a perfect world should never occur. This sequence requires that delivery is expedited before the patient herself begins to feel unwell. Thus diagnosis and management depend on the results of screening symptomless women. This is one of the central features and requirements of antenatal care.

Table 24.5 Progression of pre-eclampsia

	Stage 1	Stage 2	Stage 3
Hypertension	+	+	+
Proteinuria	0	+	+
Symptoms	0	0	+
Crisis	0	0	0
Duration	2 wk–3 mth	2 wk–3 wk	2 h–3 day
Timing of admission	Elective	Today	Emergency
Anticonvulsants	No	No	Possibly
Delivery	After 38 wk	After 34–36 wk	After stabilization

Screening for pre-eclampsia

The screening interval

Screening for pre-eclampsia begins at 20 weeks even though in rare cases pre-eclampsia has presented earlier. A critical feature of the screening procedure is the interval between examinations. The speed of progression of pre-eclampsia is variable. Some cases evolve into stage 3 in less than 2 weeks and, in unheralded crises, there is apparently no prodromal syndrome at all. However, for more typical cases, an interval of no longer than 2 weeks between examinations is necessary if symptomless pre-eclampsia is to be detected before a dangerous situation arises. Indeed, even an interval of 2 weeks may be too long. A conventional pattern of antenatal care involves monthly visits at 20, 24 and 28 weeks. This leaves two dangerous gaps where early-onset pre-eclampsia can evolve undetected, that is in the months before and after 24 weeks. This is why, for example, nearly half the cases of antenatal eclampsia seen in Oxford and an undue proportion of maternal deaths in England and Wales from eclampsia occur at this time.

To identify virtually all cases of pre-eclampsia under all circumstances, women would need to be screened at weekly intervals from 20 weeks. Clearly this is impossible and some compromise is needed. This can be achieved by reviewing expectant women at the end of the first trimester and estimating their individual risks of pre-eclampsia as low, medium or high. Low-risk women need to be screened for pre-eclampsia every 4 weeks to 32 weeks and then every 2 weeks to delivery. Medium-risk women need to be screened at 20 and 24 weeks then every 2 weeks to 36 weeks, then every week to delivery. This closes the gap between 24 and 28 weeks. High-risk women need to be seen more often, on a schedule tailored to their needs, but particularly closing the gap between 20 and 24 weeks. This determines the basic programme of observations, for women who are free of all signs of pre-eclampsia. Once these appear the risks increase and the intervals between observations need to be shortened, ultimately requiring inpatient rather than outpatient observations. In most cases, screening is best done in the community rather than in a hospital clinic.

Estimating the risks of pre-eclampsia

Some of the risk factors are listed in Table 24.6 and include fetal-specific as well as maternal-specific components.

It is universally agreed that primigravidae are several times more prone to the condition. For this reason all primigravid women are at least in a medium-risk group. The proportion of primigravidae amongst eclamptic women varies in different series, most reporting incidences around 65–75% (e.g. Templeton & Campbell 1979). The parous women who are particularly at risk are those who have had the problem before. Thus the incidence of proteinuric pre-eclampsia in a second pregnancy is 10–15 times more in those in whom it is recurrent than in those in whom the first pregnancy was normal (Davies et al 1970, Campbell et al 1985). One of the few factors that can help to identify women at risk of early-onset pre-eclampsia is a history of previous pre-eclampsia (Moore & Redman 1983). If the only previous pregnancy is non-viable the likelihood of pre-eclampsia is slightly reduced, but only if the pregnancy progressed into the second trimester (Campbell et al 1985).

The predisposition to pre-eclampsia is inherited. The daughters of eclamptic women are eight times more likely to suffer eclampsia than expected (Chesley et al 1968). The pattern of inheritance is unclear. It has been suggested that there is a single recessive gene for which the mother must be homozygous (Chesley & Cooper 1986). However identical twins do not have concordant histories (Thornton & Onwude 1991) so other factors must also be important; it has been suggested that the genotype of the fetus may be equally relevant (Liston & Kilpatrick 1991). This could imply that the father of the child could contribute. There is some evidence for this: pre-eclampsia has been reported to be more common in parous women who have changed partners (Feeney & Scott 1980) and a metabolic disorder of the fetus—long-chain 3-hydroxyacyl coenzyme A dehydrogenase deficiency—is strongly associated with the HELLP syndrome (Wilcken et al 1993). No family studies however have shown that female rela-

tives of partners of women who suffer pre-eclampsia are more likely to suffer pre-eclampsia. It is easy to take a family history of pre-eclampsia; for example, a primigravida who is the daughter of a women who suffered eclampsia, should be categorized as high rather than medium risk.

Maternal age is closely linked to parity. In most series the incidence of pre-eclampsia with age is J-shaped with higher incidences in teenage women and those more than 30 years old. The increased incidence in teenage women in mostly the result of the high proportion of primigravidae in this group, although amongst primigravidae the risk may be increased in the very young (Hauch & Lehmann 1934). Otherwise, increasing age is the key risk factor (summarized by Davies 1971). Hence if primigravidae are in a medium-risk group, older primigravidae (35 years or more) are in a high-risk group. Age is the most influential risk factor for death from pre-eclampsia or eclampsia (Lopez Llera et al 1976).

It has been believed for many years that overweight women are more prone to pre-eclampsia (MacGillivray 1961). The more stringent the diagnostic criteria the more this association tends to disappear (Lowe 1961) and is replaced by the opposite effect; that is eclampsia particularly affects underweight (Chesley 1984) and short women (Baird 1977). However even when appropriate diagnostic criteria are used, heaviness continues to be associated with pre-eclampsia in some studies (Easterling et al 1990, Eskenazi et al 1991). This issue is still unresolved.

Certain medical problems seem to predispose to pre-eclampsia. The problem is complicated because they include those that can mimic the disorder such as chronic hypertension and renal disease. In the absence of a specific diagnostic test for pre-eclampsia it is sometimes difficult or impossible to disentangle what elements of proteinuric hypertension are caused by a chronic medical problem from those arising from superimposed pre-eclampsia. The conventional definitions of pre-eclampsia cease to be applicable. If a women is permanently proteinuric there are no accepted criteria for diagnosing proteinuric pre-eclampsia.

Nevertheless it is generally agreed that chronically hypertensive women are three to seven times more likely to develop superimposed pre-eclampsia than normotensive women (Butler et al 1963, Chesley & Annitto 1947). Women with hypertension associated with chronic renal disease have a particular susceptibility to superimposed pre-eclampsia (Felding 1969) and those with diabetes about twice the incidence (Garner et al 1990). A history of migraine predisposes to pre-eclampsia (Moore & Redman 1983, Marcoux et al 1992) and eclampsia (Rotton et al 1959).

Social class is not important (Baird 1977). Lower social class is associated with shortness and a poorer diet, the former definitely and the latter possibly predisposing to

Table 24.6 Risk factors for pre-eclampsia

Maternal
   First pregnancy
   Previous severe pre-eclampsia
   Age: under 20, or over 35
   Family history of pre-eclampsia/eclampsia
   Short stature
   Migraines
   Chronic hypertension
   Chronic renal disease
   Diabetes
Fetal
   Multiple pregnancy
   Hydatidiform mole
   Placental hydrops

the problem. Another key factor is cigarette smoking, which increases in the lower social classes but is associated with a reduced incidence of pre-eclampsia in many studies, for example that by Duffus & MacGillivray (1968). Because the perinatal mortality in smokers is high it would seem likely that the effect of smoking is to diminish the maternal responses to the placental problems of pre-eclampsia. Certainly smoking cannot be prescribed to prevent pre-eclampsia.

The maternal-specific risk factors for pre-eclampsia are simple to elucidate. The fetal-specific factors only become apparent as pregnancy evolves and include some that share the common factor of an enlarged trophoblast mass: multiple pregnancy (MacGillivray 1959), hydatidiform mole (Chun et al 1964), a cause of atypical pre-eclampsia at mid-gestation and hydrops fetalis (Jeffcoate & Scott 1959) from all causes including rhesus isoimmunization.

The baseline assessment

In the first half of pregnancy the risk factors can be assessed to decide how often a woman needs to be screened for pre-eclampsia. In addition, this is the time to determine the baseline for diagnosing pre-eclampsia should it occur. That this should include a careful and accurate measurement of the arterial pressure is obvious. If proteinuria is detected, its amount and significance must be evaluated without delay; the problem cannot be avoided until the third trimester. In women who are classified in the high-risk group, for example elderly primigravidae, or primigravidae with underlying medical problems, it is worth extending the baseline to include laboratory measurements which will be used later if pre-eclampsia supervenes: platelet count, plasma creatinine and uric acid, and liver function tests. It is important to screen for symptomless bacilluria and treat any confirmed infection.

Needless to say, other baseline aspects of the pregnancy are equally important, for example, assessment of dates.

PRINCIPLES OF DIAGNOSIS

The central problem is that pre-eclampsia is only a syndrome, not a disease detected by a specific diagnostic test. The pre-eclampsia syndrome is recognized by finding the appropriate cluster of features occurring together. By convention these comprise pregnancy-induced hypertension (PIH) and pregnancy-induced proteinuria. In practice clinicians need to take a broader view and accept a wider range of combinations of the possible features of the syndrome, some of which are listed in Table 24.7. As with all syndromes, the more of the features that are clustered together the more certain is the diagnosis. It is also essential to understand that the absence of any one feature does not exclude the diagnosis. For example, eclampsia can occur without proteinuria. Even hypertension

Table 24.7 Recognition of the pre-eclampsia syndrome

A. Possible signs of the maternal syndrome
Pregnancy-induced hypertension

Excessive weight gain (> 1.0 kg/week)
Generalized oedema
Ascites

Hyperuricaemia
Proteinuria
Hypocalciuria

Raised plasma concentration of von Willebrand factor
Raised plasma concentration of cellular fibronectin
Reduced plasma concentration of anti-thrombin III
Thrombocytopenia
Increased haematocrit

Increased blood concentrations of liver enzymes

B. Possible signs of the fetal syndrome
Intrauterine growth retardation
Intrauterine hypoxaemia

does not seem to be an essential component (Schwartz & Brenner 1985). Until the specific causes are defined we cannot diagnose the disease or diseases that underlie pre-eclampsia but merely recognize potentially sinister clusters of signs. There is no logical reason why one or other feature must be present before there is the need for concern. Nor should the clinician limit the range of his search for signs of pre-eclampsia simply because they do not feature in any of the definitions.

A further problem is that pre-eclampsia cannot be stereotyped. Its different components vary from one case to the next so that one woman may have severe hypertension but little renal involvement, another severe renal involvement but little hypertension, and a third predominantly hepatic involvement. There is no simple formula to allow the clinician to stop thinking and diagnose by rote.

One consequence of these considerations is that it is impossible to diagnose stage I pre-eclampsia without resorting to additional investigations; it cannot be detected by observing changes in the blood pressure alone.

Diagnosis of pre-eclamptic hypertension

Measurement of the arterial pressure

Sphygmomanometry is a non-invasive way of estimating the true intra-arterial pressure. Phase I of the Korotkoff sounds defines the systolic pressure. Phase IV (muffling of the Korotkoff sounds) or phase V (extinction) have both been used to estimate the diastolic pressure. In non-pregnant individuals phase V is preferred (Kirkendall et al 1981). In some pregnant women, the Korotkoff sounds are heard at zero cuff pressure. In these, phase IV has to be used as the diastolic end-point. Previously it was recommended that diastolic pressure measurements in pregnancy were based on phase IV readings but now phase V is preferred, to be consistent with practice in other branches of medicine (National High Blood Pressure Education Program 1990). In pregnant women the median difference between phase IV and phase V readings is 2.7 mmHg (Perry et al 1990) compared with 0.7 mmHg in non-pregnant control subjects; in 5% the differences exceed 10 mmHg but in this survey the investigators did not find, as reported previously, that Korotkoff sounds at zero cuff pressure are a problem (MacGillivray et al 1969).

The lateral position is often used in the third trimester when the blood pressure is measured, to avoid the supine hypotension syndrome. If the blood pressure is taken in the uppermost arm it will seem to be reduced because the cuff is above the heart (van Dongen et al 1980). If the patient sits or stands, the diastolic is increased (Redman 1995) because of vasoconstriction in the lower extremities and increased peripheral resistance. There is therefore no ideal position for measuring the blood pressure in pregnancy. The semirecumbent position is to be preferred and if lateral tilt is needed to avoid supine hypotension, then care must be taken to keep the cuff level with the heart.

It is generally agreed that hypertension in obese individuals is overdiagnosed if a cuff that is too small is used. The standard cuff (12 × 23 cm) is adequate for arms with circumferences of less than 35 cm. Less than 5% of chronically hypertensive pregnant women exceed this limit, so the problem is not common. It is resolved by using a larger arm cuff (15 × 33 cm) or a thigh cuff (18 × 36 cm).

The definition and grading of hypertension The conventional dividing line is 140/90 mmHg. In the second half of pregnancy more than 20% of pregnant women have a blood pressure of 140/90 or higher at least once. However, only 1% of women reach or exceed 170/110. In the first half of pregnancy 2% of women have a blood pressure at or above 140/90 (Redman 1995).

Thus, hypertension can be graded as mild to moderate for readings in the range 140–165/90–105 mmHg, and severe for readings of 170/110 mmHg and higher. The relevance of this grading is that the case for using antihypertensive treatment is to prevent severe hypertension, however transient.

The differential diagnosis of hypertension in pregnancy In the first half of pregnancy a raised blood pressure tends to reflect a permanent state, chronic hypertension. However a normal blood pressure does not necessarily mean long-term normotension because the fall in blood pressure induced in early pregnancy may be exaggerated in some women; many with relatively severe hypertension may have normal blood pressures by 12 weeks, without treatment. In other words some women enjoy the benefits of pregnancy-induced normotension just as others suffer the disadvantages of pregnancy-induced hypertension.

In the second half, a raised blood pressure also identifies those who have an acquired pregnancy-induced hypertension, which will include cases with pre-eclampsia. An abnormal increase in blood pressure from an early baseline is important in these cases; for example, one definition specifies systolic and diastolic changes of +30 and +15 mmHg respectively (Hughes 1972). The average diastolic increment in the third trimester for all women is nearly 15 mmHg (10–12 mmHg—MacGillivray et al 1969) so a higher threshold is more appropriate for diagnosing pre-eclampsia, such as 20 mmHg, or even +25–30 mmHg (Redman & Jeffries 1988). The usual definitions of PIH have no requirement for a diastolic increment; instead an absolute level above 90 mmHg after 26 (Nelson 1955a) or 20 weeks (Butler et al 1963, Davey & MacGillivray 1988) is considered to be diagnostic provided that no previous reading reaches this limit. Individuals whose pressures rise from a diastolic pressure of 85 mmHg (mild chronic hypertension) are grouped with those whose pressures have risen from lower baselines (e.g. 70 mmHg or less (normotensive)). Even the latter category is not homogeneous. Pregnancy-induced normotension tends to be lost in the third trimester to reveal the underlying long-term hypertension. This event can easily be confused with pregnancy-induced hypertension. An extreme case has been reported of a woman whose prepregnancy readings were 224–280/140–180 mmHg; during pregnancy her arterial blood pressures fell, without treatment, which was not available at that time, to 110–130/60–80 mmHg (Chesley & Annitto 1947) which would, by convention, be regarded as normal. In the third trimester the pressure rose to attain prepregnant levels, simulating severe PIH.

Hence a rise in the arterial pressure by more than a defined amount to above a hypertensive threshold is not pathognomonic of pre-eclampsia. In other words PIH is not necessarily pre-eclampsia. It is necessary to look for other signs to confirm the diagnosis. These may include new proteinuria, hyperuricaemia or thrombocytopenia. Whereas oedema is, in general, not helpful, accelerated weight gain of more than 1.0 kg/week is. Evidence for placental disease supports the diagnosis. For example if the fetus is well-grown then pre-eclampsia is less likely, although not impossible. In many circumstances the diagnosis is beset by doubt that can be dispelled only if the disorder progresses to declare itself more clearly. Frequently delivery, induced or spontaneous, happens too soon, the sequence of events being curtailed so that the desired information is never obtained (Redman 1987). For this reason the diagnosis of mild or moderate pre-eclampsia at the end of pregnancy is always suspect.

Diagnosis of pre-eclamptic renal disease

Early involvement of the renal system (usually during Stage 1) leads to a reduced uric acid clearance whilst the glomerular filtration rate is maintained. Plasma uric acid rises, a useful change to detect Stage 1 pre-eclampsia and to distinguish pre-eclamptic from chronic hypertension. Pregnant women with chronic hypertension alone have normal plasma urate concentrations. Therefore, hyperuricaemic hypertension in the second half of pregnancy is more likely to be pre-eclamptic than not, even in the absence of proteinuria, and for that reason, to have a worse perinatal outcome (Redman et al 1976b). The normal range of plasma urate concentrations rises in the third trimester (Fig. 24.3). As a rough guide, values above 0.30, 0.35, 0.40 and 0.45 mM at 28, 32, 36 and 40 weeks respectively are likely to reflect abnormality. Just as pre-existing hypertension can muddle the presentation of pre-eclamptic hypertension so can pre-existing or constitutional hyperuricaemia. Transient hyperuricaemia may have other causes including ingestion of diuretics or acidosis. Like other signs of pre-eclampsia, hyperuricaemia is a variable component of the condition, and may not be observed even in cases of eclampsia (Dennis et al 1963).

New proteinuria of 1+ or more in all urine samples tested, combined with new hypertension, can be used to identify the onset of the second stage of the disease. Screening depends on the use of dipsticks which may give false-positive results if the urine is alkaline, and false-negative results if it is highly dilute or contains proteins other than albumin. Any positive result (1+ or more) must be immediately evaluated in a mid-stream sample of urine taken whilst a vaginal tampon is used to exclude contamination. If urinary infection can be ruled out, the amount of proteinuria should be measured—ideally over 24 hours. With a single sample, an albumin : creatinine ratio can help to correct for the degree of concentration of the urine. A 24 hour excretion of 0.5 G represents about 0.1 G albumin/mM of creatinine. Proteinuria is usually associated with glomerular dysfunction which is most simply estimated by measuring the plasma concentrations of creatinine and urea. In the absence of pre-existing renal disease a plasma creatinine above 80 μM/l is rarely normal, above 100 μM/l is always abnormal. The plasma urea is more variable but values above 6.0 mM and 7.0 mM correspond to possible and probable renal impairment. Measurement of the creatinine clearance is in theory a better approach; in practice it is so difficult to guarantee a complete collection that it is less helpful than it should be.

Once proteinuria is established, hypoalbuminaemia and other features of a nephrotic syndrome may appear, including oedema.

Diagnostic significance of oedema

Eighty-five per cent of women with proteinuric pre-eclampsia have oedema (Thomson et al 1967). This pathological oedema is easily confused with the physiological water retention found in 80% of normal pregnant women (Robertson 1971). Physiological oedema has not

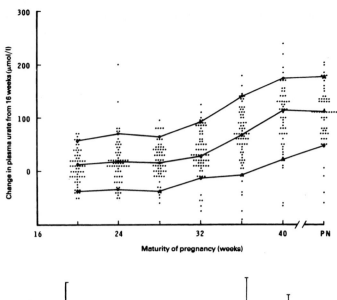

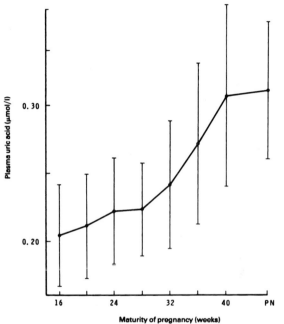

Fig. 24.3 Plasma uric acid concentration in normal pregnancy. A group of healthy primigravidae were followed serially from 16 weeks of pregnancy with measurements of plasma uric acid concentrations. The upper figure shows the increases from the baseline readings established at 16 weeks. The three lines are the 10th, 50th and 90th centiles of the changes. The lower figure shows the averages ($\pm$1 SD) of the readings.

been shown to be the precursor of pathological oedema, but will appear to be so if older definitions of pre-eclampsia are used which emphasize oedema, even in the absence of hypertension. In the best prospective study of pregnant women with no oedema, or early- or late-onset oedema, all had a similar incidence of hypertension (Robertson 1971). For all these reasons the detection of oedema is not useful clinically, nor should oedema be included in the definition of pre-eclampsia. Development of oedema is associated with a higher rate of weight gain, hence the numerous reports associating excessive weight gain with the development of pre-eclampsia. A sudden acceleration in the rate of weight gain is a useful diagnostic feature. More than 1.0 kg per week is unusual, more than 2.0 kg per week is always abnormal. In 15% of cases of pre-eclampsia and eclampsia there is no oedema—dry pre-eclampsia—a particularly dangerous variant for both mother (Eden 1922) and baby (Chesley 1978).

Diagnosis of clotting and hepatic abnormalities

The early disturbances of the clotting system are relatively inaccessible to clinical monitoring. The platelet count is the only routinely available test likely to be informative. Serial readings from a baseline early in pregnancy are more helpful than later single measurements. Counts of less than $100 \times 10^9/l$ are not normal, but should be confirmed by examination of the film to exclude clumping—a cause of spurious thrombocytopenia (Solanki et al 1985). A consistent decline by more than $100 \times 10^9/l$ from the baseline to less than $200 \times 10^9/l$ is unusual and can confirm the diagnosis if other signs are present. The platelet count should be checked at least every week once stage 2 disease is established. If the count is less than $100 \times 10^9/l$ or if the disease has progressed beyond stage 2, evidence for disseminated intravascular coagulation should be sought. A prolonged thrombin time, reduced fibrinogen concentration and evidence for haemolysis on the blood film are the simplest tests. Increased plasma concentrations of fibrin/fibrinogen degradation products, or specific components thereof, such as D-dimer (Trofatter et al 1989) can also be sought. The most sensitive test for haemolysis is to demonstrate reduced plasma concentrations of haptoglobin (Wilke et al 1992) which binds to free haemoglobin and is then rapidly cleared.

Liver dysfunction should be looked for once proteinuria is established or if there is thrombocytopenia. It is our practice to measure plasma aspartate transaminase (AST) activity as a screening test, repeated at least every week until delivery. Plasma alkaline phosphatase is not useful because it is elevated as a result of placental alkaline phosphatase.

Mistakes that are commonly made in diagnosis

The commonest mistake is to discount a raised blood pressure and ascribe it to nervousness. Systolic readings should not be ignored: a pressure of 160/80 needs to be viewed with the same caution as one of 140/90. Antenatal screening not infrequently fails to include urine testing or at least a record of the result if the test is done: this is an unacceptable omission. The importance of proteinuria is often underestimated if it is associated with moderate hypertension. Such presentations are frequently labelled as mild pre-eclampsia, whereas all proteinuric pre-eclampsia is severe. The significance of abdominal pain and vomiting may be missed, particularly by general practitioners

who encounter such symptoms every day in their non-pregnant patients with trivial problems. All too often the complaints by the patient of prodromal symptoms are not heeded, even by specialist staff; as elsewhere in clinical practice, the patient tells you the diagnosis. Jaundice is a rare and regularly misunderstood presentation. Finally, clinicians still fail to appreciate that the unseen complications of the disorder may be worse than those that are visible (hypertension and proteinuria). This is particularly true of the fetal, coagulation and hepatic complications.

When to admit to hospital

Stage 3 pre-eclampsia and eclampsia itself are both obstetric emergencies which justify admission by ambulance if the patient presents first at home, or in an outlying clinic. If new proteinuria (1+ or more) is detected in association with hypertension (diastolic of 90 mmHg or more) then the gravida should be admitted on the same day. Failure in this practice is one of the commonest causes of preventable obstetric disasters. The fact that the hypertension may be only mild does not alter this requirement. The reason for admission is that if Stage 2 pre-eclampsia has begun the disease has entered a short-lived and unstable phase. No obstetrician can guarantee the safety of a woman with proteinuric pre-eclampsia for as long as 24 hours, if she remains out of hospital.

The reason for admission is not that bed rest is therapeutic, but to achieve the aim of keeping one step ahead of events. To do this, the interval between screening observations must be shortened to at least 6 hours, with the option of immediate intervention if necessary. Thus admission to an isolated general practitioner unit is not adequate.

Some admitted with apparent Stage 2 pre-eclampsia will not have the diagnosis confirmed and can be allowed home. However, if the diagnosis is confirmed, even if her condition appears stable, it is dangerous to allow the woman home—she is now committed to staying in hospital until delivery.

Mild to moderate hypertension alone is not a reason for hospital admission, even if it is a new development in the third trimester. However, because it is commonly the earliest indication of pre-eclampsia it demands more frequent monitoring. If Stage 1 pre-eclampsia is diagnosed it may be necessary to admit to hospital non-urgently to sort out the extent of the problems, but a well-organized day care unit where the patient can be seen as often as required is all that is needed for continuing supervision thereafter.

THE TREATMENT OF PRE-ECLAMPTIC HYPERTENSION

Although the hypertension of pre-eclampsia is a secondary

feature it causes tertiary pathology and maternal death from cerebral haemorrhages. The threshold at which pressure-induced arterial injury occurs is high, varies from individual to individual, but once exceeded dangerous situations develop rapidly. Therefore good control of the blood pressure is mandatory, although it is never more than a temporary expedient pending delivery. The level at which treatment is started is a compromise between the needs for safety and the desire to avoid unnecessary medication. Our practice is to prevent all readings at or above 170 systolic or 110 diastolic, which gives a generous safety margin. If, in any 24-hour period, two measurements reach this threshold then treatment is started. Systolic hypertension is as dangerous as diastolic hypertension. There are two requirements: to gain control in the short term, and to maintain control until long enough after delivery that the risk of extreme hypertension has receded.

Acute control of hypertension

If the women presents in Stage 2 or 3 the evolution of the pre-eclampsia may be so fast that the blood pressure must be controlled within 1–3 hours. A smooth and sustained reduction is to be preferred. A number of vasodilating agents given parenterally can be used.

Hydralazine

Hydralazine has been the preferred antihypertensive agent for the treatment of acute severe pre-eclampsia (Hutton et al 1992). It may be given intravenously by either continuous infusion or intermittent boluses, or by intramuscular or subcutaneous injections. After intravenous administration there is a significant delay in the onset of action of 20–30 minutes. Hydralazine directly inhibits the contractile activity of smooth muscle. In the cerebral circulation it first dilates the capacitance vessels causing an increase in the intracranial pressure (Overgaard & Skinhoj 1975) which probably accounts for the common side-effect of severe headaches. This is an undesirable action, particularly in the context of actual or impending eclampsia where intracranial pressure may already be increased. Subsequently the resistance vessels dilate and cerebrovascular flow increases (McCall 1953, Overgaard & Skinhoj 1975). Cardiac output increases because of the increased venous return. A marked tachycardia nearly always occurs. Originally this was thought to result from stimulation of baroceptor reflexes, but hydralazine also causes a prolonged release of noradrenaline (Lin et al 1983) which correlates closely with the tachycardia, and could also explain the anxiety, restlessness and hyperreflexia which are common side-effects. These symptoms and signs, together with headaches, may affect 50% of women and simulate the features of impending eclampsia. Then the symptoms of the disease cannot be disentangled from those caused by the treatment.

It is relevant that hydralazine stimulates the release of noradrenaline which is a potent vasoconstrictor of the uteroplacental circulation in various animals, for example rhesus monkeys (Wallenburg & Hutchinson 1979), and probably in humans. Thus although it increases cardiac output, hydralazine fails to improve indices of uteroplacental perfusion in pre-eclamptic women (e.g. Jouppila et al 1985). Signs attributable to fetal distress, such as heart rate decelerations, have been noted after its use (Vink & Moodley 1982).

Thus hydralazine is not an ideal drug. It is easier to use if the sympathetic nervous system is already inhibited by methyldopa or adrenergic blocking agents. A continuous infusion is not a rational way to achieve control of the blood pressure for more than 4–6 hours. Ventricular dysrhythmias are a significant side-effect which can be avoided by using intravenous labetalol instead (Bhorat et al 1993). For longer-term control methyldopa or labetalol should be given orally. One approach is to combine intermittent intramuscular hydralazine (10 mg) with an oral loading dose of methyldopa (500–1000 mg). The hydralazine can be repeated every 2 or 3 hours until the action of methyldopa begins 6–8 hours later. Monitoring of the fetus is essential but fetal distress is rare, and more related to the severity of the pre-eclampsia than the administration of the hydralazine.

Other drugs for the acute control of hypertension

Labetalol is a combined alpha and beta adrenergic blocking agent which can be given intravenously. It lowers the blood pressure smoothly but rapidly without the tachycardia characteristic of treatment with hydralazine. A typical regimen starts with 20 mg per hour, which is doubled every 30 minutes until control has been gained. In that alpha adrenergic stimulation is thought to constrict the uteroplacental circulation, labetalol would be expected to enhance flow; in fact no effect, good or bad, has been observed (Lunell et al 1982). There are no adequate trials of its parenteral use in pregnancy to show how it might affect perinatal outcome.

Diazoxide is a powerful and rapid vasodilator; an intravenous bolus dose may cause severe hypotension, cerebral ischaemia or death from cerebral infarction (Ledingham & Rajagopalan 1979). A maternal death in this setting has been reported (Henrich et al 1977). It must therefore be given with extreme care, either as a series of miniboluses, or by slow intravenous infusion. It should not be given by obstetric staff who are unlikely to have enough experience of its use or time to monitor its administration properly.

Other vasodilators include sodium nitroprusside (Shoemaker & Meyers 1984) and nitroglycerine (Cotton et al

1985), given intravenously to severely hypertensive pregnant women. Neither is to be recommended except in extreme circumstances of specialist intensive care. Sodium nitroprusside is potentially toxic to the fetus but normal fetal survival has been associated with its use (Goodlin 1983).

The calcium channel blocking agent nifedipine is an effective vasodilator which acts rapidly when given by mouth. Two oral preparations are available: nifedipine capsules act within 10–15 minutes; nifedipine in slow-release tablets has a slower onset of action (about 60 minutes) but a more prolonged effect. The experience of nifedipine in pregnancy is limited, but so far appears to be at least as safe as hydralazine (C. W. G Redman, unpublished observations, Walters & Redman 1984) and, in some aspects of neonatal complications of prematurity with severe pre-eclampsia, possibly superior (Fenakel et al 1991). Tachycardia occurs but is less of a problem than with hydralazine. As with some other drugs the half-life is shorter than that in non-pregnant individuals (Barton et al 1991b) so that regimens need to be adjusted accordingly. In theory there could be a problem if parenteral magnesium sulphate were also used for the prophylaxis or treatment of eclampsia because of the separate effect of the magnesium ion on calcium channel functions (Iseri & French 1984); in practice there has been a report of two cases of profound hypotension in this context (Waisman et al 1988). The advantage of nifedipine over hydralazine is its ease of administration; like hydralazine it can cause severe headaches. Reports of the effects of nifedipine on the fetal or uteroplacental circulations (assessed by Doppler ultrasonography) are so far reassuring (e.g. Hanretty et al 1989). An inhibitory effect of nifedipine on platelet function (Rubin et al 1988) could be an advantage, as could a possible anticonvulsant action (Larkin et al 1988). Nifedipine can have an antitocolytic effect (Ulmsten 1984); this might lead to postpartum haemorrhage, although this complication has not been reported. Nimodipine, another calcium channel blocker, with a selective effect on the cerebral circulation, has been used to treat cerebral ischaemia in an eclamptic woman (Horn et al 1990).

Longer term control of pre-eclamptic hypertension

The control of pre-eclamptic hypertension must always be extended for a few days at the least, and frequently for longer. Therefore, once the blood pressure has been controlled acutely the effects should be prolonged by medication which will lower the blood pressure in a more sustained way. The requirements are for a drug that is safe in pregnancy, has an onset of action in 6–12 hours, allows some titration of effect and can be safely combined with a second drug if needed. The choice lies between methyldopa and various beta adrenergic blocking agents (beta blockers).

Methyldopa in adequate doses can control the blood pressure within 6–12 hours. A loading dose of 500–1000 mg is followed by 250–750 mg four times a day. Sedation is the rule for the first 48 hours and tiredness thereafter is common. Postural hypotension is rarely a problem in the antenatal patient.

The safety of methyldopa in pregnancy has been established by case-control studies (Redman 1976a, Redman et al 1977). No serious adverse fetal effects have yet been documented. Methyldopa crosses the placenta and accumulates in relatively high concentrations in amniotic fluid (Jones & Cummings 1978). Fetal heart rate variability is unaffected; there may be a slight but discernible slowing of the fetal heart rate, and neonatal blood pressure is transiently reduced for a short period after delivery (Whitelaw 1981), yet none of these effects is clinically important. The infants in one case-control study were followed up and assessed at the age of 7 years. The group exposed to methyldopa in utero were as well as their controls (Cockburn et al 1982), thus establishing the longer-term safety of methyldopa in pregnancy.

The beta blockers have the advantage of causing fewer subjective side-effects but their safety in pregnancy has not been so exhaustively investigated. A preparation such as atenolol has a slow onset of action and flat dose response curve, which make the day to day titration of blood pressure control almost impossible. However, its short-term safety for the fetus and neonate has been adequately demonstrated (Rubin et al 1983). Oxprenolol and labetalol are faster-acting alternatives. Claims that oxprenolol promotes fetal growth (Gallery et al 1985) have not been substantiated (Fidler et al 1983). Rather, there has been a tendency for the use of adrenergic beta blocking agents to be associated with smaller fetuses (Thorley 1984, Butters et al 1990, Blake & MacDonald 1991). The adverse effect was most striking with longer-term treatment starting early in the second trimester (Butters et al 1990) and is consistent enough to conclude that beta blocking agents are contraindicated in the long-term treatment of hypertension in pregnancy.

For short-term treatment, which agent is preferred probably matters less than the clinician's familiarity with its use in achieving good blood pressure control.

Postpartum hypertension

The arterial pressure progressively rises during the first 5 days after normal delivery (Walters et al 1986). This trend may be exaggerated in hypertensive women, so that the highest readings of all can be recorded during this period. Both eclampsia and the HELLP syndrome can present for the first time during this period. Inappropriately early postpartum discharge has been identified as one preventable factor associated with maternal death from pre-eclampsia or eclampsia (Hibbard 1973).

Postpartum hypertension needs to be managed, as is antepartum hypertension, with treatment titrated so that severe hypertension is avoided. It is better not to use methyldopa because of the tiredness and depression that it causes. Labetalol has a quick onset of action but postural hypotension may be a problem. Oxprenolol may cause problems with nightmares. Beta blockade can be combined with slow-release nifedipine. There are no specific contraindications to ACE inhibitors in the puerperium. The patient usually can be discharged 6–8 days after delivery. Within 2–3 weeks of discharge antihypertensive treatment can normally be reduced or stopped—a decision which can be made by the general practitioner.

Management of fluid balance and plasma volume

Salt restriction and diuretics

Oedema of pre-eclamptic women was previously treated by both salt restriction and the use of diuretics. Salt restriction can be an important part of the management of hypertension in non-pregnant patients but its use in pregnancy has been tested in only one controlled trial (Robinson 1958). Perinatal mortality in the salt-restricted group was significantly increased by nearly two-fold, and was associated with more toxaemia, in both nulliparous and parous patients.

After their introduction, the thiazide diuretics were prescribed widely for the prevention and treatment of pre-eclampsia. Nearly 7000 women were randomized in 11 controlled trials of varying size and quality. In the pooled data, the incidence of stillbirth was reduced by one-third, a difference which is not statistically significant (Collins et al 1985). Otherwise there was no evidence of benefit. Although there are a number of serious possible side-effects associated with the use of thiazide diuretics, they are rare and would not be a problem if diuretic use conferred significant benefits. Given the paucity of evidence, diuretics should be reserved for specific indications such as the rare complication of left ventricular failure.

Plasma volume expansion

Pre-eclampsia is associated with hypovolaemia. It has been claimed that if this is corrected by plasma volume expansion, renal and placental function improve (Morris et al 1979). The evidence in favour of plasma volume expansion is circumstantial, unvalidated and inconsistent. For example some (Gallery et al 1984) but not others (Belfort et al 1989, Stratta et al 1991) find that plasma

protein infusions lower blood pressure in pre-eclamptic women. The postulated improvement in uteroplacental circulation has not been demonstrated (Jouppila et al 1983).

Pre-eclamptic women are more vulnerable to blood loss but the evidence that there is a primary underfilling of the intact circulation is not good. What data are available point to an abnormal leakiness with loss of fluid and plasma proteins from the vascular compartment. This may be temporarily corrected (over 30–60 minutes for example) by infusing colloid solutions, but in the longer term, such management may simply predispose to potentially dangerous oedema formation in the lungs, brain or other tissues. Plasma volume expansion cannot therefore be considered to be a part of routine management.

Oliguria associated with pre-eclampsia or eclampsia

In Stage 2 pre-eclampsia an indwelling urinary catheter is rarely needed except during, and for about 6 hours after, Caesarean section. Oliguria (15–30 ml of urine per hour) is not necessarily abnormal. If its occurs, the most important priority is to define the reason why, before any treatment is given. The clinical reflex of giving more fluid and a diuretic without further thought is incorrect. Oliguria may be a normal response to a poor fluid intake or to the stress of surgery, and is to be expected after the arterial pressure is lowered with antihypertensive drugs. In two situations oliguria can be a cause for concern: prerenal failure associated with blood loss at delivery and renal failure associated with disseminated intravascular coagulation (DIC). The two problems may be combined with antepartum haemorrhage. Anuria is always abnormal.

To assess blood volume depletion and its correction, it may be necessary to insert a central venous pressure (CVP) line in those who have had a massive blood loss or whose pre-eclampsia has progressed beyond the second stage. If the CVP is low it is better to infuse whole blood than colloid solutions, which in turn are preferable to electrolyte solutions. Overloading with the latter carries the risk of inducing pulmonary oedema. Some advocate pulmonary artery catheterization so that the pulmonary capillary wedge pressure can be used to monitor the circulation whilst the blood volume is corrected (Clark et al 1986). In very rare cases this may be justified, but only after the patient's supervision has been transferred to an intensive care team.

Renal failure associated with renal intravascular thrombosis as a result of DIC may be prevented but will not be reversed by expanding the blood volume. The DIC can develop extremely rapidly so that in certain circumstances the situation may need to be reassessed every 4 hours. The platelet count, fibrinogen titre and thrombin time are simple screening tests, the last being prolonged when there are increased circulating fibrin/fibrinogen degradation products.

Diuretics should be reserved to control the complications of fluid overload. A single large intravenous dose of frusemide may be given as a diagnostic test in patients whose oliguria has not responded to volume replacement. If the urine output fails to increase then renal necrosis (tubular or cortical) may have already occurred.

MANAGEMENT OF THE COAGULATION DISTURBANCES

In general the only remedy for DIC is to correct the underlying problem. In pre-eclampsia this means delivery. With the knowledge that abnormal coagulation probably mediates at least some of the terminal complications of the disorder, various regimens of anticoagulation have been tried. Heparinization failed to modify the course of severe pre-eclampsia (Howie et al 1975) and although prostacyclin infusion corrected the hypertension in one case, underlying fetal problems persisted which necessitated premature delivery (Fidler et al 1980). The dangers of anticoagulation in patients at risk of cerebral haemorrhage need to be emphasized so that in routine clinical practice, anticoagulation should not be used either prophylactically or therapeutically.

Antiplatelet agents, in particular low doses of aspirin, however appear to be more promising. Given that the maternal syndrome of pre-eclampsia appears to originate from diffuse systemic endothelial dysfunction and given that it may be associated, from an early stage, with platelet disturbances (Redman et al 1978), it could be supposed that platelet activation might either amplify or even cause the endothelial problems. In either case antiplatelet therapy might have a beneficial action in preventing or retarding the progression of pre-eclampsia.

Anecdotal reports of the effectiveness of aspirin in preventing pre-eclampsia were followed by controlled trials of differing designs, using aspirin with or without another antiplatelet agent—dipyridamole. The results were promising and appear to have been confirmed by the meta-analyses of further small trials (Collins 1991, Imperiale & Petrulis 1991). However of four recent larger trials, three (Italian Study of Aspirin in Pregnancy 1993, Sibai et al 1993a, CLASP collaborative group 1994) have failed to show the expected benefits. Only one (Hauth et al 1993) has confirmed the promise of earlier studies.

The results of the Collaborative Low-dose Aspirin Study in Pregnancy (CLASP) organized by the British Medical Research Council to which nearly 9500 women were recruited world-wide have clarified some of the issues (CLASP collaborative group 1994). Low-dose aspirin had no effect in improving the outcome for women with early or established pre-eclampsia. Its ability to prevent pre-eclampsia was modest and, on its own, statistically not significant. A greater effect in preventing early-onset pre-eclampsia was discernible particularly among parous women with a previous history of early-onset pre-eclampsia. Aspirin had no effect on IUGR or perinatal survival. In short, if aspirin is beneficial its action is limited to a small group of women susceptible to early-onset pre-eclampsia. It seems that the earlier smaller trials overestimated the possible benefits of low-dose aspirin. The CLASP trial also showed that low-dose aspirin is safe to use in pregnancy. There was no increased incidence of placental bleeding, complications of epidural anaesthesia or of bleeding in the fetus or neonate.

The poor haemostasis of individuals recovering from severe DIC postpartum can, in rare circumstances, cause intractable haemorrhage. Transfusions of platelets and fresh frozen plasma may be needed in addition to the replacement of whole blood as supportive treatment.

MANAGEMENT OF ECLAMPSIA

Time of occurrence

Eclampsia has been documented as early as 16 weeks of pregnancy (Lindheimer et al 1974), but is usually confined to the second half of pregnancy, occurring more commonly towards term (Templeton & Campbell 1979). A survey of all the cases of eclampsia in the UK in 1992 (Douglas & Redman 1994) showed that most (44%) occur after delivery, more than a third (38%) antepartum, and the remainder (18%) during delivery.

Most postpartum fits happen within 24 hours of delivery but definite examples have now been described up to 23 days postpartum (Samuels 1960). Perhaps as many as half the cases of postpartum eclampsia occur more than 48 hours after delivery (Watson et al 1983).

Antepartum eclampsia tends to occur at earlier gestational ages (Douglas & Redman 1994) and, if it does, to be more dangerous (Lopez Llera 1992).

Impending eclampsia—who to treat

It is difficult, perhaps impossible, to accurately identify which patients are likely to have fits. The problem is compounded by the occurrence of unheralded eclampsia, that is convulsions without any apparent prodromal pre-eclampsia. In these women the corroborative signs of hypertension and proteinuria appear after the convulsion not before. If the current practice of curtailing pregnancies complicated by severe pre-eclampsia is effective in preventing eclampsia, then it is to be expected that the residue of cases of eclampsia would tend to comprise those with unheralded disease. This is a possible explanation why as many as 43% of cases in the UK 1992 survey were unheralded (Douglas & Redman 1994).

Hyper-reflexia is an unreliable sign of impending eclampsia, observed in most anxious individuals. Ankle clonus is possibly more useful, but only sustained clonus is likely to be informative. More important is the subjective well-being of the patient. If she feels well she is unlikely to be about to have an eclamptic fit. Headaches, vomiting or epigastric pain are ominous complaints. The symptoms are, however, non-specific and easily discounted as the consequence of viral gastroenteritis or simply flu. This should not happen in the hospitalized patient but is a diagnostic trap in the community if the symptoms are the first indication of the problem. A sudden cessation of urine output may be a premonitory sign in the catheterized patient. The level of the blood pressure, the degree of proteinuria and the presence or absence of oedema cannot be used to forecast that fits are likely in the next few hours.

In some units the problem of whom to treat is sidestepped by treating all women with Stage 2 pre-eclampsia with anticonvulsants. This is undesirable because it increases the number of treated women, and therefore the risks of major side-effects of the drugs. With strict surveillance it is possible to safely withhold anticonvulsants until convulsions begin (Chua & Redman 1991). At the moment there is no consensus as to what is right, but the evidence points to the need to be as selective as possible.

Prevention and treatment of eclamptic fits

Because eclampsia is rare few have substantial experience of its management so that individual investigators are unable to compare different regimens systematically. Different protocols have been recommended on the basis of uncontrolled case series, but only a few small controlled trials have been reported (Crowther 1990, Dommisse 1990, Friedman et al 1993).

It is disappointing that, in most instances, the first eclamptic convulsion occurs after admission to hospital (Templeton & Campbell 1979), in 77% of the cases in the 1992 UK survey (Douglas & Redman 1994); either the women who are likely to have convulsions are not identified accurately (e.g. because of the problem of unheralded eclampsia) or the treatment that is given is ineffective.

The grand mal convulsions of eclampsia are not themselves as dangerous as the underlying disturbances that they reveal. These may include cerebral microinfarcts, oedema, haemorrhages, or associated pathology such as the HELLP syndrome. The priorities are to maintain the airway; stop the convulsions; control the blood pressure, then expedite delivery.

The use of anticonvulsants

The purpose of medical treatment is to prevent or control fitting, not to sedate the patient. It is well to remember that not all sedatives are anticonvulsants, nor anticonvulsants sedatives. In general, if a patient is deemed to need anticonvulsants she also needs urgent delivery. The treatment is a short-term holding measure whilst the underlying cause of the problem—the pregnancy—is ended. It is better to consider the requirements of stopping and preventing convulsions as separate.

Intravenous diazepam is the agent of choice to stop convulsions, but is inappropriate for longer-term prevention of fits. For the latter purpose phenytoin has been used, although in the USA parenteral magnesium sulphate is preferred.

Diazepam

Diazepam was used in the treatment of nearly all (86%) cases of eclampsia in the UK in 1992 (Douglas & Redman 1994). Its anticonvulsant action is achieved by intravenous administration but its action is short-lived. Ten milligrams intravenously can be repeated intermittently as necessary with each new convulsion to a total of 50 mg. The continuous infusion of 10 mg/hour (Lean et al 1968) should not be necessary except in the most intractable cases. Diazepam impairs consciousness and in high doses may depress respiration. It crosses the placenta rapidly to cause loss of fetal heart rate variation within 2 minutes of administration (Scher et al 1972). When maternal doses exceed 30 mg neonatal side-effects become prominent including low Apgar scores, respiratory depression, poor feeding and hypothermia (Cree et al 1973). For these reasons diazepam should be used only to stop fits, not to maintain anticonvulsant treatment thereafter.

It has been claimed that the use of intravenous chlormethiazole avoids these neonatal problems. It is given as a 0.8% solution, with a loading dose of 40–100 ml to stop convulsions and then 60 mg/hour to keep the patient drowsy but easily aroused. Respiratory depression is the main maternal risk. However, it is preferable to avoid sedative preparations once fits have stopped. The choice then lies between intravenous phenytoin or parenteral magnesium sulphate.

Phenytoin

Phenytoin has been used to prevent eclampsia only relatively recently (Slater et al 1987), whereas it is routinely prescribed in medical practice. It has a long half-life so that, after loading, it needs to be given only once a day. It is absorbed slowly, variably and sometimes incompletely from the gut. To prevent recurrent fits acutely 18 mg/kg is given intravenously at the rate of not more than 50 mg/min, with an onset of action after 20 minutes. It may be better to split the dosage into two administrations separated by, for example, 2 hours (Ryan et al 1989). If given too quickly cardiovascular collapse or central nervous system depression may occur. ECG monitoring is desirable in any case. The intravenous preparation is very alkaline, irritant to veins but should not be diluted to avoid precipitation.

Apart from the difficulties of rapid intravenous administration, there is some evidence that phenytoin is not ideal for preventing eclampsia. The convulsion rate after loading in 67 women mostly with severe pre-eclampsia was 4.5% (Robson et al 1993), no lower than that reported with no treatment in a similar number of equally severely affected women (Chua & Redman 1991). Others have reported higher rates of treatment failure (Naidu et al 1992).

Magnesium sulphate

This is administered intramuscularly or intravenously, achieving therapeutic plasma concentrations of 4–7 mEq/l. Its advantage is that it does not cause depression of the cerebral nervous system of either mother or neonate (Mordes & Wacker 1978). The mode of action is not known. Vascular responsiveness is diminished in vitro, although, in vivo, the effect of magnesium administration on pre-eclamptic hypertension is transient and slight (Pritchard 1955). Cardiac and uterine muscle contractility are also impaired. The side-effect of an overdose is cardiac arrest (McCubbin et al 1981). At high concentrations it also causes a relative blockade of the neuromuscular junction which can lead to a loss of deep tendon reflexes or respiratory depression (Pritchard et al 1967).

Although in skilled hands it is safe, its side-effects include a high rate of recurrent convulsions after the start of treatment (Pritchard et al 1984, Sibai 1990), maternal death from overdosage (Hibbard 1973), hypocalcaemic tetany (Eisenbud & Lobue 1976), maternal respiratory depression (Herpolsheimer et al 1991), reduced fetal heart rate variability (Guzman et al 1993) and neonatal hypermagnesaemia associated with hyporeflexia and respiratory depression (Lipsitz 1971).

The possible case for using magnesium sulphate has been weakened by the absence not only of trial evidence of its efficacy, but also an understanding of why it should work. Now that it is thought that vasoconstriction and cerebral anoxia may cause at least part of the eclampsia syndrome, it can be postulated that magnesium sulphate may work as a cerebral vasodilator for which there is experimental (Kemp et al 1993) and clinical (Belfort & Morse 1992) evidence, not preventing the fits per se but the predisposing pathology.

CAN PRE-ECLAMPSIA BE PREVENTED?

Multiparity is the best way to avoid pre-eclampsia but this cannot be prescribed. The risk falls threefold. Clinical interventions are less effective; some such as salt restric-

tion are deleterious, having the opposite effect to that intended (Robinson 1958). As already mentioned, diuretics confer no benefit, nor does control of the blood pressure prevent superimposed pre-eclampsia in women with chronic hypertension. Calcium and other dietary supplements appear to be more effective. It has been postulated that calcium deficiency predisposes to pre-eclampsia and PIH (Belizan & Villar 1980). Just as calcium supplements reduce the blood pressure in men and non-gravid women (McCarron & Morris 1985), so they lessen the incidence of PIH but not, it should be noted, of pre-eclampsia (Belizan et al 1991).

Other dietary components may also be important—for example vitamin E, of which the blood concentration is significantly reduced in pre-eclampsia (Wang et al 1991). As an antioxidant it may help prevent the formation of free radicals which could initiate endothelial or other forms of tissue damage (Hubel et al 1989). The largest randomized controlled trial of dietary supplements did show a modest but significant reduction in the incidence of pre-eclampsia in a pre-war London population (People's League of Health 1946). The supplements comprised minerals and vitamins only, the latter including halibut liver oil to provide vitamins A and D. But fish oil, such as halibut liver oil, is also a source of long chain, n-3 unsaturated fatty acids that yield eicosapentaenoic acid for the synthesis of thromboxane A3 (TXA3) and prostacyclin I3 (PGI3) instead of TXA2 and PGI2 derived from arachidonic acid. These shift the balance of platelet reactivity towards inhibition of aggregation: in effect fish oil supplements are an alternative to antiplatelet drugs. It is possible that the benefit seen in this trial was derived from the fatty acid content of the halibut liver oil rather than the extra vitamins and minerals (Olsen & Secher 1990). The only other drug-based intervention for prevention is the use of antiplatelet agents, in particular low-dose aspirin which is discussed in the section on 'Management of coagulation disturbances'.

In summary, no consistently effective way of preventing pre-eclampsia has yet been found.

CARE OF THE FETUS

Pre-eclampsia is a placental disorder that causes a fetal as well as a maternal syndrome. The extent to which the two syndromes predominate varies from case to case. A severe maternal problem can coincide with relatively minor fetal problems or vice versa. Monitoring of the fetal state is therefore an essential part of management. As with the care of the mother it is vital to keep ahead of events, perhaps more so because the fetus, being inaccessible to direct examination, is harder and more time-consuming to assess. In Stage 1 pre-eclampsia it is necessary to know the fetal size and to monitor fetal growth. For these purposes a baseline ultrasound assessment at 16–18 weeks is helpful as a reference point. Serial abdominal circumference measurements should be done every 2 weeks. In Stage 2 pre-eclampsia it is important to monitor the fetus on a daily basis. It is not appropriate to discuss the methods here but they can include fetal heart rate analysis, ultrasound biophysical profiles and Doppler wave form analyses of the fetal circulation.

WHEN TO DELIVER

The timing of delivery is a matter of judgement, with few absolute guidelines to help the inexperienced clinician (Table 24.5). However, all women who have either Stage 3 pre-eclampsia or eclampsia should be delivered without delay, once their condition has been stabilized. This must be done regardless of gestational maturity. In the rare instances where these problems present earlier than 26 weeks the decision is, in effect, one of late termination of pregnancy.

There have to be compelling special reasons to leave women with proteinuric pre-eclampsia undelivered beyond 36 weeks. Indeed, after 34 weeks it becomes increasingly more difficult to justify conservative management. The same arguments can be transposed to women with definite non-proteinuric pre-eclampsia at 38–40 weeks. However, the practice of inducing all women with hypertension indiscriminately before term has little or no justification.

The most difficult problems arise with Stage 2 pre-eclampsia presenting between 26 and 34 weeks of pregnancy. Although delivery is desirable it is not essential. If it can be deferred for 2 weeks or longer significant maturation of the fetus may be achieved. Conservative management of proteinuric pre-eclampsia can be undertaken only by an experienced team offering continuous monitoring and care. It is not easy, and sometimes impossible, for this to be achieved in under-staffed busy units with heavy routine commitments. It is thus desirable that such patients are moved at an early stage to specialized regional centres.

The conservative approach needs to be used with discretion and in the knowledge that in some patients it will achieve little or nothing. It is essential to known how all the maternal systems are affected by the disorder and the fetal state must be reviewed continually. Delivery is necessary if the maternal blood pressure cannot be controlled, if the platelet count is less than 50×10^9/l, if the plasma creatinine has risen from normal levels to more than 120 µmol, if there is evidence for liver damage or if the pre-eclampsia progresses to Stage 3. In some cases increasing fetal problems may make extrauterine life safer. Any of these developments can happen unpredictably and suddenly, and will be missed unless the monitoring and care is maintained at a high level.

Of 122 cases of Stage 2 pre-eclampsia presenting before 32 weeks in Oxford in 1980–85, conservative management extended the life of the pregnancy beyond the onset of proteinuria by an average time of 15 days. Thirty-one per cent were delivered because of maternal problems, 48% because of fetal problems and 7% because of both. The remainder were delivered non-urgently because adequate maturation had been achieved, or because they went into spontaneous labour. Five infants all weighing less than 1000 g and all but one at less than 28 weeks died in utero. A more modest prolongation of gestational maturity has been found in a randomized controlled trial of conservative management in early pre-eclampsia (Odendaal et al 1990). However, the ability to be conservative is always limited and depends on how severely affected are the women at presentation; so conservative treatment is not always appropriate (Moodley et al 1993).

If premature delivery (before 32 weeks) is necessary then corticosteroids should be given to accelerate fetal pulmonary maturation.

The mode of delivery is determined, amongst other variables, by the speed with which it must be expedited, the ability of the fetus to withstand labour and the chances of successful induction of labour at early gestational ages. As in other circumstances, vaginal delivery is always preferred if it is safe.

Low doses of oxytocin (2–5 mu/min) are antidiuretic within 10–15 minutes of the start of the infusion (Abdul-Karim & Rizk 1970). If given intravenously with large volumes of 5% dextrose and water, this can cause hyponatraemia and convulsions (McKenna & Shaw 1979). The drug causes peripheral vasodilatation with a reflex tachycardia which may stimulate significant increases in cardiac output. If cardiac function is already compromised, which happens in rare cases of severe pre-eclampsia, myocardial failure may occur (Tepperman et al 1977).

In the management of the third stage ergometrine should be avoided because it causes hypertension; Syntocinon should be used instead. The pre-eclamptic patient is particularly prone to hypertension following ergometrine, and headaches, convulsions and death have been reported as major sequelae (Tepperman et al 1977).

A woman with a shrunken intravascular compartment is less tolerant of blood loss than is the normal pregnant woman. Blood replacement must therefore be initiated sooner, at the same time very carefully, to guard against the dangers of underfilling and overfilling.

ANALGESIA AND ANAESTHESIA FOR LABOUR AND DELIVERY

Epidural analgesia has (Moore et al 1985) and has not (Lindheimer & Katz 1985) been recommended for the management of pre-eclamptic women in labour. Those in favour point out that maternal cardiac output is unaffected (Newsome et al 1986), placental intervillous blood flow appears to be enhanced (Jouppila et al 1982) and that control of maternal blood pressure is improved (Newsome et al 1986). No controlled trials have been reported, but if the procedure is done with care, it seems to be safe for the baby. The risk is of precipitating hypovolaemia through vasodilatation and pooling of the blood in the veins of the lower extremities. These problems can be anticipated and avoided so that the benefits seem to outweigh the disadvantages. However, epidural analgesia is contraindicated if there is evidence of actual or incipient disseminated intravascular coagulation. A knowledge of at least the platelet count is essential (Ramanathan et al 1989), and if less than $100 \times 10^9/l$, further investigation of the efficiency of haemostasis is essential before proceeding. Although subdural haematoma is a rare complication of epidural anaesthesia, one case has been reported (Lao et al 1993) in relation to a Caesarean section for severe pre-eclampsia. Concern has been expressed about epidural anaesthesia in pregnant women treated with low-dose aspirin (Macdonald 1991) but in a large controlled trial there was not an excess of complications (CLASP collaborative group 1994).

A Caesarean section may have to be done too quickly to consider using epidural anaesthesia. Although general anaesthesia allows more precise control of the speed and timing of surgery there are particular risks for pre-eclamptic women. Intubation may be difficult or impossible (Heller et al 1983) because of laryngeal oedema which may also cause postoperative respiratory obstruction and cardiac arrest (Hein 1984). Laryngoscopy is a well-known cause of extreme transient reflex hypertension in all individuals. The problem is aggravated in pre-eclamptic women and may be so extreme as to cause acute pulmonary oedema (Fox et al 1977).

Anticipating these problems is the key to their management. Laryngeal oedema is one of the few indications for the use of diuretics in pre-eclampsia; if it is anticipated an experienced and well-briefed anaesthetist should do the intubation. The blood pressure swings at laryngoscopy are ameliorated if adequate control has been gained before the anaesthetic is given or by the administration of nifedipine (Kumar et al 1993), labetalol (Ramanathan et al 1988) or nitroglycerine (Longmire et al 1991) before intubation.

CHRONIC HYPERTENSION IN PREGNANCY

This group comprises women with essential or renal hypertension, or hypertension caused by miscellaneous but rare disorders. Women with essential hypertension are the commonest. They tend to be older and parous, heavier and to have a family history of hypertension. As already mentioned, an individual with chronic hypertension may appear normotensive early in the second trimester and then show a rise in the blood pressure in the third trimester simulating PIH. This causes diagnostic confusion but explains why PIH includes two groups of women: those with early pre-eclampsia (Stage 1), which tends to be non-recurrent, affect primigravidae and be associated with a raised perinatal mortality, and those with chronic hypertension enjoying the benefits of pregnancy-induced normotension. The latter presentation is usually recurrent, affects multiparae and is associated with a good perinatal outcome (MacGillivray 1982).

Thus the only sure way to confirm chronic hypertension in pregnant women is to refer to prepregnancy readings, or, if as is usual, these are not available, to reassess the blood pressure at a remote time after delivery. However, if blood pressures are consistently at or above 140/90 in the first half of pregnancy, then chronic hypertension can be inferred.

Chronic hypertension is one of the predisposing factors to pre-eclampsia so that the two conditions, which in their pure forms can be distinguished with relative ease, may commonly occur together. It used to be thought that chronic hypertension is extremely dangerous when combined with pregnancy. It is now clear that the particular risks of chronic hypertension in pregnancy can be attributed to the increased chance of developing superimposed pre-eclampsia, and that the majority of chronically hypertensive women who do not get pre-eclampsia can expect a normal perinatal outcome (Chamberlain et al 1978).

The signs of pre-eclampsia in chronically hypertensive women are the same as in other women, except that the blood pressure levels start from a higher baseline. Thus the demonstration of a rise in the blood pressure, or progressive hyperuricaemia, or abnormal activation of the clotting system is evidence of superimposed pre-eclampsia which will progress to proteinuria unless pre-empted by delivery.

Another possible complication is that of abruptio placentae. Although it is said to be commoner in women with chronic hypertension (Williams et al 1991), some disagree (Paterson 1979). The reported incidence has varied from 0.45% to 5.6% (reviewed by Sibai 1991). These data include all the unmeasured biases that depend on hospital-based populations, which would be expected to lead to an overestimate of the problem. All that can be said is that it is a relatively rare complication (about 1%), so that none of the clinical trials have been large enough to determine if antihypertensive treatment modifies the risk; nor is there an a priori reason why it should.

It is not uncommon for a woman with chronic hypertension to be on antihypertensive treatment before conception. None of the commonly used antihypertensive drugs is known to be teratogenic. However, some women treated for mild or moderate chronic hypertension can safely stop their treatment before conception to keep fetal drug exposure to a minimum.

Amongst those who must continue are some whose

blood pressures will have fallen enough by 3 months of pregnancy to be able to stop treatment at that time. In the last trimester antihypertensive treatment usually will need to be restarted to maintain blood pressure control.

In general medical practice the purpose of treating blood pressures in the range of 140–170/90–110 mm/Hg is to prevent the long-term complications of hypertension. On this time-scale, whether or not treatment is used during the brief period of gestation is irrelevant. For this reason, the indication for treatment in women with this degree of chronic hypertension would be to prevent the superimposition of pre-eclampsia—the only major short-term problem. There is evidence, based on randomized controlled trials, that the early control of moderate chronic hypertension does not confer this benefit (Redman 1980, Sibai et al 1990). Thus there is no fetal indication for the control of moderate hypertension in pregnancy—medical management can be decided solely on considerations of maternal safety.

Which antihypertensive drugs to use

The use of methyl dopa, calcium channel blockers and beta adrenergic blocking agents has already been discussed.

If diuretics are essential for good blood pressure control they can be continued throughout pregnancy but their use carries certain disadvantages if pre-eclampsia should supervene, as already discussed. Clonidine (Horvath et al 1985) and prazosin (Lubbe & Hodge 1981) have been used in pregnancy. Prenatal exposure to clonidine may cause neonatal hypertension (Boutroy et al 1988) and may be associated with longer-term hyperactivity and sleep disturbances (Huisjes et al 1986).

Angiotensin converting enzyme (ACE) inhibitors are now used widely for the treatment of various forms of long-term hypertension. Although ACE inhibitors have been given to women who have had successful pregnancies (Kreft-Jais et al 1988), there are anxieties about their safety for the fetus, based on animal experiments and the high incidence of fetal death and neonatal renal failure in the offspring of treated women (Rosa et al 1989). For this reason although they seem to be safe in the first trimester and the puerperium they should not be used during the second two trimesters.

The selection of antihypertensive drugs for use in pregnancy is summarized in Table 24.8.

POSTPARTUM FOLLOW-UP

Severe pre-eclampsia and eclampsia can cause irreversible maternal damage, particularly acute renal cortical necrosis or cerebral haemorrhage. In the absence of these complications there is no evidence that long-term health is impaired by a pre-eclamptic illness, although it may reveal medical problems for the first time.

Table 24.8 Antihypertensive drugs in pregnancy

Trimester	Relatively contraindicated drugs	Absolutely contraindicated drugs	Possible agents
First	None known	None known	Avoid all if possible
Second	Beta blockers Diuretics	ACE inhibitors	Methyl dopa Clonidine Nifedipine
Third	Diuretics	ACE inhibitors	Methyl dopa Nifedipine Beta blockers
Puerperium	Methyl dopa	None known	Beta blockers Nifedipine ACE inhibitors Diuretics

In terms of life expectancy eclamptic women (and presumably pre-eclamptic women) fall into two groups. Those who have an episode in the first pregnancy only and become normotensive soon after delivery have a normal life expectancy. The second group have recurrent pre-eclampsia in several pregnancies, or blood pressures which remain elevated in the puerperium. They have a higher incidence of later cardiovascular disorders and a reduced life expectancy compatible with the diagnosis that the initial episode of pre-eclampsia was superimposed on pre-existing hypertension (Chesley et al 1976).

The postpartum follow-up of a woman who has had severe pre-eclampsia should include assessment of the blood pressure and renal status not earlier than 6 weeks after delivery. Women with persisting renal impairment, with or without proteinuria, need an intravenous pyelogram, and possibly a renal biopsy to define the cause of their problem. Women with persisting hypertension need to have the nature of their problem fully explained. For most, all that is required is to organize a regular review of the blood pressure once or twice a year. For some, it is necessary to continue treatment indefinitely. The reasons need to be fully explained and other measures which can mitigate the problem should be emphasized: weight loss, avoidance of excessive salt intake, stopping smoking. Very rarely an individual with severe hypertension is identified who may need further investigation—for example angiography to exclude renal artery stenosis. Advice about family planning needs to be given. Oral contraceptives are a cause of hypertension which may be severe, and rarely malignant. For this reason chronic hypertension is a relative contraindication to their use. The advice given to postpartum women should be guided by whether or not hypertension persists as a chronic problem. If a pre-eclamptic woman's blood pressure returns to normal, then she need not be denied the benefits of oral contraceptives provided adequate and continuing medical supervision is available.

Women who have suffered severe pre-eclampsia want

to know the outlook for another pregnancy, an issue which is made more difficult if the recent pregnancy resulted in a perinatal death. In general, the outlook is better than the patients think, but not as good as they would like. The risk of recurrence in a second pregnancy is about 1 in 20 but higher for early-onset disease (Sibai et al 1992). The odds should be increased if there are underlying medical problems—to about 1 in 10. Rare individuals have repeated episodes of severe pre-eclampsia, often without a surviving child. Each further episode increases the risk of recurrence in another pregnancy.

CONCLUSIONS

1. Pre-eclampsia and eclampsia are the commonest causes of secondary hypertension in medical practice.
2. They are disorders primarily of the placenta and placental bed, which cause maternal and fetal syndromes.
3. The maternal syndrome is the result of diffuse maternal endothelial dysfunction.
4. It is a major cause of maternal death as well as perinatal death, prematurity and fetal growth retardation.
5. The disorder is unpredictable and variable in its onset and evolution, but is always reversed by delivery.
6. The condition is detected by screening the symptomless woman; its complications are pre-empted by well-timed delivery. However pre-eclamptic crises may be unheralded without any apparent prodromal signs.
7. The onset of proteinuria indicates advanced disease requiring admission to hospital on the day of detection, even if the blood pressure is only mildly elevated.
8. The onset of symptoms is a terminal development which precedes eclamptic convulsions. Ideally all women should be delivered before this stage is reached. However a small minority present with unheralded crises, often postpartum, apparently not preceded by prodromal signs or symptoms.
9. Control of the maternal blood pressure is an essential part of management to protect the mother from the risk of cerebral haemorrhage and generalized arteriolar injury.

REFERENCES

Abdul-Karim R, Assali N S 1961 Pressor response to angiotensin in pregnant and non-pregnant women. American Journal of Obstetrics and Gynecology 82: 246–251

Abdul-Karim R, Rizk P T 1970 The effect of oxytocin on renal hemodynamics, water and electrolyte excretion. Obstetrical and Gynecological Survey 25: 805–813

Ahmed Y, van Iddekinge B, Paul C, Sullivan H F, Elder M G 1993 Retrospective analysis of platelet numbers and volumes in normal pregnancy and in pre-eclampsia. British Journal of Obstetrics and Gynaecology 100: 216–220

Anderson J 1987 Atrial natriuretic peptide concentrations in pre-eclampsia. British Medical Journal 295: 443–444

Assali N S, Holm L W, Parker H R 1964 Systemic and regional hemodynamic alterations in toxemia. Circulation 29–30 (suppl II): 53–57

Augensen K, Bergsjo P 1984 Maternal mortality in the Nordic countries 1970–1979. Acta Obstetricia et Gynaecologica Scandinavica 63: 115–121

Baird D 1977 Epidemiological aspects of hypertensive pregnancy. Clinical Obstetrics and Gynecology 4: 531–548

Baker P N, Broughton Pipkin F, Symonds E M 1990 Platelet angiotensin II binding and plasma renin concentration, plasma renin substrate and plasma angiotensin II in human pregnancy. Clinical Science 79: 403–408

Baker P N, Broughton Pipkin F, Symonds E M 1991 Platelet angiotensin II binding sites in normotensive and hypertensive women. British Journal of Obstetrics and Gynaecology 98: 436–440

Barton J R, Hiett A K, O'Connor W N, Nissen S E, Greene J W J 1991a Endomyocardial ultrastructural findings in preeclampsia. American Journal of Obstetrics and Gynecology 165: 389–391

Barton J R, Prevost R R, Wilson D A, Whybrew W D, Sibai B M 1991b Nifedipine pharmacokinetics and pharmacodynamics during the immediate postpartum period in patients with preeclampsia. American Journal of Obstetrics and Gynecology 165: 951–954

Beck D W, Menezes A H 1981 Intracerebral hemorrhage in a patient with eclampsia. Journal of the American Medical Association 246: 1442–1443

Beeson J H, Duda E E 1982 Computed axial tomography scan demonstration of cerebral edema in eclampsia preceded by blindness. Obstetrics and Gynecology 60: 529–532

Belfort M A, Moise K J J 1992 Effect of magnesium sulfate on maternal brain blood flow in preeclampsia: a randomized, placebo-controlled study. American Journal of Obstetrics and Gynecology 167: 661–666

Belfort M A, Uys P, Dommisse J, Davey D A 1989 Haemodynamic changes in gestational proteinuric hypertension: the effects of rapid volume expansion and vasodilator therapy. British Journal of Obstetrics and Gynaecology 96: 634–641

Belizan J M, Villar J 1980 The relationship between calcium intake and edema-, proteinuria-, and hypertension-getosis: an hypothesis. American Journal of Clinical Nutrition 33: 2202–2210

Belizan J M, Villar J, Gonzalez L, Campodonico L, Bergel E 1991 Calcium supplementation to prevent hypertensive disorders of pregnancy. New England Journal of Medicine 325: 1399–1405

Benedetti T J, Carlson R W 1979 Studies of colloid osmotic pressure in pregnancy-induced hypertension. American Journal of Obstetrics and Gynecology 135: 308–311

Benedetti T J, Cotton D B, Read J C, Miller F C 1980 Hemodynamic observations in severe pre-eclampsia with a flow-directed pulmonary artery catheter. American Journal of Obstetrics and Gynecology 136: 465–470

Bhorat I E, Naidoo D P, Rout C C, Moodley J 1993 Malignant ventricular arrhythmias in eclampsia: a comparison of labetalol with dihydralazine. American Journal of Obstetrics and Gynecology 168: 1292–1296

Bing R F, Smith A J 1981 Plasma and interstitial volumes in essential hypertension: relationship to blood pressure. Clinical Science 61: 287–293

Bis K A, Waxman B 1976 Rupture of the liver associated with pregnancy: a review of the literature and report of 2 cases. Obstetrical and Gynecological Survey 31: 763–773

Blake S, MacDonald D 1991 The prevention of the maternal manifestations of pre-eclampsia by intensive antihypertensive treatment. British Journal of Obstetrics and Gynaecology 98: 244–248

Boneu B, Fournie A, Sie P, Grandjean H, Bierme R, Pontonnier G 1980 Platelet production time, uricemia, and some hemostasis tests in pre-eclampsia. European Journal of Obstetrics Gynecology and Reproductive Biology 11: 85–94

Bonnar J 1975 The blood coagulation and fibrinolytic systems during pregnancy. Clinical Obstetrics and Gynecology 2: 321–343

Bonnar J, McNicol G P 1969 Fibrinolytic enzyme system and pregnancy. British Medical Journal 3: 387–389

Boutroy M J, Gisonna C R, Legagneur M 1988 Clonidine: placental transfer and neonatal adaption. Early Human Development 17: 275–286

Brosens I A, Robertson W B, Dixon H G 1972 The role of the spiral arteries in the pathogenesis of pre-eclampsia. In: Wynn R M (ed) Obstetrics and gynecology annual. Appleton-Century-Crofts, New York, pp 177–191

Butler N R, Bonham D G 1963 Perinatal mortality. Livingstone, Edinburgh, pp 87–100

Butters L, Kennedy S, Rubin P C 1990 Atenolol in essential hypertension during pregnancy. British Medical Journal 301: 587–589

Campbell D M, MacGillivray I, Carr Hill R 1985 Pre-eclampsia in second pregnancy. British Journal of Obstetrics and Gynaecology 92: 131–140

Caron C, Goudemand J, Marey A, Beague D, Ducroux G, Drouvin F 1991 Are haemostatic and fibrinolytic parameters predictors of preeclampsia in pregnancy-associated hypertension? Thrombosis and Haemostasis 66: 410–414

Cavanagh D, Rao P S, Tsai C C, O'Connor T C 1977 Experimental toxemia in the pregnant primate. American Journal of Obstetrics and Gynecology 128: 75–85

Chamberlain G V, Philipp E, Howlett B, Masters K 1978 British births 1970, vol 2. Obstetric care. Heinemann, London, pp 39–53

Chesley L C 1978 Hypertensive disorders in pregnancy (1978c A&B). Appleton-Century-Crofts, New York, p 210

Chesley L C 1984 Habitus and eclampsia. Obstetrics and Gynecology 64: 315–318

Chesley L C, Annitto J E 1947 Pregnancy in the patient with hypertensive disease. American Journal of Obstetrics and Gynecology 53: 372–381

Chesley L C, Cooper D W 1986 Genetics of hypertension in pregnancy: possible single gene control of pre-eclampsia and eclampsia in the descendants of eclamptic women. British Journal of Obstetrics and Gynaecology 93: 898–908

Chesley L C, Williams L O 1945 Renal glomerular and tubular functions in relation to the hyperuricemia of pre-eclampsia and eclampsia. American Journal of Obstetrics and Gynecology 50: 367–375

Chesley L C, Annitto J E, Cosgrove R A 1968 The familial factor in toxemia of pregnancy. Obstetrics and Gynecology 32: 303–311

Chesley L C, Annitto J E, Cosgrove R A 1976 The remote prognosis of eclamptic women. Sixth periodic report. American Journal of Obstetrics and Gynecology 124: 446–459

Chester E M, Agamanolis D, Banker B, Victor M 1978 Hypertensive encephalopathy: a clinicopathologic study of 20 cases. Neurology 28: 928–939

Chua S, Redman C W G 1991 Are prophylactic anticonvulsants required in severe pre-eclampsia? Lancet 337: 250–251

Chun D, Braga C, Chow C, Lok L 1964 Clinical observations on some aspects of hydatidiform moles. Journal of Obstetrics and Gynaecology of the British Commonwealth 71: 180–184

Clark S L, Greenspoon J S, Aldahl D, Phelan J P 1986 Severe preeclampsia with persistent oliguria: management of hemodynamic subsets. American Journal of Obstetrics and Gynecology 154: 490–494

CLASP collaborative group 1994 Clasp—a randomised trial of low-dose aspirin for the prevention and treatment of pre-eclampsia among 9364 pregnant women. Lancet 343: 619–629

Cockburn J, Moar V A, Ounsted M, Redman C W G 1982 Final report of study on hypertension during pregnancy: the effects of specific treatment on the growth and development of the children. Lancet i: 647–649

Collins R 1991 Antiplatelet agents for IUGR and pre-eclampsia. In: Chalmers I (ed) Oxford database of perinatal trials. Version 1.2, disk issue 5.

Collins R, Yusuf S, Peto R 1985 Overview of randomised trials of diuretics in pregnancy. British Medical Journal 290: 17–23

Corkill T F 1961 Experience of toxaemia control in Australia and New Zealand. Pathology and Microbiology 24: 428–434

Cotton D B, Longmire S, Jones M M, Dorman K F, Tessen J, Joyce T H 1985 Cardiovascular alterations in severe pregnancy-induced hypertension: effects of intravenous nitroglycerin coupled with blood volume expansion. American Journal of Obstetrics and Gynecology 154: 1053–1059

Cree J E, Meyer J, Hailey D H 1973 Diazepam in labour: its metabolism and effect on the clinical condition and thermogenesis of the newborn. British Medical Journal 4: 251–255

Crowther C 1990 Magnesium sulphate versus diazepam in the management of eclampsia a randomized controlled trial. British Journal of Obstetrics and Gynaecology 97: 110–117

Davey D A, MacGillivray I 1988 The classification and definition of the hypertensive disorders of pregnancy. American Journal of Obstetrics and Gynecology 158: 892–898

Davies A M 1971 Geographical epidemiology of the toxemias of pregnancy. Israel Journal of Medical Sciences 7: 753–821

Davies A M, Czaczkes J W, Sadovsky E, Prywes R, Weiskopf P, Sterk V V 1970 Toxemia of pregnancy in Jerusalem. I. Epidemiological studies of a total community. Israel Journal of Medical Science 6: 253–266

Davies M H, Wilkinson S P, Hanid M A et al 1980 Acute liver disease with encephalopathy and renal failure in late pregnancy and the early puerperium—a study of fourteen patients. British Journal of Obstetrics and Gynaecology 87: 1005–1014

de Wolf F, Brosens I, Renaer M 1980 Fetal growth retardation and the maternal arterial supply of the human placenta in the absence of sustained hypertension. British Journal of Obstetrics and Gynaecology 87: 678–685

Dennis E J, Smythe C M, McIver F A, Howe H G 1963 Percutaneous renal biopsy in eclampsia. American Journal of Obstetrics and Gynecology 87: 364–371

Department of Health 1989 Report on confidential enquiries into maternal deaths in England and Wales 1982–84. HMSO, London, pp 10–19

Department of Health 1991 Report on confidential enquiries into maternal deaths in the United Kingdom 1985–87. HMSO, London, pp 17–27

Department of Health 1994 Report on confidential enquiries into maternal deaths in the United Kingdom 1988–1990. HMSO, London, pp 22–33

Department of Health and Social Security 1982 Report on confidential enquiries into maternal deaths in England and Wales 1976–78. HMSO, London

Department of Health and Social Security 1986 Report on confidential enquiries into maternal deaths in England and Wales 1979–81. HMSO, London, pp 13–21

Dommisse J 1990 Phenytoin sodium and magnesium sulphate in the management of eclampsia. British Journal of Obstetrics and Gynaecology 97: 104–109

Douglas J T, Shah M, Lowe G D, Belch J J, Forbes C D, Prentice C R 1982 Plasma fibrinopeptide A and beta-thromboglobulin in pre-eclampsia and pregnancy hypertension. Thrombosis and Haemostasis 47: 54–55

Douglas K A, Redman C W G 1994 Eclampsia in the United Kingdom. British Medical Journal 309: 1395–1400

Duffus G M, MacGillivray I 1968 The incidence of pre-eclamptic toxaemia in smokers and non-smokers. Lancet i: 994–995

Duffus G M, MacGillivray I, Dennis K J 1971 The relationship between baby weight and changes in maternal weight, total body water, plasma volume, electrolytes and proteins and urinary oestriol excretion. Journal of Obstetrics and Gynaecology of the British Commonwealth 78: 97–104

Duley L 1992 Maternal mortality associated with hypertensive disorders of pregnancy in Africa, Asia, Latin America and the Caribbean. British Journal of Obstetrics and Gynaecology 99: 547–553

Easterling T R, Benedetti T J, Schmucker B C, Millard S P 1990 Maternal hemodynamics in normal and preeclamptic pregnancies: a longitudinal study. Obstetrics and Gynecology 76: 1061–1069

Eden T W 1922 Eclampsia: a commentary on the reports presented to the British Congress of Obstetrics and Gynaecology. Journal of Obstetrics and Gynaecology of the British Empire 29: 386–401

Edouard L, Alberman E 1980 National trends in the certified causes of perinatal mortality. British Journal of Obstetrics and Gynaecology 87: 833–838

Eisenbud E, Lobue C C 1976 Hypocalcemia after therapeutic use of magnesium sulfate. Archives of Internal Medicine 136: 688–691

Erhard J, Lange R, Niebel W et al 1993 Acute liver necrosis in the HELLP syndrome: successful outcome after orthotopic liver transplantation. A case report. Transplantation International 6: 179–181

Eskenazi B, Fenster L, Sidney S 1991 A multivariate analysis of risk factors for preeclampsia. Journal of the American Medical Association 266: 237–241

Feeney J G, Scott J S 1980 Pre-eclampsia and changed paternity. European Journal of Obstetrics Gynecology and Reproductive Biology 11: 35–38

Felding C F 1969 Obstetric aspects in women with histories of renal disease. Acta Obstetricia et Gynecologica Scandinavica 48 (suppl 2): 1–43

Fenakel K, Fenakel G, Appelman Z, Lurie S, Katz Z, Shoham Z 1991 Nifedipine in the treatment of severe preeclampsia. Obstetrics and Gynecology 77: 331–337

Fidler J, Bennett M J, De Swiet M, Ellis C 1980 Treatment of pregnancy hypertension with prostacyclin. Lancet ii: 31–32

Fidler J, Smith V, De Swiet M 1983 Randomised controlled comparative study of methyl dopa and oxprenolol for the treatment of hypertension in pregnancy. British Medical Journal 286: 1927–1930

Filshie G M, Maynard P, Hutter C, Cooper J C, Robinson G, Rubin P C 1992 Urinary 5-hydroxyindole acetate in pregnancy induced hypertension. British Medical Journal 304: 1223

Fisher K A, Ahuja S, Luger A, Spargo B H, Lindheimer M D 1977 Nephrotic proteinuria with pre-eclampsia. American Journal of Obstetrics and Gynecology 129: 643–646

Fitzgerald D J, Mayo G, Catella F, Entman S S, Fitzgerald G A 1987 Increased thromboxane biosynthesis in normal pregnancy is mainly derived from platelets. American Journal of Obstetrics and Gynecology 157: 325–330

Fitzgerald T B, Clift A D 1958 Foetal loss in pregnancy toxaemia. Lancet i: 283–286

Fox E J, Sklar G J, Hill C H, Villanueva R, King B D 1977 Complications related to the pressor response. Anesthesiology 47: 524–525

Friedman S A, Lim K H, Baker C A, Repke J T 1993 Phenytoin versus magnesium sulfate in preeclampsia: a pilot study. American Journal of Perinatology 10: 233–238

Gaitz J P, Bamford C R 1982 Unusual computed tomographic scan in eclampsia. Archives of Neurology 39: 66

Gallery E D, Hunyor S N, Gyory A Z 1979 Plasma volume contraction: a significant factor in both pregnancy-associated hypertension (pre-eclampsia) and chronic hypertension in pregnancy. Quarterly Journal of Medicine 48: 593–602

Gallery E D, Mitchell M D, Redman C W G 1984 Fall in blood pressure in response to volume expansion associated with hypertension (preeclampsia): why does it occur? Journal of Hypertension 2: 177–182

Gallery E D, Ross M E, Gyory A Z 1985 Antihypertensive treatment in pregnancy: analysis of different responses to oxprenolol and methyldopa. British Medical Journal 291: 563–566

Gant N F, Daley G L, Chand S, Whalley P J, MacDonald P C 1973 A study of angiotensin II pressure response throughout primigravid pregnancy. Journal of Clinical Investigation 52: 2682–2689

Gant N F, Madden J D, Chand S, Worley R J, Siiteri P K, MacDonald P C 1976 Metabolic clearance rate of dehydroisoandrosterone sulfate. VI. Studies of eclampsia. Obstetrics and Gynecology 47: 327–330

Garner P R, D'Alton M E, Dudley D K, Huard P, Hardie M 1990 Preeclampsia in diabetic pregnancies. American Journal of Obstetrics and Gynecology 163: 505–508

Giles C, Inglis T C 1981 Thrombocytopenia and macrothrombocytosis in gestational hypertension. British Journal of Obstetrics and Gynaecology 88: 1115–1119

Goldby F S, Beilin L J 1972 Relationship between arterial pressure and the permeability of arterioles to carbon particles in acute hypertension in the rat. Cardiovascular Research 6: 384–390

Goodlin R C 1983 Safety of sodium nitroprusside. Obstetrics and Gynecology 62: 270

Graves S W, Moore T J, Seely E W 1992 Increased platelet angiotensin II receptor number in pregnancy-induced hypertension. Hypertension 20: 627–632

Grimes D A, Ekbladh L E, McCartney W H 1980 Cortical blindness in preeclampsia. International Journal of Gynaecology and Obstetrics 17: 601–603

Groenendijk R, Trimbos J B, Wallenburg H C S 1984 Hemodynamic measurements in preeclampsia: preliminary observations. American Journal of Obstetrics and Gynecology 150: 232–236

Gruenwald P 1966 Growth of the human fetus. II. Abnormal growth in twins and infants of mothers with diabetes, hypertension or isoimmunisation. American Journal of Obstetrics and Gynecology 94: 1120–1132

Guzman E R, Conley M, Stewart R, Ivan J, Pitter M, Kappy K 1993 Phenytoin and magnesium sulfate effects on fetal heart rate tracings assessed by computer analysis. Obstetrics and Gynecology 82: 375–379

Hanretty K P, Whittle M J, Howie C A, Rubin P C 1989 Effect of nifedipine on Doppler flow velocity waveforms in severe pre-eclampsia. British Medical Journal 299: 1205–1206

Hauch E, Lehmann K 1934 Investigations into the occurrence of eclampsia in Denmark during the years 1918–1927. Acta Obstetricia et Gynaecologica Scandinavica 14: 425–481

Hauth J C, Goldenberg R L, Parker C R et al 1993 Low-dose aspirin therapy to prevent preeclampsia. American Journal of Obstetrics and Gynecology 168: 1083–1093

Hayashi T 1956 Uric acid and endogenous creatinine clearance studies in normal pregnancy and toxemias of pregnancy. American Journal of Obstetrics and Gynecology 71: 859–870

Hein H A 1984 Cardiorespiratory arrest with laryngeal oedema in pregnancy-induced hypertension. Canadian Anaesthetists Society Journal 31: 210–212

Heller P J, Scheider E P, Marx G F 1983 Pharyngolaryngeal edema as a presenting symptom in preeclampsia. Obstetrics and Gynecology 62: 523–525

Henrich W L, Cronin R, Miller P D, Anderson R J 1977 Hypertensive sequelae of diazoxide and hydralazine therapy. Journal of the American Medical Association 237: 264–265

Herpolsheimer A, Brady K, Yancey M K, Pandian M, Duff P 1991 Pulmonary function of preeclamptic women receiving intravenous magnesium sulfate seizure prophylaxis. Obstetrics and Gynecology 78: 241–244

Hibbard L T 1973 Maternal mortality due to acute toxemia. Obstetrics and Gynecology 42: 263–270

Horn E H, Filshie M, Kerslake R W, Jaspan T, Worthington B S, Rubin P C 1990 Widespread cerebral ischaemia treated with nimodipine in a patient with eclampsia. British Medical Journal 301: 794

Horne C H W, Howie P W, Goudie R B 1970 Serum alpha$_2$-macroglobulin, transferrin, albumin and IgG levels in pre-eclampsia. Journal of Clinical Pathology 23: 514–516

Horvath J S, Phippard A F, Korda A, Henderson-Smart D J, Child A, Tiller D J 1985 Clonidine hydrochloride—a safe and effective anti-hypertensive agent in pregnancy. Obstetrics and Gynecology 66: 634–638

Howard W, Hunter C, Huber C P 1961 Intervillous blood oxygen studies. Surgery, Gynecology and Obstetrics 112: 435–438

Howie P W, Prentice C R, Forbes C D 1975 Failure of heparin therapy to affect the clinical course of severe pre-eclampsia. British Journal of Obstetrics and Gynaecology 82: 711–717

Hubel C A, Roberts J M, Taylor R N, Musci T J, Rogers G M, McLaughlin M K 1989 Lipid peroxidation in pregnancy: new perspectives on preeclampsia. American Journal of Obstetrics and Gynecology 161: 1025–1034

Hughes E C 1972 Obstetric-gynecologic terminology. Davis, Philadelphia, pp 422–423

Huisjes H J, Hadders Algra M, Touwen B C 1986 Is clonidine a behavioural teratogen in the human? Early Human Development 14: 43–48

Hutton J D, James D K, Stirrat G M, Douglas K A, Redman C W G 1992 Management of severe pre-eclampsia and eclampsia by UK consultants. British Journal of Obstetrics and Gynaecology 99: 554–556

Imperiale T F, Petrulis A S 1991 A meta-analysis of low-dose aspirin for the prevention of pregnancy-induced hypertensive disease. Journal of the American Medical Association 266: 260–264

Iseri L T, French J H 1984 Magnesium: nature's physiologic calcium blocker. American Heart Journal 108: 188–194

Italian Study of Aspirin in Pregnancy 1993 Low dose aspirin in prevention and treatment of intrauterine growth retardation and pregnancy-induced hypertension. Lancet 341: 396–400

Jeffcoate T N A, Scott J S 1959 Some observations on the placental factor in pregnancy toxemia. American Journal of Obstetrics and Gynecology 77: 475–489

Jellinek E H, Painter M, Prineas J, Russell R R 1964 Hypertensive encephalopathy with cortical disorders of vision. Quarterly Journal of Medicine 33: 239–256

Johansson B, Strandgaard S, Lassen N A 1974 On the pathogenesis of hypertensive encephalopathy. Circulation Research 34 (suppl 1): 167–171

Johnson T, Clayton C 1957 Diffusion of radioactive sodium in normotensive and pre-eclamptic pregnancies. British Medical Journal 1: 312–314

Jones H M R, Cummings A J 1978 A study of the transfer of alpha-methyldopa to the human fetus and newborn infant. British Journal of Clinical Pharmacology 6: 432–434

Jouppila R, Jouppila P, Hollmen A 1980 Laryngeal oedema as an obstetric anaesthesia complication: case reports. Acta Anaesthesiologica Scandinavica 24: 97–98

Jouppila P, Jouppila R, Hollmen A, Koivula A 1982 Lumbar epidural analgesia to improve intervillous blood flow during labor in severe preeclampsia. Obstetrics and Gynecology 59: 158–161

Jouppila P, Jouppila R, Koivula A 1983 Albumin infusion does not alter the intervillous blood flow in severe pre-eclampsia. Acta Obstetricia et Gynecologica Scandinavica 62: 345–348

Jouppila P, Kirkinen P, Koivula A, Ylikorkala O 1985 Effects of dihydralazine infusion on the fetoplacental blood flow and maternal prostanoids. Obstetrics and Gynecology 65: 115–118

Kaar K, Jouppila P, Kuikka J, Luotola H, Toivanen J, Rekonen A 1980 Intervillous blood flow in normal and complicated late pregnancy measured by means of an intravenous ^{133}Xe method. Acta Obstetricia et Gynecologica Scandinavica 59: 7–10

Katz V L, Cefalo R C 1989 Maternal death from carotid artery thrombosis associated with the syndrome of hemolysis, elevated liver function, and low platelets. American Journal of Perinatology 6: 360–362

Kaunitz A M, Hughes J M, Grimes D A, Smith J C, Rochat R W, Kafrissen M E 1985 Causes of maternal mortality in the United States. Obstetrics and Gynecology 65: 605–612

Kemp P A, Gardiner S M, Bennett T, Rubin P C 1993 Magnesium sulphate reverses the carotid vasoconstriction caused by endothelin-I, angiotensin II and neuropeptide-Y, but not that caused by NG-nitro-L-arginine methyl ester, in conscious rats. Clinical Science 85: 175–181

Kirby J C, Jaindl J J 1984 Cerebral CT findings in toxemia of pregnancy. Radiology 151: 114

Kirkendall W M, Feinleib M, Freis E D, Mark A L 1981 Recommendations for human blood pressure determination by sphygmomanometers. Sub-committee of the AHA postgraduate education committee. Hypertension 3: 510A–519A

Kreft-Jais C, Plouin P F, Tchobroutsky C, Boutry M 1988 Angiotensin converting enzyme inhibitors during pregnancy: a survey of 22 patients given captopril and nine given enalapril. British Journal of Obstetrics and Gynaecology 95: 420–422

Kumar N, Batra Y K, Bala I, Gopalan S 1993 Nifedipine attenuates the hypertensive response to tracheal intubation in pregnancy-induced hypertension. Canadian Journal of Anaesthesia 40: 329–333

Lao T T, Halpern S H, MacDonald D, Huh C 1993 Spinal subdural haematoma in a parturient after attempted epidural anaesthesia. Canadian Journal of Anaesthesia 40: 340–345

Larkin J G, Butler E, Brodie M J 1988 Nifedipine for epilepsy? A pilot study. British Medical Journal 296: 530–531

Lean T H, Ratnam S S, Sivasamboo R 1968 The use of chlordiazepoxide in patients with severe pregnancy toxaemia. Journal

of Obstetrics and Gynaecology of the British Commonwealth 75: 853–855

Ledingham J G G, Rajagopalan B 1979 Cerebral complications in the treatment of accelerated hypertension. Quarterly Journal of Medicine 48: 25–41

Leduc L, Lederer E, Lee W, Cotton D B 1991 Urinary sediment changes in severe preeclampsia. Obstetrics and Gynecology 77: 186–189

Lin M, McNay J L, Shepherd A M M, Musgrave G E, Keeton T K 1983 Increased plasma norepinephrine accompanies persistent tachycardia after hydralazine. Hypertension 5: 257–263

Lindheimer M D, Spargo B H, Katz A I 1974 Eclampsia during the 16th week. Journal of the American Medical Association 37: 1006–1008

Lindheimer M D, Katz A I 1985 Hypertension in pregnancy. New England Journal of Medicine 313: 675–680

Lipsitz P J 1971 The clinical and biochemical effects of excess magnesium in the newborn. Pediatrics 47: 501–509

Liston W A, Kilpatrick D C 1991 Is genetic susceptibility to pre-eclampsia conferred by homozygosity for the same single recessive gene in mother and fetus? British Journal of Obstetrics and Gynaecology 98: 1079–1086

Little W A 1960 Placental infarction. Obstetrics and Gynecology 15: 109–130

Lockwood C J, Peters J H 1990 Increased plasma levels of ED1$^+$ cellular fibronectin precede the clinical signs of preeclampsia. American Journal of Obstetrics and Gynecology 162: 358–362

Longmire S, Leduc L, Jones M M, Hawkins J L, Joyce T H, Cotton D B 1991 The hemodynamic effects of intubation during nitroglycerin infusion in severe preeclampsia. American Journal of Obstetrics and Gynecology 164: 551–556

Lopez Llera M 1992 Main clinical types and subtypes of eclampsia. American Journal of Obstetrics and Gynecology 166: 4–9

Lopez Llera M, Linares G R, Horta J L H 1976 Maternal mortality rates in eclampsia. American Journal of Obstetrics and Gynecology 124: 149–155

Lorentzen B, Endresen M J, Hovig T, Haug E, Henriksen T 1991 Sera from preeclamptic women increase the content of triglycerides and reduce the release of prostacyclin in cultured endothelial cells. Thrombosis Research 63: 363–372

Lowe C R 1961 Toxaemia and pre-pregnancy weight. Journal of Obstetrics and Gynaecology of the British Commonwealth 68: 622–627

Lubbe W F, Hodge J V 1981 Combined alpha- and beta-adrenoceptor antagonism with prazosin and oxprenolol in control of severe hypertension in pregnancy. New Zealand Medical Journal 94: 169–172

Lunell N O, Nylund L, Lewander R, Sarby B 1982 Acute effect of an antihypertensive drug, labetalol, on uteroplacental blood flow. British Journal of Obstetrics and Gynaecology 89: 640–644

Macdonald R 1991 Aspirin and extradural blocks. British Journal of Anaesthesiology 66: 1–3

MacGillivray I 1959 Some observations on the incidence of pre-eclampsia. Journal of Obstetrics and Gynaecology of the British Empire 65: 536–539

MacGillivray I 1961 Hypertension in pregnancy and its consequences. Journal of Obstetrics and Gynaecology of the British Commonwealth 68: 557–569

MacGillivray I 1982 Pregnancy hypertension—is it a disease? In: Sammour M B, Symonds E M, Zuspan F P (eds) Pregnancy hypertension. Ains Shams University Press, Cairo, pp 1–15

MacGillivray I, Rose G A, Rowe B 1969 Blood pressure survey in pregnancy. Clinical Science 37: 395–407

Malee M P, Malee K M, Azuma S D, Taylor R N, Roberts J M 1992 Increases in plasma atrial natriuretic peptide concentration antedate clinical evidence of preeclampsia. Journal of Clinical Endocrinology and Metabolism 74: 1095–1100

Marcoux S, Berube S, Brisson J, Fabia J 1992 History of migraine and risk of pregnancy-induced hypertension. Epidemiology 3: 53–56

Martin J N Jr, Blake P G, Lowry S L, Perry K G J, Files J C, Morrison J C 1990 Pregnancy complicated by preeclampsia-eclampsia with the syndrome of hemolysis, elevated liver enzymes, and low platelet count: how rapid is postpartum recovery? Obstetrics and Gynecology 76: 737–741

McCall M L 1953 Cerebral circulation and metabolism in toxemia of pregnancy. Observations on the effects of veratrum viride and Apresoline (1-hydrazino-phthalazine). American Journal of Obstetrics and Gynecology 66: 1015–1030

McCarron D A, Morris C D 1985 Blood pressure response to oral calcium in persons with mild to moderate hypertension. A randomized, double-blind, placebo-controlled, crossover trial. Annals of Internal Medicine 103: 825–831

McCarthy A L, Woolfson R G, Raju S K, Poston L 1993 Abnormal endothelial cell function of resistance arteries from women with preeclampsia. American Journal of Obstetrics and Gynecology 168: 1323–1330

McCubbin J H, Sibai B M, Abdella T N, Anderson G D 1981 Cardiopulmonary arrest due to acute maternal hypermagnesaemia. Lancet i: 1058

McKay D G, Merrill S J, Weiner A E, Hertig A T, Reid D E 1953 The pathologic anatomy of eclampsia, bilateral renal cortical necrosis, pituitary necrosis, and other acute fatal complications of pregnancy, and its possible relationship to the generalised Shwartzman phenomenon: American Journal of Obstetrics & Gynecology 66: 507–539

McKenna P, Shaw R W 1979 Hyponatremic fits in oxytocin—augmented labours. International Journal of Gynaecology and Obstetrics 17: 250–252

Middelkoop C M, Dekker G A, Kraayenbrink A A, Popp Snijders C 1993 Platelet-poor plasma serotonin in normal and preeclamptic pregnancy. Clinical Chemistry 39: 1675–1678

Milliez J, Dahoun A, Boudraa M 1990 Computed tomography of the brain in eclampsia. Obstetrics and Gynecology 75: 975–980

Moller B, Lindmark G 1986 Eclampsia in Sweden, 1976–1980. Acta Obstetricia et Gynaecologica Scandinavica 65: 307–314

Moodley J, Koranteng S A, Rout C 1993 Expectant management of early onset of severe pre-eclampsia in Durban. South African Medical Journal 83: 584–587

Moore M P, Redman C W G 1983 Case-control study of severe pre-eclampsia of early onset. British Medical Journal 287: 580–583

Moore T R, Key T C, Reisner L S, Resnik R 1985 Evaluation of the use of continuous lumbar epidural anesthesia for hypertensive pregnant women in labor. American Journal of Obstetrics and Gynecology 152: 404–412

Mordes J P, Wacker W E 1978 Excess magnesium. Pharmacological Reviews 29: 253–300

Morris J A, O'Grady J P 1979 Volume expansion in severe edema-proteinuria-hypertension gestosis. American Journal of Obstetrics and Gynecology 135: 276–279

Morrison R, Crawford J, MacPherson M, Heptinstall S 1985 Platelet behaviour in normal pregnancy, pregnancy complicated by essential hypertension and pregnancy-induced hypertension. Thrombosis and Haemostasis 54: 607–611

Naeye R L, Friedman E A 1979 Causes of perinatal death associated with gestational hypertension and proteinuria. American Journal of Obstetrics and Gynecology 133: 8–10

Naidu S, Moodley J, Botha J, McFadyen L 1992 The efficacy of phenytoin in relation to serum levels in severe pre-eclampsia and eclampsia. British Journal of Obstetrics and Gynaecology 99: 881–886

National High Blood Pressure Education Program 1990 National High Blood Pressure Education Program Working Group Report on High Blood Pressure in Pregnancy. American Journal of Obstetrics and Gynecology 163: 1691–1712

Nelson T R 1955a A clinical study of pre-eclampsia. Part I. Journal of Obstetrics and Gynaecology of the British Empire 62: 44–57

Nelson T R 1955b A clinical study of pre-eclampsia. Part II. Journal of Obstetrics and Gynaecology of the British Empire 62: 58–66

Newsome L R, Bramwell R S, Curling P E 1986 Severe preeclampsia: hemodynamic effects of lumbar epidural anesthesia. Anesthesia and Analgesia 65: 31–36

Norris L A, Gleeson N, Sheppard B L, Bonnar J 1993 Whole blood platelet aggregation in moderate and severe pre-eclampsia. British Journal of Obstetrics and Gynaecology 100: 684–688

Odendaal H J, Pattinson R C, Bam R, Grove D, Kotze T J 1990 Aggressive or expectant management for patients with severe preeclampsia between 28–34 weeks' gestation: a randomized

controlled trial. Obstetrics and Gynecology 76: 1070–1075

Olsen S F, Secher N J 1990 A possible preventive effect of low-dose fish oil on early delivery and pre-eclampsia: indications from a 50-year-old controlled trial. British Journal of Nutrition 64: 599–609

Overgaard J, Skinhoj E 1975 A paradoxical cerebral hemodynamic effect of hydralazine. Stroke 6: 402–404

Paterson M E 1979 The aetiology and outcome of abruptio placentae. Acta Obstetricia et Gynaecologica Scandinavica 58: 31–35

People's League of Health 1946 The nutrition of expectant and nursing mothers in relation to maternal and infant mortality and morbidity. Journal of Obstetrics and Gynaecology of the British Empire 53: 498–509

Perry I J, Stewart B A, Brockwell J et al 1990 Recording diastolic blood pressure in pregnancy. British Medical Journal 301: 1198

Pickering G 1968 High blood pressure. J and A Churchill, London, pp 1–5

Pirani B B K, Campbell D M, MacGillivray I 1973 Plasma volume in normal first pregnancy. Journal of Obstetrics and Gynaecology of the British Commonwealth 80: 884–887

Pollak V E, Nettles J B 1960 The kidney in toxemia of pregnancy: a clinical and pathologic study based on renal biopsies. Medicine 39: 469–526

Pritchard J A 1955 The use of the magnesium ion in the management of eclamptogenic toxemias. Surgery, Gynecology and Obstetrics 100: 131–140

Pritchard J A, Stone S R 1967 Clinical and laboratory observations on eclampsia. American Journal of Obstetrics and Gynecology 99: 754–765

Pritchard J A, Weisman R, Ratnoff O D, Vosburgh G J 1954 Intravascular hemolysis, thrombocytopenia and other hematologic abnormalities associated with severe toxemia of pregnancy. New England Journal of Medicine 250: 89–98

Pritchard J A, Cunningham F, Mason R A 1976 Coagulation changes in eclampsia: their frequency and pathogenesis. American Journal of Obstetrics and Gynecology 124: 855–864

Pritchard J A, Cunningham F G, Pritchard S A 1984 The Parkland Memorial Hospital protocol for treatment of eclampsia: evaluation of 245 cases. American Journal of Obstetrics and Gynecology 148: 951–963

Ramanathan J, Sibai B M, Mabie W C, Chauhan D, Ruiz A G 1988 The use of labetalol for attenuation of the hypertensive response to endotracheal intubation in preeclampsia. American Journal of Obstetrics and Gynecology 159: 650–654

Ramanathan J, Sibai B M, Vu T, Chauhan D 1989 Correlation between bleeding times and platelet counts in women with preeclampsia undergoing cesarean section. Anesthesiology 71: 188–191

Raniolo E, Phillipou G 1993 Prediction of pregnancy-induced hypertension by means of the urinary calcium : creatinine ratio. Medical Journal of Australia 158: 98–100

Redman C W G 1976 Fetal outcome in trial of antihypertensive treatment in pregnancy. Lancet ii: 753–756

Redman C W G 1980 Treatment of hypertension in pregnancy. Kidney International 18: 267–278

Redman C W G 1987 The definition of pre-eclampsia. In: Sharp F et al (eds) Hypertension in pregnancy. Perinatology Press, Ithaca, New York, pp 3–13

Redman C W G 1991 Current topic: pre-eclampsia and the placenta. Placenta 12: 301–308

Redman C W G 1995 Hypertension in pregnancy. In: de Swiet M (ed) Medical disorders in obstetric practice. Blackwell Scientific Publications, Oxford (in press)

Redman C W G, Jefferies M 1988 Revised definition of pre-eclampsia. Lancet i: 809–812

Redman C W G, Beilin L J, Bonnar J 1976a Renal function in preeclampsia. Journal of Clinical Pathology (Suppl R Coll Pathol) 91–94

Redman C W G, Beilin L J, Bonnar, J, Wilkinson R H 1976b Plasma-urate measurements in predicting fetal death in hypertensive pregnancy. Lancet i: 1370–1373

Redman C W G, Beilin L J, Bonnar J 1977 Treatment of hypertension in pregnancy with methyldopa: blood pressure control and side effects. British Journal of Obstetrics and Gynaecology 84: 419–426

Redman C W G, Bonnar J, Beilin L 1978 Early platelet consumption in pre-eclampsia. British Medical Journal 1: 467–469

Reinthaller A, Mursch-Edlmayr G, Tatra G 1990 Thrombin–antithrombin III complex levels in normal pregnancy and hypertensive disorders and after delivery. British Journal of Obstetrics and Gynaecology 97: 506–510

Roberts J M, Redman C W G 1993 Pre-eclampsia: more than pregnancy-induced hypertension. Lancet 341: 1447–1451

Roberts J M, Taylor R N, Musci T J, Rodgers G M, Hubel C A, McLaughlin M K 1989 Preeclampsia: an endothelial cell disorder. American Journal of Obstetrics and Gynecology 161: 1200–1204

Robertson E G 1971 The natural history of oedema during pregnancy. Journal of Obstetrics and Gynaecology of the British Commonwealth 78: 520–529

Robertson W B, Brosens I A, Dixon H G 1967 The pathological response of the vessels of the placental bed to hypertensive pregnancy. Journal of Pathology and Bacteriology 93: 581–592

Robinson M 1958 Salt in pregnancy. Lancet i: 178–181

Robson S C, Redfern N, Seviour J et al 1993 Phenytoin prophylaxis in severe pre-eclampsia and eclampsia. British Journal of Obstetrics and Gynaecology 100: 623–628

Rodgers G M, Taylor R N, Roberts J M 1988 Preeclampsia is associated with a serum factor cytotoxic to human endothelial cells. American Journal of Obstetrics and Gynecology 159: 908–914

Rosa F W, Bosco L A, Graham C F, Milstien J B, Dreis M, Creamer J 1989 Neonatal anuria with maternal angiotensin-converting enzyme inhibition. Obstetrics and Gynecology 74: 371–374

Rotton W N, Sachtleben M R, Friedman E A 1959 Migraine and eclampsia. Obstetrics and Gynecology 14: 322–330

Rovinsky J J, Jaffin H 1965 Cardiovascular hemodynamics in pregnancy. I. Blood and plasma volumes in multiple pregnancy. American Journal of Obstetrics and Gynecology 93: 1–15

Rubin P C, Butters L, Clark D M, Reynolds B, Sumner D J, Steedman D, Low R A, Reid J L 1983 Placebo-controlled trial of atenolol in treatment of pregnancy-associated hypertension. Lancet i: 431–434

Rubin P C, Butters L, McCabe R 1988 Nifedipine and platelets in preeclampsia. American Journal of Hypertension 1: 175–177

Rush R W, Keirse M J N C, Howat P, Baum J D, Anderson A B H, Turnbull A C 1976 Contribution of preterm delivery to perinatal mortality. British Medical Journal 2: 965–968

Ryan G, Lange I R, Naugler M A 1989 Clinical experience with phenytoin prophylaxis in severe preeclampsia. American Journal of Obstetrics and Gynecology 161: 297–304

Saftlas A F, Olson D R, Franks A L, Atrash H K, Pokras R 1990 Epidemiology of preeclampsia and eclampsia in the United States, 1979–1986. American Journal of Obstetrics and Gynecology 163: 460–465

Sagnella G A, MacGregor G A 1984 Physiology: cardiac peptides and the control of sodium excretion [news]. Nature 309: 666–667

Saleh A A, Bottoms S F, Farag A M et al 1992 Markers for endothelial injury, clotting and platelet activation in preeclampsia. Archives of Gynecology and Obstetrics 251: 105–110

Samuels B 1960 Postpartum eclampsia. Obstetrics and Gynecology 15: 748–752

Sanders T G, Clayman D A, Sanchez Ramos L, Vines F S, Russo L 1991 Brain in eclampsia: MR imaging with clinical correlation. Radiology 180: 475–478

Scher J, Hailey D M, Beard R W 1972 The effects of diazepam on the fetus. Journal of Obstetrics and Gynaecology of the British Commonwealth 79: 635–638

Schrocksnadel H, Sitte B, Steckel Berger G, Dapunt O 1992 Hemolysis in hypertensive disorders of pregnancy. Gynecologic and Obstetric Intervention 34: 211–216

Schwartz M L, Brenner W 1985 Toxemia in a patient with none of the standard signs and symptoms of preeclampsia. Obstetrics and Gynecology 66: 19S–21S

Schwartz R B, Jones K M, Kalina P et al 1992 Hypertensive encephalopathy: findings on CT, MR imaging, and SPECT imaging in 14 cases. American Journal of Roentgenology 159: 379–383

Shanklin D R, Sibai B M 1990 Ultrastructural aspects of preeclampsia. II. Mitochondrial changes. American Journal of Obstetrics and Gynecology 163: 943–953

Sheehan H L, Lynch J B 1973a Pathology of toxaemia in pregnancy.

Churchill Livingstone, London, pp 328–339

Sheehan H L, Lynch J B 1973b Pathology of toxaemia in pregnancy. Churchill Livingstone, London, pp 384–397

Sheehan H L, Lynch J B 1973c Pathology of toxaemia in pregnancy. Churchill Livingstone, London, pp 524–553

Shoemaker C T, Meyers M 1984 Sodium nitroprusside for control of severe hypertensive disease of pregnancy: a case report and discussion of potential toxicity. American Journal of Obstetrics and Gynecology 149: 171–173

Shukla P K, Sharma D, Mandal R K 1978 Serum lactate dehydrogenase in detecting liver damage associated with pre-eclampsia. British Journal of Obstetrics and Gynaecology 85: 40–42

Sibai B M 1990a The HELLP syndrome (hemolysis, elevated liver enzymes, and low platelets): much ado about nothing? American Journal of Obstetrics and Gynecology 162: 311–316

Sibai B M 1990b Magnesium sulfate is the ideal anticonvulsant in preeclampsia-eclampsia. American Journal of Obstetrics and Gynecology 162: 1141–1145

Sibai B M 1991 Diagnosis and management of chronic hypertension in pregnancy. Obstetrics and Gynecology 78: 451–461

Sibai B M, McCubbin J H, Anderson G D, Lipshitz J, Dilts P V J 1981 Eclampsia. I. Observations from 67 recent cases. Obstetrics and Gynecology 58: 609–613

Sibai B M, Mabie W C, Shamsa F, Villar M A, Anderson G D 1990 A comparison of no medication versus methyldopa or labetalol in chronic hypertension during pregnancy. American Journal of Obstetrics and Gynecology 162: 960–966

Sibai B M, Sarinoglu C, Mercer B M 1992 Eclampsia. VII. Pregnancy outcome after eclampsia and long-term prognosis. American Journal of Obstetrics and Gynecology 166: 1757–1761

Sibai B M, Caritis S N, Thom E et al 1993a Prevention of preeclampsia with low-dose aspirin in healthy, nulliparous pregnant women. New England Journal of Medicine 329: 1213–1218

Sibai B M, Ramadan M K, Usta I, Salama M, Mercer B M, Friedman S A 1993b Maternal morbidity and mortality in 442 pregnancies with hemolysis, elevated liver enzymes, and low platelets (HELLP syndrome). American Journal of Obstetrics and Gynecology 169: 1000–1006

Simanowitz M D, MacGregor W G, Hobbs J R 1973 Proteinuria in pre-eclampsia. Journal of Obstetrics and Gynaecology of the British Commonwealth 80: 103–108

Slater R M, Wilcox F L, Smith W D et al 1987 Phenytoin infusion in severe pre-eclampsia. Lancet i: 1417–1421

Smarason A K, Sargent I L, Starkey P M, Redman C W G 1993 The effect of placental syncytiotrophoblast microvillous membranes from normal and pre-eclamptic women on the growth of endothelial cells in vitro. British Journal of Obstetrics and Gynaecology 100: 943–949

Solanki D L, Blackburn B C 1985 Spurious thrombocytopenia during pregnancy. Obstetrics and Gynecology 65: 14S–17S

Spargo B H, McCartney C, Winemiller R 1959 Glomerular capillary endotheliosis in toxemia of pregnancy. Archives of Pathology 68: 593–599

Strandgaard S, Olesen J, Skinhoj E, Lassen N A 1973 Autoregulation of brain circulation in severe arterial hypertension. British Medical Journal 1: 507–510

Stratta P, Canavese C, Dogliani M et al 1991 Repeated albumin infusions do not lower blood pressure in preeclampsia. Clinical Nephrology 36: 234–239

Stubbs T M, Lazarchick J, Van Dorsten J P, Cox J, Loadholt C B 1986 Evidence of accelerated platelet production and consumption in nonthrombocytopenic preeclampsia. American Journal of Obstetrics and Gynecology 155: 263–265

Studd J W W, Blainey J, Bailey D 1970 Serum protein changes in the pre-eclampsia–eclampsia syndrome. Journal of Obstetrics and Gynaecology of the British Commonwealth 77: 796–801

Sudo N, Kamoi K, Ishibashi M, Yamaji T 1993 Plasma endothelin-1 and big endothelin-1 levels in women with pre-eclampsia. Acta Endocrinologica (Copenhagen) 129: 114–120

Sumioki H, Shimokawa H, Miyamoto S, Uezono K, Utsunomiya T, Nakano H 1989 Circadian variations of plasma atrial natriuretic peptide in four types of hypertensive disorder during pregnancy. British Journal of Obstetrics and Gynaecology 96: 922–927

Taufield P A, Ales K L, Resnick L M, Druzin M L, Gertner J M,

Laragh J H 1987 Hypocalciuria in preeclampsia. New England Journal of Medicine 316: 715–718

Templeton A, Campbell D M 1979 A retrospective study of eclampsia in the Grampian region, 1965–1977. Health Bulletin (Edinburgh) 37: 55–59

Tepperman H M, Beydoun S N, Abdul-Karim R 1977 Drugs affecting myometrial contractility in pregnancy. Clinical Obstetrics and Gynecology 28: 423–445

Terasaki K K, Quinn M F, Lundell C J, Finck E J, Pentecost M J 1990 Spontaneous hepatic hemorrhage in preeclampsia: treatment with hepatic arterial embolization. Radiology 174: 1039–1041

Thomsen J K, Storm T L, Thamsborg G, de Nully M, Bodker B, Skouby S 1987 Atrial natriuretic peptide concentrations in pre-eclampsia. British Medical Journal 294: 1508–1510

Thomson A M, Hytten R E, Billewicz W Z 1967 The epidemiology of edema during pregnancy. Journal of Obstetrics and Gynaecology of the British Commonwealth 74: 1–10

Thorley K J 1984 Randomised trial of atenolol and methyl dopa in pregnancy related hypertension. Clinical and Experimental Hypertension B3: 168

Thornton J G, Onwude J L 1991 Pre-eclampsia: discordance among identical twins. British Medical Journal 303: 1241–1242

Trofatter K F J, Howell M K, Greenberg C S, Hage M L 1989 Use of the fibrin D-dimer in screening for coagulation abnormalities in preeclampsia. Obstetrics and Gynecology 73: 435–440

Tsukimori K, Maeda H, Shingu M, Koyanagi T, Nobunaga M, Nakano H 1992 The possible role of endothelial cells in hypertensive disorders during pregnancy. Obstetrics and Gynecology 80: 229–233

Tygart S G, McRoyan D K, Spinnato J A, McRoyan C J, Kitay D Z 1986 Longitudinal study of platelet indices during normal pregnancy. American Journal of Obstetrics and Gynecology 154: 883–887

Ulmsten U 1984 Treatment of normotensive and hypertensive patients with preterm labor using oral nifedipine, a calcium antagonist. Archives of Gynecology 236: 69–72

van Dongen P W J, Eskes T K A B, Martin C B, van't Hoff M A 1980 Postural blood pressure differences in pregnancy. American Journal of Obstetrics and Gynecology 138: 1–5

Vandenplas O, Dive A, Dooms G, Mahieu P 1990 Magnetic resonance evaluation of severe neurological disorders in eclampsia. Neuroradiology 32: 47–49

Vanhoutte P M 1993 Is endothelin involved in the pathogenesis of hypertension? Hypertension 21: 747–751

Vardi J, Fields G A 1974 Microangiopathic hemolytic anemia in severe pre-eclampsia. American Journal of Obstetrics and Gynecology 119: 617–622

Vink G J, Moodley J 1982 The effect of low-dose dihydrallazine on the fetus in the emergency treatment of hypertension in pregnancy. South African Medical Journal 62: 475–477

Waisman G D, Mayorga L M, Camera M I, Vignolo C A, Martinotti A 1988 Magnesium plus nifedipine: potentiation of hypotensive effect in preeclampsia? American Journal of Obstetrics and Gynecology 159: 308–309

Wallenburg H C S, Hutchinson D L 1979 A radioangiographic study of the effects of the catecholamines on uteroplacental blood flow in the rhesus monkey. Journal of Medical Primatology 8: 57–65

Walters B N J, Redman C W G 1984 Treatment of severe pregnancy-associated hypertension with the calcium antagonist nifedipine. British Journal of Obstetrics and Gynaecology 91: 330–336

Walters B N J, Thompson M E, Lee A, De Swiet M 1986 Blood pressure in the puerperium. Clinical Science 71: 589–594

Wang Y P, Walsh S W, Guo J D, Zhang J Y 1991 Maternal levels of prostacyclin, thromboxane, vitamin E, and lipid peroxides throughout normal pregnancy. American Journal of Obstetrics and Gynecology 165: 1690–1694

Watson D L, Sibai B M, Shaver D C, Dacus J V, Anderson G D 1983 Late postpartum eclampsia: an update. Southern Medical Journal 76: 1487–1489

Weinstein L 1982 Syndrome of hemolysis, elevated liver enzymes, and low platelet count: a severe consequence of hypertension in pregnancy. American Journal of Obstetrics and Gynecology 142: 159–167

Whitelaw A 1981 Maternal methyldopa treatment and neonatal blood pressure. British Medical Journal 283: 471

Wightman H, Hibbard B M, Rosen M 1978 Perinatal mortality and morbidity associated with eclampsia. British Medical Journal 2: 235–237

Wilcken B, Leung K C, Hammond J, Kamath R, Leonard J V 1993 Pregnancy and fetal long-chain 3-hydroxyacyl coenzyme A dehydrogenase deficiency. Lancet 341: 407–408

Wilke G, Rath W, Schutz E, Armstrong V W, Kuhn W 1992 Haptoglobin as a sensitive marker of hemolysis in HELLP-syndrome. International Journal of Gynaecology and Obstetrics 39: 29–34

Williams M A, Lieberman E, Mittendorf R, Monson R R, Schoenbaum S C 1991 Risk factors for abruptio placentae. American Journal of Epidemiology 134: 965–972

Ylikorkala O, Viinikka L 1992 The role of prostaglandins in obstetrical disorders. Baillières Clinical Obstetrics and Gynaecology 6: 809–827

Zinaman M, Rubin J, Lindheimer M D 1985 Serial plasma oncotic pressure levels and echoencephalography during and after delivery in severe pre-eclampsia. Lancet i: 1245–1247

25. Infections in pregnancy

Rosalinde Hurley

GENERAL CONSIDERATIONS

Pregnancy and the puerperium

Any of the acute or chronic specific infectious diseases may be contracted during the course of pregnancy or the puerperium, and conception may occur in women already subject to infection. The coexistence of pregnancy may aggravate the risk to maternal life of the more serious of these diseases, some of which constitute a hazard to the fetus and the newborn. Fetal death may result from contagion since some viruses, bacteria and protozoa are able to cross the placental barrier, or it may be caused by placental insufficiency, hyperpyrexia or maternal exhaustion and toxaemia. The newborn may contract a transmissible disease from close contact with an infected mother shortly after birth, or as a result of maternal infection, may be born in a sickly and marasmic condition and soon succumb to intercurrent infection. In the early part of the puerperium parturient women are peculiarly susceptible to serious infections of the genital tract and childbed fever has always been one of the most important causes of maternal death.

Although serious microbial disease is well controlled in the UK, mothers of young children, particularly of those at school, are exposed to the specific infectious diseases of childhood and in addition to the common upper respiratory tract infections may contract mumps, chickenpox, measles, rubella, scarlet fever, acute bacterial tonsillitis, whooping cough, dysentery or viral diarrhoeas. As young adults the mothers may contract toxoplasmosis or poliomyelitis. Some of these diseases have important consequences in obstetric practice and pose a problem if the mother's antenatal condition necessitates admission to an obstetric unit, since isolation may be required.

The venereal diseases may be contracted at any time during pregnancy or the puerperium and those that could have fatal or crippling effects on the fetus are tested for during the antenatal period. Routine serological tests for syphilis are performed during pregnancy usually at the first visit together with other booking tests (Table 25.1).

The other venereal diseases—gonorrhoea, chancroid, granuloma inguinale and lymphogranuloma venereum— are sought during pregnancy at the routine antenatal clinical examination by eliciting the medical and social history, by physical examination and by appropriate laboratory tests.

Exacerbation of caries and dental sepsis occurs during pregnancy and women with valvular disease of the heart are at risk of infective endocarditis if dental surgery is necessitated, as well as at parturition. Endocarditis in pregnancy is discussed by Hurley (1977).

While no infection is peculiar to pregnancy, the incidence of some seems to be increased in pregnant as compared with non-pregnant women. Infections of the urinary tract are common complications and emphasis is placed

Table 25.1 Scrutiny for infectious disease at booking

History taking

General examination, especially heart, lungs and genital tract
Serological testing of booking blood*

1. for treponemal disease (TPHA, VDRL)
2. for markers of hepatitis B and C viruses
3. for rubella immune status
4. for toxoplasma immune status†
5. for HIV antibody‡

*It is important that booking serum should be stored by the laboratory until after the birth of the baby.
†In some European countries.
‡In high-risk patients, with maternal consent.

on their early diagnosis and treatment. The incidence of vulvovaginitis is increased in pregnancy and is occasioned largely by infections with members of the genus *Candida*, the fungi of thrush. The other important cause of vaginitis in pregnancy is the protozoan parasite *Trichomonas vaginalis*. Vaginosis associated with *Gardnerella vaginalis* is of less consequence.

The most notorious of the acute infections associated with the puerperium is infection of the genital tract, which formerly accounted for the majority of infectious deaths in pregnancy and the puerperium and is still the most important cause of maternal death from infection in obstetric practice in the UK. Inflammation and suppuration of the lactating breast may occur and urinary tract infections are fairly frequent. Women who have been subjected to surgery may develop bronchopneumonia or wound infections. All are common causes of elevation of the temperature in the lying-in period. Fever during pregnancy or the puerperium is likely to be infectious in origin, although drug or serum fever, fever associated with malignant or thromboembolic disease, haemolytic disease or metabolic disorder may have to be considered in its differential diagnosis. The causes of fever during pregnancy are discussed by Hurley (1989).

The newborn is peculiarly prone to certain infections and is less able to localize them than the adult. Conversely, it is immune to some other infections and immunity continues for several months after birth. The immunological status of the newborn is the result of two systems: the first is active and depends on the infant's own capacity to develop immunity; the second is passive and derived from the transfer of maternal IgG antibody during gestation. The infant is temporarily immune from certain diseases if the mother has suffered from them or is herself immune; transferred virus or protozoal antibodies may confer on the child an immunity that lasts 6–12 months, although antibodies to bacterial antigens do not persist as long.

Infections such as rubella, cytomegalic inclusion disease, toxoplasmosis and listeriosis may be disseminated and fatal in the newborn, while rarely so in the adult. Bacteria such as *Flavobacterium meningosepticum* cause meningitis in the newborn but are never isolated as pathogens in adults. The newborn infant therefore demonstrates a proclivity towards severe infections with organisms which in the adult are usually of low virulence or even non-pathogenic (e.g. some staphylococci) and is also at risk from the tendency of microbial diseases to disseminate, with fatal consequences.

The response of adults to antigen stimulation consists of production of IgM, followed quickly by production of IgG. The pattern of response in the newborn is different; IgM is elaborated as a first response, but this persists for several weeks before IgG is elaborated. The fetus elaborates IgM in response to antigen exposure in utero and detection of specific antibody in the IgM fraction of cord blood is the most useful of the diagnostic tests for congenital infections such as rubella or syphilis. Elevation of the non-specific IgM level to 18 mg/100 ml is regarded by many as indicative of intrauterine infection and is used as a screening test in sickly or debilitated infants.

The reasons for the poor response of the newborn to certain infections are not clearly understood but there is some evidence that in addition to the physiological dysglobulinaemia mentioned above, the cellular response to infection varies in the newborn and the phagocytes are less active. There is a lack of antigen-presenting macrophages.

Prematurity and low birthweight are not only prejudicial peripartum events but also predispose to serious bacterial infections with high mortality rates (neonatal sepsis). Minor sepsis of skin or conjunctivae is common. The most frequent cause of minor sepsis in the UK is *Staphylococcus aureus*. Meningitis and septicaemia may be caused by *Escherichia coli* or by other Gram-negative bacteria, including *Pseudomonas aeruginosa*, or by streptococci particularly those of Lancefield group B. The aetiology of severe forms of epidemic diarrhoea of the newborn is still disputed. Occasionally salmonella are isolated, or pathogenic *E. coli*, while other cases may have a viral aetiology.

Host–parasite interactions

With respect to microbial disease, the term immunity embraces the whole array of states that may exist between the host and indigenous or exogenous microbes—states that range from complete susceptibility with evolution of fulminant life-threatening disease to commensalism.

The indigenous flora comprise many genera and species of bacteria and to a lesser extent some of the yeasts. These commensals occupy as their habitats ecological niches determined by the physiological characteristics of the micro-organism, by local chemical and physical properties of the host and, to some extent, by the nature of other microbes inhabiting the locale. Some are members of pathogenic genera and while not exerting a harmful effect in their customary habitat, will do so if they gain ingress into the tissues of the host. Others may cause localized disease through possession of properties such as bacterial adherence and toxin production. The integrity of anatomical and physiological barriers is important in preventing microbial disease, for breaches of the integument occasioned by injury or disease provide important portals of entry for pathogenic bacteria. In order to produce disease pathogenic microbes must be capable of entering and colonizing host tissue and then of causing local or systemic damage. They must, therefore, be capable of overcoming host resistance either by specific aggressive mechanisms or by taking advantage of local or general impairment of function.

Host resistance depends on innate (genetic) as well as

environmental factors and is engineered by non-specific as wells as specific (immune) mechanisms. The principal mechanism of protection against invading micro-organisms is the immune system which is characterized by three attributes—specificity, memory and recognition of self-antigens. Its function is to protect against foreign substances. The immune status of individuals may be innate or acquired. Innate immunity is genetically or constitutionally determined and is not a function of cells of the immune system or of specific antibody, but the result of physiological, biochemical or anatomical differences principally between species. There is well defined species immunity exemplified in man by the species-specificity of microbes such as *Neisseria meningitidis*, *Treponema pallidum* and the measles (rubeola) virus, which naturally infect only man, while other species are resistant. Racial immunity also exists; a well known example is the resistance of blacks with sickle cell anaemia to disease caused by *Plasmodium falciparum*. The most outstanding example of innate immunity as it applies to obstetrics is the relative inability of *Brucella abortus* to cause abortion in man although it causes contagious abortion in cattle, formerly of considerable economic consequence in Europe. The special predilection of *B. abortus* for the reproductive system of cattle is due in part to the high concentration of erythritol, a growth-promoting substance for the microbe, in the bovine placenta and seminal vesicles; this situation is not found in man in whose tissues erythritol concentrations are low. Body temperature is an important mechanism of innate immunity. With few exceptions the optimum temperature for growth of human pathogens is around 37°C.

Immunity is acquired either passively or actively. Naturally acquired passive immunity follows the transfer of immune antibody of the IgG class from mother to fetus by the transplacental route and the ingestion of IgA antibody in colostrum. Artificially acquired passive immunity follows injection of immune products such as antitoxins, antisera or immune globulin from the same or a different species.

The microbial flora of the newborn infant and female genital tract

The origin of the different organisms in the infant is the immediate environment. During passage through the birth canal the skin and mucous membranes become contaminated with organisms from the mother and microbes are proliferating in the infant's alimentary tract within a few hours. The baby may also acquire microbes from the wider external environment. If these are virulent and the baby is disadvantaged by prematurity or low birthweight, neonatal sepsis may arise, being early onset in type with microbes derived from its own mother's genital tract and late onset with those derived from the environment. The infant's mouth becomes colonized within a few days of birth and the main source of the colonizing organisms is the maternal vagina. At birth, the intestine may contain only a few bacteria but is rapidly colonized. The flora of the breastfed infant consists largely of anaerobes such as *Lactobacillus* and *Bacteroides* (about 99%) but coliforms are also present. After weaning the flora resembles that of the adult. The upper respiratory tract is colonized soon after birth particularly after close contact with the mother at the first feed.

The vulva and vestibulum of the newborn are sterile; organisms appear in 7–8 hours. The commonest aerobic organisms are staphylococci, diphtheroids, enterococci, coliform bacilli and yeasts. Many anaerobes also occur. The vagina of the newborn is sterile and organisms appear in 12–14 hours. Staphylococci, enterococci and diphtheroids appear at first but are replaced in 2–3 days by an almost pure culture of Döderlein's bacilli. At this time the vaginal secretion is acid and glycogen is demonstrable in the vaginal epithelium. The occurrence of glycogen appears to be due to the presence of oestrogens derived from the maternal circulation. Soon this is excreted in the urine and the vaginal secretion becomes alkaline. Thereafter, until puberty, the secretion remains alkaline and staphylococci, streptococci other than *Streptococcus pyogenes*, coliforms and diphtheroid bacilli predominate.

At puberty, glycogen is again deposited in the vaginal wall, the secretion becomes acid and Döderlein's bacilli and corynebacteria are re-established as the predominant organisms. The flora is mixed and streptococci, coliforms and fungi are present. The streptococci of the vagina are varied and *Str. faecalis* (Lancefield group D) is common. Lancefield groups C, B, F and G occur but are less frequent. Other streptococci are also found. *Mycoplasma* can be demonstrated occasionally. In addition to these, numbers of Gram-negative rods, not all members of the Enterobacteriaceae, are encountered and some Gram-variable coccobacilli (*Gardnerella*) are found.

The distribution of microbes isolated from the posterior fornices of pregnant women is shown in Table 25.2 (Hurley et al 1974). The incidence of large colony mycoplasmas in pregnant women according to several authors ranges from 23 to 71% for T-mycoplasmas and from 4 to 39% for *Mycoplasma hominis*. de Louvois et al (1974) also noted an incidence of 51.6% T-mycoplasmas and of 11.7% *M. hominis* in infertile women.

After the menopause, oestrogenic activity decreases, glycogen is not deposited in the vaginal epithelium, the vaginal secretions are less acid and cocci are said to predominate amongst the vaginal flora. Many of the endogenous microbes isolated from the vagina during pregnancy are members of pathogenic genera. Some may be implicated in puerperal sepsis and others in chorioamnionitis and neonatal sepsis. Occasionally microbes are isolated that are not part of the resident flora; their presence may indicate disease of the genital tract. Those microbes exogenous to the genital tract are shown in Table 25.3.

Table 25.2 Flora of lower genital tract in 280 unselected pregnant women

Organism	% Incidence
Corynebacteria	84
Lactobacilli	82
Staphylococcus epidermidis	66
Micrococci	37
Faecal streptococci	34
Microaerophilic and anaerobic streptococci	22
Escherichia coli	19
Candida albicans	17
Mycoplasma hominis	11
Beta-haemolytic streptococci	9
Group B	5
Group C	< 1
Groups F and G	< 1
Not groupable	3
Gram-variable coccobacilli	7
Proteus mirabilis	6
Bacteroides species	5
Staphylococcus aureus	5
Non-haemolytic streptococci	4
Torulopsis glabrata	4
Trichomonas vaginalis	3
Neisseria species (pharyngis and catarrhalis)	1
Klebsiella aerogenes	< 1
Pseudomonas aeruginosa	< 1
Sought but not isolated	
Lancefield group A streptococci	Nil
Clostridium perfringens	Nil
Neisseria gonorrhoea	Nil
Listeria monocytogenes	Nil
Haemophilus species	Nil
Not sought	
Viruses, chlamydia, T-strain mycoplasmas	

Table 25.3 Abnormal pathogenic flora* of the female genital tract

Lancefield group A streptococci
Streptococcus pneumoniae
Clostridium perfringens
Clostridium tetani
Corynebacterium diphtheriae
Mycobacterium tuberculosis
Treponema pallidum
Neisseria gonorrhoeae
Neisseria meningitidis
Haemophilus ducreyi
Haemophilus influenzae
Chlamydia trachomatis
Schistosoma mansoni
Schistosoma haematobium
Enterobius vermicularis
Cytomegalovirus
Rubella virus, or vaccine virus
Herpes hominis

*Being either exogenous flora, or encountered with frequency of less than 1 in 250.

Large numbers of bacteria occur in human milk but if it is collected under strictly aseptic conditions the plate count should not exceed 2500 organisms per ml. Micrococci, diphtheroids, occasional coliforms, staphylococci, non-haemolytic streptococci and anaerobic lactobacilli are isolated and the milk of healthy nursing mothers delivered in hospital often contains appreciable numbers of *Staphylococcus aureus*.

Some commensals of man belong to the category of microbes that pathologists describe as opportunistic. Lacking genuinely invasive powers, they only occasionally exert a hostile effect on their hosts, usually when general or local resistance is lowered as a consequence of debilitating disease, trauma, haemorrhage or other conditions, or in consequence of a particular physiological state such as being newly born or pregnant. When such microbes cause disease localized to body areas where they are usually or often demonstrable as commensals, the assignment to them of a pathogenic role cannot be inferred simply from the cultural findings. Clearly, the proof that an organism, normally commensal in a given site, is responsible for disease in that particular site cannot rest solely on demonstration of the microbe but must be interpreted in conjunction with the clinical findings and the results of other laboratory tests. The reaction of the host to the microbe must be shown to be abnormal since the presence of the microbe is not.

NON-SPECIFIC INFECTIONS OCCURRING IN PREGNANCY

Urinary tract infections

These are considered in Chapter 26.

Puerperal sepsis and wound infections

Puerperal sepsis includes a series of febrile disorders of the lying-in period that share the common aetiology of being wound infections of the genital tract. Puerperal sepsis may occur after delivery or abortion and is occasioned by several genera of pathogenic bacteria, of which the most notorious and dangerous are *Clostridium* and *Streptococcus*. In the great majority of fatal cases, the microbes are introduced from without, and such infections are preventable. In general, endogenous microbes, harboured in the vagina, such as *Enterobacteriaceae* and *Staphylococcus* cause less severe forms of sepsis. Puerperal sepsis is discussed in Chapter 43.

Other wound infections

The organism most frequently found in septic wounds in gynaecological and obstetric practice is *Staph. aureus*, followed by coliform bacilli and *Proteus* spp. and streptococci, including *Str. pyogenes*, *Str. faecalis* and anaerobic cocci. Infections with *Pseudomonas aeruginosa* and non-sporing aerobes also occur.

Opinions differ on the relative importance of the operating theatre and the ward as the place of infection and this probably differs from hospital to hospital. Certainly the hands of the surgeon, the body of a member of the operating team, fomites surrounding the patient such as blankets, air sucked into the theatre from other parts of the hospital and the patient's own skin may be the source of infection. Inexpert and clumsy surgery is undoubtedly a contributory factor.

Septic abortion and shock

The availability of contraceptive techniques and legislation on abortion has led to diminution in the number of women with septic abortion but the diagnosis should be suspected in every febrile woman who is bleeding in the first trimester of pregnancy. In the majority of cases the cervical os is open and there is evidence of the passage of the products of conception. High spiking fevers and the presence of hypotension are bad prognostic signs. Pelvic examination with assessment of uterine size is important for most serious infections follow attempts to terminate pregnancy in women beyond the 12th week of gestation. As in puerperal sepsis following delivery, extension of the infection beyond the uterus is attended by correspondingly grave risks for the patient. Plain X-rays of the abdomen with the patient both in the supine and the upright positions may demonstrate the presence of intra-peritoneal or myometrial gas. Exploratory laparotomy may be required. Myometrial gas suggests *Clostridium welchii (perfringens)* infection and operative intervention may be required. Foreign bodies, such as intrauterine contraceptive devices, may require removal.

Many patients respond successfully to curettage and antibiotic therapy or even to antibiotic therapy alone. Many antibiotics have been used but the most favoured regimen is a combination of intravenous penicillin and metronidazole with intramuscular aminoglycoside in high dosage. The blood pressure and urinary output should be measured at regular intervals and antibiotic concentrations should be assayed.

The microbes causing septic abortion are similar to those causing postdelivery sepsis, but non-sporing anaerobes such as *Bacteroides fragilis* may be implicated more frequently, and with Gram-negative aerobes such as *Escherichia coli* and *Klebsiella* spp., are related to endotoxic shock. The onset of bacteraemia is accompanied by fever, rigors, nausea, vomiting, diarrhoea and prostration. Tachycardia, tachypnoea, hypotension—usually with cool, pale extremities and often with peripheral cyanosis—oliguria and mental confusion are added to the development of septic shock. The haematological manifestations of shock and the renal complication have been considered by Letsky (1989) and Davison (1989).

CHORIOAMNIONITIS

Chorioamnionitis (Charles & Hurry 1983) may be a major factor in the aetiology of preterm labour, contributing to perinatal mortality from prematurity. Prolonged rupture of the membranes is associated with a high inci-dence of chorioamnionitis and known to predispose to neonatal sepsis.

Inflammation of the fetal membranes arises in consequence of an ascending infection by microbes colonizing the lower genital tract and may result in infection of the amniotic fluid and thence the fetus. Most intrauterine infections are thought to arise in this way; the transplacental or haematogenous routes are relatively unimportant. The inflammatory reaction begins within the umbilical cord vessels or the large vessels of the chorionic plate. Leucocytes migrate, traverse the vessel walls and spread to the mesenchyme, involving the subamniotic zone of the placenta as well as the membranes and the umbilical cord. Spread of infected material to the amniotic sac may occur and fetal infection may result through swallowing or gasping or by haematogenous spread from infected fetal vessels.

Evidence favours the spread of infection through intact membranes, initiated in some cases by coitus (Naeye & Peters 1980) since seminal fluid facilitates the passage of micro-organisms through cervical mucus. Fetal membranes weakened by infection are more likely to rupture. Thus infection may precede as well as follow premature rupture of membranes.

Chorioamnionitis associated with premature rupture of membranes is aetiologically important in premature labour; premature rupture of membranes and preterm labour are associated with the presence of Group-B streptococci in the urine (Thomsen et al 1987). The evidence implicating infection as a cause of preterm labour falls broadly into two categories: the increased incidence of maternal and neonatal infection observed as attendant on preterm labour, and the reported associations between specific microbes, including genital mycoplasmas and others and prematurity and preterm premature rupture of membranes (PPROM). The evidence is marshalled by Lamont & Fisk (1993). Chorioamnionitis occurs more frequently than neonatal sepsis and is often clinically silent, being diagnosed from macroscopic and histological examination of the placenta, membranes and cord. Since these have usually been delivered through the heavily colonized vagina, bacteriological examination is unrewarding. The organisms most commonly isolated from inflamed membranes are *Escherichia coli*, staphylococci and streptococci. Clinical features in the mother include fever, leukocytosis and fetid vaginal discharge, sometimes accompanied by uterine tenderness. Rupture of membranes is invariably present.

Infection of the amniotic fluid may produce the amniotic fluid syndrome of chorioamnionitis, intrauterine and fetal lung infection (Blanc 1959). Congenital pneumonia may occur. Poor nutrition with lowering of the amniotic fluid antibacterial zinc-dependent polypeptide, may contribute to the high incidence of premature births and amniotic fluid infection in women from low socioeconomic groups. Chorioamnionitis is an important predisposing cause of neonatal sepsis. Following infection of the respiratory tree from amniotic fluid, infection of the middle ear and paranasal sinuses may occur. The onset of respiration extends the infection to the pulmonary alveoli and systemic spread may occur.

NEONATAL SEPSIS

Septicaemia and meningitis

In terms of survival and lack of crippling sequelae, the prognosis for babies of low or very low birthweight has altered completely in the last five decades. The virtual certainty of death in 1945 has been replaced by an expected survival rate in specialist centres of 30–50% for those weighing less than 1000 g and of 85% for those weighing between 1000 and 1500 g. Paradoxically, the improvement has increasingly led to more cases of neonatal septicaemia and meningitis: infection rates are between five and 100 times higher in those of low birthweight. Neonatal meningitis is less common than septicaemia and the data reported by Remington & Klein (1983) suggest overall figures of 1.8/1000 births for septicaemia and of 0.2/1000 births for meningitis, as well as rates of 13.3 and 2.6/1000 for those of birthweight less than 2500 g, and 74.5 and 18.6/1000 for those of birthweight less than 1000 g. Klein & Marcy (1990) discuss at some length, and based on many surveys and studies, the characteristics of those who develop sepsis.

Both diseases have high mortality rates which again are inversely proportional to birthweight. All available evidence suggests that neonatal meningitis is consequent on bloodstream infection since the primary site of invasion is the bloodstream with spread to meninges in 25–30% of cases. The term sepsis neonatorum or neonatal sepsis is used for both septicaemia and meningitis.

Neonatal septicaemia is a clinical syndrome characterized by signs of systemic infection and confirmed by a positive blood culture in the first 4 weeks of life. Although some commentators have distinguished primary septicaemia from septicaemia secondary to congenital anomalies, surgical procedures or debility, for epidemiological reasons it is more practical to consider neonatal sepsis in terms of early- and late-onset disease. The cardinal distinction between the two types lies in the source of the infection which in the former is the birth canal and in the latter, the environment.

Early-onset disease occurs in the first week of life as fulminant systemic illness in babies who are usually premature and of low birthweight and who have been born to women who have had abnormal pregnancies and deliveries. Premature and prolonged rupture of the membranes with premature labour, obstetric complications leading to operative or instrumental delivery, maternal or fetal distress, haemorrhage, maternal anaemia or inter-

current illness and peripartum fever are factors that should alert the neonatologist to the potential development of serious infection. The causal bacteria of early-onset sepsis are derived from the birth canal and acquired either by ascending infection in intrauterine life or during passage through the birth canal. Transplacental transmission rarely occurs but the child may be born with a true congenital bacteraemia. The bacteria associated with early-onset sepsis are usually indigenous to the maternal congenital tract but rarely, adventitious microbes such as beta-haemolytic streptococci (Lancefield group A) or *Clostridium perfringens* are isolated. The mortality rate of early-onset sepsis is high and lies between 20% and 50%.

Late-onset disease occurs after the first week of life. There are fewer prejudicial maternal peripartum events but the babies are often afflicted by congenital malformations or illness or other disease. The microbes responsible are usually those disseminated in the infant's environment, epidemiologically reflecting the distribution of pathogens at large in the particular nursery or intensive care baby unit. *Pseudomonas aeruginosa*, *Staphylococcus aureus*, *Klebsiella aerogenes*, *Enterobacter cloaceae* and others are examples of such pathogens. Group B streptococci and *Escherichia coli* are causally related both to early- and late-onset disease. Mortality is lower in late-onset neonatal sepsis: between 10% and 20%.

While it is often difficult in practice to distinguish the type of infection in individual babies, disease of late onset, originating from microbes disseminated in the environment of the susceptible newborn, must be regarded as iatrogenic and preventable by the imposition of rigorous standards of hygiene, antisepsis and asepsis. It is becoming more difficult to control, however, due to the importation of seriously ill babies, often colonized with bacteria foreign to the host centre, into special care baby units which are already overloaded and overworked from the amount of care needed for low birthweight babies. Neonatal sepsis accounts for at least 20% of all referrals of sick babies to special units. Such babies constitute an infectious hazard; necropsy studies at Queen Charlotte's Maternity Hospital showed that 80% of those with septicaemia harbour the microbe in the bronchial tree from whence during life, it may contaminate the attendant's hands and clothing, adjacent fomites, or the larger environment of the special care unit. Terminal septicaemia, whether treated or not, may thus contribute to late-onset sepsis. Dying infected babies should be nursed in isolation.

Meningitis is more frequent in the first month of life than in any other month. It is frequently undiagnosed and may not be suspected until autopsy.

The microbial aetiology of neonatal septicaemia and meningitis is similar and a full account including citations of cases associated with rare and unusual pathogens is given by Klein & Marcy (1990). Most accounts, including the first systematic study of septicaemia by Silverman &

Homan (1949), attest the pre-eminence of *Escherichia coli* and other Gram-negative rods as causative bacteria. In the past, *Str. haemolyticus*, often consequent on puerperal sepsis, seems to have caused the majority of reported cases. Davies (1971) chronicled the changing pattern of sepsis, alluding to the falling incidence of staphylococcal disease and the prominence of Gram-negative rods as causes of serious infection. Many studies in the 1960s from the USA emphasized the increasing frequency of Gram-negative rod sepsis (Gluck et al 1966, McCracken & Shinefield 1966). The group B streptococcus is also an important cause, recognized by Siegel & McCracken (1981) as the predominant pathogen in most American nurseries and together with *Escherichia coli*, accounting for 60% of all cases. Amongst the rare causes of neonatal and early infantile sepsis are *Pasteurella multocida*, *Flavobacterium meningosepticum*, *Haemophilus influenzae* and *Vibrio fetus* (now *Campylobacter*). *Neisseria meningitidis* is a rare cause although it does occur in early infancy, as does *N. gonorrhoeae*. *Candida* septicaemia is well known. Epidemics of neonatal sepsis have been associated with *Citrobacter koseri*, *Achromobacter*, *Listeria monocytogenes* and *Hansenula anomala* (Murphy et al 1986).

Fatal viral infection is rare in the newborn period and life-threatening disease is overwhelmingly of bacterial origin. Only five cases came to necropsy in 58 160 births in our hospital over a 17-year period. Disseminated candidosis is also rare; six cases were encountered over the same period.

Meningoencephalitis may be caused by *Toxoplasma gondii* and by rubella and cytomegalovirus, as well as by herpes simplex, poliomyelitis, mumps and chickenpox zoster. Coxsackieviruses also affect the central nervous system.

SPECIFIC INFECTIONS

Trichomoniasis

The protozoan parasite *Trichomonas vaginalis*, a pear-shaped, motile organism, is accepted as an aetiological agent of vaginitis. An extremely similar organism, *T. hominis*, inhabits the gastrointestinal tract. *T. vaginalis* is a less frequent cause of vaginitis than species of *Candida*. Up to 6% of pregnant women develop vaginitis with a *Trichomonas* : yeast ratio of 1 : 3 and an incidence of simultaneous infection with yeasts and trichomonads of the order of 0.8%.

The infection is diagnosed when motile trichomonads are demonstrated in the vaginal discharge and the patient has symptoms. The discharge is greenish yellow, frothy and irritant, with a musty odour.

The organism is recognized by its characteristic jerky movements in wet preparations. The vaginal secretion should be examined microscopically with low magnification and then with the 1/6-inch lens. Films stained with Leishman, Giemsa or Papanicolaou's technique may also be used to demonstrate the parasite. Cultural methods are available. Metronidazole is curative when administered both to the patient and her sexual partner.

The infection is most frequently encountered in women of reproductive age and is sexually transmitted. Studies have failed to show that it is transmitted to the newborn and it is not associated with adverse effects on the growing fetus.

Candidosis

The fungi that cause candidosis belong to the genus *Candida*, a genus of dimorphic fungi reproducing by budding but capable of filamentous growth. While some eight species are pathogenic in man, only *C. albicans*, the principal member of the genus and *C. glabrata* (formerly called *Torulopsis glabrata*) are commonly associated with vaginal thrush.

Candida species are widely spread in nature, principally as commensals in the gastrointestinal tracts of birds and animals. Numerous surveys attest to the predominant incidence of *C. albicans*, which can be found in the vaginas of up to 36% of pregnant women and up to 16% of non-pregnant women. Yeast-like fungi, predominantly *C. albicans*, have been found in the mouths of up to 54% of children aged 2–6 weeks. The organisms are rarely harboured on the skin. In spite of their occurrence as commensals, infection by these organisms can still on occasion be exogenous—in the vagina as the result of unclean instrumentation and in the mouths of babies as a result of contaminated teats or bottles. Conjugal infection can also occur. Thus although usually endemic, vaginal candidosis and thrush can occur in epidemic form.

Pregnancy and diabetes predispose to thrush vaginitis as does administration of some broad-spectrum antibiotics. Multiparous are more often infected than nulliparous women. The incidence of vaginal yeasts rises in pregnancy but there is general agreement that the number is greatly diminished after parturition, possibly as a consequence of the cleansing effect of the lochia. The overall incidence of vaginal thrush in pregnant women is about 16%. The incidence is highest in the third trimester and in the summer months. In non-pregnant women, the incidence is higher in the summer months and exacerbations occur in the premenstrual period. *Candida* vulvovaginitis rarely occurs in little girls but is fairly frequent after the menopause. Although typically white and curd-like, the discharge may be thick and often highly acid in the acute stages; vulvitis is a concomitant feature.

The diagnosis of candidosis is made on clinical grounds but positive culture is required for confirmation. The criteria for diagnosis include the observation of plaques or of cheesy debris in the vagina; signs of vaginitis or vulvovaginitis accompanied by isolation of fungus, or isolation of the fungus alone which in 84% of instances is associated with the first two criteria. Clinically, the disease is characterized by pruritus and discharge.

Polyene antifungal antibiotics such as nystatin or amphotericin B are effective in vaginal thrush, as are drugs of the imidazole group. The cure rate with specific drugs in vaginal candidosis is of the order of 90% although more than one course may have to be given. A small but appreciable number of women suffer from long-standing thrush which is refractory to ordinary regimens of treatment.

Syphilis

Syphilis is the most notorious of the congenital infections; the ready transmissibility of *Treponema pallidum* to the fetus led Stokes et al (1944) to include this feature in their definition of the disease. Syphilis appeared to be under some measure of control in the late 1960s and early 1970s but since then there has been a rise in the number of cases of infectious syphilis throughout the world. Ingall et al (1990) discuss possible reasons for the rise and emphasize the risk factors, including promiscuity and drug abuse, that may lead to increases in reported cases of congenital disease. Transmission of spirochaete to the fetus is always from the infected mother since direct transmission to the fetus via spermatozoa does not occur. Traditionally it is held that infection of the fetus does not occur before the fourth month of pregnancy and that it is most likely after the sixth month, since this accords with observed pathological change in the fetus. The Langhans' cells of the early placenta are thought to be impenetrable by the spirochaete. Infection involves the placenta with haematogenous spread, resulting in widespread involvement of fetal tissues.

The risk to the fetus varies with the stage of untreated syphilis in the mother. In general, the outcome of earlier pregnancies will be miscarriages or stillbirths and subsequently, living syphilitic children will be born. After many years healthy non-infected children may be born. This sequence of events is called Kassowitz' law but according to Catterall (1979) it seldom occurs. More usually miscarriages alternate with stillbirths or live syphilitic children and healthy babies may be born between two infected babies. Fiumara et al (1952) assessed the risk to the fetus according to the stage of untreated syphilis in the mother. In primary or secondary syphilis the risk of transmission approaches 100% and normal full-term infants are not to be expected. Some 50% are born prematurely or die in the perinatal period and 50% have congenital syphilis. The risk is lower in early and late latent syphilis; in the former 20% will be normal infants and in the latter 70%.

The clinical manifestations of congenital syphilis have been well described (Ingall & Norins 1976, Catterall 1979) and can be considered in three groups. Those of *early infectious syphilis* include skin rashes (syphilitic pemphigus or rashes typical of secondary syphilis), mucous patches (snuffles), hepatosplenomegaly, lymphadenopathy, osteochondritis (pseudoparalysis of Parrot) and meningovascular syphilis. Definitive diagnosis is based on dark ground microscopy; lesions of the skin and mucous membranes are teeming with spirochaetes. Serological tests establish a presumptive diagnosis, particularly if specific IgM is demonstrable in the infant's blood.

The *late, non-infectious manifestations of congenital syphilis* occur after the second year of life, most commonly between the ages of 7 and 15. Interstitial keratitis is the most common of these lesions but nerve deafness, Clutton's joints, gummata and neurosyphilis may all occur.

The *stigmata of congenital syphilis* are occasioned by structural abnormalities consequent on fetal infection and include Parrot's nodes, frontal bossing and the 'hot cross bun' skull, saddle nose, high arched palate, bulldog facies and anomalies of secondary dentition (Hutchinson's teeth and Moon's molars). Hutchinson's triad (interstitial keratitis, Hutchinson's teeth and eighth nerve deafness) is pathognomonic of congenital syphilis. The diagnosis of late congenital syphilis can be confirmed by serological tests in the majority of instances.

Congenital syphilis can be prevented and its prevention is one of the aims of antenatal care. Serological tests for treponemal disease should be made on serum taken at the booking visit; retesting later in pregnancy may also be advisable. In the UK those with serological evidence of treponemal disease should be referred to the care of a genitourinary physician; Ingall & Norins (1976) state the guidelines that should be followed by American physicians. A full account of diagnosis and treatment is given by Ingall et al (1990).

Gonorrhoea

This is an acute, specific infectious disease, usually transmitted during sexual intercourse and characterized in adults primarily by invasion of the genitourinary tract although secondary disturbances may complicate its course. In women the disease begins with an acute urethritis, infection of Skene's ducts and spread to the cervix. After a few days it becomes subacute and the infection may spread to Bartholin's glands, the bladder, the Fallopian tubes and the pelvic peritoneum. Unless treated promptly the infection becomes chronic, resulting in Bartholin cyst or abscess, chronic cervicitis, chronic salpingo-oophoritis and occasionally through bloodstream dissemination, in arthritis, tenosynovitis or ophthalmia. Rarely the disease is disseminated and fatal from the beginning. Venereal warts affecting the thighs and labia are probably of viral aetiology but are often associated with gonorrhoea.

Salpingitis may cause non-occlusive scarring and loss of ciliary action in the Fallopian tubes leading to ectopic pregnancy, an appreciable cause of maternal death. The risk of endometritis following termination of pregnancy is increased threefold in those with gonorrhoea, and infected women are more likely to have prolonged rupture of membranes or premature labour.

In neonates gonococcal ophthalmia, which is rare in adults, is the most common manifestation of infection but skin infections and infections of the anus, rectum and pharynx may occur, and, occasionally, disseminated infection may result in meningitis (Jephcott 1992). Vulvovaginitis also occurs in infants, spreading by contact with imperfectly sterilized fomites such as napkins, and assuming epidemic proportions in institutions. The gonococcus is not, however, the only cause of epidemic vulvovaginitis; it can also be caused by streptococci or staphylococci.

The diagnosis depends in the main on demonstration of the parasite and in acute infections with typical signs and symptoms direct examination of a Gram-stained smear will often show the characteristic kidney- or bean-shaped Gram-negative intracellular diplococci. However, these may be concealed by a heavy flora of commensal organisms and the resemblance of some of these to *Neisseria gonorrhoeae* may give rise to difficulty. Experience is needed in identifying *N. gonorrhoeae* in stained films. Wherever possible cultures must be made. In chronic cases the gonococcus is less easy to demonstrate and to cultivate and specimens sent to the laboratory must be taken from the sites most likely to be the seat of chronic infection, such as Bartholin's glands and the cervical glands. Fluid withdrawn from joint lesions and pus from chronically inflamed Fallopian tubes are frequently sterile. The gonococcus is extremely susceptible to drying and care must be taken with swabs sent to distant laboratories; these swabs should be placed in transport medium. Procaine penicillin or ampicillin with probenecid, or spectinomycin, co-trimoxazole or cefuroxime are used in treatment. Penicillin resistance occurs in some strains.

Chlamydial infections

Evidence has accumulated that isolates from lymphogranuloma venereum, trachoma, inclusion conjunctivitis and milder infections of the genital tract are related, justifying their inclusion in the genus *Chlamydia*. *Chlamydia trachomatis* has been isolated from various clinical conditions including non-specific urethritis, cervicitis and Reiter's disease.

The chlamydiae are a group of obligate intracellular parasites lying between bacteria and viruses which do not grow on artificial media but can be propagated in fertile eggs and by tissue culture. The inclusion bodies associated with *C. trachomatis* contain glycogen and stain with iodine. The organisms can be serotyped and those isolated from the genital tract and eye in the UK are serotypes D, E, F and G. *C. trachomatis* is an important cause of non-specific infection of the genital tract and its role in pelvic inflammatory disease is established. The agent is sensitive to sulphonamides, tetracycline and erythromycin. The latter is the agent of choice for treating chlamydial cervicitis during pregnancy.

C. psittaci, the cause of psittacosis, mainly affects birds and non-primate mammals and is responsible for enzootic and epizootic ovine and bovine abortion. Pregnant women coming into contact with sheep at lambing time may contract the infection and abort. *C. psittaci* may be isolated from the fetus (Johnson et al 1985).

Toxoplasmosis

Toxoplasmosis is probably unique amongst the parasitic diseases of man in that its congenital form was recognized before the postnatally acquired form. There is little difference in the prevalence rates between sexes although the disease is clearly more important and more frequently diagnosed in women of childbearing age. There are few data from which to derive morbidity, mortality or case fatality rates.

Serological surveys show that infection with the protozoan parasite *Toxoplasma gondii* is common and widespread in man. The organism is an obligatory intracellular parasite, elongated or sickle-shaped and approximately $3-4 \times 6-7\ \mu m$. The coccidian parasite exists in three forms—the trophozoite, the tissue cyst and the cat-associated oocyst. The latter two are the principal forms implicated in transmission. Pregnant women should avoid the consumption or handling of raw meat and wear gloves gardening or if it is necessary for them to handle cat litter. Of great importance in obstetrics is the fact that infection can be passed congenitally from mother to fetus, in some species through several generations. The disease may be acquired during intrauterine life if the mother is infected during pregnancy.

Illness is a rare accompaniment of this common infection and the best known manifestation of acquired toxoplasmosis is lymphadenopathy, which may be accompanied by the presence of glandular fever-like cells in the blood. The disease affects both sexes and the peak incidence is between 25 and 35 years.

Although placental transmission has been demonstrated in chronically infected mice, in humans congenital infection is believed to follow primary infection and the prognosis for subsequent pregnancies is good. The risk to the fetus appears to be related to the gestational age at which primary maternal infection occurs, with transmission being less likely in the first trimester but if it does occur, resulting in more severe disease. Infection leading to stillbirth or neonatal death, or to survival with ocular and cerebral involvement, occurs only in the offspring of mothers who acquire primary infection in the first or second trimester.

Although transmission rates as high as 33% have been reported following primary maternal infection, 72% of the infected newborn were spared overt clinical infection. Such asymptomatic infants may suffer no serious consequences or may later develop chorioretinitis, blindness, strabismus, hydrocephaly or microcephaly, cerebral calcification, psychomotor or mental retardation, epilepsy, or deafness. Children known to have had congenital toxoplasmosis must therefore be kept under observation for months or years.

The available data are insufficient to support or to refute the hypothesis that *T. gondii* causes malformations during the period of organogenesis. The infected infant should be treated with spiramycin or pyrimethamine/sulphonamide and folinic acid. There is some evidence that treatment of the mother who has an acute attack in pregnancy with spiramycin decreases the fetal risk.

T. gondii may be isolated from ventricular or cerebrospinal fluid, blood, lymph node or other tissue. Mice or multimammate rats are inoculated by the intracerebral, intraperitoneal or subcutaneous routes and left for 6–8 weeks. Their sera are tested for antibodies and finally after killing, a saline emulsion of brain is examined for *Toxoplasma* cysts. Fertile hen's eggs or tissue cultures may be inoculated but these methods are less sensitive. The histological appearance of excised lymph nodes may suggest toxoplasmosis.

Serological tests include the cytoplasm-modifying (dye) test of Sabin and Feldman, complement fixation, haemagglutination and fluorescence inhibition. Enzyme linked immunosorbent assay (ELISA) and enzyme linked immunosorbent agglutination assay are now widely used, and the IgG avidity test is promising as a possible indicator of early acquired infection. The interpretation of serological tests can be very difficult as latent infection is so common. Demonstration of a rising titre or the presence of specific IgM antibody indicates active infection. When it is not possible to demonstrate a rise a dye test titre of 1 : 1000 is probably reliable evidence of current infection.

The risk to the fetus of primary maternal toxoplasmosis is of the order of 50%, some 15% in the first trimester and 70% in the third. In early gestational life abortion is the likely outcome. Since 1975 in Austria, all women have been screened for *Toxoplasma* antibody during pregnancy (Aspock 1985). If seroconversion (primary infection) occurs the mother is treated. Spiramycin is used if infection occurs in the first trimester; otherwise pyrimethamine and sulphametoxydiazine are given. It is believed that congenital infection has been reduced by 50–70% in consequence of these measures. Prenatal diagnosis of toxoplasmosis was discussed by Desmonts et al (1985). The results of a 20-year follow-up of those with congenital toxoplasmosis demonstrated that subclinical infection at birth could have severe consequences and persuaded Koppe et al (1986) that women should be screened before marriage and during pregnancy.

In the UK, screening for *Toxoplasma* antibodies is not routinely performed during pregnancy because the incidence of infection is low.

Listeriosis

Listeria monocytogenes is one of few pathogens that can form colonies at 4°C and it can survive in nature in hay, straw and earth for many months. It has been isolated from many species of domestic birds, insects and crustaceans. The infective cycle is probably based on its survival in soil or vegetation, multiplication in silage, establishment of carrier or diseased state in animals or fowls, and for man, growth in food derived from these sources and consumed after inadequate heating. Its localization in the genital tracts of many vertebrates and its transmission to the fetus characterize its importance in obstetrics. A large outbreak of listeriosis occurred in 1981 in the Atlantic provinces of Canada, including many perinatal cases, and was attributed to cabbage fertilized with infected sheep manure. Of 25 cases of maternal and perinatal listeriosis in Nova Scotia, 17 infants were born alive although five died; there were three stillbirths and five spontaneous abortions.

Characteristically, infection in pregnant women is associated with two or more febrile episodes. The first, recognized in retrospect as the primary infection, is associated with malaise, headache, fever, backache, pharyngitis, conjunctivitis, diarrhoea and abdominal or loin pain. The condition may be diagnosed as pyelonephritis since the kidneys may be involved in the listeric process but the true nature of the infection will be recognized if the often slowly growing *L. monocytogenes* is actively sought in cultures of blood and of other sites, such as the genital tract and urine. Resolution of fever may occur if antibacterial therapy has been given but relapse is likely. Within 1–20 days of delivery, often of an infected premature baby, there is a further febrile episode regarded as a manifestation of reinfection from the placenta. In about 40% of cases fever is not marked at any time; the disease presents as an influenza-like illness or is completely unremarked by the patient. There is a suggestion that recurrent or persistent genital listeric infection may be a cause of habitual abortion in man as in domestic or wild animals. Due to difficulties in isolation of the microbe and in the performance and interpretation of serological tests, the aetiological diagnosis may be difficult to substantiate in abortion.

The incidence of listeric infection in the perinatal

period in the UK is about 1 in 30 000 births and in the USA in the early 1980s about 3.7 in 1000 000 population. Neonatal septicaemia may occur in epidemic form in cattle and epidemics in man have been reported from East Germany and New Zealand. Cross-infection in neonatal units has also occurred.

Listeric infection of the newborn occurs in two forms. The early-onset type results from infection in utero, whether by the haematogenous transplacental route or following the inhalation of contaminated amniotic fluid, and is manifest as septicaemia within 2 days of birth. There is meconium staining of the amniotic fluid and the usually prematurely born infant has signs of respiratory distress and sometimes a rash. The late form of the disease presents predominantly as a meningoencephalitis, sometimes with slow hydrocephalus developing after the fifth day. This type may be transmitted from the environment. About one-quarter to one-third of babies with early-onset disease are born dead; necropsy demonstrates typical appearances of granulomatosis infantiseptica with miliary microabscesses and granulomata in the liver, spleen, adrenal glands, lungs, pharynx, gastrointestinal tract, central nervous system and skin. The disease is more frequent in continental Europe than in the British Isles and *L. monocytogenes* is thought to rank third after *Escherichia coli* and the group B streptococcus as a cause of neonatal sepsis in France. Mortality rates of 90% used to be recorded for infantile listeriosis but given early diagnosis and prompt treatment with bactericidal agents in high dosage, an overall mortality of 50% is more likely. If a surviving infant is more than 36 weeks of gestation at birth there are likely to be adverse sequelae. Combination therapy with ampicillin and gentamicin is the treatment of choice.

Avoidance of food or pet acquired infections during pregnancy

Both toxoplasmosis and listeriosis may arise in consequence of eating contaminated food, as may food poisoning (salmonellosis). Some types of food such as ripened soft cheeses and paté may contain large numbers of *L. monocytogenes* and are best avoided during pregnancy. It is important that prepacked cook-chill foods should be eaten piping hot, and that chickens and other meat should be thoroughly cooked to destroy vegetative bacteria and toxoplasma cysts. Pet food, if prepared from raw meat, should be handled with scrupulous hygiene, and cat litter should be disposed and gardening done using the gloved hand (HMSO 1992).

VIRAL DISEASES

Some viral diseases in pregnancy are important because of the deleterious effects they may have on the developing fetus and in the newborn. The main complications of these diseases are shown in Table 25.4. Only major diseases will be discussed here.

Rubella

Although more severe disease may occur in adults, rubella is a mild infection characterized by a generalized rash which may be preceded by catarrh and enlargement of the posterior cervical lymph nodes. Constitutional disturbance is slight and complications apart from those affecting the fetus in utero are uncommon. The brief and evanescent rash of rubella starts as a faint macular erythema which first involves the face and neck, spreads rapidly to the trunk and extremities and disappears from one site even as the next becomes involved. The eruption has vanished by the third day and sometimes does not occur at all. The rash of rubella is traditionally regarded as characteristic but similar rashes may be caused by other viruses. The incubation period is usually 17–18 days. Patients are infectious during the last week of the incubation period and for about a week after the disappearance of the rash.

The incubation period, the date of known contact, the degree of contact and the duration of infectivity are all factors that must be considered by the pathologist and obstetrician when interpreting the results of serological tests for rubella in early pregnancy. An accurate history is of paramount importance. The disease is rarely acquired by children under the age of 6 months except by the intrauterine route and it is also rare in persons over 40 years old.

Rubella virus is carried in the nasopharynx and the disease is spread by droplets emanating from persons in the last week of the incubation period or who have had the rash 7–14 days previously. Susceptible people who wish to work in units where they will contact women in the first trimester of pregnancy should be actively encouraged to accept rubella vaccine, as should susceptible women contemplating pregnancy, for example those attending infertility clinics.

The disease is often clinically inapparent because there is no rash. In the UK over 90% of women of childbearing age have serological evidence of past rubella infection or of vaccination, and are immune. This percentage is rising as those who have been immunized in early adolescence enter their childbearing years. Serologically demonstrable reinfection is possible but viraemia is not detectable in such cases and in its absence the products of conception should remain uninfected. Congenital rubella is documented after reinfection (Ross et al 1992) and it is important to remember that the effect of vaccination given in infancy may wane as women enter childbearing years. Susceptibility or immunity to rubella cannot be adduced from evidence of the past history and must be based on serological examination.

Table 25.4 Viral infections during pregnancy implicated in fetal or neonatal disease

Virus	Potential effect on mother	Potential effect on fetus or newborn
Coxsackie A	Herpangina, hand, foot and month disease; myocardiopathy	Transplacental transmission; abortion
Coxsackie A$_9$		?Gastrointestinal defects
Coxsackie B	Often unnoticeable; aseptic meningitis; Bornholm disease	Myocarditis-meningoencephalitis; neonatal sepsis
B$_2$ and B$_4$		?Urogenital anomalies
B$_3$ and B$_4$		?Cardiovascular lesions
B$_2$ B$_3$ and B$_4$		Late stillbirth
B$_1$–B$_5$		Nosocomial neonatal sepsis
Cytomegalovirus	Usually asymptomatic but sometimes moderate to high fever in primary infection	Chronic infection; acute disease; late-onset sequelae
ECHO virus	Rash of ECHO$_9$ may resemble rubella; maternal disease may mimic appendicitis or abruptio placentae, as in other enterovirus infections	Neonatal sepsis; fatal disseminated infection (hepatic necrosis); late stillbirth (ECHO II); nosocomial neonatal sepsis (ECHO 5, 11, 18, 19, 31)
Enterovirus	Usually non-specific febrile illness; abdominal pain	Neonatal sepsis
Hepatitis A	Acute or subclinical disease; flu-like illness; chills and high fever; constitutional symptoms and jaundice; increased severity in pregnancy	Vertical transmission; nosocomial spread
Hepatitis B	Asymptomatic chronic carrier state; acute hepatitis	Vertical transmission; chronic carrier state; rarely acute or fulminant neonatal hepatitis
Hepatitis C	Acute hepatitis	Vertical transmission as yet little studied
Hepatitis D (delta agent)	Superinfection in those with HBV	
Hepatitis E	High mortality in pregnant women	
Herpes simplex	Oral or genital infection; more severe in pregnancy	Abortion following primary infection; ?prematurity; fatal disseminated infections (HSV2 > HSV1); ?congenital malformations
HIV	Acceleration of disease; asymptomatic; AIDS or PGL	Vertical transmission; infantile disease; ?central nervous system malformations
Human T-cell leukaemia virus (HTLV-l)	Adult T-cell leukaemia/lymphoma; tropical spastic paresis	Vertical or perinatal transmission and persistent infection leading to ATLL
Influenza	Increased mortality in pandemics	?Increased fetal mortality; ???congenital malformations; ?increase in childhood leukaemia
Lymphocytic choriomeningitis	Meningitis/meningoencephalitis	Congenital disease
Measles	May be complicated by pneumonia and CCF; more severe and may be fatal	Probably increased mortality; congenital measles
Mumps	No special effect	Increased fetal mortality; ?endocardial fibroelastosis
Parvovirus B19	Asymptomatic; erythema infectiosum	Second trimester abortion; hydrops fetalis with severe anaemia; vertical transmission; haematological effects following late infection in pregnancy
Poliomyelitis	Increased severity and mortality	Fetal death; late stillbirth; neonatal disease
Polyoma	Asymptomatic	?Increased risk of jaundice
Rubella	No special effect	Fetal death; chronic persisting infection; congenital malformations
Varicella-zoster	Often more severe; maternal death	Neonatal chickenpox; congenital varicella syndrome; infantile zoster
Vaccinia and variola	Increased severity and mortality	Fetal death; intrauterine or neonatal disease
Venezuelan and western equine encephalomyelitides	Meningoencephalitis	Neonatal encephalitis

HSV = herpes simplex virus, HIV = human immunodeficiency virus, CCF = chronic congestive failure.

Before laboratory diagnosis was possible rubella was diagnosed on clinical grounds, as are the majority of cases today. Not all rubella-like rashes are caused by the rubella virus however, and recourse to a diagnostic virology laboratory should be made wherever feasible. During pregnancy this must always be done because of the serious consequences of misdiagnosis. The presence of a transient arthralgia as the rash begins to fade, which occurs in 60–70% of postpubertal females, supports the clinical diagnosis of rubella.

Rubella in pregnancy is uncommon. It is probably less infectious than measles or varicella and the chance of contracting if from brief or casual exposure is small. The risk is five times greater when the contact is within the family group than when the contact is outside it, which emphasizes the importance of eliciting an accurate history of the nature of the contact during pregnancy.

Maternal virus is transmitted to the fetus transplacentally and maternal viraemia is postulated as the factor essential for the genesis of fetal infection. Rubella causes spontaneous abortion and stillbirth; the incidence is about double that in control populations—10% compared with 5%. The virus produces an antimitotic effect upon infected cells which leads to retardation in cell division and results in major malformations if it occurs during a critical phase of organogenesis. Chronic infection may persist throughout gestation and may cause further damage. The perinatal mortality rate varies from 110 to 290 per 1000 total births (Horstmann et al 1965, Banatvala 1971).

Prospective studies have shown that when rubella is acquired in early pregnancy the incidence of congenital malformations varies from 15% to 35%. If it is acquired during the first month of gestation, the incidence of defects may approach 50–60% and such defects may be multiple. Thereafter the incidence of malformations declines until by the 16th week it is about 5%. Even if infection is acquired after the first trimester, up to the 31st week, the babies may show evidence of intrauterine infection since, when followed up for 2–3 years, poor communicative ability, poor physical growth and developmental retardation may be noted.

It is important that babies born to women known to have had rubella even late in pregnancy should be regularly surveyed for physical or other defects before reaching school age. Congenitally infected children may themselves act as vectors of infection. At 6 months of age, 20–30% of them may still be excreting virus from the nasopharynx and even at 1 year of age, 7–9% still do so. Susceptible women of childbearing age who nurse or attend such children should be protected by vaccination.

The diagnosis of rubella in pregnancy is established by serological tests. Since rubella antibodies persist indefinitely, antibody detected within 14 days of contact when the contact date is certain indicates that the patient has previously had rubella. If serum can be obtained during the acute phase of the illness paired sera are examined to detect a significant rise in antibody. If serum cannot be obtained during the acute phase or if only one sample is available but the duration of pregnancy necessitates rapid diagnosis, the presence of rubella-specific IgM, which does not usually persist for more than 2 months, indicates active or recent infection. Serological tests made on patients presenting well after the incubation period are difficult to interpret, although the presence of high titres may suggest the diagnosis.

Virus isolation is a lengthy and exacting procedure and is not usually feasible in pregnancy when rapid diagnosis is desirable. At birth, congenitally infected infants generally have high rubella antibody levels which persist for longer than would be expected if such antibody was maternally derived—that is, longer than 4–6 months. Rubella-specific IgM can usually be detected during the first year of life and since the IgM class of immunoglobulins cannot cross the placenta the presence of this antibody in cord blood indicates intrauterine infection. Virus may be detected in the nasopharynx, urine and stools.

Protective antibodies, whether acquired in response to a naturally occurring infection or in response to vaccine, persist and afford clinical protection of an extremely high order. It is therefore desirable that vaccine should be offered to girls before they reach childbearing years. There is a case for also giving an effective rubella vaccine to mature women as 15–20% are susceptible to rubella, gamma globulin offers no appreciable protection and subclinical infection is common. Measles/mumps/rubella vaccine offered to young children in the UK since 1988 has interrupted the epidemic cycle and reduced the incidence of rubella reported in pregnancy to single figures. Susceptible women may be offered single antigen vaccine provided they are advised to avoid pregnancy for at least 3 months. The puerperium offers a good opportunity for vaccination in women who are susceptible but have not yet completed their families. The menstrual period is also said to offer a good opportunity.

Women who are to be offered vaccine in the puerperium are usually tested for susceptibility by appropriate serological tests on serum obtained at booking. The baseline value obtained then is also useful if they are exposed to a rubella-like illness later in pregnancy. The suggestion that termination of pregnancy should be offered to those who are inadvertently vaccinated just before or during early pregnancy is not supported by clinical observations, although the theoretical risk that the vaccine is itself teratogenic remains and vaccine virus can cross the placenta.

Cytomegalovirus infections

Cytomegalovirus is a member of the herpesvirus group; these viruses are characterized by their tendency to cause latent as well as acute infections. Cytomegalovirus is probably transmitted in urine and saliva, requiring close and prolonged contact. Up to 12% of healthy women excrete virus during pregnancy and it is possible that pregnancy enhances susceptibility to infection or reactivation of virus. However, about half the female population in the western hemisphere are without antibody by the time they reach childbearing years and as the highest seroconversion rate occurs between the ages of 15 and 35, the chances of primary infection coinciding with pregnancy are high.

Since 0.5–3% of newborn infants excrete virus, congenital infection is by no means rare. The majority of babies excreting virus escape serious disease or even outward signs of infection although in the past it was thought that intrauterine infection invariably resulted in central nervous system damage in a high proportion of cases. The outcome of primary infection during pregnancy probably depends upon its virulence and duration. Peckham et al (1983) noted an incidence of 3 per 1000 of the congenital infection in 14 789 pregnancies. A total of 7% of the 42 infected babies were seriously handicapped; 33% had minor or transient problems and 60% were unscathed. Sixty-seven per cent were born to women who had developed primary infection during pregnancy.

Infection during pregnancy may cause abortion or congenital defects and late in pregnancy it may cause severe fetal disease with stillbirth, either preterm or at term. The child may be born alive, often of low birthweight, only to die in the neonatal period with fulminating disease of which the extraneural symptoms are jaundice, often with hepatosplenomegaly, thrombocytopenic purpura, choroidoretinitis and anaemia. Others may develop symptoms after an apparently normal neonatal period. A number show spasticity, microcephaly and mental retardation. Hydrocephalus, optic atrophy and epilepsy have also been reported.

There is no case for screening for cytomegalovirus infection during pregnancy. Since primary infection during pregnancy is more hazardous to the fetus, some encouragement should be given to avoid possible sources; this would include good hygiene in the workplace and at home, and the avoidance of contact with infectious body fluids. There is at present no licensed vaccine for CMV available in the UK.

Herpes simplex

Herpes virus hominis infection of the female genital tract is the most common viral disease in gynaecology and the most common cause of ulcerative lesions of the female genital tract in England. Many cases are asymptomatic. More than 90% of the genital infections are caused by type 2 virus while the majority of infections of the oral mucosa, cornea and brain are caused by type 1. With the prevalence of oral sex, type 1 genital infections are becoming more frequent. Primary genital infection is caused most frequently by venereal contact but non-venereal infection has been described. After initial infection the condition can be reactivated by temperature change, emotional trauma, premenstrual tension, menstruation and the use of oral contraceptives.

Clinically apparent infections of the vulva or perineum may be accompanied by pain, burning, malaise, ulceration, inguinal adenopathy and fever but infections of the cervix and those high in the vagina produce few subjective symptoms. Vesicular vulvovaginitis is not the main feature of the infection and 50% or more of all genital herpes infections may be asymptomatic. Asymptomatic infections of the vulva are rare but cervical lesions may present as diffuse cervicitis with multiple tiny superficial ulcers or more rarely as a necrotizing cervicitis resembling squamous carcinoma.

There is some evidence that the virus may be transmitted transplacentally but most neonatal infections are caused by type 2 virus which is probably transmitted during the second stage of labour and more often in consequence of primary infection rather than recurrence. Neonatal herpes is rare in the UK, with an overall reported incidence of about one in 40 000 live births and an incidence of severe disease of about one in 200 000. The incidence of disseminated herpes is greater among premature infants. The liver and adrenals are involved,

with focal coagulative necrosis as the characteristic lesion. The virus may be recovered from many organs and infection of the central nervous system may be the dominant clinical feature. The diagnosis can be made clinically if typical vesicular eruption of the skin occurs during the first week of life but about half the infants who go on to develop disseminated infection do not have vesicles in the early stages of the disease. Diagnosis is confirmed by examination of cells scraped from the base of local lesions by electron or light microscopy. The virus may be cultured within 2–4 days.

If virus is known to be present in the genital tract at or near term Caesarean section should be considered and the case for section is strengthened if lesions are present. There is no real evidence that Caesarean section reduces the probability of neonatal disease unless it is performed within 4 hours of rupture of membranes. Monif and Hardt (1984) discuss the management of herpetic vulvovaginitis during pregnancy, basing it on the recommendations of the American Academy of Pediatrics (Committee on Fetus and Newborn 1980). Repeated viriculture is not favoured in the UK (Kelly 1988). Infants exposed at delivery should be observed closely and early treatment with acyclovir can be instituted if symptoms develop. The prognosis is very poor in those with disseminated herpes, whether treated or untreated.

Varicella-zoster

Women of childbearing age are rarely affected by varicella-zoster virus since most are already immune as a result of childhood infection. Pregnant women in close contact should be tested for varicella-zoster antibody; prophylactic immune globulin (ZIG) can be offered to those susceptible (Department of Health 1990). However, even if given within 72 hours of exposure, overt infection still occurs in about two-thirds. Abortion and intrauterine infection resulting in disseminated disease have been reported. If maternal infection occurs near or at term neonatal chickenpox presents at birth or within the first 2–3 weeks of life, depending on the interval between maternal infection and birth.

The fetus may be infected in the early weeks of pregnancy and still survive to term; brain damage is the main feature. Cerebral complications and pneumonitis are common in neonatal chickenpox although generalized rash and local eruption along a dermatome may be seen, as in zoster. Early treatment with immunoglobulins may be of value in the case of women with chickenpox in early pregnancy and immunoglobulin may be administered prophylactically to the offspring of women who have varicella at or about term. The mortality rate of neonatal varicella is variously reported as 0–23%. Zoster immune globulin should be given to newborn babies exposed within 5 days of delivery. Acyclovir may be given to the mother before delivery.

Congenital malformation (varicella embryopathy) may

follow maternal varicella-zoster infection in the first trimester of pregnancy. The syndrome is characterized by fetal growth retardation, aplasia and scarring of a limb, neurological damage or eye abnormalities and is fully described by Brunell (1984). The magnitude of the risk is not known but is believed to be less than one in a hundred. Varicella-zoster infection in pregnancy is reviewed by Craddock-Watson (1990).

The hepatitis viruses

The hepatitis viruses are responsible for much morbidity and mortality worldwide from acute infections and their damaging sequelae. They include a range of unrelated pathogens: hepatitis A, B, C, D and E, of which the hepatitis B virus has been most studied in relation to pregnancy. Hepatitis A is transmitted by the faeco-oral route by person to person spread and through contaminated food; it is endemic in most of the world causing acute usually mild or subclinical infection without sequelae. Immunity probably persists for life and an inactivated vaccine is available. Human normal immunoglobulin may be used for short-term protection and probably prevents secondary cases. There is evidence that the virus can be vertically transmitted and that it can spread in neonatal intensive care units (Watson et al 1993).

Hepatitis B virus is an important endemic virus, evidence of carriage varying from 0.5–1% in Northern Europe, North America and Australia to 2–7% in Eastern Europe, the Mediterranean and the Middle East and up to 35% in the Far East and tropical Africa. Thus, worldwide, there may be 300 million carriers. Infection may lead to persistent infection, marked by HB_sAg in 2–10% of cases, and sometimes progressing to chronic persistent or chronic active hepatitis, cirrhosis or hepatocellular carcinoma. Among carriers of the virus, those with HB_eAg are the most infectious. Hepatitis B is transmitted parenterally, through blood-to-blood contact, including traumatic sexual intercourse, injury with contaminated sharps, instruments like needles, sharing of impedimenta of mainline drug addiction and by vertical transmission. Transfusion-associated infection is now rare in parts of the world where transfusion services are well organized and donors are screened. The risks of transmission from mother to child are shown in Table 25.5. Infants born to hepatitis B carriers, especially carriers of e antigen, should be protected by active and passive immunization shortly after birth. In the UK, most women are tested for HB_sAg during pregnancy and, if positive for e markers, vaccine plus immunoglobulin is offered to those children born to women who are e antigen positive, surface antigen positive without e markers, or who have had acute hepatitis B during pregnancy (HMSO 1992). Hepatitis B vaccine is of good efficacy, but the recent appearance of virus-induced escape mutants (Carman et al 1990) is worrying, and may jeopardize vaccination strategy.

Table 25.5 Risks of hepatitis B virus transfer from mother to child (from Mowat 1980)

Mother HBsAG-positive	Infant infection rate
Acute hepatitis 3 months before to 1 month after delivery	80–90%
Acute hepatitis in early pregnancy	10–30%
Asymptomatic carrier mother	10%
HBeAg-positive	90%
HBeAg-negative	30%
HBeAg-negative, HBeAg-positive	0%

Hepatitis C virus is a cause of non A non B hepatitis, responsible for some 20–40% of cases of recognized acute viral hepatitis. It is readily transmitted by the parenteral route and is a risk of blood transfusion and needle sharing in intravenous drug abusers. Its epidemiology is, as yet, not fully understood as tests for antibody have only recently been introduced. There is little evidence for spread by the sexual route, or within families. Vertical transmission occurs, but seemingly at a fairly low level. For example Lam et al (1993) reported only four of 66 children at risk. Half those infected with hepatitis C virus progress to chronic liver disease, and infection may go on to hepatocellular carcinoma. Screening in pregnancy is proceeding in some centres to assess the risks of transmission more fully.

Hepatitis D virus (delta agent) can only replicate in the presence of hepatitis B. If it superinfects, fulminant hepatitis or serious chronic liver disease may result. Immunization against hepatitis B is protective but the agent has been little studied in pregnancy.

Hepatitis E virus is transmitted by the faeco-oral route, causing usually an acute and self-limiting infection. It has a high mortality in pregnant women, of the order of 17–30%, and occurs in epidemic form in India, Central and South East Asia, the Middle East and North Africa.

Acquired immune deficiency syndrome

The acquired immune deficiency syndrome (AIDS) is the late effect of a lymphocytopathic retrovirus, human immunodeficiency virus (HIV) types I and II. The virus is transmitted sexually, predominantly by anal intercourse and traumatic sexual practices, particularly in homosexual males although it can be transmitted heterosexually. It is also transmitted by blood-to-blood contact, especially through the shared syringes and needles used by intravenous drug abusers. Recipients of blood and blood products are at risk of transmission if control measures have not been undertaken. The disease is transmissible from mother to fetus.

Fever, weight loss, diarrhoea and lymphadenopathy are the major presenting signs of AIDS together with pneumonia, thrombocytopenic purpura and others. Opportunist infections include amongst the viruses cytomegalovirus (pulmonary, central nervous system or gastrointestinal involvement) and herpes simplex virus (mucocutaneous, pulmonary, gastrointestinal or disseminated disease). Progressive multifocal leukoencephalopathy (papovavirus-induced) may occur. Overwhelming bacterial sepsis may be associated inter alia with *Salmonella* or *Mycobacteria*, especially *M. avium intracellulare*. As with other conditions associated with severe immune defects, candidosis is frequent and infections by *Aspergillus* species, *Cryptococcus* and other fungi occur. Dissemination or extensive local involvement by parasites including *Toxoplasma gondii*, *Cryptosporidium*, *Strongyloides* and *Pneumocystis carinii* is frequent.

Tumours other than Kaposi's sarcoma especially Hodgkin's and non-Hodgkin's lymphomas are also associated, together with squamous carcinoma of the rectum and other tumours. Other disorders such as enteropathy and progressive encephalopathy or myelopathy may also occur. The latter seems to be separate from the immune deficiency. Neurological manifestations are reviewed by Carne & Adler (1986).

The cytopathic virus is a retrovirus of the subfamily Lentiviridae, a group of viruses rapidly lethal to the domestic animals they infect (Seale 1985). It attacks T-cell subsets as well as macrophages and cells throughout the brain. In a proportion of infected persons, infection with virus after an incubation period of 15–57 months as determined in recipients of infected blood, or of 4.5 years with a range of 2.6–14.2 years as more recently calculated, causes symptoms of AIDS (12%) or AIDS-related complex (48%; Weber et al 1986). It is calculated that the proportion developing AIDS will increase with time.

The route of spread is similar to that of hepatitis B virus—by sexual transmission especially by homosexual anal intercourse, by blood-to-blood contact through transfusion of whole blood or blood components, by semen and by maternal–fetal or neonatal transmission. Certain groups of individuals are thus at high risk. These include homosexual or bisexual males, recipients of unscreened or untreated blood or blood products, intravenous drug abusers and those whose consorts have AIDS or are HIV-antibody positive. Preventive measures include education of the public in safer sex, guidance to health care personnel from the Department of Health and Social Security (1985a,b 1986a), donor selection and antibody screening for blood donors (Barbara et al 1986) and for potential semen donors (Department of Health and Social Security 1986b).

Transplacental transmission of HIV occurs in early pregnancy (Jovaisas et al 1985, Sprecher et al 1986). Abnormal development in such fetuses includes growth failure, a prominent box-like forehead, wide-set eyes, short nose and patulous lips such as occur in the fetal alcohol syndrome which may have been associated. (Marion et al 1986). Children of infected mothers probably acquired the infection in utero but may also acquire it from maternal blood at birth or postnatally or from breast milk. The risk of transmission is not known but may be as high as 65% in children of mothers who have already given birth to an infected child (Centers for Disease Control 1985). It is considerably less in those born to mothers who are antibody positive but not ill (Lancet 1988). The results of the European Collaborative Study (1992) give an overall risk of transmission of 14%, with breastfeeding doubling this figure. In relatively wealthy communities with sound health services infants of HIV-infected mothers should not be breastfed (Cutting 1992).

As the AIDS epidemic gains ground in the UK there is a case for screening those in high-risk categories for antibody to the virus. A positive test denotes exposure to the virus and because the infection persists, probably for life, it is presumptive evidence of infectiousness (Curran et al 1985). If screening tests are to be undertaken during pregnancy, maternal consent for counselling will be required. Obstetricians who need to advise mothers with AIDS of the risk of vertical transmission will find help from a useful Royal College of Obstetricians and Gynaecologists document on the subject of AIDS in children (Hudson 1987). Termination of pregnancy would have to be considered.

Parvovirus

Parvovirus B 19 was discovered in sera from healthy blood donors in 1975 and is the cause of erythema infectiosum (slapped cheek syndrome, fifth disease) and of transient aplastic crisis in those with chronic haemolytic anaemia. It is associated with acute arthralgia and arthritis and with chronic anaemia in immunodeficient patients. Acute infection in pregnancy may cause abortion or stillbirth and is associated with non-immune hydrops. An estimated 10% of confirmed B19-infected fetuses will not survive, although less than a third of women who are infected transmit infection vertically to the fetus. A prospective study by the Public Health Laboratory Service showed a fetal loss rate of 16% in a group of 186 women (PHLS 1990). The rate of loss was most marked in the second trimester. The interval between maternal infection and fetal loss may be as long as 11 weeks, but is usually 4–5 weeks. Perinatal and neonatal infection has been observed occasionally. A good account of B19 infection in pregnancy is given by Cohen & Hall (1992). The diagnosis in pregnancy is established by serological demonstration of B19 IgM.

CONCLUSIONS

Life-threatening microbial disease is currently rare in pregnant and parturient women in the UK. With advances in paediatric intensive care, the emphasis on serious infections has shifted to the unborn or recently born child, particularly if the latter is of low, or very low birthweight. Great advances have been made in the prevention of congenitally acquired infections, notably through the introduction of rubella virus vaccine.

As knowledge of microbial pathogens increases, newly recognized disease entities emerge or older observations are re-emphasized. Such are the apparent adverse effects on the fetus of Lyme disease (Markowitz et al 1986), the role of *Chlamydia psittaci* of ovine origin and of *Streptococ-*
cus milleri in spontaneous abortion (Roberts et al 1967, Johnson et al 1985, MacGowan & Terry 1987), fetal distress associated with *Cryptosporidium* infection (Dale et al 1987), maternal and fetal death caused by *Pasteurella multocida* (Rasaiah et al 1986) and hydrops fetalis associated with human parvovirus infection (Anand et al 1987, Thurn 1988). Many of these infections are currently receiving intense study. Some will remain rarities; others may be important as causes of maternal and fetal morbidity or mortality.

REFERENCES

Anand A, Gray E S, Brown T et al 1987 Human parvovirus infection in pregnancy and hydrops fetalis. New England Journal of Medicine 316: 183–186

Aspock H 1985 Toxoplasmosis in prenatal and perinatal infections. WHO, Geneva

Banatvala J E (ed) 1971 Current problems in clinical virology. Churchill Livingstone, Edinburgh

Barbara J A J, Contreras M, Hewitt P 1986 AIDS: a problem for the transfusion service? British Journal of Hospital Medicine 36: 178–184

Blanc W A 1959 Amniotic infection syndrome: pathogenesis, morphology and significance in circumnatal mortality. Clinics in Obstetrics and Gynaecology 2: 704–734

Brunell P A 1984 Fetal and neonatal varicella-zoster infections. In: Amstey M S (ed) Virus infections in pregnancy. Grune & Stratton, New York

Carman W F, Zanetti A, Karayiannis P et al 1990 Vaccine induced escape mutant of hepatitis B virus. Lancet ii: 325–329

Carne C A, Adler M W 1986 Neurological manifestations of human immunodeficiency virus infection. Lancet 293: 462–463

Catterall R D 1979 Venereology and genitourinary medicine, 2nd edn. Hodder & Stoughton, London

Centers for Disease Control 1985 Recommendations for assisting in the prevention of perinatal transmission of human T-lymphotropic virus type III/lymphadenopathy associated virus and acquired immunodeficiency syndrome. Communicable Disease Center: Mortality and Morbidity Weekly Reports 34: 721–726, 731–732

Charles D, Hurry D J 1983 Chorioamnionitis. In: Charles D (ed) Clinics in obstetrics and gynaecology, vol 10. WB Saunders, London

Cohen B J, Hall S 1992 Parvovirus B19. In: Greenough A, Osborne J, Sutherland S (eds) Congenital, perinatal and neonatal infections. Churchill Livingstone, London

Committee on Fetus and Newborn, Committee on Infectious Diseases 1980 Perinatal herpes simplex virus infections. Pediatrics 66: 142

Craddock-Watson J E 1990 Varicella-zoster virus infection during pregnancy. In: Morgan-Capner P (ed) Current topics in clinical virology. Public Health Laboratory Service

Curran J W, Morgan W M, Hardy A M, Jaffe H W, Darrow W W, Dowdle W R 1985 The epidemiology of AIDS: current status and future prospects. Science 229: 1352–1357

Cutting W A M 1992 Breast feeding and HIV infection. British Medical Journal 305: 788

Dale B A S, Gordon G, Thomson R, Urquhart R 1987 Perinatal infection with cryptosporidium. Lancet i: 1042–1043

Davies P A 1971 Bacterial infection in the fetus and newborn. Archives of Disease in Childhood 46: 1–27

Davison J 1989 Renal disease. In: de Swiet M (ed) Medical disorders in obstetric practice. Blackwell Scientific Publications, Oxford

de Louvois J, Blades M, Harrison R F, Hurley R, Stanley V C 1974 Frequency of mycoplasmas in fertile and infertile couples. Lancet i: 1073

Department of Health and Social Security 1985a Acquired immune deficiency syndrome AIDS. General information for doctors. DHSS, London

Department of Health and Social Security 1985b Acquired immune deficiency syndrome AIDS. Information for doctors concerning the introduction of the HTLV-III antibody test. DHSS, London

Department of Health 1990 Immunisation against infectious disease. HMSO, London

Department of Health and Social Security 1986a Acquired immune deficiency syndrome AIDS. Guidance for surgeons, anaesthetists, dentists and their teams in dealing with patients infected with HTLV-III. DHSS, London

Department of Health and Social Security 1986b Acquired immune deficiency syndrome AIDS. Guidance for doctors and AI clinics concerning AIDS and artificial insemination. DHSS, London

Desmonts G, Forestier F, Thulliez P H et al 1985 Prenatal diagnosis of congenital toxoplasmosis. Lancet i: 500–504

European Collaborative Study 1992 Risk factors for mother to child of HIV-1. Lancet 339: 1007–1012

Fiumara N J, Bleming W L, Downing J G, Good F L 1952 The incidence of prenatal syphilis at the Boston City Hospital. New England Journal of Medicine 247: 48

Gluck L, Wood H F, Fousek M D 1966 Septicemia of the newborn. Pediatric Clinics of North America 13: 1131–1148

HMSO 4/92 1992 While you are pregnant: safe eating and how to avoid infection from food and animals. HMSO, London

Horstmann D M, Banatvala J E, Riordan J R et al 1965 Maternal rubella syndrome in infants. American Journal of Diseases of Children 110: 408

Hudson C (ed) 1987 Report of the subcommittee on problems associated with AIDS in relation to obstetrics and gynaecology. Royal College of Obstetrics and Gynaecology, London

Hurley R 1977 Heart disease, parturition and antibiotic prophylaxis. In: Lewis P (ed) Therapeutic problems in pregnancy. MTP Press, Lancaster

Hurley R 1989 Fever and infectious diseases In: de Swiet M (ed) Medical disorders in obstetric practice. Blackwell Scientific Publications, Oxford

Hurley R, Stanley V C, Leask B G S, de Louvois J 1974 Microflora of the vagina during pregnancy In: Skinner F A, Carr J G (eds) The normal microbial flora of man. Academic Press, London

Ingall D, Norins L 1976 Syphilis In: Remington J S, Klein J O (eds) Infectious diseases of the fetus and newborn infant. WB Saunders, London

Ingall D, Dobson S R M, Musher D 1990 In: Remington J S, Klein J O (eds) Infectious diseases of the fetus and newborn infant, 3rd edn. WB Saunders, London, pp 367–394

Jephcott A E 1992 *Neisseria gonorrhoea*. In: Greenough A, Osborne J, Sutherland S (eds) Congenital perinatal and neonatal infections. Churchill Livingstone, Edinburgh

Johnson F W A, Matheson B A, Williams H et al 1985 Abortion due to infection with *Chlamydia psittaci* in a sheep farmer's wife. British Medical Journal 290: 592–594

Jovaisas E, Koch M A, Schafer A, Stauber M, Lowenthal D 1985 LAV/HTLV-III in 20-week fetus. Lancet ii: 1129

Kelly J 1988 Genital herpes during pregnancy. British Medical Journal 297: 1146–1147

Klein J O, Marcy S M 1990 Bacterial sepsis and meningitis. In: Remington J S, Klein J O (eds) Infectious diseases of the fetus and newborn infant, 3rd edn. W B Saunders, London, pp 601–656

Koppe J G, Loewer-Sieger D H, de Roever-Bonnet 1986 Results

of a 20 year follow-up of congenital toxoplasmosis. Lancet i: 254–256

Lam J P H, McOmish F, Burns S M, Yap P L, Mok J Y Q, Simmonds P 1993 Infrequent vertical transmission of hepatitis C virus. Journal of Infectious Diseases 167: 572–576

Lamont R F, Fisk N 1993 The role of infection in the pathogenesis of preterm labour. In: Studd J (ed) Progress in obstetrics and gynaecology, vol 10. Churchill Livingstone, Edinburgh

Lancet 1988 Vertical transmission of HIV. Lancet ii: 1057–1058

Letsky E 1989 Haemostasis and haemorrhage In: de Swiet M (ed) Medical disorders in obstetric practice. Blackwell Scientific Publications, Oxford

MacGowan A P, Terry P B 1987 Streptococcus milleri and second trimester abortion. Journal of Clinical Pathology 40: 292–293

Marion R W, Wiznia A A, Hutcheon R G, Rubinstein A 1986 Human T-cell lymphotropic virus type III (HTLV-III) embryopathy. A new dysmorphic syndrome associated with intrauterine HTLV-III infection. American Journal of Diseases of Children 140: 638–640

Markowitz L E, Steere A C, Benach J L, Slade J D, Broom C V 1986 Lyme disease during pregnancy. Journal of the American Medical Association 255: 3394–3396

McCracken G H, Shinefield H R 1966 Changes in the pattern of neonatal septicaemia and meningitis. American Journal of Diseases of Children 112: 33–39

Monif G R G, Hardt N S 1984 Management of herpetic vulvovaginitis in pregnancy. In: Amstey M S (ed) Virus infection in pregnancy. Grune & Stratton, New York

Mowat A P 1980 Viral hepatitis in infancy and childhood. In: Sherlock S (ed) Virus hepatitis. W B Saunders, London

Murphy N, Damjanovi C V, Hart C A, Buchanan C R, Whittaker R, Cooke R W 1986 Infection and colonisation of neonates by Hansenula anomala. Lancet i: 291–293

Naeye R L, Peters E C 1980 Causes and consequences of premature rupture of fetal membranes. Lancet i: 192–194

Peckham C S, Chin K S, Coleman J C et al 1983 Cytomegalovirus infection in pregnancy: preliminary findings from a prospective study. Lancet ii: 352

Public Health Laboratory Service Working Party on Fifth Disease 1990 Prospective study of human parvovirus (B19) infection in pregnancy. British Medical Journal 300: 1166–1170

Rasaiah B, Otero J G, Russell I J et al 1986 Pasteurella multocida septicaemia during pregnancy. Canadian Medical Association Journal 135: 1369–1372

Remington J S, Klein J O (eds) 1983 Infectious diseases of the fetus and newborn infant, 2nd edn. W B Saunders, London

Roberts W, Grist N R, Giroud P 1967 Human abortion associated with infection by ovine abortion agent. British Medical Journal 4: 36

Ross R, Harvey D R, Hurley Rosalinde 1992 Reinfection and congenital rubella syndrome. The Practitioner 236: 246–271

Seale J 1985 AIDS Virus infection: prognosis and transmission. Journal of the Royal Society of Medicine 78: 613–615

Siegel J D, McCracken G H Jr 1981 Sepsis neonatorum. New England Journal of Medicine 1: 642–647

Silverman W A, Homan W E 1949 Sepsis of obscure origin in the newborn. Pediatrics 3: 157–176

Sprecher S, Soumenkoff G, Puissant F, Degueldre M 1986 Vertical transmission of HIV in 15-week fetus. Lancet ii: 288

Stokes J H, Beerman H, Ingraham N R Jr (eds) 1944 Modern clinical syphilogy, 3rd edn. W B Saunders, London

Thomsen A C, Morup L, Brogaard Hansen K 1987 Antibiotic elimination of Group B streptococci in urine in prevention of preterm labour. Lancet i: 591

Thurn J 1988 Human parvovirus B19: historical and critical review. Reviews of Infectious Diseases 10: 1005–1011

Watson J C, Fleming D W, Borella A J, Olcott E S, Conrad R E, Baron R C 1993 Vertical transmission of hepatitis A resulting in an outbreak in a neonatal intensive care unit. Journal of Infectious Diseases 167: 567–571

Weber J N, Wadsworth J, Rogers L A et al 1986 Three year prospective study of HTLV-II/LAV infection in homosexual men. Lancet i: 1179

26. Urinary tract in pregnancy

John M. Davison   William Dunlop

INTRODUCTION

Few aspects of maternal physiology change more profoundly during pregnancy than those affecting the urinary tract. An understanding of these changes is of fundamental importance since abnormalities must be assessed against basal values inappropriate for the non-pregnant state. For these reasons, a brief account of the most significant alterations in renal physiology must be considered before discussing urinary disorders which may complicate pregnancy.

PREGNANCY-INDUCED ALTERATIONS IN THE URINARY TRACT

Pregnancy is associated with substantial dilatation of the urinary tract (Peake et al 1983). By the third trimester some 97% of women show evidence of stasis or hydronephrosis (Cietak & Newton 1985a). Dilatation is more pronounced on the right than the left at all stages of pregnancy (Fig. 26.1), perhaps because of the customary dextrorotation of the uterus. Nephrosonographic studies suggest that renal parenchymal volumes also increase during pregnancy (Cietak & Newton 1985b), probably the result of increases in intrarenal fluid predominantly (Davison & Lindheimer 1980). It appears that a 70% increment has occurred by the beginning of the third trimester but that there may be a slight reduction during the latter weeks of pregnancy (Cietak & Newton 1985b). Very occasionally these cause massive urethral and renal pelvis dilatation (as well as slight reducion in cortical width), but this is without ill-effect in the long term

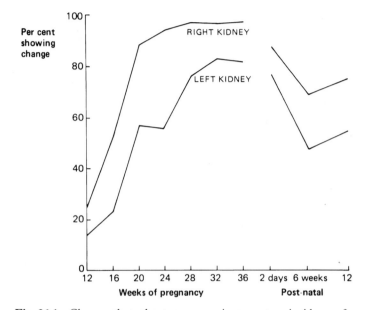

Fig. 26.1 Changes throughout pregnancy in percentage incidences for both kidneys of stasis and hydronephrosis with or without clubbing. Derived from the nephrosonographic data of Cietak & Newton (1985a).

(Brown 1990). Rarely, the changes may be extreme and precipitate the overdistension syndrome (see later) and hypertension (Satin et al 1993).

Renal haemodynamics

By the second trimester, renal blood flow (assessed indirectly as effective renal plasma flow) has increased, probably by as much as 70–80% (Davison & Dunlop 1984). During the third trimester a significant reduction has been described (Dunlop 1981). This cannot be attributed solely to the effects of maternal posture (Dunlop 1976, Ezimokhai et al 1981), although posture may have a substantial effect upon the results of investigations during late pregnancy (Chesley & Sloan 1984). Since renal blood flow is one of the most important influences on the rate of filtration by the kidney, substantial increases in glomerular

489

filtration rate (GFR) occur during pregnancy (Davison & Hytten 1974). However the 50% increase is rather less than renal blood flow (Dunlop 1981); in consequence the filtration fraction, the proportion of renal plasma flow filtered at the glomerulus, decreases during early pregnancy (Davison & Dunlop 1980).

In clinical practice, it is convenient to assess the glomerular filtration rate by means of the creatinine clearance, usually over a 24-hour period in order to ensure reasonable accuracy. Serial investigations of groups of healthy women suggest that this has increased by 45% by the eighth week of pregnancy (6 weeks after conception; Davison & Noble 1981); this increase is maintained throughout the second trimester (Davison & Hytten 1974) but a significant and consistent decrease in values equivalent to the non-pregnant occurs during the last weeks of pregnancy (Davison et al 1980). Since the renal clearance of a substance bears a reciprocal relationship to its plasma concentrations, plasma creatinine concentration falls during early pregnancy but rises progressively during the third trimester. During pregnancy significant renal impairment may be present in women who have plasma concentrations of creatinine within the normal non-pregnant range, but on the other hand, increases in plasma creatinine concentrations (or decreases in creatinine clearance) during the third trimester of pregnancy may not imply pathological changes.

The augmented glomerular filtration rate (GFR) of pregnancy is probably due exclusively to increased renal blood flow, without coexistent glomerular hypertension and the evidence so far, albeit limited, argues against hyperfiltration sclerosis in normal human pregnancy (Davison 1989). Elegant studies of glomerular function and morphology in the rat have revealed no sustained increases in glomerular capillary blood pressure, no loss of nephrons, no persistent proteinuria and no morphological changes in animals which had completed five consecutive cycles of pregnancy, lactation, a long period in the lifespan of this species, compared with age-matched virgin controls (Baylis 1994).

Tubular function

Few constituents of the urine are excreted at the same rate as they are filtered at the glomerulus. Some substances, such as hippurate derivatives, are actively secreted into the urine but most are partially reabsorbed during passage through the nephron. In many cases of apparent tubular reabsorption a degree of secretion by the kidney is also present, although it is difficult to determine the relative contributions of these two processes in human subjects. Virtually no reliable information is available about the changes associated with human pregnancy.

Glucose is so avidly reabsorbed by the kidney that none is detectable by routine clinical testing in the urine of healthy non-pregnant individuals. However, during normal pregnancy, glucose excretion increases soon after conception (Davison & Dunlop 1980). Excretion rates may be as much as 10 times those of non-pregnant women (20–100 mg/day) and there is marked variability both within and between days, the pattern bearing no demonstrable relationship to blood sugar concentrations. Some two-thirds of apparently healthy pregnant women will exhibit glycosuria to a degree conventionally considered clinically significant on repeated urinalysis (Lind & Hytten 1972); conversely, not all women with impaired glucose tolerance during pregnancy are significantly glycosuric on routine testing (Lind 1975). Glycosuria does not therefore provide reliable information about carbohydrate metabolism during pregnancy.

The extent to which glycosuria is provoked by pregnancy bears a significant relationship to the extent to which glucose is reabsorbed from the glomerular filtrate, not only during pregnancy but also in the same subjects in the non-pregnant state (Davison & Hytten 1975, Davison & Dunlop 1984). It has been suggested that this phenomenon may be related to unsuspected renal tubular damage caused by previous urinary tract infections (Davison & Dunlop 1980, Davison et al 1984). Within a week of delivery, glucose excretion has returned to non-pregnant patterns (Davison & Lovedale 1974). This is almost certainly due to the reduction of the glomerular filtration rate, for defects in glucose reabsorption can still be demonstrated by appropriate infusion protocols in women who have previously been severely glycosuric (Davison & Dunlop 1984).

Changes in glomerular filtration rate are also partly responsible for the increased renal clearances of other urinary constituents and for reductions in their circulating concentrations. Of particular note in clinical practice are urea and uric acid, both of which decrease considerably during the first trimester of pregnancy (Davison & Dunlop 1984, Lind et al 1984). However, during late pregnancy, the circulating concentrations of uric acid tend to increase. Part of this increase may reflect decreasing glomerular filtration (Davison et al 1980) but there is also convincing evidence of altered renal handling. Renal reabsorption of uric acid decreases significantly during early pregnancy and rises gradually towards non-pregnant values thereafter (Dunlop & Davison 1977). The increased excretions of calcium (along with an inhibition of crystalluria) and protein are due to alteration in tubular function as well as augmented renal haemodynamics (Sturgiss et al 1994). Increased total protein excretion should not be considered abnormal until it exceeds 400–500 mg in 24 hours.

The distal renal tubule is actively concerned with volume homeostasis. Once again there is evidence of substantial change in this area of physiology during human pregnancy (Brown & Gallery 1994). Total body water increases by between 6 and 8 litres and there is a net retention of some 900 mmol of sodium. Although plasma osmolality is markedly reduced (by about 10 mosmol/l) from the early weeks of pregnancy (Davison et al 1981), it is not associated with the water diuresis which would occur in the non-pregnant individual. While the process of osmoregulation is effective during pregnancy, there must be important changes in the osmotic thresholds which trigger control mechanisms, such as the sensation of thirst and the release of the antidiuretic hormone, arginine vasopressin (AVP) (Davison et al 1988). Other changes include a substantial increase in the metabolic clearance rate (MCR) of AVP, which rises four-fold after the first trimester, paralleling the appearance of, and marked increases in, circulating levels of a placental enzyme, vasopressinase (also called oxytocinase), which is a cystine aminopeptidase capable of inactivating large quantities of AVP in vitro. The MCR of l-deamino-8-D-AVP (desmopressin acetate, dDAVP), an analogue of AVP that is resistant to enzyme degradation, is unchanged suggesting that the aminopeptidase enzymes are also active in vivo (Lindheimer et al 1989, Davison et al 1993, Lindheimer & Barron 1994). The osmoregulatory changes must be taken into account when managing women with known central diabetes insipidus (DI) and when diagnosing the rare syndrome of transient DI of pregnancy, which usually presents during the second trimester of pregnancy and remits postpartum.

These substantial alterations in physiological norms affect the interpretation of disordered renal function during pregnancy. A brief account of the changes of greatest clinical significance is provided in Table 26.1.

INFECTION OF THE URINARY TRACT

Definitions

The analysis of urine specimens during pregnancy is especially likely to be hampered by contamination at the time of collection with bacteria from urethra, vagina or perineum. This problem can be overcome by suprapubic aspiration of bladder urine (McFadyen et al 1973), but this inconvenient procedure is distasteful to most patients and obstetricians. Another approach is to use the number of colony counts obtained upon culture of a fresh midstream urine specimen collected by a clean-catch technique involving anteroposterior swabbing of the vulva with water or a soap solution (not antiseptic) at least three times before starting micturition. True bacteriuria may then be defined as more than 100 000 bacteria of the same species per millilitre of urine, present in two consecutive specimens. Bacteriuria is frequently associated with discomfort on voiding, urgency and increased frequency of micturition but these symptoms are common in pregnancy even in the absence of urinary tract infection. Conversely, asymptomatic (covert) bacteriuria, in which true bacteriuria is present without subjective evidence of urinary tract infection, may be of considerable clinical significance.

Bacteriuria originating from the upper urinary tract is more likely to recur and requires more rigorous surveillance and treatment (Fairley et al 1966). Numerous techniques have been used to investigate this problem without great success. The identification of antibody-coated bacteria in urine seemed promising but its precise value remains controversial (see Cunningham & Lucas 1994).

Pathogenesis

Bacteria originating in the large bowel probably colonize the urinary tract transperineally. By far the commonest infecting organism is *Escherichia coli*, responsible for 75–90% of bacteriuria during pregnancy. The pathogenic virulence of this organism, which is not the most plentiful in faeces, appears to derive from a number of factors, including resistance to vaginal acidity, rapid division in urine, adherence to cells and the production of chemicals which decrease ureteric peristalsis and inhibit phagocytosis (McFadyen 1986). Other organisms frequently responsible for urinary tract infection include *Klebsiella*, *Proteus*, coagulase-negative staphylococci and *Pseudomonas*. The interaction between host and infection is an exciting area of research and much is being discovered about the roles of uroepithelial receptors, bacterial adhesions

Table 26.1 Physiological changes in common indices of renal function associated with human pregnancy: mean value (± 1 standard deviation)

Measurement	Units	Non-pregnant	Early pregnancy	Late pregnancy	Source
Effective renal plasma flow	ml/min	480 (72)	841 (144)	771 (175)	1
Glomerular filtration rate					
Inulin clearance	ml/min	105 (24)	163 (19)	169 (22)	2
24-h creatinine clearance	ml/min	94 (8)	136 (11)	114 (10)	3, 4
Plasma					
Creatinine	μmol/l	77 (10)	60 (8)	64 (9)	5
Urea	mmol/l	4.3 (0.8)	3.0 (0.7)	2.8 (0.7)	5
Uric acid	μmol/l	246 (59)	189 (48)	269 (56)	6
Osmolality	mosmol/kg	288 (2.5)	278 (2.0)	280 (2.0)	7, 8

Sources: 1. Dunlop 1981; 2. Davison & Hytten 1974; 3. Davison & Noble 1981; 4. Davison et al 1980; 5. Lind, unpublished observations; 6. Lind et al 1984; 7. Davison et al 1981; 8. Davison et al 1988.

and induction of inflammatory responses (Lomberg et al 1992, Roche & Alexander 1992).

Asymptomatic bacteriuria

About 5% of young women are susceptible to bacteriuria. This is approximately the proportion found to be bacteriuric on routine screening during pregnancy (Whalley 1967). Of those found to be non-bacteriuric on screening, only 1.5% develop bacteriuria later in pregnancy. However, since the number of women in the initially uninfected group greatly exceeds the number with initial bacteriuria, this small percentage contributes substantially to the total population of pregnant women with urinary tract infection, accounting for some 30% of cases (Fig. 26.2). Of interest, a recent antenatal study (Stenquist et al 1989), in which 99% of women took part in at least one screening, suggested that bacteriuria was highest between the 9th and 17th weeks of pregnancy. The 16th week was the optimal time for a single screen of bacteriuria calculated calculated on the number of bacteria-free gestational weeks gained by treatment.

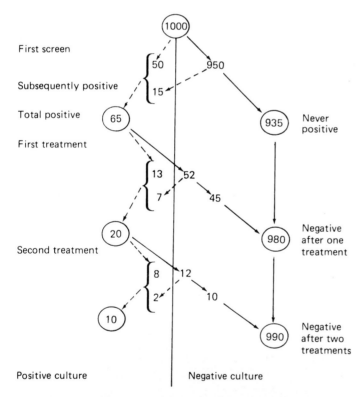

Fig. 26.2 Approximate outcome of screening and treatment for asymptomatic bacteriuria in 1000 women during pregnancy. Continuous arrows represent a change from positive to negative culture; interrupted arrows represent change towards positive culture. The 6.5% total positive rate comprises 5.0% positive on first culture and 1.5% subsequently positive. The first course of treatment produces a negative culture in 80% of bacteriuric women, but 15% of these develop recurrent bacteriuria. Second and subsequent courses of treatment produce negative cultures in only 40% of remaining bacteriuric women.

Asymptomatic bacteriuria has been implicated in several complications of pregnancy, including low birthweight, fetal loss, pre-eclampsia and maternal anaemia (Kass 1962). Several of these apparent relationships may have resulted from inaccuracies in matching cases and controls (Beard & Roberts 1968) and none is usually supported by subsequent studies (Gilstrap et al 1981, Davison et al 1984, Martinell et al 1990). A meta-analysis of the better studies by Romero et al (1989) conclude that there was an association between untreated asymptomatic bacteriuria and low birthweight preterm delivery and that therapy did reduce the incidence of low birthweight neonates. When evidence of previous parenchymal damage is present, however, there may be a greater propensity to hypertension (McGladerry et al 1992). Also, there is some evidence of an association between any type of urinary infection in pregnancy and sudden unexpected postperinatal death (Gardner 1985).

Not all untreated bacteriuric women develop symptoms of acute urinary tract infection during pregnancy and those found to have sterile urine when screened at antenatal booking will later contribute substantially to the pool of symptomatic women. Some therefore argued that screening programmes are not cost-effective (Lawson & Miller 1973, Campbell-Brown et al 1987). Chng & Hall (1982) found that as a predictor of symptomatic urinary infection, bacteriuria had a specificity of 89% but a sensitivity of only 33% and a false positive rate of almost 90%. However, when their population was screened only by a single urine test an unusually high prevalence (11.8%) of bacteriuria was detected. Interestingly, they suggested that women with a history of previous urinary tract infection and current bacteriuria were 10 times more likely to develop symptoms during pregnancy than women without either feature.

Most obstetricians still treat asymptomatic bacteriuria. The agent chosen must not only be effective against the organism identified but also acceptable for use during pregnancy. Ampicillin and cephalosporins are commonly prescribed but short-acting sulphonamides may be equally effective. However, sulphonamides should be avoided during the last few weeks of pregnancy since they competitively inhibit the binding of bilirubin to albumin and can increase the risk of neonatal hyperbilirubinaemia. Nitrofurantoin, which often causes nausea, may not be readily tolerated by pregnant women and should also be avoided during late pregnancy because of the risk of haemolysis due to deficiency of erythrocyte phosphate dehydrogenase in the newborn. The tetracyclines are not recommended during pregnancy because they predispose to dental staining in the child and (rarely) to acute fatty liver in the mother.

A 2-week course of therapy is usually adequate and there is much controversy about short (especially single-dose) courses (Zinner 1992). Recurrent infection is common, however, affecting some 30% of bacteriuric women; after two courses of treatment about 15% will continue to have positive urinary cultures (Fig. 26.2). Recurrence may be due either to relapse, when the same organism is found within 6 weeks of the initial infection, or to reinfection, when a different organism is detected more than 6 weeks after treatment. Treatment during pregnancy has little effect on the subsequent prevalence of bacteriuria, nor does persistent bacteriuria in women with normal urinary tracts contribute to chronic renal disease. Some 20% of bacteriuric women have some abnormality of the urinary tract (Fowler & Pulaski 1982), but in most this is minor and not clearly related to the disease. Postpartum intravenous urography is probably best reserved for bacteriuric women with a history of acute symptomatic infections before or during pregnancy, for those in whom bacteriuria is difficult to eradicate or for those in whom there is postpartum recurrence of disease (Davison & Lindheimer 1985).

Symptomatic urinary tract infection

In the series of Chng & Hall (1982) 11.8% of bacteriuric women developed symptoms of urinary tract infection during pregnancy, whereas only 3.2% of women with sterile urine at initial screening did so. In the pregnant population as a whole, the incidence of symptoms was 4%. The upper urinary tract appears to be involved in a substantial proportion of cases: other workers estimate that acute pyelonephritis occurs in 1–2% of pregnancies, making it the most common renal complication of pregnancy (Davison & Lindheimer 1985, Cunningham & Lucas 1994).

Acute pyelonephritis classically presents as a febrile illness associated with loin pain and vomiting, but there is considerable individual variation. The differential diagnosis includes other urinary tract pathology such as renal calculus or acute hydronephrosis (which can be recognized on ultrasound scanning or limited excretory urography), other causes of pyrexia such as respiratory tract infection, viraemia or toxoplasmosis (appropriate serological screening should be performed) and other causes of acute abdominal pain such as acute appendicitis, biliary colic, gastroenteritis, necrobiosis of a uterine fibroid or abruption of the placenta (Cunningham et al 1987). Acute pyelonephritis is associated with an increased incidence of premature labour and possibly also with intrauterine growth retardation or fetal death. The glomerular filtration rate may be reduced at the time of an acute episode during pregnancy (Whalley et al 1975) in contradistinction to the usual lack of impairment of renal haemodynamics in non-pregnant patients.

Perhaps 20% of women with severe pyelonephritis develop complications in addition to renal dysfunction, including urinary obstruction, haematological dysfunction, perinephric cellulitis and abscess, septicaemic shock and pulmonary injury (Cunningham & Lucas 1994). Respiratory distress syndrome can be life-threatening (Cunningham et al 1987) and occurs in 8% of acute urinary infection patients if beta-mimetic tocolysis is given (Towers et al 1991). Prompt recognition and appropriate respiration support prevent severe hypoxaemia that may cause fetal death (Weinberger 1993).

Women with acute pyelonephritis should be managed in hospital. On admission, a midstream urine sample should be obtained, together with blood cultures in severely ill patients, but it will usually be necessary to begin antibiotic treatment before microbiological results are available. Recently it has been argued that urine and blood culture results are so rarely used to guide empirical therapy that the practice should be discontinued (MacMillan & Grimes 1991), thus saving much revenue. However, the cost of urine culture and sensitivities is trivial compared to the cost of hospitalization, which is also admittedly unnecessary for many patients with an uncomplicated infection.

The chosen antibiotic must achieve high concentrations both in blood and in renal parenchyma. Ampicillin and the cephalosporins are widely favoured but an aminoglycoside such as gentamicin may be of value in the acutely ill patient. The intravenous route of administration is preferred until pyrexia resolves, when oral therapy may be substituted. Antibiotic therapy should be continued for at least 1 month after an episode of acute pyelonephritis; thereafter urine culture should be arranged at each antenatal visit.

Ultrasonic examination of the renal tract of pregnant women with pyelonephritis usually reveals significantly increased pelvicalyceal dilatation compared to normal physiological dilatation of pregnancy but as treatment does not necessarily produce a consistent decrease, the anomaly may antedate the acute infection (Twickler et al 1991).

Acute hydoureter and hydronephrosis

Very occasionally pregnancy can precipitate the overdistension syndrome, with obstruction occurring at varying levels at or above the pelvic brim (Eckford et at 1991, Satin et al 1993). There is a recurrent loin pain with increments in plasma creatinine but urinalysis reveals few or no red cells and repeat midstream urine specimens are negative. If positioning on the unaffected side, with appropriate antibiotics if needed, fails to resolve the situation, then urethral catheterization on ultrasound-guided percutaneous nephrostomy may be required (van Sonnenberg et al 1992).

CHRONIC RENAL DISEASE

There are conflicting views regarding pregnancy in

women with renal disease (Katz & Lindheimer 1994). The majority view is that, with the exception of certain specific disease entities such as systemic lupus erythematosus, renal polyarteritis nodosa, scleroderma, perhaps IgA nephropathy, membranoproliferative glomerulonephritis and reflux nephropathy, the obstetric outcome is usually successful provided renal function is at most moderately compromised and hypertension is absent or minimal. If hypertension is present and it requires more than one drug for its control, the obstetric success becomes substantially less. In general, pregnancy does not have an adverse effect on the natural history of the renal disease (Davison et al 1985a, Davison & Baylis 1994).

Renal dysfunction and its obstetric implications

It is inadvisable to assess renal function by plasma creatinine levels alone, as an individual may lose up to 50% of renal function, be symptom-free and still have a deceptively normal plasma creatinine level. Although a plasma creatinine of 75 µmol/l and a urea of 4.5 mmol/l, would be acceptable in non-pregnant subjects; they are suspect in pregnant women (Table 26.1).

The ability to conceive and sustain a viable pregnancy is reduced more by the degree of functional impairment than by the nature of the underlying renal lesion. Fertility is diminished as renal function falls. When prepregnancy plasma creatinine and urea levels exceed 275 µmol/l and 10 mmol/l respectively, normal pregnancy is rare. There are exceptions and successes have been documented in women with moderate to severe disease, including some treated by chronic ambulatory peritoneal dialysis as well as by haemodialysis (Hou 1994).

Prepregnancy counselling

Ideally, pregnancy is probably best restricted to women whose prepregnancy plasma creatinine levels are 200 µmol/l or less and whose diastolic blood pressure is 90 mmHg or less. Some clinicians recommend that pregnancy should not be undertaken if blood creatinine exceeds 135 µmol/l (Bear 1978). Whatever level is chosen, it should be recognized that degrees of impairment which do not cause symptoms or appear to disrupt homeostasis in non-pregnant individuals can certainly jeopardize pregnancy. The question has to be asked: 'Is pregnancy advisable?' (Table 26.2). In a woman with chronic renal disease who wishes to have a family, the sooner she conceives the better because in some, renal function will decline as they get older.

Effect of renal disease on pregnancy versus effect of pregnancy on renal disease

Clinicians do not always have the opportunity to counsel

Table 26.2 Prepregnancy assessment: Is pregnancy advisable?

Factors to be considered
Type of chronic renal disease (see Table 26.6)
General health considerations
Diastolic blood pressure < 90 mmHg
Renal function
Plasma creatinine < 250 µmol/l
Plasma urea < 10 mmol/l
Presence or absence of proteinuria
Review of all drug therapy

Table 26.3 Antenatal assessment: Should pregnancy continue?

Factors to be considered
Type of chronic renal disease (see Table 26.6)
General health considerations
Gestational age
Effect of pregnancy on blood pressure
Effect of pregnancy on renal function or plasma biochemistry
Review of all drug therapy
Past obstetric history

Table 26.4 Prepregnancy assessment: categories of renal functional status

Classification	Plasma creatinine (µmol/l)
Intact or mildly impaired renal function	≤ 125
Moderate renal insufficiency	≥ 125
Severe renal insufficiency	≥ 250

women with chronic renal disease before pregnancy (see Lindheimer & Katz 1994). A patient with suspected or known renal disease often presents with pregnancy as a *fait accompli* and then the question is: 'Should pregnancy continue?' (Table 26.3). Also, think about the diagnosis of renal artery stenosis (Haybourne et al 1991). In view of the radically different obstetric and long-term outlooks in women with different degrees of renal insufficiency (Abe et al 1985, Davison et al 1985b), it is important to consider the impact of pregnancy by categories of renal functional status prior to conception (Table 26.4) (Cunningham et al 1990, Abe 1991, 1994, Imbascati & Ponticelli 1991, Jungers et al 1991).

Intact or mildly impaired renal function with minimal hypertension

Women with chronic renal disease but normal or only mildly decreased renal function at conception usually have a successful obstetric outcome and pregnancy does not adversely affect the course of their disease (Surian et al 1984, Hayslett 1985). Some authors suggest that this statement, although generally correct, should be tempered somewhat in lupus nephropathy, membranoproliferative glomerulonephritis and perhaps IgA and reflux nephropathies, which may be adversely affected by intercurrent pregnancy (Becker et al, 1985, Nicklin 1991, Abe 1994). When renal disease is detected or suspected for the first time during pregnancy (often because proteinuria or hypertension is first detected at the booking antenatal examination), it is usually surmised that renal function had been satisfactorily maintained until pregnancy brought an underlying mild lesion to clinical expression (Lindheimer & Katz 1994).

In most women with renal disease the glomerular filtration rate increases during pregnancy, but the increases are usually less than those in normal pregnant women. Increased proteinuria is the most common effect of pregnancy in chronic renal disease, occurring in almost 50% of pregnancies (although rarely in women with chronic pyelonephritis), and can be massive (often exceeding 3 g in 24 hours), frequently leading to nephrotic oedema. Between pregnancies and during long-term follow-up, hypertension, renal functional abnormalities and proteinuria are less common and less severe. When renal failure does supervene, it usually reflects the inexorable course of a particular renal disease.

Moderate renal insufficiency

Prognosis has to be more guarded when renal function is moderately impaired before pregnancy (plasma creatinine 125–250 μmol/l but the number of cases reported is still small. In one series, renal morbidity often occurred early in pregnancy; five of 11 developed serious deterioration in renal function culminating in terminal renal failure several months postpartum (Kincaid-Smith et al 1980). Because of this experience and the fact that deterioration was also seen in an occasional patient with apparently stable renal function, these investigators are rather pessimistic about pregnancy in women with either mild or moderate renal disease.

Another study of the influence of pregnancy on chronic renal disease specifically examined the influence of the level of kidney function before pregnancy or when first seen in pregnancy (Bear 1976). No immediate loss of renal function could be detected in 29 patients whose plasma creatinine levels were less than 170 μmol/l. In four of eight patients whose initial plasma creatinine level was above 180 μmol/l, however, there was a further significant increase in plasma creatinine during pregnancy, which was complicated in virtually every case. Four patients in this group progressed to end-stage renal failure within 18 months of delivery. These and other workers have emphasized that uncontrolled hypertension is a very important factor in the overall deterioration (Imbasciati et al 1984, Hou et al 1985, Imbasciati & Ponticelli 1991, Abe 1994, Jungers 1994).

We generally recommend that pregnancy is best avoided in women who have lost 50% of their kidney function but recent studies question this. Hou et al (1985) recorded a successful obstetrical outcome in 92% of the pregnancies in 22 women with plasma creatinine levels of 190–300 μmol/l whose pregnancies were allowed to go beyond the second trimester. Many of these patients had hectic blood pressure and in 25% there was an accelerated decline in renal function. Thus, although fetal survival is now improved in such women (Hou 1994), maternal risks, especially complications of poorly controlled hypertension, preclude encouraging such women to conceive or continue pregnancies which are already in progress.

Severe renal insufficiency

Most women in this category (plasma creatinine > 250 μmol/l) are amenorrhoeic or anovulatory (Lim 1994). The likelihood of conceiving, let alone having a normal pregnancy and delivery, is therefore low but not impossible. As data on such patients are very limited, it is difficult to evaluate whether pregnancy has an adverse effect on their disease (Hou 1994). In our opinion the risk of maternal complications (severe pre-eclampsia or bleeding) is greater than the probability of a successful obstetric outcome.

Antenatal assessment

Patients should be seen at 2-week intervals until 32 weeks' gestation and weekly thereafter. Routine serial antenatal observations should be supplemented by:

1. assessment of 24-hour creatinine clearance and protein excretion
2. careful monitoring of blood pressure for early detection of hypertension and assessment of its severity
3. early detection of pregnancy-induced hypertension (pre-eclampsia)
4. assessment of fetal size, development and well-being
5. early detection of asymptomatic bacteriuria or urinary tract infection.

Renal function

If renal function deteriorates, reversible causes should be sought, such as urinary tract infection, subtle dehydration, or electrolyte imbalance, occasionally precipitated by inadvertent diuretic therapy. Near term, a 15–20% decrement in function, which affects plasma creatine minimally, is permissible. Failure to detect a reversible cause of a significant decrement is reason to end the pregnancy by elective delivery. When proteinuria occurs and persists but blood pressure is normal and renal function is preserved the pregnancy can be allowed to continue.

Blood pressure

Most of the specific risks of hypertension appear to be mediated through superimposed pre-eclampsia. There is still controversy about the incidence of pre-eclampsia in those women with pre-existing renal disease. The diagnosis cannot be made with certainty on clinical grounds alone, because hypertension and proteinuria may be manifestations of the underlying renal disease (Gaber et al 1994). Treatment with hypertension usually awaits diastolic pressure > 110 mmHg (see Ch. 24), but many would treat women with underlying renal disease more aggressively, believing this preserves function. Without doubt, perinatal outcome is poor in the presence of poorly controlled hypertension, nephrotic range proteinuria in early pregnancy and/or GFR ≤ 70 ml/minute prior to pregnancy or in the first trimester, whatever the type of renal disease (Abe 1991, Jungers et al 1991).

Fetal surveillance and timing of delivery

Serial assessment of fetal well-being is essential because renal disease can be associated with intrauterine growth retardation and, when complications do arise, the judicious moment for intervention is influenced by fetal status. Current management should minimize intrauterine fetal death as well as neonatal morbidity and mortality (Table 26.5). Regardless of gestational age, most babies weighing 1500 g or more survive better in a special care nursery than in a hostile intrauterine environment. Delivery before 38 weeks may be necessary if there are signs of impending intrauterine fetal death, if renal function deteriorates substantially, if uncontrollable hypertension supervenes or if eclampsia occurs.

Problems with particular renal diseases

Specific problems are associated with particular renal diseases (Table 26.6). The crux of the clinical situation is the balance between maternal prognosis and fetal prognosis—the effect of pregnancy on that disease and the effect of that disease on pregnancy. This balance is influenced by factors such as the degree of renal insufficiency,

Table 26.5 Renal disease and pregnancy: improvements in perinatal mortality over the past four decades

Renal disease	1950s	1960s	1970s	1980s	1990s
Mild					
Preterm delivery	8%	10%	19%	25%	28%
Perinatal mortality	18%	15%	7%	< 5%	< 3%
Moderate					
Preterm delivery	15%	21%	40%	52%	57%
Perinatal mortality	58%	45%	23%	10%	10%

These estimates are based on studies reviewed in Davison & Baylis (1994) and do not include cases of systemic lupus erythematosus.

the presence or absence of hypertension as well as the type of disease.

Acute and chronic glomerulonephritis

The acute disease is very rare as a complication of pregnancy and it can be mistaken for pre-eclampsia.

Table 26.6 Effects of pregnancy on established chronic renal disease

Renal disease	Effects
Chronic glomerulonephritis	Usually no adverse effect in the absence of hypertension. One view is that glomerulonephritis is adversely affected by the coagulation changes of pregnancy. Urinary tract infections may occur more frequently
IgA nephropathy	Risks of uncontrolled and/or sudden escalating hypertension and worsening of renal function
Pyelonephritis	Bacteriuria in pregnancy can lead to exacerbation. Multiple organ system derangements may ensue including adult RDS
Reflux nephropathy	Risks of sudden escalating hypertension and worsening of renal function
Urolithiasis	Infections can be more frequent, but ureteral dilatation and stasis do not seem to affect natural history
Polycystic disease (PKD)	Functional impairment and hypertension usually minimal in childbearing years
Diabetic nephropathy	Usually no adverse effect on the renal lesion, but there is increased frequency of infection, oedema, and/or pre-eclampsia
Systemic lupus erythematosus (SLE)	Controversial; prognosis most favourable if disease in remission > 6 months prior to conception. Steroid dosage should be increased postpartum
Periarteritis nodosa	Fetal prognosis is dismal and maternal death often occurs
Scleroderma (SS)	If onset during pregnancy then can be rapid overall deterioration. Reactivation of quiescent scleroderma may occur postpartum
Previous urinary tract surgery	Might be associated with other malformations of the urogenital tract. Urinary tract infection common during pregnancy. Renal function may undergo reversible decrease. No significant obstructive problem but Caesarean section often needed for abnormal presentation and/or to avoid disruption of the continence mechanism if artificial sphincter present
After nephrectomy, solitary kidney and pelvic kidney	Might be associated with other malformations of urogenital tract. Pregnancy well tolerated, dystocia rarely occurs with a pelvic kidney
Wegener's granulomatosis	Limited information. Proteinuria (± hypertension) is common from early in pregnancy. Immunosuppressives are safe but cytotoxic drugs are best avoided
Renal artery stenosis	May present as chronic hypertension or as recurrent isolated pre-eclampsia. If diagnosed then transluminal angioplasty can be undertaken in pregnancy if appropriate

The prognosis of chronic glomerulonephritis during pregnancy is hard to evaluate primarily because most reports are poorly documented, often failing to list the degree of functional impairment, the blood pressure prior to conception and the histological characteristics of the glomerulonephritis. One view is that most glomerular diseases are aggravated because of the hypercoagulable state that accompanies pregnancy, and patients are more prone to superimposed pre-eclampsia or hypertensive crises earlier in pregnancy (Fairley et al 1973). Our experience is that renal function decreases most often in patients with diffuse glomerulonephritis in whom hypertension is invariably both more common and severe; nonetheless, most of the pregnancies are successful (Katz et al 1980).

Hereditary nephritis, an uncommon disorder which may first manifest itself or exacerbate during pregnancy, is a variant of hereditary nephritis in which the patient has disordered platelet morphology and function. Pregnancy in women with this disorder has been successful from a renal viewpoint, but their pregnancies can be complicated by bleeding problems.

Pyelonephritis (tubulointerstitial disease)

The prognosis of pregnancy in women with chronic pyelonephritis seems similar to that of patients with glomerular disease in that its outcome is most favourable in normotensive patients with adequate renal function. Disease of an infectious nature has a propensity to exacerbate during pregnancy, and may be minimized if the patient is well hydrated and rests frequently, positioned in lateral recumbency (ureteral obstruction by the enlarged uterus probably does not occur in this position). It has been suggested that patients with this condition are more prone to hypertensive complications during pregnancy, but in our experience they have a more benign antenatal course than women with glomerular disease.

Recurrent infection might be superimposed on vesicoureteric and intrarenal reflux and the resultant renal changes are termed reflux nephropathy. It is one of the most frequent diseases in women of childbearing age: a third of cases are clinically unmarked by pregnancy, up to 30% of women developing end-stage renal failure have reflux nephropathy and this is usually present before 40 years (Bailey 1992, Jungers 1994).

Polycystic renal disease (PKD)

This entity may remain undetected during pregnancy, but careful questioning of pregnant women for a history of familial problems and the use of ultrasonography may lead to earlier detection. These patients do well when functional impairment is minimal and hypertension absent, which is often the case during childbearing years (Gabow 1993). They do, however, have an increased incidence of hypertension late in pregnancy, when their pregnancies are compared with those of sisters unaffected by this autosomal dominant disease.

There are other much rarer inherited renal disorders, some of which have an earlier onset than hereditary nephritis and PKD. These include cystinosis, nephronophthisis, tuberous sclerosis, Von Hippel–Landau disease, in some of which antenatal diagnosis is technically possible (Davison & Baylis 1994, Krebelmann et al 1994).

Diabetic nephropathy

Because many patients have been diabetic since childhood, they probably already have microscopic changes in their kidneys. During pregnancy, diabetic women have an increased prevalence of bacteriuria and may be more susceptible to symptomatic urinary tract infection. They also have an increased frequency of peripheral oedema and pre-eclampsia. Most women with diabetic nephropathy demonstrate the normal increments in renal function, and pregnancy does not accelerate deterioration of diabetic nephropathy (Coombs & Kitzmiller 1991, Hayslett & Reece 1994). It should be remembered, however, that the condition of non-pregnant diabetes with plasma creatinine levels > 125 µmol/l too often progresses to renal failure.

Systemic lupus erythematosus

Systemic lupus erythematosus is a relatively common disease; its predilection to childbearing age makes the coincidence of systemic lupus erythematosus and pregnancy an important clinical problem (Grimes et al 1985). The profound disturbance of the immunological system in systemic lupus erythematosus, the complicated immunology of pregnancy, the multiple organ involvement and the complex clinical picture are just a few reasons for the vast literature (Mor-Yosef et al 1984).

There are differing opinions regarding the effects of pregnancy on lupus nephropathy. Transient improvements, no change, and a tendency to relapse have all been reported. Decisions regarding the status of the disease, as well as the assessment of the importance of having a baby to the patient and her partner, should be made on an individual basis. The majority of pregnancies succeed, especially when the maternal disease is in sustained, complete clinical remission for at least 6 months prior to conception. This applies even if the patient has severe pathological changes in her original renal biopsy and heavy proteinuria in the early stages of her disease. Continued signs of disease activity or increasing renal dysfunction certainly reduce the likelihood of an uncomplicated pregnancy (Jungers et al 1982). From recent reviews of the literature it appears that as many as 19% experience decrements in GFR (progressive in 8%) and 42% have hypertension. The figures are worse if renal insufficiency (plasma creatinine > 125 μmol/l) antedates the pregnancy (Imbasciati & Ponticelli 1991, Nicklin 1991).

Lupus nephropathy may sometimes become manifest during pregnancy and when accompanied by hypertension and renal dysfunction in late pregnancy may be mistaken for pre-eclampsia. Some patients have a definite tendency to relapse, occasionally severely in the puerperium, and many advise steroids or an increase in steroid dosage at this time. The concept of the stormy puerperium is disputed, so others merely observe postpartum patients and do not institute or increase steroids unless signs of decreased activity are noticed (Petri et al 1991).

SLE sera may contain a bewildering array of autoantibodies against nucleic acids, nucleoproteins, cell surface antigens and phospholipids. Antiphospholipid antibodies (APA) exert a complicated effect on the coagulation system. This led to the rather enigmatic description of a lupus (LE) anticoagulant found in 5–10% of patients with SLE. It has since been observed in patients with other conditions and even in patients without any identifiable disorder. Placental transmission of lupus serum factor can occur (Lancet Editorial 1984).

Although the LE-anticoagulant was first described in patients with systemic lupus erythematosus, it has since been observed in patients with other conditions and even in patients without any identifiable disorder (Hughes 1983, Lubbe et al 1984). Intrauterine death is common in women with circulating LE-anticoagulant and/or anticardiolipin antibodies (ACA or anti-LE), these latter active against certain phospholipid components of cell walls. The fetus can be at hazard in all three trimesters, the level of risk overall having been put at 80–90% (Love & Santoro 1990). It is known that the placentas in such cases shown extensive thrombotic and arteriosclerotic changes. Because treatment with steroids and aspirin can lead to successful pregnancies, it is important to screen for LE-anticoagulant in all women with systemic lupus erythematosus in order to identify this particular cohort, and perhaps also in women with a history of recurrent intrauterine death or thrombotic episodes.

An increased incidence of congenital cardiac anomalies (with or without arythmias or even heart block) has been described in the offspring of women with systemic lupus erythematosus and other maternal connective tissue disease, even when maternal pathology appears quiescent (Singsen et al 1985). This association appears to be related to the transplacental passage of a maternal antibody to soluble tissue ribonucleoprotein. This maternal antibody (anti-Ro (SS-A)) is detectable in almost all cases of isolated congenital complete heart block (Scott et al 1983). The prevalence of anti-Ro (SS-A) in patients with systemic lupus erythematosus is 25–30%, where it may also have other untoward associations, particularly recurrent abortion. Paradoxically, the mother's heart is usually unaffected, even though the antibody is present in her system at a higher concentration than in the fetus. The fetal heart may therefore be more vulnerable to antibody-mediated damage than the mature heart, or it may possess phase-specific antigens (Taylor et al 1986). Alternatively, blocking maternal antibodies of the IgA or IgM class (not transferred to the fetus) could prevent an IgG antibody causing maternal damage.

Interestingly, maternal lupus may become apparent, clinically and serologically, many years after the birth of a baby with heart block (Kasinath & Katz 1982).

Periarteritis nodosa

In contrast to lupus nephropathy, the outcome of pregnancy in women with renal involvement due to periarteritis nodosa is very poor, largely because of the associated hypertension which is frequently of a malignant nature (Mor-Yosef et al 1984). Although a few successful gestations have been reported, in most cases fetal prognosis is dismal and many pregnancies have ended with maternal deaths. This may merely reflect the nature of the disease itself, but it must nevertheless be taken into consideration when making a decision to go on with a pregnancy. It appears that therapeutic termination of pregnancy (as an alternative form of management) has less risk to the mother (Nagey et al 1983).

Scleroderma

This term includes a heterogeneous group of limited and systemic conditions causing hardening of the skin. Systemic sclerosis implies involvement of both skin and other sites, particularly certain internal organs. Renal involvement occurs in about 60% of patients, usually within 3–4 years of diagnosis. The combination of pregnancy and scleroderma is unusual because this infrequent disease occurs most often during the fourth and fifth decades and because patients with scleroderma tend to be relatively infertile. Whenever scleroderma has its onset during pregnancy, there is a greater tendency for deterioration. Even after an uneventful and successful pregnancy reactivation in the puerperium, with the use of converting enzyme inhibitors being necessary (Steen et al 1989), can be unexpected.

Most maternal deaths have involved rapidly progressive scleroderma with pulmonary complications, infection, hypertension and/or heart failure (Magmon & Fejgin 1989).

Previous urinary tract surgery

Permanent urinary diversion is still used in the management of patients with congenital lower urinary tract defects; but since the introduction of self-catheterization for neurogenic bladders, its use in this group has declined in these patients. The most common complication of pregnancy is urinary infection, ranging from asymptomatic bacteriuria to severe pyelonephritis (Barrett & Peters 1983). Preterm labour occurs in 20% and there is some evidence that the use of prophylactic antibiotics throughout pregnancy reduces the incidence of this complication.

Renal function during pregnancy may decline, usually related to underlying infection or intermittent obstruction. With an ileal conduit, elevation and compression by the expanding uterus can cause outflow obstruction whereas with a ureterosigmoid anastomosis, actual ureteral obstruction may occur. The changes usually reverse after delivery.

The mode of delivery is dictated by obstetric factors and not the presence of the urinary diversion. Abnormal presentation mainly accounts for a Caesarean section rate of 25%, but of course minor genital tract abnormalities may contribute. Vaginal delivery is safe for women with an ileal conduit, augmentation cystoplasty or an ureterosigmoid anastomosis if one bears in mind that in the latter group, continence is dependent on an intact anal sphincter, which should be protected during vaginal delivery with an adequate mediolateral episiotomy.

Solitary kidney

Some patients have either a congenital absence of one kidney or marked unilateral hypoplasia. The majority that we know about, however, have had a previous nephrectomy because of pyelonephritis with abscess or hydronephrosis, unilateral tuberculosis, congenital abnormalities or tumour (Klein 1984). When counselling women with a single-kidney, one should known the indication for and the time since the nephrectomy. In patients who had an infectious or structural renal problem sequential prepregnancy investigation is needed for detection of any persistent infection.

There is no difference whether the right or left kidney remains as long as it is located in the normal anatomical position: if function is normal and stable, women with this problem seem to tolerate pregnancy well despite the superimposition of increases in glomerular filtration rate on the already hyperfiltering nephrons. Ectopic kidneys, usually pelvic, are more vulnerable to infection and are associated with decreased fetal salvage, probably because of an association with other malformations of the urogenital tract. If infection occurs in a solitary kidney during pregnancy and does not quickly respond to antibiotics, then termination may have to be considered for preservation of renal function.

Urolithiasis

The prevalence of urolithiasis in pregnancy ranges from 0.3 to 0.35 per 1000 women (Coe et al 1978). Renal and uteric calculi are one of the most common causes of non-uterine abdominal pain severe enough to necessitate hospital admission during pregnancy. When there are complications that need surgical intervention, pregnancy should not be a deterrent to intravenous urography, although there may be valid reluctance on the part of the clinician to consider radiological reinvestigation. Recently it was proposed that specific clinical criteria should be met before the undertaking of an intravenous urogram, as follows:

1. microscopic haematuria
2. recurrent urinary tract symptoms
3. sterile urine culture when pyelonephritis is suspected.

The presence of two of these criteria points to a diagnosis of calculi in approximately 50% of gravidas, and an intravenous urogram is advised (Miller & Kakkis 1982).

Management should be conservative in the first instance, consisting primarily of adequate hydration, appropriate antibiotic therapy and pain relief with systemic analgesics (Maikranz et al 1987). The use of continuous segmental epidural block (T11 and L2) has been advocated, an approach that has long been used in non-pregnant patients with ureteric colic and which may even favourably influence spontaneous passage of the calculi. When the block is carefully confined to the relevant segments for pain relief, the patient micturates without difficulty, moves without assistance, and is at lower risk from thromboembolic problems than a drowsy patient immobilized in bed with pain, nausea and vomiting (Maikranz et al 1994).

An alternative approach involves placement of internal ureteral tubes or stents, between bladder and kidneys, under local anaesthesia, using cystoscopy or endoluminal ultrasound (Wolf et al 1992). The stent retains its position because it has a pig-tail or J-like curve at each end, and to prevent encrustation it can be changed every 8 weeks. Also ultrasound-guided nephrostomy is a safe and effective method of relieving ureteric colic, or symptomatic obstructive hydronephrosis (von Sonnenberg et al 1992).

Wegener's granulomatosis

There is a paucity of information on pregnancy course and outcome in women with this disorder. Proteinuria (± hypertension) is very common from early in pregnancy (Fields et al 1991) and the reports to date have described both complicated and uneventful pregnancies, including women taking either azathioprine or cyclophosphamide (Murty et al 1991).

Nephrotic syndrome

The most common cause of nephrotic syndrome in late

pregnancy is pre-eclampsia (Fisher et al 1981). This form has a poorer fetal prognosis than pre-eclampsia with less heavy proteinuria, but the maternal prognosis is similar. Other causes of nephrotic syndrome in pregnancy include proliferative or membranoproliferative glomerulonephritis, lipid nephrosis, lupus nephropathy, hereditary nephritis, diabetic nephropathy, renal vein thrombosis, amyloidosis and secondary syphilis. Some of these conditions do not respond to, and may even be seriously aggravated by steroids, serving to emphasize the importance of establishing a tissue diagnosis before initiating steroid therapy.

The term nephrotic syndrome denotes the triad of heavy proteinuria, hypoalbuminaemia and generalized oedema, often associated with hyperlipidaemia. Since most of its manifestations derive from the excessive loss of protein in the urine, a more liberal definition is often used by nephrologists. This includes any renal disease characterized by proteinuria in excess of 3.5 g/24 h in the absence of depressed glomerular filtration rate. The prognosis of this syndrome is usually determined by the nature of the underlying glomerular problem. Of course, the most common cause of nephrotic syndrome in late pregnancy is pre-eclampsia (Fisher et al 1981).

If renal function is adequate and hypertension is absent, there should be few complications during pregnancy. Several of the physiological changes occurring during pregnancy may, however, simulate aggravation or exacerbation of the disease. For example, increments in renal haemodynamics as well as increase in renal vein pressure may enhance protein excretion. Levels of serum albumin usually decrease by 5–10 g/l during normal pregnancy, and the further decreases that can occur in the nephrotic syndrome may enhance the tendency toward fluid retention. Despite oedema, diuretics should not be given, because these patients have a decreased intravascular volume and diuretics could compromise uteroplacental perfusion or aggravate the increased tendency to thrombotic episodes.

Questions that patients ask

Patient expectation is higher than ever. The questions are usually quite simple. 'Is pregnancy advisable? Will the pregnancy be complicated? Will I have a live and healthy baby? Will I come to long-term term harm?' (Table 26.7) (see Davison & Baylis 1994, Lindheimer & Katz 1994).

For any patient a balance must be struck between pregnancy outcome and the impact pregnancy has in the long term. Crucial determinants are the functional status of the kidneys at conception, the presence or absence of hypertension, and the nature of the renal lesion. If a patient wants to know if pregnancy will have a successful outcome, the answer is a qualified yes, provided her renal dysfunction is minimal. If dysfunction is moderate, there is still a fair chance that pregnancy will succeed,

Table 26.7 Renal disease and pregnancy: renal functional status, complications and outcome

Prospects	Disease severity		
	Mild	Moderate	Severe
Pregnancy complications	26%	47%	86%
Successful obstetric outcome	96%	89%	46%
Long-term sequelae	< 3%	25%	53%

These estimates are based on data reviewed in Davison & Baylis (1994) and do not include cases of systemic lupus erythematosus.

but the risks are much greater than in normal pregnancy. These statements have to be tempered somewhat in certain nephropathies which appear to have a more problematical outcome during pregnancy. This is most true of collagen disorders affecting the kidney. Pregnancy outcome in the presence of focal glomerular sclerosis, reflux nephropathy, IgA nephropathy and mesangioproliferative glomerulonephritis is disputed.

Pregnancy does not adversely affect the natural history of the underlying renal lesion if kidney dysfunction is minimal and hypertension is absent at conception, again with the exception of certain collagen disorders. An important factor to be considered in long-term prognosis is the sclerotic effect that hyperfiltration might have in the residual (intact) glomeruli in kidneys of patients with moderate renal insufficiency, which could cause further progressive loss of renal function. Similarly, the compensatory changes in a woman with a single kidney are another form of hyperfiltration which might over many years lessen the lifespan of that kidney. At the centre of this hypothesis is the implication that increases in glomerular pressure or glomerular plasma flow lead to sclerosis within the glomerulus (Brenner et al 1982), a concept that certainly cannot be ignored, since a pregnant woman with renal disease, like any healthy pregnant woman, experiences months of physiological hyperfiltration as part of the overall maternal adaptation to pregnancy. It seems unlikely, however, that there are any long-term sequelae in normal pregnancy (Baylis & Rennke 1985) and reassuring data are accruing from clinical practice (Dawson & Baylis 1994) and with research with animal models which has rigorously examined the mechanism controlling renal function in health and disease (Baylis 1994).

RENAL TRANSPLANT PATIENTS

After transplantation, renal and endocrine functions return rapidly and normal sexual activity invariably ensues. About one in 50 women of childbearing age with a functioning renal transplant becomes pregnant. A total of 35% of all conceptions do not go beyond the initial trimester largely due to spontaneous or therapeutic abortions. Over 90% of pregnancies that do continue past the first trimester end successfully (Davison 1994). Over 5000 pregnancies are on record in women with a renal allograft, but of course many pregnancies, successful and unsuccessful, go unreported.

There are reports of transplants performed with the surgeons unaware that the recipient was in the second trimester of pregnancy (Sola et al 1988). The fact that mother, baby and kidneys came to no harm does not negate the importance of contraception counselling for all renal failure patients and the exclusion of pregnancy prior to transplantation.

Counselling and clinical considerations

The return of fertility and the possibility of conception in women of childbearing age who have transplants dictate appropriate counselling for all such patients. Contraceptive advice should be routine. Couples who want a child should be encouraged to discuss all the implications, including the harsh realities of maternal prospects of survival. All involved must appreciate the possibility that the woman may not live to participate in the long-term care of her child (Table 26.8).

Prepregnancy guidelines

Individual centres formulate their own specific guidelines, but certain basic considerations cannot be ignored. Most advise that it is best to wait 18 months to 2 years post-transplant. This has turned out to be good advice because by then the patient will certainly have recovered from the major surgery and any sequelae, graft function will have stabilized and immunosuppression will be at maintenance levels (Davison et al 1985c). Thus potential teratogenic and suppressive effects and the risks of low birthweight or small-for-dates babies will be minimal.

A suitable set of guidelines is given here, bearing in mind that these criteria are only relative indications:

1. good general health for about 2 years since transplantation
2. stature compatible with good obstetric outcome
3. no proteinuria
4. no significant hypertension
5. no evidence of graft rejection
6. no evidence of pelvicalyceal distension on a recent intravenous urogram
7. stable renal function plasma creatinine of 200 μmol/l or less
8. drug therapy reduced to maintenance levels: prednisone, 15 mg/day or less and azathioprine, 2 mg/kg body weight/day or less. Safe doses of cyclosporin A have not yet been established because of limited clinical experience but quoted anecdotally in 5 mg/kg bodyweight/day or less, or even a change from cyclosporin A to azathioprine before or in early pregnancy.

Antenatal assessment

Pregnant renal transplant patients must be considered at high risk (Table 26.9). Antenatal care should be hospital-based and supplemented with attention to renal function surveillance, blood pressure control, bone disease, anaemia, detection of any infection (however trivial) and assessment of fetal well-being (see Davison, 1994).

Graft rejection and immunosuppressive therapy

Serious rejection episodes occur in 9% of pregnant renal allograft recipients where pregnancy is beyond the second trimester (Davison & Lindheimer 1984). This incidence of rejection is no greater than that expected for non-pregnant allograft recipients, but it might be considered high because it is generally assumed that the privileged immunological state of pregnancy benefits the transplant. Furthermore, there are reports of reduction or cessation of immunosuppressive therapy during pregnancy without rejection episodes.

Whether pregnancy influences the course of subclinical chronic rejection, a problem present in most recipients, is unknown. No factors consistently predict which patients will develop rejection during pregnancy. There may also be a non-immune contribution to chronic graft failure due to the damaging effect of hyperfiltration through remnant nephrons, perhaps even exacerbated during pregnancy (Feehally et al 1986).

Difficulties can arise in distinguishing rejection from acute pyelonephritis, recurrent glomerulopathy, possibly

Table 26.8 Renal transplants and pregnancy: complications and outcome

Prospects	Incidence (%)
Pregnancy complications	49
Successful obstetric outcome	93 (70)
Long-term sequelae	12 (25)

These estimates are based on data reviewed in Davison (1994) for pregnancies which attained at least 28 weeks' gestation (1961–94). Figures in parentheses refer to prospects when pregnancy complications developed prior to 28 weeks' gestation.

Table 26.9 Pregnancy in renal allograft recipients: antenatal watchpoints

Serial surveillance of renal function
Hypertension or pre-eclampsia
Graft rejection
Maternal infection
Fetal surveillance: intrauterine growth retardation
Premature rupture of membranes
Preterm labour
Decision of timing and method of delivery
Effects of drugs on fetus and neonate

severe pre-eclampsia and even cyclosporin A nephrotoxicity. Renal biopsy, which can be undertaken safely during pregnancy, might be necessary for definitive diagnosis. Ultrasonography alone may be very helpful because alterations in the echogenicity of the renal parenchyma and the presence of an indistinct corticomedullary boundary are indications of rejection (Levzow 1982).

Immunosuppressive therapy is usually maintained at prepregnancy levels, but adjustments may be needed if maternal leucocyte or platelet counts decrease. When white blood cell counts are maintained within physiological limits for pregnancy, the neonate is usually born with a normal blood count (Davison et al 1985c). Azathioprine liver toxicity has been noted occasionally during pregnancy and responds to dose reduction (Campos et al 1984). The most sensitive method of monitoring azathioprine dosage is measurement of red blood cell 6-thioguanine nucleotide. This metabolite of both azathioprine and 6-mercaptopurine is the best index of bioavailability (Lennard et al 1984).

Cyclosporin A is supposedly more effective than conventional immunosuppression, but evaluations are urgently needed in pregnancy because numerous adverse effects are attributed to this drug in non-pregnant transplant recipients, including renal and hepatic toxicity, tremor, convulsions, neoplasia, hypertension and thromboembolism. Theoretically some of the maternal physiological adaptations of pregnancy could be blunted by cyclosporin A: for example, its depressive effects on extracellular volume and renal haemodynamics may reduce a woman's ability to cope with the challenge of pregnancy on renal function and the placental circulation. More information is emerging (see Davison 1994) and overall the pregnancy success rate seems comparable to that with routine immunosuppression. Reports from the recently established US National Transplantation Pregnancy Register are particularly enlightening (Ahlswede et al 1992, Armenti et al 1992, 1993), with over 300 patients by 1993 and in 154 pregnancies in 115 women on cyclosporin A (54% of whom needed antihypertensive medication(s) prior to conception), birthweights overall were reduced and specifically intrauterine growth retardation was greater. This, however, may relate more to hypertension and/or renal dysfunction than to cyclosporin A.

Renal function

The better the renal function before pregnancy the more satisfactory the obstetrical outcome (Davison 1985), although one study indicates that increments in glomerular filtration rate in pregnancy are highest in women with lowest initial glomerular filtration rate (Tegzess et al 1985). In patients with satisfactory renal function before pregnancy, there may be a decline in glomerular filtration rate as well as appearance of significant proteinuria during the third trimester. These are usually transient and normal function returns postpartum. Permanent impairment of renal function is seen occasionally, especially where compromised prior to conception.

Hypertension

Hypertension, particularly before 28 weeks' gestation, is associated with adverse perinatal outcome (Sturgiss & Davison 1991). This may be due to covert cardiovascular changes that accompany or are aggravated by chronic hypertension.

There is a 30% incidence of pre-eclampsia but, since the diagnosis is usually made by clinical criteria, it may be incorrect. In the absence of a renal biopsy, it may be difficult to distinguish pre-eclampsia from rejection and even recurrent glomerulopathy. Blood uric acid levels and 24-hour urinary protein excretion are often well above the norms for pregnancy in normotensive pregnant transplant patients. Increased values do not necessarily signify pre-eclampsia or herald its onset. Furthermore, although many of the hypertensive syndromes occurring in pregnant transplant recipients are quite severe, there is only one report of a patient in whom the condition progressed rapidly to eclampsia (Williams & Jelen 1979). Incidentally, a subsequent pregnancy was normotensive and uneventful (Williams & Johnstone 1982).

Diabetes mellitus

The results of renal transplantations have been progressively improving in those patients whose end-stage renal failure was caused by juvenile onset diabetes mellitus (Remuzzi et al 1994). Inevitably pregnancies are now occurring in such women and the problems experienced are at least double those in other pregnant renal allograft recipients, perhaps related to the widespread, often covert, cardiovascular changes that accompany severe diabetes (Castro et al 1986).

When women have received a pancreas as well as a kidney allograft the outlook may be considerably better (Calne et al 1988, Tyden et al 1989). For the future, the consensus is that simultaneous kidney/pancreas transplants are the treatment of choice for women with diabetic nephropathy (Light 1993), and inevitably these women will be potential mothers.

Timing and method of delivery

The factors previously discussed in relation to chronic renal disease also apply here. Timing depends on balancing fetal intrauterine jeopardy against neonatal morbidity and mortality, bearing in mind the mother's well-being at all times.

The transplanted kidney very rarely produces mechanical dystocia during labour and does not sustain mechanical injury during vaginal delivery. Caesarean section is usually necessary only for purely obstetrical reasons. Regardless of the route of delivery, steroids must be augmented. Prophylactic antibiotics should be used for any surgical procedure, however trivial; for example, episiotomy.

Neonatal problems

There are hazards for the newborn (Table 26.10). Preterm delivery occurs in 50% and intrauterine growth retardation in at least 20% (range 8–40%), lower birthweights are seen in infants born to recipients less than 2 years post-transplant (Cunningham et al 1983, Ahlswede et al 1992) and cyclosporin A in some series is associated with severe birthweight depression (Pickrell et al 1988, Haugen et al 1991).

Although there are no frequent or predominant congenital anomalies (Raine et al 1992), one or more complications occur in about 40% of babies including respiratory distress syndrome, adrenocortical insufficiency, thrombocytopenia, leukopenia, cytomegalovirus and other infection, as well as development of hepatitis B surface antigen (HB Ag) carrier state (Davison et al 1985b).

Infectious hepatitis

These patients may have been exposed to multiple transfusions when on haemodialysis, and some may carry hepatitis B virus. Whereas women developing acute hepatitis in late pregnancy or within 2 months after delivery often transmit HB Ag to their offspring, the risk to children of asymptomatic carriers is much lower, and antigenicity is most likely to occur in infants whose mothers were also HB Ag-positive (Beasley et al 1983, Lil et al 1986).

When HB Ag is transmitted to the baby, the antigen invariably disappears within a few weeks after birth, only to be found later in life if active infection develops. This suggests that many HB Ag-positive neonates have been infected with their mother's blood or vaginal secretions at delivery and that this maternally acquired antigen is

Table 26.10 Neonatal problems in offspring of renal allograft recipients

Preterm delivery/small for gestational age
Respiratory distress syndrome
Depressed haematopoiesis
Lymphoid/thymic hypoplasia
Adrenocortical insufficiency
Septicaemia
Cytomegalovirus infection
Hepatitis B surface antigen carrier state
Congenital abnormalities
Immunological problems
   Reduced lymphocyte phytohaemagglutin-reactivity
   Reduced T-lymphocyte
   Reduced immunoglobulin levels
   Chromosome aberrations in lymphocytes

cleared before a fresh infection is contracted (alternatively, it may incubate outside the blood system). Further evidence of perinatal infection is that most cord blood specimens are HB Ag-negative or have very low AB Ag titres, even among infants who become HB Ag carriers.

Without prophylaxis, a high percentage of infants of HB Ag-positive mothers become carriers within 2–3 months of birth—an interval that again suggests that infection first occurred during labour or delivery. Furthermore, if infection occurs during pregnancy, immunoprophylaxis initiated at birth would be unlikely to prevent acquisition of the carrier state by the infant (Flewett 1986). However, hepatitis B immune globulin (HBIG) or hepatitis B virus vaccine (HBVV) given within a few hours of birth is highly effective in reducing the HB Ag carrier state in 50–70% of infants, but not if administration is delayed beyond 48 hours. HBIG and HBVV combined are highly effective in preventing perinatal transmission of HB Ag infection. Over 90% of infants born to HB Ag-positive carrier mothers are protected—a much better rate than achieved with either HBIG or HBVV alone. Most of the remaining 10% who become carriers, despite combined therapy, are presumed to have had in utero infections that were already established at birth.

Breastfeeding

As there are substantial benefits to breastfeeding and it can be argued that the baby has already been exposed to azathioprine and its metabolites throughout pregnancy and that their concentrations in mothers' milk are minimal, then breastfeeding should be allowed. Little is known, however, about the quantities of azathioprine and its metabolites in breast milk and about which levels are biologically trivial or substantial (Fagerholm et al 1980). Even fewer data are available about cyclosporin A in breast milk except that levels are usually greater than those in a simultaneously taken blood sample (Flechner et al 1985). Until these many uncertainties are resolved, breastfeeding should not be encouraged.

Long-term assessment

Azathioprine can cause transient gaps and breaks in the chromosomes of leucocytes. These defects may take almost 2 years to disappear spontaneously but in tissues not yet studied these anomalies may not be as temporary. The sequelae could be eventual development of malignancies in affected offspring or abnormalities in the reproductive performance in the next generation. There are some disturbing animal observations. For instance, fertility problems affect the female offspring of mice that have received low doses of 6-mercaptopurine, the major metabolite of azathioprine (equivalent to 3 mg/kg, Reimers & Sluss 1978). These offspring subsequently prove sterile, or if they conceive, have smaller litters and more dead fetuses than do unexposed dams. Thus, exposure in utero may not affect otherwise normal females until they embark on their reproductive careers.

Maternal follow-up after pregnancy

General outlook

The long-term impact, in terms of general well-being and renal prognosis, is difficult to quantify. The consensus is that it is safest to wait 2 years after transplantation before becoming pregnant. Pregnancy does occasionally and sometimes unpredictably cause irreversible declines in renal function. Recent studies, however, based on a comparison of groups of renal cadaver transplant recipients who did and did not become pregnant, concluded that pregnancy had no effect on graft function or survival (Whetam et al 1983, Rizzoni et al 1992, Sturgiss & Davison 1992). One exception, however, is a study from Finland which concludes that pregnancy does carry an increased risk of long-term reduced renal function and shorter graft survival and, furthermore, success in one post-transplant pregnancy does not guarantee success in repeated pregnancies (Salmela et al 1993). In this study, strangely, there were no graft losses in the controls and a low (36%) preterm delivery rate compared to the rest of the literature, possibly indicating longer pregnancies which theoretically might contribute to the long-term problems if time was bought at the expense of persistent hypertension and slowly dwindling renal function, which occurs even in late pregnancy in healthy women. More long-term studies are needed to assess this area, especially with the advent of new immunosupressive drugs.

Contraception

Oral contraceptives can produce subtle changes in the immune system, but this does not necessarily contraindicate their use. Low-dose oestrogen-progestogen preparations can be prescribed, although some authorities avoid them because of the possibility of causing or aggravating hypertension or further increasing the incidence of thrombo-embolism. If oral contraceptives are prescribed, careful and frequent surveillance is needed.

An intrauterine contraceptive device (IUCD) may aggravate menstrual problems, which in turn, may obfuscate signs and symptoms of abnormalities of early pregnancy, such as threatened abortion or ectopic pregnancy. The increased risk of pelvic infection associated with the IUCD makes this method worrisome in an immunosuppressed patient. In any case, the efficacy of these devices may be reduced by immunosuppressive and anti-inflammatory agents, possibly due to modification of the leucocyte response (Buhler & Papiernik 1983). Nevertheless, many patients request this method. Careful counselling and follow-up are essential.

Gynaecological problems

Long-term immunosuppression increases the risk of developing malignancy a hundred-fold (Penn 1990). This is probably due to loss of immune resistance, chronic immunosuppression allowing tumour proliferation or prolonged antigenic stimulation of the reticuloendothelial system. The genital tract is an important site for cancer (Halpert et al 1986). Reports of cervical change range from cellular atypia to invasive squamous cell carcinoma. Carcinoma of the vulva has also been noted in young patients. Regular pelvic examinations and cervical cytology are essential in these women. Lastly, unusual malignancies have been reported and include reactivation of latent choriocarcinoma (Lelievre et al 1978) and metastases from occult choriocarcinoma in a cadaver kidney (Manifold et al 1983).

REFERENCES

Abe S 1991 An overview of pregnancy in women with underlying renal disease. American Journal of Kidney Disease 17: 112–115

Abe S 1994 The influence of pregnancy on the long-term renal prognosis of IgA nephropathy. Clinical Nephrology 41: 61–64

Abe S, Amagasaki Y, Konishi K et al 1985 The influence of antecedent renal disease on pregnancy. American Journal of Obstetrics and Gynecology 153: 508–514

Ahlswede K M, Armenti V T, Mokritz M J 1992 Premature births in female transplant recipients: degree and effect of immunosuppressive regimen. Surgical Forum 43: 524–525

Armenti V T, Ahlswede K M, Ahlswede B A et al 1992 The National Transplant Registry: an analysis of 325 pregnancies in female kidney recipients. Journal of American Society of Nephrology 3: 851P

Armenti V T, Ahlswede B A, Moritz M J et al 1993 National Transplantation Registry: analysis of pregnancy outcomes of female kidney recipients with relation to time interval from transplantation to conception. Transplantation Proceedings 25: 1036–1037

Armenti V, Ahlswede K M, Ahlswede B et al 1994 National Transplantation Pregnancy Register — outcome of 154 pregnancies in cyclosporine-treated female transplant recipients. Transplantation 57: 502–506

Bailey R R 1992 Vesicoureteric reflux and reflux nephropathy. In: Cameron J S, Davison A M, Grunfeld J P, Kerr D, Ritz E (eds) Oxford textbook of clinical nephrology. Oxford University Press, Oxford, pp 1983–2001

Barret R J, Peters W A 1983 Pregnancy following urinary diversion. Obstetrics and Gynaecology 62: 582–586

Baylis C 1994 Glomerular filtration and volume regulation in gravid animal models. Clinical Obstetrics and Gynecology (Baillière) 8: 235–264

Baylis C, Rennke H G 1985 Renal hemodynamics and glomerular morphology in repetitively pregnant aging rats. Kidney International 28: 140–145

Bear R A 1976 Pregnancy in patients with renal disease: study of 44 cases. Obstetrics and Gynecology 48: 13–18

Bear R A 1978 Pregnancy in patients with chronic renal disease. Canadian Medical Association Journal 18: 663–665

Beard R W, Roberts A P 1968 Asymptomatic bacteriuria during pregnancy. British Medical Bulletin 24: 44–48

Beasley R P, Hwang L-U, Lee G Y 1983 Prevention of perinatally transmitted hepatitis B virus infections with hepatitis B immune globulin and hepatitis B vaccine. Lancet ii: 1099–1102

Becker G J, Fairley K F, Whitworth J A 1985 Pregnancy exacerbates glomerular disease. American Journal of Kidney Disorders 6: 266–272

Brenner B M, Meyer T W, Hostetter T H 1982 Dietary protein intake and the progressive nature of kidney disease: the role of hemodynamically mediated glomerular injury in the pathogenesis of progressive glomerular sclerosis in aging, renal ablation and intrinsic renal disease. New England Journal of Medicine 307: 652–659

Brown M A 1990 Urinary tract dilatation in pregnancy. American Journal of Obstetrics and Gynecology 164: 641–643

Brown M A, Gallery E A M 1994 Volume homeostasis in normal pregnancy and pre-eclampsia: physiology and clinical implications. Clinical Obstetrics and Gynecology (Ballière) 8: 287–310

Buhler M, Papiernik E 1983 Successive pregnancies in women fitted with intrauterine devices who take anti-inflammatory drugs. Lancet i: 483

Burleson R L, Sunderji S G, Aubry R H et al 1983 Renal allotransplantation during pregnancy. Transplantation 36: 334–335

Calne R Y, Brons E G M, Williams P F 1988 Successful pregnancy after paratopic segmental pancreas and kidney transplantation. British Medical Journal 296: 1709

Campbell-Brown M, McFadyen I R, Seal D V, Stephenson M L 1987 Is screening for bacteriuria in pregnancy worthwhile? British Medical Journal 294: 1579–1582

Campos H, Kreiss H A, Rioux P et al 1984 Azathioprine withdrawal in renal transplant recipients. Transplantation 38: 29–31

Castro L A, Baltzer U, Hillebrand G et al 1986 Pregnancy in juvenile diabetes mellitus under cyclosporine treatment after combined kidney and pancreas transplantation. Transplantation Proceedings 18: 80–81

Chesley L C, Sloan D M 1964 The effect of posture on renal function in late pregnancy. American Journal of Obstetrics and Gynecology 89: 754–759

Chng P K, Hall M H 1982 Antenatal prediction of urinary tract infection in pregnancy. British Journal of Obstetrics and Gynaecology 89: 8–11

Cietak K A, Newton J R 1985a Serial qualitative maternal nephrosonography in pregnancy. British Journal of Radiology 58: 399–404

Cietak K A, Newton J R 1985b Serial quantitative maternal nephrosonography in pregnancy. British Journal of Radiology 58: 405–413

Coc F L, Parks J H, Lindheimer M D 1978 Nephrolithiasis during pregnancy. New England Journal of Medicine 298: 324–326

Coombs G A, Kitzmiller J L 1991 Diabetic nephropathy and pregnancy. Clinical Obstetrics and Gynecology 13: 505–515

Cunningham F G, Lucas M J 1994 Urinary tract infections complicating pregnancy. Clinical Obstetrics and Gynecology (Baillière) 8: 353–373

Cunningham G F, Lucas M J, Hankins G D V 1987 Pulmonary injury complicating antepartum pyelonephritis. American Journal of Obstetrics and Gynecology 156: 797–807

Cunningham G F, Cox S M, Harstad T W et al 1990 Chronic renal disease and pregnancy outcome. American Journal of Obstetrics and Gynecology 163: 453–459

Cunningham R J, Buszta C, Braun W E et al 1983 Pregnancy in renal allograft recipients and longterm follow-up of their offspring. Transplantation Proceedings 15: 1067–1070

Davison J M 1985 The effect of pregnancy on renal function in renal allograft recipients. Kidney International 27: 74–79

Davison J M 1988 The effect of pregnancy on longterm renal function in women with chronic renal disease and single kidneys. Clinical and Experimental Hypertension B8: 222A

Davison J M 1994 Pregnancy in renal allograft recipients: problems, prognosis and practicalities. Clinical Obstetrics and Gynecology (Baillière) 8: 501–525

Davison J M, Baylis C 1995 Renal disease. In: de Swiet M (ed) Medical disorders in obstetric practice, 3rd edn. Blackwell Scientific Publications, Oxford (in press)

Davison J M, Dunlop W 1980 Renal hemodynamics and tubular function in normal human pregnancy. Kidney International 18: 152–161

Davison J M, Dunlop W 1984 Changes in renal hemodynamics and tubular function induced by normal human pregnancy. Seminars in Nephrology 4: 198–207

Davison J M, Hytten F E 1974 Glomerular filtration during and after pregnancy. Journal of Obstetrics and Gynaecology of the British Commonwealth 81: 588–595

Davison J M, Hytten F E 1975 The effect of pregnancy on the renal handling of glucose. Journal of Obstetrics and Gynaecology of the British Commonwealth 82: 374–381

Davison J M, Lindheimer M D 1980 Changes in renal haemodynamics and kidney weight during pregnancy in the unanaesthetised rat. Journal of Physiology, London 301: 129–136

Davison J M, Lindheimer M D 1984 Pregnancy in women with renal allografts. Seminars in Nephrology 4: 240–251

Davison J M, Lindheimer M D 1985 Pregnancy and the kidney: an update. In: Pitkin R M, Zlantnik F J (eds) The yearbook of obstetrics and gynecology. Year Book Medical Publishers, Chicago, pp 55–83

Davison J M, Lovedale C 1974 The excretion of glucose during normal pregnancy and after delivery. Journal of Obstetrics and Gynaecology of the British Commonwealth 81: 30–34

Davison J M, Noble M C B 1981 Serial changes in 24 hour creatinine clearance during normal menstrual cycles and the first trimester of pregnancy. British Journal of Obstetrics and Gynaecology 88: 10–17

Davison J M, Dunlop W, Ezimokhai M 1980 24 hour creatinine clearance during the third trimester of normal pregnancy. British Journal of Obstetrics and Gynaecology 87: 106–109

Davison J M, Vallotton M B, Lindheimer M D 1981 Plasma osmolality and urinary concentration and dilution during and after pregnancy: evidence that lateral recumbency inhibits maximal urinary concentrating ability. British Journal of Obstetrics and Gynaecology 88: 472–479

Davison J M, Sprott M S, Selkon J B 1984 The effect of covert bacteriuria in schoolgirls on renal function at 18 years and during pregnancy. Lancet ii: 651–655

Davison J M, Katz A I, Lindheimer M D 1985a Obstetric outcome and longterm renal prognosis. Clinics in Perinatology 12: 497–519

Davison J M, Katz A I, Lindheimer M D 1985b Pregnancy in women with renal disease and renal transplantation. Proceedings of the European Dialysis and Transport Association and European Renal Association 22: 439–459

Davison J M, Dellagrammatikas H, Parkin J M 1985c Maternal azathioprine therapy and depressed haemopoiesis in the babies of renal allograft recipients. British Journal of Obstetrics and Gynaecology 92: 233–239

Davison J M, Shiells E A, Philips P R et al 1988 Serial evaluation of vasopressin release and thirst in human pregnancy: role of human chorionic gonadotrophin in the osmoregulatory changes of gestation. Journal of Clinical Investigation 81: 798–806

Davison J M, Shiells E A, Philips P R et al 1993 Metabolic clearance of vasopressin and an analogue resistant to vasopressinase in human pregnancy. American Journal of Physiology 264: F348–353

Dunlop W 1976 Investigations into the influence of posture on renal plasma flow and glomerular filtration rate during late pregnancy. British Journal of Obstetrics and Gynaecology 83: 17–23

Dunlop W 1981 Serial changes in renal haemodynamics during normal human pregnancy. British Journal of Obstetrics and Gynaecology 88: 1–9

Dunlop W, Davison J M 1977 The effect of normal pregnancy upon the renal handling of uric acid. British Journal of Obstetrics and Gynaecology 84: 13–21

Eckford S D, Gigngnell J C 1991 Ureteric obstruction in pregnancy—diagnosis and management. British Journal of Obstetrics and Gynecology 98: 1337–1340

Ezimokhai M, Davison J M, Philips P R et al 1981 Non-postural serial changes in renal function during the third trimester of normal human pregnancy. British Journal of Obstetrics and Gynaecology 88: 465–471

Fagerholm M I, Coulan C G, Moyer T P 1980 Breast feeding after renal transplantation. 6-Mercaptopurine content of human breast milk. Surgical Forum 31: 447–449

Fairley K F, Bond A G, Adey F 1966 The site of infection in pregnancy bacteriuria. Lancet i: 939–941

Fairley K F, Whitworth J A, Kincaid-Smith P 1973 Glomerulonephritis: II. In: Kincaid-Smith P, Mathew T H, Becker E L (eds) Glomerulonephritis and pregnancy. New York, John Wiley, pp 997–1011

Feehally J, Bennett S E, Harris K P G et al 1986 Is chronic renal transplant rejection a non-immunological phenomenon? Lancet ii: 486–488

Fields C L, Ossorio M A, Roy T M et al 1991 Wegener's granulomatosis complicated by pregnancy: a case report. Journal of Reproductive Medicine 36: 463–466

First M R, Combs C A, Weiskittel P et al 1995 Lack of effect of pregnancy on renal allograft survival or function. Transplantation 59: 472–476.

Fisher K, Luger A, Spargo B H et al 1981 Hypertension in pregnancy: clinical–pathological correlations and remote prognosis. Medicine 60: 267–274

Flechner S M, Katz A R, Rogers A J et al 1985 The presence of cyclosporine in body tissues and fluids during pregnancy. American Journal of Kidney Diseases 5: 60–63

Flewett T H 1986 Can we eradicate hepatitis B? British Medical Journal 293: 404

Fowler J E, Pulaski E T 1982 Excretion urography, cystography and cystoscopy in the evaluation of women with urinary tract infection. New England Journal of Medicine 304: 462–464

Gaber L W, Spargo B H, Lindheimer M D 1994 Renal pathology in pre-eclampsia. Clinical Obstetrics and Gynecology (Baillière) 8: 443–468

Gabow P A 1993 Autosomal dominant polycystic kidney disease. New England Journal of Medicine 329: 332–342

Gardner A 1985 Urinary tract infection during pregnancy and sudden unexpected infant death. Lancet ii: 495

Gilstrap L C, Leveno K J, Cunningham F G et al 1981 Renal infection and pregnancy outcome. American Journal of Obstetrics and Gynecology 141: 709–716

Grimes D A, Le Bolt S A, Grimes K R et al 1985 Systemic lupus erythematosus and reproductive function: a case control study. American Journal of Obstetrics and Gynecology 153: 179–186

Halpert R, Fruchter R G, Sedlis A et al 1986 Human papillomavirus and lower genital neoplasia in renal transplant patients. Obstetrics and Gynecology 68: 251–258

Haugen G, Fauchald P, Sodal G 1991 Pregnancy outcome in renal allograft recipients: influence of cyclosporin A. European Journal of Obstetrics Gynecology and Reproductive Biology 29: 25–29

Hayslett J P 1985 Pregnancy does not exacerbate primary glomerular disease. American Journal of Kidney Disorders 6: 273–277

Hayslett J P, Reece E A 1994 Managing diabetic patients with nephropathy and other vascular complications. Clinical Obstetrics and Gynecology (Baillière) 8: 405–424

Heybourne K D, Schultz M F, Goodlin R C et al 1991 Renal artery stenosis during pregnancy: a review. Obstetrical and Gynecological Survey 46: 509–514

Hou S 1994 Pregnancy in women on haemodialysis and peritoneal dialysis. Clinical Obstetrics and Gynecology (Baillière) (in press)

Hou S H, Grossman S D, Madias N E 1985 Pregnancy in women with renal disease and moderate renal insufficiency. American Journal of Medicine 78: 185–194

Imbasciati E, Ponticelli C 1991 Pregnancy and renal disease: predictors for fetal and maternal outcome. American Journal of Nephrology 11: 353–362

Imbasciati E, Pardi G, Bozetti P et al 1984 Pregnancy in women with chronic renal failure. Proceedings of the 4th World Congress of the International Society for the Study of Hypertension in Pregnancy: 78

Jungers P 1994 Reflux nephropathy and pregnancy. Clinical Obstetrics and Gynaecology (Baillière) (in press)

Jungers P, Dougados M, Pelissies C et al 1982 Lupus nephropathy and pregnancy. Archives of Internal Medicine 142: 771–776

Jungers P, Houillier P, Forget D 1991 Specific controversies concerning the natural history of renal disease in pregnancy. American Journal of Kidney Diseases 17: 166–122

Kasinath B S, Katz A I 1982 Delayed maternal lupus after delivery of offspring with congenital heart block. Archives of Internal Medicine 142: 2317

Kass E H 1962 Pyelonephritis and bacteriuria. Annals of Internal Medicine 56: 46–53

Kincaid-Smith P, Whitworth J A, Fairley K F 1980 Mesangial IgA nephropathy in pregnancy. Clinical and Experimental Hypertension 2: 821–838

Klein E A 1984 Urologic problems of pregnancy. Obstetrical and Gynecological Surveys 39: 605–615

Knebelmann B, Antiganac C, Gubler M C et al 1994 A molecular approach to inherited kidney disorders. Kidney International (in press)

Lancet Editorial 1984 Lupus anticoagulant. Lancet i: 1157–1158

Lawson D H, Miller A W F 1973 Screening for bacteriuria in pregnancy: a critical reappraisal. Archives of Internal Medicine 132: 904–908

Leikin J B, Arof H M, Pearlman L M 1986 Acute lupus pneumonitis in the postpartum period: a case history and review of the literature. Obstetrics and Gynecology 68: 298–318

Lelievre R, Ribet M, Gosselin B et al 1978 Chorio-carcinoma après transplantation. Journal of Urological Nephrology (Paris) 84: 345–346

Lennard L, Brown C B, Fox M et al 1984 Azathioprine metabolism in kidney transplant recipients. British Journal of Clinical Pharmacology 18: 693–700

Levzow B L 1982 The appearance of renal transplant rejection with ultrasound. Medicine and Ultrasound 6: 43–52

Lewis G J, Lamont C A R, Lee H A et al 1983 Successful pregnancy in a renal transplant recipient taking cyclosporin A. British Medical Journal 286: 603

Light J A 1993 Experience with 50 kidney/pancreas transplants at the Washington Hospital Center. Dialysis and Transplantation 22: 522–532

Lil L, Sheng M H, Tong S P 1986 Transplacental transmission of hepatitis B virus. Lancet ii: 872

Lim V S 1987 Reproductive function in patients with renal insufficiency. American Journal of Kidney Diseases 9: 363–367

Lim V S 1994 Reproductive endocrinology in uraemia. Clinical Obstetrics and Gynecology (Baillière) 8: 469–480

Lind T 1975 Changes in carbohydrate metabolism during pregnancy. Clinics in Obstetrics and Gynaecology 2: 395–412

Lind T, Hytten F E 1972 The excretion of glucose during normal pregnancy. Journal of Obstetrics and Gynaecology of the British Commonwealth 79: 961–965

Lind T, Godfrey K A, Otum H et al 1984 Changes in serum uric acid concentrations during normal pregnancy. British Journal of Obstetrics and Gynaecology 91: 128–132

Lindheimer M D, Katz A I 1987 Gestation in women with kidney disease: prognosis and management. Clinical Obstetrics and Gynecology 1: 921–967

Lindheimer M D, Barron W M 1994 Water metabolism and vasopressin secretion during pregnancy. Clinical Obstetrics and Gynecology (Baillière) 8: 311–331

Lindheimer M D, Katz A I 1994 Gestation in women with kidney disease: prognosis and management. Clinical Obstetrics and Gynecology (Baillière) 8: 387–404

Lindheimer M D, Barron W M, Davison J M 1989 Osmoregulation and vasopressin release in pregnancy. American Journal of Physiology 257: F159–F169

Lomberg H, Jodal U, Leffler H et al 1992 Blood group non-secretors have an increased inflammatory response to urinary tract infection. Scandinavian Journal of Infectious Diseases 24: 77

Love P E, Santoro S A 1990 Antephospholipid antibodies: anticardiolipin and the lupus anticoagulant in systemic lupus erythematosus (SLE) and in non-SLE disorders. Annals of Internal Medicine 112: 682–698

Lubbe W F, Butler W S, Palmer S J et al 1984 Lupus anticoagulant in pregnancy. British Journal of Obstetrics and Gynaecology 91: 357–363

Manifold I H, Champion A E, Goepel J R et al 1983 Pregnancy complicated by gestational trophoblastic disease in a renal transplant recipient. British Journal of Medicine 287: 1025–1026

McFadyen I R 1986 Urinary tract infection in pregnancy.

In: Andreucci V E (ed) The kidney in pregnancy. Martinus Nijhoff, Boston, pp 195–229

McFadyen I R, Eknyn S J, Gardner N H N et al 1973 Bacteriuria of pregnancy. Journal of Obstetrics and Gynaecology of the British Commonwealth 80: 385–405

McGladdery S L, Aparicio S, Verrier-Jones K 1992 Outcome of pregnancy in an Oxford–Cardiff cohort of women with previous bacteriuria. Quarterly Journal of Medicine 303: 533–539

MacMillan M C, Grimes D A 1991 The limited usefulness of urine and blood cultures in treating pyelonephritis in pregnancy. Obstetrics and Gynecology 78: 745

Magmon R, Fejgin M 1989 Scleroderma in pregnancy. Obstetrical and Gynecological Survey 44: 530–534

Maikranz P, Lindheimer M D, Coe F C 1994 Nephrolithiasis. Clinical Obstetrics and Gynecology (Baillière) (in press)

Martinell J, Jodall U, Lipiu-Janson G 1990 Pregnancies in women with and without renal seaming after urinary infections in childhood. British Medical Journal 300: 840–844

Miller D R, Kakkis J 1982 Prognosis, management and outcome of obstructive renal disease in pregnancy. Journal of Reproductive Medicine 27: 199–201

Mor-Yosef S, Navot D, Rabinowitz R et al 1984 Collagen disease in pregnancy. Obstetrical and Gynecological Surveys 39: 67–83

Murty G E, Davison J M, Cameron D S 1991 Wegener's granulomatosis complicating pregnancy: first report of a case with a tracheostomy. Journal of Obstetrics and Gynecology 10: 399–403

Nagey D A, Fortier K J, Linder J 1983 Pregnancy complicated by periarteritis nodosa: induced abortion as an alternative. American Journal of Obstetrics and Gynecology 147: 103–105

Nicklin J L 1991 Systemic lupus erythematosus and pregnancy at the Royal Women's Hospital, Brisbane 1979–1989. Australian and New Zealand Journal of Obstetrics and Gynecology 31: 128–133

Peake S L, Roxburgh H B, Langlois S 1983 Ultrasonic assessment or hydronephrosis of pregnancy. Radiology 128: 167–170

Penn I 1990 Cancers complicating organ transplantation. New England Journal of Medicine 323: 1767–1768

Petri M, Howard D, Repke J 1991 Frequency of lupus flare in pregnancy: the Hopkins Lupus Pregnancy Center experience. Arthritis and Rheumatism 34: 1538–1545

Pickrell M D, Sawers R, Michael J 1988 Pregnancy after renal transplantation: severe intrauterine growth retardation during treatment with cyclosporin A. British Medical Journal 296: 825

Powers R D 1991 New directions in the diagnosis and therapy of urinary tract infection. American Journal of Obstetrics and Gynecology 164: 1387–1389

Raine A E G, Margreiter R, Brunner F P et al 1992 Report on management of renal failure in Europe XXII, 1991. Nephrology, Dialysis and Transplantation 7 (suppl 2): 7–35

Reimers T J, Sluss P M 1978 6-Mercaptopurine treatment of pregnant mice: effects on second and third generations. Science 201: 65–67

Remuzzi G, Ruggenenti P, Mauer S M 1994 Pancreas and kidney/pancreas transplants: experimental medicines or real impairment? Lancet 343: 27–31

Rizzoni G, Ehrich J H H, Broyer M et al 1992 Successful pregnancies in women on renal replacement therapy: report from the EDTA Registry. Nephrology, Dialysis and Transplantation 7: 1–9

Roche R J, Moxon E R 1992 The molecular study of bacterial virulence: a view of current approaches illustrated by the study of adhesion in uropathogenic E. coli. Pediatric Nephrology 6: 587–596

Romero R, Oyazun E, Mazar M et al 1989 Meta-analysis of the relationship between asymptomatic bacteriuria and preterm delivery/low birthweight. Obstetrics and Gynecology 73: 576–582

Romero J C, Lahera V, Salom M G et al 1992 Role of endothelium dependent relaxing factor nitric oxide on renal function. Journal of American Society of Nephrology 2: 1371–1387

Salmela K, Kyllonen L E J, Holmberg C et al 1993 Impaired renal function after pregnancy in renal transplant recipients. Transplantation 56: 1372–1375

Satin A J, Seikin G L, Cunningham F G 1993 Reversible hypertension in pregnancy caused by obstructive uropathy. Obstetrics and Gynecology 81: 823–825

Scott J S, Maddison P J, Taylor P V et al 1983 Connective-tissue disease, antibodies to ribonucleoprotein and congenital heart block. New England Journal of Medicine 309: 209–212

Singsen B H, Akhter J E, Weinstein M M et al 1985 Congenital complete heart block and SSA antibodies: obstetric implications. American Journal of Obstetrics and Gynecology 152: 655–658

Smith C A 1982 Progressive systemic sclerosis and post-partum renal failure complicated by peripheral gangrene. Journal of Rheumatology 9: 455–460

Sola R, Ballarin J, Castrol et al 1988 Renal transplantation during pregnancy. Transplantation Proceeding 20: 270

Steen V D, Conte C, Day N 1989 Pregnancy in women with systemic sclerosis. Arthritis and Rheumatism 32: 151–157

Stenquist K, Dahlin-Nilsson I, Lidin-Janson G 1989 Bacteriuria in pregnancy. Frequency and risk of acquisition. American Journal of Epidemiology 129: 372–379

Sturgiss S N, Davison J M 1991 Perinatal outcome in renal allograft recipients: prognostic significance of hypertension and renal function before and during pregnancy. Obstetrics and Gynecology 78: 573–577

Sturgiss S N, Davison J M Effect of pregnancy on longterm function of renal allografts. American Journal of Kidney Diseases: An update (in press)

Sturgiss S N, Dunlop W, Davison J M 1994 Renal haemodynamics and tubular function in human pregnancy. Clinical Obstetrics and Gynecology (Baillière) 8: 209–234

Surian M, Imbasciati E, Cosci P et al 1984 Glomerular disease and pregnancy: a study of 123 pregnancies in patients with primary and secondary glomerular diseases. Nephron 36: 101–105

Taylor P V, Scott J S, Gerlis L M et al 1986 Maternal antibodies against fetal cardiac antigens in congenital complete heart block. New England Journal of Medicine 315: 667–672

Tegzess A M, Meijer S, Visser G H et al 1985 Improvements of renal function during pregnancy in patients with a cadaveric allograft. Proceedings EDTA-ERA 22: 503–507

Towers C V, Kaminskas C M, Garite T J et al 1991 Pulmonary injury with antepartum pyelonephritis: can patients at risk be identified? American Journal of Obstetrics and Gynecology 164: 974

Twickler D, Little B B, Satin A J et al 1991 Renal pelvicalyceal dilation in antepartum pyelonephritis: ultrasonographic findings. American Journal of Obstetrics and Gynecology 165: 1115–1119

Tyden G, Brattstrom C, Bjorkman U et al 1989 Pregnancy after combined pancreas–kidney transplantation. Diabetes 38 (suppl 1): 43–45

Van Sonnenberg E, Casola G, Talner L B et al 1992 Symptomatic renal obstruction or urosepsis during pregnancy: treatment by sonographically guided percutaneous nephrostomy. American Journal of Roentgenology 158: 91–94

Weinberger S E 1993 Recent advances in pulmonary medicine (Part II). New England Journal of Medicine 328: 1462–1470

Whalley P J 1967 Bacteriuria of pregnancy. American Journal of Obstetrics and Gynecology 97: 723–738

Whalley P J, Cunningham F G, Martin F G 1975 Transient renal dysfunction associated with acute pyelonephritis of pregnancy. Obstetrics and Gynaeceology 46: 174–179

Whetam J C G, Cardelle C, Harding M 1983 Effect of pregnancy on graft function and graft survival in renal cadaver transplant patients. American Journal of Obstetrics and Gynecology 145: 193–197

Williams P F, Jelen J 1979 Eclampsia in a patient who had had a renal transplant. British Medical Journal 2: 972

Williams P F, Johnstone M 1982 Normal pregnancy in renal transplant recipient with a history of eclampsia and intrauterine death. British Medical Journal 285: 1535

Wolf M C, Hollander J B, Salisz J A 1992 A new technique of ureteral stent placement during pregnancy using endoluminal ultrasound. Surgical Gynecology and Obstetrics 175: 575–576

Zinner S H 1992 Management of urinary tract infections in pregnancy: a review with comments on single dose therapy. Infection 4: S280–S285

Normal labour

27. The labouring mother

Ann Oakley

In modern industrial societies the last 100 years have brought enormous changes in the reproductive roles of women in general, and in the management of childbirth in particular. Average family size has decreased substantially—between 1840 and 1980 fertility (live births per 1000 women aged 15–44) fell by almost half (Macfarlane & Mugford 1984). The losses that women incurred during the Victorian era in the world of paid work and civil rights have been largely recovered. In 1984, 41% of the labour force in the UK were women. Although this percentage is not much higher than it was in the 1880s, it hides a large change in the proportion of married women employed—while 1 in 10 held a job in 1911 (Klein 1965), 6 in every 10 did so in 1980. In 1980, 52% of women with dependent children were in the labour force—27% of those with children aged 4 or under (Martin & Roberts 1984).

Accompanying these changes has been an increased social emphasis on sex equality, though in many ways the social and economic positions of men and women remain different. For example, in 1980 average earnings of women in full-time work were 59% of men's (Martin & Roberts 1984). Other social changes have profoundly affected the reproductive roles of women. There has been a very large rise in the number of one-parent families: from 474 000 in 1961 to 975 000 in 1981 (National Council for One-Parent Families 1983). One consequence of the economic recession of the 1980s is that some 28% of the population in Britain now lives in poverty (Mack & Lansley 1985). Whereas in the 1970s the elderly formed the largest group in poverty, that group is now families with children and especially female-headed one-parent families (Department of Health and Social Security 1983). There has also been a growing awareness of the different needs and situations of different ethnic groups.

These facts form the backdrop against which women's experiences of obstetric care need to be seen. As far as childbirth is concerned, the greatest change that has occurred over the last century is that reproduction has become a medical specialty and its control has been removed from the community and from women and is now vested with medical professionals instead.

One consequence of this transformation is that the point of view of mothers themselves may be forgotten. Thus it has become necessary to articulate and make visible their perspective—an exercise which is considerably aided by two important 20th-century social movements—feminism and the consumer movement in health care.

MOTHERS AND THE MEDICALIZATION OF CHILDBIRTH

In the 19th century doctors played a minor role in the care of pregnant women. This was partly because medical care was expensive and most people could not afford it, but there were other important reasons. Before the era of laboratory pregnancy tests and ultrasound scanning, it was difficult for doctors and midwives to diagnose pregnancy. The morality of the time made clinical examination of the patient difficult; it was rarely done, and when it was the textbooks advised the doctor to keep his eyes on the ceiling (Smith 1979). The lack of specialist medical knowledge about childbearing forced practitioners to rely antenatally almost wholly on lifestyle advice—healthy babies would be secured if the mother slept with the window open, ate meat sparingly and occupied her mind with pleasant thoughts. Until the late 19th century and even early 20th century, a popular therapy for reproductive problems was bloodletting, based on the old Hippocratean theory of pregnancy as a state of plethora, in which the body contained too much blood (Oakley 1984). Nevertheless the predominant view was that pregnancy was not in itself a pathological condition but 'a natural physiological state' (Johnstone 1913).

Prior to the modern obstetric era, most women would never have seen a doctor in pregnancy, and most had their babies with the help of midwives—either the trained or untrained variety. As one historian has put it: 'It is not generally realized that until the seventeenth century, midwifery in England had been a strictly non-medical lay craft which was quite marginal to the existing framework of medical practice and medical training, and medical corporate control ... No medical licences were granted in midwifery and the care of women in labour was in no sense a medical responsibility' (Versluysen 1981). For centuries the main requirement for the office of midwife in Europe was that the woman should be married, of mature age and a mother herself (Donnison 1977). Even after the state intervened to regulate the work of midwives, untrained but experienced (bona fide) midwives were allowed to continue practising. It was not until 1947 that the roll of the Central Midwives Board in England no longer contained names of women admitted under the bona fide practice clause.

This practice of women caring for women in childbirth was part of a long tradition of women's community health care (Oakley 1976). In preindustrialized Europe and colonial America, ordinary people turned to the *good woman*, *cunning woman* or *wise woman* for help with illness. Healing the sick and caring for the dependent was part of women's domestic role. Women's domestic knowledge embraced the recognition and use of pain-killers, digestive aids, anti-inflammatory agents, ergot, belladonna and digitalis; it was within this context that lay midwifery flourished (Clark 1968, Chamberlain 1981).

The story of the male medical takeover of childbirth is relatively well known. At its centre is the apocryphal story of the Chamberlen family who, in the 17th century, negotiated their way into upper-class homes with a magic box containing forceps, blindfolded the labouring woman and locked the door in order to guard their technological secret. Although some medical historians have argued that the invention of the obstetric forceps was the single most important factor in the successful medicalization of midwifery, this would appear to be largely wishful thinking. Even contemporary proponents of the forceps contended that they were needed in only some 0.1–0.2% of cases (Smellie 1752, Bland 1781). Without effective antiseptics forceps carried a high risk of untreatable—sometimes fatal—infection.

In reality the aspiring male midwives of the 18th and 19th centuries were not popular with labouring women or with doctors. Women were afraid of instruments and unhappy about permitting male access to their bodies during birth. Male midwives not only used the technology of the forceps, but also carried out destructive surgery of the fetus in obstructed labour, which did not increase their appeal as childbirth attendants (though it was undoubtedly sometimes useful). At one end of the social continuum the male midwife William Smellie paid his working-class clients for the privilege of delivering them and allowing his male apprentices to watch (Glaister 1894). At the other end of the spectrum, upper-class households paid physicians to hang around outside the labour room, in case they were needed, thereby preventing them from any access to knowledge of normal labour. Midwifery was stereotyped as women's work and so those men who wanted to enter it had to contend with the dismissive attitudes of the medical profession, who regarded midwifery as something doctors ought not to get themselves embroiled in. In line with this attitude hospital-based physicians and surgeons refused to admit maternity patients to hospital at all. Labouring women were placed with small children, the insane, those infected with venereal disease, and the dying and incurable as categories of people whose claim to medical importance was so tenuous that they were said to have no place in hospital at all.

This was an important factor in the development of the early lying-in hospitals in the 18th century; gaining control over client preferences by hospitalizing them was much more of an influential factor in the increasing medicalization of childbirth than the invention of the forceps. One of the explicit aims behind the founding of the early maternity institutions was that medical men ought to be able to gain more experience of normal deliveries. The lying-in hospitals provided hospitalized delivery for poor women. Table 27.1 shows some figures for deliveries during 1818 at one of the early dispensaries providing maternity care. The physician–accoucheur of the Westminster General Dispensary was an unusual man, Augustus Bozzi Granville, who had been present when Laennec had first demonstrated his use of the stethoscope in 1816. Granville's analysis of midwifery at the Westminster General Dispensary showed that the bulk of labours were normal, and instruments were used in little more than 1% of all deliveries.

It is very hard to know how labouring women felt

Table 27.1   Labour and delivery in 1818 (from Granville 1819)

Normal* % (n)	Abnormal† % (n)	Total % (n)
96.7 (619)	3.3 (21)	100 (640)

* Defined as 'terminated without the slightest interference, by nature alone' (84% of these labours took 12 hours or less).
† 'When nature becomes passive ... and the assistance either of the *hand* or instruments, is absolutely necessary to terminate the labour' (in 38% of these 21 deliveries instruments were used—1.3% of the grand total of all deliveries).

about the care available to them during these years of fundamental changes in the management of childbirth. Granville himself was of the opinion, in 1819, that 'however distressed the poor mother may be, she will always prefer her own habitation, and the unbought, soothing cares of her own family, during her time of trial, to the spacious ward, and the precise attention of a hired matron and strange nurses' (Granville 1819). He also noted 'a decided aversion amongst lying-in women, against the interference of the Accoucheur, and the use of the most harmless instruments'. At this time the mother's risk of dying in childbirth was probably around 1 in 200. Puerperal fever accounted for about 40% of these deaths (Farr 1885). Infant mortality was around 150 per 1000 livebirths throughout the 19th century (incomplete registration makes it impossible to compile an accurate figure for stillbirths and other perinatal deaths). Death of mother and child was therefore a real risk, but we cannot assume that women necessarily approached childbirth with fatalism or great fear, because cultural attitudes to birth were not the same then as they are now.

If hospitals were needed by the obstetrical specialists to build up their knowledge and control of clients, they had, by the late 19th century, a particular attraction for women also: they offered the possibility of pain relief in labour. Midwives delivering babies at home had no analgesia to offer mothers until R. J. Minnitt at Liverpool Maternity Hospital designed a portable apparatus for delivering gas and air in 1932. This fact may have been partly responsible for the move among middle-class mothers to have babies in hospital in the early decades of the 20th century, a move which was associated with the unusual epidemiological picture of higher social class temporarily going hand-in-hand with higher maternal mortality (Registrar-General 1930).

Place of delivery was first documented by the British Registrar-General in 1927, when 15% of all livebirths occurred in institutions: he thought the main reason for hospital birth was lack of home facilities. By 1954 the figure for institutional deliveries was 64% and in that year, whatever mothers thought, the British Medical Journal was still able to declare that 'the proper place for the confinement is the patient's own home' (British Medical Journal Editorial 1954). By 1960 the proportion of babies delivered in institutions had risen by only 1% since 1954 and this, not coincidentally, was the year in which one of Britain's most energetic consumer pressure groups in the maternity care field was born: the Association for Improvements in Maternity Services (AIMS), originally named the Society for the Prevention of Cruelty to Pregnant Women.

CONSUMERS' REVOLT?

Table 27.2 compares the objectives of AIMS when it was first founded with those formulated 21 years later in 1981.

Table 27.2 Aims of AIMS 1960–1981

1960	1981
More money for the NHS, especially hospital maternity services	Midwife control of maternity care for low-risk women
More midwives, and improvements in their working conditions	Antenatal care for low-risk women to be community-based
More home helps (for home births)	Antenatal care to include evaluation and information related to mother's diet
No woman in labour should be left alone against her will	Nutritional assistance for women with poor diets
More research on pain relief and the psychology of childbirth	Increase in the maternity grant to be given to all pregnant women

It is apparent that interpreting the rights of women to make choices in childbirth in 1960 meant an emphasis on hospital delivery: in its early years AIMS campaigned to increase the number of hospital maternity beds, because at the time there was a demand by women for them. By 1981 the emphasis had shifted to an increase in community care. Midwives remained important. The research called for on analgesia and psychological aspects of childbirth in 1960 became, in 1981, a demand for attention to diet as a component of good maternity care. Financial support for childbearing women has emerged as a priority.

The rise of groups such as AIMS, the National Childbirth Trust (NCT), the Maternity Alliance and a host of others has given prominence to the maternal (and parental) point of view. Collectively they have provided a voice for what is incorrectly dubbed the consumer's perspective (Stacey 1976). Although many women belong to these organizations, many do not; membership is likely to be weighted towards the informed middle classes, which means that these pressure groups cannot be assumed to speak for all women. Having said that, it is of course necessary to query the assumption that all women share a single viewpoint on any specific issue, such as analgesia or position in labour, or more generally as to the overall management of childbirth. There is no reason to assume this. Women having babies do not form a homogeneous group (Riley 1977). In the same way not all obstetricians are in agreement about how to treat women in childbirth—there is a wide range of attitudes and great variation in clinical practice.

Consumer groups in the maternity care field have nevertheless stressed certain themes, and continue to do so. From a historical viewpoint the existence of these organizations is a response to the situation that had evolved by the mid 20th century—one in which control of childbirth had passed into the hands of the professionals. It became necessary for those using the maternity services to reclaim their own rights to have a voice in the shaping of these services. Comparing the situation in Britain with that in other countries, it appears that protest of this kind is much more likely to happen when services have been increasingly centralized in hospital and there has been an erosion of community care (Houd & Oakley 1986), hence the AIMS appeal for more community-based care (Table 27.2). For example, in some northern European countries such as Sweden and Finland, antenatal care remains community-based and there are few organizations of client groups. Conversely, countries with fee-for-service private health care systems such as the USA seem to make client protest more likely.

The consumers' revolt in childbirth has everywhere emphasized the same key themes: the right to information, the right to choose, respect for social and psychological aspects of childbearing and for the integrity and privacy and individuality of childbearing women and their families, and pregnancy and birth as normal physiological events. Over the last 10 years there has also been increasing stress on the need for obstetric procedures to be properly evaluated for effectiveness and safety before they enter routine practice. These themes are closely intermeshed, as is evident in the following editorial entitled 'Safety first?' from a 1984 edition of the AIMS newsletter:

Our health care, like other aspects of our lives, has been fragmented, specialised and with increasing specialisation comes loss of an overall vision of purpose. Pregnancy and birth have been removed from the continuum of normal women's health care; pregnancy is regarded as an abnormal state and the line between the abnormal and the pathological is very thin. Obstetricians' responses to pregnancy and birth are conditioned by their training: they specialise in the abnormal, and seek to discover and cure the pathological. The more tests and procedures that are deemed necessary in their searching, the more reason there is to believe that pregnancy is indeed fraught with danger. The more interventions that become accepted as standard practice, the further we move away from the baseline of a truly normal birth—a strong, healthy woman giving birth to a strong, healthy child.

Much of the data needed for a thorough evaluation of many procedures is not even collected, far less published in an accessible form for prospective parents. If it is 'all for your own good', it should be demonstrably so. (AIMS Editorial 1984.)

Two other factors have contributed to the assertiveness of organizations such as AIMS. One is the women's movement, which has entailed an emphasis on appropriate health care for women, and the other is medical sociology, which, as an academic-based discipline, has sought (among many other enterprises) to highlight the social within medicine (Stacey & Homans 1978).

As a result of these forces, there are now systematic data which can be marshalled to answer questions about what women want in obstetric care—bearing in mind, naturally, the need to be sceptical about the formulation of the question itself. Although it is tempting to regard these data as new, the omission from obstetric data of the childbearing woman's point of view is a relatively recent development. Many of the government reports on maternity care published in the first half of this century, for instance, gave a good deal of prominence to women's experiences and attitudes and stressed the desirability of considering the implications for the maternity services of the social and economic position of women (see Ministry of Health 1927). If one compares the three national birth surveys carried out in 1946, 1958 and 1970 (Joint Committee 1948, Butler & Bonham 1963, Chamberlain et al 1978), it is clear that the first of these was sensitive to these issues in a way in which the later two were not. (For example, in 1946 there was concern about the costs of childbearing to women, about women's views of their care and the relationship between household work and pregnancy outcome.)

The rest of this chapter will explore some of what is known about the point of view of mothers in relation to specific topics in the maternity care debate today. The following will be considered: place of birth, delivery personnel, natural childbirth, analgesia, induction of labour, instrumental delivery, Caesarean section, monitoring in labour, client–professional communication, and mother–infant bonding.

PLACE OF BIRTH

Where do women want to have their babies? This is a complicated question, because it lacks meaning in the abstract. People's wants are the outcome of many factors, including their own personalities and psychologies, the information they have about different options and the long-term implications of settling for one option rather than another, and the pressures on them to want certain things. On the whole people want what they have. If they did not do so, society would be in a constant state of flux and change. To want something very different requires a vision of an alternative, and most people's daily lives do not encourage visions.

These generalizations apply to maternity care. But given this generally conservative impulse, a number of statements can be made on the basis of available surveys about women's preferences for place of delivery. Table 27.3, which is taken from Ann Cartwright's national study of induction, certainly shows that most women would prefer the place of delivery in which their last child was born. This applies both to the group whose last baby was born

Table 27.3 Preferences for place of birth in the next pregnancy (from Cartwright 1979)

	Place of birth in the last pregnancy	
	Home birth (%)	Hospital birth (%)
Prefer same as last time	91	83
Prefer not to have same as last time	9	15
Other comment	—	2
Number of mothers (= 100%)	97	2083

in hospital and to the group who had a home birth. But the table also shows a preference for a second home birth in the group who have already experienced one, which is considerably stronger than the preference expressed for a second hospital delivery among women whose last baby was delivered in hospital. Whereas 9% of women who had a home birth last time said they would not want one again, 15% of those who had a hospital birth last time would not choose to repeat this. Cartwright also asked the women in the sample who had had one baby at home and one in hospital to compare their experiences; 76% preferred it at home and 15% in hospital—the remainder had no preference (Cartwright 1979).

Reviewing studies of preferences for place of birth, Macintyre (1977) has shown that the proportion of women who would like to have a baby at home is always higher than the proportion booked to do so. The preference for home delivery appears to rise with parity and also with the experience of home delivery. The best evidence for this latter point is Goldthorpe & Richman's (1974) study of unintended home delivery due to a strike by hospital ancillary staff. The sample consisted of 65 women who had their babies at home because of the strike, although they had been booked for hospital delivery. When told that they could not have their babies as planned, 22% of the women said they felt pleased, 40% did not mind, and 38% were disappointed or very disappointed. However, after having the baby, 80% said they wanted to have their next baby at home, and this was independent of whether the labour at home had been easy or difficult (Goldthorpe & Richman 1974).

Preferences for place of birth, even if comprehensive information can be obtained about them, are fairly meaningless unless we can also find out what it is about a home or hospital delivery that renders it attractive. From a policy point of view, this is important information. Going back to the Cartwright survey, some of its findings are suggestive. Comparing home and hospital experiences, it was found that labour lasted a significantly shorter time at home, fewer women were left alone during labour and significantly fewer had episiotomies. In the home group, 76% of husbands were present at the birth compared with 30% in hospital. Of the mothers at home, 57% held their babies as long as they wanted, compared with 29% in hospital. Table 27.4 shows reactions to pain relief. Again, the home birth group seem to do better, perhaps because

it is easier for women to receive individualized care at home. This is reflected in the findings relating to communication between mothers and their attendants. Mothers in home and hospital groups were equally likely to have had worries during their labour and to have discussed these worries with someone. But those at home were more likely to say that the person they talked to was helpful (89% compared with 59% of the hospital group). Overall, 44% of the home group as against 34% of the hospital group said labour and delivery had been pleasurable experiences (O'Brien 1978).

The economic costs to the mother and the family of maternity care are frequently forgotten in debates about the best form of care. In 1979 Stilwell calculated the average cost per birth of home, general practitioner unit and consultant unit deliveries (Table 27.5). The cost of a home delivery is lower than the other two options, although the family costs are actually lowest for a general practitioner unit delivery.

Women having babies are people with a variety of other roles and responsibilities. Commonly they have households to run and other children to look after. These considerations may push some women towards hospital delivery, where they will be able to have a temporary break from these responsibilities and others towards home, so that they can continue to assume them. However none of these reasons may apply, and one important issue remains to be mentioned: safety.

Safety is a concept that can be interpreted in many ways. It has at least two dimensions: physical and psychological. In thinking about the idea of safety we often split these two meanings, but to do so is really nonsensical because the psyche and the soma are closely related. There is a vast body of evidence demonstrating that stress is bad for successful reproduction and that psychologically felt stress has physiological manifestations in childbearing women (Oakley et al 1982). It is difficult to attach a precise value to findings such as the white coat effect—the impact on fetal heart rates of physicians' arrival in the labour room (Myers 1979), but the links between the mother's environment and her behaviour are none the less real.

Whereas the supposedly superior physical safety of hospital delivery is constantly emphasized, the greater psychological safety of home birth is a message that emerges clearly from women's accounts of having a baby

Table 27.4 Reactions to pain relief (from O'Brien 1978)

	Hospital birth (%)	Home birth (%)
First given pain relief at right time	69	82
Given enough pain relief	72	87
On balance, felt glad about what they had	74	87
Number given pain relief	1730	60

Table 27.5 Average cost per birth by place of delivery (from Stilwell 1979)

	Home (£)	GP/Hospital (£)	Consultant unit (£)
Public sector costs	196.69	216.87	241.02
Family costs	60.67	53.80	89.15
Total	257.36	270.67	330.17

at home (Kitzinger 1979). In part this is because the chances of maternal psychological stress are generally lower at home, and this, as Richards has pointed out in a discussion of the risks of hospital delivery, is related to the fact that:

the mother's attendants are visitors in her home; she is not staying temporarily in the institution *they* run. This means that many of the procedures and routines that a mother is forced to accept by social pressures in hospital are avoided in the home. At home social relationships are not influenced by the demands of a large bureaucratic structure dominated by an ethos of technical efficiency; instead they result from the needs and wishes of the individuals concerned. This is a point of overwhelming importance . . . (Richards 1979).

It is not an invariable rule that what benefits the mother also benefits the baby. However, it is undoubtedly true that it is easier for mother and baby to feel close after the birth when both are in their own home: the phenomenon of mother–infant bonding could only have been discovered as a necessity under conditions of near universal hospital delivery.

As well as emphasizing the enhanced psychological safety of home birth, consumer groups in the childbirth field have of course also tangled with the epidemiologists and statisticians on the question of comparative perinatal mortality rates at home and in hospital. In doing so, they have made the point that many parents wish to be informed about the relative risks of different places of birth and are intelligent enough to understand the basic statistical arguments. It is the case that no one has yet successfully proved that hospital birth is a physically safer alternative for most mothers and babies (Campbell & Macfarlane 1987). It is equally clear that many obstetricians do not regard home delivery as a sensible option, though perhaps few would go so far as to say, along with the President of the American College of Obstetricians and Gynecologists (ACOG) in 1979, that: 'home delivery is the earliest form of child abuse' (ACOG 1979). On the contrary, it is worth noting that when a select committee in Britain investigated the topic of violence in the family in 1977, one of its recommendations was for more home deliveries, since this was seen to facilitate the making of a good mother–baby relationship, thereby making child abuse less likely (Select Committee on Violence in the Family 1977).

As Alberman wrote in 1977:

the opportunity to examine the relative safeties of home and hospital delivery without bias has been lost . . . as is the case with so many innovations . . . the rapid expansion of hospital confinement was carried out without regard to well-planned trials, and now, with a confinement rate of over 94% it is too late for such trials to be performed . . . In addition, a true comparison of home versus institutional delivery will never be achieved until it is possible to study outcomes such as the long-term quality of births in terms of physical, psychological and mental health, the benefit to the mother of relief of pain or anxiety, the long-term benefit in terms of incidence of complications such as prolapse or urinary incontinence, and other similar measures (Alberman 1977).

In this situation, the fact that some women are asking for the right to choose where they have their babies hardly seems unreasonable. Surveys show that the maternity services function in such a way that relatively few women are able to exercise choice about where they have their antenatal care or their babies. In a study carried out in London in the mid 1970s, 58% of the women interviewed were simply told by their general practitioners where they would have their babies and 61% were given no choice about shared or hospital-only antenatal care (Oakley 1981). In the Cartwright study (1979) the women who were happy about their initial booking for delivery were asked: 'Did you feel you had a choice about this?' A total of 87% of women who had their babies at home said yes, compared with 56% of those who had their babies in hospital (O'Brien 1978).

WHO SHOULD DELIVER?

In Britain in 1985 a midwife was the senior person present at 76% of births. There is very little information available about women's preferences for attendants during labour and delivery. Perhaps the first preference is that there should be *someone* there: many complaints in the 1950s and 1960s highlighted the loneliness of labouring mothers in hospitals where staff were too busy or not sufficiently sensitive to stay with the mother during labour. Continuous support during labour is not irreconcilable with high-technology obstetrics. For example, the policy pioneered by O'Driscoll at the National Maternity Hospital in Dublin combines active management of labour with the provision of a personal nurse (O'Driscoll & Meagher 1980).

A second commonly stated preference is for the birth attendant to be someone the mother already knows. When the mother delivers in hospital this is not very likely to happen: the London study already referred to found that 75% of the women had never seen the person who delivered their baby before. As one of the women said:

It was *horrific* that the midwife and the pupil midwife who were there I'd never seen in my life before and I've never seen them again since. And yet they were *the* people in about the most vital and powerful experience of my life so far (Oakley 1981).

In historical and cross-cultural terms this is an unusual situation (Mead & Newton 1967). Whilst it may be reassuring to feel that the person helping the mother to deliver the baby is technically expert, yet the impact of a familiar deliverer is likely to be considerable.

A Know-your-Midwife (KYM) scheme conducted in London looked at the effect of continuity of care on labour and delivery, and found some interesting differences. One group of women (the KYM group) were looked after throughout the pregnancy, labour and the postnatal period by a team of four midwives. The other group received the standard pattern of hospital care. The KYM group were less often admitted to hospital antenatally than the control group; they used less analgesia in labour although they had longer labours; they had more normal deliveries; were more likely to deliver in an alternative position; they found motherhood easier and were more satisfied with their care than women in the control group (Flint & Poulengris 1987).

These findings are consistent with other evidence showing that midwifery care leads to more normal results for low-risk women than specialist care (Runnerstrom 1969). On these grounds, those women who want a normal labour and delivery should prefer care by midwives; however, nothing is simple in the maternity care field, and a preference for doctors may often be expressed. This is congruent with the professional claim that obstetricians are the people who know best how to secure healthy babies, which is itself part of the medicalization of life we are all socialized to accept (McKeown 1979).

The question of who should be with the labouring mother was tackled in a different way by Sosa and his colleagues in a randomized controlled trial (RCT) carried out in Guatemala some years ago. In this study, women randomized to the intervention group received the support of a lay companion throughout labour, whereas the control group (as in the KYM scheme) received the standard pattern of care. There were impressive differences in some labour and delivery variables in favour of the supported group (Sosa et al 1980). A more recent application of this approach by Klaus et al (1986) resulted in the findings shown in Table 27.6. All the differences in the incidence of perinatal problems were in favour of the supported group. As Table 27.6 shows, the findings for the comparative incidence of Caesarean section and oxytocin and the overall incidence of problems were statistically significant. Another finding not shown in the table was that mean duration of labour was significantly

shorter in the supported group (7.7 versus 15.5 hours; $P < 0.001$).

NATURAL CHILDBIRTH?

Both natural and technological forms of childbirth are capable of breeding their own orthodoxies. The modern conflict between users and providers of maternity care is often seen as centring on this notion of the natural as opposed to the unnatural medicalized, technological version of childbirth. There is a sense in which this is clearly true, and it is the sense in which medical services and therapies have the status of a cultural accretion. Human beings invented them, but they did not invent childbirth. The impact of this on women having babies is sometimes to make them believe in childbirth as an unnatural activity because it, like illness, has become the province of hospitals and doctors (Oakley 1977).

The equation between the unnatural and the medicalized derives its meaning from the very fact that pregnancy and birth are taken to hospitals and doctors, just as are other forms of illness. While this is clearly appropriate for those mothers and fetuses who develop problems, many consumer groups contend that it is not appropriate care for most mothers and fetuses, because it enhances the risk of complications arising. This was the substance of one of the early books in the present alternative childbirth movement—Suzanne Arms' 'Immaculate Deception' (1975). Arms argues that women have been deceived by obstetricians into believing in an unobtainable ideal—the no-risk birth. They have been co-opted by the obstetrical establishment into accepting a hospitalized and interventionist management of childbirth whereby a structure said to minimize the risks of childbearing actually inflates these risks by leading to iatrogenic complications.

Anthropologists point out that no human society provides for childbirth as a purely natural event. Everywhere childbirth is defined and hedged about with rules, rituals and prescriptions dictating how labouring women, their families and helpers should behave (Ford 1945). The stereotype of primitive childbirth as an unattended birth behind a bush describes an event 'as rare and remarkable as an American birth taking place in a taxi cab' (Mead & Newton 1967). Most importantly, the lack of modern medical facilities and therapies does not necessarily mean an attitude of non-interference; for example, herbs may be used to accelerate labour, abdominal stimulation, including external version, may be used, and manual removal of the placenta is by no means unknown (Oakley 1982).

In modern obstetric practice, the question is often asked whether women really want natural childbirth. This issue causes heated reactions on both sides. Obstetricians condemn women's viewpoints as cranky, whimsical and dangerous and women object that obstetricians are trying

Table 27.6 Percentage of patients who experienced perinatal problems during labour and delivery (from Klaus et al 1986)

Problems	No support (n = 249) (%)	Support (n = 168) (%)
Caesarean section	17	7 (P < 0.01)
Meconium staining	18	13
Asphyxia	3	2
Oxytocin	13	2 (P < 0.001)
Analgesia	4	1
Forceps	3	1
Other	1	1
Total	59	27 (P < 0.001)

to frighten them into submission. It may be objected (by obstetricians) that they should not have to contend with something called 'The Good Birth Guide'; neurosurgeons, after all, do not have to grapple with 'The Good Neurosurgery Guide'. Total lack of comprehension may be expressed about instances such as the mother whose pregnancy was initiated by in vitro fertilization but who chose to have her baby at home and whose baby died during the second stage of labour: how could someone be so foolish as to risk such a precious hard-won pregnancy through the selfish desire for a familiar place of birth? (Francis 1985).

One explanation of these patterns is the fact that by and large women and obstetricians do have different perspectives on childbirth. A pooled analysis of data from two research projects in York and London showed that obstetricians and mothers see the nature, context, control and criteria of success of childbirth differently. These differences in the frames of reference of the two groups are responsible for at least some of the conflicts that develop (Graham & Oakley 1981).

Is there any systematic evidence about the proportion of women who support natural (i.e. non-interventionist) childbirth? No research has exclusively and directly tackled this question, but partial answers can be gleaned from a variety of sources. Macintyre (1981) approached this question by asking how the women in her Scottish study felt about the prospect of intervention during labour or delivery; her findings are shown in Table 27.7. Negative feelings were expressed by a third of the women; a very small proportion said they felt positively about the prospect.

In Cartwright's study of induction (1979), the main reason women gave for not wanting an induction was that they wanted the baby to come naturally. A study of British Asian women in Warwickshire found that 48% of mothers expressed a desire that nature would determine the timing and mode of birth. This desire was voiced most strongly by women who had experienced an unwelcome level of medical intervention in a previous birth. The chief reasons given for preferring a natural birth were twofold: firstly, that women who had had induced labours with epidural analgesia and perhaps an instrumental delivery tended to feel they had not really given birth; secondly, they were concerned that elective delivery led to a disturbed mother–child relationship (Homans 1980). In London in the mid 1970s, 96% of a sample of women interviewed before delivery said they would prefer a labour and delivery without medical intervention because such a birth would be more natural. Specifically, 73% said they would not like to have an induction on these grounds—but 21% of these women did experience an induction (Oakley 1981).

It is commonly said that the desire for natural childbirth is limited to middle-class women, and it may also be objected that some women actually campaign for medical interventions. The latter point is undoubtedly true—indeed, it follows from the point made earlier, that not all women want the same kind of birth experience. The question of social class is more complex. In a study done in New England, Nelson (1983) found that there were two client models of childbirth; both were in competition with the medical model. Table 27.8 shows some dimensions of the two client models identified in this study. Quite large differences exist between the two groups with respect to medication, artificial rupture of membranes (ARM) and fetal monitoring, but not for the other procedures shown in the table. Nelson summed up the differences thus:

The working class women ... favoured intervention because they thought it could bring the product easily, quickly and safely. The middle class women favoured a process which entailed safety (as they defined it) and personal participation, but excluded medical intervention in a natural process (Nelson 1983).

As Nelson points out, the preferences of working-class women in such settings may reflect inhibition, due to a feeling of not being able to control the birth process. In addition, middle-class women may have access to more information about childbirth. But account must also be taken of the fact that the social and economic position of the two groups is different. Working-class women have children younger, have more accidental pregnancies and more limited material resources for childbearing. The pursuit of natural childbirth requires time, money and

Table 27.7 Women's feelings at 34 weeks' gestation about intervention during labour or delivery (from Macintyre 1981)

Feelings	% Women ($n = 45$)
Positive feelings about intervention	2
Accepting or indifferent	58
Negative feelings	36
Not asked	4
Total	100

Table 27.8 Planning for childbirth—choices about procedures by social class (from Nelson 1983)

	Percentage of women who wanted each procedure*	
	Working class (%)	Middle class (%)
Shave	20	20
Enema	42	46
Labour medication	57	11
Delivery medication	58	17
ARM†	59	4
Episiotomy	64	62
Fetal monitoring	90	55
Hold baby at birth	92	97

* Calculated on number in each group who expressed a choice. Total number of subjects in study = 322.
†Artificial rupture of membranes.

assertiveness, and will not be pursued at all unless it is seen to be a priority. It is clear that some women do not see it as a priority.

PAIN: THE CURSE OF WOMEN?

There are many views on the subject of pain in childbirth. How much pain do women feel? How much should they feel? What are the best methods for relieving pain? Who should determine how much pain relief should be available? From a biblical position, the pain of childbirth is part of the meaning of womanhood. A more recent rendering of this is its psychoanalytic reworking, according to which masochism is to be regarded as a feminine personality trait. As an editorial in the British Medical Journal (1973) put it: 'The assumption that man is born to suffer and that woman is born to suffer more than man is found in the earliest human literature'. However, there is a continuum of views on the matter of pain in childbirth. There are those who say that relaxation and information are the main analgesics necessary; others assert that every appropriate modern analgesic method should be applied to its relief. Care-providers and their clients are divided on this topic, and a political ideology such as feminism is compatible with opposing points of view.

There is surprisingly little research directly tapping the views of labouring women about pain. In 1982, 1000 women delivering at Queen Charlotte's Maternity Hospital were asked to grade the pain they felt in labour on a linear analogue scale (Morgan et al 1982). Those who had felt the most pain were mothers who had not received any analgesia and those who felt the least were those who had been given an epidural. One in three mothers experienced more pain than they had expected and this proportion was the same in all analgesic groups (Morgan et al 1982). Other surveys provide similar kinds of information although, unfortunately, there has been no standard way of eliciting the information, so it is difficult to make direct comparisons between different studies. Cartwright (1979) looked at pain relief in her study of induction: Table 27.9 gives data for her study according to whether the labour was induced or not, and for all labours. About one in four women said that they had not been given the right amount of pain relief. It is important to note that a drug or procedure given to alleviate pain may have other physical effects for the mother: thus Cartwright found that the proportion of women who felt sick or were sick during labour was considerably higher for the epidural than for any other group.

Other surveys demonstrate some of the regional and subcultural differences in attitudes to pain and pain relief. Analysis of data from the National Birthday Trust Fund survey of pain Relief in Labour (Social Science Record Unit 1992, unpublished report) found significant differ-

Table 27.9 Pain relief and induced and spontaneous labours (from Cartwright 1979)

	Induced labours (%)	Labours starting spontaneously (%)	All labours (%)
Pain relief			
None	11	21	19
Epidural/spinal anaesthesia	9	4	5
Other injection	72	62	64
Inhalant analgesia	4	6	5
Other	4	6	5
Amount of pain relief			
Enough	70	73	72
Would have liked more	7	7	7
Too much	9	7	8
Mixed views/other	14	13	13
Number of labours	522	1599	2134

ences between ethnic groups, with Asian women being more likely to describe the pain experienced as unbearable, and also more likely than other women to feel they had not been free to choose their method of pain relief. Comparison of mothers' and health professionals' perceptions of the same labours showed that health professionals were more likely than mothers to judge pain relief as effective; in other words, the professionals tended to underestimate the women's pain. Again, these differences were sharper for ethnic minority women. A study carried out in Oxford found that 26% of women assessed their labour pain as greater and 65% as less than expected: for 9% it was as they had expected (Ounstead & Simons 1979). Macintyre's prospective interview study of married primigravidae in Aberdeen found that the overall experience of childbirth, in which pain was a prominent component, was worse than expected for one in three mothers, but also better than expected for one in three; the rest had no particular expectations, were not able to remember them, or found the experience similar to what they had expected (Macintyre 1981). Two of the comments quoted by Macintyre were:

(It's) totally different. It's really, well, it's a pain you can never realise until you have it yourself . . . it's something that you don't realise until you have a baby of your own.

and

Well, with having an epidural I couldn't really say if it was worse than I expected because I was hoping to have a normal delivery.

The picture with respect to pain and its relief during labour is considerably more complicated than it may at first appear. An important consideration is that different analgesic experiences are associated with different rates of intervention, and both analgesic and intervention experiences are combined in the mothers' recollections.

In the Queen Charlotte's survey, for example, 11%

of the mothers having no analgesia had their labours induced, and 1% had an assisted delivery, compared with a 35% induction and 51% assisted delivery rate in the epidural group (Morgan et al 1982). Secondly, satisfaction with childbirth, including feelings about the amount of pain experienced and relieved, evolves over time. It is necessary to know not only how mothers feel immediately or soon after delivery, but also what they make of the experience months or years later. The Queen Charlotte's study showed that the proportion of mothers dissatisfied with the experience of childbirth 1 year later was lowest in the no analgesia group, and highest in the miscellaneous combinations group, and at a point in between for the group of women who had had epidurals alone or in combination with another method. One reason for this differential increase in dissatisfaction over time may be the long-term health effects of childbirth. For example, MacArthur and colleagues' (1991) recent study of 11 701 women delivering between 1978 and 1985 found a significant association between epidural anaesthesia and persistent backache between 1 and 9 years after giving birth; other specific features of labour and delivery were also associated with particular adverse health outcomes. As regards the long-term recall of childbirth, a recent American study which examined mothers' recollections of their birth experiences with a 14–21-year period of follow-up found a striking consistency of recall over time. However, the significance attached to negative effects seemed to intensify over time, whereas the positive aspects tended to be recalled in a similar way at the different time points (Simkin 1992).

There are also methods aside from medical ones for relieving labour pain. Fear, as described by Grantly Dick-Read (1942) and others, can lead to pain; thus the alleviation of fear by information and relaxation may directly affect pain. Contrary to some of its claims, however, there is no evidence that childbirth preparation classes on their own have an appreciable effect (Enkin 1982). There is some evidence that childbirth preparation classes reduce the need for analgesia, though they do not necessarily have all the dramatic effects claimed for them. Other relaxation strategies such as music may be seen as helpful: the music of Barry Manilow (in this context said to be relaxing) became fashionable in 1984 as an aid to childbirth by Caesarean section (Guardian 4 April 1984). Flynn et al (1978) found that ambulation in labour reduced the need for analgesia and had other effects, including higher Apgar scores and a reduced need for augmentation of labour with oxytoxic drugs.

The pain of childbirth may be different in important ways from other types of pain—in having the achievable end-product of a baby, for example—yet important connections can be made between its experience and management and those of other types of pain. For example, giving information to surgical patients has been shown to reduce postoperative pain (Janis 1985). It is known that individual pain thresholds vary, and although some health professionals and others may tend to see patterned differences between social groups in terms of attitudes to pain, at least for the British population, the notion that people in lower social classes have a high perception of pain and a greater prevalence of neuroticism has been shown to be false (Larson & Mercer 1984).

ELECTIVE DELIVERY

The present wave of consumer criticism in obstetrics was provoked by concern in the mid 1970s about rising induction rates (Gillie & Gillie 1974) and the same wave is now riding the tide of critical attitudes towards rising Caesarean section rates (Maternity Alliance 1983). The issues involved in induction of labour and Caesarean section relate both to what may be seen as the prevention of natural childbirth, and to the unwarranted promotion of medical and technological control, unwarranted in the sense that high induction and Caesarean section rates may carry more hazards than they provide benefits for mothers and babies.

Induction

It is clear from studies of women's attitudes that a number of different components are involved. The main ones are pain, medical interventions associated with induction, and patterns of interaction and communication with medical staff. Overall, induction appears to mean more pain for mothers, more medical interventions and a less satisfying mode of staff–patient communication.

In an NCT study of women attending NCT antenatal classes, 64% of the multiparae who had the opportunity to compare their induced labour with a previous non-induced one reported induction as worse because of its greater pain and discomfort (Kitzinger 1975). On the same basis of a comparison with previous labours, the mothers in Cartwright's (1979) study found induction more painful than a spontaneous labour. Stewart's (1979) survey of attitudes to induction in women delivering in the Nuneaton Maternity Hospital found that in 45% of induced patients the pain of labour was greater than they had expected; the same figure was reported in the study of Lewis et al (1975) which also contained a control group of women having spontaneous labours: 33% of the spontaneous group said the pain of labour had exceeded their expectations.

The question of the degree of pain felt is, of course, intimately linked to the question of the degree of pain relief offered and accepted. All available studies concur in the conclusion that women whose labours are induced receive more pain relief. In the retrospective study by Yudkin et al (1979) 32% of a spontaneous onset group of

200 women received no pain relief or Entonox (nitrous oxide and oxygen) only, as against only 6% in an induced group of a further 200 women—findings not dissimilar from those of the NCT report (Kitzinger 1975); 49% of inductions were accompanied by epidural analgesia, while the figure was 14% for the spontaneous group.

In Stewart's (1979) study, twice as many women who were induced had epidurals. The increased use of analgesic drugs with induction is likely to have negative effects on the baby (Richards 1977, 1979) and induced labours tend to be shorter than those that begin spontaneously (Cartwright 1979). Indeed, shortening the length of labour sometimes appears to be a carrot held out by obstetricians to women to persuade them of the advantages of induced labour specifically, and the active management of labour in general. According to the active management of labour policy, as advocated and practised by O'Driscoll, it is important to assure women that their babies will be born within a definite time period 'because the prospect of prolonged labour is often a cause of serious concern' (O'Driscoll & Meagher 1980). In fact no one appears to have asked women which of the two alternatives they would prefer: a shorter more painful labour or a longer, possibly less painful one.

In many places routine fetal heart rate monitoring is practised in all induced labours. The women in Cartwright's national sample (1979) who had their babies in 1975 reported a rate of electronic fetal heart rate monitoring of 32% for induced and 17% for spontaneous labours; the sample in the study by Yudkin et al (1979) of women delivering in Oxford in the same year yielded rates of 65 and 19% respectively. The procedures involved in attaching scalp electrodes to the fetus are experienced by some women as painful (Oakley 1981) but maternal reactions to continuous fetal heart rate monitoring have in general received scant investigation. Of more than 500 articles on this topic published between 1970 and 1980, only two considered maternal attitudes. The following range of reactions was reported in one of these:

The monitor was seen as a protector, sometimes with quasimagical powers; as an extension of their own bodies; as an aid to communication; as an extension of the baby; as a distraction; as an aid to recognising the onset of contractions; as a mechanical monster; as a competitor for the husband's attention—or the midwife's, or the doctor's—as a facilitator of husband participation in labour and as a source of anxiety (Lumley & Astbury 1980).

A more recent randomized controlled trial of electronic fetal heart rate monitoring compared mothers' views of this technique with their views about intermittent auscultation: the electronically monitored women experienced more restriction of movement and were not more reassured by this method of monitoring than women exposed to the traditional alternative (Garcia et al 1985a).

It is not entirely clear why induced labours attract more epidurals. Are epidurals administered more often in these cases because women request them, because medical staff expect an induced labour to be more painful and advise the mother accordingly, or because it is more convenient to organize an epidural at the same time as the other procedures required for an induction? Another possibility is that the greater use of epidurals in induced labour may be the consequence of a more general attitude to intervention among obstetricians, so that those who favour induction are also likely to favour epidurals. Obstetricians regard epidurals as increasing their job satisfaction—and that of midwives; though most midwives in fact hold the view that this is not so (Cartwright 1979).

The more common use of epidural analgesia in induced as opposed to spontaneous labours is part of the explanation of the higher rate of instrumental delivery associated with induced labours (Cartwright 1979, Yudkin et al 1979). Cartwright found differences in the incidence of instrumental delivery according to whether or not the husband was present (a higher rate characterized the husband-present group), and she suggests that 'possibly husbands agitate for something to be done—or possibly forceps are occasionally used as a reason for asking the husband to leave?' Yudkin et al (1979) present the following interpretation:

It could be that the high rate of forceps deliveries among the induced women reflects not so much the inability of these women to deliver spontaneously, but rather the close attention of the supervising obstetrician. Having started a woman's labour electively and closely followed it through to full dilation with fetal monitoring the obstetrician may well feel that he can ensure a successful delivery by intervening in the second stage as well.

Kirke (1975), in one of the very few studies of consumer attitudes carried out by doctors, reports that 'almost three quarters of those who had forceps deliveries said they either did not mind or were pleased about it, and one quarter were disappointed because they had wanted a natural birth'. It is difficult to know how to regard those who were pleased at having a forceps delivery. Would they have been very pleased if they had been offered a Caesarean section instead? Without some assessment of the meaning of the use of techniques like these for the mothers the recording of simple votes is not very illuminating. A randomized controlled trial designed to compare the consequences for mothers and babies of the vacuum extractor versus forceps found that women allocated to vacuum extraction reported less pain at delivery, but had more worries about their babies (Garcia et al 1985b).

There is some evidence that, not unreasonably, and as is the case with fetal monitoring (Starkman 1976), instrumental deliveries are more positively evaluated by mothers when they are seen as a solution to real obstetric problems rather than as a routine procedure (Oakley 1981). The same probably holds for episiotomy, a procedure which has become more common in recent years, and which appears to be considerably more painful and problematic for mothers than is usually recognized (Kitzinger 1981).

In a leading article on induction in labour in 1976, the British Medical Journal attempted to disentangle the main points emerging from the media debate on induction. The article took the view that since induction was only practised by clinicians 'in good faith for the good of the mother and the baby' its misrepresentation in the media must be 'disquieting evidence that doctors were not adequately communicating their intentions to their patients' (British Medical Journal Editorial 1976).

Lack of information and inadequate discussion are certainly major themes in the studies that have been done of women's attitudes to induction. The most detailed data on this are given by Cartwright (1979). Only 57% of women whose labours were induced had discussed induction at all in pregnancy. Two out of five said they would have liked more information about it. Whereas middle-class women were more likely to have discussed induction beforehand, working-class women were more likely to feel deprived of adequate information about pregnancy and birth in general. The more middle-class sample described in the NCT report appear to have had a similar experience: only 56% of the induced group had discussed induction.

The situation with respect to induction is a prime example of that described by Friedson as liable to promote overt conflict between doctor and patient. Friedson (1975) notes that 'the very nature of professional practice seems to stimulate the patient on occasions to be especially wary and questioning'. In the first place, professional knowledge is never complete, and procedures applied to parents may eventually turn out to be incorrect or hazardous; professional knowledge tends to disregard the validity of the patient's definitions of her condition. Secondly, there is the tendency towards the routinization of cases that constitute clinical material, so that patients become mere instances of a class, each individual instance being considered the same as every other in its class. Given that the variation between different practitioners and institutions in induction rates is a matter of relatively public knowledge, and that hazards of the procedure are fairly openly discussed, it is hardly surprising that many women feel these days that induction of labour is not a purely clinical matter to be left to obstetricians, but one in which they themselves should be able to exercise choice. Indeed, 81% of the women in Cartwright's study indicated that in circumstances where a doctor was uncertain about what clinical course to adopt in their case, they would like the situation explained to them so that they could choose what should be done. This is surely a very important point. Despite the fact that four-fifths of mothers would

prefer to be involved in the decision-making process, only a third of those whose labours were induced felt they had had any kind of choice.

The desire of many women to take part in decisions about induction does not necessarily mean that they are opposed to induction. As Ounsted & Simons (1979) somewhat provocatively phrase it: 'in addition to those women who insist on natural childbirth at all costs, there appears to be another group who may exert pressure on their obstetricians to induce labour in the absence of clear-cut medical reasons'. Although 6% of Cartwright's sample had tried to arrange not to have an induction, 2% recorded an attempt to have one. Both adequate discussion of induction beforehand and good emotional support from medical staff during labour and delivery contribute to relatively comfortable experiences of induction (Kitzinger 1975, Cartwright 1979). Attitudes and reactions to childbirth are, in this sense, a function of many different variables, including women's prior experiences of birth and obstetric care, their confidence (or lack of it) in their body's ability to labour spontaneously, and the degree of unpredictability their social circumstances are able to support concerning the time of birth. Tables 27.10 and 27.11 from Cartwright's study show the same pattern as Table 27.3: the proportions of women who would prefer the same pattern of care for their next baby as they had for the last one are highest for the natural alternative in each case, i.e. no induction, no epidural, home birth.

No study has been done to date on the specific topic of women's attitudes to post-term pregnancy, although there is evidence that such pregnancy may often be experienced as 'tedious, frustrating and uncomfortable' (Cartwright 1979). The issue of elective induction of labour also

Table 27.10 Preferences for induction in the next labour (from Cartwright 1979)

	Labour last time	
	Induced (%)	Not induced (%)
Prefer same as last time	17	93
Prefer not to have same as last time	78	5
Other comments	5	2
Number of mothers (= 100%)	552	1593

Table 27.11 Preferences for epidural analgesia in the next labour (from Cartwright 1979)

	Analgesia in the last labour	
	Epidural (%)	No epidural (%)
Prefer same as last time	63	82
Prefer not to have same as last time	34	13
Other comments	3	5
Number of mothers (= 100%)	110	2053

involves the matter of a correct expected date of delivery; many mothers feel quite strongly about the negotiation of this as an area in which they possess personal knowledge (Oakley 1981). From the point of view of obstetricians exercising control over the timing of women's deliveries, the development and routine application of ultrasonic scanning have, of course, been extremely important; this is yet another field in which maternal attitudes have not been adequately investigated.

Caesarean section

More research has been done in the USA than in the UK on the social and psychological costs of a Caesarean section (Marieskind 1979). It is interesting to note that a Consensus Development Task Force set up in 1979 by the National Institutes of Health to examine Caesarean childbirth numbered a sociologist and a psychologist among its members; one of its assignments was to consider the 'psychological effects of Caesarean delivery on the mother, infant and family' (Shearer 1981).

It is significant that the operation of Caesarean section is referred to in a different way from other forms of abdominal surgery; it is not called an operation, or surgery, but a section. Following this terminology, while it is accepted among surgeons that depression is a common consequence of major surgery, especially if it is carried out as an emergency procedure, the same assumption is not made about a Caesarean section. Many of the psychological consequences of surgery in general also apply to Caesarean section. These include a temporary response of emotional relief and elation at having survived the operation, worry about the mutilating effects of the operation on the body and its attractiveness to others, and a long drawn-out period of physical and psychological discomfort (Janis 1958). It is worth noting that the kinds of demands that the care of the newborn may make involve activities that are likely to be forbidden to any patient on a surgical ward for some days (if not weeks) after abdominal surgery. It is presumably factors of this kind that account for the association between an admission to a psychiatric hospital in the first 90 days after childbirth and a Caesarean delivery (Kendell et al 1981).

In one British study, Trowell (1978) compared 16 mothers who had emergency Caesarean sections under general anaesthetic with a control group of spontaneously vaginally delivered women. All were having first babies and the babies weighed over 2.49 kg (5.5 lb) and were not admitted to a special care unit. No sections were performed for pressing obstetric reasons. At 1 month, observations showed that mothers who had had a Caesarean section looked more but smiled less at their babies and the Caesarean babies were rated as being more tense. Striking differences emerged from the questioning of the mothers.

Those who had had sections more often remembered birth as a bad experience, expressed doubts about their capacity to care for the baby and were depressed or anxious. As the author comments:

These women had expected a normal vaginal delivery and had prepared themselves for this. They tended to feel a failure as a woman, unable to have a normal delivery and angry with the baby for not 'coming out', and there was some anger towards the hospital, although at the same time, an acknowledgement of the crisis that had occurred and a belief that the hospital had saved their and their baby's lives. Perhaps because of these feelings the Caesarean mothers were more anxious and apprehensive about parenthood and its responsibilities (Trowell 1978).

These sorts of attitudes were still present at a year, with the mothers who had had a Caesarean section more likely to describe motherhood in negative terms, more likely to delay responding to their child's crying and reporting a late age at which they first felt their child responded to them as a person. The group of mothers who had had a Caesarean section expressed more anger in their handling of their children by shouting, smacking and losing their tempers. There were indications that the babies born by Caesarean section had a slower motor development (age of sitting unaided), and some interaction measures from the observations showed continuing differences between the groups. The groups in this study are small and as the author herself emphasizes, it was intended to be a pilot study.

Another study comparing perceptions of childbirth among socially similar groups of women having Caesarean and vaginal deliveries found a generalized loss of self-esteem among the former mothers (Marut & Mercer 1979).

The profound effects that can follow a Caesarean section are recognized among women, and one of the more striking developments in recent years has been the growth of self-health groups offering support to mothers. The very existence of these groups is, of course, a clear indication of the psychological and social needs for support which women who have undergone these procedures may feel. As with induction there are situations in which some women prefer an elective delivery by Caesarean section to a vaginal one. Section rates are very high among private patients (Richards 1979) which may in part reflect a movement of women who request Caesarean sections into the private sector where they may be more likely to get them on demand.

In conclusion, out of this discussion of specific topics from the general viewpoint of the labouring mother, certain key themes emerge about women's perspectives on the management of childbirth today. These themes are:

1. *Control*: who should be in control of labour and delivery—the health professional or the mother? What

is the appropriate time perspective for measuring success-delivery and its immediate aftermath at one extreme, or the long-term development of the child at one extreme and the family on the other?

2. *Evaluation*: have obstetric procedures been systematically evaluated and has this evaluation represented the consumer's perspective within it?

3. *Success*: how is the success of childbearing to be measured?' What relative weighting should be given to hard versus soft measures of outcomes: mortality and physical morbidity versus depression and dissatisfaction, for example?

4. *Communication*: what kind of communication marks the interaction of the labouring mother with those who care for her? In particular, to what extent are information and support of mothers by health professionals part of this communication?

This chapter ends with a brief consideration of each of these themes.

WHOSE BABY IS IT ANYWAY?

This is the title of an editorial in the Lancet in 1980 which considered professional responses to women's assertion of the right to make informed choices about childbirth. The editorial observed that there is a spectrum of response—from the declared goal of seeking to help parents to free themselves of dependence on the medical profession, through to condemning the consumer protest as dangerous faddism.

However professionals respond, it remains true that it is the mother who is having the baby and who will live with the consequences of the management of her particular childbirth for the rest of her life. Whereas professionals might wish to control childbirth (Beazley 1975) so, on the whole, do mothers; at least, they wish to remain in control within the parameters of what that means to them (Humenick 1981). To have a feeling of control is not the same as having a labour and delivery free of medical intervention. Much more important is the extent to which a woman feels that her own wishes have been respected.

COMMUNICATION: THE GOLDEN RULE

In order to respect the wishes of the labouring mother, it is a prerequisite for those caring for her to find out how she approaches birth and her own role in it. There is a substantial literature on communication problems in obstetric and midwifery practice: much of the debate within consumer groups concerns what is wrong with the way professionals relate to childbearing women, and what can be done about it. There is not enough communication; staff treat mothers as cases and not as individuals; they offer patronizing reassurance when what has been asked for is information, and so forth. Richards (1981)

has drawn attention to one dimension of communication failure as perceived by mothers:

Characteristic of many conversations between doctor and mother is the use of that peculiar 'we' by the doctor. 'We would not want to do anything that might jeopardise the baby'. In one way there is the correct implication that everyone is, or should be united in the wish to see the mother delivered safely of a healthy baby. But, especially if the mother does not sound too keen to submit to whatever is being proposed, there is also an implicit message that it is only the doctor who has the true interests of mother or, more especially, the child at heart. It is a patronising and paternalistic 'we' that is often used. There is the hint that the mother is not only an incompetent vessel for her baby (labours are only safe in retrospect) but that she may be selfishly uncaring and not doing what is best for her baby (Richards 1981).

Under the busy and understaffed conditions of many care-settings today, it is often difficult for staff to convey an attitude of caring and sensitivity to each mother's preferences and status as a person. Also, medical and midwifery training contain very little in the way of lessons in human interaction. Medical ideologies proscribe, rather than prescribe, involvement with the patient, and this may mean that emotional distance between mother and professionals is felt to be preferable.

These difficulties have led to the suggestion from at least one childbirth activist that what is needed is verbal disarmament: mothers must practise techniques of verbally disarming professionals in order to get across their point of view to them. Thus, for example, the following remark of an obstetrician:

I find your wish for a home birth selfish and irresponsible. You are just looking for a fulfilling experience for yourself and not thinking about your baby

might be countered by the mother saying:

I am sorry you find it necessary to say such things, doctor. *Pause.* I want you to know that it will damage our relationship (Wright 1983).

Whether or not such suggestions are being taken up by women using the maternity services today, there is clearly enormous scope for improving professional–client communication.

A HEALTHY BABY OR A GOOD EXPERIENCE?

Within the medical model of childbirth, there is an overwhelming emphasis on mortality and its avoidance and on physical morbidity. Within the social model of childbirth on the one hand, more holistic criteria of success are stressed: the mother's experience of birth is part of this, as is her emotional condition during the early years and months of motherhood, her relationship with the baby, the baby's long-term development and the whole nexus of relationships—the nuclear family, the extended family, the household—into which the baby is born.

The conflict between these two ways of assessing success in childbirth is evident in the question above, which poses a healthy baby and a good experience as opposing aims. If the consumer movement in maternity care has succeeded in saying anything loudly and clearly then it is surely this: that a healthy baby and a good experience are, for the majority of mothers, not different goals, but the same one. This message is brought out most sharply in the literature on mother–infant bonding which has stressed the fact that childbirth does not end with the delivery of the baby; a relationship, begun prenatally, has to be forged between mother and neonate, and in the forging of this relationship obstetric procedures either may or may not help. Table 27.12 shows the association between some such procedures and breastfeeding as one indicator of the mothers' and babies' relationships with one another. Mothers who have Caesarean deliveries and any type of analgesia or anaesthesia in labour and whose babies go into special care are more likely than other mothers to have stopped breastfeeding within 2 weeks of delivery. Of course these factors are interrelated but the statistical analysis showed that any factor causing a delay of more than 4 hours between delivery and the first breastfeed was likely to jeopardize the success of breastfeeding (Martin & Monk 1982). It is obvious that what

Table 27.12 Proportion of mothers who had stopped breastfeeding within 2 weeks by type of delivery, analgesia or anaesthesia and baby's postpartum care (from Martin & Monk 1982)

	Proportion (%) of mothers who had stopped breastfeeding within 2 weeks in England and Wales (*n = 2499*)
Delivery type	
Normal	19
Forceps/vacuum	19
Caesarean section	28
All mothers	19
Analgesia/anaesthesia	
Nothing	11
Gas and air	20
Injection (excluding epidural)	20
Epidural	22
General anaesthetic	28
All mothers	19
Baby's care	
No special care	18
Special care	23
All babies	19

obstetricians do may have long-term effects, especially when the link between early feeding and adult health is considered (Faulkner 1980). When childbirth is not successful and a perinatal death occurs, then the behaviour of obstetricians and paediatricians is not necessarily less important. Seeing and touching the dead baby are often important, and it is rare for those parents who have done so to regret it, while fantasies about the dead child's appearance may be a real obstacle to grieving for those who are not given this opportunity (Stringham et al 1982).

EVALUATION

As Haggerty (1980) has commented in relation to early interventions designed to improve mother–infant bonding: 'there are no quick fixes for parenting difficulties arising from generational inadequacies and poverty'. Thus while some professional attempts to improve bonding may be relatively successful, the total amount of variance attributable to such interventions is small compared to that explained by background social characteristics (2–23% versus 10–25%). Doctors and other health professionals are, fortunately, not gods.

One meaning of evaluation is therefore an attempt to assess the boundaries of obstetric care in its claim to expertise in childbearing. Another meaning, which runs through many of the points made in this chapter about the experiences of mothers, is to locate these experiences more centrally within studies designed to answer questions about the effectiveness and safety of specific therapies and procedures. What is effective and safe physiologically may not be so psychosocially, and vice versa. There is no doubt that at least part of the recent critique highlighting the experiences of labouring mothers themselves has concerned the anxiety women can feel about being subjected to procedures which have not been shown to be effective. Like the dormouse and the doctor in A. A. Milne's poem of that name, women and those who care for them in labour are engaged in a dispute about the kind of scenario that is good for health. Whereas the doctor took the view that chrysanthemums were what the dormouse needed, the dormouse himself felt that geraniums and delphiniums were better. In the end, the dormouse gave up, closed his eyes and resigned himself merely to dreaming about what he wanted. There is, however, no sign that women are likely to do that.

REFERENCES

ACOG 1979 American College of Obstetricians and Gynecologists Newsletter, 4 May

Alberman E 1977 Facts and figures. In: Chard T, Richards M (eds) Benefits and hazards of the new obstetrics. Spastics International Publications, London

Arms S 1975 Immaculate deception. Bantam Books, New York

Beazley J 1975 The active management of labor. American Journal of Obstetrics and Gynecology 122: 161–168

Bland R 1781 Some calculations from the Midwifery Reports of the Westminster General Dispensary, London

British Medical Journal Editorial 1954 24(4): 54

British Medical Journal Editorial 1976 1: 729

Butler N R, Bonham D 1963 Perinatal mortality. E & S Livingstone, Edinburgh

Campbell R, Macfarlane A 1987 Where to be born? The debate and the evidence. National Perinatal Epidemiology Unit, Oxford

Cartwright A 1979 The dignity of labour. Tavistock, London

Chamberlain G, Howlett B, Philipp E, Masters K 1978 British births 1970. Obstetric care. Heinemann, London

Chamberlain M 1981 Old wives' tales. Virago, London

Clark A 1968 The working life of women in the seventeenth century. Frank Cass, London

Department of Health and Social Security 1983 Low income families 1981. DHSS, London

Dick-Read G 1942 Childbirth without fear. Heinemann, London

Donnison J 1977 Midwives and medical men. Heinemann, London

Enkin M 1982 Antenatal classes. In: Enkin M, Chalmers I (eds) Effectiveness and satisfaction in antenatal care. Spastics International Medical Publications, London

Farr W 1885 Vital statistics. Edward Stanford, London

Faulkner F 1980 Prevention in childhood of health problems in adult life. WHO, Geneva

Flint C, Poulengris P 1987 The 'know your midwife' report. Private publication, 49 Peckerman's Wood, London SE26 6RZ

Flynn A M, Kelly J, Hollins G, Lynch P F 1978 Ambulation in labour. British Medical Journal 2: 591–593

Ford C S 1945 A comparative study of human reproduction. Yale University Publications in Anthropology no 32, New York

Francis H H 1985 Obstetrics: a consumer-oriented service? Journal of Maternal and Child Health March: 69–72

Friedson E 1975 Dilemmas in the doctor–patient relationship. In: Cox C, Mead A (eds) A sociology of medical practice. Collier-Macmillan, London

Garcia J, Corry M, MacDonald D, Elbourne D, Grant A 1985a Mothers' views of continuous electronic fetal heart rate monitoring and intermittent auscultation in a randomized controlled trial. Birth 12: 79–85

Garcia J, Anderson J, Vacca A, Elbourne D, Grant A, Chalmers I 1985b Views of women and their medical and midwifery attendants about instrumental delivery using vacuum extraction and forceps. Journal of Psychosomatic Obstetrics and Gynaecology 4: 1–9

Gillie L, Gillie O 1974 The childbirth revolution and the vital first hours. Sunday Times 13 October, 20 October

Glaister J 1894 Dr W Smellie and his contemporaries. James Nackhose, Glasgow

Goldthorpe W O, Richman J 1974 Maternal attitudes to unintended home confinement. Practitioner 212: 845

Graham H, Oakley A 1981 Competing ideologies of reproduction: medical and maternal perspective on pregnancy. In: Roberts H (ed) Women, health and reproduction. Routledge & Kegan Paul, London

Granville A B 1819 A report of the practice of the midwifery at the Westminster General Dispensary during 1818. Burgess and Hill, London

Haggerty R J 1980 Damn the simplicities. Pediatrics 66: 323–324

Homans H 1980 Pregnant in Britain: a sociological approach to Asian and British women's experiences. PhD thesis, University of Warwick

Houd S, Oakley A 1986 Alternative perinatal services. In: Phaff J M L (ed) Perinatal health services in Europe: searching for better childbirth. Croom Helm, London

Humenich S S 1981 Mastery: the key to childbirth satisfaction? A review. Birth and the Family Journal 8: 79–90

Janis I 1958 Psychological stress: psychoanalytic and behavioural studies of surgical patients. John Wiley, New York

Johnstone R W 1913 A textbook of midwifery. Adam & Charles Black, London

Joint Committee of the Royal College of Gynaecologists and the Population Investigation Committee 1948 Maternity in Great Britain. Oxford University Press, Oxford

Kendell R E, Rennie D, Clarke J A, Dean C 1981 The social and obstetric correlates of psychiatric admissions in the puerperum. Psychological Medicine 11: 341–350

Kirke P 1975 The consumer's view of the management of labour. In: Beard R, Brudenell M, Dunn P, Fairweather D (eds) The management of labour. Proceedings of the 3rd study group of the RCOG. RCOG, London

Kitzinger S 1975 Some mothers' experiences of induced labour. NCT, London

Kitzinger S 1979 Birth at home. Oxford University Press, Oxford

Kitzinger S (ed) 1981 Episiotomy. NCT, London

Klaus M H, Kennell J H, Robertson S S, Sosa R 1986 Effects of social support during parturition on maternal and infant morbidity. British Medical Journal 293: 585–587

Klein V 1965 Britain's married women workers. Routledge & Kegan Paul, London

Lancet Editorial 1980 Whose baby is it? i: 1284–1285

Larson A G, Mercer D 1984 The who and why of pain: analysing social class. British Medical Journal 288: 883–886

Lewis B V, Rana S, Crook E 1975 Patient response to induction. Lancet i: 1197

Lumley J, Astbury J 1980 Birth rites. Sphere Books, Melbourne

MacArthur C, Lewis M, Knox E G 1991 Health after childbirth. HMSO, London

Macfarlane A, Mugford M 1984 Birth counts: statistics of pregnancy and childbirth. HMSO, London

Macintyre S 1977 The management of childbirth: a review of sociological research issues. Social Science and Medicine 11: 477–484

Macintyre S 1981 Expectations and experiences of first pregnancy. Report on a prospective interview study of married primigravidae in Aberdeen. Occasional paper no 5. University of Aberdeen, Aberdeen

Mack J, Lansley S 1985 Poor Britain. Allen & Unwin, London

Marieskind H I 1979 An evaluation of Caesarean section in the United States. Report submitted to the US Department of Health, Education and Welfare

Martin J, Monk J 1982 Infant feeding 1980. OPCS Social Survey Division, HMSO, London

Martin J, Roberts C 1984 Women and employment: a lifetime perspective. HMSO, London

Maternity Alliance 1983 One birth in nine—trends in Caesarean sections since 1978. Maternity Alliance, London

Marut J S, Mercer R T 1979 The Caesarean birth experience. Nursing Research 28: 260–266

McKeown T 1979 The role of medicine. Basil Blackwell, Oxford

Mead M, Newton N 1967 Cultural patterning of perinatal behaviour. In: Richardson S A, Guttmacher A F (eds) Childbearing—its social and psychological aspects. Williams and Wilkins, Baltimore

Ministry of Health 1927 The protection of motherhood (by Campbell J M). Reports on Public Health and Medical Subjects no 48. HMSO, London

Morgan B, Bulpitt C, Clifton P, Lewis P J 1982 Effectiveness of pain relief in labour: survey of 1000 mothers. British Medical Journal 285: 689–690

Myers R E 1979 Maternal anxiety and fetal death. In: Zichella Pancheri L (ed) Psychoneuroendocrinology in reproduction. North Holland Biomedical Press, Elsevier, Holland

National Council for One-Parent Families 1983 One parent families. NCOPF, London

Nelson M K 1983 Working class women, middle class women and models of childbirth. Social Problems 30: 285–296

Oakley A 1976 Wisewoman and medicine man: changes in the management of childbirth. In: Mitchell J, Oakley A (eds) The rights and wrongs of women. Penguin, Harmondsworth

Oakley A 1977 Cross-cultural practices. In: Chard J, Richards M (eds) Benefits and hazards of the new obstetrics. Spastics International Medical Publications, London

Oakley A 1981 From here to maternity. Penguin, Harmondsworth

Oakley A 1982 Obstetric practice: cross-cultural comparisons. In: Stratton P (ed) Psychobiology of the human newborn. Wiley, New York

Oakley A 1984 The captured womb: a history of the medical care of pregnant women. Basil Blackwell, Oxford

Oakley A, Macfarlane A, Chalmers I 1982 Social class, stress and reproduction. In: Rees A R, Purcell H (eds) Disease and the environment. John Wiley, Chichester

O'Brien M 1978 Home and hospital: a comparison of the experiences of mothers having home and hospital confinements. Journal of the Royal College of General Practitioners 28: 460–466

O'Driscoll K, Meagher D 1980 Active management of labour. WB Saunders, London

Ounstead M, Simons C 1979 Maternal attitudes to their obstetric care. Early Human Development 3: 201–204

Registrar-General 1930 Decennial supplement on occupational mortality. HMSO, London

Richards M P M 1977 The induction and acceleration of labour: some benefits and complications. Early Human Development 1: 3–17

Richards M P M 1978 A place of safety? An examination of the risks of hospital delivery. In: Kitzinger A, Davis J A (eds) The place of birth. Oxford University Press, Oxford

Richards M P M 1979 Perinatal morbidity and mortality in private obstetric practice. Journal of Maternal and Child Health September: 341–345

Richards M P M 1981 Whose choice in childbirth? Unpublished paper presented at National Childbirth Trust Silver Jubilee Conference, 10 October 1981

Riley E D M 1977 What do women want? The question of choice in the conduct of labour. In: Chard T, Richards M P M (eds) Benefits and hazards of the new obstetrics. Spastics International Medical Publications, London

Runnerstrom L R 1969 The effectiveness of nurse-midwifery in a supervised hospital environment. American College of Nurse Midwives Bulletin 14: 40

Select Committee on Violence in the Family 1977 Violence to children, vol 1. HMSO, London

Shearer E 1981 National Institutes of Health consensus development task force on Caesarean childbirth. The process and the result. Birth and the Family Journal 8: 25–30

Simkin P 1992 Just another day in a woman's life: Part II: nature and consistency of women's long-term memories of their first birth experiences. Birth 19(2): 64–81

Smellie W 1752 A treatise on the theory and practice of midwifery. London

Smith F B 1979 The people's health 1830–1910. Croom Helm, London

Sosa R, Kennell, Klaus M, Robertson S 1980 The effect of a supportive companion on perinatal problems, length of labour and mother–infant interaction. New England Journal of Medicine 303: 597–600

Stacey M 1976 The health service consumer: a sociological misconception. In: Stacey M (ed) The sociology of the National Health Service. Monograph no 22. University of Keele, Staffordshire

Stacey M, Homans H 1978 The sociology of health and illness: its present state, future prospects and potential for health research. Sociology 12: 281–307

Starkman M 1976 Psychological responses to the use of the fetal monitor during labour. Psychosomatic Medicine 38: 269–277

Stewart P 1979 Patients' attitudes to induction and labour. British Medical Journal 2: 749–752

Stilwell J A 1979 Relative costs of home and hospital confinement. British Medical Journal 2: 257–259

Stringham J G, Riley J H, Ross A 1982 Silent birth: mourning a stillborn baby. Social Work July: 322–327

Trowell J 1978 The effects of obstetric procedures on the mother/child relationship. A pilot study of emergency Caesarean section. Unpublished paper. Department for Children and Parents, Tavistock Clinic, London

Versluysen J C 1981 Midwives, medical men and 'poor women labouring of child'—lying-in hospitals in eighteenth century London. In: Roberts H (ed) Women, health and reproduction. Routledge & Kegan Paul, London

Wright M 1983 Verbal disarmament. New Generation 1: 8–9

Yudkin P, Frumar A M, Anderson A B M, Turnbull A C, Yudkin P 1979 A retrospective study of the induction of labour. British Journal of Obstetrics and Gynaecology 86: 257–263

28. The endocrine control of labour

Alec Turnbull

PRELIMINARY NOTE TO CHAPTER

This volume is dedicated to the work of Sir Alec Turnbull. In order to give those who never knew him a flavour of the clarity of his writing, Professor Chamberlain has kept one of Alec Turnbull's chapters from the 1987 edition intact. The endocrine control of labour was one of Professor Turnbull's favourite subjects and exemplifies his work.

As 9 years have gone by since it was written, Professor Philip Steer and colleagues have been asked to add an update to the subject in 1994. This they have done willingly and well. The Editor is grateful to them.

An update on the endocrine control of labour

The birth of a mature and healthy infant depends on the mechanism which ensures that the uterus stays quiescent during pregnancy while the fetus is developing and then at the appropriate time initiates the powerful and co-ordinated uterine activity and the softening of the cervix which cause cervical dilatation and ultimately delivery of the mature infant. The vital importance of this control mechanism working as reliably as it does is illustrated by the fact that 95% of human infants are born at term. Although only 5% are born preterm, they account for 85% of early neonatal deaths not due to lethal deformity (Rush et al 1976).

It is remarkable how, in each species, the uterus remains quiescent throughout a pregnancy of whatever duration is necessary for the full development of the fetus. Then, and normally only when the fetus is fully mature, the quiescent uterus becomes contractile, the cervix softens and dilates and the transition from an intrauterine to an extrauterine existence is completed by the expulsion of a fetus capable of maintaining its own existence.

There is substantial evidence in many animals implicating the fetus in the timing of the onset of labour (Thorburn et al 1977) and this applies whether pregnancy is maintained by the placenta, as in the sheep, or by the corpus luteum, as in the goat. In the human it is difficult to obtain direct evidence because of the inaccessibility of the normal intrauterine fetus in late pregnancy. In the first instance, therefore, it seems helpful to review the now well known cascade of hormonal events associated with the initiation of labour in the sheep and then proceed to consider the evidence for and against a similar control mechanism in man.

PARTURITION IN THE SHEEP

The earliest well defined event in ovine parturition is a sharp rise in the concentration of cortisol in the fetal circulation 7–10 days before delivery (Bassett & Thorburn 1969), due mainly to an increase in cortisol secretion (Liggins et al 1973). The increased cortisol secretion probably reflects an increased adrenocortical sensitivity to adrenocorticotrophin (ACTH), since fetal ACTH levels rise at the same time, rather than before the levels of cortisol (Liggins et al 1977a). The increased cortisol secretion may also depend on the process of maturation in the character of fetal pituitary ACTH secretion. Silman et al (1976) have demonstrated quality of difference between fetal and adult sheep which may develop to some extent before birth.

The importance of fetal adrenal activity in the sheep rests, of course, on the original observation that fetal hypophysectomy prevents the onset of labour (Liggins et al 1967), while intrafetal infusion of ACTH, cortisol or dexamethasone all induce labour, bringing about the endocrine changes found in the spontaneous onset of labour in this species (Liggins 1969a,b). Figure 28.1, taken from studies published by Flint et al (1975a), demonstrates that following the intrafetal injection of dexamethasone, measurements in serial blood samples from the uteroovarian vein show a marked fall in progesterone concentration, followed by an increase in oestrogen and then a sharp increase in prostaglandin F, which reaches a peak with delivery of the fetus.

The mechanism by which increased levels of glucocorticoids in the sheep fetus bring about changes in placental steroids and prostaglandin F was clarified by Anderson et al (1975) and Steele et al (1976) when they showed that fetal cortisol induced increased activity of the enzymes 17α-hydroxylase and $C_{17,20}$-lyase in the fetal placenta. With the progesterone being metabolized its level falls, while that of 17α-hydroxyprogesterone, androstenedione, oestrone and oestrone sulphate all increase. Figure 28.2 shows the enzymatic steps in which fetal cortisol can apparently increase activity and thus bring about the synthesis of oestrogens from C_{21} precursors.

Placental steroids and prostaglandin F

Figure 28.1 shows how in sheep parturition increased synthesis of prostaglandin F (PGF) immediately follows the sharp increase in oestrogen level in the uteroovarian vein. Liggins et al (1977a) showed that PGF synthesis

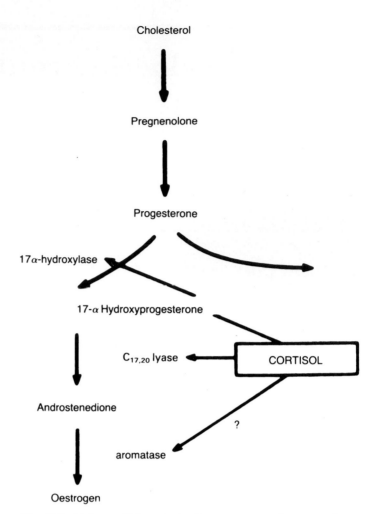

Fig. 28.2 Pathway of biosynthesis of progesterone and oestrogen in sheep placenta, indicating the possible sites of action of fetal cortisol on 17α-hydroxylase, $C_{17,20}$-lyase and aromatase. From Liggins et al (1977a).

may be stimulated by the raised oestrogens, but PGF can also be released and parturition induced without an increase in oestrogen levels by administering inhibitors of 3β-hydroxysteroid dehydrogenase, such as cyanoketone (Mitchell & Flint 1977), trilostane (Taylor et al 1982) or epostane (Ledger et al 1985a) which all reduce the blood level of progesterone.

Oxytocin, prostaglandins and the Ferguson reflex

As labour progresses, pressure of the fetal presenting part on the cervix and vagina activates a neurohumoral reflex (Ferguson reflex) by which a neural afferent pathway from the dilating cervix or the distending vagina reaches the hypothalamus via the spinal cord, and results in a humoral efferent, the secretion of oxytocin from the posterior pituitary (Flint et al 1975b). As well as stimulating uterine contractility, oxytocin also causes a release of PGF from uterine tissues (Mitchell et al 1976) which in turn stimulates more uterine contractions and thus further oxytocin

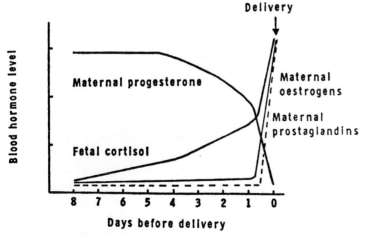

Fig. 28.1 Diagrammatic representation of the hormonal changes in the fetal and maternal circulation associated with parturition in the sheep. After Flint et al (1975a).

release, so that the process of parturition, once established, accelerates until the fetus is delivered.

Local prostaglandin production, cervical softening and dilatation

Prostaglandin production within the uterine cervix itself appears to play an important part in the process of cervical softening, dilatation and effacement (Ellwood et al 1979, 1981). The studies by Ellwood et al suggest that in the sheep cervix, increased prostaglandin E (PGE) and prostacyclin synthesis in the cervix may be more important than PGF in bringing about the remarkably rapid connective tissue changes in the cervix associated with parturition (Fig. 28.3) with breakdown of collagen fibres into fibrils, activation of fibrocytes and increased tissue fluid, all

predisposing to greater extensibility. The sheep cervix changes from being long, hard and tightly closed, to being fully dilated with a few hours of a labour in which amniotic fluid pressure changes are much less marked than in human labour (Ellwood et al 1980a). The possibility that these changes depend more on the effects of local prostaglandins on the cervical tissues than on traction on the cervix from myometrial contractions is supported by the findings of Ledger et al (1985b) who found that the usual changes in cervical extensibility occurred during labour in sheep even when the cervix was surgically isolated from the uterus.

Thus, the process of parturition in the sheep is initiated by a maturational process in the fetus leading to activation of the pituitary–adrenal axis and increasing cortisol in the fetal circulation. This initiates the whole cascade of

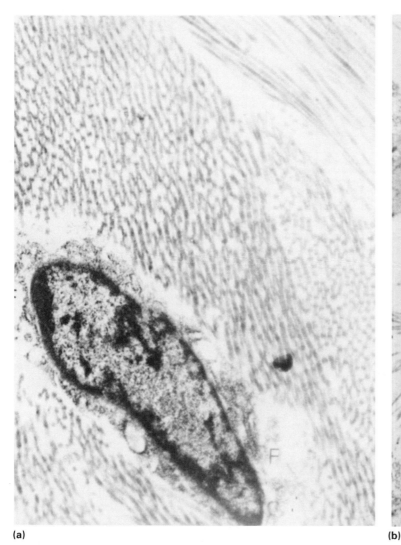
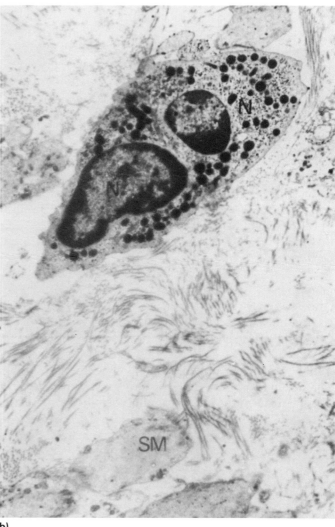

(a)   (b)

Fig. 28.3 (a) High power micrograph of tissue from a sheep cervix in late pregnancy (105 days' gestation) showing the highly organized collagen fibrils arranged in dense bundles running in a number of directions. Fibroblast cells (F) are found within and between fibril bundles (×26 000). (b) Micrograph of tissue from a sheep cervix immediately after spontaneous vaginal delivery at 140 days' gestation. Collagen fibrils are no longer arranged in compact bundles and the arrangement of the extracellular materials is now apparently random. Increased tissue fluid spaces are present. A polymorphonuclear leucocyte (N) has invaded the tissue. A group of smooth muscle cells are also visible (SM) (×11 480). From Ellwood (1981).

hormonal events involving changes in the secretion of placental steroid hormones, PGF, oxytocin activation of the Ferguson reflex and softening and dilatation of the uterine cervix.

Although pregnancy maintenance in other ruminants such as the goat and the cow depends on the corpus luteum, parturition is also controlled by a mechanism similar to that in the sheep, in which fetal cortisol acts as a trigger. On the other hand, different mechanisms control parturition in small mammals and the fetus does not seem to play a critical role. In the rat, removing the fetus or aspirating the fetal brain during pregnancy has no effect on the duration of pregnancy, at which the uterus empties its remaining contents, although labour may be protracted (Challis & Nathanielsz 1979). While the monkey fetus may play a small part in controlling the time of its own birth (Kittinger 1977, Novy 1977), Challis et al (1977) could find no progesterone withdrawal before labour in this species. The main factor in common with sheep labour was increased PGF in amniotic fluid and unconjugated oestrogens in maternal venous blood.

What mechanisms control human parturition?

INITIATION OF PARTURITION IN HUMAN PREGNANCY

Fetal pituitary–adrenal activity

In the absence of uterine distension by polyhydramnios, anencephaly of the human fetus with absence of the cerebrum, malformation of the pituitary and hypoplasia of the adrenal glands is associated with an increased range of gestation at delivery following spontaneous onset of labour, compared with pregnancies with a normal fetus (Fig. 28.4). About one-third delivered preterm, one-third at term and one third past term. Although most other studies of pregnancy complicated by anencephaly without hydramnios have reported an increased proportion with extreme prolongation of gestation, the study of Honnebier & Swaab (1973) was by far the largest and their findings imply that in man the fetal pituitary–adrenal axis acts as a fine tuner of the time of onset of labour, rather than acting as the on/off switch as it does for sheep parturition.

Silman et al (1976) have demonstrated maturational changes in the function of the human fetal anterior pituitary during the last few weeks of gestation, when secretion of real ACTH 1–39 apparently supersedes that of fragments similar to α-melanotrophin (α-MSH) and corticotrophin-like intermediate peptide (CLIP). Rising concentrations of cortisol have been demonstrated in amniotic fluid during late pregnancy (Gautray et al 1974, Fencl & Tulchinsky 1975, Murphy et al 1975, Turnbull et al 1977) and cortisol levels are higher in cord blood from infants born following the spontaneous onset of labour than in infants delivered following induced labour

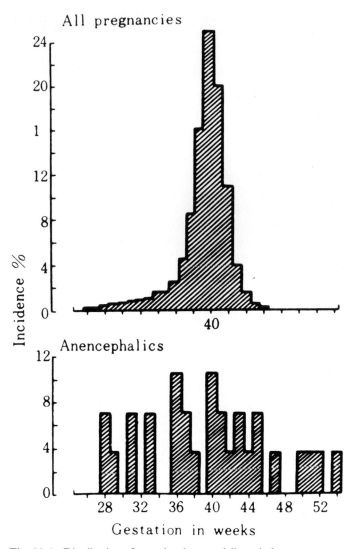

Fig. 28.4 Distribution of gestational age at delivery in human pregnancy comparing all pregnancies with those complicated by an anencephalic fetus without hydramnios. Adapted from Honnebier & Swaab (1973).

or elective Caesarean section (Cawson et al 1974, Murphy 1975, Leong & Murphy 1976). Such findings suggest that fetal cortisol secretion increases before the spontaneous onset of human labour but in a critically important study, Gennser et al (1977) found no difference between the levels of cortisol in human fetal blood samples obtained before and soon after spontaneous onset of labour at term, disproving any surge of fetal cortisol secretion before the onset of human labour.

There is no 17α-hydroxylation in the human placenta delivered following spontaneous onset labour (A. P. F. Flint, unpublished observations). Administration of potent synthetic glucocorticoids to the mother in late human pregnancy simply suppresses maternal and fetal adrenal activity and reduces maternal levels of cortisol, dehydro-epiandrosterone (DHEA) and oestriol (Anderson 1976).

Cortisol crosses the human placenta more readily than

it does that of the sheep. High cortisol levels in the human fetus after delivery seem to have resulted from transfer from the high levels in the mother during labour. When the pain of labour is prevented by lumbar epidural block in human labour, neither maternal nor fetal cortisol levels increase (Thornton et al 1976, Cawson et al 1974). Glucocorticoid administration to human mothers does not reduce progesterone or increase oestrogen levels as it does in the sheep.

If increased fetal adrenal activity has any role in human parturition, its mechanism of action remains unknown. DHEA sulphate (DHEAS) is a fetal adrenal steroid of major importance which could have a potential role in human labour as an oestrogen precursor. DHEAS of both maternal and fetal origin contributes equally to placental oestradiol-17β synthesis, whereas the contribution of maternal DHEAS to oestriol production is less than 10% (Siiteri & Macdonald 1966). During pregnancy, maternal metabolic clearance of DHEAS increases (Gant et al 1971) with a progressive fall in maternal plasma DHEAS, although the level in amniotic fluid tends to increase (Turnbull et al 1977). Mochizuki & Tojo (1980) have demonstrated that intravenous injection of DHEAS in late human pregnancy seems to accelerate softening and dilatation of the cervix in comparison with controls, probably by causing increased concentrations of oestradiol-17β in the maternal serum, myometrium and cervix, and perhaps also by activating collagenolytic activity in the cervix.

These findings suggest gradually increasing fetal adrenal activity with effects on placental biosynthesis over the last few weeks of human pregnancy, rather than a relatively sudden change like that in sheep pregnancy. Decreased maternal levels of progesterone before human labour have been reported in only two studies (Caspo et al 1971, Turnbull et al 1974), both conducted serially in primigravidae and collected with the strictest possible criteria of normality. Progesterone withdrawal did not occur in every case before labour, however, and oestradiol and progesterone levels during labour were the same as those 1 week before labour (Turnbull et al 1974). Further studies by Bibby (1980) demonstrated the same continuing increase in progesterone and oestradiol in late human pregnancy found in most other studies. Figures 28.5 and 28.6 show how the findings in his cases compared with those of Turnbull et al (1974). In human peripheral venous blood, the levels of both oestrogens and progesterone seem to increase up to the onset of term and preterm labour. Salivary steroid concentrations are thought to reflect the circulating concentrations of the free hormone and hence may be more biologically relevant than the total plasma concentration or the urinary excretion of a metabolite. Recently, Darne et al (1987) reported an increase in the salivary oestriol : progesterone ratio most marked in the 5 weeks before spontaneous human labour.

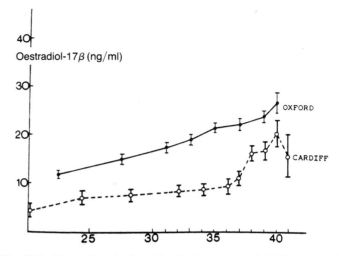

Fig. 28.5 Mean (± SEM) of peripheral plasma oestradiol-17β measured serially during pregnancy in 23 normal women of mixed parity in Oxford and 33 normal Cardiff primigravidae, from 20 weeks until the spontaneous onset of labour. Oxford women were investigated by Bibby (1980); Cardiff women were investigated by Turnbull et al (1974).

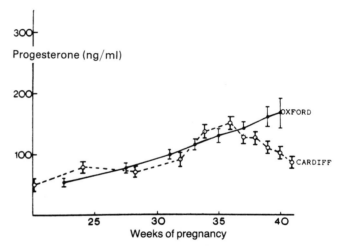

Fig. 28.6 Mean (± SEM) levels of peripheral plasma progesterone measured serially in 23 normal women of mixed parity in Oxford and 33 normal Cardiff primigravidae from 20 weeks' gestation until the spontaneous onset of labour. Oxford women were investigated by Bibby (1980); Cardiff women were investigated by Turnbull et al (1974).

However, these findings were not confirmed in another study in Australian women by Lewis et al (1987).

These findings do not exclude the possibility that changes in oestrogens or progesterone in target tissues may play a crucial role in the initiation of labour. As will be described later, increased prostaglandin secretion plays a key role in the initiation of parturition. Prostaglandins are synthesized in the amnion, chorion and decidua; Mitchell et al (1982) have shown that unconjugated oestrogens and DHEA may be capable both of stimulating the synthesis of prostaglandins in dispersed cell preparations of fetal membranes and also of inhibiting progesterone synthesis in the decidua and chorion. Thus, these tissues could be subjected to local progesterone withdrawal and increased oestrogen action great enough to initiate labour without any detectable change in peripheral hormone levels. Lopez-Bernal et al (1986b) demonstrated that Epostane, which inhibits the conversion of pregnenolone to progesterone, will almost completely inhibit progesterone synthesis both by the human placenta and the choriodecidua. Tissues obtained at term are more sensitive than those obtained early in pregnancy. In adequate dosage, Epostane can induce abortion or facilitate the effect of prostaglandins (Pattison et al 1985, Webster et al 1985, Selinger et al 1987). However, no reduction in progesterone production by the chorion or decidua was demonstrated in relation to the spontaneous onset of human labour by Lopez-Bernal et al (1987b). Nevertheless, progesterone withdrawal is such an important feature of the initiation of labour in so many species that local progesterone inhibition and its release remain a regulatory option for human pregnancy maintenance and the initiation of labour. This possible mechanism has not been finally excluded although it is now largely discounted. It appears that progesterone is essential for the maintenance of human pregnancy but that human parturition begins and progresses to the birth of the fetus without progesterone being withdrawn as occurs in some other species.

MYOMETRIAL GAP JUNCTIONS

Garfield et al (1979) demonstrated myometrial cell contacts termed gap junctions, which are thought to represent low-resistance pathways to the flow of excitation, in uterine muscle obtained from guinea-pigs and sheep at delivery or post-partum. In human tissues, they were also present in a much higher proportion of samples after the onset of spontaneous labour than before it. Gap junctions are composed of symmetrical portions of the plasma membrane from two opposing cells; intermembranous protein particles protrude through each membrane to span the gap between the membranes. The structure of myometrial gap junctions is similar to that described in other cells (Fig. 28.7).

Garfield et al (1979) proposed that gap junctions between myometrial cells were essential for the development of the effective uterine muscle contractility which leads to the expulsion of the uterine contents in pregnancy in all animals, including man. In rats and sheep, progesterone withdrawal appears necessary for their formation, again raising the possibility that in some subtle way progesterone withdrawal may initiate human labour. Alternatively, and probably more likely with human parturition, prostaglandins can stimulate gap junction formation, according to Garfield et al (1979). The authors claim that oxytocin does not possess this ability and cannot stimulate

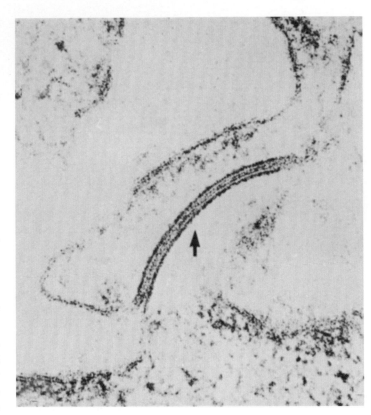

Fig. 28.7 Gap junction (arrow) between two muscle cells from the myometrium of a ewe obtained during parturition (thin section ×200 000). From Verhoeff & Garfield (1986).

myometrium in the absence of gap junctions. Additional support for the hypothesis of increased prostaglandin alone being enough to activate the uterus and expel its contents is provided by the work of Manabe et al (1981) who investigated the Japanese method for inducing midtrimester abortion—inserting a balloon catheter into the lower uterine cavity through the cervix and applying prolonged traction. This method, which reliably causes abortion, often of a live fetus, has no effect on plasma levels of oestradiol, oestriol or progesterone. Although Manabe et al (1981) did not measure prostaglandin levels in their cases, studies by Mitchell et al (1977b) and by Keirse et al (1983), which demonstrated that cervical manipulation increases levels of prostaglandin metabolites in peripheral blood, suggest that the Japanese technique probably induces abortion by causing prolonged or repeated release of PGF, which must also lead to the formation of gap junctions, since abortion occurs.

Prostaglandins

The mechanism which controls prostaglandin synthesis in the pregnant human uterus and initiates the onset of labour remains unknown. This may seem surprising, considering how much the phenomenon has been

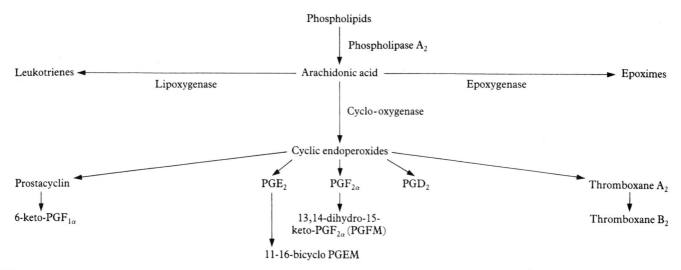

Fig. 28.8 Pathways from phospholipids to prostaglandins, prostacyclin, thromboxane, and their major metabolites and to leukotrienes and epoximes.

investigated and the importance of prostaglandins in labour in most species (Liggins 1979). The difficulty in elucidating the regulation of human labour is that it seems to be of a paracrine nature; that is, it resides largely within the uterus and is determined by interactions between contiguous cells (Liggins 1981) rather than by changes in circulating levels of hormones. It is therefore a paracrine rather than an endocrine control system, and shares with other paracrine systems the problems of complexity and inaccessibility.

Biosynthesis of prostaglandins

Figure 28.8 illustrates the main pathways of synthesis and metabolism of prostanoids from arachidonic acid—the arachidonic acid cascade. Measurement of PGE and PGF in peripheral plasma is hampered by their low concentrations, due to their rapid clearance, especially in the lungs. Measurement of the main, stable PGF metabolite, 13,14-dihydro-15-keto-PGF (PGFM) in peripheral plasma is a better measurement of PGF production. Measurement of the same PGE metabolite (PGEM) is hindered by its instability. While the 11–16 bicyclo-PGEM metabolite is stable, its concentration does not change significantly during pregnancy or with the onset of progression of labour to delivery, in contrast to the several-fold increase in the plasma concentration of PGFM during human labour (Demers et al 1983). However, bicyclo-PGEM assay can be reliably used to detect and measure increases in plasma following administration of exogenous prostaglandins (Brennecke et al 1985).

Arachidonic acid is converted into prostaglandin endoperoxides, from which are formed all the prostaglandins of the 2 series, as well as thromboxane A_2. Cyclo-oxygenase, the enzyme catalysing the formation of prostaglandins

from arachidonic acid, is present in cells either in an active form, or is readily activated. The rate of prostaglandin synthesis is controlled more by the rate of release of arachidonic acid than the activity of cyclo-oxygenase. Factors which activate phospholipase A_2 are therefore likely to be of greater importance in stimulating the increased prostaglandin which initiates labour than those which activate cyclo-oxygenase. Little is so far known of the factors which determine the extent to which free arachidonic acid is metabolized via cyclo-oxygenase to prostaglandin or by lipoxygenase to leukotrienes.

During pregnancy, peripheral blood levels of PGFM show little change but increase massively during labour (Fig. 28.9; Sellers et al 1981a, Mitchell 1984). This demonstrates the importance of metabolite assays in revealing prostaglandin production in labour. By contrast, there were no significant increases in peripheral plasma concentrations of PGE or PGF during labour (Mitchell et al 1978a).

Measurements made in amniotic fluid first demonstrated the increase in prostaglandins during labour. Since

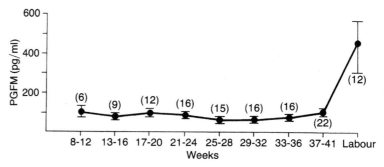

Fig. 28.9 Peripheral plasma concentrations (mean ± SEM) number of samples (in parentheses) of 13,14-dihydro-15-keto-PGF (PGFM) in 16 women throughout pregnancy and labour. From Mitchell (1984).

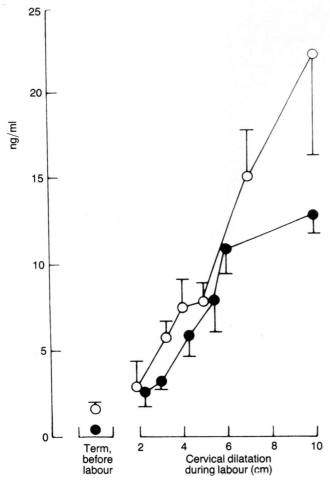

Fig. 28.10 Mean concentrations (± SEM) of PGE$_2$ (●) and PGF$_{2\alpha}$ (○) in amniotic fluid during late pregnancy and labour at term. After data from Keirse & Turnbull (1973) and Keirse et al (1974).

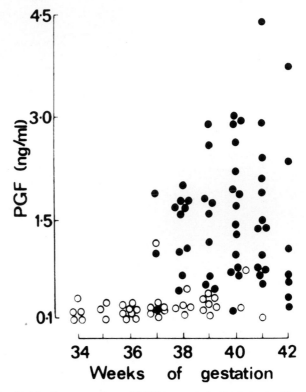

Fig. 28.11 Concentrations of PGF in amniotic fluid obtained by amniocentesis (●) and by amniotomy (○) before the onset of labour. Adapted from Mitchell et al (1977a).

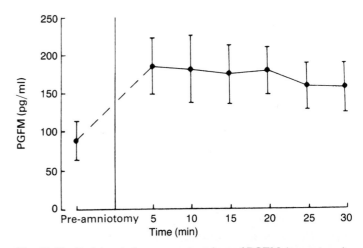

Fig. 28.12 Peripheral plasma concentrations of PGFM (mean ± SEM) before and for 30 min after amniotomy. Adapted from Sellers et al (1980).

none of the tissues which surround it contain prostaglandin-metabolizing enzymes, amniotic fluid concentrations of prostaglandins are high and increase rapidly as labour progresses. The concentration of PGF increases more rapidly than that of PGE (Fig. 28.10).

An early publication (Hibbard et al 1974) suggested that prostaglandin levels in amniotic fluid increased progressively from 36 weeks towards term. We could not demonstrate this trend when samples obtained by amniotomy at rupture of the membranes were separated from those obtained by amniocentesis (Fig. 28.11).

The raised levels of PGF in amniotic fluid obtained by amniotomy in comparison with amniocentesis were among the first observations to suggest a local intrauterine control of prostaglandin biosynthesis. This concept was also favoured by subsequent findings that peripheral plasma levels of PGFM were elevated within 5 minutes of amniotomy and remained high for at least 30 minutes thereafter (Fig. 28.12). This initial increase in PGFM is not associated with the onset of labour, which seems to depend on a secondary and continuing increase in PGFM (Sellers et al 1981c).

Regulation of prostaglandins for the initiation of human labour

At present, the mechanism which brings about the increased levels of prostaglandins found in association with human labour remains unknown. Even the source of the increased prostaglandins is not entirely resolved. In reviewing the whole field, however, Casey & MacDonald (1986) concluded: 'increased synthesis of PGE_2 in amnion is the key event in the onset of labour'. The authors suggest that increased prostaglandin synthesis in the amnion results either from an increase in the rate of release of arachidonic acid from glycerophospholipids, or an increase in the activity of the prostaglandin synthetase in amnion, or from both. They believed that these changes depended on a fetal signal, possibly reaching the amnion through fetal urine which stimulates increased PGE_2 synthesis by amnion (Casey et al 1983). Since fetal urine samples obtained before labour also exert this effect, other regulatory mechanisms must be involved. More recently, Casey & MacDonald (1988) have suggested that human pregnancy maintenance depends on the inhibition of $PGF_{2\alpha}$ formation in decidua, and that the onset of labour therefore results from release of inhibition of decidual $PGF_{2\alpha}$ synthesis.

Sites of prostaglandin synthesis

Early studies of prostaglandin production from the uterus usually assumed that the main source of $PGF_{2\alpha}$ was the myometrium. However, early studies in the pregnant sheep by Liggins & Greaves (1971) showed that at the onset of parturition when the concentration of $PGF_{2\alpha}$ was rising in the uterine vein, the concentration of $PGF_{2\alpha}$ was elevated in the maternal component of the placental cotyledon but only later in the myometrium. This suggested that the prostaglandin in the myometrium had diffused there from the uterine epithelium. Both in the pregnant sheep uterus (Campos et al 1980) and in the non-pregnant human uterus (Abel et al 1980) the uterine epithelium or endometrium predominantly converts arachidonic acid to $PGF_{2\alpha}$ and PGE_2, whereas the myometrium produces mainly prostacyclin (PGI_2). An additional site of prostaglandin synthesis is the cervix. During incubation of sheep cervical tissues, substantial quantities of prostanoids are released into the medium, predominantly PGE_2 and PGI_2 (Ellwood et al 1981). The parturient cervix releases greater quantities than the non-parturient. The concentration of PGE_2 and PGI_2 in the cervical vein of sheep increases sharply at the time when cervical ripening begins. Ellwood et al (1980b) also investigated the potential of the pregnant human cervix to produce prostaglandins. Tissues obtained during the first trimester of pregnancy produced PGE, PGF, PGFM and 6-keto-$PGF_{1\alpha}$ when superfused in vitro. Thromboxane B_2 (TXB_2) production was minimal. Preliminary evidence from tissues taken at Caesarean hysterectomy during the third trimester of human pregnancy suggested that at this stage the cervix may exhibit greater production of prostaglandin production (Fig. 28.13). Hence, the human cervix may

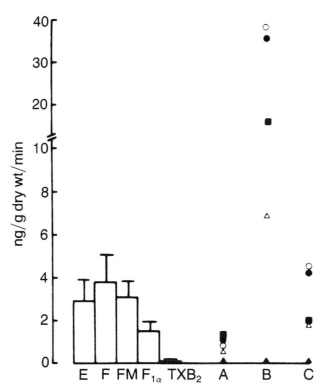

Fig. 28.13 Prostanoid production rates in cervical tissues obtained from three women in the third trimester of pregnancy are shown in comparison with the mean rates found in cervical tissues from women in the first trimester. Patient A: elective Caesarean section at 37 weeks; patient B: emergency Caesarean section at 34 weeks, 6–7 cm dilatation; patient C: emergency Caesarean section at 40 weeks, full dilatation. For each patient, the production rates are shown for PGE (●), PGF (○), PGFM (△), 6-oxo-$PGF_{1\alpha}$ (■) and TBX_2 (▲). Each point represents the mean of between four and six measurements. Adapted from Ellwood et al (1980b).

produce prostaglandins in vivo which could act locally during pregnancy and contribute to cervical softening and dilatation over the last few weeks of pregnancy—unlike the sheep—as well as contributing to the accelerating dilatation which characterizes labour.

In reviewing prostaglandin synthesis in human parturition, Casey & MacDonald (1986) agree that prostaglandin synthesis in the fetal membranes and decidua plays a central role in the initiation of labour. In the amnion, PGE_2 is by far the most important prostaglandin produced and since there is little or no 15-keto-prostaglandin dehydrogenase (PGDH) in amnion, the large quantities of PGE_2 formed are not metabolized. However, the human myometrium is capable of actively metabolizing PGE_2 to $PGF_{2\alpha}$ because it is an important source of PG-9-oxo-reductase activity (Canete Soler et al 1987). While the chorion also synthesizes PGE_2 and the decidua synthesizes PGE_2 and $PGF_{2\alpha}$, both tissues show considerable prostaglandin dehydrogenase activity which tends quickly to inactivate the prostaglandins synthesized.

The availability of free arachidonic acid also appears to be an important rate-limiting factor in the synthesis of prostaglandins. Table 28.1 shows the result of studies of

Table 28.1   Prostaglandin E production by collagenase-dispersed amnion cells (pmol/10^6 cells/3 h) (from Lopez Bernal et al 1987a)

	Spontaneous labour ($n = 14$)	Elective Caesarean section ($n = 9$)	Induced labour ($n = 6$)
Basal	27.5 ± 5.5	13.6 ± 2.7	10 ± 3.1
	└── $P = 0.05$ ──┘		
	└──────── $P = 0.02$ ────────┘		
$\pm 10\ \mu mol/l$ Arachidonic acid	$46.6+ \pm 5.8$	39.3 ± 7.8	32.9 ± 6.5

Mean $\pm$ SEM.

PGE_2 synthesis of collagenase-dispersed amnion cells in culture, comparing samples obtained from women during continuing pregnancy and those during labour at delivery (Lopez-Bernal et al 1987a). The rate of PGE_2 synthesis is greater in the amnion samples obtained from women in labour. When arachidonic acid is added to these cultures, however, the differences between samples obtained from continuing late pregnancy and labour almost disappear, indicating that the previous difference simply depended on the greater availability of arachidonic acid during labour.

Regulation of increased prostaglandin biosynthesis in labour

Gustavii (1978) suggested that phospholipase A_2 was released from decidual lysosomes destabilized by the local withdrawal of progesterone and increase of oestrogens. Increased phospholipase A_2 activity would stimulate the release of free arachidonic acid from membranes as well as phospholipids. In fact, human amniotic fluid contains much more arachidonic acid than is required for the amount of prostaglandin synthesized in labour and the same is true of uterine muscle (Keirse et al 1977). However, as these workers point out, the intracellular availability of arachidonic acid for prostaglandin-synthesizing enzymes is unknown and could be an important regulatory factor.

Inhibition of prostaglandin biosynthesis during pregnancy

Maathius & Kelly (1978) demonstrated that the concentration of prostaglandins in human pregnancy decidua is lower in pregnancy than that in the endometrium at any stage of the normal menstrual cycle. Apparently the human conceptus somehow interferes with endometrial synthesis or metabolism of PGE and PGF soon after plantation. There were extremely low levels of both PGF and PGE in endometrium early in pregnancy at a conceptual age of about 17 days. The prostaglandin levels in normal late secretory endometrium were about 200 times greater than in early pregnancy. Increased oestrogen and progesterone levels do not suppress prostaglandin synthesis, for in non-pregnant endometrium, high levels of oestradiol and progesterone are associated with high prostaglandin levels.

These findings, coupled with the great excess of arachidonic acid over PGE and PGF in amniotic fluid and uterine tissues in late human pregnancy (Keirse et al 1977), suggest that human pregnancy maintenance may depend on inhibition of prostaglandin synthesis in intrauterine tissues, particularly decidua. The fact that decidual prostaglandins are suppressed even when the pregnancy is extrauterine (Abel et al 1980) suggests that the factors may have a systemic rather than a local action.

Saeed et al (1977) discovered that mammalian plasma inhibited bovine seminal vesical prostaglandin synthase because it contained endogenous inhibitors of prostaglandin synthesis (EIPS) in blood protein fractions rich in haptoglobin and albumin, respectively. Brennecke et al (1982, 1985) investigated EIPS in human pregnancy but found similar activities in the plasma of non-pregnant women; men; women in the first and second trimesters of pregnancy, and at full term and postpartum. There appeared to be a small but significant decrease in EIPS activities in plasma samples obtained from women in the third trimester and from those at full term, but since this was not maintained in labour or the puerperium, a decrease in EIPS is not the cause of the increased prostaglandin formation during labour.

Although measurement of EIPS activity has not clarified the mechanism which inhibits prostaglandin synthesis effectively in human pregnancy, Mortimer et al (1985) demonstrated that amnion obtained from pregnant women could contain an endogenous prostaglandin synthetase inhibitor which was no longer present in amnion obtained from women during labour. Wilson et al (1985) have demonstrated in amniotic fluid two proteins which can inhibit PGF synthesis in human endometrial cells. These proved to be novel endogenous proteins which inhibited endometrial cell phospholipase A_2. These inhibitors could be identified in amniotic fluid from women with continuing pregnancy but not from fluid obtained in labour. Wilson (1988) has recently reviewed progress in this field. One of the proteins is a dimer of the other and had been called chorionic inhibitor of phospholipase. It resembles lipocortin in many ways and is not glucocorticoid-dependent. Work continues in this exciting area.

Prostanoids in the fetal and neonatal circulation

This topic has been reviewed by Turnbull et al (1981). Table 28.2 shows the levels of prostaglandins in the maternal circulation in late pregnancy and late labour and in the umbilical circulation after spontaneous delivery. The concentrations of PGE, PGF and PGFM are much higher in the umbilical than in the maternal circulation in either pregnancy or labour. Prostaglandin levels

Table 28.2 Prostaglandins in maternal and umbilical circulation at term (pg/ml) (after Mitchell et al 1978a,b)

	Maternal circulation		Umbilical (spontaneous labour)	
	Late pregnancy ($n = 13$)	Late labour (cervix 5–8 cm) ($n = 5$)	Artery ($n = 12$)	Vein ($n = 12$)
PGE	4.8 ± 1.0	5.4 ± 2.2	109.3 ± 26.9	241.9 ± 24.9
PGF	6.2 ± 0.5	12.4 ± 3.5	79.7 ± 10.4	87.8 ± 11.1
PGFM	59.0 ± 6.7	282.7 ± 55.3	639.9 ± 180.2	630.8 ± 107.3

Mean ± SEM.

are higher in the umbilical vein than in the artery, indicating that the increased PGE must be of maternal rather than fetal origin.

Prostaglandins have a role in the control of fetal and placental haemodynamics and influence the fetal circulation. Respiratory distress syndrome is associated with high levels of PGF in the infant's circulation, and patent ductus arteriosus with high levels of PGE (Turnbull et al 1981). The fact that PGE can open the ductus and that inhibitors of PG synthesis (PGSI) can close the ductus indicates the importance of prostaglandins in the fetus and also shows that use of PGSI in pregnancy or labour can lead to potentially dangerous intrauterine ductal closure. This may occur if PGSI are given to treat preterm labour. They could cross the placenta, cause in utero closure of the ductus arteriosus and lead to increased pulmonary arterial pressure, associated with hyperplasia of the fetal pulmonary vascular smooth muscle and leading eventually to persistent pulmonary hypertension of the newborn (Wilkinson et al 1979). This complication can result from unusually low circulating levels of PGE in the neonate caused by excessive levels of PGSI (Wilkinson et al 1979). Great caution must therefore be exercised before prescribing treatment with PGSI during pregnancy. Nowadays, however, the benefit of prolonging intrauterine existence for even a few days more may be vital when preterm delivery threatens at 25–26 weeks. The benefits may outweigh the potential hazards of PGSI as additional tocolytics. The human ductus arteriosus does not contain prostaglandin receptors before 21 weeks and the gestational age at which these receptors develop is not known, but probably varies to some extent from one fetus to another (Lopez-Bernal et al 1986a).

OXYTOCIN

Although oxytocin has been extensively used for the induction and augmentation of labour, there has been much uncertainty about its importance in the normal physiological onset and maintenance of human labour. Maternal oxytocin levels are only of the order of a few microunits and show little or no change before labour. Fetal oxytocin by comparison increases significantly in association with spontaneous labour (Chard et al 1971). Since the increase is greater in umbilical arterial than

venous plasma (Chard 1977), oxytocin must be synthesized by the fetus and seems to be transferred from fetus to mother (Dawood et al 1978a).

Of critical importance has been the discovery that the concentration of oxytocin receptors in human myometrium and decidua increases during late pregnancy and also considerably in relation to labour, indicating that labour results from increasing sensitivity of the uterus to oxytocin, so that the uterus can be stimulated by an oxytocin level in maternal blood which would have had no effect previously when the concentration of myometrial oxytocin receptors was low (Fuchs et al 1982, Husslein 1985).

Maternal oxytocin

Oxytocin levels have been investigated increasingly in recent years, with the development of sensitive radioimmunoassays. The earlier data were reported by Chard et al (1970), who were initially unable to detect oxytocin in maternal plasma during pregnancy or labour, but found measurable amounts in 40% of mixed umbilical cord plasma samples. Subsequently, Chard et al (1971) identified oxytocin in the peripheral circulation of some women during labour. The frequency of positive values gradually increased during the first stage and reached a maximum of 60% of positive values during delivery, implying spurt release of oxytocin from the posterior pituitary gland (Gibbens et al 1972). Several recent studies have detected oxytocin in maternal plasma throughout pregnancy and labour (Kumaresan et al 1974, Dawood et al 1978b, Vasicka et al 1978, Leake et al 1979). The studies in Oxford by Sellers et al (1981b) showed measurable concentrations of oxytocin in 93% of maternal plasma samples during pregnancy (Fig. 28.14). Values varied widely between patients throughout pregnancy, ranging from less than 1 to 27 pg/ml. There was no change in maternal plasma oxytocin concentration during early or late labour. These findings agreed with those of Kumaresan et al (1974), Gazárek et al (1976) and Vasicka et al (1978). However, Dawood et al (1978b) found higher levels in second-stage labour and Leake et al (1979) found high levels at delivery of the fetal head. Disparity in the results may be due to the spurt release of oxytocin; blood may not have been sampled frequently enough during labour to demonstrate a change in levels.

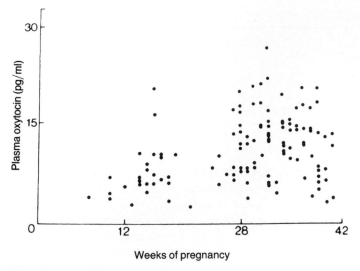

Fig. 28.14 Maternal plasma oxytocin concentrations during pregnancy. From Sellers et al (1981b).

Oxytocin receptors

The concentration of oxytocin receptors in the myometrium correlates well with the sensitivity of the uterus to oxytocin. Table 28.3 shows the concentration of oxytocin receptors in the human myometrium in the non-pregnant state, during early and late pregnancy and in early labour, and demonstrates the dramatic increase in labour found by Fuchs et al (1982). There are also marked increases in oxytocin receptors in the decidua. Treating decidual cells with oxytocin causes release of prostaglandins (Fuchs et al 1981), confirming the mechanism which had earlier been demonstrated by Mitchell et al (1977b) that vaginal examination in late human pregnancy causes increased blood levels of prostaglandins in maternal blood, reaching a peak 5 minutes after examination. Examination stimulates the Ferguson reflex, by which a neural afferent from the cervix causes oxytocin release from the posterior pituitary. The humoral effect depends on the oxytocin being taken up by decidual oxytocin receptors which promote decidual prostaglandin release.

Table 28.3 Oxytocin receptors in the myometrium and decidua (fmol/ng DNA) (from Fuchs et al 1982)

	Myometrium		Decidua	
	n	Receptor concentration	n	Receptor concentration
Non-pregnant: menstruating	14	27.6 ± 7.97	6	24.9 ± 5.59
Pregnant: 13–17 weeks	5	171.6 ± 67.4	1	629
Pre-term labour: 28–36 weeks	8	2353 ± 358	8	3673 ± 947
Before labour: 37–43 weeks	6	1391 ± 180	6	1510 ± 302
Early labour: 37–43 weeks	5	3458 ± 886	3	3177 ± 1426
Advanced labour*: 37–43 weeks	7	257 ± 104	2	786

*Samples taken from lower uterine segment.
Mean ± SEM.

Clearly, the initiation of labour depends not so much on the oxytocin level itself as on the mechanism which induces oxytocin receptors in the myometrium. Liggins (1973) showed in the sheep that continuous intravenous infusion of relatively small doses of prostaglandins in late pregnancy caused increasing myometrial responsiveness both to prostaglandins and to oxytocin after several hours. A similar response has been observed in human pregnancy (Liggins et al 1977b). The basis of this sensitization is unknown, but could result from the formation of gap junctions. Liggins' observations suggest that gap junctions could be formed by continuous myometrial stimulation with low levels of prostaglandins. Indomethacin, a prostaglandin synthase inhibitor, partly inhibits gap junction formation in vitro (Garfield et al 1980).

Fetal oxytocin

Fetal oxytocin has been investigated by Chard et al (1970, 1971) and more recently by Dawood et al (1978a) and Sellers et al (1981b). The mean oxytocin concentrations in umbilical arterial and venous plasma collected after labour following spontaneous vaginal delivery, and before labour at elective Caesarean section, reported by Sellers et al (1981b) are shown in Figure 28.15. These levels are very similar to those found both by Dawood et al (1978a) and Chard et al (1971), with a significant arteriovenous oxytocin difference in samples obtained before and after labour. Umbilical arterial plasma oxytocin levels are consistently higher than umbilical venous levels. The levels in both fetal umbilical arterial and venous plasma are significantly higher than in maternal plasma. Initiation and maintenance of human labour may therefore be influenced by fetal oxytocin. Dawood et al (1978a) calculated

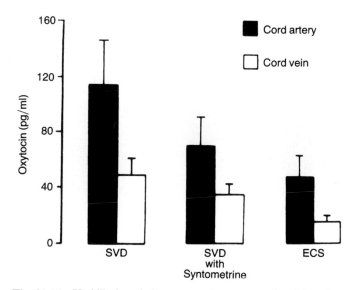

Fig. 28.15 Umbilical cord plasma oxytocin concentration. Mean ± SEM. SVD = spontaneous vaginal delivery; ECS = elective Caesarean section. From Sellers et al (1981b).

that the fetal oxytocin secretion rate could be as high as 2.75 ± 0.5 mu/min (mean ± SEM) in infants delivered by Caesarean section after the spontaneous onset of labour. By contrast, in infants delivered by elective Caesarean section before labour, the calculated oxytocin secretion rate was only 1.0 ± 0.2 mu/min. Fetal oxytocin secretion rates in infants delivered after spontaneous labour were around 3 mu/min, similar to the dose of oxytocin of around 2–8 mu/min, which is normally administered to women to induce labour at term.

The situation should not be over-simplified. Chard et al (1971) showed that spontaneous labour was also associated with an even greater increase in vasopressin than oxytocin in the fetal circulation. Furthermore, the possible influence of low and unchanging maternal oxytocin levels on human uterine contractility may be of primary importance in initiating labour, since the uterus will become increasingly sensitive to its potential effects as the concentration of myometrial oxytocin receptors increases.

Relaxin, prolactin and prostaglandins

Relaxin, prolactin and prostaglandins all appear to be paracrine hormones of the human amnion, chorion and decidua and to be involved in parturition. While the role of prostaglandins is well established, the specific effects of relaxin and prolactin remain to be established (Bryant-Greenwood et al 1987). According to MacLennan (1983), the polypeptide hormone relaxin is thought in mammals to promote connective tissue remodelling during reproduction, inhibition of myometrial contractility until late pregnancy and cervical ripening at parturition. In fact, little is known about the actions of relaxin and it is only recently that an analogue of human relaxin has been synthesized and used to develop a radioimmunoassay with which Eddie et al (1986) measured blood levels of relaxin in human pregnancy. Relaxin was not detectable in men or in non-pregnant women, but was present in all serial blood samples collected from three pregnant women. Concentrations ranged from 0.9 to 1.18 ng/ml; the highest levels were in the first trimester and almost all the readings after 24 weeks were under 0.5 ng/ml and showed no consistent rising or falling trend. MacLennan et al (1986) measured relaxin blood levels in 368 samples from 302 pregnant women between 6 and 41 weeks' gestation, using a guinea-pig relaxin antiserum utilizing a porcine label and a porcine standard. The levels they found were similar to those of Eddie et al (1986) and significantly lower levels were also found in the third trimester than in the first or second. In one woman in whom the subsequent onset of labour was preterm, relaxin levels fell steadily, below the 95% confidence levels for normal pregnancy.

Relaxin appears to be produced particularly by the cells of the chorionic cytotrophoblast (Bryant-Greenwood et al 1987) and only half the tissues after spontaneous delivery contained positive relaxin-stained cells, whereas all the tissues from elective Caesarean section contained cells positively stained with antiserum to relaxin.

Prolactin was positively localized in the decidua and occasionally also in the amnion (Bryant-Greenwood et al 1987). Prostaglandin synthase was previously localized in the amnion and chorion. Recently Lopez-Bernal et al (1987b) have demonstrated that relaxin, present in the chorion laeve and decidua at term, may have a paracrine effect on the amnion, inhibiting PGE production during continuing pregnancy but favouring its production during spontaneous labour. These findings may help to explain the mechanism by which local vaginal application of purified porcine relaxin facilitates cervical ripening and induction of labour (MacLennan et al 1980).

CONCLUSIONS

Parturition in human pregnancy, unlike that in the sheep and some other species, is not preceded by dramatic changes in maternal peripheral plasma levels of oestradiol or progesterone. Fetal cortisol secretion does not suddenly increase before labour, nor does it have any effects on the endocrine function of the fetal placenta as it does in the sheep. Maternal administration of corticosteroids in human pregnancy simply suppresses maternal and fetal adrenocortical function, causing a fall in maternal oestrogen levels.

The maintenance of human pregnancy may depend on a mechanism which tonically inhibits prostaglandin synthesis in uterine tissues. Unlike the sheep, human myometrium is relatively sensitive to prostaglandins throughout pregnancy. Human amnion and decidua are capable of synthesizing prostaglandins in vitro at any stage of pregnancy and labour may depend on the withdrawal of potent inhibitors of prostaglandin synthesis from these tissues. The inhibitory process normally seems to be particularly effective in early pregnancy and may lessen as pregnancy advances. It may involve the presence in intrauterine tissues of lipocortins capable of synthesizing prostaglandins. We have been unable to demonstrate obvious effects of oestrogen or progesterone on PGE production by fetal membranes or decidua (Lopez-Bernal et al 1987c).

In late human pregnancy, the prostaglandin-synthesizing mechanism seems to be readily, if transiently, activated by minor local stimuli such as vaginal examination, sweeping the membranes or amniotomy. The stable PGFM increases markedly within 5 minutes of amniotomy and the increase persists for 30 minutes afterwards. While Sellers et al (1980) could not show this increase to be associated with oxytocin release, as in the sheep, Chard & Gibbens (1983) demonstrated that amniotomy does cause a transient increase in maternal plasma oxytocin levels, indicating that the Ferguson reflex may be involved in human as well as in sheep pregnancy.

It has been shown (Sellers et al 1981c) that an increase in maternal PGFM levels occurs in all patients immediately following amniotomy, but that this increase is transient. The onset of progressive labour depends on a subsequent continuing increase in PGFM, usually associated with a steady increase in uterine contractility.

It has proved difficult to measure the changes in PGE at the onset of labour in human pregnancy. PGEM proved to be unstable (Granström et al 1980). Radioimmunoassay of a stable metabolite (biocyclo-PGEM) was developed (Demers et al 1983). Although this effectively measured increased blood levels when exogenous PGE was administered, it showed no change in level during human pregnancy, labour or the puerperium, implying that if increased PGE_2 is secreted by uterine tissues during labour, it must somehow be retained with the uterus. There is, however, indirect evidence that PGE_2 increases in the fetal circulation in the 48–72 hours before the onset of labour. Boddy et al (1974) showed that fetal breathing movements ceased during that period and Castle & Turnbull (1983) have reviewed the evidence that in man and animals, increasing the level of PGE in the fetal circulation inhibits fetal breathing, while intrafetal infusion of a prostaglandin synthetase inhibitor stimulates breathing. It is possible that a local increase in PGE levels occurring in uterine tissues 48–72 hours before labour may therefore initiate the whole process of human parturition.

The increasing synthesis of PGE and PGF in the human uterus at term can undoubtedly bring about all the features of progressive labour—in the uterine muscle, powerful coordinated contractions; in the cervix, breakdown and fibrillation of collagen fibres and other connective tissue changes associated with cervical softening and increased extensibility (Ellwood et al 1979, 1980b, Ellwood 1981). Working together, these factors can bring about dilatation and effacement of the cervix, formation of the lower uterine segment, rupture of the membranes and the whole process of labour and parturition, culminating in the safe and effective delivery of the infant and placenta.

The action of oxytocin has, in recent years, been shown to play an important role in human labour. This is not due to elevation of the oxytocin level in the maternal circulation but to a large increase in the concentration of oxytocin receptors in the myometrium and in the decidua, sensitizing the uterus to the effects of oxytocin already present in maternal blood. Stimulating decidual cells with oxytocin causes prostaglandin release. In labour, dilatation of the cervix and vagina can stimulate oxytocin secretion through the Ferguson reflex, causing increased prostaglandin release from the decidua. Once the excitation system has been activated, it therefore leads to accelerating labour progress as in other species.

In the human fetus, high levels of oxytocin are found in the umbilical arterial blood after vaginal delivery—higher than in the umbilical vein blood—indicating a fetal origin for the oxytocin. Cord blood oxytocin levels are much lower before the onset of labour but it is not known if the increased fetal production of oxytocin (and vasopressin) plays a part in the initiation or maintenance of human labour.

Prostaglandins are also involved in the third stage of labour. PGFM levels in the maternal circulation rise in the first and second stages of labour but much more after delivery of the baby, reaching their highest levels 5 min after delivery (Sellers et al 1982). While these prostaglandins probably originate in the uterus, the factors controlling their release are unknown. The surge of prostaglandins after delivery of the fetus is likely to influence expulsion of the placenta and fetal membranes.

Although intramuscular administration of a mixture of ergometrine and oxytocin (Syntometrine) has been used in the UK for many years to facilitate delivery of the placenta by controlled traction and to reduce postpartum haemorrhage, there have been several reports in which severe postpartum haemorrhage could not be controlled until PGF or PGE was administered by intravenous or intramyometrial injection (Henson et al 1983).

While there is increased understanding of the factors which maintain human pregnancy and initiate labour at term, much remains to be done before full understanding is achieved.

REFERENCES

Abel M H, Smith S K, Baird D T 1980 Suppression of concentration of endometrial prostaglandin in early intrauterine and ectopic pregnancy in women. Journal of Endocrinology 85: 379–386

Anderson A B M 1976 Hormone changes preceding premature labour. In: Turnbull A C, Woodford F P (eds) Prevention of fetal handicap through antenatal care, vol 3. Associated Scientific Publishers, Amsterdam, pp 137–148

Anderson A B M, Flint A P F, Turnbull A C 1975 Mechanism of action of glucocorticoids in induction of ovine parturition: effect on placental steroid metabolism. Journal of Endocrinology 66: 61–70

Bassett J M, Thorburn G D 1969 Fetal plasma corticosteroids and the initiation of parturition in sheep. Journal of Endocrinology 44: 285–288

Bibby J G 1980 Studies in human pregnancy and parturition with particular reference to the role of prostaglandins and steroid hormones. Thesis for MD, University of Otago, Dunedin, New Zealand

Boddy K, Dawes G S, Robinson J 1974 Intra uterine fetal breathing movements. In: Gluck L (ed) Modern perinatal medicine. Year Book Publishers, Chicago, pp 381–390

Brennecke S P, Bryce R L, Turnbull A C 1982 The prostaglandin synthase inhibiting ability of maternal plasma and the onset of human labour. European Journal of Obstetrics and Gynecology and Reproductive Biology 14: 81–88

Brennecke S P, Castle B M, Demers L M. Turnbull A C 1985 Maternal plasma prostaglandin E_2 metabolite levels during human pregnancy and parturition. British Journal of Obstetrics and Gynaecology 92: 345–349

Bryant-Greenwood G D, Rees M C P, Turnbull A C 1987 Immunohistochemical localisation of relaxin, prolactin and prostaglandin synthase in human amnion, chorion and decidua. Journal of Endocrinology 114: 491–496

Campos G A, Liggins G C, Seamark R F 1980 Differential production of PGF and 6-keto-PGF$_{1\alpha}$ by the rat endometrium and myometrium in response to oxytocin, catecholamines and calcium ionophore. Prostaglandins 20: 297–310

Canete Soler R, Lopez-Bernal A, Turnbull A C 1987 Conversion of prostaglandin E$_2$ to prostaglandin F$_{2\alpha}$ by human myometrium. Hormone and Metabolism Research 19: 515–516

Casey M L, MacDonald P C 1986 Initiation of labor in women. In: Huszar G (ed) The physiology and biochemistry of the uterus in pregnancy and labor. CRC Press, Boca Raton, Florida, pp 155–161

Casey M L, MacDonald P C 1988 The role of a fetal–maternal paracrine system in the maintenance of pregnancy and the initiation of parturition. In: Jones C T (ed) Fetal and neonatal development. Perinatology Press, Ithaca, New York

Casey M L, MacDonald P C, Mitchell M D 1983 Stimulation of prostaglandin E$_2$ production in amnion cells in culture by a substance(s) in human fetal and adult urine. Biochemical and Biophysical Research Communications 114: 1056–1063

Castle B M, Turnbull A C 1983 The presence or absence of fetal breathing movements predicts the outcome of preterm labour. Lancet ii: 471–472

Cawson M J, Anderson A B M, Turnbull A C, Lampe L 1974 Cortisol, cortisone and 11-deoxycortisol levels in human umbilical and maternal plasma in relation to the onset of labour. Journal of Obstetrics and Gynaecology of the British Commonwealth 81: 737–745

Challis J R G, Nathanielsz P W 1979 Parturition in small mammals. In: Keirse M J N C, Anderson A B M, Bennebroek Gravenhorst (eds) Human parturition. Leiden University Press, Leiden, pp 1–10

Challis J R G, Robinson J S, Thorburn G D 1977 Fetal and maternal endocrine changes during pregnancy and parturition in the Rhesus monkey. In: Knight J, O'Connor M (eds) The fetus and birth vol 47. Ciba Foundation Symposium. Elsevier/Excerpta Medica/North Holland, Amsterdam, pp 211–228

Chard T 1977 The posterior pituitary gland. In: Fuchs F, Klopper A (eds) Endocrinology of pregnancy. Harper & Row, New York, pp 271–290

Chard T, Gibbens G L D 1983 Spurt release of oxytocin during surgical induction of labor in women. American Journal of Obstetrics and Gynecology 147: 678–680

Chard T, Boyd N R H, Forsling M L, McNeilly A S, London J 1970 The development of a radioimmunoassay for oxytocin: the extraction of oxytocin from plasma and its measurement during parturition in human and goat blood. Journal of Endocrinology 48: 223–234

Chard T, Hudson C N, Edwards C R N 1971 Release of oxytocin and vasopressin by the human fetus during labour. Nature 234: 352–354

Caspo A I, Knobil E, van der Molan H J, Wiest W G 1971 Peripheral plasma progesterone levels during human pregnancy and labor. American Journal of Obstetrics and Gynecology 110: 630–632

Darne J, McGarrigle H H G, Lachelin G C L 1987 Saliva oestriol, oestradiol, oestrone and progesterone levels in pregnancy: spontaneous labour at term is preceded by a rise in the saliva oestriol:progesterone ratio. British Journal of Obstetrics and Gynaecology 94: 227–235

Dawood M Y, Wang C F, Gupta R, Fuchs F 1978a Fetal contribution to oxytocin in human labor. Obstetrics and Gynecology 52: 205–209

Dawood M Y, Raghavan K S, Pociask C, Fuchs F 1978b Oxytocin in human pregnancy and parturition. Obstetrics and Gynecology 51: 138–143

Demers L M, Brennecke S P, Mountford L A, Brunt J D, Turnbull A C 1983 Development and validation of a radioimmunoassay for prostaglandin E$_2$ metabolite levels in plasma. Journal of Clinical Endocrinology and Metabolism 57: 101–106

Eddie L N, Bell R J, Lester A et al 1986 Radioimmunoassay of relaxin in pregnancy with an analogue of human relaxin. Lancet i: 1344–1346

Ellwood D A 1981 The uterine cervix in pregnancy and at parturition. DPhil Thesis, University of Oxford

Ellwood D A, Anderson A B M, Mitchell M D, Turnbull A C 1979 A significant increase in the in-vitro production of prostaglandin E by ovine cervical tissue at delivery. Journal of Endocrinology 81: 133P–134P

Ellwood D A, Mitchell M D, Anderson A B M, Turnbull A C 1980a Specific changes in the in vitro production of prostanoids by the ovine cervix at parturition. Prostaglandins 19: 479–488

Ellwood D A, Mitchell M D, Anderson A B M, Turnbull A C 1980b The in vitro production of prostanoids by the human cervix during pregnancy; preliminary observations. British Journal of Obstetrics and Gynaecology 87: 210–214

Ellwood D A, Anderson A B M, Mitchell M D, Turnbull A C 1981 Prostanoids, collagenase and cervical softening in the sheep. In: Ellwood D A, Anderson A B M (eds) The cervix in pregnancy and labour. Churchill Livingstone, Edinburgh, pp 57–73

Fencl M, Tulchinsky D 1975 Total cortisol in amniotic fluid and fetal lung maturation. New England Journal of Medicine 292: 133–136

Flint A P F, Anderson A B M, Steele P A, Turnbull A C 1975a The mechanism by which fetal cortisol controls the onset of parturition in the sheep. Biochemical Society Transactions 3: 1189–1194

Flint A P F, Forsling M L, Mitchell M D, Turnbull A C 1975b Temporal relationship between changes in oxytocin and prostaglandin F levels in response to vaginal distension in the pregnant and puerperal ewe. Journal of Reproduction and Fertility 43: 551–554

Fuchs A R, Husslein P, Fuchs F 1981 Oxytocin and the initiation of human parturition. II. Stimulation of prostaglandin production in human decidua by oxytocin. American Journal of Obstetrics and Gynecology 141: 694–697

Fuchs A R, Fuchs F, Husslein P, Soloff M S, Fernstrom M J 1982 Oxytocin receptors and parturition, a dual role for oxytocin in the initiation of labor. Science 215: 1396–1398

Gant N F, Hutchinson H T, Siiteri P K, MacDonald P C 1971 Study of the metabolic clearance rate of dehydroisoandrosterone sulfate in pregnancy. American Journal of Obstetrics and Gynecology 111: 555–563

Garfield R E, Rabidean S, Challis J R G, Daniel E E 1979 Ultrastructural basis for maintenance and termination of pregnancy. American Journal of Obstetrics and Gynecology 133: 308–315

Garfield R E, Kannan M S, Daniel E E 1980 Gap junction formation in myometrium; control by oestrogens, progesterone and prostaglandins. American Journal of Physiology 238: C81–C89

Gautray I-P, Jolivet A, Dhem N, Vielk J-P, Tajchner G 1974 Reflexion sur le rôle du foetus dans le déclenchement du travail à terme: exploration du liquide amniotique. In: Bose M J, Palmer R, Savean Cl (eds) Avortement et parturition provoqués. Masson, Paris, pp 227–238

Gazárek F, Polanka J, Talaš M et al 1976 Plasma oxytocin and oxytocinase levels in third trimester of pregnancy and at labour. Endocrinologia Experimentalis 10: 283–287

Gennser G, Ohrlander S, Eneroth P 1977 Fetal cortisol and the initiation of labour in the human. In: Knight J, O'Connor M (eds) The fetus and birth. Elsevier/Excerpta Medica/North Holland, Amsterdam, pp 401–420

Gibbens D, Boyd N R H, Chard T 1972 Spurt release of oxytocin during human labour. Journal of Endocrinology 53: LIV–LV

Granström E, Hamberg M, Hamsson C, Kindhal H 1980 Chemical instability of 15-keto-13,14-dihydro-PGE$_2$. The reason for low assay reliability. Prostaglandins 19: 933–957

Gustavii B 1978 Local membrane mechanism in the onset of labor in humans. In: Prenatal endocrinology and parturition. Inserm Symposium, INSERM, Paris, p 93

Henson G, Gough J D, Gillmer M D G 1983 The control of persistent primary post-partum haemorrhage due to uterine atony with intravenous prostaglandin E$_2$. British Journal of Obstetrics and Gynaecology 90: 280–282

Hibbard B M, Sharma S C, Fitzpatrick R I, Hamlett J D 1974 Prostaglandin F$_{2\alpha}$ concentrations in amniotic fluid in late pregnancy. Journal of Obstetrics and Gynaecology of the British Commonwealth 81: 35–38

Honnebier W I, Swaab D F 1973 The influence of anencephaly upon intrauterine growth of fetus and placenta and upon gestation length.

Journal of Obstetrics and Gynaecology of the British Commonwealth 80: 577–588

Husslein P 1985 Mode of action of oxytocin and the role of its receptor in the production of prostaglandins. In: Wood C (ed) The role of prostaglandins in labour. Royal Society of Medicine Services, International Congress and Symposium Series, London, no. 92, pp 15–23

Keirse M J N C, Turnbull A C 1973 Prostaglandins in amniotic fluid during late pregnancy and labour. Journal of Obstetrics and Gynaecology of the British Commonwealth 80: 970–973

Keirse M J N C, Flint A P F, Turnbull A C 1974 Prostaglandins in amniotic fluid during pregnancy and labour. Journal of Obstetrics and Gynaecology of the British Commonwealth 81: 131–135

Keirse M J N C, Hicks B R, Mitchell M D, Turnbull A C 1977 Increase of the prostaglandin precursor, arachidonic acid, in amniotic fluid during spontaneous labour. British Journal of Obstetrics and Gynaecology 84: 937–940

Keirse M J N C, Thiery M, Parevijck W, Mitchell M D 1983 Chronic stimulation of uterine prostaglandin synthesis during cervical ripening before the onset of labour. Prostaglandins 25: 671–682

Kittinger G W 1977 Endocrine regulation of fetal development and its relation to parturition in the rhesus monkey. In: Knight J, O'Connor M (eds) The fetus and birth. Ciba Foundation Symposium 47, Elsevier/Excerpta Medica/North Holland, Amsterdam, pp 235–249

Kumaresan P, Anandagarangam P B, Dianzon W, Vasicka A 1974 Plasma oxytocin levels during human pregnancy and labor as determined by radioimmunoassay. American Journal of Obstetrics and Gynecology 119: 215–223

Leake R D, Weitsman R E, Glatz T H, Fisher D A 1979 Stimulation of oxytocin secretion in the human. Clinical Research 27: 99A

Ledger W L, Webster M A, Anderson A B M, Turnbull A C 1985a Effect of inhibition of prostaglandin synthesis on cervical softening and uterine activity during ovine parturition resulting from progesterone withdrawal induced by epostane. Journal of Endocrinology 105: 227–233

Ledger W L, Webster M, Harrison L P, Anderson A B M, Turnbull A C 1985b Increase in cervical extensibility during labor induced after isolation of the cervix from the uterus in pregnant ewes. American Journal of Obstetrics and Gynecology 151: 397–402

Leong M K H, Murphy B E P 1976 Cortisol levels in maternal venous and umbilical cord arterial and venous serum at vaginal delivery. American Journal of Obstetrics and Gynecology 124: 471–473

Lewis P R, Galvin P M, Short R V 1987 Salivary oestriol and progesterone concentrations in women during late pregnancy, parturition and the puerperium. Journal of Endocrinology 115: 177–181

Liggins G C 1969a Premature parturition after infusion of corticotrophin or cortisol into fetal lambs. Journal of Endocrinology 42: 323–329

Liggins G C 1969b The fetal role in the initiation of parturition in the ewe. In: Foetal autonomy. Ciba Foundation Symposium 14. Associated Scientific Publishers, Amsterdam, pp 218–231

Liggins G C 1973 Hormonal interactions in the mechanisms of parturition. Memoirs of the Society of Endocrinology 20: 119–139

Liggins G C 1979 Initiation of parturition. British Medical Bulletin 35: 145–150

Liggins G C 1981 Initiation of parturition. In: Novy M J, Resko J A (eds) Fetal endocrinology. Academic Press, New York, pp 211–238

Liggins G C, Grieves S A 1971 Possible role for prostaglandin $F_{2\alpha}$ in parturition in sheep. Nature, London 232: 629–631

Liggins G C, Kennedy P C, Holen L W 1967 Failure of initiation of parturition after electrocoagulation of the pituitary of the fetal lamb. American Journal of Obstetrics and Gynecology 98: 1080–1086

Liggins G C, Fairclough R J, Grieves S A, Kendall J Z, Knox B S 1973 The mechanism of parturition in the ewe. Recent Progress in Hormone Research 29: 111–150

Liggins G C, Fairclough R J, Grieves S A, Forster C S, Knox B S 1977a Parturition in the sheep. In: Knight J, O'Connor M (eds) The fetus and birth. Elsevier/Excerpta Medica/North Holland, Amsterdam, pp 5–25

Liggins G C, Forster C S, Grieves S A, Schwarz A L 1977b Control of parturition in man. Biology and Reproduction 16: 39–56

Lopez-Bernal A, Castle B, Turnbull A C 1986a Prostaglandin binding

by human fetal ducts arteriosus at mid gestation. Hormone and Metabolic Research 18: 214–215

Lopez-Bernal A, Tindell D J, Selinger M, Turnbull A C 1986b Local inhibition of progesterone production in human chorio-decidua by Epostane. Hormone and Metabolic Research 18: 503

Lopez-Bernal A, Hansell D J, Alexander S, Turnbull A C 1987a Prostaglandin E production by amniotic cells in relation to term and pre-term labour. British Journal of Obstetrics and Gynaecology 94: 864–869

Lopez-Bernal A, Gryant-Greenwood G D, Hansell D J, Hicks B R, Greenwood F C, Turnbull A C 1987b Effect of relaxin on prostaglandin E production by human amnion: changes in relation to the onset of labour. British Journal of Obstetrics and Gynaecology 94: 1045–1051

Lopez-Bernal A, Hansell D J, Alexander S, Turnbull A C 1987c Steroid conversion and prostaglandin production by chorionic and decidual cells in relation to term and pre-term labour. British Journal of Obstetrics and Gynaecology 94: 1052–1058

Maathius J B, Kelly R W 1978 Concentrations of prostaglandins $F_{2\alpha}$ and E_2 in the endometrium throughout the human menstrual cycle after the administration of clomiphene or an oestrogen-progesterone pill and in early pregnancy. Journal of Endocrinology 77: 361–371

MacLennan A H 1983 The role of relaxin in human reproduction. Clinics in Reproduction and Fertility 2: 77–95

MacLennan A H, Green R C, Bryant-Greenwood G D, Greenwood F C, Seamark R F 1980 Ripening of the human cervix and induction of labour with purified relaxin. Lancet i: 220–223

MacLennan A H, Nicholson R, Green R C 1986 Serum relaxin in pregnancy. Lancet ii: 241–243

Manabe Y, Manabe A, Aso T 1981 Plasma concentrations of oestrone, oestradiol, oestriol and progesterone during mechanical stretch-induced abortion at mid-trimester. Journal of Endocrinology 91: 385–389

Mitchell B, Cruikshank B, McLean D, Challis J R G 1982 Local modulation of progesterone production in human fetal membranes. Journal of Clinical Endocrinology and Metabolism 55: 1237–1239

Mitchell M D 1984 Role of prostaglandins in parturition. In: Ridge J, Freedman P S, Brierly C A (eds) Prostaglandin perspectives. Media Medica, Wiley, Chichester, pp 1–4

Mitchell M D, Flint A P F 1977 Progesterone withdrawal: effects on prostaglandins and parturition. Prostaglandins 14: 611–614

Mitchell M D, Flint A P F, Turnbull A C 1976 Stimulation by oxytocin of prostaglandins F levels in uterine venous effluent in pregnant and puerperal sheep. Prostaglandins 9: 47–56

Mitchell M D, Keirse M J N C, Anderson A B M, Turnbull A C 1977a Evidence for local control of prostaglandins within the human uterus. British Journal of Obstetrics and Gynaecology 84: 35–38

Mitchell M D, Flint A P F, Bibby J, Brunt J, Arnold J M, Anderson A B M, Turnbull A C 1977b Rapid increases in plasma prostaglandin concentrations after vaginal examination and amniotomy. British Medical Journal 2: 1183–1185

Mitchell M D, Flint A P F, Bibby et al 1978a Plasma concentrations of prostaglandins during late human pregnancy: influence of normal and pre-term labor. Journal of Clinical Endocrinology and Metabolism 46: 947–951

Mitchell M D, Brunt J, Bibby J, Flint A P F, Anderson A B M, Turnbull A C 1978b Prostaglandins in the human umbilical circulation at birth. British Journal of Obstetrics and Gynaecology 85: 114–118

Mochizuki M, Tojo S 1980 Effects of dehydroepiandrosterone sulfate on softening and dilatation of the uterine cervix in pregnant women. In: Naftolin F, Stubblefield P G (eds) Dilatation of the uterine cervix. Raven Press, New York, pp 267–286

Mortimer G, Stimson W H, Hunter I C, Govan A D T 1985 A role for amniotic epithelium in the control of human parturition. Lancet i: 1074–1075

Murphy B E P 1975 Does the human fetal adrenal play a role in parturition? American Journal of Obstetrics and Gynecology 115: 521–525

Murphy B E P, Patrick J, Denton R L 1975 Cortisol in amniotic fluid during human gestation. Journal of Clinical Endocrinology and Metabolism 40: 164–167

Novy M J 1977 Endocrine and pharmacological factors which influence the onset of labour in rhesus monkeys. In: Knight J, O'Connor M (eds) The fetus and birth. Ciba Foundation Symposium 47, Elsevier/Excerpta Medica/North Holland, Amsterdam, pp 259–288

Pattison N S, Webster M A, Phipps S L, Anderson A B M, Gillmer M D G 1985 Inhibition of 3β-hydroxysteroid dehydrogenase activity in first and second trimester human pregnancy and the luteal phase using Epostane. Fertility and Sterility 42: 875–881

Rush R W, Keirse M J N C, Howat P, Baum J D, Anderson A B M, Turnbull A C 1976 Contribution of pre-term delivery to perinatal mortality. British Medical Journal 2: 965–968

Saeed S A, McDonald Gibson W J, Cuthbert J et al 1977 Endogenous inhibitor of prostaglandin synthetase. Nature (London) 270: 32–36

Selinger M, MacKenzie I Z, Gillmer M D G, Phipps S L, Ferguson J 1987 Progesterone inhibition in mid-trimester termination of pregnancy: physiological and clinical effects. British Journal of Obstetrics and Gynaecology 94: 1218–1222

Sellers S M, Hodgson H T, Mitchell M D, Anderson A B M, Turnbull A C 1980 Release of prostaglandins following amniotomy is not mediated by oxytocin. British Journal of Obstetrics and Gynaecology 87: 43–46

Sellers S M, Mitchell M D, Bibby J G, Anderson A B M, Turnbull A C 1981a A comparison of plasma prostaglandin levels in term and pre-term labour. British Journal of Obstetrics and Gynaecology 88: 362–366

Sellers S M, Hodgson H T, Mountford L A, Mitchell M D, Anderson A B M, Turnbull A C 1981b Is oxytocin involved in parturition? British Journal of Obstetrics and Gynaecology 88: 725–729

Sellers S M, Mitchell M D, Anderson A B M, Turnbull A C 1981c The relation between the release of prostaglandins at amniotomy and the subsequent onset of labour. British Journal of Obstetrics and Gynaecology 88: 1211–1216

Sellers S M, Hodgson H T, Mitchell M D, Anderson A B M, Turnbull A C 1982 Raised prostaglandin levels in the third stage of labor. American Journal of Obstetrics and Gynecology 144: 209–212

Siiteri P K, MacDonald P C 1966 Placental oestrogen biosynthesis during human pregnancy. Journal of Clinical Endocrinology 26: 751–761

Silman R E, Chard T, Lowry P J, Smith I, Young I M 1976 Human foetal pituitary peptides and parturition. Nature (London) 260L: 716–718

Steele P A, Flint A P F, Turnbull A C 1976 Activity of steroid C17,20 lyase in the ovine placenta: effect of exposure to foetal glucocorticoid. Journal of Endocrinology 69: 239–246

Taylor M J, Webb R, Mitchell M D, Robinson J S 1982 Effect of progesterone withdrawal in sheep during late pregnancy. Journal of Endocrinology 92: 85–93

Thorburn G D, Challis J R G, Robinson J S 1977 The endocrinology of parturition. In: Wynn R M (ed) Cellular biology of the uterus. Plenum Press, New York, pp 653–732

Thornton C A, Carrie L E S, Sayers L, Anderson A B M, Turnbull A C 1976 A comparison of the effect of extradural and parenteral analgesia on maternal plasma cortisol concentrations during labour and the puerperium. British Journal of Obstetrics and Gynaecology 83: 631–635

Turnbull A C, Patten P T, Flint A P F, Keirse M J N C, Jeremy J Y, Anderson A B M 1974 Significant fall in progesterone and rise in oestradiol levels in human peripheral plasma before the onset of labour. Lancet i: 101–104

Turnbull A C, Anderson A B M, Flint A P F, Jeremy J Y, Keirse M J N C, Mitchell M D 1977 Human parturition. In: Knight J, O'Connor M (eds) The fetus and birth. Elsevier/Excerpta Medica/North Holland, Amsterdam, pp 427–452

Turnbull A C, Lucas A, Mitchell M D 1981 Prostaglandins in the perinatal period. In: Scarpelli E M, Cosmi E V (eds) Reviews in perinatal medicine, vol 4. Raven Press, New York, pp 273–297

Vasicka A, Kumaresan P, Han G S, Kumaresan M 1978 Plasma oxytocin in initiation of labor. American Journal of Obstetrics and Gynecology 130: 263–273

Verhoeff A, Garfield R A 1986 Ultrastructure of the myometrium and the role of gap junctions in myometrial function. In: Huszar G (ed) The physiology and biochemistry of the uterus. CRC Press, Boca Raton, pp 73–91

Webster M A, Phipps S L, Gillmer M D G 1985 Interruption of first trimester human pregnancy following Epostane therapy. Effect of prostaglandin E2 pessaries. British Journal of Obstetics and Gynaecology 92: 963–968

Wilkinson A R, Aynsley-Green A, Mitchell M D 1979 Persistent pulmonary hypertension with abnormal prostaglandin E levels in preterm infants after maternal treatment with naproxan. Archives of Disease in Childhood 54: 942–945

Wilson T 1988 Lipocortins and their possible role in the onset of labour. In: Brierley C A (ed) Prostaglandin perspectives. Media Medica, Wiley, Chichester, pp 1–3

Wilson T, Liggins G C, Aimer G P, Skinner S J M 1985 Partial purification and characterisation of two compounds from amniotic fluid which inhibit phospholipase activity in human endometrial cells. Biochemical and Biophysical Research Communications 131: 22–29

AN UPDATE ON THE ENDOCRINE CONTROL OF LABOUR

Mark R. Johnson   Phil R. Bennett   Philip J. Steer

The mechanisms underlying the onset and progression of labour in the human are complex and remain poorly understood. One thing is certain and that is the important role played by the prostaglandins. Our appreciation of this is largely due to work carried out in Alec Turnbull's laboratories in Oxford during the 1970s and 1980s. His team included Murray Mitchell, John Challis and Marc Kierse; all are now established experts in their own right. Affectionately known as the Oxford Circus, they have continued to work in various parts of the world on the mechanisms involved in the onset of labour. Therefore, the work initiated by Alec Turnbull continues and his legacy will continue to deepen our understanding of the mechanisms of parturition for many decades to come.

In the first edition of this book in 1987, Alec Turnbull's chapter, 'The endocrine control of labour', comprehensively reviewed the literature up to that date. In many areas, little has changed, but in some, particularly those of prostaglandin, oxytocin and relaxin, the field has advanced, in addition novel roles for corticotrophin releasing hormone, nitric oxide and several cytokines have been suggested.

THE ROLE OF THE PLACENTAL HORMONES

Changes in the oestrogen to progesterone ratio and absolute reductions in the circulating levels of progesterone have long been thought to be important in the genesis of labour. However, the reported findings up to 1987 were not consistent (Turnbull et al 1974, Biddy et al 1980, Darne et al 1987, Lewis et al 1987). More recently, the ability of the progesterone antagonist, RU486, to induce labour has given arguments for the role of progesterone new force. It suggests that high levels of progesterone play an active role in the maintenance of human pregnancy.

Moreover, around the time of labour, the changes in the fetal membrane metabolism of steroids increase the ratio of oestrogens to progesterone at the tissue level and this may not be apparent systemically (Chibbar et al 1986). The change in ratio promotes oxytocin and oxytocin receptor mRNA expression, and prostaglandin synthesis. Oestrogens promote gap junction formation, an effect which is also antagonized by progesterone (Garfield et al 1980). In addition, the in vitro effects of RU486 suggest that progesterone not only inhibits prostaglandin synthesis, but also enhances prostaglandin dehydrogenase activity.

PROSTAGLANDINS

Increased prostaglandin synthesis within the uterus is probably a prerequisite for the onset of labour. However, the main site of production remains controversial. The amnion is a major site of storage of arachidonic acid, and large increases in prostaglandin synthesis have been demonstrated to occur in the amnion at the onset of labour. To reach their target tissues, the decidua, cervix and myometrium, prostaglandins from the amnion must cross the chorion. Paradoxically, the chorion is rich in prostaglandin dehydrogenases and might therefore be expected to be a barrier to prostaglandin transfer. However, many individual cells have been shown by immunohistochemistry to lack prostaglandin dehydrogenase (Challis et al 1991). They may provide a passage for prostaglandins and several groups have suggested that this enables prostaglandins to cross the chorion unaltered (Nackla et al 1986, Bennett et al 1990). Although some have disputed these findings (Roseblade et al 1990), it is clear that prostaglandins injected into the amniotic cavity are able to induce labour, suggesting that at least some of the injected prostaglandins remain in an active form. Several workers have suggested that prostaglandin synthesis in the amnion is increased by a fetal signal acting through the amniotic fluid.

An alternative source of prostaglandins is the decidua. Increases in prostaglandin synthesis, similar to those seen in the amnion, are seen within the decidua in association with labour (Skinner & Challis 1985). Although the decidua is not in intimate contact with the amniotic fluid it is possible that fetal signals may cross the chorion to reach the decidua or that the signal for the onset of labour is carried in the maternal circulation.

Alec Turnbull suggested that the cyclo-oxygenase (COX) enzyme is ready and waiting in the fetal membranes for its substrate arachidonic acid and that it is the activity of phospholipase A2 (PLA2) which controls overall prostaglandin synthesis. However, it is now apparent that COX activity may be more important than originally thought. Any stimulus to prostaglandin synthesis must also increase COX activity as it has a short half-life and, in addition, undergoes destruction after a limited number of reactions (Marshall et al 1987). The amnion appears to produce only lipoxygenase metabolites of arachidonic acid before the onset of labour, but with the onset of labour the ratio of cyclo-oxygenase/lipoxygenase metabolites alters, suggesting that the activities of COX and PLA2 must be controlled independently. Enzyme kinetic studies suggest that the increase in COX activity with the onset of labour is due entirely to the synthesis of new enzyme (Smeija et al 1993). This implies an increase in activity of its genes, or an increase in the translation of its mRNA. The existence of two COX genes has been reported, COX-1, on chromosome 1, with an mRNA of approximately 2.8 kb (DeWitt & Smith 1988, Yokoyama & Tanabe 1989) and COX-2 on chromosome 9, with an mRNA of approximately 4.0 kb (due to a long untranslated portion on the 5' end) (O'Banion 1991). Although not identical, the two COX enzymes are of a similar size and show a high degree of homology. COX-1 is expressed in tissues which synthesize prostaglandin continuously, while COX-2 is expressed in tissues in which prostaglandin synthesis is induced by an external signal. It is the COX-2 enzyme which is responsible for the increased prostaglandin synthesis with the onset of labour (Slater et al 1994). It is likely that fetal prostaglandin synthesis is mediated by COX-1, and this raises the possibility that it may be possible to use specific COX-2 inhibitors to prevent or inhibit preterm labour without the fetal side-effects of oliguria or closure of the ductus seen with COX inhibitors such as indomethacin which affect both COX-1 and COX-2.

Although it is likely that COX activity is important in the regulation of fetal membrane prostaglandin synthesis, there must also be an increase in substrate availability, implying an increase in PLA2 activity. Until recently, it was thought that PLA2 would be a cellular homologue of pancreatic PLA2 (Bennett et al 1993), and it was debated as to whether its activity was regulated by changes in expression (Aitkin et al 1990) or by post-transcriptional factors (Bennett et al 1994). Indeed, the decrease in the expression of lipocortin-1 before the onset of labour suggests that it may be the inhibitor of PLA2 activity (Bennett et al 1994). However, the discovery of a novel PLA2 which is more active at the relevant calcium concentrations and with a 20-fold selectivity for arachidonyl-phospholipids (Clark et al 1991), has superseded the debate on the factors involved in the regulation of cellular pancreatic PLA2.

The primary stimulus to increased prostaglandin synthesis is uncertain. It is possible that amniotic fluid contains inhibitors of arachidonic metabolism which are withdrawn near to term. The ability of amniotic fluid to inhibit prostaglandin synthesis in amnion cells falls by 25% between early pregnancy and term, and by more than 50% in samples taken before and after the onset of labour at term (Saeed et al 1982). Alternatively, the fetus may excrete substances in the urine and so into the amniotic fluid which stimulate prostaglandin synthesis in the amnion (Strickland et al 1983).

Prostaglandin receptors have been studied using both pharmacological and receptor binding studies. However, the recent cloning of the prostanoid receptors will allow their tissue distribution and regulation to be investigated more fully. Studies of their concentration and activity will allow their role to be more fully determined in the near future.

OXYTOCIN (MATERNAL)

The demonstration that extracts of the posterior pituitary stimulated uterine contraction, and the isolation of oxytocin as the active component, made it seem likely that oxytocin is important in the onset and progression of labour in the human. However, failure to demonstrate an increase in the circulating levels of oxytocin with the onset of labour (Vasicka et al 1977), even in the presence of oxytocinase inhibitors (Yusoff Dawood et al 1978), raised doubts as to its importance in the process of parturition. These doubts were to some extent allayed by the observation of increased myometrial sensitivity to oxytocin with advancing gestation (Takahashi et al 1980), resulting from an increase in the myometrial expression of the oxytocin receptor (Fuchs et al 1984). This suggested that changes in plasma levels were not a necessary prerequisite for oxytocin to have a significant role in the onset of labour. Moreover, the demonstration of decidual oxytocin synthesis with the onset of labour suggests that oxytocin released from the decidua may act in a paracrine manner to stimulate myometrial contractility (Miller et al 1993). Changes in the local oestrogen : progesterone ratio may be important in the regulation of the synthesis of oxytocin (Richard & Zingg 1990) and the expression of the oxytocin receptor (Maggi et al 1992). Coincident with increases in myometrial receptor expression, decidual and fetal membrane oxytocin receptor mRNA expression is also increased during labour (Takemura et al 1994). Oxytocin binding to these tissues results in prostaglandin synthesis and release (Fuchs et al 1981, Moore et al 1988). The effects of oxytocin are probably mediated through activation of phospholipase C and protein kinase C (Moore et al 1988), which with prostaglandins acts to increase ovarian oxytocin release (Flint et al 1981, Hirst et al 1990). The local synthesis of oxytocin may be increased by local inflammatory factors such as cytokines, which may be of aetiological significance in preterm labour associated with chorioamnionitis. Indeed, that oxytocin antagonists stop preterm labour suggests that oxytocin does have an important role in labour (Akerlund et al 1986, Goodwin et al 1994). Recently, more detailed studies (sampling at 1-minute intervals) have demonstrated an increase in frequency and duration (but not amplitude)

of oxytocin secretion pulses during normal labour, supporting the possibility that oxytocin may be acting in an endocrine as well as a paracrine mechanism during labour (Fuchs et al 1991). Thus, at the onset of normal term labour, changes in the oestrogen : progesterone ratio may result in increased expression of both myometrial oxytocin receptors and decidual synthesis of oxytocin. The increased tissue levels of oxytocin may stimulate the release of prostaglandins from the fetal membranes and decidua, which may enhance oxytocin further release and set in train a positive feedback loop, with oxytocin and prostaglandins stimulating myometrial contractility and the prostaglandins acting in addition to promote cervical compliance.

OXYTOCIN (FETAL)

Although the fetal neurohypophysis contains significant amounts of oxytocin and higher levels have been reported in the umbilical artery than in the vein, its role during labour remains at best uncertain. Moreover, there is increasing evidence that fetal oxytocin does not reach the maternal circulation (Hirst et al 1993) and that the umbilical artery/vein difference may be due to placental aminopeptidase activity.

RELAXIN

A major role for relaxin during labour has not been accepted widely. However, recent data suggest that it may have several minor roles in the onset and progression of labour, with interactions between prostaglandins, oxytocin and the mechanical forces of labour.

During pregnancy in the rat, relaxin infusions have variable effects depending on their temporal relation to the time of onset of labour. Labour starting during a relaxin infusion is longer and is associated with lower levels of oxytocin than control labours, but labour after the cessation of the infusion is faster and associated with higher levels of oxytocin (Jones et al 1986). As, during parturition, the decidua is the main source of circulating oxytocin, these data suggest that relaxin increases the expression, but inhibits the release of decidual oxytocin. During lactation, relaxin infusion prevents the episodic release of oxytocin (essential to evoke a rise in intramammary pressure) (O'Byrne et al 1986), but increases the baseline release of oxytocin (Way et al 1992). In the human, the relationship between relaxin and oxytocin is not known. Oxytocin infusions during the menstrual cycle (Johnson et al unpublished observation) or during pregnancy at term (Hochman et al 1978) have no effect on circulating relaxin levels. Although relaxin levels appear to increase during breastfeeding, no relationship between relaxin and oxytocin is seen either at this time or during labour (Johnson et al unpublished observation). (Johnson et al 1992). The administration of PGE_2 for the induction of second-trimester abortion results in an increase in circulating levels of relaxin (Seki et al 1987). In contrast, at term, the administration of $PGF_{2\alpha}$ has no effect on circulating relaxin levels (Hochman et al 1978). The addition of relaxin to cultures of fetal membranes obtained before the onset of labour inhibited prostaglandin release. However, the addition of relaxin to similar cultures of membranes obtained during labour increased prostaglandin release if the membranes were intact. (López Bernal et al 1987). These data suggest that the response of relaxin to prostaglandins and the response of prostaglandin synthesis to relaxin is dependent on the stage of gestation. Indeed, relaxin immunoreactivity observed in the fetal membranes prior to the onset of labour disappears after labour has begun (Bryant-Greenwood 1987).

Porcine relaxin consistently inhibits spontaneous and induced myometrial contractions in vitro and in vivo in animal studies (Porter et al 1979, Goldsmith et al 1989). In the human, in vitro data conflict. Extracts of human corpora lutea and porcine relaxin have been demonstrated to inhibit both stimulated and spontaneous contractions of human myometrium in vitro (Szlachter et al 1982), but human relaxin (H2) has no effect (Petersen et al 1991). There are no data relating the in vivo administration of relaxin, whether porcine or human, to myometrial contractility. However, high mean levels of plasma relaxin during labour are related to low levels of the mean uterine activity integral (Johnson et al 1992). These data suggest that relaxin has a negative effect on myometrial contractility in the human.

In rats and pigs, removal of the activity of relaxin, either by ovariectomy or the administration of neutralizing antibodies, results in labour, which is prolonged and attended by a high fetal mortality rate (Downing & Sherwood 1985). These findings are associated with reduced cervical elasticity (Downing & Sherwood 1985). This suggests that relaxin is important for normal cervical ripening. In the human, such studies have not been performed, but an analogous situation exists. Women with premature ovarian failure can only become pregnant after ovum donation. Such women do not have functional ovarian tissue and, consequently, no relaxin in their circulation (Johnson et al 1991). In cases where labour is allowed to start spontaneously cervical dilatation occurs successfully, although it may be slower than normal (Eddie et al 1990). This suggests that in the human relaxin is not essential for cervical dilatation. However, normal human pregnancy may be a relatively relaxin-deficient state as the circulating levels of relaxin are, at their peak, two orders of magnitude less than those in the rat and the pig. Thus, the comparison of a spontaneously conceived pregnancy with one conceived following ovum donation may be that of a relaxin-deficient state with an absolute absence of relaxin. Indeed, there is evidence to suggest that relaxin does affect cervical compliance during labour in the human. Measurements of head–cervix force have been obtained using specially designed force sensors. The ratio of active force to active pressure gives an indication of cervical compliance. High mean levels of relaxin are associated with improved force levels for a given intrauterine pressure in spontaneous and induced labour (a high force to pressure ratio is associated with more rapid cervical dilatation) (Johnson et al 1992).

CORTICOTROPHIN RELEASING HORMONE

Circulating levels of corticotrophin releasing hormone (CRH) increase progressively throughout pregnancy, especially during the weeks prior to the onset of labour. CRH has no direct effect on myometrial contractility. However, in vitro, it enhances both the contractile response to oxytocin (Quartero et al 1992) and oxytocin-induced prostaglandin production from the fetal membranes and placenta (Jones et al 1989). The affinity of the myometrial CRH receptor is low until term, when it increases markedly (Hillhouse et al 1993). In addition, although the affinity of the binding protein remains constant, its levels fall with advancing gestation (Lowry 1993). These changes mean that while in early pregnancy CRH is bound exclusively to the binding protein, towards term the increased affinity of the myometrial receptor, the reduced levels of the binding protein and the higher circulating levels of CRH favour binding to the myometrial receptor. In addition. CRH may affect the fetal hypothalamic–pituitary–adrenal axis, increasing the production of cortisol (Riley & Challis 1991). This may lead to a reduction in the production of progesterone by the fetoplacental unit, and to the changes described above.

CYTOKINES

Platelet activating factor (PAF) (Hoffman et al 1990), interleukin-1 (IL-1), interleukin-6 (IL-6), and tumour necrosis factor (TNF) have all been suggested to be responsible for increased prostaglandin synthesis in the amnion (Romero & Mazor 1988, Romero et al 1992). All are present in amniotic fluid in increased concentrations after the onset of labour and are able to stimulate prostaglandin synthesis in amnion cells in vitro. Whether the changes in cytokines are the cause or effect of labour is uncertain, but the secretion of PAF by the fetus correlates with its lung maturity. This supports a role of PAF in the onset of labour.

While the exact mechanism for the onset of labour remain mysterious, some shapes emerge from the gloom. Some, such as the recently suggested role for nitric oxide, may prove to be evanescent as morning mist, whereas others yet to be discovered could prove to be the links we need to establish the chain of causation, so many of whose links have already been provided by Alec Turnbull.

REFERENCES

Aitkin M A, Rice G E, Brennocke S P 1990 Gestational tissue phospholipase A2 mRNA content and onset of spontaneous labour in human. Reproduction, Fertility and Development 2: 575–581

Akerlund M, Hauksson A, Lundin S, Melin P, Trojanar J 1986 Vasotocin analogues which competatively inhibit vasopressin stimulated contractions in healthy women. British Journal of Obstetrics and Gynaecology 93: 22–24

Bennett P R, Chamberlain G V P, Patel L, Elder M C, Myatt L 1990 Mechanisms of parturition: the transfer of prostaglandin E2 and 5-HETE across fetal membranes. American Journal of Obstetrics and Gynaecology 162: 683–687

Bennett P R, Slater D, Moore G E 1993 Expression of a common cellular phospholipase A2 by human intrauterine tissues. Prostaglandins 45: 121–125

Bennett P R, Slater D, Berger L, Moore G E 1994 The expression of phospholipase A2 and lipocortins (annexins), I, II and V in human fetal membranes and placenta in association with labour. Prostaglandins 478: 81–90

Bibby J G 1980 Studies in human pregnancy and parturition with particular reference to the role of prostaglandins and steroid hormones. MD thesis, University of Otago, Dunedin, New Zealand

Bryant-Greenwood G D, Rees M C, Turnbull A C 1987 Immunohistochemical localisation of relaxin, prolactin and prostaglandin synthase in human amnion, chorion and decidiua. Journal of Endocrinology 114: 491–496

Challis J R G, Riley S C, Yang K 1991 Endocrinology of labour. Fetal Medicine Reviews 3: 47–66

Chibbar R, Hobkirk R, Mitchell B F 1986 Sulfohydrolase activity for estrone sulfate and dehydroepiandrosterone sulfate in human fetal membranes and decidua around the time of parturition. Journal of Clinical Endocrinology and Metabolism 62: 90–94

Clark J D, Lin L, Kriz R W et al 1991 A novel arachidonic acid selective cytosolic phospholipase A2 from human monocytic cell line. Cell 65: 1043–1045

Darne J, McGarrigle H H G, Lachelin G C L 1987 Saliva oestriol, oestradiol, oestrone and progesterone levels in pregnancy; spontaneous labour at term is preceded by a rise in the saliva oestriol : progesterone ratio. British Journal of Obstetrics and Gynaecology 94: 227–235

DeWitt D L, Smith W L 1988 Primary structure of prostaglandin G/H synthase from sheep vesicular gland determined from the complimentary DNA sequence. Proceedings of the National Academy of Sciences of the USA 85: 1412–1417

Downing S J, Sherwood O D 1985 The physiological role of relaxin in the pregnant rat. 1. The influence of relaxin on parturition. Endocrinology 116: 1200–1205

Eddie L W, Cameron I T, Leeton J F, Healy D L, Renou P 1990 Ovarian relaxin is not essential for dilatation of the cervix. Lancet i: 243

Flint A P F, Sheldrick E L 1982 Ovarian secretion of oxytocin is stimulated by prostaglandin. Nature 356: 526–529

Fuchs A R, Husslein P, Fuchs F 1981 Oxytocin and the initiation of human parturition II. Stimulation of prostaglandin production in human decidual cells by oxytocin. American Journal of Obstetrics and Gynecology 141: 694–698

Fuchs A R, Fuchs F, Husslein P, Soloff M S 1984 Oxytocin receptors in pregnant human uterus. American Journal of Obstetrics and Gynecology 150: 734–741

Fuchs A R, Romero R, Keefe D, Parra M, Oyarzun E, Behnke E 1991 Oxytocin secretion and human parturition: pulse frequency and duration increase during spontaneous labor in women. American Journal of Obstetrics and Gynecology 165: 1515–1523

Garfield R E, Kannan M S, Daniel E E 1980 Gap junction formation in myometrium: control by estrogens, progesterone, and prostaglandins. American Journal of Physiology 238: C81–C89

Goldsmith L T, Skurnick J H, Wojtczuk A S, Linden M, Kuhar M J, Weiss G 1989 The antagonistic effect of oxytocin and relaxin on rat uterine segment contractility. American Journal of Obstetrics and Gynecology 161: 1644–1649

Goodwin T M, Paul R, Silver H 1994 The effect of the oxytocin anatagonist atosiban on preterm uterine activity in the human. American Journal of Obstetrics and Gynecology 170: 474–478

Hillhouse E W, Milton N, Grammatopoulos D, Quartero H W P 1993 The identification of a human myometrial corticotrophin-releasing hormone receptor that increases in affinity during pregnancy. Journal of Clinical Endocrinology and Metabolism 76: 736–741

Hirst J J, Rice G D, Jenkin D, Thorburn G D 1990 Regulation of oxytocin secretion by the ovine corpus luteum: effect of activators of protein kinase C. Journal of Endocrinology 124: 225–232

Hirst J J, Haluska G J, Cook M J, Novy M J 1993 Plasma oxytocin and nocturnal uterine activity: maternal, but not fetal concentrations increase progressively during late pregnancy and delivery in rhesus monkey. American Journal of Obstetrics and Gynecology 169: 414–422

Hochman J, Weiss G, Steinetz B G, O'Byrne E M 1978 Serum relaxin concentrations in prostaglandin- and oxytocin-induced labor in women. American Journal of Obstetrics and Gynecology 130: 473–474

Hoffman D R, Romero R, Johnston J M 1990 Detection of platelet activating factor in amniotic fluid of complicated pregnancies. American Journal of Obstetrics and Gynecology 162: 525–531

Johnson M R, Abdalla H, Allman A C J, Wren M E, Kirkland A, Lightman S L 1991 Relaxin levels in ovum donation pregnancies. Fertility and Sterility 56: 59–61

Johnson M R, Allman A C J, Steer P J, Lightman S L 1992 Circulating levels of relaxin may influence the time of onset and progression of labour. Journal of Endocrinology 135: 31

Jones S A, Summerlee A J S 1986 Relaxin acts contrally to inhibit oxytocin release during parturition: an effect that is reversed by naloxone. Journal of Endocrinology 111: 99–102

Jones S A, Challis J R G 1989 Local stimulation of prostaglandin production by corticotrophin releasing hormone in fetal membranes and placenta. Biochemical and Biophysical Research Communication 159: 964–970

Lewis P R, Galvin P M, Short R V 1987 Salivary oestriol and progesterone concentrations in women during late pregnancy, parturition and the puerperium. Journal of Endocrinology 115: 177–181

López Bernal A, Bryant-Greenwood G D, Hansell D J, Hicks B R, Greenwood F C, Turnbull A C 1987 Effect of relaxin on prostaglandin E production by human amnion: changes in relation to the onset of labour. British Journal of Obstetrics and Gynaecology 94: 1045–1051

Lowry P J 1993 Corticotrophin-releasing factor and its binding protein in human plasma. Ciba Foundation Symposia 172: 108–128

Maggi M, Magini A, Fiscella A et al 1992 Sex steroid modulation of neurohypophysial hormone receptors in human nonpregnant myometrium. Journal of Clinical Endocrinology and Metabolism 74: 385–392

Marshall P J, Kulmacz R J, Lands W E M 1987 Constraints on prostaglandin synthesis in tissues. Journal of Biological Chemistry 262: 3510–3514

Miller F D, Chibbar R, Mitchell B F 1993 Synthesis of oxytocin in amnion, chorion and decidua: a potential paracrine role for oxytocin in the onset of human parturition. Regulatory Peptides 45: 247–251

Moore J J, Moore R M, Vander Kooy D 1988 Protein kinase C activation is required for oxytocin induced prostaglandin production in human amnion cells. Journal of Endocrinology 72: 1073–1080

Nackla S, Skinner K, Mitchell B F, Challis J R G 1986 Changes in prostaglandin transfer across human fetal membranes following spontaneous labour. American Journal of Obstetrics and Gynecology 155: 1337–1341

O'Banion M K, Sadowski H B, Winn W, Young D A 1991 A serum and glucocorticoid regulated 4 kb mRNA encodes a cyclo-oxygenase related protein. Journal of Biological Chemistry 266: 23261–23266

O'Byrne K T, Eltringham L, Clarke G, Summerlee A J S 1986 Effects of porcine relaxin on oxytocin release from the neurohypophysis in the anaesthetised lactating rat. Journal of Endocrinology 109: 393–397

Petersen L K, Svane D, Uldbjerg N, Forman A 1991 Effects of human relaxin on isolated rat and human myometrium and uteroplacental arteries. Obstetrics and Gynecology 78: 757–762

Porter D G, Downing S J, Bradshaw J M C 1979 Relaxin inhibits spontaneous and prostaglandin-induced myometrial activity in anaesthetized rats. Journal of Endocrinology 83: 183–192

Quartero H W P, Srivatsa G, Gillham B 1992 Role for cyclic adenosine-monophosphate in the synergistic interaction between oxytocin and corticotrophin releasing factor in isolated human gestational myometrium. Journal of Clinical Endocrinology 36: 141–145

Richard S, Zingg H H 1990 The human oxytocin gene promoter is regulated by estrogens. Journal of Biological Chemistry 265: 6098–6103

Riley, S C, Challis, J R G 1991 Corticotrophin-releasing hormone production by the placenta and fetal membranes. Placenta 12: 105–119

Romero R, Mazor M, 1988 Infection and preterm labour. Clinical Obstetrics and Gynecology 31: 553–584

Romero R, Mazor M, Sepulveda W, Anila A, Copeland D, Williams J 1992 Tumor necrosis factor in preterm and term labour. American Journal of Obstetrics and Gynecology 166: 1576–1587

Roseblade C K, Sullivan M F, Khan F, Lumb M R, Elder M G 1990 Limited transfer of prostaglandin E2 across fetal membranes before and after labour. Acta Obstetrica et Gynecologica Scandinavica 69: 399–403

Saeed S A, Strickland D M, Young D C, Dang A, Mitchell M D 1982 Inhibition of prostaglandin synthesis by human amniotic fluid: acute reduction in labor. Journal of Clinical Endocrinology and Metabolism 55: 801–805

Seki K, Uesato T, Kato K 1987 Serum relaxin concentrations in women following the administration of 16,16-dimethyl-trans-Δ2-prostaglandin l methyl ester during early pregnancy. Prostaglandins 33: 739–742

Skinner K A, Challis J R G 1985 Changes in synthesis and metabolism of prostaglandins by human fetal membranes and decidua at labor. American Journal of Obstetrics and Gynecology 151: 159–165

Slater D, Berger L, Newton R, Moore G E, Bennett P R 1994 The relative abundance of type 1 to type 2 cyclo-oxygenase mRNA in human amnion at term. Biochemical and Biophysical Research Communication 198: 304–308

Smieja Z, Zakar T, Walton J, Olson P 1993 Prostaglandin endoperoxide synthase kinetics in human amnion before and after labor at term and following prterm labor. Placenta 14: 163–175

Strickland D M, Saeed S A, Casey M L, Mitchell M D 1983 Stimulation of prostaglandin synthesis by urine of human fetus may serve as a trigger for human parturition. Science 220: 521–523

Szlachter N, O'Byrne E, Goldsmith L, Steinetz B G, Weiss G 1980 Myometrial inhibiting activity of relaxin-containing extracts of human corpora lutea of pregnancy. American Journal of Obstetrics and Gynecology 136: 584–586

Takahashi K, Diamond F, Bieniarz J, Yen H, Burd L 1980 Uterine contractility and oxytocin sensitivity in preterm, term and postterm pregnancy. American Journal of Obstetrics and Gynecology 136: 774–779

Takemura M, Kimura T, Nomura S et al 1994 Expression and localisation of human oxytocin receptor mRNA and its protein in chorion and decidua during parturition. Journal of Clinical Investigation 93: 2319–2323

Turnbull A C, Patten P T, Flint A P F, Keirse M J N C, Jeremy J Y, Anderson A B M 1974 Significant fall in progesterone and rise in oestradiol levels in human peripheral plasma before the onset of labour. Lancet i: 101–104

Vasicka A, Kumarsan P, Han G S, Kumaresan M 1977 Plasma oxytocin in initiation of labor. American Journal of Obstetrics and Gynecology 130: 263–273

Way S A, Leng G 1992 Relaxin increases the firing rate of supraoptic neurones and increases oxytocin secretion in the rat. Journal of Endocrinology 132: 149–158

Yokoyama C, Tanabe O 1989 Cloning of the human gene prostaglandin endoperoxide synthase and primary structure of the enzyme. Biochemical and Biophysical Research Communications 165: 888–895

Yusoff Dawood M, Raghavan K S, Pociask C, Fuchs F 1978 Oxytocin in human pregnancy and parturition. Obstetrics and Gynecology 51: 138–143

29. The physiology and biochemistry of labour

Ian A. Greer

Material in this chapter contains contributions from the first edition and we are grateful to the previous author for the work done.

INTRODUCTION

Labour represents the transition of the uterus from a quiescent capacitance vessel into an efficient contractile unit capable of effecting birth. Traditionally this process is divided into three stages:

The first stage—from the onset of regular uterine contractions to full dilatation of the cervix.
The second stage—from full cervical dilatation to delivery of the baby.
The third stage—from delivery of the baby until the delivery of the placenta.

However the transition from capacitance vessel to contractile unit is not as sudden as these traditional definitions might suggest. Rather, it evolves gradually over the last few weeks of pregnancy during the phase termed prelabour, and from a physiological perspective this component of the process perhaps should be added to our traditional categorization of the process.

Prelabour and labour consist of two distinct but nonetheless interlinked processes: cervical ripening and increasing myometrial excitement. The increased myometrial excitement of prelabour is perhaps best documented by the work of Caldeyro Barcia (1959) in the 1950s. Using intramyometrial balloon catheters to record contractions, he showed that the uterus is never entirely quiescent. Its spontaneous contractility during pregnancy, first described in 1872 by Braxton Hicks, increases both in frequency and intensity over the last 5–6 weeks of pregnancy, climaxing in labour and delivery per se. This is illustrated schematically in Figure 29.1, however, this might also be used to show the increase in uterine sensi-

tivity to oxytocin or development of intermyometrial cell gap junctions, which develop over the same time period. Cervical ripening is the conversion of the firm sphincter associated with maintenance of pregnancy to a compliant and easily dilating structure which allows uterine contractility easily to effect the transport of the fetus through the birth canal. These changes are perhaps best illustrated by the work of the late Dr Anne Anderson and the late Professor Sir Alexander Turnbull (Anderson & Turnbull 1969). Their results from a longitudinal study of 90 primigravidae are also shown in Figure 29.1, where it can be seen that effacement occurs over the same time period as the development of myometrial excitement. Bishop (1964) also illustrated that the ripeness of the cervix increases as term approaches and developed a scoring system for ripeness which can guide the success of induction of labour, as the more ripe the cervix the greater is the likelihood of spontaneous labour. Cervical ripening and myometrial excitement develop in synchrony and progress to the regular uterine contractility and cervical dilatation of labour. This chapter will consider each of these events separately.

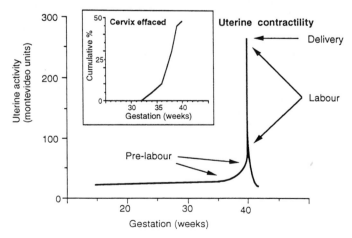

Fig. 29.1 Schematic representation of changes in uterine contractility and cervical effacement towards the end of pregnancy.

CERVICAL RIPENING

Connective tissue remodelling

Cervical composition

Unlike the uterine corpus, the cervix contains very little smooth muscle. It is composed of collagen fibrils (mainly of collagen types I and III) bound together into dense bundles which confers on the cervix the rigidity which is characteristic of its non-pregnant and early pregnant state (Fig. 29.2). The ground substance consists of large molecular weight proteoglycan complexes. Proteoglycans consist of a protein core to which are attached glycosaminoglycan branches. Glycosaminoglycans (GAG) are long chains of highly negatively charged repeating disaccharides containing one hexosamine (glucosamine or galactosamine) and one uronic acid (glucuronic or iduronic). There are a variety of GAG, such as heparin and heparan sulphate and dermatan and chondroitin sulphate. These vary in their composition with regard to the exact combination of hexosamine and uronic acid residues and each varies intrinsically with regard to chain length. The predominant GAG found in the cervix are chondroitin and dermatan sulphate (Uldbjerg et al 1983a). In turn the proteoglycans are attached covalently by a link protein to hyaluronic acid, another long glycosaminoglycan (Fig. 29.3). In addition to forming the ground substance of the tissue, proteoglycans invest collagen fibrils with their protein cores attaching to the collagen. The GAG side-chains of the proteoglycan can then interact with further collagen molecules and with each other. This relationship is important in orientating the collagen fibrils and thus providing mechanical strength (Scott & Orford 1981).

The binding affinity of GAG to collagen increases with increasing chain length and charge density. Hyaluronic

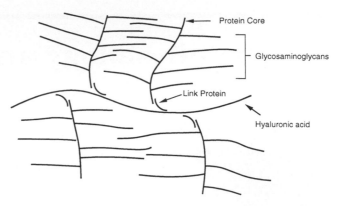

Fig. 29.3 Glycosaminoglycans making up proteoglycan complexes which interact with each other and bind to collagen fibrils.

acid, which is not found in proteoglycans, but rather exists as a free GAG or linked to proteoglycans forming proteoglycan complexes typical of cartilage, therefore binds least strongly of the GAG molecules and will act to destabilize the collagen fibrils. In contrast, dermatan sulphate binds strongly to collagen because of its ability to bind in orthoganol positions at the d- and e-bands of collagen fibrils and promote tissue stability. Changes in the proteoglycans/GAG composition can therefore alter the collagen binding and facilitate collagen breakdown. In the non-pregnant state, the cervix consists of around 80% water (Liggins 1978), which increases to around 86% in late pregnancy (Uldbjerg et al 1983a). As GAG are hydrophilic, these molecules may be important in controlling tissue hydration, with increased hydration destabilizing the collagen fibrils and promoting ripening. The collagen fibrils and GAG are produced by fibroblasts which constitute the major cellular component of the cervical connective tissue. A small amount of elastin is also present within the cervix. However, the changes in elastin fibre concentration and distribution associated with cervical ripening have yet to be established. Elastin may also be important in returning the cervix to a non-pregnant shape following delivery.

The changes associated with cervical ripening include a reduced collagen concentration within the tissue, an increase in water content, and a change in the proteoglycan/GAG content. Fibroblast activation occurs and local prostaglandin production increases. An inflammatory infiltrate also occurs at term in parallel with this ripening process and the stroma becomes oedematous and highly vascularized. However, the mechanism whereby these changes occur is unclear.

Collagen and cervical ripening

Although there is an increase in the total collagen content of the cervix at term, the collagen concentration is reduced (Fosang et al 1984, Kokenyesi & Woessner 1990,

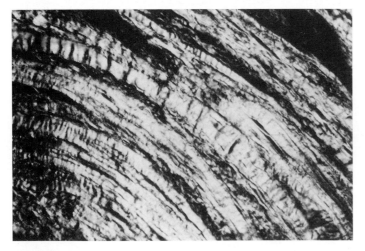

Fig. 29.2 Photomicrograph of a cervical biopsy from a normal pregnant uterine cervix at 10 weeks gestation Stained with Picrosirius Red which selectively stains polymerized collagen making the fibrils birefringent. As can be seen these are densely packed collagen fibrils characteristic of the early pregnant state (×24).

Jeffrey 1991) and the cervical connective tissue at term shows widely scattered and dissociated collagen fibrils with an increase in the ground substance when compared to the early pregnant or non-pregnant cervix (Danforth et al 1960). In addition, the collagen fibrils are reduced in size (Danforth et al 1960). The cervical collagen concentration measured biochemically also decreases (Danforth et al 1974, Uldbjerg et al 1983b, Granstrom et al 1989), but this change in collagen concentration appears to be more marked when studied histologically using stains specific for polymerized collagen, as it seems that a much lower proportion of the collagen exists as intact fibres in the dilated cervix at term (Junqueira et al 1980). Several mechanisms have been postulated to explain these changes in collagen composition; essentially, these are increased enzymatic collagen degradation and alteration in the proteoglycan/GAG composition of the ground substance.

Collagen is amenable to breakdown by collagenase produced by fibroblasts and leucocytes and leucocyte elastase produced by macrophages, polymorphs and eosinophils. Collagenase is secreted in a latent form, procollagenase, and is activated by cleavage of the proenzyme by plasmin or stromelysin to the active form which specifically breaks down the triple helix of the collagen fibril by hydrolysing peptide bonds, while elastase acts on the telopeptide non-helical domains (Wooley 1984, Stricklin & Hibbs 1988). Collagenase will degrade collagen types I, II and III and the predominant types of collagen found in the human cervix are type I (66%) and type III (33%) (Kleissl et al 1978). Elastase can break down not only elastin and collagen, but also proteoglycans. It may act synergistically with collagenase on collagen. The collagen fragments produced by these enzymes can be further broken down by non-specific proteases. As the cervical collagen content decreases through pregnancy, the leucocyte elastase and collagenase activity increase (Uldbjerg et al 1983b). In addition, the amount of soluble collagen, reflecting partly degraded collagen, in the tissue increases in parallel with the increased enzyme activities (Ito et al 1979, Uldbjerg et al 1983b). There is evidence from animal models that collagen degradation fragments are found in the cervix at parturition (Rajabi et al 1991a). Thus there appears to be a remodelling of collagen during pregnancy and parturition. The mature collagen with many cross links may be broken down during pregnancy and replaced with new collagen which is more amenable to rapid breakdown at the time of parturition having fewer cross links. The importance of collagen content to the progress of labour is illustrated by Ekman et al (1986) who showed that among women in spontaneous labour there were significantly higher cervical collagen concentrations in those with low cervical scores (i.e. less cervical ripeness) compared to those with high cervical scores. Furthermore, this group (Granstrom et al 1991) has shown that women making slow progress in labour have increased cervical collagen concentration and less collagen extractability than women in normal labour, although there was no difference in collagenolytic activity between the groups.

Once labour is established, there is a major increase in circulating collagenase (Rajabi et al 1985) and collagenase activity in cervical tissue. Increased levels of collagenase activity have been reported in cervical biopsies obtained at 6–8 cm dilatation during labour compared to biopsies from non-pregnant and pregnant non-labouring subjects (Osmers et al 1990), and Rajabi et al (1988) have reported an increase in cervical collagenase activity of 13–14 times over that obtained in tissue from women at term not in labour. Procollagenase production in the cervix, at least in animal models, appears to be under the control of steroid hormones and prostaglandins, with increased procollagenase production and gene expression being found in response to physiological (10^{-7}–10^{-9} M) concentrations of oestrogen and progesterone (Rajabi et al 1991b). Furthermore, there is evidence that this oestrogen-stimulated increase in procollagenase is associated with an increase in collagen degradation reflecting active collagenase activity (Rajabi et al 1991a). Prostaglandins, as well as having a direct effect on procollagenase production (Goshowaki et al 1988), may act as the intermediary in oestrogen-induced procollagenase production as indomethacin (an inhibitor of prostaglandin production) inhibits the effect of oestrogen (Rajabi et al 1991b). Paradoxically, progesterone, which might have been expected to inhibit procollagenase production, increased the production of this protease at physiological concentrations, however, this may be important for tissue remodelling during pregnancy or to increase stores of this latent form of the protease in anticipation of activation at the time of parturition. Pharmacological concentrations of progesterone (10^{-4} M) inhibit procollagenase production and gene expression in response to oestrogen (Rajabi et al 1991b). This change in collagenolytic activity may also be reflected in the further increase in soluble collagen seen at term and during labour (von Maillot & Zimmermann 1976, Granstrom et al 1989). However, Granstrom et al (1989) have shown no difference in collagenolytic activity between women at term not in labour and women at term in labour, although both groups had significantly and substantially higher collagenolytic activities compared to the non-pregnant cervix. Although there are conflicting data on collagenase activity in the cervix in relation to parturition, it would appear that there is a remodelling of collagen in the cervical connective tissue which occurs as pregnancy advances. The physiological basis of this would appear to be to facilitate ripening during the processes of parturition.

Glycosaminoglycans and proteoglycans

The changes of cervical ripening do not appear to be due

simply to collagen breakdown as a change in proteo-glycan, GAG and water content also occurs. The total GAG content of the cervix increases substantially by term, indicating active synthesis (Osmers et al 1993), however, the concentration of GAG may remain relatively constant (Golichowski 1980). The increase in total GAG is likely to reflect increased production by fibroblasts which become increasingly active as pregnancy advances (Junqueira et al 1980, Parry & Ellwood 1981). There is a relative increase in hyaluronic acid and a relative de-crease in chondroitin and dermatan sulphate, compared to both the non-pregnant cervix and the cervix in the third trimester of pregnancy (von Maillot et al 1979, Golichowski 1980, Osmers et al 1993), although other studies have not found any increase in hyaluronic acid concentration (Uldbjerg et al 1983a, Fosang et al 1984, Uldbjerg & Malmstrom 1991). Granstrom et al (1991) have found increased concentrations of hyaluronic acid in cervical biopsies taken from women in normal labour compared to women in protracted labour, although there was no difference in sulphated GAG which would include dermatan and chondroitin sulphates. Such a change in hyaluronic acid concentration/availability could at least partly explain the increased water content of the cervix which is seen during pregnancy (Ito et al 1979, Uldbjerg et al 1983a) and more particularly the marked increase seen just prior to term (Fitzpatrick & Dobson, 1981). The accumulation of hyaluronic acid and water between colla-gen fibrils will disperse them and increase distensibility. In addition, in view of the role of GAG in orientating the collagen fibrils and protecting them from breakdown, a decrease in dermatan sulphate concentration is likely to reduce the mechanical strength of the collagen fibrils, and make them more amenable to breakdown by proteo-lytic enzymes. Alternatively (or additionally), the increased hyaluronic acid content and associated increase in hydra-tion could reflect breakdown of the proteoglycan com-plexes to provide free hyaluronic acid and proteoglycans. The proteases required for this could come from the activated fibroblasts, or the leucocytes which infiltrate the cervical connective tissue. In addition to providing these proteases, leucocytes could increase vascular dilatation and permeability and thereby enhance tissue hydration.

Although there are some conflicting reports on changes in cervical glycosaminoglycans in association with labour, the available data appear to support a major increase in hyaluronic acid and a reduction in dermatan sulphate. In addition the relative concentration of chondroitin sulphate may fall as ripening occurs. As collagen is tightly bound by dermatan sulphate, a reduction in dermatan sulphate is likely to lead to a reduction in the rigidity of the tissue due to destabilization of the collagen fibrils while increased hyaluronic acid, or an increase in the hyaluronic acid available to bind water, may be associated with an increase in tissue hydration, and increased tissue deformability. The change in dermatan and chondroitin sulphates may antedate the increase in hyaluronic acid and may act to set the scene for destabilization of colla-gen, while the hyaluronic acid is associated with the major change in the cervix with substantial dispersal of collagen fibrils and increased tissue deformability immediately prior to ripening.

The lack of agreement as to the precise changes in GAG concentrations during ripening, perhaps suggests that the alteration in the ground substance may be more subtle. It could reflect a change in the proteoglycan com-position of the tissue which may not require a significant change in the concentration of GAG, but rather in their organization relative to proteoglycans. There are at least three proteoglycans relevant to cervical connective tissue; two small proteoglycans substituted with one (decorin) or two (biglycan) dermatan sulphate chains, and a large proteoglycan (PG-L) with chondroitin/dermatan sulphate side-chains. Decorin is the predominant proteoglycan found in cervical tissue and avidly binds collagen (Uldbjerg & Danielsen 1988, Uldbjerg & Malmstrom 1991). Biglycan appears not to bind collagen well due to its biglycan struc-ture and could destabilize collagen fibrils. PG-L forms proteoglycan complexes linking to hyaluronic acid in a similar way as in cartilage and could control tissue hydra-tion. At term there is an increase in the ratio of decorin to collagen and an increase in production of biglycan and PG-L (Uldbjerg & Ulmsten 1990, Uldbjerg & Malmstrom 1991). Such an alteration in the proteoglycan composition of the ground substance could easily result in a major alteration of the biomechanical properties of the cervix. In the rat, a strong correlation exists between the cervical linear circumference and the small dermatan sulphate proteoglycan : collagen ratio (Kokenyesi & Woessner 1990) supporting this contention. There is evidence from in vitro studies with human tissue that pregnancy is associated with increased proteoglycan production with increases in PGL, decorin and biglycan with the decorin increasing least (Norman et al 1991), but this is accom-panied by an increase in proteoglycan degradation as the proteoglycan concentration falls. Nonetheless the new collagen formed through pregnancy may be secreted into a different proteoglycan milieu which, with biglycan and PGL predominating, would lead to the organization of the collagen fibrils. This work is supported by analysis of cervical biopsies taken after delivery where the relative tissue production of biglycan and PGL were increased while decorin was reduced compared to non-pregnant and term pregnant tissues (Norman et al 1993).

Control of cervical ripening

Cervical ripening appears to be an active process rather than a passive process consequent upon increased uterine activity. The latter possibility seems improbable in view of the changes which occur within the connective tissue and cellular components of the cervix during ripening, as these changes suggest significant activity within the tissue. Furthermore, in animal studies cervical ripening occurs even when the cervix is physically isolated from the uterus (Stys et al 1980, Ledger et al 1985), and ripening can also occur in the absence of detectable uterine activity.

Prostaglandins and other arachidonic acid metabolites

Prostaglandins undoubtedly play a role in the control of cervical ripening in the human. They are synthesized from arachidonic acid, which is stored in the cell membrane in a phospholipid complex, and released from tissues on demand. When cells are activated they will produce free arachidonic acid by the action of phospholipases, either phospholipase A_2 or phospholipase C acting in concert with diacylglyceride lipase. The free arachidonic acid can then be converted via the cyclo-oxygenase pathway to produce prostaglandins or via the lipoxygenase pathway to produce leukotrienes which are important inflammatory mediators (Fig. 29.4). Which of these pathways predominate and which prostaglandin is produced depends on the cell type. For example prostacyclin is the main prostaglandin produced by the vascular endothelium while thromboxane A_2 is the major product in platelets and PGE_2 and $PGF_{2\alpha}$ are the major products in the uterus and cervix.

The main prostaglandins produced by the cervix are PGE_2, PGI_2, and to a lesser extent $PGF_{2\alpha}$, and their production increases at term (Ellwood et al 1980). In addition, amniotic fluid concentrations of PGE_2 and $PGF_{2\alpha}$ correlate directly with the cervical score in women at term who are not in labour (Calder 1980). Receptors for PGE_2 and $PGF_{2\alpha}$ can also be demonstrated in the cervix (Crankshaw et al 1979). These data suggest that

prostaglandins have a physiological role in ripening and a further sharp increase in production accompanies parturition per se. There is no doubt that prostaglandins are effective pharmacological agents for ripening the cervix and natural and synthetic prostaglandins can ripen the cervix at any stage in pregnancy (Calder 1980, Calder & Greer 1991). Much of our knowledge regarding the physiological properties of prostaglandins in cervical ripening has been inferred from pharmacological observations. There are essentially two possible ways in which prostaglandins might bring about ripening: first, they could induce collagen breakdown and, secondly, they could alter collagen binding and tissue hydration by altering the GAG/proteoglycan composition.

There is little doubt that PGE_2 treatment will reduce collagen concentration promoting changes similar to those seen during physiological ripening (Uldbjerg et al 1981, Ekman et al 1986, Johnston et al 1992). In addition, PGE_2 metabolite concentrations in plasma following PGE_2 administration for induction of labour correlate with the change in cervical score (Greer et al 1990). However, there is disagreement as to whether PGE_2 will induce collagenolysis. Some studies have reported an increase in collagenase or collagenase-like hydrolytic activity following PGE_2 administration (Szalay et al 1981, Ding et al 1990) and prostaglandins, as discussed above, appear to be involved in the control of procollagenase production in animal models (Goshowaki et al 1988, Rajabi et al 1991b), while other studies have reported no change or a reduction in collagenase (Ellwood et al 1981, Uldbjerg et al 1983c, Rath et al 1987). This may to some extent reflect methodological problems in assessing collagenase activity. The study by Rath et al (1987), however, not only showed no change in collagenase activity, but also round an absence of collagen breakdown fragments on electrophoresis of tissue extracts taken from pregnant human cervices treated with the prostaglandin analogue sulprostone compared to placebo-treated cervices. In this study significant cervical ripening occurred in the treated group. This evidence suggests that prostaglandin treatment may have no direct stimulatory effect on collagenase activity, at least in the human, in vivo. Furthermore, Hillier & Wallis (1981) have shown that PGE_2 and $PGF_{2\alpha}$ have no effect on collagen breakdown in vitro. In contrast, however, arachidonic acid, the substrate for prostaglandins and leukotrienes, increased collagen breakdown in similar experiments, and phospholipase inhibitors blocked this response, while cyclo-oxygenase inhibitors were ineffective at concentrations which blocked prostaglandin production (Hillier & Wallis 1981).

Despite this, cervical ripening in terms of tissue compliance occurs rapidly in vitro following PGE_2 treatment (Conrad & Ueland 1976). This discrepancy may be explained by the finding of Christensen & Bygdeman (1985) and Christensen et al (1985), who showed that

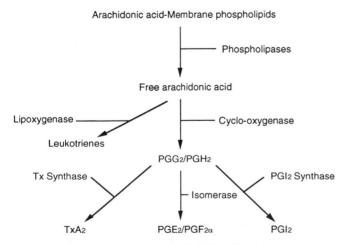

Fig. 29.4 Biosynthetic pathways for prostaglandins, thromboxane and leukotrienes.

PGE$_2$- and arachidonic acid-treated cervical tissues produced an increase in unidentified arachidonic acid products which were not prostaglandins.

Thus, arachidonic acid-induced ripening may be a non-prostaglandin-mediated effect perhaps due to leukotriene production which may also be stimulated by PGE$_2$. This possibility, however, remains speculative, but would be in keeping with the hypothesis (Liggins 1981) that cervical ripening is an inflammatory type process. Such an hypothesis is supported by the work of Ito et al (1987, 1990); they have shown that cytokines will markedly stimulate collagenase synthesis from macrophages and monocytes, that cervical explants from pregnant rats but not non-pregnant rats produce interleukin-1-like factors and that interleukin 1 can stimulate the production of elastase-like enzymes in human uterine cervical fibroblasts. Prostaglandins might also act in this manner by stimulating production of, or augmenting (Colditz 1990), the effect of chemotactic cytokines such as interleukin 8. This would induce a neutrophil influx and possibly release of leucocyte collagenase from storage granules within the neutrophil. As such a process is dependent on neutrophils being recruited to the tissue it would not be evident in vitro. It is also of interest that hyaluronic acid can induce interleukin 1 production from human monocytes (Hiro et al 1986) and thus the increase in hyaluronic acid production may also stimulate activation of an inflammatory response to facilitate tissue remodelling.

Prostaglandins may also act on the GAG composition and proteoglycan complexes in the cervical tissue (Uldbjerg et al 1981, 1983c). In animal studies PGE$_2$ has been shown to induce an increase in hydration and hyaluronic acid concentration. Paradoxically Cabrol et al (1990) found that in a rat model inhibition of prostaglandin production resulted in an increase in hyaluronic acid and suggested that this may be due to diversion of substrate towards the lipoxygenase pathway. PGE$_2$ can influence cervical fibroblast production of collagen and GAG. The production of these two substances is inversely related so that when collagen synthesis is reduced, an increase in GAG production occurs (Norstrom 1984, Norstrom et al 1985). This increase in GAG production by prostaglandins may be due to induction of the enzyme hyaluronic acid synthetase within the fibroblasts resulting in a substantial increase in hyaluronic acid (Murota et al 1977). A further possible mechanism is that PGE$_2$ may induce proteolytic breakdown of proteoglycan complexes which could also cause the increase in free hyaluronic acid content, although some studies do not support an increase in hyaluronic acid production in response to prostaglandins (Uldbjerg et al 1983c). Thus, PGE$_2$ mediated cervical ripening might easily be explained by changes in GAG/proteoglycan content or composition which will disperse and destabilize the collagen fibrils and increase tissue compliance as discussed above.

Oestrogen and progesterone

Other agents also act to control cervical structural changes. Oestradiol can stimulate prostaglandin production where there has been previous exposure to progesterone (Horton & Poyser 1976), and has been used to bring about cervical ripening in the clinical situation (Gordon & Calder 1977, Allen et al 1989). The mechanism underlying the effect of oestradiol on the cervix may be due, at least in part, to induction of prostaglandin synthesis. These findings have also been reported in the sheep where oestradiol-induced ripening has been associated with increased cervical prostaglandin production along with an alteration in GAG synthesis (Fitzpatrick & Dobson 1981). In addition, oestradiol has been linked to an increase in collagenase activity (Mochizuki & Tojo 1980), although this has not been confirmed by others (Ellwood et al 1981, Wallis & Hillier, 1981). Oestradiol might also be responsible for the influx of protease-producing leucocytes which could induce ripening and which would not be evident in vitro.

Progesterone appears to have an inhibitory effect on cervical ripening and parturition in animals where a fall in progesterone at term results in ripening and labour. Such a fall does not occur in the human, but progesterone is a potent anti-inflammatory agent (Siiteri et al 1977) and could still be an important physiological inhibitor of the ripening process in vivo by inhibiting neutrophil influx and activation (Jeffrey & Koob 1980). This possibility is supported by the ripening effects of antiprogestins on the cervix prior to termination of pregnancy (Gupta & Johnston 1990, Radestad et al 1990) and which is associated with a neutrophil influx in animal models (Chwalisz et al 1991). Kelly et al (1992) have recently shown that choriodecidua and chorion can synthesize interleukin 8, a neutrophil chemotactic and activating factor, and that this production is inhibited by progesterone and stimulated by antiprogestogens. PGE$_2$ acts synergistically with interleukin 8 to reduce by 100-fold the threshold for interleukin 8's effect in terms of neutrophil influx (Colditz et al 1990).

Thus endogenous or exogenous PGE$_2$ may destabilize the cervical and choriodecidual tissue and attract neutrophils. However, antiprogestins might exert their effects through prostaglandins as they appear to stimulate prostaglandin synthesis and reduce catabolism in vitro (Kelly et al 1986, Kelly & Bukman 1990). This may also be the mechanism of uterine sensitization to oxytocin seen with antiprogestin treatment. However, ex vivo studies with cervical biopsies treated with the antiprogestin RU 486 have shown no difference in prostaglandin production from radiolabelled arachidonic acid compared to placebo-treated cervices despite a significant objectively assessed ripening effect in the treated group (Radestad et al 1990). Nonetheless, the marked success of antiprogestins in effecting cervical ripening and abortion suggest that they will provide a useful tool to help dissect out the physiological control of cervical ripening and perhaps eventually also an effective agent for cervical ripening and induction of labour in clinical practice (Frydman et al 1991).

Relaxin

Relaxin has been shown to have some effect on cervical ripening in women (MacLennan 1981) and it has been reported to increase collagenase activity (von Maillot et al 1977). Human fibroblasts exhibit relaxin receptors and relaxin has a mitogenic effect on fibroblasts (McMurtry et al 1980). Relaxin may therefore be involved in the ripening process but our understanding of this possible mechanism is far from clear. However, if relaxin were to prove an effective pharmacological agent for ripening in the clinical situation, it may, unlike the prostaglandins, be selective on the cervix and devoid of stimulatory effects on uterine contractility. Such a selective effect would be of value in the process of induction of labour, avoiding the stimulation of uterine activity prior to adequate cervical ripening. Recently recombinant human relaxin has become available and has been used in clinical studies. It has been administered as a vaginal gel; however, this did not alter serum relaxin concentrations and there was no effect on cervical score or labour outcome (Bell et al 1993). This lack of effect may reflect an inadequate dose of relaxin, failure of significant absorption from the vagina into the cervix or simply that relaxin has no effect on the human cervix. These possibilities have not been addressed and it is impossible to say whether or not relaxin has a role in the physiology or pharmacology of cervical ripening. The availability of human relaxin does provide a tool to assess its role and such investigations would be of value to our understanding of the mechanism of cervical ripening.

UTERINE CONTRACTILITY

The myometrium consists predominantly of smooth muscle cells arranged in bundles embedded in a connective tissue matrix, made up principally of collagen, which helps to transmit the generated tension throughout the tissue. As with all smooth muscle cells, they contract in a calcium-dependent manner by the interaction of myosin and actin filaments within each smooth muscle cell. When intracellular free calcium increases it interacts with calmodulin to activate myosin light chain kinase which in turn phosphorylates the light chains of myosin. The phosphorylated myosin interacts with actin and results in contraction. A fall in calcium results in dephosphorylation and relaxation. The calcium may be made available from extracellular sources or can be released from the sarcoplasmic reticulum of the smooth muscle cells through a variety of receptor-operated and voltage-dependent calcium channels.

The myometrium is not richly innervated (Garfield 1986), thus nervous stimulation does not appear to be essential for uterine activity. This suggests that the myometrium is under hormonal control. Despite the lack of innervation, uterine contractions are usually coordinated in a cohesive manner during parturition. This is brought about by the development of intercellular connections termed gap junctions which develop during the last few weeks of pregnancy and become most numerous during labour (Garfield et al 1977, 1980a, Garfield & Hayashi 1981, Garfield et al 1990). Gap junctions form when a mirror image of protein units, termed connexons, sited within adjacent cell membranes fuse to form an aqueous pore which allows the free passage of small molecules and ions. Thus, these junctions allow the cells to communicate both metabolically and electrophysiologically (Cole et al 1985, 1986) with a low resistance pathway for electrical signals which are critical for the development of the powerful, coordinated contractions of labour. This transforms the myometrium into a functional syncitium. The spontaneous electrical activity of the uterus originates from pacemaker cells in the myometrium which have a lower resting membrane potential than the other smooth muscle cells. There appears to be no constant pacemaker area within the human uterus (Wolfs & van Leeuwan 1979) and each myometrial cell is capable of becoming a pacemaker, thus allowing pacemaker areas to move within the tissue (Osa et al 1983). The control of myometrial activity therefore depends both on the development of gap junctions which are essential for coordinated uterine action and also changes in free intracellular calcium to activate the myometrial cells and induce contractions

Prostaglandins and uterine contractility

As in cervical ripening, prostaglandins appear to play a major role in the physiology and pharmacology of uterine contractility. This similarity is more likely to be by nature's design than by accident to allow ripening and contractility to develop in synchrony using similar physiological mechanisms. Pharmacologically, we can stimulate labour using prostaglandins and parturition can be delayed by inhibitors of prostaglandin production such as indomethacin (Creasy 1990). Prostaglandins E_2 and $F_{2\alpha}$ increase in amniotic fluid (Hillier et al 1974, Keirse 1979) and their metabolites increase in the peripheral circulation (Mitchell et al 1978a, 1982, 1984, Brennecke et al 1985, Johnston et al 1993) during the course of spontaneous labour. However, the major increase in PGE_2 metabolites appears to occur prior to established labour, while the major increase in $PGF_{2\alpha}$ metabolites occurs during labour correlating directly with the duration of labour (Johnston et al 1993). Furthermore, the increase in $PGF_{2\alpha}$

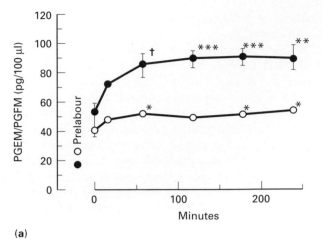

(a)

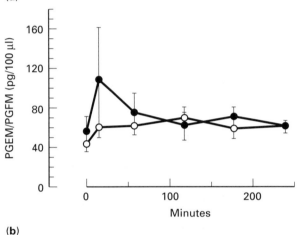

(b)

Fig. 29.5 Mean (SE) PGEM and PGFM concentrations in peripheral plasma during normal labour in 11 primigravid women (**a**) and dysfunctional labour in six primigravid women (**b**). ○ = PGEM; ● = PGFM. *$P < 0.02$, compared to pre-amniotomy (time 0) value; **$P < 0.008$, compared to pre-amniotomy (time 0) value; ***$P < 0.0006$, compared to pre-amniotomy (time 0) value; †$P < 0.05$, compared to immediately preceding value. Reproduced with permission from Johnston et al (1993).

metabolites failed to occur in women with dysfunctional labour (Johnston et al 1993) (Fig. 29.5). This suggests that $PGF_{2\alpha}$ is more important for generating and maintaining uterine contractility and this is supported by the work of Reddi et al (1984) who showed that amniotic fluid levels of $PGF_{2\alpha}$ were also reduced in dysfunctional labour. It is interesting that following PGE_2 administration for induction of labour an increase in the endogenous production of $PGF_{2\alpha}$ occurs which coincides with the onset of uterine contractility (Greer et al 1990). This suggests that PGE_2 production may activate $PGF_{2\alpha}$ production and thereby uterine contractility, but the mechanism behind this is unclear. As PGE_2 metabolite concentrations in plasma following PGE_2 administration for induction of labour correlate with the change in cervical score, it may be that PGE_2 is more important for cervical ripening.

Myometrial receptors for these prostaglandins may increase at term (Hertelendy & Molnar 1990). Both PGE_2

and $PGF_{2\alpha}$ can stimulate uterine contractility and sensitize the uterus to oxytocin (Hertelendy & Molnar 1990). At a cellular level these prostaglandins can cause both a phasic contraction and an increase in tonic tension with phasic contractions superimposed on this (Chamley & Parkington 1984). The phasic contraction appears to reflect a sodium influx into the cell while the tonic tension seems to be due to increased intracellular calcium induced by the prostaglandins (Reiner & Marshall 1976).

In vitro studies have shown that some prostaglandins will induce gap junction formation while cyclo-oxygenase inhibitors will inhibit gap junction formation (Garfield et al 1980a, 1980b). Oestradiol, however, has also been shown to induce gap junction formation, yet this effect is enhanced by cyclo-oxygenase inhibitors (MacKenzie & Garfield 1985). This apparent paradox can be explained by the fact that some prostaglandins such as PGE_2 and $PGF_{2\alpha}$ can stimulate gap junction formation, while others possibly including PGI_2 will inhibit their formation (Garfield et al 1980a, 1980b), although the mechanism behind this is unclear. Such an inhibitory effect by a prostaglandin like PGI_2 might be brought about by preventing the oestradiol-induced development of gap junctions, so that when its production is inhibited by a cyclo-oxygenase inhibitor, gap junction formation will increase as observed by MacKenzie & Garfield (1985). An alternative explanation is that cyclo-oxygenase inhibitors divert the arachidonic acid substrate into the leukotriene pathway and so may be effective by this route. However, there is no information on the effect of leukotrienes on gap junction formation to support or refute this hypothesis, and a recent study by Lopez Bernal et al (1989) has suggested that leukotrienes have little direct effect on human myometrial contractility.

The prostaglandins involved in stimulating uterine activity appear to be produced mainly in the amnion and decidua and not the myometrium. The myometrium does have the ability to produce prostaglandins. During pregnancy this ability is enhanced, due to increased levels of cyclo-oxygenase, but there is always an excess of PGI_2 synthase present, so that PGI_2 is the major prostaglandin product of myometrium (Christensen & Green 1983). This has been shown to reflect smooth muscle PGI_2 production rather than vascular endothelial PGI_2 production (Keirse et al 1984, Moonen et al 1985). The precise role of PGI_2 on myometrial activity is unclear, but it appears to be inhibitory (Lye & Challis 1982). In addition, no change in PGI_2 synthase occurs in relation to the time of parturition (Moonen et al 1984, Keirse, 1985). Thus, we must look towards the amnion and decidua as sources of stimulatory prostaglandins for the myometrium.

The major prostaglandin produced by the amnion and chorion is PGE_2 (Kinoshita et al 1977, Mitchell et al 1978b, Okazaki et al 1981, Olson et al 1983a) while the decidua will produce both PGE_2 and $PGF_{2\alpha}$ although the latter tends to predominate (Kinoshita et al 1977, Okazaki et al 1981, Skinner & Challis 1985). The ability of the amnion to produce PGE_2 appears to increase towards term (Lopez Bernal et al 1987a) and amnion obtained after labour has a higher rate of prostaglandin production (Olson et al 1983a, Okazaki et al 1981, Lopez Bernal et al 1987a) and a lower content of arachidonic acid (Mitchell & Lundin-Schiller 1990). Prostaglandin production appears to be controlled by the availability of substrate, i.e. arachidonic acid (Lopez Bernal et al 1987b). Labour does not appear to alter the incorporation of arachidonic acid into membrane phospholipids (Olson & Smieja 1988). However, amnion cells obtained from patients before labour and following labour can both respond to exogenous arachidonic acid while only cells obtained after labour can utilize arachidonic acid incorporated into intracellular pools (Rose et al 1990). This suggests that at the time of parturition, there is a switching on of an enzyme system to generate free arachidonic acid from membrane phospholipids (phospholipases) or alternatively coupling of such a system to the cyclo-oxygenase pathway. Alternatively, increased phospholipase activity could be brought about by means of the loss of an inhibitory mechanism. Recently, a protein which inhibits phospholipase activity has been characterized in fetal membranes. The activity of this protein, termed gravidin, may decrease in labour (Wilson et al 1989) and may be under the control of progesterone (Schuster-Woldan & Wilson 1993).

As there are specific high-affinity PGE_2 receptors in the myometrium (Adelantado et al 1985), it would appear that PGE_2 must play a role in myometrial contractility and therefore must be able to cross the chorion and decidua to reach the myometrium. Paradoxically however, $PGF_{2\alpha}$ increases more than PGE_2 in labour and the chorion contains high content and activity of 15-prostaglandin dehydrogenase activity (Challis et al 1990) and 13,14 reductase activity and therefore possesses an enormous capacity for prostaglandin metabolism (Okazaki et al 1981, Skinner & Challis 1985). Despite this high metabolic activity of chorion, PGE_2 has been shown to be able to cross the fetal membranes with significant quantities escaping metabolism (Nakla et al 1986), although other studies have been unable to confirm significant transfer (Roseblade et al 1990). As PGE_2 is the major prostaglandin produced by the amnion during parturition, while $PGF_{2\alpha}$ is the one which is seen to rise more markedly during the active phase of labour, it has been suggested that the $PGF_{2\alpha}$ might be produced by the conversion of PGE_2 through 9-keto-reductase, an enzyme which is present in the decidua. This hypothesis has been examined and while PGE_2 can be converted by 9-keto-reductase to $PGF_{2\alpha}$, it does not appear to proceed at a rate sufficient to explain the increase in $PGF_{2\alpha}$ seen in spontaneous

labour (Niesert et al 1986b, Cheung & Challis 1989). So it appears that the amnion produces the majority of PGE_2 which is seen in spontaneous labour and this can cross the fetal membranes to the myometrium; the likely source of $PGF_{2\alpha}$ is decidua, although a small amount may be formed from PGE_2 via the 9-keto-reductase pathway as discussed above.

Oxytocin

Oxytocin has traditionally been thought to have a role in the control of myometrial activity. It will induce contractions in a previously sensitized uterus and will also increase the force and frequency of contractions in uteri which are already contracting (Fuchs 1990). These effects have been exploited pharmacologically by obstetricians for induction and augmentation of labour since the seminal work of Turnbull & Anderson in the 1960s (Turnbull & Anderson 1968). At a cellular level oxytocin appears to act by enhancing the frequency and duration of electrical discharges from the myometrial cells by increasing intracellular calcium availability. The increase in cytosolic calcium ion concentration is brought about by calcium ion influx through specific agonist-operated calcium channels and also by the release of intracellular calcium stores and this may be mediated by generation of the second messenger inositol trisphosphate (Schrey et al 1986, 1988). This is in contrast to prostaglandins which cause calcium influx through voltage-operated channels and do not release intracellular calcium stores (Molnar & Hertelendy 1990, Thornton 1992a).

Despite these established effects of oxytocin, and especially the use of escalating oxytocin administration for induction and augmentation of labour by titrating administration against contraction frequency and intensity (Turnbull & Anderson 1968), plasma concentrations of oxytocin are not increased during late pregnancy or the first or second stage of labour (Thornton et al 1988, 1992b). Furthermore there is no evidence of any deficiency of oxytocin production being associated with inefficient uterine activity (Thornton et al 1992b). There may, however, be an increase in the pulse frequency of oxytocin release associated with labour (Fuchs 1990). Oxytocin, therefore, cannot mediate its effects on the myometrium by simply increasing its plasma concentration. It is known that the uterine sensitivity to oxytocin increases with advancing gestation and is maximal at the time of parturition (Fuchs 1990) and this may be the result of an increased number of receptors for oxytocin within the myometrium (Alexandrova & Soloff 1980, Fuchs et al 1982). Alternatively, or additionally, the change in sensitivity could be related to the membrane potential in the myometrium as the uterus has its lowest sensitivity to oxytocin when the resting membrane potential is highest in mid pregnancy and vice versa (Kao

1977). The control of the number and development of oxytocin receptors in the myometrium is unclear. Oestrogens have been shown to be able to stimulate oxytocin receptors while progesterone will inhibit this effect (Soloff et al 1979, Alexandrova & Soloff 1980, Fuchs 1983). Clinical practice suggests that pretreatment with prostaglandins increases uterine sensitivity to oxytocin. This may be due to the development of oxytocin receptors in a similar way to prostaglandin-induced gap junction formation. There is some evidence to suggest that oxytocin can stimulate decidual and amniotic prostaglandin production which could also contribute to the efficacy of oxytocin (Husslein 1985), however, administration of oxytocin in dysfunctional labour is not associated with any increase in PGE_2 or $PGF_{2\alpha}$ metabolites in plasma (Johnston et al 1993). Oxytocin concentrations in plasma do increase in the third stage of labour but this is not a consistent event. It is possible that oxytocin is a third-stage hormone which is important physiologically for the delivery of placenta and the prevention of postpartum haemorrhage in the human and that it is being harnessed artificially to drive contractions pharmacologically in the first stage of labour.

Oestrogen and progesterone

The steroid hormones are also of importance in the control of myometrial activity. While much of our information on the role of these hormones comes from animal studies, they remain relevant in the human, although unlike animals such as the sheep, human labour cannot be explained simply by alterations in steroid hormone concentrations. Oestrogens have a stimulatory effect on uterine contractility by reducing the resting membrane potential of the cells and increasing the formation of gap junctions (Garfield et al 1977, 1980a, 1980b, Fuchs 1985). The latter effect appears to be due to stimulation of messenger RNA (Lye et al 1993, Petrocelli & Lye 1993) and subsequent synthesis of connexin-43, the protein which makes up the gap junctions, and this effect can be inhibited by anti-oestrogens and inhibitors of protein synthesis (Garfield et al 1980a, Mackenzie & Garfield 1985). Oestrogens may also stimulate prostaglandin production (Olson et al 1983b) and oxytocin receptors (Alexandrova & Soloff 1980). The inhibitory effects of progesterone are mediated via a decrease in electrical conductiveness between cells by inhibiting the formation of gap junctions (Garfield et al 1980a, 1980b) via reduction in mRNA production for connexin-43 (Petrocelli & Lye 1993). Furthermore, progesterone will antagonize the stimulatory effect of oestrogen on connexin-43 mRNA (Petrocelli & Lye 1993). Conversely, antiprogesterones such as RU486 will induce gap junction formation (Garfield & Baulieu 1987) by stimulating mRNA for connexin-43 (Petrocelli & Lye 1993).

CONTROL OF PARTURITION

While we are aware of several components of the physiological systems controlling labour, the mechanism behind human parturition remains enigmatic. Much of our knowledge on mammalian parturition stems from the progesterone block theory of labour which was first proposed by Csapo in 1961. This theory suggests that there is a balance between myometrial stimulants, including oestrogen and prostaglandins, and myometrial relaxants such as progesterone. During pregnancy this balance would be tipped in favour of progesterone, but in parturition progesterone levels would fall and the balance would then tip in favour of the myometrial stimulants and labour would ensue. While this theory holds true for parturition in the sheep, in the human there is no change in progesterone concentration at the time of labour. Paradoxically however, antiprogestogens are effective abortificients both in animals and humans and increase the myometrial sensitivity to prostaglandins (Baulieu 1985, Garfield & Baulieu 1987, Rodger & Baird 1987, Rodger et al 1988). This effect suggests that progesterone must play a major role in maintaining pregnancy in the human. Thus, despite the lack of any change in progesterone levels at term in the human, there may still be a change at cellular level in receptors or receptor occupancy. This raises the possibility that an endogenous antiprogestogenic steroid exists in the human which could compete at receptor level with progesterone, so reducing the effects of progesterone at a cellular level without any change in the plasma levels of this hormone being apparent.

In contrast to the human, parturition in the sheep is reasonably well understood now and while there are many substantial differences from the human situation, it is unlikely phylogenetically that two entirely separate mechanisms exist in mammals, and there appear to be several common and parallel components between both these species. As much of our understanding of human parturition stems from investigations in ovine models, we should first consider how parturition is controlled in the sheep.

Ovine parturition

The control of parturition in the sheep appears to be mediated through maturation of the fetal hypothalamo–pituitary–adrenal axis (Challis & Brooks 1989). The fetal hypothalamus releases corticotrophin releasing factor (CRF) which in turn stimulates adrenocorticotrophic hormone (ACTH) in the pituitary over the last few weeks of gestation (Brooks & Challis 1988). The ACTH in turn stimulates fetal adrenal cortisol production which acts in the placenta to stimulate activity of 17-hydroxylase which is required to convert progesterone to oestrogen (Flint et al 1975). Thus, the balance between myometrial stimulants and myometrial relaxants is disturbed with a reduction in the myometrial relaxant progesterone and an increase in the myometrial stimulant oestrogen. This change in placental steroid production will stimulate prostaglandin production, gap junction formation and myometrial excitability and enhance uterine sensitivity to oxytocin which culminates in parturition.

This theory is supported by the increase in ACTH (Norman et al 1985) and subsequently cortisol (Bassett & Thorburn 1969) in the fetal circulation towards term. Activation of the hypothalamo–pituitary–adrenal axis with the resultant cortisol production is also likely to play a major role in organ maturation by enhancing enzyme activities (Liggins 1976). This ensures that organ maturation is satisfactory prior to parturition and so not only stimulates labour, which might be regarded as the ultimate maturational process in the fetus, but prepares the fetus for extrauterine survival. This theory is supported by the evidence that fetal hypophysectomy (Liggins et al 1967), bilateral destruction of the paraventicular nuclei (the location of the CRF producing neurones) (McDonald & Nathanielsz 1991) or adrenalectomy (Drost & Holm 1968) will upset the timing of parturition. In addition CRF (Wintour et al 1986), ACTH, cortisol (Liggins 1968, Lye et al 1983) and oestrogen (Liggins 1983) can all stimulate parturition while progesterone will inhibit it in the ovine model (Liggins 1983).

Within the activation of the hypothalamo–pituitary–adrenal axis which occurs and results in the stimulation of uterine activity, there are a number of positive feedback loops which will amplify the process (Challis & Brooks 1989). Cortisol appears to stimulate production of cortisol binding globulin thus preventing or reducing the negative feedback of cortisol at hypothalamic and pituitary levels so allowing CRF and ACTH to increase despite high levels of cortisol (Challis & Brooks 1989). Furthermore, cortisol also appears to be able to enhance its own production in response to ACTH at the level of the fetal adrenal (Challis et al 1985, Challis & Roberts 1988). This may be a result of increasing ACTH receptors or induction of enzymes essential for steroid production. There is also some evidence that PGE_2 may feedback in a positive manner to stimulate ACTH and cortisol levels (Thorburn et al 1988), so augmenting the whole process.

Human parturition

In the human just as in the sheep, prostaglandins appear to constitute the final common pathway for both cervical ripening and uterine contractility as discussed above. Their production appears to be controlled by the fetus. This may be due to activation of the hypothalamo–pituitary–adrenal axis, again linking fetal maturation

with parturition. However, the major difference between these species is that the human placenta is deficient in 17α-hydroxylase. This means that it cannot convert progesterone to oestrogen and no change in progesterone or oestrogen levels are found at the onset of human labour (Liggins 1983). The presence of aromatase in the human placenta does, however, allow it to convert androgens to oestrogens and so may alter the oestrogen/progesterone ratio, although this does not appear to be under the direct control of the cortisol cascade. The major androgen produced by the human fetal adrenal is DHEA sulphate which placental aromatase will convert to oestradiol.

Despite the seeming lack of evidence suggesting that the hypothalamo–pituitary–adrenal axis in the human fetus is unable to alter the steroid hormone milieu at placental level, there is much evidence supporting activation of this axis in the initiation of human labour. Maternal plasma levels of CRF increase exponentially during the second half of pregnancy peaking at delivery and high concentrations of this substance are also found in umbilical cord plasma and amniotic fluid at term (Goland et al 1986, Sasaki et al 1987, Campbell et al 1987, Petraglia et al 1987). An increase in CRF can also be found in the amniotic fluid in the third trimester (Laatikainen et al 1988). Furthermore, high levels of CRF have also been associated with the onset of preterm labour (Frim et al 1988). The source of CRF, however, is not from the fetal or the maternal hypothalamus but from the placenta. The CRF will disappear from the maternal circulation within 24 hours of delivery (Goland et al 1986, Campbell et al 1987) and gestationally related mRNA for CRF is also present in placental cells and parallels the increase in plasma CRF (Frim et al 1988) Further support for placental production comes from the finding that umbilical venous plasma has a higher CRF concentration than arterial plasma (Goland et al 1986, 1988). The cell origin of CRF appears to be in the syncitiotrophoblast which has been localized by immunocytochemistry (Riley et al 1991). In addition the amnion, the chorion and the decidua have all been shown to produce CRF and to produce it in greater quantities after spontaneous labour than after elective Caesarean section (Jones et al 1989).

This production of CRF is regulated by steroid hormones as progesterone will inhibit it while corticosteroids will increase its production, the latter forming a positive feedback loop (Jones et al 1989, Robinson et al 1988). In vitro studies suggest that CRF will act by stimulating ACTH production (Petraglia et al 1987) and ACTH increases in concentration during the third trimester (Cart et al 1981). Like CRF, ACTH can be produced by the fetal membranes as mRNA for proopiomelanocortin (POMC), the ACTH prehormone, is present in placental cells and is stimulated by CRF (Margioris et al 1988). Thus placental CRF and ACTH production will feedback to further stimulate the fetal adrenal to produce cortisol and DHEA-sulphate, the latter being converted to oestradiol by placental aromatase, and so facilitate uterine activity. There is also evidence linking hypothalamo–pituitary–adrenal axis activation with organ maturation in the human with high levels of CRF being associated with lung maturation in vivo (Laatikainen et al 1988).

The hypothalamo–pituitary–adrenal axis is also involved in the control of prostaglandin production. PGE_2 and $PGF_{2\alpha}$ are able to stimulate ACTH production, an effect which can be blocked by CRF antagonists (Petraglia et al 1987), indicating that CRF is an intermediary in this process. In addition, there is evidence to support an interaction in the opposite direction as CRF appears to be able to stimulate PGE_2 and $PGF_{2\alpha}$ production from the human placenta and fetal membranes (Jones & Challis 1989). Thus within the fetal membranes a positive feedback loop exists between the prostaglandins, CRF and ACTH.

From the above discussion it appears that there is evidence implicating the hypothalamo–pituitary–adrenal axis in human labour. However, this cannot be the whole story as human labour cannot be induced by cortisol administration and it is known that cortisol will inhibit prostaglandin production by inhibiting the actions of phospholipases, through lipocortins, which provide the arachidonic acid from the cell membrane necessary for prostaglandin production (Flower & Blackwell 1979, Hong & Levine 1979, Blackwell et al 1986, Flower 1986). So there must be some other factor involved in human parturition. Indeed the complexity of the process of parturition may represent a physiological safeguard against preterm labour with no single factor being able to initiate labour, but rather a series of interrelated and interdependent factors. It appears that in human labour a direct stimulus may be present which could bypass the inhibitory effects of corticosteroids on prostaglandin production. This could help drive the system with regard to the production of prostaglandins, which act as the final common mediators in parturition. There is evidence that fetal urine at term contains a substance able to stimulate production of prostaglandins from the fetal membranes,

with urine obtained after spontaneous vaginal delivery having a greater stimulatory effect than that obtained following elective Caesarean section (Casey et al 1983, Niesert et al 1986a). There is also evidence to suggest that the arachidonic acid utilized for prostaglandin production in response to stimulation by fetal urine comes from extracellular sources (Niesert et al 1986a). Recently Takahashi et al (1988) have shown that phospholipase C activity increases in the amniotic fluid towards term and that this appears to be derived from fetal urine. They also showed that phosphotidylinositol increases in amniotic fluid between 30 and 37 weeks' gestation then decreases toward term. The source of this phosphotidylinositol is likely to be the fetal lung. As this phospholipid is rich in arachidonic acid it could supply the extracellular source of arachidonic acid for prostaglandin production, with the fall in phosphotidylinositol after 37 weeks reflecting the breakdown of this phospholipid for subsequent prostaglandin production. Again, the availability of substrate possibly from fetal lung and the stimulatory factor to drive prostaglandin production in fetal urine could be related to organ maturation.

In conclusion, the control of human parturition appears to be due to activation of the hypothalamo–pituitary–adrenal axis and this is linked to organ maturation. There are several positive feedback loops driving this pathway in the fetoplacental unit and in addition there are interactions between this pathway and prostaglandins. CRF will stimulate prostaglandin production from fetal membranes and prostaglandins in turn can stimulate CRF. However, this system may be more facilitatory than stimulatory, priming the membranes for prostaglandin production when the appropriate stimulus is provided by the fetus, with the stimulus being linked to organ maturation. This hypothesis however remains speculative, being derived from the fragmented evidence for the role of these systems in human parturition. Undoubtedly this is a gross oversimplification of a complex process which in view of its key role in the survival of the species may have multiple interacting and interdependent mechanisms aimed at safeguarding the timing of labour which is crucial for survival.

REFERENCES

Adelantado J M, Humphrey S J, Lopez Bernal A, Turnbull A C 1985 Is there a topographical distribution of prostaglandin E_2 receptors in the pregnant human uterus? In: Jones C, Nathanielsz P W (eds) The physiological development of the fetus and newborn. Academic Press, London, pp 489–492

Alexandrova M, Soloff M A 1980 Oxytocin receptors and parturition I. Control of oxytocin receptor concentration in the rat myometrium at term. Endocrinology 106: 730–735

Allen J, Uldberg N, Petersen L K et al 1989 Intracervical 17-β-oestradiol before induction of second trimester abortion with a prostaglandin E_1 analogue. European Journal of Obstetrics Gynecology and Reproductive Biology 32: 123–127

Anderson A M, Turnbull A C 1969 Relationship between length of gestation and cervical dilatation, uterine contractility and other factors during pregnancy. American Journal of Obstetrics and Gynecology 105: 1207–1215

Bassett J M, Thorburn G D 1969 Foetal plasma corticosteroids and initiation of parturition in sheep. Journal of Endocrinology 44: 285–286

Baulieu E E 1985 RU486: an antiprogestin with contragestive activity in women. In: Baulieu E E, Segal S J (eds) The antiprogestin steroid RU486 and human fertility control. Plenum, New York pp 1–25

Bell R J, Permezel M, MacLennan A, Hughes C, Healy D, Brennecke S 1993 A randomized double blind placebo controlled trial of the safety of vaginal recombinant human relaxin for cervical ripening. Obstetrics and Gynecology 82: 328–333

Bishop E H 1964 Pelvic scoring for elective induction. Obstetrics and Gynecology 24: 266–268

Blackwell G J, Carnuccio R, Di Rosa M, Flowers R J, Parente L, Persico P 1986 Macrocortin: a polypeptide causing the antiphospholipase effect of glucocorticoids Nature (London) 287: 147–148

Braxton Hicks J 1872 On the contractions of the uterus throughout pregnancy: their physiological effects and their value in the diagnosis of pregnancy. Transactions of the Obstetric Society XIII: 216–231

Brennecke S, Castle B M, Demers L M, Turnbull A C 1985 Maternal plasma prostaglandin E_2 metabolite levels during human pregnancy and parturition. British Journal of Obstetrics and Gynaecology 92: 345–349

Brooks A N, Challis J R G 1988 Regulation of the hypothalamic–pituitary–adrenal axis at birth. Canadian Journal of Physiology and Pharmacology 66: 1106–1111

Cabrol D, Dallot E, Bienkiewicz A, El Alj A, Sedbon E, Cedard L 1990 Cyco-oxygenase and lipoxygenase inhibitors induce changes in the distribution of glycosaminoglycans in the pregnant rat uterine cervix. Prostaglandins 39: 515–523

Calder A A 1980 Pharmacological management of the unripe cervix in the human. In: Naftolin F, Stubblefield P G (eds) Dilatation of the uterine cervix. Raven, New York, pp 317–333

Calder A A, Greer I A 1991 Pharmacological modulation of cervical compliance in the first and second trimesters of pregnancy. Seminars in Perinatology 15: 162–171

Caldeyro-Barcia R 1959 Uterine contractility in obstetrics. Proceedings of the Second International Congress of Gynecology and Obstetrics, vol 1, Montreal, pp 65–78

Campbell E A, Linton E A, Wolfe C D A, Scraggs P R, Jones M T, Lowery J P 1987 Plasma corticotrophin-releasing hormone concentrations during pregnancy and parturition. Journal of Clinical Endocrinology and Metabolism 64: 1054–1059

Carr B R, Parker C R, Madden J D, Macdonald P C, Porter J C 1981 Maternal plasma adrenocorticotrophin and cortisol relationships throughout human pregnancy. American Journal of Obstetrics and Gynecology 139: 416–422

Casey M L, Macdonald P C, Mitchell M D 1983 Stimulation of prostaglandin in culture by a substance(s) in human fetal and adult urine. Biochemical and Biophysical Research Communications 114: 1056

Challis J R G, Roberts J 1988 Adenylate cyclase activity in adrenal membrane preparation from fetal sheep after in-vivo treatment with ACTG metopirone and cortisol. Medical Sciences Research 16: 353

Challis J R G, Brooks A N 1989 Maturation and activation of hypothalamic–pituitary–adrenal function in fetal sheep. Endocrine Reviews 10: 182–204

Challis J R G, Huhtanen D, Sprague C, Mitchell B F, Lye S J 1985 Modulation by cortisol of adrenocorticotrophin-induced activation of adrenal function in fetal sheep. Endocrinology 116: 2267–2272

Challis J R G, Jacobs R, Riley S C et al 1990 Distribution of prostaglandin synthesizing and metabolizing enzymes in intrauterine tissues. In: Garfield R E (eds) Uterine contractility. Serono Symposia. Massachusetts, Norwell, pp 143–152

Chamley W A, Parkington H C 1984 Relaxin inhibits the plateau component of the action potential in the circular myometrium of the rat. Journal of Physiology (London) 353: 51–65

Cheung P Y C, Challis J R G 1989 Prostaglandin E_2 metabolism in the human fetal membranes. American Journal of Obstetrics and Gynecology 161: 1580–1585

Christensen N J, Green K 1983 Bioconversion of arachidonic acid in human pregnant reproductive tissues. Biochemical Medicine 30: 162

Christensen N J, Bygdeman M 1985 The effect of prostaglandin on the bioconversion of arachidonic acid in the cervical tissue in early pregnancy. Prostaglandins 29: 291–302

Chwalisz K, Hegele Hartung C, Schulz R, Qing S S, Louton P T, Elger W 1991 Progesterone control of cervical ripening— experimental studies with the progesterone antagonists onapristone, lilopristone and mefipristone. In: Leppert P C, Woessner J F (eds) The extracellular matrix of the uterus cervix and fetal membranes:

synthesis, degradation and hormonal regulation. Perinatology Press, Ithaca, New York, pp 119–131

Colditz I G 1990 Effect of exogenous prostaglandin E_2 and actinomycin D on plasma leakage induced by neutrophil activating peptide-1/interleukin 8. Immunology and Cell Biology 68: 397–403

Cole W C, Garfield R E 1986 Evidence for physiological regulation of gap junction permeability. American Journal of Physiology 251: C411–C420

Cole W C, Garfield R E, Kirkcaldy J S 1985 Gap junctions and direct intercellular communication between rat uterine smooth muscle cells. American Journal of Physiology 249: C20–C31

Conrad J T, Ueland K 1976 Mediation of the stretch modulus of human cervical tissue by prostaglandin E_2. American Journal of Obstetrics and Gynecology 126: 218

Crankshaw D J, Crankshaw J, Branda L A, Daniel E E 1979 Receptors for E type prostaglandins in the plasma membrane of non-pregnant myometrium. Archives of Biochemistry and Biophysics 198: 459–465

Creasy R 1990 Preterm inhibition of myometrial contractility: clinical considerations. In: Garfield R E (eds) Uterine constractility. Serono Symposia. Norwell, Massachusetts, pp 371–380

Csapo A I 1961 Defence mechanisms in pregnancy. In: Progesterone and the defence mechanisms of pregnancy. CIBA Foundation Study Group No 9. Little Brown, Boston, no 9, pp 1–22

Danforth N D, Buckingham J C, Roddick J W 1960 Connective tissue changes incident to cervical effacement. American Journal of Obstetrics and Gynecology 86: 939–945

Danforth D N, Veis A, Breen M, Weinstein H G, Buckingham J C, Manalo P 1974 The effect of pregnancy and labor on the human cervix: changes in collagen, glycoproteins and glycosaminoglycans. American Journal of Obstetrics and Gynecology 120: 641–649

Ding J Q, Granberg S, Norstrom A 1990 Clinical effects and cervical tissue changes after treatment with 16, 16 dimethyl-trans delta 2 PGE1 methylester. Prostaglandins 39: 281–285

Drost M, Holm L W 1968 Prolonged gestation in ewes after foetal adrenalectomy. Journal of Endocrinology 40: 293–296

Ekman G, Malmstrom A, Uldbjerg N, Ulmsten U 1986 Cervical collagen: an important regulator of cervical function in term labour. Obstetrics and Gynaecology 67: 633–636

Ellwood D A, Mitchell M D, Anderson A B M, Turnbull A C 1980 The in-vitro production of prostanoids by the human cervix during pregnancy: preliminary observations. British Journal of Obstetrics and Gynaecology 87: 210–214

Ellwood D A, Anderson A B M, Mitchell M D, Murphy G, Turnbull A C 1981 Prostanoids, collagenase and cervical softening in sheep. In: Ellwood D A, Anderson A B M (eds) The cervix in pregnancy and labour: clinical and biochemical investigations. Churchill Livingstone, Edinburgh, pp 57–73

Fitzpatrick R J, Dobson H 1981 Softening of the ovine cervix at parturition. In: Ellwood D A, Anderson A B M (eds) The cervix in pregnancy and labour: clinical and biochemical investigations. Churchill Livingstone, Edinburgh, pp 40–56

Flint A P F, Anderson A B M, Steel P A, Turnbull A C 1975 The mechanism by which foetal cortisol controls the onset of parturition in the sheep. Biochemistry Society Transactions 3: 1189

Flower R J 1986 The mediators of steroid action. Nature (London) 320: 20

Flower R J, Blackwell G J 1979 Anti-inflammatory steroids induce biosynthesis of a phospholipase A_2 inhibitor which prevents prostaglandin generation. Nature (London) 278: 456–459

Fosang A J, Handley C J, Santer V 1984 Pregnancy related changes in the connective tissue of the ovine cervix. Biology of Reproduction 30: 1223–1235

Frim D, Emanuel R, Robinson B et al 1988 Characterization and gestational regulation of corticotrophin-releasing hormone messenger RNA in human placenta. Journal of Clinical Investigation 82: 287–292

Frydman R, Baton C, Lelaidier C, Vial M, Bourget P H, Fernandex H 1991 Mefipristone for induction of labour. Lancet 337: 488–489

Fuchs A R 1983 The role of oxytocin in parturition. Current Topics in Experimental Endocrinology 4: 231–265

Fuchs A R 1985 Oxytocin in animal parturition. In: Amico J A, Robinson A G (eds) Oxytocin: clinical and laboratory studies. Elsevier, Amsterdam, pp 277–235

Fuchs A R 1990 Oxytocin and oxytocin receptors: maternal signals for parturition. In: Garfield R E (eds) Uterine contractility. Serono Symposia. Massachusetts, Norwell, pp 177–190

Fuchs A R, Fuchs F, Hurstein P, Soloff M S, Fernstrom M J 1982 Oxytocin receptors and human parturition: a dual role for oxytocin in the initiation of labor. Science (New York) 215: 1396–1398

Garfield R A 1986 Structural studies of innervation on non pregnant rat uterus. American Journal of Physiology 251: C41–V56

Garfield R E, Baulieu E E 1987 The antiprogesterone steroid RU 486: a short pharmacological and clinical review with emphasis on the interruption of pregnancy. Baillières Clinical Endocrinology and Metabolism 1: 207–221

Garfield R A, Hayashi R H 1981 Appearance of gap junctions in the myometrium of women during labor. American Journal of Obstetrics and Gynecology 140: 254–260

Garfield R E, Kannan M S, Daniel E E 1980a Gap junction formation in myometrium: control by estrogens, progesterone and prostaglandins. American Journal of Physiology 238: C81–C89

Garfield R E, Merrett D, Groven A K 1980b Gap junction formation and regulation in myometrium. American Journal of Physiology 239: C217–C228

Garfield R E, Sims S, Daniel E E 1977 Gap junctions: their presence and necessity in myometrium during gestation. Science (New York) 198: 958–960

Garfield R E, Tabb T, Thilander G 1990 Intercellular coupling and modulation of uterine contractility. In: Garfield R E (ed) Uterine contractility. Serono Symposia. Massachusetts, Norwell, pp 21–40

Goland R S, Wardlaw S L, Stark R I, Brown L S, Frantz A G 1986 High levels of corticotrophin-releasing hormone immunoactivity in maternal and fetal plasma during pregnancy. Journal of Clinical Endocrinology and Metabolism 63: 1199–1203

Goland R S, Wardlaw S L, Blum M, Tropper R J, Stark R I 1988 Biologically active corticotrophin-releasing hormone in maternal and fetal plasma during pregnancy. American Journal of Obstetrics and Gynecology 159: 884–890

Golichowski A 1980 Cervical stromal interstitial polysaccharide metabolism in pregnancy. In: Naftolin F, Stubblefield P G (eds) Dilatation of the uterine cervix: connective tissue biology and clinical management. Raven, New York, pp 99–112

Gordon A J, Calder A A 1977 Oestradiol applied locally to ripen the unfavourable cervix. Lancet ii: 1319–1321

Goshowaki H, Ito A, Mori Y 1988 Effects of prostaglandins on the production of collagenase by rabbit uterine cervical fibroblasts. Prostaglandins 36: 107–114

Granstrom L, Ekman G, Ulmsten U, Malstrom A 1989 Changes in the connective tissue of corpus and cervix uteri during ripening and labour in term pregnancy. British Journal of Obstetrics and Gynaecology 96: 1198–1202

Granstrom L, Ekman G, Malmstrom A 1991 Insufficient remodelling of the uterine connective tissue in women with protracted labour. British Journal of Obstetrics and Gynaecology 98: 1212–1216

Greer I A, McLaren M, Calder A A 1990 Plasma prostaglandin E_2 and prostaglandin $F_{2\alpha}$ metabolite levels following vaginal administration of prostaglandin E_2 for induction of labor. Acta Obstetricia et Gynecologica Scandinavica 69: 621–626

Gupta J K, Johnston N 1990 Effect of mifepristone on dilatation of the pregnant and non-pregnant cervix. Lancet i: 1238–1240

Hertelendy F, Molnar M 1990 Mode of action of prostaglandins on myometrial cells. In: Garfield R E (ed) Uterine contractility. Serono Symposia. Massachusetts, Norwell, pp 221–236

Hillier K, Wallis R M 1981 Prostaglandins, steroids and the human cervix. In: Ellwood D A, Anderson A B M (eds) The cervix in pregnancy and labour. Churchill Livingstone, Edinburgh, pp 144–162

Hillier K, Calder A A, Embrey M P 1974 Concentrations of prostaglandin $F_{2\alpha}$ in amniotic fluid and plasma in spontaneous and induced labours. Journal of Obstetrics and Gynaecology of the British Empire 81: 257–263

Hiro D, Ito A, Matsuta K, Mori Y 1986 Hyaluronic acid is an endogenous inducer of interleukin 1 production by human monocytes and rabbit macrophages. Biochemical and Biophysical Research Communications 140: 715–722

Hong S L, Levine L 1979 Inhibition of arachidonic acid release from cells as the biochemical action of anti-inflammatory corticosteroids. Proceedings of the National Academy of Sciences of the USA 73: 1730

Horton E W, Poyser N 1976 Uterine luteolytic hormone: a physiological role for prostaglandin $F_{2\alpha}$. Physiological Reviews 56: 595–561

Husslein P 1985 Mode of action of oxytocin and the role of its receptor in the production of prostaglandins In: Wood C (ed) The role of prostaglandins in labour. Royal Society of Medicine, London, pp 15–24

Ito A, Kitamira K, Mori Y, Hirakowa S 1979 The change in solubility of type I collagen in human cervix in pregnancy at term. Biochemical Medicine 21: 262

Ito A, Hiro D, Sakyo K, Mori Y 1987 The role of leukocyte factors on uterine cervical ripening and dilatation. Biology Reproduction 37: 511–517

Ito A, Lippert P, Mori Y 1990 Human recombinant interleukin-1a increases elastase-like enzyme in human uterine cervical fibroblasts. Gynecological and Obstetrical Investigation 30: 239–241

Jeffrey J J 1991 Collagen and collagenase: pregnancy and parturition. Seminars in Perinatology 15: 118–126

Jeffrey J J, Koob T J 1980 Endocrine control of collagen degradation in the uterus In: Naftolin F, Stubblefield P G (eds) Dilatation of the uterine cervix. Raven, New York, pp 135–145

Johnston T A, Greer I A, Kelly R W, Calder A A 1992 The effect of pH on the release of PGE_2 from vaginal and endocervical preparations for induction of labour. An in-vitro study. British Journal of Obstetrics and Gynaecology 99: 877–880

Johnston T A, Greer I A, Kelly R W, Calder A A 1993 Plasma prostaglandin metabolite concentrations in normal and dysfunctional labour. British Journal of Obstetrics and Gynaecology 100: 483–488

Jones S A, Challis J R G 1989 Local stimulation of prostaglandin production by corticotrophin-releasing hormone in human fetal membranes and placenta. Biochemical and Biophysical Research Communications 159: 192–199

Jones S A, Brooks A N, Challir J R G 1989 Steroids modulate corticotrophin-releasing hormone production in human fetal membranes and placenta. Journal of Clinical Endocrinology and Metabolism 68: 825–830

Junqueira L C U, Zugaib M, Montes G S, Toledo D M S, Krisztan R M, Shigihara K M 1980 Morphological and histochemical evidence for the occurrence of collagenolysis and for the role of neutrophilic polymorphonuclear leukocytes during cervical dilatation. American Journal of Obstetrics and Gynecology 138: 273–281

Kao C Y 1977 Electrical properties of uterine smooth muscle. In: Wynn R M (ed) Biology of the uterus. Plenum, New York, pp 423–496

Keirse M J N C 1979 Endogenous prostaglandins in human parturition. In: Kerise M J N C, Anderson A B M, Bennebroek Gravenhorst J (eds) Human parturition. Leiden University Press, The Hague, pp 101–104

Keirse M J N C 1985 Biosynthesis and metabolism of prostaglandins within the human uterus in early and late pregnancy. In: Wood C (ed) The role of prostaglandin in labour. Royal Society of Medicine, London

Keirse M J N C, Moonen P, Klok G 1984 Prostaglandin synthase in pregnant human myometrium is not confined to the uteroplacental vasculature. IRCS Medical Science 12: 824

Kelly R W, Bukman A 1990 Antiprogestagenic inhibition of uterine prostaglandin inactivation: a permissive mechanism for uterine stimulation. Journal of Steroid Biochemistry and Molecular Biology 37: 97–101

Kelly R W, Healy D L, Cameron I T et al 1986 The stimulation of prostaglandin production by two antiprogesterone steroids in human endometrial cells. Journal of Clinical Endocrinology Metabolism 62: 1116–1123

Kelly R W, Leask R, Calder A A 1992 Choriodecidual production of interleukin 8 and mechanism of parturition. Lancet 339: 776–777

Kinoshita K, Satoh K, Sakamoto S 1977 Biosynthesis of prostaglandin in human decidua amnion chorion and villi. Endocrinologica Japanocia 24: 343–350

Kleissl H P, Van der Rest M, Naftolin F, Glorieux F H, De Leon A

1978 Collagen changes in the human cervix at parturition. American Journal of Obstetrics and Gynecology 130: 748–753

Kokenyesi R, Woessner J F 1990 Relationship between dilatation of the rat uterine cervix and a small dermatan sulphate proteoglycan. Biology of Reproduction 42: 87–97

Laatikainen T J, Raisanen I J, Salmiren K R 1988 Corticotrophin-releasing hormone in amniotic fluid during gestation and labor and in relation to fetal lung maturation. American Journal of Obstetrics and Gynecology 159: 891–895

Ledger W L, Webster M, Harrison L P, Anderson A B M, Turnbull A C 1985 Increase in cervical extensibility during labour induced after isolation of the cervix from the uterus in the pregnant sheep. American Journal of Obstetrics and Gynecology 151: 397–402

Liggins G C 1968 Premature parturition after infusion of corticotrophin or cortisol into foetal lambs. Journal of Endocrinology 42: 323–329

Liggins G C 1976 Adrenocortical-related maturational events in the fetus. American Journal of Obstetrics and Gynecology 126: 931

Liggins G C 1978 Ripening of the cervix. Seminars in Perinatology 2: 261–271

Liggins G C 1981 Cervical ripening as an inflammatory process. In: Ellwood D A, Anderson A B M (eds) The cervix in pregnancy and labour. Clinical and biochemical investigations. Churchill Livingstone, Edinburgh, pp 1–12

Liggins G C 1983 Initiation of spontaneous labour. Clinical Obstetrics and Gynecology 26: 47–55

Liggins G C, Kennedy P C, Holm L W 1967 Failure of initiation of parturition after electrocoagulation of the pituitary of the fetal lamb. American Journal of Obstetrics and Gynecology 98: 1080–1086

Lopez Bernal A M, Hansell D J, Alexander S, Turnbull A C 1987a Prostaglandin E production by amniotic cells in relation to term and preterm labour. British Journal of Obstetrics and Gynaecology 94: 864–869

Lopez Bernal A M, Hansell D J, Alexander S, Turnbull A C 1987b Steroid conversion and prostaglandin production by chorionic and decidual cells in relation to term and preterm labour. British Journal of Obstetrics and Gynaecology 94: 1052–1058

Lopez Bernal A M, Canete Soler R, Turnbull A C 1989 Are leukotrienes involved in human uterine contractility? British Journal of Obstetrics and Gynaecology 96: 568–573

Lye S J, Challis J R G 1982 Inhibition by PGI_2 of myometrial activity in-vivo in non-pregnant ovariectomized sheep. Journal of Reproduction and Fertility 66: 311

Lye S J, Prague C L, Mitchell B F, Challis J R G 1983 Activation of ovine fetal adrenal function by pulsatile or continuous administration of adrenocorticotrophin (1–24) 1. Effects on fetal plasma corticosteroids. Endocrinology 113: 770–776

Lye S J, Nicholson B J, Mascarenhas M, MacKenzie L, Petrocelli T 1993 Increased expression of connexin-43 in the rat myometrium during labor is associated with an increase in the plasma estrogen : progesterone ratio. Journal of Endocrinology 132: 2380–2386

McDonald T J, Nathanielsz P W 1991 Bilateral destruction of the fetal paraventricular nuclei prolongs gestation in sheep. American Journal of Obstetrics and Gynecology 165: 764–770

MacKenzie L W, Garfield R E 1985 Hormonal control of gap junctions in the myometrium. American Journal of Physiology 248: C296–C308

MacLennan A H 1981 Cervical ripening and the induction of labour by vaginal prostaglandin $F_{2\alpha}$ and relaxin. In: Ellwood D A, Anderson A B M (eds) The cervix in pregnancy and labour: clinical and biochemical investigations. Churchill Livingstone, Edinburgh, pp 187–196

McMurty J P, Floersheim G L, Bryant-Greenwood G D 1980 Characterization of the binding of ^{125}I-labelled syccinylated porcine relaxin in human and mouse fibroblasts. Journal of Reproduction and Fertility 58: 43–49

Margioris A N, Grino M, Protos P, Gold P W, Chrousos G P 1988 Corticotrophin-releasing hormone and oxytocin stimulate the release of placental proopiomelonocortin peptides. Journal of Clinical Endocrinology and Metabolism 66: 922–926

Mitchell M D 1984 The mechanism(s) of human parturition. Journal of Developmental Physiology 6: 107–118

Mitchell M D, Lundin-Schiller S 1990 The regulation of arachidonic acid metabolism in pregnancy. In: Garfield R E (ed) Uterine contractility. Serono Symposia. Massachusetts, Norwell, pp 205–220

Mitchell M D, Flint A D F, Bibby J et al 1978a Plasma concentrations of prostaglandin during late human pregnancy: influence of normal and preterm labour. Journal of Clinical Endocrinology and Metabolism 46: 947–951

Mitchell M D, Bibby J, Hicks B R, Turnbull A C 1978b Specific production of prostaglandin E by human amnion in-vitro. Prostaglandins 15: 377–382

Mitchell M D, Ebenhack K, Kraemar D L, Cox K, Cutrer S, Strickland D M 1982 A sensitive radioimmunoassay for 11-deoxy-13,14 dihydro-15-keto 11,16-cyclo prostaglandin E_2: application as an index of prostaglandin E_2 biosynthesis during human pregnancy and parturition. Prostaglandins and Leukotrienes in Medicine 9: 549–557

Mochizuki M, Tojo S 1980 Effect of dehydroepiandrosterone sulfate on softening and dilatation of the uterine cervix in pregnant women. In: Naftolin F, Stubblefield P G (eds) Dilatation of the uterine cervix: connective tissue biology and clinical management. Raven, New York, pp 267–286

Moonen P, Klok G, Keirse M J N C 1984 Immunohistochemical localisation of prostaglandin endoperoxide synthase and prostacyclin synthase in pregnant human myometrium. European Journal of Obstetrics Gynecology and Reproductive Biology 19: 151

Moonen P, Klok G, Keirse M J N C 1985 Increase in concentration of prostaglandin endoperoxide synthase and prostacyclin synthase in late pregnancy. Prostaglandins 28: 309

Murota S, Abe M, Otsuka K 1977 Stimulatory effect of prostaglandins on the production of hexosamine-containing substances by cultured fibroblasts (3) induction of hyaluronic acid synthetase by prostaglandin $F_{2\alpha}$. Prostaglandins 14: 983–991

Nakla S, Skinner K, Mitchell B F, Challis J R G 1986 Changes in prostaglandin transfer across human fetal membranes obtained after spontaneous labor. American Journal of Obstetrics and Gynecology 155: 1337–1341

Niesert S, Mitchell M D, MacDonald P C, Casey M L 1986a The effect of fetal urine on arachidonic acid metabolism in human amnion cells in monolayer culture. American Journal of Obstetrics and Gynecology 155: 1310–1316

Niesert S, Christopherson W, Korte K, Mitchell M D, MacDonald P C, Casey M L 1986b Prostaglandin E_2 9-ketoreductase activity in human decidua vera tissue. American Journal of Obstetrics and Gynecology 155: 1348–1352

Norman L J, Lye S J, Wlodek M E, Challis J R G 1985 Changes in pituitary response to synthetic ovine corticotrophin-releasing factor in fetal sheep. Canadian Journal of Physiology and Pharmacology 63: 1398–1403

Norman M, Ekman G, Malmstrom A 1993 Changed proteoglycan metabolism in human cervix immediately after spontaneous vaginal delivery. Obstetrics and Gynecology 81: 217–223

Norman M, Ekman G, Ulmsten U, Barchan K, Malmstrom A 1991 Proteoglycan metabolism in the connective tissue of pregnant and non-pregnant human cervix. An in-vitro study. Biochemical Journal 275: 5155–5200

Norstrom A 1984 The effects of prostaglandins on the biosynthesis of connective tissue constituants in the non-pregnant human cervix uteri. Acta Obstetricia et Gynecologica Scandinavica 63: 169–173

Norstrom A, Bergman I, Lindblom B, Christensen N J 1985 Effects of 9 deoxo-16, 16 dimethyl-9-methylene PGE_2 on muscle contractile activity and collagen synthesis in the human cervix. Prostaglandins 29: 337–346

Okazaki T, Casey M L, Ikita J R, Macdonald P C, Johnston J M 1981 Initiation of human parturition XII. Biosynthesis and metabolism of prostaglandins in human fetal membranes and uterine decidua. American Journal of Obstetrics and Gynecology 139: 373

Olson D M, Smieja Z 1988 Arachidonic acid incorporation into lipids of term human amnion. American Journal of Obstetrics and Gynecology 159: 995–1001

Olson D M, Skinner K, Challis J R G 1983a Prostaglandin output in relation to parturition by cells dispersed from intrauterine tissues. Journal of Clinical Endocrinology and Metabolism 57: 694–699

Olson D M, Skinner K, Challis J R G 1983b Estradiol-17β and

20-hydroxyestradiol induced differential production of prostaglandins by cells dispersed from human intrauterine tissues at parturition. Prostaglandins 25: 639

Osa T, Ogasawara T, Kato S 1983 Effects of magnesium, oxytocin and prostaglandin $F_{2\alpha}$ on the generation and propagation of excitation in the longitudinal muscle of rat myometrium during late pregnancy. Japanese Journal of Physiology 33: 51–67

Osmers R, Rath W, Adelmann-Grill B C, Fittkow C, Szeverenyi M, Kuhn W 1990 Collagenase activity in the cervix of non-pregnant and pregnant women. Archives of Gynecology and Obstetrics 248: 75–80

Osmers R, Rath W, Pflanz M A, Kuhn W, Stuhlsatz H W, Szeverenyi M 1993 Glycosaminoglycans in cervical connective tissue during pregnancy and parturition. Obstetrics and Gynecology 81: 88–92

Parry D S, Ellwood D A 1981 Ultrastructural aspects of cervical softening in sheep. In: Ellwood D A, Anderson A B M (eds) The cervix in pregnancy and labour: clinical and biochemical investigations. Churchill Livingstone, Edinburgh, pp 74–84

Petraglia F, Sawchenk P E, Rivier J, Vale W 1987 Evidence for local stimulation of ACTH secretion by corticotrophin-releasing factor in human placenta. Nature (London) 328: 717–719

Petrocelli T, Lye S J 1993 Regulation of transcripts encoding the myometrial gap junction protein connexin-43 by estrogen and progesterone. Journal of Endocrinology 133: 284–290

Radestad A, Bygdeman M, Green K 1990 Induced cervical ripening with mifepristone (RU 486) and bioconversion of arachidonic acid in human pregnant uterine cervix in the first trimester. Contraception 41: 283–292

Rajabi M R, Dean D D, Woessner Jr J F 1985 Serum collagenase activity in pregnant parturient and postpartum women. Annals of the New York Academy of Science 460: 492–493

Rajabi M R, Dean D D, Beydoun S N, Woessner J F 1988 Elevated tissue levels of collagenase during dilatation of uterine cervix in human parturition. American Journal of Obstetrics and Gynecology 159: 971–976

Rajabi M R, Dodge G R, Solomon S, Poole A R 1991a Immunochemical and immunohistochemical evidence of estrogen-mediated collagenolysis as a mechanism of cervical dilatation in the guinea pig at parturition. Endocrinology 128: 371–378

Rajabi M R, Solomon S, Poole A R 1991b Hormonal regulation of interstitial collagenase in the uterine cervix of the guinea pig. Endocrinology 128: 863–871

Rath W, Adelmann-Grill B C, Pieper U, Kuhn W 1987 The role of collagenases and proteases in prostaglandin induced cervical ripening. Prostaglandins 34: 119–127

Reddi K, Kambaran S R, Norman R J, Joubert S M, Philpott R H 1984 Abnormal concentrations of prostaglandins in amniotic fluid during labour in multigravid patients. British Journal of Obstetrics and Gynaecology 91: 781–787

Reiner O, Marshall J M 1976 Action of D-60 on spontaneous and electrically stimulated activity of the parturient rat uterus. Naunyn-Schmiedeberg's Archives of Pharmacology 290: 21–28

Riley S C, Walton J C, Herlick J M, Challis J R G 1991 The localization and distribution of corticotrophin-releasing hormone in the human placenta and fetal membranes throughout gestation. Journal of Clinical Endocrinology and Metabolism 72: 1001–1007

Rodger M W, Baird D T 1987 Induction of therapeutic abortion in pregnancy and mifepristone in combination with prostaglandin pessary. Lancet ii: 1415–1418

Rodger M W, Logan A F, Baird D T 1988 Induction of early abortion with mifepristone (RU486) and two different doses of prostaglandin pessary (gemeprost). Contraception 39: 497–502

Rose M P, Myatt L, Elder M G 1990 Pathways of arachidonic acid metabolism in human amnion cells at term. Prostaglandins Leukotrienes and Essential Fatty Acids 39: 303–309

Roseblade C K, Sullivan M H F, Khan H, Lumb M R, Elder M G 1990 Limited transfer of prostaglandin E_2 across the fetal membranes before and after labor. Acta Obstetrica et Gynecologica Scandinavica 69: 399–404

Sasaki A, Shinkawa O, Margioris A N et al 1987 Immunoreactive corticotrophin-releasing hormone in human plasma during pregnancy, labor and delivery. Journal of Clinical Endocrinology and Metabolism 64: 224

Schrey P, Read A M, Steer P J 1986 Oxytocin and vasopression stimulate inositol phosphate production in human gestational myometrium and decidual cells. Bioscience Reproduction 6: 613–619

Schrey P, Cornford P A, Read A M, Steer P J 1988 A role for phosphonositide hydrolysis in human uterine smooth muscle during parturition. American Journal of Obstetrics and Gynecology 159: 964–970

Schuster-Woldan N, Wilson T 1993 The control of gravidin production. In: 3rd European Congress Prostaglandins in Reproduction Edinburgh, p 40

Scott J E, Orford C R 1981 Dermatan sulphate rich proteoglycan associated with rat tail tendon collagen at the d band in the gap region. Biochemical Journal 197: 213

Skinner K A, Challis J R G 1985 Changes in the synthesis and metabolism of prostaglandins by human fetal membranes and decidua at labor. American Journal of Obstetrics and Gynecology 151: 519

Soloff M S, Alexandrova M, Fernstrom M J 1979 Oxytocin receptors: triggers for parturition and lactation? Science (New York) 204: 1313–1315

Stricklin G P, Hibbs M S 1988 Biochemistry and physiology of mammalian collagenases. In: Nimni M E (ed) Collagen biochemistry, vol 1. CRC Press, Boca Raton, Florida, pp 187–205

Stys S J, Clarke K E, Clewell W M et al 1980 Hormonal effects on cervical compliance in sheep. In: Naftolin F, Stubblefield P G (eds) Dilatation of the uterine cervix. Raven, New York, pp 147–156

Szalay S, Husslein P, Grunberger W 1981 Local application of prostaglandin E_2 and its influence on collagenolytic activity of cervical tissue. Singapore Journal of Obstetrics and Gynecology 12: 15

Takahashi H, Murata M, Maki M 1988 Phospholipase C activity and phosphotidylinositol in amniotic fluid. Gynecologic and Obstetrical Investigation 25: 23–30

Thorburn G D, Hooper S B, Rice G E, Fowden A L 1988 Luteal regression and parturition: a comparison. In: McNeillis D, Challis J R G, Macdonald P C, Nathanielsz P, Roberts J (eds) The onset of labour: cellular and integrative mechanisms. Ithaca Perinataology Press, New York, pp 185–206

Thornton S, Davison J M, Baylis P M 1988 Plasma oxytocin during third stage of labour: comparison of natural and active management. British Medical Journal 297: 167–169

Thornton S, Gillespie S I, Greenwell J R, Dunlop W 1992a Mobilisation of calcium by the brief application of oxytocin and prostaglandin E_2 in single cultured human myometrial cells. Experimental Physiology 77: 293–305

Thornton S, Davison J M, Baylis P H 1992b Plasma oxytocin during the first and second stages of spontaneous human labour. Acta Endocrinologica 126: 425–429

Turnbull A C, Anderson A B M 1968 Induction of labour II intravenous oxytocin titration. Journal of Obstetrics and Gynaecology of the British Commonwealth 75: 24–31

Uldbjerg N, Danielsen C C 1988 A study of the interaction between type I collagen and a small dermatan sulphate proteoglycan. Biochemical Journal 251: 643–648

Uldbjerg N, Ulmsten U 1990 The physiology of cervical ripening and cervical dilatation and the effect of abortificient drugs. Baillières Clinics in Obstetrics and Gynaecology 4: 263–282

Uldbjerg N, Malmstrom A 1991 The physiology of proteoglycans in cervical dilatation. Seminars in Perinatology 15: 127–132

Uldbjerg N, Ekman G, Malmstrom A, Sporring B, Ulmsten U, Wingerup L 1981 Biochemical and morphological changes of human cervix after local application of prostaglandin E_2 in pregnancy. Lancet i: 267–268

Ulbjerg N, Ekman G, Malmstrom A, Olson K, Ulmsten J 1983a Ripening of the human uterine cervix related to changes in collagen, glycosaminoglycans and collagenolytic activity. American Journal of Obstetrics and Gynecology 147: 662–666

Uldbjerg N, Ulmsten U, Ekman G 1983b Ripening of the human uterine cervix in terms of connective tissue biochemistry. Clinical Obstetrics and Gynecology 26: 14–26

Uldbjerg N, Ekman G, Malmstrom A, Ulmsten U, Wingerup L 1983c

Biochemical changes in human cervical connective tissue after local application of prostaglandin E$_2$. Gynecologic and Obstetric Investigation 15: 219–299

von Maillot K, Zimmermann B K 1976 The solubility of collagen of the uterine cervix during pregnancy and labour. Archive fur Gynakologie 220: 275–280

von Maillot K, Weiss M, Nagelschmidt M, Struck H J 1977 Relaxin and cervical dilatation during parturition. Archive fur Gynakologie 223: 323–334

von Maillot K, Stuhlsatz H W, Mohanaradhkrishan V, Grieling H 1979 Changes in the glycosaminoglycan distribution pattern in the human uterine cervix during pregnancy and labour. American Journal of Obstetrics and Gynecology 135: 503–506

Wallis R M, Hillier K 1981 Regulation of collagen dissolution in the human uterine cervix by oestradiol-17β and progesterone. Journal of Reproduction and Fertility 62: 55–61

Wilson T, Liggins G C, Joe L 1989 Purification and characterisation of a uterine phospholipase inhibitor that loses activity after labor onset in women. American Journal of Obstetrics and Gynecology 160: 602–606

Wintour E M, Bell R J, Carson R S et al 1986 Effect of long term infusion of ovine corticotrophin-releasing factor in the immature ovine fetus. Journal of Endocrinology 111: 469–475

Wolfs G M J A, van Leeuwan M 1979 Electromyographic observations on the human uterus during labour. Acta Obstetricia et Gynecologica Scandinavica (Supplement) 90: 1–61

30. The management and monitoring of labour

Martin J. Whittle

Material in this chapter contains contributions from the first edition and we are grateful to the previous author for the work done.

INTRODUCTION

Recent years have seen the development of conflict in delivery units, not only as a result of the debate about who should look after women in labour but also because of uncertainties about what constitutes optimal care. In many countries outside the UK, labour is managed primarily by doctors, although often with nursing assistance to oversee the hour to hour care of the mother and fetus. Under these circumstances, delivery is nearly always the preserve of medical staff, nurses acting very much as hand-maidens. One of the reasons for this is financial, he who delivers being he who is paid, an arrangement which, in some countries, also applies to midwives.

The midwifery service in the UK aims to provide a holistic approach to the care of the mother, the midwife having antenatal, intrapartum and postpartum responsibilities. Difficulties between obstetricians and midwives have arisen for a number of reasons. First there was feeling that the management of pregnancy, and particularly labour, is too mechanistic when medically driven, and that midwives provided a more humane approach. Secondly the two professional groups have different philosophies which probably reflect their training as much as anything. Whilst midwives believe that pregnancy and labour are essentially normal events and that care can be as natural as possible, obstetricians have a more pessimistic view, regarding pregnancy as a potentially pathological condition in which timely intervention may be necessary to prevent serious complications.

The Cumberlege Report reaffirms the importance of the midwives' role (Report of the Expert Maternity Group 1993), going further to suggest that medical participation may be unnecessary in many circumstances. Whilst recognizing that the reduction of medical involvement may be desirable, it is still important to realize that complications can arise in pregnancy and labour with alarming rapidity and that the identification of a low-risk case is only possible, with confidence, retrospectively. Clearly there is a need to resolve the extreme views which have been expressed and the next few years are going to be challenging for us all. A failure of the different professional groups to reach a realistic compromise will undoubtedly prejudice the standards of care available to our patients.

The considerable discussion about how labour should be managed has arisen from an increasingly self-critical philosophy amongst obstetricians. It is true that much of what is done has been handed from one generation of doctors (and midwives) to another, but the publication of *Effective Care in Pregnancy and Childbirth* (Chalmers et al 1989) raised important questions about current practice. A further development of this work has appeared (Cochrane Pregnancy and Childbirth Database) and both these help to encourage discussion about different management strategies and provide a guide as to those areas in which local testing of protocols and subsequent audit may seem appropriate. However their contents should not be accepted without question, a current, rather disturbing tendency.

This chapter will discuss the management and monitoring of labour, both of which need to be clearly understood if inappropriate decisions are to be avoided. In spite of comments made above, the vast majority of normal labours will be, quite rightly, cared for by midwives and their vast accumulated experience and knowledge should be shared with young doctors in training so that all may benefit.

MANAGEMENT OF LABOUR

Aims

The aim of successful labour management is to ensure

the safe delivery of a healthy baby to a fit, satisfied mother using the minimum of interference. At the same time it is necessary to provide appropriate choices for analgesia, position in labour and a pleasant environment in which to give birth.

To achieve these aims within the context of the often busy delivery unit is not easy. Many units are themselves cramped, unwelcoming places providing little in the way of privacy. Staffing levels, both midwifery and obstetric, are sometimes inadequate, particularly when the natural ebb and flow of work in the delivery unit is considered. The need for experienced, resident anaesthetic staff immediately available in the delivery unit is essential not only to provide various forms of conduction anaesthesia but also to be on hand if emergency situations, such as acute fetal distress or major maternal haemorrhage, arise. Finally the potential need for neonatal resuscitation requires that both midwives and obstetricians have adequate skills and training in this procedure. In busy units and especially those dealing with high-risk cases, the availability of experienced paediatric support is essential; in fact one study suggests that it is important even in low-risk circumstances, the services of a paediatrician being found necessary at about 20% of deliveries (MacVicar et al 1993).

The often unsatisfactory environment of the hospital delivery unit has led to a search for other models of care in labour and delivery such as DOMINO (DOMiciliary IN and Out) and home confinements. The DOMINO model seems to offer the best compromise between care at home, when in early labour, but with delivery itself in hospital where all the necessary support is potentially available. It also appears to be the most cost-effective method of providing care to low-risk mothers (Scottish Office Home and Health Department 1993). The mother can leave the hospital along with her midwife soon after the baby has been born. The main disadvantage of a home confinement is the difficulty of reaching the mother if things go wrong. Resources do not generally allow the development of a comprehensive and robust transfer system and in any case the numbers of midwives willing and able to conduct home confinements would be insufficient if demand rose substantially (Murphy-Black 1993).

The three main components to labour management involve the assessment of the progress of labour, the care of the woman and the monitoring of the fetal condition.

General assessment

In many cases the initial assessment will be by the admitting midwife, who ideally should be the individual who will be with the woman throughout her labour (Report of the Expert Maternity Group 1993). The environment of the admission room is important and it should not give the impression of a wartime casualty clearing station. There should be regard to privacy and the area should be adequately equipped and staffed by appropriately trained personnel.

Diagnosis of labour

This is one of the more difficult diagnoses to make in obstetrics and a lack of awareness of this fact in the past sometimes led to inappropriate action, such that women who were merely having uterine tightenings were deemed in early labour. Augmentation was attempted by stimulating uterine contractions by membrane rupture and oxytocin, a course of action which often resulted in a prolonged and ineffectual labour.

The symptoms of labour are:

1. Regular, painful uterine contractions.
2. Passing a blood-streaked mucous plug—the operculum of mucus from the cervical canal.

Unfortunately these symptoms are not necessarily reliable and the only certain way of diagnosing labour is when there is progressive cervical change in the form of effacement, dilatation or both.

Following admission it is necessary to confirm that both mother and baby are healthy and to review past and current obstetric history to exclude the existence of risk factors. The woman requires the usual routine checks on her blood pressure, urine analysis and general well-being, physical and psychological.

Palpation will reveal the presentation and state of engagement of the presenting part, fetal size and amniotic fluid status; fetal condition will often be established from cardiotocography, combined if necessary by ultrasound examination. All these investigations should, ideally, be performed in the admission room.

Once the diagnosis has been made the woman can be admitted to the delivery unit. If considered to be at low risk, the continuing care during labour should become the responsibility of a midwife. The level of medical involvement will depend on local arrangements and it is important that agreed guidelines are established by individual units. These should be an amalgam of ideas from both midwives and obstetricians—it is inappropriate for medical staff to impose plans and ideas without prior discussion with midwives.

Progress of labour

First stage

The time of onset of labour is judged retrospectively and as described above is not always easy to identify. Some take the onset to be at the time of admission to the delivery unit but this is fallacious since labour may have commenced some time before. The first stage is divided into latent and active phases.

The *latent phase* of labour can be said to occupy the time from the onset of labour until the point at which progressive cervical dilatation occurs, usually after the cervix has reached about 3–4 cm. It is an important period in which significant changes occur in both the physical and biochemical characteristics of the cervix in preparation for dilatation. During this time the function of the cervix is being modified from that of a sphincter, which retained the baby in the uterus for 9 months, to a structure with the capacity to dilate sufficiently to allow delivery.

These fundamental changes in the cervix, which can undoubtedly take hours or even days to occur, probably involve alterations in the collagen within the cervical matrix and alterations in hydration state. During the latent phase the proportions of glycoaminoglycans (GAG) change with a fall in dermatan sulphate and a rise in hyaluronic acid (Gee 1994), a shift which brings about a change in the physical characteristics of the cervix.

Recognition by the attendants that the latent phase may be of considerable duration is important, and interference by inappropriate artificial rupture of the membranes or injudicious use of oxytocin may well produce an unsatisfactory outcome with a long labour, terminating possibly in abdominal delivery. Hence, it is vital to ensure that labour is well established before attempting augmentation by oxytocin or rupture of membranes.

Although the biochemical changes in the cervix are of fundamental importance to the progress of labour, the fetal presenting part has a significant mechanical role and difficult labours are often experienced in malpositions when the presenting part fits poorly into the lower segment.

Unsatisfactory labour often follows formal induction because it is nearly always undertaken in the *latent phase* of labour, all of which must be traversed before active progress commences. The favourability of the cervix prior to induction, semiquantified by the Bishop's score, provides a crude estimate of the likely duration of the latent phase. One study suggested that when the Bishop's score (Table 30.1) was low (< 3) the eventual Caesarean section rate in primigravidae was 42% (Sims 1985), but this was reduced to 18% by prior use of prostaglandins to ripen the cervix. This process presumably goes some way to induce the biochemical changes in the cervix which otherwise occur naturally during the latent phase of labour.

Table 30.1 Modified Bishop's cervical score

Factor	Score			
	0	1	2	3
Cervical dilatation	< 1 cm	1–2 cm	2–4 cm	> 4 cm
Length of cervix	> 4 cm	2–4 cm	1–2 cm	< 1 cm
Consistency of cervix	Firm	Average	Soft	—
Position of cervix	Posterior	Mid/anterior	—	—
Position of head to ishial spines	3 cm ↑	2 cm ↑	< 1 cm ↑	> 1 cm ↓

During the *active phase* of labour the cervix should dilate at a rate of at least 1 cm/hour and if not then failure to progress in labour is diagnosed. By setting a minimum rate of dilatation it is possible, in contrast to the latent phase, to calculate the likely maximum duration of the active phase. Thus if the active phase commences at 4 cm the cervix should be fully dilated within 6 hours.

The active phase is characterized by steadily increasing uterine work, components of which comprise intrauterine pressure and both the duration and frequency of contractions. There have been many attempts to quantify uterine work and a number of different units have been devised such as Alexandria and Montevideo units, uterine activity units (UAU) and uterine work described in kilopascals (Fig. 30.1). Some tocodynamometers calculate mean work over a 15-minute period, and although the individual range is very large, a typical reading would be about 1500 kPa/15 minutes.

Assessment of uterine activity is traditionally from manual palpation by an experienced midwife. Although frequency and duration can be timed reasonably accurately, the

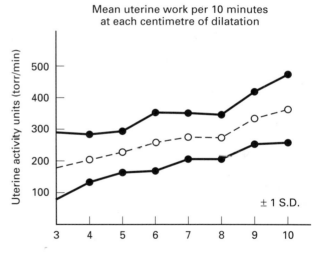

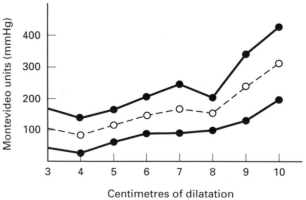

Fig. 30.1 Uterine work during labour measured in Uterine Activity Units and Montevideo Units. Both show increasing 'uterine work' as labour proceeds.

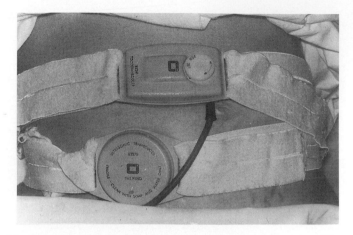

Fig. 30.2 External tocodynamometer positioned over the uterus. The lower transducer detects the fetal heart rate using Doppler ultrasound.

strength of contraction is very subjective and impressions can undoubtedly be influenced by the mother's own response to her pains; maternal obesity will also contribute to the difficulties.

Objective evidence concerning uterine activity is best obtained with either an external tocodynamometer (Fig. 30.2) or by an internally placed pressure catheter. The former only gives an indication of the timing and duration of the uterine contractions and even though the contraction shape appears on the trace, the amplitude gives no information about intrauterine pressure. The continuous information provided by the pictorial representation of uterine activity aids interpretation of the fetal heart rate pattern and, indeed, should be regarded as an important component.

The quantitation of uterine activity can only be achieved from intrauterine pressure monitoring which is achieved by the passage of a fluid-filled catheter or, preferably, a pressure tip transducer, via the cervix and into the amniotic space. This enables intrauterine pressure to be monitored directly but is in itself an invasive procedure which should be reserved for those cases in which problems with labour have arisen or are anticipated.

Although knowledge of uterine work is important the main evidence that the contractions are effective is that the cervix is progressively dilating at an appropriate rate and that there is descent of the presenting part. This fact emphasizes the importance of carefully monitoring the changes in the cervix and the crucial role that the partogram has in the management of labour.

A typical partogram is shown in Figure 30.3 and in the vast majority of units only one type will be used regardless of the woman's parity. However, in the National Maternity Hospital, Dublin different colour partograms are used depending on whether the woman is primiparous or multiparous, emphasizing the difference between these two groups and how they perform in labour. Thus, whereas it may be acceptable that a woman in her first

pregnancy shows a cervical dilatation in the active phase of labour of 1 cm/hour, it most certainly is not if she is multiparous when dilatation of perhaps 2–3 cm/hour may be expected.

The difference between spontaneous and induced labour is also significant, the woman in induced labour having the potential for a long latent phase (see above). Staff working on units with high induction rates may become so used to long and difficult labours that they may fail to recognize as abnormal the spontaneously labouring woman whose labour is truly making slow progress.

The partogram was developed to provide a pictorial view of the individual labour so that progress could be assessed at a glance and appropriate action taken. The use of the method in Africa transformed the problem of delay in labour. Various schemes were devised; but alert and action lines drawn to the right of an optimal progress line helped attendants decide the point at which transfer for poor progress was required. Different methods were used to achieve this aim and sets of stencils as devised by Studd (1973) proved of value (Fig. 30.4).

In addition to details of the cervical changes, the partogram provides information concerning other components of progress such as descent of the presenting part and uterine activity in terms of frequency and strength of contractions. The maternal and fetal condition can also be seen at a glance.

Second stage

The duration of the second stage of labour has been restricted traditionally to about 2 hours. Epidural anaesthesia has allowed views about this restraint to be modified, although it is important to ensure that women are not left for endless periods of time in the second stage without assessment and it is important that progress, in the form of steady descent of the presenting part, is being made.

The reasons for restricting the length of this stage of labour relate to the health of both mother and baby. As far as the mother is concerned excessive bearing down in an attempt to overcome a serious obstruction may possibly weaken the pelvic floor leading to later urinary and vaginal problems or, at the very worse, cause a vesicovaginal fistula. It has been shown that the likelihood of subsequent urinary stress incontinence may be higher when the second stage extends beyond 2 hours regardless of type of analgesia (MacArthur et al 1991). Excessive straining by the mother will cause exhaustion, dehydration and increase the risk of postpartum haemorrhage. The skilled and experienced midwife can often persuade the woman to conserve her efforts until the presenting part has descended to the perineum. The use of epidural anaesthesia contributes to the problem by abolishing the bearing-down reflexes and will also increase the need for

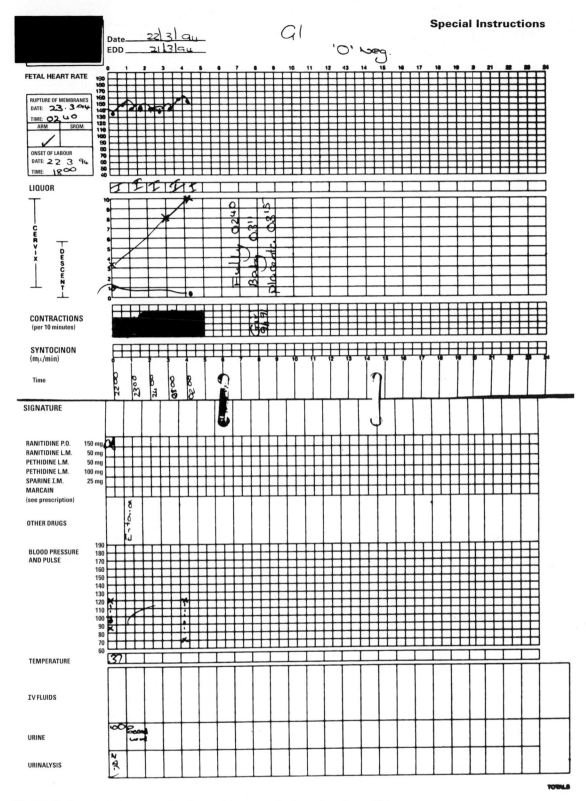

Fig. 30.3   A typical partogram showing rapid progress in the active phase of labour.

operative assistance in the form of forceps or vacuum extraction but usually only as a low cavity lift-out procedure.

The fetal acid–base status can change quite rapidly in the second stage but usually only when the mother is actively bearing down. This is a result of respiratory acidosis from rising carbon dioxide levels rather than oxygen lack producing a metabolic acidosis. Fetal heart rate patterns are difficult to interpret at this time but

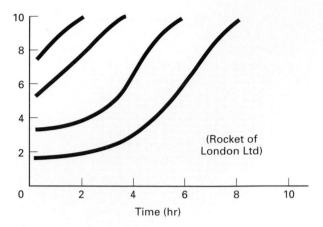

Fig. 30.4 A set of Studd stencils.

should not be ignored, especially if abnormal traces have occurred in the first stage (see below).

Abnormal progress in labour

Different patterns of progress are described. Figure 30.5 shows primary dysfunctional labour in which the cervix dilates at less than the optimal rate. This pattern may occur in about 25% of primiparous woman in spontaneous labour and just under 10% of multiparous woman; its frequency is naturally much greater when labour has been induced. This pattern is also familiar when the fetal head is in the occipito-posterior position and undergoing rotation, which once completed allows normal progress to be made. Primary dysfunctional labour is often associated with inadequate uterine activity (poor powers—see below) and treatment is with oxytocin to augment contractions; the majority will respond favourably with progress being re-established.

Figure 30.5 gives an example of secondary arrest; when this occurs in primiparous woman the usual require-

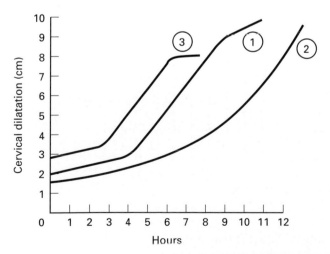

Fig. 30.5 Different patterns of cervical dilatation. 1 = Normal labour; 2 = primary dysfunctional labour; 3 = secondary arrest in labour.

ment is to increase uterine contractions using oxytocin. However in the multigravid mother the possibility of disproportion should be considered and the pelvis carefully evaluated before augmentation.

When the partogram indicates that progress in labour is suboptimal the simplest method of establishing the cause is to identify which of the three components determining progress in labour, namely the Powers, Passenger and Passages, are responsible.

Powers

Insufficient uterine power, or work, is probably the most likely cause of inadequate progress. Although the midwife will be able to indicate the palpated strength and frequency of contractions on the partogram, the presence of poor progress demands that an objective assessment of contraction power is obtained by use of intrauterine pressure monitoring. If the evidence suggests that in spite of good uterine activity, inadequate progress is being made, the decision to perform a Caesarean section can be taken sooner and certainly before both mother and baby become exhausted. Too often labour becomes unnecessarily protracted because the clinician does not have the necessary relevant information on uterine activity with which to make an appropriate decision. It is impossible to overemphasize the need to continually foward-plan in labour management, it being a prerequisite that the clinician considers what he will need to know in 3 or 4 hours time to make a clinical decision.

Should inadequate uterine activity be suspected, correction by use of oxytocin is the appropriate therapy with reassessment in 2–3 hours. Once a decision to start oxytocin has been taken it is imperative that the obstetrician ensures that the order is initiated immediately since in time-limited situations, such as labour, any unnecessary delay becomes highly significant.

Poor progress in the second stage of labour should be considered in the same way as that in the first stage and it can also occur as the result of ineffective uterine activity. Nevertheless when there is delay at full dilatation it is even more vital that the woman is carefully assessed to ensure that vaginal delivery is feasible before oxytocin is used.

Passenger

Whilst it is possible for a baby to be too large to be delivered vaginally this is not often the case, although cephalopelvic disproportion is frequently given as the indication for Caesarean section. More commonly the fetus has a malposition, usually occipitoposterior, which leads to relative disproportion. This occurs because deflexion of the fetal head presents the larger occipitofrontal diameter, which is on average 11.5 cm, to the pelvis, compared with the usual 9.5 cm of the suboccipitobregmatic diameter when the vertex leads. This deflexion must be corrected before descent and rotation can occur, a process which will be usually achieved only by adequate uterine activity.

Malpresentation is a different problem which must be excluded as a cause of failure to progress before oxytocin is administered. This is particularly important in multiparous women, who may be at high risk for malpresentation, since use of oxytocin in these women can result in uterine rupture.

If the baby is considered to be particularly large then a careful evaluation of the progress of labour is required and the potential for vaginal delivery reassessed. It should be remembered that multiparous mothers may be especially at risk since inappropriate assumptions are often made about their ability to deliver normally based on their previous performance.

Although shoulder dystocia can be difficult to anticipate, slow progress, particularly in late first stage of labour, can provide an important clue. Careful evaluation of the size of the baby at this time may save more serious problems later.

Passages

The pelvis is rarely responsible for failure to progress, at least in the first stage of labour when delay due to the passages is most likely to be due to deficiencies at the pelvic brim, a rare problem in the UK. Nevertheless regard should be given to the clinical indicators that pelvic disproportion may be a potential factor, namely maternal height and general appearance. There is virtually never an indication, if the presentation is cephalic, for X-ray pelvimetry during or just before labour. Although a deficient pelvis is uncommon in women from the Western world (0.5%–1.0%), it does occasionally occur and must be recognized if serious consequences are to be avoided.

Resistance to progress from the soft passages is a common cause for delay in the second stage of labour which can be relieved by episiotomy, a procedure which divides the perineal body along with skin overlying this structure. Excessive use of episiotomy is to be deprecated but, conversely it can prevent not only serious trauma to the perineal body, attached muscles and perineum but also occasionally fetal compromise.

MATERNAL WELL-BEING

The improvements in the general health of the population in the UK mean that the vast majority can cope physiologically with the dynamic changes of pregnancy. In addition, the fact that pregnancy occurs in the UK usually in younger women, only about 7% being older than 35 years, means that serious, debilitating illness is un-

common. In spite of this all mothers should be carefully assessed at the start of labour. Many activities which were a matter of routine in the early stage of labour, such as enemas and pubic shaving, are no longer practised.

During labour regular observations are made of blood pressure, pulse, temperature and urine output. These are non-intrusive but important since deviations may indicate developing problems. Should labour become prolonged, and therefore abnormal, they provide a vital baseline against which to observe changes in the mother's condition.

Psychological support is essential and this can best be achieved by the continual presence of a partner or a single midwife who the woman has come to know, preferably in the antenatal period. This embodies one of the recommendations in the Cumberlege Report and must be considered highly desirable if it is achievable. Randomized controlled trials do seem to suggest that the presence of a single carer throughout labour will improve outcome in terms of a reduced need for pain relief and also fewer instrumental deliveries (Hodnett 1993).

The presence of the woman's partner will also be supportive but it is important that he is there because he wants to be rather than as a result of coercion. For the unmarried teenager the presence of a sister or aunt, for example, may help although this is no guarantee.

The availability of adequate pain relief is particularly desirable and although good psychological help and careful antenatal preparation will reduce the need for pharmacological support, this must be available on demand when required.

Pethidine given intramuscularly is still probably the commonest prescription but other agents, such as pentazocine, also find favour. The use of opiates such as heroin would be very rarely used now and only under special circumstances.

The most effective method of pain relief is now by conduction anaesthesia and epidural anaesthetic technology has been considerably refined over recent years.

FETAL WELL-BEING

The preferred method of monitoring the fetus in labour has remained a controversial issue for many years and more recently has led to a view that monitoring may cause more trouble than it is worth. The first description of the fetal heart sounds was by Mayor in 1818, an observation confirmed by Kergaradec in 1821. The latter observed that a slowing of the fetal heart rate was often associated with a poor outcome. Evory Kennedy in Dublin in 1843 enhanced these observations by adding meconium staining of the amniotic fluid as a further feature of fetal distress. The definition of fetal distress—alterations in fetal heart rate and meconium-stained amniotic fluid—has been in existence, therefore, for many years.

The use of the fetal heart rate alone as a marker of fetal distress clearly has its limitations but intelligent use of the information derived from the continuous trace and judicious use of fetal blood sampling to establish the fetal acid–base status does produce a system which will reasonably exclude the fetal compromise that arises from oxygen deprivation. Unfortunately there is a tendency to overcall fetal distress and this has led to a higher than desirable incidence of operative delivery for this indication.

The relatively poor results from the use of fetal heart rate monitoring arise from three main factors:

1. The technique is somewhat crude and the physiology uncertain.
2. The training of staff, both midwives and obstetricians, in the use of the technique is almost uniformly poor.
3. The fear of litigious consequences if the baby is born in poor condition or subsequently develops mental or physical handicap, may lead to the defensive use of an inappropriately high Caesarean section rate for supposed fetal distress.

Undoubtedly not all babies require continuous heart rate monitoring in labour; the results of the Dublin study tend to suggest this (MacDonald et al 1985). However the situation in Dublin is not one which necessarily applies in other units. The midwife virtually never leaves the mother throughout her labour and there is a very short and well-defined obstetric chain of medical command. Under these circumstances it is easy to ensure that regular auscultation will be both undertaken and recorded and in the low-risk case with clear amniotic fluid it should, and probably does, suffice. While it can be argued that there are few advantages to any fetal heart rate monitoring in low-risk women in spontaneous labour, the Dublin study did suggest that even in this group, if labour was prolonged, continuous electronic fetal monitoring identified more babies with milder acidosis than did traditional auscultation alone; convulsions following delivery were also more common in the latter group.

In the more usual circumstances that exist in labour wards elsewhere, in which staff are often heavily pressed, continuous fetal heart rate monitoring ensures that, whatever else is happening, the fetus is under constant supervision. Certainly there is a need to monitor all fetuses for which a risk factor is present, when the labour is being induced or augmented and probably when an epidural anaesthetic is in place.

Detection of the fetal heart rate

Intermittent fetal heart rate monitoring

This is the traditional method of heart rate monitoring, the rate being determined either from the heart sounds heard through a Pinard stethoscope or using a simple Doppler heart detector. The number of beats is usually counted over a minute and the heart rate calculated. This procedure is performed about 30–45 seconds after a uterine contraction and usually every 15 minutes in the first stage of labour and every 5 minutes in the second stage. The aim is to detect the ominous late decelerations associated with fetal hypoxia and as a technique it seems adequate when there are no complications. However, fetal status using this method is determined using just tiny snatches of the overall heart rate which provides only crude information about the fetus and gives no indication of impending or developing problems.

Continuous fetal heart rate monitoring

The benefit of continuous monitoring is that it offers sequential information concerning the fetal condition. Indeed one of the mistakes that the tyro of fetal monitoring often makes is not to assess the whole trace, merely concentrating on the 20 minutes or so placed in front of him.

The detection of the fetal heart electronically demands that the automatic counter is presented with a clear signal. When the fetal ECG is used from a scalp clip (Fig. 30.6) it is the R wave which forms the counting source. The signal is usually electronically clean and provides accurate information, the rate being determined from the R–R interval. The continuous fetal heart rate trace will reflect both short- and long-term variability in the baseline rate (see below).

Ultrasound using the Doppler principle can also be used as a continuous fetal heart rate detector. Various filtering techniques allow a reproduction close to that of the fetal ECG but spurious variability can produce interpretation difficulties so caution is needed. Further,

Computation of heart rate

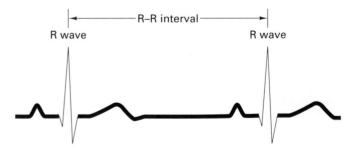

Heart rate is inversely related to the duration of the R–R interval
i.e., the longer the R–R interval, the slower the rate and vice versa

Hence, heart rate (beats per min) $= \dfrac{1}{\text{R–R interval (s)}} \times 60$

e.g., for an R–R interval of 0.5 s.
heart rate (beats per min) $= \dfrac{1}{0.5} \times 60 = 120$

Fig. 30.6 Fetal ECG complex and the R–R interval.

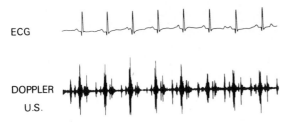

Fig. 30.7 Comparison between fetal ECG and ultrasound signals.

Table 30.2 Classification (after Hon) of fetal heart rate deceleration patterns

1 Early decelerations (head compression)
    Occur with contractions
    Uniform onset and recovery
    Amplitude rarely greater than 40 bpm
    Probably benign
2 Variable decelerations (cord compression)
    Variable relationship to contractions
    'Ragged' waveform
    Variable amplitude
    Potentially dangerous to the fetus
3 Late decelerations (uteroplacental insufficiency)
    Occur late in relationship to the contractions
    Uniform onset and recovery
    Initially may be of low amplitude
    Indicate fetal hypoxia (50%)

there is group averaging so the beat to beat variation cannot be observed (Fig. 30.7).

Phonocardiography is rarely if ever used in this country although is more frequent in Europe and especially Germany. The advantage of the technique is that the heart sounds are reasonably discernible from the background noise so that the method allows the fetal heart rate variability to be established with some reliability.

Indications for fetal monitoring

Continuous fetal heart rate monitoring should be considered whenever risk factors exist. There are five circumstances under which continuous monitoring may be particularly valuable:

1. preterm labour
2. post-term pregnancy
3. meconium staining of the amniotic fluid
4. fetal growth retardation/small for dates
5. breech presentation.

The use of an admission test has been proposed as a method of ascertaining fetal status prior to, or early in, labour. Abnormalities in the baseline rate or the presence of decelerations indicate either that the baby would be unable to withstand labour (Arulkumaran & Ingemarsson 1990) or is at risk of adverse condition at delivery.

Others (Fairlie et al 1989) have used Doppler waveform studies of the umbilical artery as an assessment of fetal condition; again abnormal results are frequently associated with the development of fetal distress during labour.

In the absence of these factors, a compromise which most women find acceptable is the strategy of running short traces intermittently, perhaps of 30 minutes' duration every 2 hours, backed by regular auscultation.

Fetal heart rate patterns

The fetal heart rate trace is analysed in terms of its baseline rate, baseline variability and periodic changes. The classification of fetal heart rate patterns developed by Hon is the only one now acceptable and terms such as Type 1 and Type 2 decelerations should be discarded. The FIGO classification is complex and the one shown in Table 30.2 is suggested.

Baseline fetal heart rate (Fig. 30.8)

The overall baseline rate is usually regarded as lying between 120 and 160 beats per minute (b.p.m.) although with the fetus at or close to term, a range between 110 and 150 b.p.m. is now considered more acceptable (FIGO 1987). This rate probably represents a balance between the sympathetic and parasympathetic components of the autonomic nervous system. The variability of the baseline rate is derived from the continually changing beat to beat rate inherent in both fetus and adults. Loss of the variability can occur as a natural phenomenon associated with normal rest/activity cycles but it can also indicate cerebral depression arising from hypoxia. Certain drugs, particularly the opiates, can reduce variability.

Changes in the baseline rate over time can be important indicators of developing hypoxia, the rate rising probably in response to increasing sympathetic drive.

Periodic changes (Fig. 30.9)

Early decelerations These are relatively rare decelerations which are probably the result of fetal head compression. They are subtle with the amplitude of the

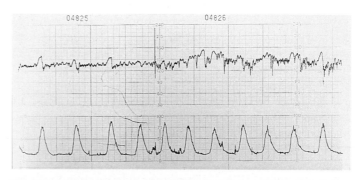

Fig. 30.8 Normal fetal heart rate pattern showing stable baseline rate with accelerations. Paper speed 1 cm/min.

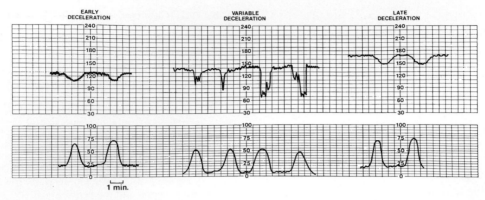

Fig. 30.9 Periodic deceleration patterns (schematic).

deceleration falling no lower than by 40 b.p.m. and the waveform occurs coincidentally with contractions. It is thought that they do not have any particular significance as far as the fetal condition is concerned and may arise from increased fetal intracranial pressure during a uterine contraction.

Variable decelerations These are common and can be found at some time or another in almost all traces. They have not only erratic shapes and appearances but also a variable relationship to contractions, so that on occasions they can be late in timing. It is thought that they arise from compression of the umbilical cord, their inconsistent appearances resulting from differential compression of artery and vein. The former causes fetal blood pressure to rise and, via the baroreceptors, heart rate to fall. The latter reduces blood flow returning to the heart and lowers blood pressure resulting in a compensatory acceleration in heart rate. Shallow or even deep but brief, decelerations have little consequence for the fetus; persistent variable decelerations will eventually cause hypoxia. Often the pattern can be relieved by turning the woman on her side and certainly oxytocin should be discontinued if they persist. The use of an amnioinfusion to relieve compression has been found effective in some circumstances.

Complete cord compression will result in the development of profound respiratory and metabolic acidosis within 10 or 20 minutes (Smith 1987). These sudden problems are difficult to predict but can result in acute hypoxic damage which may arise not only from the low oxygen levels in the fetal blood but also perhaps from major haemodynamic changes in the fetal cerebral vasculature. Unfortunately events may occur so quickly that any action to deliver the baby may still result in death or damage. Conversely, the majority of babies can withstand, perhaps, up to 5 minutes of severe cord compression without significant damage, although a fairly profound respiratory acidosis may result.

Late decelerations These are uncommon and repre-

sent the fetal response to hypoxia. Why the fetus responds in this way, in contrast to adults who develop tachycardia, is uncertain. The initial responses are the results of the effect of hypoxia on the fetal chemoreceptors in the aortic arch which, when activated, cause fetal blood pressure to rise and, as a baroreceptor response, the fetal heart rate to fall. Thus in the initial stages the changes are entirely reflex driven and physiological—blood flow to the brain, heart and adrenals is maintained or increased at the expense of carcass, kidney and gut. If hypoxia deepens the fetal response changes such that fetal blood pressure falls rather than rises and the fetal heart rate pattern shows deep meandering decelerations probably as a result of hypoxia on the myocardium.

It is important to emphasize that only about 50% of fetuses showing late decelerations will be acidotic. This is often held as evidence that the technique of fetal heart rate monitoring is worthless but in actual fact the observation reflects the underlying physiology, a fetus not developing acidosis until lengthy hypoxia has eroded its buffering systems.

Fetal acid–base measurement

Whenever fetal heart rate monitoring is being employed it is vital that fetal acid–base status can be established from a scalp blood sample (Fig. 30.10). Ideally it should be possible to measure pH, PCO$_2$, PO$_2$ and base excess so that the underlying cause of the acidosis can be established. Because of the limitations in interpreting fetal heart rate traces the diagnosis of fetal distress should be confirmed in usually all cases by fetal blood pH prior to Caesarean section for this indication. The usually accepted critical pH of 7.20 is probably too high and 7.15 may be more realistic. However falling scalp blood pH levels, if respiratory acidosis can be excluded, indicate that an impending problem exists and that action aimed at delivering the baby will probably be necessary. Cord blood samples indicate a surprisingly wide normal range

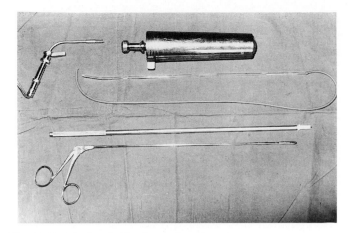

Fig. 30.10 Fetal scalp blood sampling kit.

Table 30.3 Cord blood gases—normal range (2.5th to 97.5th centiles) (from Westgate 1993)

	Artery	Vein
pH	7.26 (7.04–7.38)	7.35 (7.16–7.47)
P_{CO_2} (mmHg)	55.0 (37–81)	40.0 (27–59)
BD blood (mmol/l)	3.7 (−1.7–12.4)	2.9 (−1.5–9.6)

for pH which can only be interpreted if the gases are known (Table 30.3) (Westgate 1993).

Other monitoring techniques

One of the weaknesses of continuous fetal heart rate monitoring is that it does not provide much quantitative information about the fetal condition so that in some circumstances relatively minor heart rate changes may be found in a profoundly hypoxic baby while severe abnormalities may occur when the baby is only mildly affected. Dissatisfaction has led to a search for other techniques which may provide a more precise measure of the baby's condition.

Some techniques have concentrated on the measurement of fetal blood gases with a view to positively detecting whether or not hypoxia exists. Recent attempts at this using near infrared spectroscopy have proved interesting but widespread application may prove difficult.

More detailed analysis of the ECG complex itself may prove advantageous although it would also require use of the continuous heart rate trace. Preliminary data using the ST segment changes of the ECG waveform does seem to provide a guide to the significance of certain fetal heart rate patterns and in a randomized study certainly was found to reduce Caesarean section rates for fetal distress (Westgate et al 1992).

One major problem is in the interpretation of fetal heart rate traces themselves. Computer assistance may

be an answer and would at least help to reduce the inconsistencies in interpretation which are observed in everyday practice. The ability to fit the fetal heart rate trace into the context of the labour requires skill and experience and artificial intelligence systems may prove valuable.

Management of the fetal heart rate in labour

Often the fetal heart rate changes are taken out of the context of the woman's labour whereas they should be regarded as an integral part of the decision-making process. Thus if labour is progressing rapidly but the deterioration in the fetal heart rate patterns is gradual then it is quite likely that a safe vaginal delivery is going to be possible. Conversely deterioration in the face of slow progress in labour will almost certainly result in the need for operative delivery, probably by Caesarean section. Likewise the presence of abnormal fetal heart rate patterns in the face of minimal uterine activity is unlikely to result in a successful vaginal delivery. The presence of other risk factors, such as suspected growth retardation or prematurity, will also influence how the information from the fetal heart rate traces is used.

The main requirement for the fetus during labour is the maintenance of an adequate supply of oxygen. Figure 30.11 shows the components responsible, namely the uterine blood flow, the placenta and the umbilical circulation.

The *uterine blood flow* will be influenced by a number of factors including uterine contractions and the maternal

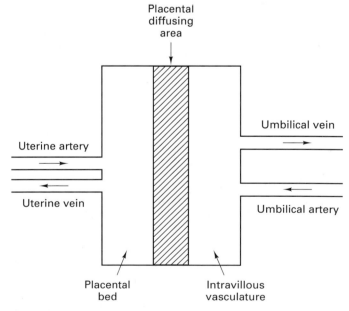

Fig. 30.11 The components responsible for maintaining an adequate oxygen supply to the fetus in labour.

blood pressure which can be lowered by supine posture or conduction anaesthesia. The effects of reduced uterine blood flow on the fetal heart rate pattern often develop fairly slowly and in the early stages will produce only subtle changes. Further deterioration is not, in itself, an indication for an immediate Caesarean section but rather demands a search for the underlying cause which can often be iatrogenic. Thus reduction in the oxytocin infusion to lessen the uterine activity or the repositioning of the woman to relieve hypotension will usually improve matters. Evaluation of the fetal condition by scalp blood sampling will indicate the current acid–base status and allow more rational decision making.

The *placenta*, which gets the blame for much that goes amiss in obstetrics, will only rarely be implicated in the development of fetal heart rate abnormalities because so long as it is still appropriately attached, it will continue to function well as a gas-exchange organ. Abruption will, of course, produce dramatic changes in the fetal heart rate but this is a relatively rare event.

Compression of the *umbilical cord* will cause rapid and sometimes dramatic fetal heart rate changes, in contrast to events in the uterine circulation. Most often these are temporary effects that will usually resolve spontaneously but alteration of the woman's position and the more recently described use of amnioinfusion may also help. The assessment of the fetal acid–base status in the presence of variable decelerations can be unrewarding since rapid changes in pH can arise from the respiratory acidosis which develops during cord compression. Occasionally severe cord compression will produce dramatic effects, occasionally resulting in death and damage, before intervention is possible.

The importance of devising a clear management plan for these differing clinical circumstances cannot be over-emphasized. Usually serious problems arise in the management of labour because of prevarication and lack of forward thinking. Explicit action plans are required so that all members of the team, and the woman herself, know what is going is to happen. The obstetrician must learn to anticipate what information he might need to make his decision. It takes time and experience to develop these skills but they are vital if appropriate management of labour is to be achieved.

CONCLUSIONS

The successful management of labour is only possible when midwives and obstetricians work as a team rather than in conflict. The basic skill required in providing adequate care in labour is the ability to recognize abnormality when it occurs and to have a clear plan of corrective action. The use of protocols or guidelines is essential but these must be devised by a representative group of carers with regard for local facilities and problems. Often an unsatisfactory outcome in labour will arise from poor communication and planning, both of which are potentially avoidable and, parenthetically, do not cost money.

REFERENCES

Arulkumaran S, Ingemarsson I 1990 Appropriate technology in intrapartum fetal surveillance. In: Studd J (ed) Progress in obstetrics and gynaecology, vol 8. Churchill Livingstone, Edinburgh, pp 127–140

Chalmers I, Enkin M, Keirse M J N C (eds) 1989 Effective care in pregnancy and childbirth. Oxford University Press, Oxford

Fairlie F M, Lang G D, Sheldon C D 1989 Umbilical artery velocity waveforms in labour. British Journal of Obstetrics and Gynaecology 96: 151–157

FIGO 1987 International Journal of Gynaecology and Obstetrics 25: 159–167

Gee H 1994 Biochemistry and physiology of the cervix in late pregnancy. In: Symonds M (ed) Current obstetrics and gynaecology. Churchill Livingstone, Edinburgh, pp 68–73

Hodnett E D 1993 Support from caregivers during childbirth. In: Enkin M W, Kierse M J N C, Renfrew M J, Neilson J P (eds) Childbirth and pregnancy module. Cochrane database of systematic review. Review No 03871 April 1993. Cochrane updates on disk, Oxford Update, Software, Spring 1993

MacArthur C, Lewis M, Knox E G 1991 Health after childbirth. HMSO, London, pp 125–152

MacDonald D, Grant A, Sheridan-Pereira M, Boylan P, Chalmers I 1985 The Dublin randomised controlled trial of intrapartum fetal monitoring. American Journal of Obstetricis and Gynecology 152: 524–539

MacVicar J B, Dobbie H G, Owen-Johnson L, Jagger C, Hopkins M, Kennedy J 1993 Simulated home delivery in hospital; a randomised control trial. British Journal of Obstetrics and Gynaecology 100: 316–323

Murphy-Black T 1993 Home birth; can we offer women choices for childbirth? British Journal of Midwifery 1(4): 166–168

Report of the Expert Maternity Group 1993 Changing childbirth. HMSO, London

Scottish Office Home and Health Department 1993 Provision of maternity services in Scotland. HMSO, Edinburgh

Simms C D 1985 Induction of labour—methods. In: Studd J (ed) The management of labour. Blackwells, London, pp 133–145

Smith N C 1987 Assessment of fetal acid–base status. In: Whittle M J (ed) Clinical obstetrics and gynaecology, vol 1. Ballière Tindall, London, pp 97–109

Studd J W W 1973 Partograms and normograms of cervical dilatation in the management of primigravid labour. British Medical Journal 4: 451–484

Westgate J 1993 The assessment of acid–base status at birth. MD Thesis, University of Plymouth, pp 114–143

Westgate J, Harris M, Curnow J S H, Greene K R 1992 Plymouth randomised trial of cardiotocogram only versus ST waveform analysis plus cardiotogram for intrapartum monitoring. Lancet 340: 194–198

31. The midwife's role in the management of normal labour

Rowena J. Davies

Material in this chapter contains contributions from the first edition and we are grateful to the previous author for the work done.

INTRODUCTION

In the UK the dangers of childbirth for both mother and baby have now largely disappeared, thanks to better nutrition, hygiene and the development of safer anaesthetics, surgical techniques, pharmacology, blood transfusions, radiology, and the expertise of the many professionals interested in reproductive medicine.

Legislation restricts those who may attend a mother in childbirth to medical practitioners and practising midwives. Persons undergoing training to become either a midwife or a medical practitioner may attend under supervision, but the practising midwife or medical practitioner remains accountable for the care given (UKCC 1991a).

Mothers choose when they have their children and can control their fertility as no previous generation has, and so each child becomes very special—a planned delight rather than a yearly chore. The birth of a baby is now a social event not a medical problem. The child is born into a family who will be responsible for its health, well-being and introduction into society as a member of the next generation. The fear of death or damage having been removed from societies' collective mind means that the process of childbirth may be looked forward to as an experience to be enjoyed.

With a greater understanding about childbirth and with the choices now available, parents are interested in taking control of their pregnancy and labour rather than acquiescing to medical doctrine or custom and practice.

Mothers increasingly are no longer content to take part in treatment or management if they believe that it is not necessary or is merely a device to speed them through the system. Thus the midwife and obstetrician have been on occasion seen as an adversary rather than an ally, support and guide in the process. Indeed in the past, conflict between midwives and doctors was not unknown, and has to be guarded against even today, as each practitioner may perceive the care of the pregnant woman as their own bailiwick not to be usurped by anyone else. This conflict between the professions was of longstanding and perhaps did not serve the best interests of mothers and babies. Thankfully the respective roles of doctor and midwife today serve to compliment each other, each respecting the other's particular expertise.

The Midwife's Code of Practice clearly states the duties, responsibilities and limits of the midwife:

A midwife is a person who having been regularly admitted to a midwifery education programme duly recognised in the country in which it is located has successfully completed the prescribed course of studies in midwifery and has acquired the requisite qualifications to be registered and legally licensed to practice midwifery. She must be able to give the necessary supervision, care and advice to women during pregnancy, labour and the post-partum period, to conduct deliveries on her own responsibility and to care for the newborn and the infant. This care includes preventative measures, the detection of abnormal conditions in mother and child, procurement of medical assistance and the execution of emergency measures in the absence of medical help. She has an important task in health counselling and education, not only for the patients but also within the family and the community. The work should involve antenatal education and preparation for parenthood and extends to certain areas of gynaecology, family planning and child care. She may practice in hospitals, clinics, health units, domiciliary conditions or in any other service (UKCC 1991a).

The activities of midwives are defined in the European Community Midwives Directive 80/155/EEC article as follows:

Member States shall ensure that midwives are at least entitled to take up and pursue the following activities—to provide sound family planning information and advice—to diagnose pregnancies and monitor normal pregnancies; to carry out examinations necessary for the monitoring of the development of normal pregnancies—to prescribe or advise on the examination necessary for the earliest possible diagnosis of pregnancies at risk—to provide a programme of parenthood preparation and a complete preparation for childbirth, including advice on hygiene and nutrition—to care for and assist a mother during labour and to monitor the condition of the fetus in utero by the appropriate clinical and technical means—to conduct spontaneous deliveries including where required an episiotomy and in urgent cases a breech delivery—to recognise the warning signs of abnormality in the mother or infant, which necessitates the referral to a doctor and to assist the latter where appropriate, to take the necessary emergency measures in the doctors absence, in particular the manual removal of the placenta, possibly followed by manual examination of the uterus—to examine and care for the newborn infant, take all initiatives which are necessary in case of need and to carry out where necessary immediate resuscitation—to care for and monitor the progress of the mother in the post-natal period and to give all necessary advice to the mother on infant care to enable her to ensure that optimum progress of the newborn infant—to carry out treatment prescribed by a doctor—to maintain all necessary records. (UKCC 1991a)

Todays midwives are expected and qualified to be autonomous practitioners of midwifery and are held accountable for their own practice. They may be employed by the health service, by private health organizations or may practice independently.

Historically, matters concerning women and childbirth were the main responsibility of the midwife, and there have probably always been midwives. Their art has been described since at least the times of the Old Testament. In the pre-Christian era midwives were educated and enjoyed a high social standing. Unfortunately by the middle ages, with the control that the priests had over society, the healing arts of women including that of midwifery fell into disrepute and even to practise midwifery was to court the risk of being accused of witchcraft.

Soranus, a Roman physician of the second century, described his prerequisites for a good midwife which perhaps are not so different from those laid down in the several Acts and codes agreed today. They include literacy, good memory, industry, patience and morality, good health and intelligence and long delicate fingers with nails cut short. Also the midwife should be educated in both theory and practice not merely in midwifery but in all related branches of medicine in order that she could give good advice both concerning diet and she should have also a knowledge of the psychological aspects of childbirth and also keep a cool head in any obstetric emergency (Towler 1986).

In comparison with the definition of a midwife adopted by the International Confederation of Midwives and International Confederation of Gynaecologists and Obstetricians in 1972 and 1973 following the amendment of the definition formulated by the World Health Organization, it would appear that to some extent the role perceived for the midwife has now come full circle.

By the beginning of the twentieth century it had been realized that the best interests of mothers and babies were not being served by the then current arrangements. Whereas those who could afford to pay were able to choose which physician and midwife would attend them and also procure aftercare in the guise of a *monthly nurse*, the poor had to make do with an uneducated largely untrained midwife who would be prepared to attend the mother for a minimal fee. The consequence of poverty might produce complications best managed by a doctor but as the mother would not be able to afford his fee and as there were few doctors willing to work for nothing, morbidity and mortality rates were consequently high.

The medical profession was already developing the mechanisms and restrictions by which doctors were approved to attend pregnant women, and had approved academic standards that had to be adhered to. Eventually in July 1902 the first Midwives Act received Royal assent and came into force in 1903. Its purpose was to secure better training for midwives and to regulate their practice. Gradually through successive legislation midwives were required to undergo more and more formalized training, to be placed on a roll later a register, to notify their intention to practice yearly, to undertake theoretical refreshment at 5 yearly intervals and to have their practice supervised by suitably qualified persons appointed by the local supervising authority (UKCC 1991b).

The Standing Maternity & Midwifery Advisory Committee (Department of Health 1970) recommended that all deliveries should take place in or adjacent to consultant obstetric units. This was to reduce further the mortality and morbidity rates of mother and baby. Home deliveries were seen as potentially dangerous and any mother choosing home delivery was seen as foolhardy. The centralization of maternity services led to increased medicalization and the loss of the expertise of some general practitioners in intrapartum care, and the loss of continuity of care given by the community midwife. Mothers were delivered in a sterile theatre-like environment by people they did not know and who would then pass their care on to yet another stranger. Labour seemed to be an experience best got through very quickly. Various techniques of active management of labour were developed to hasten the process and were applied to most mothers sometimes whether or not agreement with the mother had first been obtained.

Every facet of childbirth tended to be controlled by the professionals to ensure uniformity and to aid in the management of the organization rather than meeting the needs of the individual. This mode of management eventually led to much dissatisfaction among mothers, who felt that they were being processed through the system rather than being supported as individuals, and led to a diminution of midwifery skills, as midwives were employed mainly in one area of the hospital maternity unit and tended to lose their comprehensive midwifery skills as a result.

During the late 1970s and 1980s mothers and some practitioners of midwifery came to the view that mothers had lost control of the management of their pregnancies and strove to redress the balance by supporting and campaigning for more natural childbirth and the regaining of parental control. In the management of labour there should be a safe and sensible middle course that can be found and adopted, that does encompass the necessary measures to monitor the well-being of mother and baby whilst respecting and supporting the mother's needs and aspirations.

The increase in intervention, diagnostic ultrasound and invasive fetal monitoring had failed to eliminate intra-parturn fetal morbity and mortality as was expected. However the expectation of parents that any failure to produce a healthy baby was because of negligence may have been reinforced if every known test and procedure has not been performed which would lead them to take legal action against the midwife or doctor concerned.

In 1987 Flint's report on the outcomes of the Know your Midwife Scheme (Flint & Poulengris 1987) stated that mothers offered continuity of care by a small team of midwives throughout the antenatal intrapartum and postnatal period benefited by having less time to wait in clinics, had fewer antenatal admissions, requested less analgesia and had less intervention with no detriment in clinical outcome and an increased feeling of satisfaction. The concept of team midwifery designed to address many of the concerns raised by parents about the fragmentation of care they received has been adopted using different models. Their success has been variable and some hospitals have abandoned their projects because of lack of support, staffing issues and other difficulties of implementation (Wraight et al 1993).

More recently the Health Service Committee Report on Maternity Services (House of Commons 1992) indicated strong support for the concept of mothers being offered continuity of care by small teams of midwives and for the return towards more community-based care for the majority of women with low-risk pregnancies, and for the mother to have more choice concerning her birth attendants and her place of delivery.

In 1993 The Department of Health published the Report of the Expert Maternity Group (Department of Health 1993) chaired by Baroness Cumberledge. 'Changing Childbirth' reviewed current policy and made recommendations for changes in the now traditional pattern of maternity care; many maternity units and purchasing authorities are making this a priority in their business plans and most midwives have received these changes with enthusiasm because they focus on the mother's needs and wishes rather than organizational or on operational priorities.

Primarily, the expert committee supported the philosophy of 'Choice, Continuity and Control' for the mother in all aspects of her maternity care. She should have:

Choice: The mother should have choice in place of care and carer and type of care, and be offered information that enables her to make the best choices for herself and her baby.

Continuity: The mother should have continuity of care offered by the lead professional throughout pregnancy and childbirth (general practitioner, midwife or obstetrician).

Control: The mother should be in control of her own experience and be given information that enables her to be a partner in her care rather than be a passive recipient of the service.

In addition, there were recommendations made concerning the training necessary to ensure delivery of a high quality of service to mothers and babies, particularly with reference to obstetric and neonatal emergencies. The requirements of women with different needs, cultural, ethnic, ability and age related, have been highlighted for special consideration, as has the necessity for the development of excellent communication systems between the mother and her carer.

Maternity services also are now incorporated into the Patient's Charter (Department of Health 1994), with 14 charter standards that mothers can expect maternity units and the health professionals offering care to comply with.

PREPARATION FOR CHILDBIRTH AND PARENTHOOD

Part of the midwives role is to 'provide a programme of parenthood preparation and complete preparation of childbirth including advice on hygiene and nutrition' (UKCC 1991a). Antenatal classes are provided by most maternity units either within the hospital setting or within the community or both.

The composition of classes varies but usually incorporates dietary advice, exercises (sometimes aquatic), basic child care and advice on feeding, and are an introduction to the types of pain relief available varying from the more common entonox (nitrous oxide and oxygen), pethidine and epidural to TENS (transcutaneous electronic nerve stimulation), acupuncture, hypnosis, psychoprophylaxis and relaxation. Education concerning the different stages of labour is given, including different types of delivery.

There is a fine balance to be made between the reassurance that most labours will be uncomplicated and will not need medical intervention and the need to explain in advance the procedures that may be necessary if the labour develops complications.

A tour of the maternity unit is usually offered so that parents may meet some of the staff and be familiar with their surroundings. The courses are in the main run by midwives, but often include physiotherapists, health visitors, obstetricians, anaesthetists, dentists and dieticians. Importantly, the classes provide a forum for parents to elicit information and express their fears or anxieties and to aid successful less painful labour by reducing fear and tension (Wilberg 1992).

Attendance at the classes is optional, and so not all mothers and their partners attend. The most motivated will attend, whereas those most in need of support, education and information may not have the time or interest to attend. This may be especially so if access to classes is restricted by locality or timing or if there are language or cultural difficulties in attendance.

As many pregnant women are in full-time employment they may find it difficult to get time off from work during the day to attend classes. Evening and even weekend classes prove very popular and should be considered where at all possible.

Some units hold classes especially designed for one particular group, for example young mothers. The classes designed to inform about labour may concentrate on one or more aspects of possible outcomes. There should be a sensible path taken between explaining the usual course of labour emphasizing the normal but also explaining the possibilities that may necessitate intervention. There is also a fine line between overexplanation that may be interpreted as scare mongering and keeping parents in the dark; perhaps it is impossible to satisfy all parents' needs and expectations all the time. In addition, there is the danger of raising the expectations of mothers if those teaching are not going to be involved in the labour and therefore make incorrect assumptions about the facilities that exist.

Some mothers choose to attend classes run by the National Childbirth Trust, Lemaze, other organizations or individual teachers. Usually husbands or partners are welcome to participate in the classes, and some units hold specific sessions for fathers to be.

LABOUR

The definition of normality is debatable. A large body of those caring for pregnant women would say that no pregnancy can be said to be normal until after the third stage has been completed. Others will assert that normal women will labour normally and have normal babies. As certain technologies have become more commonplace they have become embraced within the definitions of normal labour. Performing episiotomies, suturing perineums and topping up epidurals are all now part of the midwife's role, and a mother choosing an epidural as her method of pain relief in labour would not be considered to be experiencing an abnormal labour.

The onset of labour may be diagnosed by the effacement and dilatation of the cervix and the commencement of regular (painful) contractions, sometimes accompanied by a show or spontaneous rupture of the membranes.

As the estimated date of the delivery draws nearer the parents may become anxious about whether they will be able to recognize the signs of labour or whether they will reach hospital or contact the midwife in time. They do not wish to embarrass themselves by going to hospital when labour is not in progress. The presence of contractions in themselves are not a conclusive diagnosis of labour and many mothers will experience periods of regular painful contractions and still not be in labour for many hours or even days.

Some mothers believe that labour will follow a set sequence of events and become confused when their particular labour does not follow what the textbooks, classes or peer advice may have indicated.

Ideally, the mother will have been well prepared for all eventualities by attendance at antenatal classes and will have been cared for antenatally by the midwife(s) who will also be delivering her. However, in many units the mother must rely on advice concerning the confirmation of labour from contact with a midwife in the delivery suite who will not have met her before.

In some maternity units the mother may contact their team midwife who will give advice, or who may even visit at home to diagnose labour or assess when transfer into hospital is necessary.

There are some indicative factors which will prompt the midwife to advise immediate attendance for assessment. These may include rupture of membranes, blood loss, lack of fetal activity or very frequent painful contractions.

Whatever the situation the midwife must do her best to assess the physical and psychological condition of the mother. An anxious mother may benefit from early transfer into hospital, similarly a mother with a long distance to travel or a history of short labour will need to think about coming in sooner rather than later. Where possible and if the management of the service is so designed the mother may be visited at home by her midwife who then may assess mother and babys' condition, confirm whether labour has commenced and thus enable the mother to remain in her own familiar relaxed home surroundings for as long as possible.

If the mother is delivering at home she will have been given the telephone number of a midwife or have a contact number so that the on-call community midwife will attend.

The ambience of the delivery suite and the welcome given to the mother on her arrival in labour may colour the mothers' perception of the entire experience of labour. As Flint asserts: 'mothers remember their midwives, and this will be for good or bad'. If the concept of continuity of care for mothers throughout pregnancy, labour and the puerperium has been adopted the mother may already know the midwife who will care for her and should have had the opportunity to discuss her fears, anxieties or wishes; the mother should be more relaxed and confident that her needs will be met and her wishes be respected.

If the midwife is unknown to the mother she will have to use her communication skills and professional expertise to put the mother and her partner at ease and reduce the anxiety often brought about by unfamiliar surroundings.

It is customary for the mother to be accompanied by her partner, mother, sister or a friend. Indeed in some cultures several members may be expected to be involved in the birth process. On occasion the mother will wish also an additional birth attendant to be present—her NCT teacher, an acupuncturist or hypnotherapist.

The assessment to diagnose the onset of labour is very important. First if wrongly diagnosed, any future management decisions, such as artificial rupture of membranes or a Syntocinon infusion, will be made on an incorrect basis and may lead to unnecessary further intervention or instrumental delivery if the labour is incorrectly diagnosed as being prolonged. Secondly if the mother is told that she is in labour and she is not, she, and others, will make the presumption that within a short period she will have delivered her baby. To then be told that she is not in labour will be demoralising to her, and may decrease whatever trust she may have had in her midwife.

Usually the antenatal notes will be at hand so that the midwife can ensure that there are no untoward aspects of either the pregnancy or of the present situation that are a potential cause for concern. The midwife should then discuss with the mother how she feels, assess the degree of any anxiety or distress and any wishes the mother has about the management of her labour. If the mother has a written birth plan this should be reviewed at this stage. The midwife should take a short history of the labour, noting the time that contractions started, their frequency, strength and duration, if the membranes have ruptured, colour and odour of the liquor or if there has been a show. Baseline observations of temperature, pulse and blood pressure are taken and her urine is tested.

An abdominal examination should confirm the late pregnancy status of longitudinal lie, cephalic presentation and the degree of engagement of the fetal head, the fetal heart rate is checked either by Pinard's stethoscope or a hand-held ultrasound monitor.

The midwife will then confirm that labour has commenced by performing a vaginal examination to assess the effacement and dilatation of the cervix, whether the membranes are intact, the position of the fetal head in relation to the pelvis and the level of the fetal head in the pelvis.

Until comparatively recently the custom and practice in many units dictated that mothers were given enemas and had their pubic hair shaved. Both these practices are unnecessary, and at the very least uncomfortable and distasteful. If it is found that the mother is very constipated a suppository may be offered.

Often mothers like to take a warm bath or shower to ease contractions, and may use warm water as their main method of pain relief in the first stage of labour.

The first stage

During the first stage of labour the midwife's role is to observe mother and babys' progress and to offer support and encouragement. Regular observation of the mother's condition will include temperature, pulse and blood pressure, with a check of the frequency, strength and duration of uterine contractions. The frequency of observations will vary from unit to unit, and also the method of their recording. However, the midwife must make accurate and contemporaneous records whatever mode she chooses. The well-being of the mother is also noted. How she is managing her labour, her level of relaxation or anxiety, her wishes as to pain relief, activity or environment. She may have made a detailed birth plan, or may have preferred to adopt a wait and see strategy. Whatever the case each mother's labour is unique to her, and to fulfil her needs and wishes at the time must be the midwife's main objective.

If, as it is hoped, the midwife is already known to the mother through antenatal visits or classes there should be little difficulty in strengthening the relationship of trust and regard that the midwife should be held in. However, if the midwife has not met the mother previously this relationship will have to be made as rapidly as possible.

The continued good health of the fetus during the stress of labour is one of the midwife's main objectives. Most fetuses will withstand the stresses placed upon them by the labour very well; it is for the midwife however to be constantly alert for any indication that the fetus is becoming distressed. The midwife should auscultate the fetal heart regularly throughout labour, perhaps hourly in the early stages then much more frequently as contractions increase in frequency, strength and duration.

The necessity for continuous electronic fetal monitoring is debatable. Some units have adopted the policy of monitoring the fetal heart by cardiotocography on admission for 20 or 30 minutes, then discontinuing if all is normal. Some units use telemetry, which enables the mother freedom of movement whilst still being continuously monitored. If telemetry is not available, continuous cardiotocography restricts the mother to bed or at best a small area around her bed, and for many women this can prove distressing and may disrupt their own plans for labour.

Mobility in labour aids progress by using the weight of the uterus and the fetus to assist in dilating the cervix, and pressure on the lower segment stimulates the uterus to contract further aiding the process.

If in hospital, the mother should be provided with comfortable, pleasant surroundings and must be afforded as much privacy as she desires. Many hospitals are now converting the delivery suites into more home-like rooms that contain comfortable rocking chairs, bean bags and floor mats, aiming to provide a relaxed warm and welcoming atmosphere together with the close proximity of all the technological equipment and facilities necessary should they be needed. Once the onset of labour has been confirmed, progress will be assessed by regular vaginal examinations. Policies and guidelines vary from unit to unit, however each examination must be for a particular purpose, that is acted upon when necessary, and must be performed in a sterile manner.

Until quite recently it was universally considered to be unwise for the mother to eat and drink more than a very minimal amount of water in labour because of the risk of Mendelson's syndrome should general anaesthesia be necessary. This view has been relaxed in some units, and mothers in the latent stage of labour may drink and even have small amounts of food without undue risk after consulting the midwife about the style of food.

Throughout the labour the midwife may have to remind the mother to empty her bladder at reasonably frequent intervals. A full bladder may be displaced from the pelvis into the abdomen and the urethra become stretched. This may lead to urinary retention and subsequent urogynaecological problems. Where necessary if the mother cannot void urine herself, the midwife will have to pass a catheter.

As mentioned previously the mother may have strong views about what she will need with regards to pain relief or may wish to avoid analgesia completely. She may have expressed these views in her birth plan, in the clinic or on admission to the delivery suite. At all times the midwife must respect these wishes and support the mother in achieving her aim.

However, if the labour proves more painful than expected or if the nature of the discomfort is not that which was expected (e.g. backache), the mother may need to be supported through a change of mind. In her book *Sensitive Midwifery*, Flint (1986) expresses the belief that many mothers feel more fulfilled if they have managed labour without analgesia, and that part of the role of the midwife is to support her in this achievement. However, Flint also asserts that another important skill of the midwife is to help mothers know and understand that they may in fact need analgesia (Flint 1986).

Towards the end of the first stage of labour contractions often become very frequent, strong and lengthy and the mother may feel that she is getting no respite between them. She may feel that she is losing control of the situation and find that there is no comfortable position which she can adopt. She may also become very distressed. She may experience the desire to push even if the cervix is not yet fully dilated. The danger of this is that it causes the cervix to become oedematous and will delay full dilatation and will also tire the mother unnecessarily. The midwife will need all her expertise to persuade the mother to desist until full dilatation is achieved (Chamberlain et al 1991).

The second stage

The second stage of labour begins with the full dilatation of the cervix and is completed once the baby is born. It is the stage that requires the mother to be active and may last a few minutes or a few hours. During this stage the contractions are frequent and are typically expulsive in type. Usually the mother will have an uncontrollable urge to bear down during contractions and this will assist in the descent of the fetus through the birth canal.

Usually the mother will enter the second stage of labour well nourished and not too tired. She may have had some form of pain relief and will have rested in between contractions. The baby will also be in good condition. The midwife's role during this time is to encourage and support the mother so that she can successfully and safely deliver her baby.

It is important that the condition of the fetus is checked frequently throughout this stage and usually the fetal heart rate is auscultated immediately after each contraction. The descent of the presenting part is palpated and signs of descent such as distending vulva, pouting anus and visible occiput are watched for and noted.

The midwife should assist the mother to adopt the most comfortable position possible. This may mean frequent position changes. It is unlikely that any mother today would be asked to adopt the stranded beetle position, supine with her feet in stirrups or held immovable by the attendant. This is the worst position possible as the uterus compresses the descending aorta and the inferior vena cava causing a reduced blood flow and thus oxygenation to the placental bed.

Most mothers will at least wish to sit up well supported by pillows or their partner, perhaps squatting in the birthing chair or cushion on hands and knees, the left lateral position, or in water. There is a popular move towards water birth, and whereas many mothers find that warm water is very relaxing and gives effective pain relief, often they will choose to deliver in bed or on a mat on the floor.

Whatever the method chosen by the mother the midwife must be a constant observer, making sure of the baby's well-being, that the second stage is progressing and that the mother is encouraged and supported throughout, always communicating with the mother and her partner giving information about the progress, boosting morale and allaying anxieties.

As delivery become imminent it is very important that the midwife has prepared to receive the baby and has all the necessary equipment ready for any emergency measure that may be necessary. It is helpful to have an assistant present but not strictly necessary. Birth is a highly intimate event and gone, it is hoped, are the births when the delivery room was packed with students or any other interested onlookers all giving advice and exhorting the mother to push. Most mothers do not need to be taught to push. As long as they do not commence pushing too early or have an epidural anaesthetic usually all that is necessary will be for the midwife to encourage and reassure the mother to keep her confident in her own abilities.

It is not considered necessary today for midwives to be masked and gowned as though in theatre in order to deliver the mother. Sterile precautions are taken to protect both mother and baby from contamination by the midwife and today unfortunately midwives must ensure that they take precautions against accidental contamination with blood or body fluids from the mother.

The delivery should be conducted in peaceful, quiet and calm surroundings with any advice or instruction being given by the midwife assisting the mother. All efforts must be made to prevent perineal or vaginal damage, by first watching and assessing the perineal stretch and perhaps gently keeping the fetal head flexed until it is crowned by gentle pressure on the occiput.

Once the head has been delivered it is customary to feel gently for any cord which sometimes may be looped round the baby's neck. If found it is either drawn over the baby's head or if tight round the neck it must be clamped using two artery forceps and cut. During this time the mother should be encouraged not to push if at all possible. Once the shoulders have rotated to present at the pelvic outlet in a anterior posterior position the midwife will gently guide the baby's head backwards and downwards towards the mother's anus, thus aiding the freeing of the anterior shoulder from under the symphysis pubis. Then the baby's head is lifted upwards towards the mother's abdomen to allow the posterior shoulder to be born.

The babys' trunk should be supported as soon as possible and the baby delivered. The posterior shoulder can cause much damage to the posterior wall of the vagina and great care must be taken to prevent this. Some parents will have requested to delay cutting the cord until it has stopped pulsating. Some partners will also request that they may cut the cord.

Routine episiotomies are not necessary, and each situation must be assessed individually. If the midwife considers that there is a need for an episiotomy she should first explain the reasons for this to the mother. Local anaesthesia is administered as 10 ml of 1% xylocaine along the line of the proposed line of incision and a (right) mediolateral episiotomy performed at the height of contraction once the xylocaine has become effective.

The third stage

The third stage of labour can be defined as the time following delivery of the baby to the expulsion of the placenta. This process is normally completed within about 20 minutes if active management is not employed.

The normal physiological process is that the uterine contractions continue after delivery of the baby and reduce the surface area of the uterine cavity causing the placenta to shear off the wall. Further contractions cause the placenta to be forced into the lower segment then into the vagina and finally expelled, together with the amnion and chorion.

There are two methods of delivering the placenta and membranes. The first is to wait until signs of separation and descent have occurred. The midwife places the ulna border of her left hand just above the fundus and waits for the signs of separation which are:

1. a small gush of blood
2. lengthening of the umbilical cord
3. the fundus rises, is harder and more mobile.

During this time it is very important not to fiddle with the fundus or pull on the cord, because this may interfere with the physiological process, and cause a partial separation to occur. The midwife may then instruct the mother to push out the placenta or assist by using fundal pressure using the fundus as a piston to assist in expulsion. The placenta is supported and twisted round to cause the membranes to form a rope. This aids in their complete removal.

The alternative, and more common method of delivery of the third stage, is by active management. An intramuscular injection of Syntometrine is given to the mother with the birth of the anterior shoulder of the baby. This causes the placenta to separate rapidly and the placenta is delivered by controlled cord traction.

Active management of the third stage shortens this stage, and reduces blood loss. Whichever method of management is chosen the midwife must be alert to prevent or reduce postparturm haemorrhage, and must ensure that she has examined the placenta for completeness. Retention of part of the placenta or membranes can cause primary or secondary postpartum haemorrhage or uterine infection. Other abnormalities of placenta, membranes or cord may be noted and reported if felt appropriate. After delivery of the placenta and membranes, any blood and clots are collected and the blood loss measured and recorded (Sweet 1988).

As soon as is practicable, and as soon as possible, the genital tract should be examined for lacerations or tears and sutured where appropriate.

The first hour following delivery is sometimes called the fourth stage of labour and this is the time during which the new family are getting to know each other. The baby may be put to the breast, the mother's temperature, pulse and blood pressure are taken, her uterus and lochia checked, and she may shower or be assisted to bathe and a light meal be offered. During this time the midwife's role is to remain observant, ensure the safety of mother and baby but encourage the close contact between the baby and his/her new family.

THE CARE OF THE NEWBORN BABY

These days the baby is often given to the mother as soon as the cord has been separated. However, the wishes of the mother in this must be respected. Sometimes the mother wishes the baby to be cleaned and checked before she holds him. The midwife's responsibilities are to assess the baby's condition and initiate resuscitation if necessary.

If antenatal or labour factors have indicated that resuscitation may be necessary, the midwife must prepare the room accordingly with the necessary equipment and call for medical aid—a neonatologist if in hospital, the general practitioner if at home or the paediatric emergency unit if help from the general practitioner is not available.

Mucus extraction may be necessary—though by no means do all babies need this. The unexpected appearance of meconium, however, will need mucus extraction before the delivery of the thorax. If mucus extraction is necessary it should be carried out gently, without undue force and without removing the baby from the mother's arms if at all possible. Overstimulation can produce a reflex apnoea.

The baby should be kept from becoming chilled by being wrapped or covered in a warm towel whilst in the mother's arms. The baby can lose heat extraordinarily quickly, especially through the head, and all efforts must be made to prevent this.

During the first few minutes after delivery while the mother is holding the baby the midwife will be observing the baby's condition and making an initial Apgar score. The Apgar score devised by the late Dr Virginia Apgar in 1953 (O'Dowd & Phillip 1994) gives a basic assessment of the baby at 1 and 5 minutes of life based on the evaluation of five clinical features—heart rate, respiration, muscle tone, reflex irritability and colour. The highest and best score is 10; there are limitations to the accuracy of this method of assessment but its appeal lies in its lack of invasiveness and its relative simplicity.

As soon as is practicable the baby is examined, weighed and his/her head circumference and length measured.

Examination aims to identify any minor or major abnormalities and includes examination of the baby's skull, fontanelles and sutures, placement of the ears and eyes. Examination of the mouth is made to exclude soft and hard palate deformities and is essential. The limbs must be examined, fingers and toes counted, the chest and abdomen examined and also the site of insertion of the cord. The cord is usually clamped using a Hollister clamp placed about 2 cm from the umbilicus. The entire length of the spine is examined to exclude neural tube defects. The external genitalia are inspected and the general skin tone and skeletal system noted. Note whether urine or meconium has been passed. The baby's temperature is taken either per axilla or per anus. The examination should be performed with the mother's agreement and in a place where she may watch and participate if she wishes.

It is not necessary to bathe the baby at this stage unless the parents specifically wish this. There is a risk that the baby may become chilled unnecessarily and it is unlikely that the newly delivered mother will be able to learn any useful parenting tips at this early stage.

The baby should be dressed and if delivered in hospital, labelled with two name labels which record the baby's name, date and time of birth and hospital number (if given). This label must be checked with the mother or father.

Phytomendione (vitamin K) is offered almost universally to babies orally or by injection, to prevent haemorrhagic disease of the newborn.

The mother may have decided how she will feed her baby, and may have decided to try breastfeeding. Unfortunately, many women have never seen another woman breastfeed and will have heard stories about the difficulty of breastfeeding and may fear that it will prove restricting, messy and painful. Some partners too do not approve of their wives breastfeeding (Renfrew et al 1990).

Whereas breastfeeding is a natural instinct, to be successfully established it must be learned. Putting the baby to the breast within the first 10 minutes after delivery has been shown to contribute to successful feeding, positioning of the baby correctly and ensuring the mother is comfortable and pain free are also vital for success (White et al 1990).

As soon as is practicable the midwife should complete her record of the delivery and complete the Birth Notification form. This is actually a duty of the father or any other person in attendance upon the mother at birth, but usually it is the midwife who does this.

The midwife should complete her notes immediately after delivery. The method of record keeping varies between hospitals, computerized systems being increasingly used by some units. The independent midwife must keep her own register of cases.

After an hour once the mother has bathed, the mother

and baby can be transferred to the postnatal ward by the midwife who may continue the care or will hand over care to a colleague.

If the mother has elected to be part of the DOMiciliary Midwife IN and Out scheme (DOMINO), she may remain in the delivery suite or postnatal ward for a minimal period and then transfer with her community midwife to have her care continued at home.

ABNORMAL SITUATIONS

One of the purposes of antenatal care is to assess, monitor, detect and prevent complications or abnormalities in both mother and baby to ultimately ensure safe delivery of both mother and baby.

During labour similarly the aim is to support and encourage the mother and to assess and monitor her progress and that of the baby. The duties of the midwife are to call for medical aid if an abnormal condition is detected in mother or child (UKCC 1991a).

In the hospital environment the lines of communication concerning referral to medical advice and assistance are usually well established and follow an agreed protocol. For mothers delivering at home, the midwife will refer any cause for concern to the general practitioner with whom the mother has booked for pregnancy and delivery care (who may not be her usual general practitioner). Where the mother has not found a general practitioner to undertake this care, the midwife has the duty to contact her local supervisor of midwives and to contact if at all possible a medical practitioner on call for emergencies.

The arrangements for many maternity units include the facility for the community midwife to contact the delivery suite of the local hospital for advice, there may be a designated consultant obstetrician who will provide medical cover for mothers without general practitioner support, and some maternity units still have an emergency obstetric unit (the old flying squad) that the midwife may call out.

In the situation where the midwife considers either home confinement is no longer appropriate or in the situation that the mother refuses to have a medical practitioner in attendance even though the midwife deems it advisable, the midwife has the duty to continue to care for the mother and baby, and consult with her supervisor of midwives in each of the health authorities in which she give's care. When she books a mother for home delivery it is also customary to notify the local supervisor who will be available for consultation, support and guidance should any difficulties arise.

It is sad that litigation or the threat of being the subject of a claim is a cause of concern for most obstetricians and midwives. The temptation to practice defensive obstetrics is great and the midwife is increasingly having to be aware of her duties and responsibilities and the possible conflict between the wishes of the mother and the possible danger to the baby (Douglas 1991).

Trust hospitals are now liable to find the 'costs of any successful claims against them and awards of £2 million are not unknown. This amount would, if payable, effectively remove most if not all of many maternity units' yearly budget. The changes in the rule concerning legal aid in 1990 means that claims made on behalf of the infant are now state funded (Mason & Edwards 1993). This has meant a large increase in the number of claims made.

The natural response to this may be to practise defensive midwifery and ensure that all possible methods of invasive monitoring of the baby are used. Intervention to hasten delivery by forceps, ventouse or Caesarean section may be justified on the grounds that the damage to the baby happened despite all possible means of monitoring and active management and therefore could not have been caused by negligence.

The midwife may find herself in conflict with the mother if the mother wishes limited monitoring and no intervention when the midwife recommends electronic monitoring or episiotomy. She may find herself in the unenviable situation of being sued for assault if she performs an episiotomy to expedite delivery in the case of fetal distress, or being sued because the baby suffered intrapartum hypoxia and subsequent damage because delivery was prolonged as a result of the midwife acquiescing to the mother's express wishes not to have an episiotomy.

The midwife's best defences are clear, explicit and meticulous contemporaneous record keeping, excellent communication skills and a determination to build a good relationship on mutual trust with the mother and her partner from the moment the midwife meets them.

Before birth legally the baby has no rights, but after birth may be awarded enormous damages if negligence can be proved (Dimond 1990).

CONCLUSION

Today's midwife practises her art in a multicultural society. She will if she is fortunate meet women and their partners from all over the world and learn much about the needs, wishes and birth traditions of the women she cares for. To be effective she will need to maintain a flexible attitude and to ensure that her practice remains up to date and be prepared to learn new skills, whilst refining her old ones. She must also gain the trust and respect of mothers and their families and in addition the professional respect of her obstetrician, general practitioner and other colleagues that she must work with to ensure that the mother and her family receive the quality of care that they have come to expect.

REFERENCES

Chamberlain G, Dewhurst J, Harvey D 1991 Obstetrics, 2nd edn. Gover Medical, London, 1991

Department of Health 1970 Standing Maternity and Midwifery Advisory Committee. Domiciliary midwifery and maternity bed needs report of the subcommittee. HMSO, London

Department of Health 1993 Changing Childbirth. Part 1—report of the expert maternity group—UK. HMSO, London

Department of Health 1994 NHS—The Patient's Charter—maternity services—UK. HMSO, London

Dimond B 1990 Legal aspects of nursing. Prentice Hall International, Cambridge

Douglas G 1991 Law fertility and reproduction. Sweet & Maxwell, London

Flint C 1986 (reprinted 1991) Sensitive midwifery. Butterworth-Heinemann, Oxford

Flint C, Poulengris P 1987 The know your midwife's report. C Flint, 49 Peckermans Wood, London

House of Commons 1992 Health Committee Second Report—maternity services vol 1. HMSO, London

Mason D, Edwards P 1993 Litigation: a risk management guide for midwives. Capstick, Kent

O'Dowd M J, Phillip E E 1994 The history of obstetrics and gynaecology. The Parthenon Publishing Group

Renfrew M, Fisher C, Arms S 1990 Best feeding—getting it right for you. Celestial Arts, California

Sweet B R 1988 Mayes' midwifery—a textbook for midwives, 11th edn. Baillière Tindall, London

Towler J, Bramall J 1986 Midwives in history & society. Croom Helm, London

UKCC 1991a Midwife's' code of practice. United Kingdom Central Council for Nursing Midwifery and Health Visiting, London

UKCC 1991b Midwives rules. United Kingdom Central Council for Nursing Midwifery and Health Visiting, London

White A, Freeth S, O'Brien M 1990 Infant feeding. OPCS. HMSO, London

Wilberg G M 1992 Preparing for birth and parenthood. Butterworth-Heinemann, Oxford

Wraight A, Ball J, Seccombe I, Stock J 1993 Mapping team midwifery—a report to the Department of Health. IMS, Brighton

32. Analgesia and anaesthesia

Michael Harmer

Material in this chapter contains contributions from the first edition and we are grateful to the previous authors for the work done.

INTRODUCTION

The knowledge that it is possible to alleviate the pain of labour dates far back. Early Chinese writings describe the use of opiates and soporifics during childbirth, whilst in the Middle Ages they seemed to depend more upon self-administration of alcoholic drinks. However, in some groups the relief of childbirth pain was considered evil and had led to the execution of those attempting to help the mother, a practice which fortunately is no longer in fashion. The first recognized obstetric anaesthetic, using ether, was administered by Dr James Young Simpson in 1847 but perhaps it was not until John Snow in 1853 administered chloroform to Queen Victoria for the birth of Prince Leopold that obstetric anaesthesia and analgesia gained respectability.

Of the agents still in current use, nitrous oxide was first used as an obstetric analgesic by Klikowitsch in 1881, but did not become widely available until the introduction of the Minnit apparatus in 1934 which delivered a mixture of nitrous oxide in air. In 1961, the currently used 50 : 50 mixture of nitrous oxide and oxygen was described by Tunstall. While nitrous oxide has remained in use, other inhalational agents (trichloroethylene and methoxyflurane) administered in air via drawover vaporizers have come and gone.

The use of systemic analgesics in labour was not seen until 1902 when von Steinbuchel introduced the combination of morphine and scopolamine. In 1940, pethidine was first used and has remained the most commonly used systemic analgesic in obstetric practice in the UK to this day.

The earliest use of local anaesthetics in labour dates from 1910 when Stiasny applied cocaine to the vagina and vulva. Although spinal subarachnoid analgesia had first been performed in 1885, it was not until 1928 that Pitkin popularized its use in obstetric practice. Lumbar epidural analgesia was described by Dogliotti in the 1940s but continuous lumbar epidural analgesia only became popular in the UK in the late 1960s.

Whilst the provision of general anaesthesia in obstetrics has a degree of inherent risk, due in part to the changes in maternal physiology consequent upon pregnancy, the provision of analgesia in labour should be absolutely safe. The longstanding methods of intermittent inhalation of analgesic agents and the use of intermittent intramuscular injections of narcotic analgesics have shown themselves in millions of pregnancies to be safe procedures. Newer techniques, which have the advantage of providing a better quality of analgesia, must also prove themselves as safe. Therefore, concern must be expressed that epidural analgesia has been associated with more than one maternal death (Department of Health and Social Security 1982).

The variety of techniques available for relieving labour pain should mean that every mother can find a method that will suit her. However, the actual technique used will vary according to local availability and other pressures; the provision of a full range of techniques may be hampered by lack of staff or funds. The current situation with regard to availability and choice of analgesic method is covered later.

NON-PHARMACOLOGICAL METHODS

Psychophysical methods

Psychoprophylaxis is often wrongly considered as a simple distraction technique when in fact it is far more widely based; the total package consisting of antenatal preparation and education along with the development of various techniques of relaxation. In preparation for labour the mother requires careful explanation of events that may happen and, hopefully, allaying of fear. This form of instruction has formed part of the basis of *natural childbirth* as first introduced by Dick-Read in the 1930s (Dick-Read 1944). Fundamental to this philosophy is the belief that pain is the result of fear and misinterpretation of sensations associated with uterine contractions. If the mother learns how to relax fully and how to dissociate herself from the episode of contraction, labour can become an enjoyable experience. Whilst some may scorn the aims of natural childbirth, it is prudent to remember that a relaxed and fully prepared mother is likely to be easier to manage should problems arise in labour.

Whilst psychoprophylaxis may be of value in early labour it is seldom satisfactory for the whole of labour. Studies on the efficacy of psychoprophylaxis are often difficult to compare with other approaches but one well conducted study has been reported (Scott & Rose 1976). Two matched groups were compared; one had attended a full course of psychoprophylaxis classes based on the Lamaze method (Lamaze 1956) whilst the other had not. The results showed that the prepared group had a higher frequency of spontaneous vaginal delivery which possibly related to the lower rate of epidural block employed in this group. In other aspects—length of labour, Apgar scores and incidence of fetal distress—there was no difference between the groups. In UK hospitals, where a wide range of pain relief methods is available, less than 5% of mothers use only psychophysical techniques.

Hypnosis

Hypnosis is helpful in a small minority of patients but the reported success rate has varied from 23 to 59% amongst selected subjects of successful relief of pain during labour (Moya & James 1960, Davidson 1962, Gross & Posner 1963). Analgesics were required during delivery in most of the mothers in two of these studies (Moya & James 1960, Gross & Posner 1963). The major problem with hypnosis is that for a high success rate a great deal of time is needed in antenatal preparation.

Acupuncture

Although this technique has been of value in the management of certain painful conditions, particularly chronic pain, what little evidence there is available suggests that it has only limited efficacy for the pain of labour. Wallis et al (1974) found that even when an experienced acupuncturist was employed, the technique failed to give pain relief in 19 of 21 cases so treated. Another study using

electroacupuncture (Abouleish & Depp 1975) found the method time-consuming and restrictive and the analgesia to be inconsistent and unpredictable.

Transcutaneous nerve stimulation

This technique involves the application of a variable electrical stimulus to the skin at the site of pain and is based upon the gate theory of pain control (Melzack & Wall 1965). Studies have shown there to be great or considerable relief of labour pain in 20–24% of mothers with about 60% having slight relief (Robson 1979, Stewart 1979). It is said to be most helpful for backache. A controlled study of two parity groups comparing transcutaneous nerve stimulation (TNS) and a placebo (Harrison et al 1986) showed that in terms of pain relief there was no difference between the groups. However, mothers did find the apparatus reassuring and the study concludes that TNS may have a part to play in short labour.

Audioanalgesia

The use of white sound as a dissociative technique has been reported by one or two enthusiasts (Burt & Korn 1964, Barbe & Sattenspiel 1965) as helpful during labour but not appropriate for use during delivery.

Abdominal decompression

The technique of abdominal decompression as a method of reducing the pain of labour was introduced by Heyns (1959). The apparatus required is large and cumbersome. The hypothesis for its efficacy rests upon the contention that if the muscles of the anterior and posterior abdominal walls are held in a state of contraction, the pregnant uterus is flattened and excessive contraction of the upper segment of the uterus leads to pain. If the excessive tone in the abdominal walls is reduced, pain should be reduced also. There have been conflicting reports of the technique's success (Scott & Loudon 1960) and its failure (Shulman & Birnbaum 1966). The claim that abdominal decompression improves the acid–base status and oxygenation of the fetus has been denied (Newman & Wood 1967). As a technique it would seem to have little place in modern practice.

INHALATION ANALGESIA

Until 1983 when the Central Midwives Board withdrew approval for the use of trichloroethylene by unsupervised midwives there were three agents available for use: nitrous oxide, trichloroethylene and methoxyflurane. Currently only nitrous oxide is available in the UK, the other inhalational agents having been withdrawn. However, there has been some interest in the use of newer anaesthetic agents.

Nitrous oxide

Nitrous oxide was first used as an obstetric analgesic by Klikowitsch in 1881. It became widely used with the introduction of the Minnitt apparatus (1934) which delivered a mixture of nitrous oxide in air but there was always unease about its use in this apparatus as mixtures containing as little as 10% oxygen could be produced. In addition there were reports of machines in use that delivered even lower concentrations of oxygen (Cole & Nainby-Luxmore 1962). In the early 1960s the currently available 50 : 50 preprepared mixture of nitrous oxide and oxygen (Entonox) was described by Tunstall (1961). The composition of the gas in the cylinder remains constant throughout the time when it is in use. The one exception to this being if the contents of the cylinder are allowed to cool below $-7°C$, when the constituent gases separate. This would lead to pure oxygen being available initially until it was exhausted, when pure nitrous oxide would be delivered. Temperatures of $-7°C$ are not exceptional in some parts of the British Isles (Crawford et al 1967) and recommendations have been made on the storage and use of Entonox cylinders based on the advice of a Medical Research Council committee which considered the problem (Cole et al 1970).

Entonox is employed as a self-administered, intermittent inhalation which, if used in the correct manner, can produce acceptable levels of analgesia. It takes some 20–30 seconds of Entonox inhalation to achieve effective blood concentrations of nitrous oxide, so it is important that pain is anticipated and inhalation started when the contraction is first felt. In the first stage of labour, where the initial part of the contraction is not always very painful, it may be tempting for the mother to wait until the pain is fully established before using the Entonox. However, if she breathes Entonox early she has an effective blood concentration of nitrous oxide when the peak of the contraction occurs. Delay in utilization is one of the major reasons for dissatisfaction with inhalational analgesia. The problem of this lag period before analgesia is achieved can be partly overcome by continually breathing a low concentration of Entonox as a background so that intermittent inhalation takes less time to reach the peak concentration, and is therefore more effective (Davies et al 1978, Arthurs & Rosen 1981).

One factor that influences the use of the Entonox apparatus is that about 30% of mothers have a horror of anaesthetic masks. A simple mouthpiece provides an acceptable alternative to over 95% of mothers with no loss of efficacy (Dolan & Rosen 1975).

The effectiveness of Entonox in preventing the pain of labour is of approximately the same order as pethidine. This has been stated by Beazley et al (1967) as 23% total success but 40% total failure. Other studies on the efficacy of nitrous oxide have produced similar results (Report to the Medical Research Council 1970, Holdcroft & Morgan 1974). It should be possible for 80% of mothers to obtain substantial benefit from inhalational analgesia when properly managed by the midwife.

Other inhalational analgesics

The alternative forms of inhalation analgesia to Entonox have been powerful volatile anaesthetic agents given at low concentrations in air using a drawover vaporizer. These are not currently in widespread use but newer agents may yet have a place in clinical practice.

Trichloroethylene is no longer available for use in obstetric analgesic practice but deserves mention as an historic landmark. It was introduced as an alternative to nitrous oxide, which at that time was administered via the Minnitt apparatus, and was approved for use by the unsupervised midwife in two temperature-compensated vaporizers, the Emotril (*E*pstein, *M*acintosh, *O*xford, *Tril*ene) and the Tecota (*Te*mperature *co*mpensated *t*richloroethylene *a*ir) which produced a concentration of 0.35 or 0.5% trichloroethylene in air within a narrow range.

The uptake, distribution and elimination of trichloroethylene was slow in comparison with nitrous oxide and analgesia did not occur until about 4 minutes of inhalation (Dundee & Moore 1960). However, because elimination was also slow it allowed the development of a resting level of analgesia, sometimes accompanied by drowsiness; the quality of analgesia achieved was similar to Entonox.

Methoxyflurane had similar characteristics to trichloroethylene and was administered as a 0.35% mixture in air delivered from an automatically temperature-compensated drawover vaporizer, the Cardiff Inhaler (Jones et al 1971). Reservations were expressed about the possibility of renal damage associated with its use but most authorities deny any renal damage when it is used at a concentration of 0.35% (Rosen et al 1972, Creasser et al 1974). Use of methoxyflurane declined when the British Standards Institution found it was no longer feasible annually to test Cardiff Inhalers.

Enflurane in a 1% concentration in air has been shown to be more effective than Entonox for obstetric analgesia during labour (McGuinness & Rosen 1984). However, this enhanced analgesia was associated with excessive drowsiness.

Isoflurane, the most recently introduced volatile anaesthetic agent, has been used in a 0.75% concentration in oxygen (McLeod et al 1985) where it produced good analgesia but with a high degree of drowsiness. More recently, it has been used in a 0.2% concentration in Entonox (Wee et al 1993) where it produced superior analgesia to Entonox alone with no increase in drowsiness.

NARCOTIC ANALGESICS

Pethidine

The mainstay of systemically administered analgesics has been pethidine since its introduction into obstetric practice in the 1940s. The reason for the popularity of pethidine has been ascribed to the fact that it is less soporific than the alternatives of morphine or heroin. The standard method of administration is for the labouring mother to receive a dose of pethidine (100–150 mg), given intramuscularly. The onset of analgesia takes some 10–15 minutes. This dose of pethidine is normally repeated as necessary every 3–4 hours. In modern obstetric practice it is rare for a mother to receive more than two doses. Due to its side-effects of nausea and vomiting, it is best administered with an antiemetic. There may be benefits to using lower doses (pethidine 50 mg) repeated as necessary to reduce the incidence of side-effects.

Placental transfer of pethidine is rapid with changes being seen in the fetal EEG shortly after maternal administration (Rosen et al 1970). The depressant effects on the fetus appear to be greatest around 2–3 hours after maternal administration (Shnider & Moya 1964) and least if delivery occurs within an hour (Belfrage et al 1981) or after more than 6 hours (Morrison et al 1973). The depressant effects of pethidine on neurobehavioural functions and feeding in the neonate persist for 48 hours (Wiener et al 1979).

The effectiveness of intermittently administered intramuscular pethidine was studied by Beazley et al (1967) who revealed that less than 25% of mothers so treated had pain-free labour whilst 40% had not experienced any relief.

Other analgesics

Morphine and diamorphine

Whilst morphine was the first opioid analgesic used in labour, its contemporary use is uncommon, mainly because it has been said to produce 10-fold greater respiratory depression in the newborn than equipotent doses of pethidine (Way et al 1965). Diamorphine is occasionally used, often for an anxiolytic effect, but studies suggest that it too tends to be concentrated in fetal nervous tissue (Scanner & Woods 1965).

Pentazocine

Studies have shown that this partial agonist analgesic, when used in multiple doses, produces fewer low Apgar scores in babies as compared to pethidine (Refstad & Lindbaek 1980). In addition, the fetal heart rate is not so effected by pentazocine as it is with pethidine. The chief drawback to pentazocine is unpleasant hallucinogenic side-effects and the limited pain relief that it can produce.

Meptazinol

Meptazinol, a partial agonist analgesic, is free of strict prescribing restrictions. Given intramuscularly, it was initially believed to be equipotent with pethidine (Paymaster 1977) but administered intravenously by a patient-controlled method was only half as potent as pethidine (Slattery et al 1981). It has also been said to have less respiratory-depressant effects than pethidine but this has been questioned (Slattery et al 1983). Meptazinol produces less neonatal respiratory depression and acidosis than pethidine (De Boer et al 1987). This advantage is probably not related to the rate of placental transfer as meptazinol and pethidine have similar transfer characteristics (Carson & Reynolds 1988). However, a high degree of nausea and vomiting—an uncomfortable side-effect—may limit its use.

Patient-controlled analgesia

The effect of biological variation on a fixed dose schedule for pain relief by the intramuscular route leads to many dissatisfied mothers. Administration of small doses of drug intravenously should enable titration to an adequate level of analgesia. Scott (1970) used an infusion of dilute pethidine administered intravenously by a simple patient-controlled clamp on the infusion line to control labour pain in a problem mother. A more sophisticated approach was developed by Evans et al (1976a)—a patient-activated syringe pump, the Cardiff Palliator, which included electronic controls. Other more sophisticated, micro-processor-controlled machines have since become available. Most devices incorporate safety features designed to avoid the possibility of overdose and have been used with good effect in obstetric units, particularly those unable to provide a full epidural service (Harper et al 1983). The effectiveness of patient-controlled analgesia is greater than standard intramuscular injection (Evans et al 1976a, Robinson et al 1980). Such apparatus shows wide variation in the demand by mothers for analgesics, indicating the necessity for a system which will allow for considerable interindividual variation.

Epidural and spinal opiates

In recent years, morphine receptors in the spinal cord have been identified. Morphine and other analgesic drugs placed in the epidural space have been shown to produce good pain relief in the postoperative period. Trials in obstetrics, however, have shown great variability in effectiveness (Skjoldebrand et al 1982). Many factors have been proposed to explain the non-effectiveness in obstetrics, including the type of pain associated with labour and the site of morphine receptors involved in uterine pain. Single injections of opiates into the subarachnoid space have been effective in obstetric practice (Scott et al 1980) but the technique has a potential problem of late-onset respiratory depression. There has been some interest in the use of pethidine in the epidural space. Pethidine is known to have local anaesthetic (Tham et al 1993) as well as analgesic activity and has been shown to have analgesic effects when given epidurally in labour (Edwards et al 1992).

Opiate antagonists

A major concern with any narcotic agent used in labour is that respiratory depression in the neonate will result. It is believed that if narcotic analgesics have been given to the mother within 2 hours of delivery, neonatal depression is more likely. However, this is by no means an unbreakable rule. The use of patient-controlled analgesia up to delivery has not been associated with problems of respiratory depression in the newborn (Evans et al 1976a).

If there is concern about opioid-induced neonatal depression, a narcotic antagonist (naloxone) may be administered. It is not advisable to administer naloxone to the mother before delivery as this would also reverse analgesia, but it is best administered to the infant as necessary at birth. The intravenous dose of naloxone for rapid reversal of respiratory depression in the neonate is 40 µg (Evans et al 1976b). Administered intramuscularly in a 200 µg dose, it works within a few minutes (Wiener et al 1977). Pethidine has been shown to have long-term depressant effects on feeding and neurobehavioural status and naloxone has been shown to prevent or considerably diminish such effects (Wiener et al 1977, 1979). No adverse effects have been reported in the use of naloxone in these dosages in the newborn.

CONDUCTION ANALGESIA

Local anaesthesia

The increased use of local anaesthesia, especially for epidural analgesia, has been a major development in obstetric practice in the last few decades. It is essential therefore to review the toxicity and side-effects of local anaesthetics in both the mother and the fetus.

Effects on the mother

The most serious side-effects affect the central nervous system. Moderate overdose may only lead to drowsiness but a large overdose may cause a convulsion or even a series of convulsions. The possibility of a local anaesthetic as the cause of a convulsion should always be considered. Whilst central nervous system effects are the most likely following overdose, serious cardiovascular responses also occur. They consist of bradycardia and hypertension which may be followed by cardiac arrest, especially if an inadvertent intravenous injection of bupivacaine has been administered. Local anaesthetics affect the heart by blocking sodium channels and hence slowing conduction. Whilst the heart tolerates lignocaine well (it is used as an antiarrhythmic), Clarkson et al (1984) found that bupivacaine appears to cause a prolonged blockade. Such toxicity is further enhanced by existing acidosis, hypoxia or hypercarbia (Thigpen et al 1983).

The exact doses of local anaesthetics which are toxic is not agreed but the figures presented in Table 32.1 may act as a guideline to safe dosage.

Side-effects from local anaesthetics are much more likely to occur if the dose of drug is inadvertently injected intravenously. They rarely occur as a result of repeated administration, particularly if doses are only given when the analgesic effect of the preceding dose has worn off.

Effects on the fetus

Local anaesthetics can indirectly affect the fetus by blocking sympathetic activity and causing hypotension in the mother, leading to a reduction in placental blood flow. All local anaesthetics cross the placental barrier and can have direct effects upon the fetus. Changes in beat-to-beat variability have been reported following injection of local anaesthetic into the mother's epidural space (Lavin et al 1981, Abboud et al 1982). These changes due to the uptake of drug into the fetal myocardium, are not considered to be of great importance. The most serious toxic reactions are associated with misplaced injections

Table 32.1 Safe doses and concentrations of local anaesthetics

Drug used	Dose/concentration
Lignocaine	
With adrenaline	500 mg (7 mg/kg)
Without adrenaline	200 mg (3 mg/kg)
For infiltration	0.25–0.5%
For nerve block	1–2%
Prilocaine	
With adrenaline	600 mg
Without adrenaline	400 mg
For infiltration	0.25–0.5%
For nerve block	1%
Bupivacaine	
Without adrenaline	150 mg (2 mg/kg)
For infiltration	0.25%
For nerve block	0.25–0.5%

of local anaesthetics, such as into the fetal scalp during perineal infiltration (Kim et al 1979).

There has been much interest in the long-term effects on the fetus of local anaesthetics. These studies are based upon changes in neurobehavioural patterns. Lignocaine or mepivacaine cause a slight diminution of responsiveness and muscle tone persisting for more than a week after delivery (Tronick et al 1976), whilst bupivacaine was not considered to have these problems (Scanlon et al 1976). Other work shows that, depending upon the dose, bupivacaine causes similar neurobehavioural changes to the other local anaesthetic agents (Wiener et al 1979). Overall, the effects of local anaesthetics on the fetus are minor and appear to be of little clinical importance.

Infiltration with local anaesthetic

The most commonly administered form of local anaesthesia is infiltration of the perineum with a local anaesthetic such as lignocaine prior to performing an episiotomy incision at the time of delivery. Large amounts of local anaesthetic are not necessary, therefore side-effects from this block are rare so long as misplaced or intravenous injections are avoided.

Nerve blocks

Only two nerve blocks are commonly used: the pudendal nerve block and the paracervical block.

Pudendal nerve block

Pudendal nerve block is almost always used to facilitate operative vaginal delivery and is usually performed by the obstetrician. The nerve is blocked in, or close to, the pudendal canal on the lateral wall of the ischiorectal fossa where it is closely associated with the pudendal artery and vein. There are two methods of performing bilateral pudendal block: the transvaginal or the transperineal approach.

Transvaginal approach This is performed with the mother in the lithotomy position. A pudendal block needle some 12.5 cm in length is attached to a 20 ml syringe containing local anaesthetic solution. The needle is placed along the second and third fingers of one hand and introduced carefully into the vagina. The region of the ischial spine is palpated with the tips of the fingers and the needle advanced through the vaginal wall immediately behind the ischial spine to a depth of about 1.25 cm, with the needle passing through the sarcospinous ligament. Following aspiration to check that the needle is not in a vein, an injection of 10 ml of local anaesthetic solution is made. The procedure is repeated on the other side.

Transperineal approach This is only used when the presenting part of the fetus is too low to permit the use of the transvaginal approach. An unguarded needle is inserted through the perineal skin at a point halfway between the fourchette and the ischial tuberosity. Two fingers of the other hand are placed within the vagina and the ischial spine is identified and the needle advanced until its point lies just behind the ischial spine. After careful aspiration, 10 ml of local anaesthetic solution is injected. The procedure is repeated on the other side.

Paracervical block

Paracervical block can be of value in the first stage of labour. It is performed by inserting a special sheathed needle 1–2 cm through the epithelium of each lateral fornix of the vagina (Fig. 32.1) and depositing 5–10 ml of local anaesthetic solution into each paracervical region. This is a highly vascular area and an inadvertent intravascular injection is possible. It provides successful analgesia in approximately 80% of mothers (Belfrage & Floberg 1983).

Paracervical block enjoyed a period of popularity but as a single-short technique, analgesia lasts only 1 hour, though the duration of action has been extended by the use of catheter techniques. Doubts have been expressed concerning the safety of paracervical block for the fetus. In the first few minutes after initiating a block a high incidence of fetal bradycardia associated with a falling pH and oxygen tension has been seen (Baxi et al 1979). These changes have been investigated by Cibils (1976)

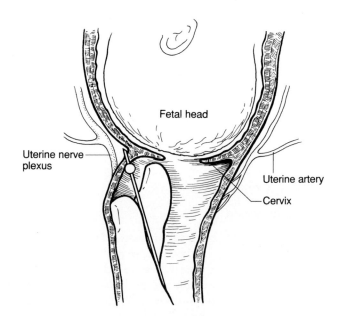

Fig. 32.1 Placement of paracervical block needle. Note the close proximity of the uterine artery. Reproduced with permission from Moir & Thorburn (1986).

who demonstrated that if local anaesthetic solution at a concentration similar to that attained during paracervical block is applied to a segment of uterine artery it causes marked vasoconstriction. So fetal asphyxia may be caused by a reduction in uteroplacental blood flow secondary to uterine artery vasoconstriction. It has been suggested that the block should be administered in well spaced stages in order to minimize these effects (Van Dorsten et al 1981). This complication has led to a marked diminution of its use worldwide, although its success and simplicity might justify reinvestigation.

Subarachnoid (spinal) block

The use of a subarachnoid (or spinal) injection of local anaesthetic has been widely used for anaesthesia in the second stage of labour. Its use for analgesia in the first stage of labour is limited by the fact that it is usually a single injection and therefore of limited duration. The development of very fine spinal catheters introduced the possibility of their use to provide a continuous block. However, they have been associated with the development, in a few patients, of a cauda equina syndrome (Rigler et al 1991) and their use in all fields of anaesthesia has been suspended. A low spinal anaesthetic (a saddle block) may be achieved by injecting a small amount of local anaesthetic (10 mg bupivacaine) prepared as a hyperbaric solution into the subarachnoid space with the mother sitting up. This produces good anaesthesia for operative vaginal delivery or removal of retained placenta. The resurgence of spinal anaesthesia for Caesarean section is discussed later.

Epidural block

The epidural (extradural) space, which contains arteries, veins, lymphatics and fat, extends from the foramen magnum to the sacrococcygeal membrane. It is the space between the dura mater internally and the bony vertebral canal externally (Fig. 32.2). Anteriorly, the bony vertebral canal is bounded by the posterior ligament of the vertebrae and posteriorly by the ligamentum flavum covering the vertebral laminae. The lateral aspect of the epidural space is limited by the vertebral pedicles and, between these, the intervertebral foramina.

When local anaesthetic is injected into the epidural space its penetrates the dural cuffs surrounding the nerves and blocks the fully formed spinal nerves. In addition, there is evidence of spread of local anaesthetic into the cerebrospinal fluid, though the importance of this is questionable. However, it is accepted that, for effective anaesthesia, the local anaesthetic must gain direct access to the appropriate spinal nerve in the vicinity of the intervertebral foramen.

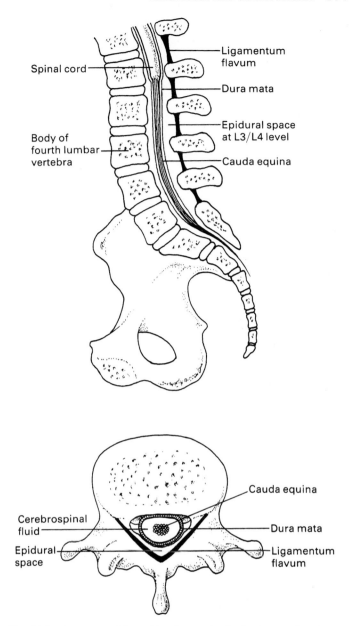

Fig. 32.2 Anatomy of the epidural space in the lumbosacral region. From Crawford (1984).

The nerve supply involved in the pain of labour is derived from two distinct areas which require to be blocked. In the first stage of labour, nerves from T10 to L1 must be blocked, whilst the lower sacral nerves (S2–5) are involved in the second stage of labour (Fig. 32.3). For this reason optimal positioning of mothers for epidural block is important to achieve best results as labour progresses.

The epidural space can be approached from two directions: through the sacrococcygeal membrane (the caudal approach) or between two adjacent vertebral spines. The lumbar region is usually selected to allow blockade to an adequate level with the added safety factor that the spinal cord normally stops at L1–2.

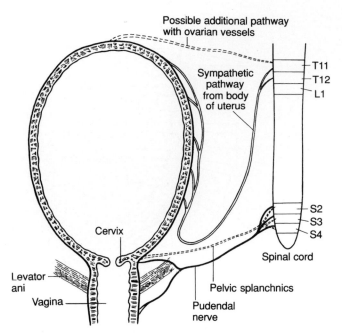

Fig. 32.3   The nerve pathways involved in pain in labour. The pain of uterine contractions enters the spinal cord at segments T11, T12 and L1. The pain of the second stage is transmitted to the cord at the level of S2–4. In addition to the main pathways, pain may also be transmitted through secondary pathways. Reproduced with permission from Moir & Thorburn (1986).

Caudal epidural block

The caudal epidural space is accessible through the sacrococcygeal membrane found at the lower end of the sacral vertebrae where the posterior laminae are not fused. The membrane is located by careful palpation in the midline down the back of the sacrum. At the lower end of the sacrum a gap is appreciated which can be likened to palpating the space between the knuckles of the clenched hand. Once located, suitable preparation of the skin and superficial infiltration with local anaesthetic should be performed. The caudal epidural block is usually a single-shot procedure and a disposable 20 gauge needle may be used.

The needle is inserted pointing slightly cephalad through the sacrococcygeal membrane until it abuts against the posterior aspect of the sacral vertebrae (Fig. 32.4). The needle is then slightly withdrawn and turned in a much more cephalad direction so that the hub of the needle lies in the natal cleft when the needle can easily be advanced up the sacral canal for a distance of 1–2 cm. A syringe should be attached to the needle and careful aspiration carried out. In order to reduce the risk of inadvertent intravascular injection of local anaesthetic, an intravenous cannula can be used in place of a needle. If blood is present, the procedure to this point should be repeated. If clear fluid is obtained it can be assumed that the dural sac extends below its normal level of S2 and has

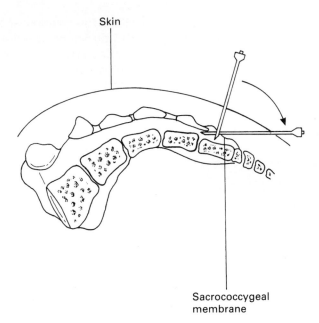

Fig. 32.4   Insertion of needle for caudal anaesthesia. From Cotton (1985).

been pierced. In this case the procedure is best abandoned. If there is no aspiration of liquid, 1–2 ml of air should be injected through the needle with the fingers of the operator's other hand placed lightly over the sacral hiatus. If injection is easy and no crepitus is felt, the needle is in position. Further confirmation of correct needle placement can be obtained by listening over the lumbar spine whilst injecting a small amount of air (Lewis et al 1992). Local anaesthetic is then administered through the needle in increments of about 50 mg lignocaine or 20 mg bupivacaine.

A continuous technique can be used via the caudal approach using a suitable needle and catheter but is best avoided because of the possibility of infection from the gastrointestinal tract and in any event it has no advantages over the lumbar approach. As a single injection it is of more value in the second stage of labour. To achieve a block high enough to relieve first-stage pain a large volume of local anaesthetic has to be used.

Although this is a simple technique it is not without serious complications. Inadvertent dural puncture can occur due to wide variability in the distance between the upper limit of the sacral hiatus and the lower extremity of the dural sac, which may range from 16 to 75 mm (Trotter 1947). If during initial insertion the needle is inadvertently advanced too far and passed through the sacrococcygeal joint it may pierce the rectum, which in itself would not be a great problem, but it may also enter the fetal head if it is pressed on to the perineum at the same time. This complication has been reported on several occasions, and in two reports led to fetal death

(Finster et al 1965, Sinclair et al 1965). Referring to this complication, Bonica (1970) suggests that caudal block should not be initiated after the presenting part has descended to the perineum whilst Moore (1966), in addition, advocates that a rectal examination of the mother should always be performed before solution is injected in order to ensure that the needle has not penetrated deep to the sacrum.

Continuous lumbar epidural block

By far the most commonly used local anaesthetic technique for labour pain is the continuous lumbar epidural block. Whilst the vast majority of such blocks provide excellent analgesia, it is important to bear in mind that one cannot guarantee that an epidural will be successful, a fact that should be explained to the mother before the procedure is embarked upon. It is equally important to differentiate for the mother between sensation and pain, for in an ideal epidural uterine contraction should be felt without pain. In addition to analgesia some degree of motor paralysis is likely but the use of mixed drug infusions has gone far towards reducing the severity of such motor block (see later).

An epidural in labour is normally inserted with the mother in the lateral position as this is most comfortable. It is also possible in the sitting position, which can be particularly advantageous in the obese in allowing better identification of bony landmarks. The approach to the epidural space is usually in the midline although a more lateral approach has been advocated (Carrie 1977) to avoid trauma to the ligaments of the spine and to run less risk of dural puncture.

Prior to initiation of the epidural block an intravenous infusion of Hartmann's solution is set up to ensure circulatory preloading, the function of which is to limit the fall in blood pressure that may occur when sympathetic blockade is produced by the epidural. Preloading should be cautious in mothers at risk of fluid overload. Full resuscitation facilities for the mother must always be readily available.

The mother is usually turned into the left lateral position and her back aligned with the edge of the bed or trolley. Her back should be flexed only as far as is comfortable. The operator, after a full scrub-up, dons sterile gown and gloves. The skin is cleaned carefully over the lower thoracic and lumbar region and the area draped. The skin, subcutaneous tissue and supraspinous ligament are infiltrated with local anaesthetic. The most commonly used epidural needle is a Tuohy (Fig. 32.5); this is advanced through the ligaments to reach the ligamentum flavum.

Once the ligamentum flavum has been reached a technique is employed to identify accurately the epidural

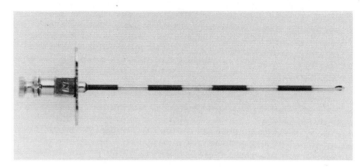

Fig. 32.5   A winged Tuohy epidural needle.

space. The most commonly used technique relies upon the loss of resistance to injected air or saline. Using a freely moving syringe containing a small amount of air or saline, it is not possible to inject whilst the needle tip is in the ligament but injection becomes easy when the epidural space is entered. When the ligamentum flavum is punctured it is often possible to sense a slight click at the same time as loss of resistance to injection occurs. Careful aspiration through the needle confirms that the dura mater has not been punctured; if any fluid is aspirated, and air was used in the syringe, it can be assumed to be cerebrospinal fluid. However, if saline was used it may be necessary to differentiate it from cerebrospinal fluid by testing for sugar. If cerebrospinal fluid is aspirated the needle should be withdrawn and resited in a different interspace. If there is no fluid aspirated, a fine catheter is threaded down the needle into the epidural space.

The catheter employed for epidural block may have a single end-hole or a number of side-holes. In the case of the side-hole catheter, this should be inserted 3 cm into the epidural space for most reliable results (Kumar et al 1985) whilst only 2 cm of an end-hole catheter should be inserted (Gough et al 1986). If problems are encountered in passing the catheter it is important that it should never be pulled back through the needle as it could be severed by the needle tip.

Once the catheter is satisfactorily sited, the puncture site is sprayed with antibiotic and an occlusive dressing applied. A bacterial filter is attached to the hub of the catheter and a small test dose of local anaesthetic is injected (10 mg bupivacaine). This small test dose is intended to confirm that the catheter has not penetrated the dura mater. If there is no sign of nerve blockade after 5 minutes, it is safe to inject a further dose of local anaesthetic to produce the epidural block. Ideally, only small boluses (3–4 ml) of local anaesthetic should be given at a time. An initial total dose of around 10 ml of 0.25% bupivacaine is usual and depending upon its effectiveness, the dose is adjusted in volume of concentration in future top-ups. In addition to misplacement of the catheter in the subarachnoid space it is also possible for it to be passed intravascularly. To identify this problem, some feel that the test dose should contain adrenaline which if accidently injected intravascularly will produce maternal tachycardia.

Contraindications to epidural block

The contraindications of epidural block may be considered as either absolute or relative.

Absolute contraindications The first absolute contraindication is when the mother refuses permission for the epidural. The second is when there is sepsis in the lumbosacral region involving the area through which the epidural needle will pass. Thirdly, epidural block is absolutely contraindicated when there is any condition that will lead to a maternal coagulopathy. The fear in these last two situations is that the formation of an abscess or haematoma may cause spinal cord compression. Scott & Hibbard (1990) in a survey of over half a million obstetric epidurals, found only one case of an epidural abscess and one of an epidural haematoma. In both cases surgical decompression was performed and there was a degree of neurological recovery.

Obstetric conditions that predispose to coagulopathy include moderate or severe pre-eclampsia, placental abruptions, prolonged retention of products of conception, recent spontaneous abortion and thrombocytopenia. If it is deemed necessary or desirable to use epidural analgesia in any mother in these groups, it is essential that coagulation studies should confirm normal clotting. Such tests must have been performed immediately (less than 30 minutes) before commencement of the procedure.

The use of anticoagulants (but not low-dose heparin: Minihep) should be considered an absolute contraindication to epidural analgesia. If it is necessary to give anticoagulants to a mother with an epidural in situ a period of 30 minutes should pass after insertion of the catheter in order to ensure that any traumatized vessel has time to seal.

In any mother with coagulopathy, whether of pathological or therapeutic origin, it is also important that normal coagulation is present prior to the withdrawal of the catheter as damage can also be caused.

Maternal hypotension and active substantial haemorrhage must be considered temporary absolute contraindications. If an epidural is to be used after such occurrences it is important to consider the effects that haemorrhage may have on coagulation and the guidelines mentioned above should be followed.

Relative contraindications Progressive neurological disease has traditionally been considered a relative contraindication on the grounds that such disease may be unpredictable, leading to relapse at any time. If a relapse coincides with the use of an epidural there could be

a dispute over the possibility of damage having been caused by the epidural. It is advisable in any mother with such disease to explain the situation at length (and document the explanation) prior to embarking upon epidural analgesia.

Complications of epidural block

In a review of maternal complications of epidural analgesia for labour (Crawford 1985), covering some 27 000 lumbar epidurals, there were nine potentially life-threatening complications, of which only three caused real concern for the mother's safety.

Complications can be considered as problems associated with the siting of the catheter and those associated with the use of epidural block. In general if a problem is encountered in inserting the epidural needle and catheter, the attempt should be abandoned and another attempt made at a different interspace.

Aspiration of blood Blood may be aspirated through the needle or catheter from a traumatized epidural vein. If blood is continually aspirated it must be assumed that the catheter lies in a vein and it should be removed and resited.

Dural puncture The needle may be accidently advanced through the dura mater into the cerebrospinal fluid (CSF). In order to avoid the development of low CSF pressure, it is important to prevent fluid leaking out of the epidural needle. If dural puncture has occurred the needle should be withdrawn and resited at a different interspace. If a catheter is sited in a new interspace, there does not appear to be any substantial entry of local anaesthetic through the puncture hole into CSF. There is some evidence, at present rather limited, to show that if a dural tap should occur, the best treatment is to insert the epidural catheter deliberately into the subarachnoid space. This allows the provision of good analgesia and may plug the hole in the dura.

In the postdelivery period, headaches are a common complication occurring in 70% of dural taps (Crawford 1972). These may initially be treated with an epidural drip consisting of an infusion through a bacterial filter of Hartmann's solution into the epidural space. In addition, sitting and standing in the immediate postdelivery period should be discouraged. A laxative is useful to prevent excessive straining at defaecation, which may aggrevate the leak of CSF. If symptoms continue after the use of these procedures then an epidural blood patch should be performed (Crawford 1980). This consists of injecting 15–20 ml of blood, freshly taken from the patient, into the epidural space. This appears to be safe and generally does not interfere with any subsequent epidural (Abouleish et al 1975). However, one case has been reported in which it was found to be impossible to extend a block—administered 3 years subsequent to blood patching—above the L2 level (Rainbird & Pfitzner 1983). The authors of this last report postulate that the organized clot following blood patching may have led to fibrous tethering of the dura to the wall of the spinal canal, hence interferring with local anaesthetic spread.

Sympathetic block The most common finding after initiation of epidural block is a fall in maternal blood pressure. In general, if the fall in systolic blood pressure is greater than 20 mmHg some effective action should be taken. Normally the drip rate of the intravenous Hartmann's infusion is increased and the possibility of aortocaval compression excluded. If the fall in blood pressure does not respond to these simple measures, a vasopressor may be administered—usually ephedrine in increments of 5 mg repeated as necessary. Ephedrine is used as it causes less effect on uterine blood flow than other sympathomimetics (Ralston et al 1974). More recently, there has been increased interest in the use of phenylephrine as a vasopressor as it has less chronotropic effects on the maternal heart and is not detrimental to the fetus (Ramanathan & Grant 1988).

Inadvertent subarachnoid block (total spinal) The misplacement of epidural catheters into the CSF is possible with consequent inadvertent subarachnoid injection of a large dose of local anaesthetic; a widespread spinal block will occur with cardiovascular and respiratory collapse. Full resuscitation measures must be employed promptly to support ventilation and circulation, but cardiopulmonary resuscitation is not easy in the pregnant woman at term and standard resuscitation techniques require some adaptation to prevent aortocaval compression (Rees & Willis 1988, Goodwin 1992).

Partial block A unilateral block is a not infrequent result of the initial injection of local anaesthetic. It can usually be corrected by having the mother lie on the unblocked side whilst another dose is injected. If the problem persists the catheter has probably been advanced too far and withdrawal by 2–3 cm may overcome the problem. If the initial block is confined to a single nerve root this suggests that the catheter has passed into or through an intervertebral foramen and slight withdrawal of the catheter will frequently correct the situation. A missed segment occurs in about 6–7% of epidurals and is persistent throughout labour in 1.5% (Ducrow 1971, Bromage 1972). It typically involves the first lumbar nerve root and can often be relieved by varying the mother's position and the drug concentration.

Top-up doses and infusions

Good continuous analgesia is only possible by ensuring top-up doses of local anaesthetic are given promptly as pain returns. It is also important to note the pattern of return of pain as this allows optimal positioning of the mother prior to top-up and hence the best quality block can be obtained.

The use of an intermittent top-up regimen requires regular doses at intervals of about 2 hours, the average labour requiring between three and six top-ups. There has been increasing interest in the use of epidural infusions of local anaesthetics to reduce this need. Bupivacaine infusions at different concentrations have been reported (Glover 1977, Evans & Carrie 1979). More recently Li et al (1985) showed that using a 0.125% solution of bupivacaine at 10 ml/h extended the median interval between top-ups from 145 to 245 minutes. However, there can still be some breakthrough pain with plain bupivacaine solutions and this has led to increasing interest in the use of a combination of low concentrations of bupivacaine with analgesics. Almost every analgesic has been used but the most common is fentanyl (Chestnut et al 1988, Murphy et al 1991). By reducing the dose of local anaesthetic there is also the added benefit of a reduction in motor block, even to the extreme of allowing the mother with an epidural in place to mobilize.

The rate of epidural infusions has also been studied but there has been no agreed figure because of the wide degree of interpatient variability. The introduction of patient-controlled epidural analgesia (PCEA) has allowed the individual patient to titrate themselves to a suitable degree of analgesia (Gambling et al 1988). Such a system has the added benefit of allowing the patient to be actively involved in their own pain management and hence have an enhanced degree of satisfaction (Gambling et al 1990). Although originally used in North America, this technique is gaining popularity in the UK.

Epidural analgesia and delivery

The characteristics of the second stage of labour and delivery are altered by the provision of an epidural. There will be a reduction in pelvic floor tone which may reduce the ability of the presenting part to rotate to the anteroposterior position. There will be a reduction in lower abdominal muscle power which will affect maternal expulsive effort. The degree that these are affected will depend upon the amount of motor blockade produced by the epidural. With full sensory loss, the bearing-down reflex will be lost but this should not influence the mother's ability to bear down.

The combination of these effects is to attenuate the interval between full dilatation of the cervix and delivery. In addition, there has been a deal of interest in the assertion that the normal oxytocic surge associated with the descent of the fetal head is lost under epidural analgesia (Goodfellow et al 1983). Some workers have shown that stopping the epidural in the second stage will lead to a shortened full dilatation to delivery time and a reduced incidence of instrumental delivery (Chestnut et al 1987), whilst others have strangely found the converse (Philips & Thomas 1983). Alternatively, augmentation with oxytocin in the second stage has been shown to reduce the incidence of forceps delivery in mothers having an epidural (Saunders et al 1989, Carli et al 1993).

Overall the incidence of forceps delivery should not be higher in mothers having an epidural if the preceding points are taken into consideration. However, if a forceps delivery is considered advantageous, the quality of analgesia achieved with an epidural allows for easy instrumentation.

THE AVAILABILITY AND USE OF ANALGESIC TECHNIQUES

Whilst there are a number of analgesic techniques available to the mother, not all delivery units are able to offer the full range and as each mother is an individual, it is not surprising that there is wide variability in the type of analgesia used. The current situation about availability and maternal usage has recently been investigated in a national survey conducted by the National Birthday Trust (Chamberlain et al 1993). This survey was conducted over one week in 1990 and covers data from 15 900 mothers throughout the UK. In total, 293 obstetric units participated in the survey.

The availability of non-drug methods for pain relief is shown in Table 32.2. There was a high, possibly media-driven, availability of TENS. The relative unavailability of acupuncture and hypnosis probably reflects the time-consuming nature of this method of analgesia.

The availability of drugs for pain relief is shown in Table 32.3. An epidural service was available in over 70% of units with approximately three-quarters of these providing a 24-hour service; in the other units availability was limited. Pethidine and Entonox were available in 97.6% and 99% of units respectively.

The actual main method of pain relief used by mothers

Table 32.2 The availability of non-drug methods for pain relief (reproduced with permission from Chamberlain et al 1993)

Method	Units No.	%
TENS and relaxation	146	54.3
Relaxation	71	26.4
TENS alone	18	6.7
TENS, relaxation and hypnosis	12	4.5
TENS, relaxation and acupuncture	10	3.7
Acupuncture alone	3	1.1
All of above	3	1.1
Acupuncture and relaxation	2	0.7
Hypnosis and relaxation	2	0.7
Acupuncture and hypnosis	1	0.4
Hypnosis alone	1	0.4

Table 32.3 The availability of drugs for pain relief (reproduced with permission from Chamberlain et al 1993)

	Units No.	%
Entonox, pethidine and epidural	151	52.4
Entonox and pethidine	60	20.8
Entonox, pethidine, epidural and other	56	19.4
Entonox, pethidine and other	13	4.5
Entonox, epidural and other	3	1
Entonox only	2	0.7
Epidural only	1	0.3
Pethidine only	1	0.3
Other only	1	0.3

in the survey, as recorded by the midwife, is presented in Table 32.4. The figures presented are not mutually exclusive as some mothers had significant use of more than one type of analgesia. The overall findings show that more than 50% of mothers had Entonox and about 40% received pethidine. Approximately 18% of mothers used an epidural in labour, a figure almost identical to a previous study on epidural usage (Hibbard & Scott 1990). Despite the high media profile of non-drug methods of pain relief, they were seldom used as the main method.

The effectiveness of the various methods of analgesia used may be assessed by using the mothers' opinion as to whether a method was helpful or unhelpful. The benefit of the various methods is presented in Table 32.5. If one considers the ratio of helpful to unhelpful as a

Table 32.4 The frequency of main analgesic method used as recorded by the midwife (adapted with permission from Chamberlain et al 1993)

Method	No.	%
Entonox	5706	55.1
Pethidine	3916	37.8
Other narcotic analgesics	712	3.4
Relaxation	406	3.9
Epidural	1834	17.7
TENS	428	4.1
Massage	515	5.0
Other (homeopathy, hypnosis and acupuncture)	24	0.2
Study population	10 352	100

Table 32.5 Methods of pain relief identified as helpful and unhelpful as a percentage of their use (reproduced with permission from Chamberlain et al 1993)

Method	Helpful (%)	Unhelpful (%)
Relaxation	32	13
Massage	22	12
TENS	22	20
Pethidine	28	14
Entonox	43	13
Epidural	73	4

measure of the effectiveness of a method, it is clear that epidural analgesia is by far the most effective.

ANAESTHESIA FOR OPERATIVE DELIVERY

The provision of anaesthesia for operative delivery has seen major changes in the last decade with the gradual decrease in the use of general anaesthesia and the more widespread use of regional anaesthesia, in particular the increased popularity of spinal (subarachnoid) anaesthesia. This change is probably one of, if not the, major reasons for the dramatic improvement seen in anaesthetically related maternal deaths (Department of Health 1989, Department of Health, Welsh Office, Scottish Home and Health Department, Department of Health and Social Services, Northern Ireland 1991). However, such improvements should not lead to a sense of complacency and the risks inherent in obstetric anaesthesia, largely as a result of altered maternal physiology, must still be borne in mind whenever an anaesthetic is given, be it for a Caesarean section or for a more minor procedure.

Whichever type of anaesthetic is to be used for whatever procedure, there are some basic points in maternal preparation that are common to all anaesthetics.

Maternal starvation and antacid therapy

It has been traditional for mothers in labour to be kept starved just in case they should require an anaesthetic. However, current attitudes are changing to allow the oral intake of clear fluids throughout labour and some consider it safe to allow mothers to eat bland foods in the early part of labour; the outcome of such proposals remains unclear.

Whilst there may be some controversy regarding the necessity of starvation of all labouring mothers, it is universally accepted that prior to an anaesthetic, be it general or regional, something should be given to reduce the acidity of the stomach contents. Gastric acid production can be eliminated by giving an H_2 receptor antagonist. Ranitidine is the most commonly used drug in the UK. It can be given intravenously when it takes about 45–60 minutes to have its effect (McCaughey et al 1981), or, if time allows, and particularly in the elective situation, oral dosing has been shown to be effective (Gillett et al 1984). Whether every mother in labour should be given prophylactic ranitidine or just those perceived as being at particular risk of requiring operative delivery varies between individual units. The newer agent, omeprazole, a proton pump inhibitor, has also been shown to be effective in reducing the volume of gastric acid (Yau et al 1992) and awaits further evaluation.

Even if gastric acid production is eliminated, there will always be a residual volume of acid present in the stomach. Before anaesthesia this acid must be neutralized,

and 0.3 M sodium citrate given at least 10 minutes before anaesthesia has been shown to be effective (Gibbs et al 1982) and is now the accepted standard.

Aortocaval compression

Aortocaval compression has long been appreciated as a cause of both maternal and fetal morbidity (Crawford et al 1973). It is routinely avoided by ensuring that the mother is never allowed to lie flat on her back, but is always kept in a lateral or tilted position prior to and during surgery. The increased use of spinal anaesthesia, with its coincident sympathetic blockade, makes the meticulous avoidance of aortocaval compression even more important.

Intravenous access

Massive haemorrhage in obstetrics often occurs with little warning and the importance of inserting a large bore intravenous cannula (at least 16 G) before starting any form of anaesthetic cannot be overstressed.

Anaesthetic techniques

It is beyond the scope of this chapter to cover in detail all anaesthetic techniques employed in obstetric practice. If detailed information is required, the reader should consult any standard obstetric anaesthesia textbook. However, a few points of interest regarding current practice are perhaps appropriate.

General anaesthesia

The basic principle of the rapid sequence induction of anaesthesia has changed little over the years but recently there has been some concern regarding the sympathetic response to laryngoscopy and intubation. This causes a marked rise in maternal blood pressure and may also affect placental blood flow. For these reasons it is advantageous to obtund this response, particularly in the pre-eclamptic mother. The most commonly used method is the administration of an ultra-short-acting opioid just before induction of anaesthesia (Black et al 1984). This effectively prevents the rise in blood pressure and has only limited effects on the neonate; naloxone can be given to the baby to reverse any more serious adverse effects.

With the at-risk fetus in mind, there is some evidence to suggest that 100% oxygen supplemented with isoflurane is the preferred maintenance technique for emergency Caesarean section (Piggott et al 1990).

The increasing popularity of local anaesthesia means that there are less mothers being given general anaesthetics. Whilst this has seemed to have beneficial effects with regard to maternal deaths, it may rebound as trainees have less exposure to general anaesthesia, and may subsequently be less able to cope with an unexpected problem.

Local anaesthesia

As previously mentioned there has been a great increase in the use of local anaesthesia (both epidural and spinal block) for operative deliveries; the advantages being obvious. The use of spinal anaesthesia in particular has allowed the rapid establishment of good operating conditions. The traditional drawbacks of this technique have been that it is a 'single-shot' injection and hence has only a finite duration. As a consequence of this it has not been advised for difficult or repeat procedures. In addition, the incidence of severe postdural puncture headache has weighed against spinal anaesthesia. The first problem has been largely overcome by the use of a combined spinal-epidural technique (Carrie 1990) and the second by the introduction into practice of pencil-point spinal needles which are less traumatic and have a much reduced postdural puncture headache rate (Shutt et al 1992). Added to this, the modern more aggressive approach to managing such headaches has made spinal anaesthesia a highly acceptable technique to mother, anaesthetist and surgeon.

POSTOPERATIVE PAIN

Whilst there are great steps being made to improve postoperative pain relief in general patients by the introduction of acute pain services (Gould et al 1992), it is a sad fact that the postoperative obstetric patient does not always receive such care. This inequality is particularly unfortunate, as in all other respects, those working in obstetrics have great experience and ability in relieving pain. Techniques used in general patients such as patient controlled analgesia and epidural opioids should be just as readily available in the obstetric unit.

REFERENCES

Abboud T K, Khoo S S, Miller F, Doan T, Henriksen E M 1982 Maternal, fetal and neonatal responses after epidural anaesthesia with bupivacaine, 2-chloroprocaine or lidocaine. Anesthesia and Analgesia 61: 638

Abouleish E, Depp R 1975 Acupuncture in obstetrics. Anesthesia and Analgesia 54: 83

Abouleish E, Wadhwa R K, De La Vega S, Tan R N, Uy N T L 1975 Regional analgesia following epidural blood patch. Anesthesia and Analgesia 54: 634

Arthurs G J, Rosen M 1981 Acceptability of continuous nasal nitrous oxide during labour—a field trial in six maternity hospitals. Anaesthesia 36: 384

Barbe D P, Sattenspiel E 1965 Audioanalgesia in labor and delivery. Obstetrics and Gynecology 25: 683

Baxi L V, Petrie R H, James L S 1979 Human fetal oxygenation following paracervical block. American Journal of Obstetrics and Gynecology 135: 1109

Beazley J M, Leaver E P, Morewood J H M, Bircumshaw J 1967 Relief of pain in labour. Lancet i: 1033

Belfrage P, Floberg J 1983 Obstetrical paracervical block with chloroprocaine or bupivacaine. Acta Obstetrica et Gynecologica Scandinavica 62: 245

Belfrage P, Boreus L O, Hartvig P, Irestedt L, Raabe N 1981 Neonatal depression after obstetrical analgesia with pethidine. Acta Obstetrica et Gynaecologica Scandinavica 60: 43

Bembridge M, MacDonald R, Lyons G 1986 Spinal anaesthesia with hyperbaric lignocaine for elective caesarian section. Anaesthesia 41: 906

Black T E, Kay B, Healy T E J 1984 Reducing the haemodynamic responses to laryngoscopy and intubation. A comparison of alfentanil with fentanyl. Anaesthesia 39: 883

Bonica J J 1970 Lumbar epidural versus caudal anesthesia. In: Shnider S M (ed) Obstetrical anesthesia. Williams & Wilkins, Baltimore

Bromage P R 1972 Unblocked segments in epidural analgesia for relief of pain in labour. British Journal of Anaesthesia 44: 676

Burt R K, Korn G W 1964 Audioanalgesia in obstetrics. American Journal of Obstetrics and Gynecology 88: 361

Carli F, Creagh-Barry P, Gordon H, Logue M M, Dore C J 1993 Does epidural analgesia influence the mode of delivery in primiparae managed actively? A preliminary study of 1250 women. International Journal of Obstetric Anesthesia 2: 15

Carrie L E S 1977 The paramedian approach to the epidural space. Anaesthesia 32: 670

Carrie L E S 1990 Extradural, spinal or combined block for obstetric surgical anaesthesia. British Journal of Anaesthesia 65: 225

Carson R J, Reynolds F 1988 Placental transfer of meptazinol in the rabbit. British Journal of Pharmacology 95: 582

Chamberlain G, Gunn P 1987 Birthplace. Report of the National Birthday Trust national survey. John Wiley, Chichester

Chamberlain G, Wraight A, Steer P (eds) 1993 Pain and its relief in childbirth. The results of a national survey conducted by the National Birthday Trust. Churchill Livingstone, London

Chestnut D H, van de Walker G E, Owen C L, Bates J N, Choi W W 1987 The influence of continuous epidural bupivacaine on the second stage of labour and method of delivery in nulliparous women. Anesthesiology 66: 774

Chestnut D H, Owen C L, Bates J N, Ostman L G, Choi W W, Geiger M W 1988 Continuous infusion epidural analgesia in labor: a randomized, double-blind comparison of 0.0625% bupivacaine/0.0002% fentanyl versus 0.125% bupivacaine. Anesthesiology 68: 754

Cibils L A 1976 Response of human uterine arteries to local anaesthetics. American Journal of Obstetrics and Gynecology 126: 202

Clarkson C W, Hondeghem L, Matsubara T et al 1984 Possible mechanism of bupivacaine toxicity: fast inactivation block with slow diastolic recovery. Anesthesia and Analgesia 63: 199

Cole P V, Nainby-Luxmore R C 1962 The hazards of gas and air in obstetrics. Anaesthesia 17: 505

Cole P V, Crawford J S, Doughty A G et al 1970 Specifications and recommendations for nitrous oxide/oxygen apparatus to be used in obstetric analgesia. Anaesthesia 25: 317

Cotton B R 1985 Obstetric anaesthesia. In: Smith G, Aitkenhead A R (eds) Textbook of Anaesthesia. Churchill Livingstone, Edinburgh, pp 407–418

Crawford J S 1972 The prevention of headache consequent upon dural puncture. British Journal of Anaesthesia 44: 588

Crawford J S 1980 Experiences with epidural blood patch. Anaesthesia 35: 513

Crawford J S 1985 Some maternal complications of epidural analgesia for labour. Anaesthesia 40: 1219

Crawford J S, Ellis D B, Hill D W, Payne J P 1967 Effects of cooling on the safety of premixed gases. British Medical Journal 2: 138

Crawford J S, Burton M, Davies P 1973 Anaesthesia for section: further refinements of a technique. British Journal of Anaesthesia 45: 726

Creasser C W, Stoelting R K, Krishma G, Peterson C 1974 Methoxyflurane metabolism and renal function after methoxyflurane analgesia during labor and delivery. Anesthesiology 41: 62

Davidson J A 1962 An assessment of the value of hypnosis in pregnancy and labour. British Medical Journal 2: 951

Davies J M, Willis B A, Rosen M 1978 Entonox analgesia in labour. A pilot study to reduce the delay between demand and supply. Anaesthesia 33: 545

De Boer F, Shortland D, Simpson R L, Clifford W A, Cately D M 1987 A comparison of the effects of maternally administered meptazinol and pethidine on neonatal acid–base status. British Journal of Obstetrics and Gynaecology 94: 256

Department of Health 1989 Report of Health and Social Subjects 34. Report on Confidential Enquiries into Maternal Deaths in England and Wales 1982–4. HMSO, London

Department of Health and Social Security 1982 Report on Health and Social Subjects 26. Report on Confidential Enquiries into Maternal Deaths in England and Wales 1976–1978. HMSO, London

Department of Health, Welsh Office, Scottish Home and Health Department, Department of Health and Social Services, Northern Ireland 1991 Report on Confidential Enquiries into Maternal Deaths in the United Kingdom 1985–7. HMSO, London

Dick-Read G 1944 Childbirth without fear. Heinemann, London

Dolan P F, Rosen M 1975 Inhalation analgesia in labour: facemask or mouthpiece. Lancet ii: 1030

Ducrow M 1971 The occurrence of unblocked segments during continuous lumbar epidural analgesia. British Journal of Anaesthesia 43: 1172

Dundee J W, Moore J 1960 Alterations in response to somatic pain associated with anaesthesia. IV. Effect of sub-anaesthetic concentration of inhalational agents. British Journal of Anaesthesia 32: 453

Edwards N D, Hartley M, Clyburn P, Harmer M 1992 Epidural pethidine and bupivacaine in labour. Anaesthesia 47: 435

Evans K R L, Carrie L E S 1979 Continuous epidural infusion of bupivacaine in labour. Anaesthesia 34: 310

Evans J M, Rosen M, MacCarthy J, Hogg M I J 1976a Apparatus for patient-controlled administration of intravenous narcotics during labour. Lancet i: 17

Evans J M, Hogg M I J, Rosen M 1976b Reversal of narcotic depression in the neonate by naloxone. British Medical Journal 2: 1098

Finster M, Poppers P J, Sinclair J C, Morishima H O, Daniel S S 1965 Accidental intoxication of the fetus with local anesthetic drug during caudal anesthesia. American Journal of Obstetrics and Gynecology 92: 922

Gambling D R, Yu P, Cole C, McMorland G H, Palmer L 1988 A comparative study of patient controlled epidural analgesia (PCEA) and continuous infusion epidural analgesia (CIEA) during labour. Canadian Journal of Anaesthesia 35: 249

Gambling D R, McMorland G H, Yu P, Lazlo C 1990 Comparison of patient-controlled epidural analgesia and conventional intermittent 'top-up' injections during labour. Anesthesia and Analgesia 70: 256

Gibbs C P, Spohr L, Schmidt D 1982 The effectiveness of sodium citrate as an antacid. Anesthesiology 57: 44

Gillett G B, Watson J D, Langford R M 1984 Ranitidine and single-dose antacid therapy as prophylaxis against acid aspiration syndrome in the obstetric patient. Anaesthesia 39: 638

Glover D J 1977 Continuous epidural analgesia in the obstetric patient: a feasibility study using a mechanical infusion pump. Anaesthesia 32: 499

Goodfellow C F, Hull M G R, Swaab D F, Dogterom J, Buijs R M 1983 Oxytocin deficiency at delivery with epidural anaesthesia. British Journal of Obstetrics and Gynaecology 90: 214

Goodwin A P L, Pearce A J 1992 The human wedge. A manoeuvre to relieve aortocaval compression during resuscitation in late pregnancy. Anaesthesia 47: 433

Gough J D, Johnston K R, Harmer M 1986 Kinking of epidural catheters. Anaesthesia 41: 1060

Gould T H, Crosby D L, Harmer M et al 1992 Policy for controlling pain after surgery: effect of sequential changes in management. British Medical Journal 305: 1187

Gross H N, Posner N A 1963 Evaluation of hypnosis for obstetric delivery. Medical Journal of Australia 43: 819

Harper N J N, Thomson J, Brayshaw S A 1983 Experience with self-administered pethidine with special reference to the general practitioner obstetric unit. Anaesthesia 38: 52

Harrison R F, Woods T, Shore M, Mathews G, Unwin A 1986 Pain relief in labour using transcutaneous electrical nerve stimulation (TENS). A TENS/TENS placebo controlled study in two parity groups. British Journal of Obstetrics and Gynaecology 93: 739

Heyns O S 1959 Abdominal decompression in the first stage of labour. Journal of Obstetrics and Gynaecology of the British Empire 66: 220

Hibbard B M, Scott D B 1990 The availability of epidural anaesthesia and analgesia in obstetrics. British Journal of Obstetrics and Gynaecology 97: 402

Holdcroft A, Morgan M 1974 Assessment of the analgesic effect in labour of pethidine and 50% nitrous oxide in oxygen (Entonox). Journal of Obstetrics and Gynaecology of the British Commonwealth 81: 603

Johnson J R, Moore J, McCaughey W et al 1983 Use of cimetidine as an oral antacid in obstetric anaesthesia. Anesthesia and Analgesia 62: 720

Jones P L, Molloy M J, Rosen M 1971 The Cardiff Penthrane inhaler. A vaporiser for the administration of methoxyflurane as an obstetric analgesic. British Journal of Anaesthesia 43: 190

Kim W Y, Pomerace J J, Miller A A 1979 Lidocaine intoxication in a newborn following local anesthesia for episiotomy. Pediatrics 64: 643

Kumar C M, Dennison B, Lawler P G P 1985 Excessive dose requirements of local anaesthetic for epidural analgesia. How far should an epidural catheter be inserted? Anaesthesia 40: 1100

Lamaze F 1956 Qu'est ce quel l'accouchement sans douleur, 1st edn. La Farandale, Paris

Lavin J P, Samuels S V, Miodovnik M, Holroyde J, Loon M, Joyce T 1981 The effects of bupivacaine and chloroprocaine as local anesthetic for epidural anesthesia on fetal heart rate monitoring patterns. American Journal of Obstetrics and Gynecology 141: 717

Lewis M P N, Thomas P, Wilson L F, Mulholland R C 1992 The 'whoosh' test. A clinical test to confirm correct needle placement in caudal epidural injections. Anaesthesia 47: 57

Li D F, Rees G A D, Rosen M 1985 Continuous extradural infusion of 0.0625% or 0.125% bupivacaine for pain relief in primigravid labour. British Journal of Anaesthesia 57: 264

Lussos S A, Datta S 1993 Anesthesia for cesarean section Part III: General anesthesia. International Journal of Obstetric Anesthesia 2: 109

McCaughey W, Howe J P, Moore J, Dundee J W 1981 Cimetidine in elective caesarian section. Anaesthesia 36: 167

McGuinness C, Rosen M 1984 Enflurane as an analgesic in labour. Anaesthesia 39: 24

McLeod D D, Ramayya G P, Tunstall M E 1985 Self-administered isoflurane in labour. A comparison study with Entonox. Anaesthesia 40: 424

Melzack R, Wall P D 1965 Pain mechanism: a new theory. Science 150: 971

Minnitt R J 1934 Self-administered analgesia for the midwifery of general practice. Proceedings of the Royal Society of Medicine 27: 1313

Moir D D, Thorburn J 1986 Obstetric anaesthesia and analgesia, 3rd edn. Baillière Tindall, Eastbourne

Moore D C 1966 Caudal anesthesia in obstetrics. New England Journal of Medicine 274: 749

Morrison J C, Wiser W L, Rosser S I et al 1973 Metabolites of meperidine related to fetal depression. American Journal of Obstetrics and Gynecology 115: 1132

Moya F, James L S 1960 Medical hypnosis for obstetrics. Journal of the American Medical Association 174: 2026

Murphy J D, Henderson K, Bowden M I, Lewis M, Cooper G M 1991 Bupivacaine versus bupivacaine and fentanyl for epidural analgesia; effects on maternal satisfaction. British Medical Journal 302: 564

Newman J W, Wood E C 1967 Abdominal decompression and foetal blood gases. British Medical Journal 3: 368

Paymaster N J 1977 Analgesia after operation—a controlled comparison of meptazinol, pentazocine and pethidine. British Journal of Anaesthesia 49: 1139

Philips K C, Thomas T A 1983 Second stage of labour with or without extradural analgesia. Anaesthesia 38: 972

Piggott S E, Bogod D, Harmer M, Rees G A D, Rosen M 1990 The use of 100% oxygen for emergency Caesarean section. British Journal of Anaesthesia 65: 325

Rainbird A, Pfitzner J 1983 Restricted spread of analgesia following epidural blood patch. Case report with a review of possible complications. Anaesthesia 38: 481

Ralston D H, Shnider S M, DeLorimar A A 1974 Effects of equipotent ephedrine, metaraminol, mephentamine and methoxamine on uterine blood flow in the pregnant ewe. Anesthesiology 40: 354

Ramanathan S, Grant G J 1988 Vasopressor therapy for hypotension due to epidural anesthesia for cesarean section. Acta Anaesthesiologica Scandinavica 32: 559

Rees G A D, Willis B A 1988 Resuscitation in late pregnancy. Anaesthesia 43: 347

Refstad S O, Lindbaek E 1980 Ventilatory depression of the newborn of women receiving pethidine or pentazocine. A double-blind comparative trial. British Journal of Anaesthesia 52: 265

Report to the Medical Research Council of the committee on nitrous oxide and oxygen analgesia in midwifery 1970 Clinical trials of different concentration of oxygen and nitrous oxide for obstetric analgesia. British Medical Journal 1: 709

Rigler M L, Drasner K, Krejcie T C et al 1991 Cauda equina syndrome after continuous spinal anesthesia. Anesthesia and Analgesia 72: 275

Robinson O, Rosen M, Evans J M, Revill S I, David H, Rees G A D 1980 Self-administered intravenous and intramuscular pethidine: controlled trial in labour. Anaesthesia 35: 763

Robson J E 1979 Transcutaneous nerve stimulation for pain relief in labour. Anaesthesia 34: 357

Rosen M G, Scibetta J J, Hochberg C J 1970 Human fetal EEG III: pattern changes in presence of fetal heart rate alterations and after use of maternal medication. Obstetrics and Gynecology 36: 132

Rosen M, Latto I P, Asscher A W 1972 Kidney function after methoxyflurane analgesia during labour. British Medical Journal 1: 81

Saunders N J, Spiby H, Gilbert L et al 1989 Oxytocin infusion during second stage of labour in primiparous women using epidural analgesia: a randomised double blind placebo controlled trial. British Medical Journal 299: 1423

Scanlon J W, Ostheimer G W, Lurie A D, Brown W U, Weiss J B, Alper M H 1976 Neurobehavioural responses and drug concentrations in newborns after maternal epidural anesthesia with bupivacaine. Anesthesiology 45: 400

Scanner J H, Woods L A 1965 Comparative distribution of titanium-labelled dihydromorphine between maternal and fetal rats. Journal of Pharmacology and Experimental Therapy 148: 176

Scott D B, Hibbard B M 1990 Serious non-fatal complications associated with epidural block in obstetric practice. British Journal of Anaesthesia 64: 537

Scott D P, Loudon J D O 1960 A method of abdominal decompression in labour. Lancet i: 1181

Scott J R, Rose N B 1976 Effect of psychoprophylaxis (Lamaze preparation) on labor and delivery in primipara. New England Journal of Medicine 294: 1205

Scott J S 1970 Obstetric analgesia. A consideration of labor pain and a patient-controlled technique for its relief with meperidine. American Journal of Obstetrics and Gynecology 106: 959

Scott P V, Bowen F E, Cartwright P et al 1980 Intrathecal morphine as sole analgesic during labour. British Medical Journal 2: 351

Shnider S M, Moya F 1964 Effects of meperidine on the newborn infant. American Journal of Obstetrics and Gynecology 89: 1009

Shulman H, Birnbaum S J 1966 Evaluation of abdominal decompression during first stage of labor. American Journal of Obstetrics and Gynecology 95: 421

Shutt L E, Valentine S J, Wee M Y K, Page R J, Prosser A, Thomas T A 1992 Spinal anaesthesia for Caesarean section: comparison of 22-gauge and 25-gauge Whitacre needles with 26-gauge Quinke needles. British Journal of Anaesthesia 69: 589

Sinclair J C, Fox H A, Lentz J F, Fuld C L, Murphy J 1965 Intoxication of the fetus by a local anesthetic. A newly recognised complication of maternal caudal anesthesia. New England Journal of Medicine 273: 1173

Skjoldebrand A, Garle M, Gustafsson L L, Johansson H, Lunell N O, Rane A 1982 Extradural pethidine with and without adrenaline during labour: wide variation in effect. British Journal of Anaesthesia 54: 415

Slattery P J, Harmer M, Rosen M, Vickers M D 1981 A comparison between meptazinol and pethidine given intravenously on demand in the management of postoperative pain. British Journal of Anaesthesia 53: 927

Slattery P J, Harmer M, Rosen M, Vickers M D 1983 Comparison of the respiratory depressant effects of IV meptazinol and pethidine. British Journal of Anaesthesia 55: 245P

Stewart P 1979 Transcutaneous nerve stimulation as a method of analgesia in labour. Anaesthesia 34: 361

Tham E J, Oldroyd G J, Power I 1993 An investigation of the local anaesthetic effects of pethidine in IV regional anaesthesia in volunteers. British Journal of Anaesthesia 71: 309P

Thigpen J W, Kotelko D M, Shnider S M et al 1983 Bupivacaine cardiotoxicity in hypoxic–acidiotic sheep. Anesthesiology 59: A204

Tronick E, Wise S, Als H, Adamson R, Scanlon J, Brazelton T B 1976 Regional obstetric anesthesia and newborn behaviour. Effect over the first 10 days of life. Pediatrics 58: 94

Trotter M 1947 Variations of the sacral canal: their significance in the administration of caudal analgesia. Current Researches in Analgesia and Anesthesia 26: 192

Tunstall M E 1961 Use of a fixed nitrous oxide and oxygen mixture from one cylinder. Lancet ii: 964

Van Dorsten J P, Miller F C, Yeh S-Y 1981 Spacing the injection interval with paracervical block: a randomised study. Obstetrics and Gynecology 58: 696

Wallis L, Shnider S M, Palahnuik R J, Spivey H T 1974 An evaluation of acupuncture analgesia in obstetrics. Anesthesiology 41: 506

Way W L, Costley C E, Way E L 1965 Respiratory sensitivity of the newborn infant to meperidine and morphine. Clinical Pharmacology and Therapeutics 6: 454

Wee M Y K, Hasan M A, Thomas T A 1993 Isoflurane in labour. Anaesthesia 48: 369

Wiener P C, Hogg M I J, Rosen M 1977 Effects of naloxone on pethidine-induced neonatal depression. British Medical Journal 2: 228

Wiener P C, Hogg M I J, Rosen M 1979 Neonatal respiration, feeding and neurobehavioural state. Effects of intrapartum bupivacaine, pethidine and pethidine reversed by naloxone. Anaesthesia 34: 996

Yau G, Kan A F, Gin T, Oh T E 1992 A comparison of omeprazole and ranitidine for prophylaxis against aspiration pneumonitis in emergency Caesarean section. Anaesthesia 47: 101

Abnormal labour

33. Preterm labour and delivery of the preterm infant

Stephen A. Walkinshaw

Material in this chapter contains contributions from the first edition and we are grateful to the previous authors for the work done.

Prematurity and its consequences remain a major health problem. The mortality following preterm birth has fallen steadily over the last two decades, and particularly over the last 5 years (Cooke 1992). However, the long-term consequences, both respiratory and neurological, have not improved at the same rate in recent years.

DEFINITION

A preterm infant is defined as one who is born at less than 259 days (37 completed weeks) of pregnancy (WHO 1977). As menstrual dating may be inaccurate in up to 20% of women, then gestation should be based on the best clinical estimate including ultrasound. Extreme prematurity is usually defined as gestations less than 28 completed weeks. The lower limit of preterm birth varies dependent on national definitions of stillbirth; in the UK this is 24 weeks, but in many countries this is 20 or 22 weeks. This, and underreporting of livebirths of very immature infants (Powell et al 1987), makes comparison of preterm birth rates between countries and even within countries difficult.

Because of these difficulties, much epidemiological work has used birthweight as a standard. Low birthweight is defined as less than 2501 g, very low birthweight (VLBW)

as less than 1501 g, and extremely low birthweight (ELBW) as less than 1000 g.

Preterm labour is defined as the occurrence of regular uterine activity which produces either cervical effacement or dilatation prior to 37 completed weeks of gestation (Anderson 1977). The term threatened preterm labour is often used to describe pregnancies complicated by episodes of clinically significant uterine activity but without cervical change.

INCIDENCE

In developed countries the incidence of preterm birth varies between 5% and 10% (Rush et al 1976, Editorial 1991) and has altered little over the past 20 years. Over long periods, some areas have shown a decline, such as in Aberdeen, from 9.3% in 1951–55, to 6.8% in 1976–80 (Hall 1985). Over shorter periods, rates in Haguenau in France have fallen from 8.2% in 1972 to 5.6% in 1981 (Papiernik et al 1985).

In practical terms preterm births at the mature end of the gestation range are less important although numerically high. Deliveries under 32 weeks account for around 1.5% of births (van der Berg & Oeschli 1984, Wariyar et al 1989), and deliveries under 28 weeks account for 0.26–0.6% (van der Berg & Oeschli 1984, Macfarlane et al 1988), with perhaps a recent increase due to more complete reporting. These distinctions are important as two-thirds of deaths in preterm infants occur in infants born at less than 28 weeks.

The incidence of preterm labour, because of problems of definition, is not available, but is likely to be higher than that of spontaneous preterm delivery. In one study, one-third of women with preterm uterine activity went home undelivered within 48 hours (Kragt & Kierse 1990).

Preterm premature rupture of the membranes (preterm PROM) occurs in 1% of all pregnant women (Gibbs & Blanco 1982) but with appropriate exclusions occurs in 40–60% of women eventually delivering spontaneously preterm.

EPIDEMIOLOGY

Preterm labour and delivery are not homogeneous entities. Four major categories can be identified: elective preterm delivery such as for alloimmunization or growth retardation, complicated emergency delivery such as abruptio placentae, preterm PROM, and uncomplicated spontaneous preterm delivery. The latter two account for around half of all preterm births, with elective delivery occurring in 16–18%, and complicated emergency delivery in one-quarter (Halliday 1988, Wariyar et al 1989).

The classic epidemiological associations of preterm labour and preterm PROM are those of poverty and social disadvantage (Table 33.1).

Maternal characteristics

There is an increased risk of preterm delivery in women under 20 years of age (Lumley 1993) and in women over 35 years of age. Primiparity is associated with a higher rate of preterm delivery independent of age (Bakketeig & Hoffman 1981). Marital status is certainly a strong risk factor in North American populations (Wen et al 1990) but is only significantly associated with preterm birth in Australian women over the age of 25 years (Lumley 1993). The relationship is strongest in deliveries under 28 weeks (relative risk 1.7).

Table 33.1 Associations with preterm labour

Maternal characteristics
  Social class
  Age (under 20 or over 35)
  Primiparity
  Ethnicity
  Weight and weight gain
  Marital status
  Cigarette smoking
  Substance abuse
  Heavy or stressful work
  Psychological stress
Past reproductive history
  Previous spontaneous miscarriage
  Previous preterm birth
  Uterine abnormalities
  Previous pregnancy bleeding
Present pregnancy complications
  Multiple gestation
  Assisted conception pregnancy
  Pre-existing maternal illness
  Asymptomatic bacteriuria
  Gestational hypertension
  Antepartum haemorrhage
  Disorders of amniotic fluid volume
  Fetal malformation
  Cervical incompetence
Genital tract infection/colonization
  N. gonorrhoea
  Beta-haemolytic streptococci
  Bacterial vaginosis
  Mycoplasmas and ureoplasmas
  C. trachomatis
  Anaerobic species

Ethnicity has always been an issue in preterm labour and delivery. Much of the difference in the incidence of low birthweight between developed and developing areas is due to the excess of growth-retarded infants, with the rate of preterm births being similar. In North American studies however (Garn et al 1977, Wen et al 1990) there is a consistently increased risk for black women independent of social class. The magnitude of the risk is greatest for extremely preterm deliveries (Schoendorf et al 1992).

Although maternal nutritional studies have not shown any clear relationship with preterm births, low maternal prepregnancy weight (less than 50 kg) and poor weight gain (less than 0.24 kg per week) are associated with an increased risk (Wen et al 1990, Barros et al 1992). Maternal height does not appear to be a factor.

Cigarette smoking results in an excess of births under 34 weeks' gestation, the greatest risk being to those smoking more than 20 cigarettes per day (Meyer 1977). This appears to be due to an excess of abruptio placentae, placenta praevia and preterm PROM. The relative risk of preterm birth lies between 1.1 and 1.65 (Lumley 1987). An increased risk as a consequence of alcohol consumption remains unproven. Cocaine use increases the rate of preterm delivery (2.4), in part a consequence of a higher risk of abruptio placentae (Volpe 1992). Opiate use has persistently been implicated in preterm birth but it has been difficult to disentangle their effect from that of confounding social factors. More recent data (Boer et al 1993, Walkinshaw et al 1993), controlling for social circumstances, confirms an excess of preterm births in opiate users.

Regular moderate exercise may actually reduce the incidence of preterm delivery (Berkowitz et al 1982). Vigorous activity into the third trimester may increase the risk (Kulpa et al 1987). Sexual activity is not implicated in preterm birth (Lumley & Astbury 1989). The physical and psychological stress of work itself has been implicated, the clearest evidence deriving from French work demonstrating an association between preterm birth and an index of occupational fatigue based on posture, machine work, physical effort, repetition and workplace environment (Mamelle et al 1984). Others have subsequently demonstrated similar, but less marked, associations for both heavy manual and highly stressful work (Launer et al 1990, Klebanoff et al 1990), and the latter emphasized that the association only became significant at the extremes, in this study defined as female medical staff working in excess of 100 hours weekly. Psychological stress per se has been implicated, but randomized trials of social support during pregnancy have not demonstrated any reduction in preterm births.

The lack of antenatal care has been suggested as a primary risk factor, even allowing for differences in access and utilization (Murray & Bernfield 1988), but others have challenged this assumption (Tyson et al 1990). Considering what occurs in antenatal clinics and parent education classes in the UK, it is difficult to identify which components of prenatal care prior to 34 weeks would be likely to have an impact on preterm delivery

Past reproductive history

Previous second-trimester spontaneous miscarriage carries an increased risk of subsequent preterm labour, but the risk following induced or spontaneous early miscarriage is more contentious (Keirse et al 1978). Lumley (1993) has demonstrated relative risks of 1.7, 2.9 and 5.9 for preterm labour less than 28 weeks for one, two and three prior spontaneous miscarriages. Holbrook et al (1989) suggest that there is no increase in risk unless there are more than two preceding early losses.

Previous preterm birth is the single best predictor of preterm delivery, with a relative risk of around three (Wen et al 1990). The risk increases if there has been more than one previous preterm birth and the more preterm the first birth, the less likely the subsequent pregnancy is to go to term (Hoffman & Bakketeig 1984).

Uterine abnormalities such as uterus didelphus, unicornus, or women with Asherman's syndrome or leiomyomas are less likely to deliver at term, but are rare causes of preterm birth.

Women with a past history of antepartum bleeding, especially abruptio placentae, are at increased risk of recurrence (Crenshaw et al 1973) and therefore are at increased risk of repeated preterm delivery.

Current pregnancy complications

Many pregnancy complications are associated with preterm birth, and many of these are included in complex risk scores for the prediction of preterm labour (Creasy et al 1980). Their precise relationship with prematurity is considered in their individual chapters.

Multiple gestation makes up the largest single group, accounting for just over 2% of all births, with almost half being born preterm. For similar reasons polyhydramnios frequently results in preterm delivery (Kirbinen & Jouppila 1978).

Any severe maternal medical condition may result in preterm birth, as often for maternal reasons as for fetal. Similarly, acute maternal illness, especially systemic infection, can precipitate labour. Together these groups contribute substantially to elective preterm delivery.

Bleeding in pregnancy carries a risk irrespective of timing (Turnbull 1977). Threatened first- or early second-trimester miscarriage doubles the risk of subsequent preterm labour.

Pregnancies complicated by fetal malformation, in particular multiple anomalies, renal anomalies and anterior abdominal wall defects, deliver preterm more often than expected. Some preterm births in this group are iatrogenic, often without clear advantage to the fetus.

The association between asymptomatic bacteriuria and preterm labour remains unclear (Wang & Smaill 1989), although recent work is more supportive (Romero et al 1991). Randomized trials of antibiotics for this condition appear to demonstrate a reduction in preterm delivery (Smaill 1993).

The putative relationship between preterm delivery and assisted conception is interesting in so far as it raises interesting speculation on links between the aetiology of difficult reproduction and that of preterm labour. The relationship persists even after correcting for age and multiple pregnancy.

Genital tract infection or colonization

Evidence to support a role for infection in preterm labour

There is now a considerable body of evidence linking many preterm births following preterm labour and preterm PROM is associated with genital tract infection.

1. Clinical and histological chorioamnionitis is more common in the placenta and membranes of preterm deliveries (Russell 1979, Hillier et al 1988). This relationship is maintained after adjustment for socioeconomic confounding variables.
2. Maternal and neonatal sepsis is more common following preterm delivery than term delivery.
3. Amniotic fluid cultures are more frequently positive in preterm labour (Romero et al 1988a), with an average rate of 16%. Those with positive cultures are more likely to develop chorioamnionitis, to be refractory to tocolytics and to rupture the membranes spontaneously compared with those with negative cultures. The incidence of positive cultures is higher in cases of preterm PROM (28%).
4. Amniotic fluid in preterm labour contains other biochemical evidence of inflammation such as increased leucocyte counts, lower glucose levels, higher prostaglandin levels, and evidence of increased cytokine activity (interleukin 1, tumour necrosis factor, platelet activating factor).
5. Studies demonstrate associations between specific microorganisms and preterm labour. These include *Neisseria gonorrhoea*, Group B streptococci, *Chlamydia trachomatis* (Alger et al 1988), *Mycoplasma hominis* and *Ureoplasma ureolyticum* (Lamont et al 1987), *Gardnerella vaginalis*, *Bacteroides* species and *Haemophilus* species (McDonald et al 1991, Kurki et al 1992). Some of these associations have been challenged (Romero & Mazor 1988). The most convincing study remains that of Macdonald and colleagues who demonstrated significant independent risk of preterm delivery for two groups of organisms, namely those associated with bacterial vaginosis and a group of virulent enteropathogens. This risk is most marked in preterm deliveries under 34 weeks.

6. Randomized trials of antibiotic treatment of asymptomatic bacteriuria, preterm labour and preterm PROM show reductions in maternal and neonatal infectious morbidity.

7. Experimental evidence demonstrating interplay between bacterial products and initiation of prostaglandin synthesis.

Mechanisms for bacteria as a cause of preterm labour

Microorganisms must first breach the cervical barrier before initiating changes in the membranes and structures in the lower uterine segment. Defence is initially maintained by the physical mucous cervical plug and the presence of secretory IgA in cervical fluid. Proteases are produced in abundance by many bacteria inhabiting the female genital tract (McGregor et al 1986). IgA-specific proteases are produced by both *N. gonorrhoea* and ureoplasmas (Plaut 1978, Kapatais-Zoumbos et al 1985). Mucinase and neuraminidase are also produced by many genital microorganisms (McGregor 1988) and may disrupt the mucin plug.

Once through the initial barrier, bacteria may initiate preterm labour via a number of routes. The key processes are the stimulation of the production of prostaglandins and the release of a number of immune mediators such as platelet-activating factor or 5-HT which stimulate smooth muscle cells directly.

The prostaglandin pathways are accessed via several routes. Bacteria may directly metabolize arachidonic acid. Both phospholipase A$_2$ and C can be released from microorganisms (Bejar et al 1981, McGregor 1988) and these may be able to release arachidonic acid from appropriate stores in the amnion. However the major route is via the effects of released bacterial toxins in initiation of the inflammatory process in the decidua and chorioamnion. These endotoxins may directly stimulate prostaglandin synthesis in the amnion and chorion (Lamont et al 1985), or via the release from the chorion of cytokines such as IL-6 (Dudley et al 1992). The most dramatic effects of these endotoxins are on the decidua, and particularly on cells of bone marrow origin, such as monocytes and macrophages, which make up half of all decidual cells (Vince et al 1990). These cells are stimulated to produce large quantities of cytokines, particularly IL-1, TNF and IL-6 (Casey et al 1989, Romero et al 1990a). These in turn stimulate prostaglandin synthesis in both decidua and amnion (Romero et al 1989, Mitchell et al 1991). Once activated, this complex cycle of cytokine stimulation becomes established, with mutual enhancement of the differing immune mediators which is difficult to reverse.

Other econasoids are produced such as thromboxane and the leukotrienes. These may cause local circulatory disturbance, and the leukotrienes are potent chemotactic agents (Lopez-Bernal et al 1990), thus fuelling the inflammatory process. Free radical damage occurs and other mediating substances derived from decidual cells, and which can directly stimulate myometrial cells, are released. Other released cytokines, such as IL-2 and IL-4, have important roles in cell-mediated immune processes. It is easy to see that once bacterial products have initiated this complex immunological, endocrinological and biochemical process, labour may be inevitable.

The final route by which microorganisms may initiate labour is by membrane disruption. Proteases are produced by both decidual cells and bacteria. Bacterial proteases are often very non-selective but some genital bacteria produce elastase and collagenase. Such enzymes could reduce tensile strength of membranes (McGregor et al 1987) and there is good evidence that the proteases produced by some genital organisms have this capability (Sbarra et al 1987). Once the membranes are ruptured, labour is initiated by a combination of normal factors and by the processes outlined above. The potential pathways and interactions are outlined in Figure 33.1.

DIAGNOSIS OF PRETERM LABOUR AND PRETERM PREMATURE RUPTURE OF MEMBRANES

It is often difficult to distinguish between threatened

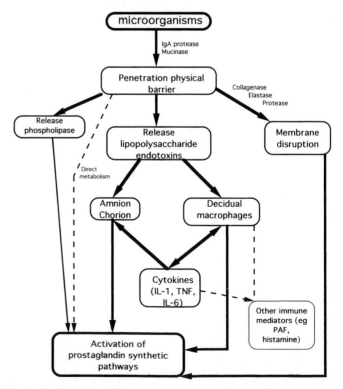

Fig. 33.1 Mechanisms by which infection could cause preterm labour.

preterm labour and actual preterm labour. Many women present with uterine activity in the third trimester, with up to 10% of women with normal pregnancies progressing to term complaining of painful uterine activity preterm (Iams et al 1990a). Up to one-third of women subsequently presenting with preterm labour reported no prodromal symptoms (Iams et al 1990b).

Attempts have been made to define a group of symptoms likely to result in preterm delivery based on the placebo arms of randomized trials to prevent preterm labour (Ingemarrson et al 1976). These all include regular contractions (at intervals of less than 10 minutes for 30 minutes, or eight in 60 minutes) accompanied by either cervical effacement or change in dilatation and effacement. Changes in parameters assessed by digital vaginal examination are best quantitated using the Bishop score. By any method, a clinical diagnosis of preterm labour will be an overestimate.

Preterm PROM can sometimes present a similar diagnostic dilemma. Here the differential diagnosis lies between PROM, watery vaginal discharge and urinary incontinence. A careful history may help, but commonly other tests are required after speculum examination to examine and sample the fluid present in the vagina. These include ferning of amniotic fluid on a glass slide, with an accuracy of 96% and a false-negative rate of 5–10% (Friedman & Macelin 1969); the use of the alkalinity of amniotic fluid to alter the colour of nitrazine paper, with a maximum accuracy of over 90%, but a false-positive rate of up to 15% and false-negative rate of 10%; or the use of newer but less extensively evaluated tests such as alphafetoprotein (AFP), diamine oxidase and fibronectin. If no fluid is seen, then often it is best to re-examine after the woman has been supine for a few hours. Amniotic fluid volume assessment by ultrasound may aid clarification, but is yet to be appropriately assessed. Instillation of dye into the amniotic cavity is rarely justified, but has a place where a diagnosis cannot be made in the extremely preterm, to prevent prolonged hospitalization. Methylene blue is to be avoided as it may cause fetal methaemoglobinaemia.

PREDICTION OF PRETERM DELIVERY

Much effort has been expended in attempts to identify groups of women at high risk of preterm delivery who might benefit from increased surveillance and the potential early use of therapy to abort threatened preterm labour. A number of different approaches have been used.

Risk factor scoring

Many scoring systems have been constructed, all based on epidemiological risk factors such as those outlined in Table 33.1. In all past reproductive history plays the major role, with a history of previous preterm births, second-trimester miscarriages and cone biopsy all scoring highly (Creasy et al 1980, Holbrook et al 1989). Many other risk factors such as abdominal surgical procedure in pregnancy, stilboestrol exposure and uterine malformation are rare and are poor predictors of the bulk of preterm delivery. Overall the peformance of risk scoring, though easily applied, has been poor. Pooled results give a sensitivity of only 40% and a false-positive rate of almost 80% (see McLean et al 1993). Such results fail to identify most women at risk and falsely label many normal pregnancies as at risk, exposing them to potential interventions, some of which, for example cerclage or tocolysis, carry risks themselves.

Cervical assessment

It has been widely assumed that premature effacement or dilatation of the cervix is related to an increased risk of preterm delivery. The evidence to support this is poor. Positive predictive values of cervical changes range from 4% to 30% (Leveno et al 1986, Mortensen et al 1987), and sensitivities are less than 50%. Others have reported no additional advantage over risk factor scoring (Blondel et al 1990). The largest study is from France and considers length and dilatation of the cervix (see Papiernik 1993). Between 19 and 31 weeks' gestation in nulliparae, dilatation of the os was associated with an adjusted relative risk of 1.8 to 3.6, and a short cervix with an adjusted risk of 2.2 to 2.8.

Vaginal ultrasound assessment of cervical length offers another potential screening tool, although difficulties in determining the normal range have hampered its use in prospective screening. Overall cervical assessment is unlikely to be of value in low risk screening, but there may be value in considering a single digital or ultrasound assessment of cervical length at around 28 weeks in women with a history of previous preterm delivery.

Uterine activity monitoring

The development of non-invasive sensing devices and computer technology have made it possible to detect uterine activity in the home, with data being transmitted by telephone. Its use is based on measurement of contraction frequency, and the documented increase in this in the 24–48 hours prior to delivery. Initial work suggested sensitivities of 57–80% (Katz et al 1986, Main et al 1988) in high-risk groups, with positive predictive values of 32–72%. Subsequent studies (Hill et al 1990, Knuppel et al 1990) have confirmed the possibility that this type of monitoring with daily nursing support and intensive obstetric supervision may reduce the incidence of preterm birth.

Biochemical markers

Attempts to utilize progesterone, oestradiol and newer mediators of the inflammatory process have not shown any promise as screening tests. Plasma corticotrophin releasing factor (CRH), a peptide produced by the placenta, has recently been implicated in human parturition (Quatero et al 1989) and preliminary studies are promising as a marker. Of recent interest is fetal fibronectin, a protein present in the extracellular matrix of the decidua basalis. Preliminary studies have suggested that in women presenting with preterm uterine activity, measurement of fetal fibronectin levels by means of a simple vaginal swab has a 82% sensitivity in the prediction of those going on to deliver preterm with a positive predictive value of 83% (Lockwood et al 1991). Further preliminary studies indicate sensitivities of 70–80% in the prediction of preterm delivery from antenatally obtained samples, although the false-positive rates remain high (Lockwood et al 1993, Nageotte et al 1994). The positive test pre-dated preterm delivery by 3.4 weeks. Further studies are awaited.

PREVENTION OF PRETERM LABOUR

Identification of women at risk by some sort of screening is important, but even 100% sensitivity would be ineffective if appropriate therapy is not available to either prevent preterm labour or to modify its outcome. Prevention would be the primary aim, but another approach would be early identification which would allow time for administration of drugs which might modify neonatal outcome. The major approaches have been by education, by the use of home uterine monitoring and by pharmacological means.

Education programmes

This approach depends on the premise that groups of women can be taught to recognize early symptoms of preterm labour, and that earlier presentation may modify outcome. In addition frequent contact with health care providers may have other effects. The most widely quoted study is that from France where an entire population was subjected to an education programme which focused both on an appreciation that excess physical effort or heavy work may predispose to preterm uterine activity and on the ability to recognize early the features of early preterm labour. Although none of the work was carried out as a controlled trial, representative samples of the French population have been studied at intervals (see Papiernik 1993 for review of this work). The preterm delivery rate declined from 7.9% in 1972 to 4.1% in 1988–89. Delivery under 34 weeks' gestation declined from 3.3% to 1.3% over this period. Similar reductions in very preterm births were demonstrated in the more detailed study in Haguenau carried out as part of the assessment of this programme (Papiernik et al 1985), with a fall in deliveries under 32 weeks from 1.5% to 0.5% over 10 years. Some of this fall may be due to well-documented changes in the population over this period, including a reduction in parity, and reductions in births at both extremes of age.

Although two other large population studies have shown a reduction in preterm delivery over time (Herron et al 1982, Meis et al 1987), randomized trials of high-risk women have shown no reduction in preterm births by use of education programmes (Main et al 1985, Mueller-Huebach et al 1989, Goldenberg et al 1990). The largest trial (Collaborative Group on Preterm Birth Prevention 1993) did not show any reliable benefit from an education programme although there was considerable heterogeneity in the effect on preterm births amongst centres participating, with some centres having more preterm births in the intervention arm. It therefore remains debatable whether such education/intervention programmes truly influence the prevalence of this complication in the population.

Home uterine activity monitoring

Ambulatory monitoring is expensive both in time and in committment from individual families. Five appropriate randomized trials have addressed the issue of whether early diagnosis of preterm uterine activity using these techniques will reduce preterm deliveries (Keirse 1993a). There was a reduction (odds ratio 0.67, 95% confidence intervals 0.49–0.91) in preterm births but the quality of the trials is poor. What remains unclear is to what extent extra support helps, and some studies (Iams et al 1987) have suggested no additional benefit from home monitoring over support. Clearly further work is required but the technique has promise.

Pharmacological intervention

Trials of prophylactic oral beta-mimetics, now five in number, have not demonstrated any effect on preterm delivery, birthweight or death. Studies using fish oil supplementation show prolongation of pregnancy (Olsen et al 1992) but it is too soon to tell if preterm delivery will be affected by such therapy.

Treatment of asymptomatic bacteriuria with antibiotics appears to reduce the likelihood of delivery of an infant weighing less than 2500 g, odds ratio 0.6 (CI 0.45–0.80) (Smaill 1993). One of the trials involving specifically group B streptococci also demonstrated a reduction in preterm PROM (Thomsen et al 1987). Although the overall impact on preterm delivery within the population will be small, such therapy should be offered where screening for bacteriuria takes place.

Two interesting interventions have received less notice, namely the use of magnesium supplementation and the use of progesterone.

Magnesium sulphate is a well-established tocolytic in established preterm labour and probably acts by interfering with the uptake, binding and distribution of intracellular calcium in smooth muscle (Altura et al 1987). Three trials with 1700 women (Kovacs et al 1988, Spatling et al 1988, Sibai et al 1989) examined the effects of routine oral magnesium supplementation on preterm delivery. The odds ratio for premature delivery in the supplemented group was 0.67 (95% Cl 0.47–0.94). Reduction of preterm births by one-third would be a major achievement for such simple and safe therapy and more large studies are required.

Trials of 17α hydroxyprogesterone caproate in the prevention of miscarriage have demonstrated an unexpected benefit in reduction in preterm birth, with an odds ratio of 0.5 (Cl 0.3–0.85) (Prendeville 1993), which similarly demands further more detailed study although weekly intramuscular injections are required.

Cervical cerclage

Cerclage may have a place in the prevention of preterm birth in very high risk women (three or more previous preterm deliveries). Subanalysis of the large European trial (MRC/RCOG Working Party 1993) suggests reduction of the risk of delivery before 33 weeks in these women by about one-quarter by the use of cerclage. Overall there is a trend to a reduction in preterm birth in all women with previous second-trimester loss or preterm delivery.

Clearly preventative measures have far to go but some easily applied measures show sufficient promise to warrant further study.

MANAGEMENT OF PRETERM LABOUR

Once a diagnosis of putative preterm labour is made, management is centred on a number of questions.

1. Why is the woman in preterm labour?
2. How is the fetus (and its parents)?
3. What therapy is indicated?
4. What monitoring should be used in labour?
5. How should the fetus be delivered?

1. Why is the woman in preterm labour?

This is essentially an aetiological work-up (Table 33.2). It will include a full history and clinical examination,

Table 33.2 Investigations for suspected preterm labour

Full blood count, C-reactive protein
Kleihauer test and/or AFP
Plasma urea and electrolytes
Urine microscopy/culture
High vaginal/endocervical swabs for group B streptocooci, *E. coli* and other known aetiological organisms
Amniocentesis
Ultrasound examination

including ultrasound examination. The key clinical diagnoses to be excluded are fetal death, multiple pregnancy, uterine malformation, cervical incompetence, maternal systemic disease, infection and placental abruption.

All investigative modalities require to be available 24 hours a day, and individuals skilled in ultrasound and third-trimester amniocentesis must be similarly available. Maternal white blood cell counts and C-reactive protein estimates may give an index of general infection, although results must be interpreted using normal pregnancy ranges. Particular care is needed if glucocorticoid therapy has already been initiated as the leucocyte count may be markedly elevated. CRP levels below 30 mg/l may be normal, although persistent values above 20 mg/l are highly suggestive of chorioamnionitis (Fisk 1988). Kleihauer testing may detect occult fetomaternal haemorrhage suggestive of concealed abruption. More recently it has been suggested that AFP is a more sensitive index of fetomaternal haemorrhage although third-trimester normal ranges are less well described.

Urine microscopy is essential to exclude urinary tract infection as a cause of preterm labour, as appropriate antibiotics will be required before successful suppression of labour is achieved. Genital tract infection, especially group B streptococcal infection, should be excluded quickly.

Although popular in North America, amniocentesis is less practised on labour wards in the UK. With intact membranes, the incidence of positive culture is around 16% (Romero & Mazor 1988). In experienced hands it is not associated with significant risk of ruptured membranes (Dunlow & Duff 1990). There is good evidence that the presence of organisms in the amniotic cavity is associated with an increased risk of ruptured membranes and of failed tocolysis (Romero & Mazor 1988). Such information would be useful clinically in determining a subset of women likely to deliver in order to maximize care, for example by ensuring transfer to units with appropriate neonatal facilities. This may be especially important in the very preterm, with the suggestion recently that outcome for these is best in very large tertiary units (International Neonatal Network 1993). Culture results take too long for clinical use and gram staining is the acute gold standard (Romero et al 1988b). Other easily obtained rapid tests may supplement gram staining, such as white cell counts (Romero et al 1991), glucose levels (Romero et al 1990b) and leucocyte esterase activity (Egley et al 1988). All of these tests are applicable to any labour ward, and should perhaps be more widely utilized.

Ultrasound plays a key role in the assessment of preterm labour. Its diagnostic functions include the diagnosis of multiple pregnancy, confirmation and quantitation of polyhydramnios, determination of fetal presentation, diagnosis of previously unsuspected malformation, and, in skilled hands, identification of subchorionic haemorrhage. Maternity units delivering preterm infants need to ensure the availability at all times of someone skilled enough to perform these complex assessments.

2. How is the fetus?

The next question to be addressed before deciding on therapy is that of fetal well-being. This is approached using conventional cardiotocography and by ultrasound assessment.

Accurate knowledge of gestation is central to the management of preterm labour and it may be necessary to assess gestational age where this is uncertain. Given the social class and age-related associations of preterm labour, late presentation for antenatal care and concealed pregnancy are more common than in the general obstetric population. Gestational assessment is less accurate in the late second and early third trimester. Routine measurements of biparietal diameter (BPD), femur length, head circumference and abdominal circumference should be made. Where possible transcerebellar diameter or foot length should be assessed, as these measurements are less affected by deviations in fetal growth (Mercer et al 1987, Reece et al 1987) and are the most accurate measures of gestation at this stage.

Liquor volume should be assessed as this may help differentiate the growth-retarded from the preterm fetus. Maximum pool depth or amniotic fluid index may be used and it is better to utilize gestationally adjusted reference ranges (Nwosu et al 1993) rather than absolute values. Growth is difficult to assess in the absence of good gestational data, and is made more so by the view that growth retardation is more common than expected in preterm deliveries (Tamura et al 1984). Weight can be estimated using a number of formulae but no single formula stands out (Robson et al 1993); however, those of Hadlock (Hadlock et al 1985) and Shepard (Shepard et al 1982) are most commonly used. More sophisticated methods of determining appropriateness of growth relative to maternal characteristics (Wilcox et al 1993) or relative to previous ultrasound measurements (Deter et al 1986) are possible but may not yet be applicable in the labour ward. Strenuous efforts to determine gestation and weight accurately are important at the lower limits of

viability in order to prevent fetuses from being erroneously labelled previable.

Whilst carrying out such assessment, some impression of fetal activity and general behaviour can be made. Fetal breathing activity is not as useful a test of well-being under these conditions as its absence has been proposed as a predictor of true preterm labour (Agustsson & Patel 1987).

Well-being is normally assessed by cardiotocography. This is evaluated using standard criteria modified for use in the preterm fetus. Both fetal heart rate reactivity and amplitude of accelerations are reduced prior to 32 weeks (Natale et al 1984). Isolated variable decelerations are common and not of pathological significance. Caution is required in defining fetal distress by cardiotocography alone in the preterm fetus, and recourse to other biophysical assessment and even fetal cord blood sampling may be necessary in the extremely preterm to use the best management.

Following these extensive investigations, clinicians are in a position to determine which therapies, including immediate delivery, are appropriate to maximize outcome.

3a. Therapies to improve outcome: delaying delivery

Several drugs are now available to delay delivery in spontaneous preterm labour and where possible these should be utilized to allow other therapies which may improve outcome to be given. There are few complete contraindications to the inhibition of preterm labour (Table 33.3). Current drugs used are beta-mimetics, prostaglandin synthetase inhibitors, magnesium sulphate, calcium channel blockers and antibiotics.

Beta-adrenergic agonists

Mechanism of action   The action of the commonly used drugs (ritodrine, salbutamol, terbutaline) is dependent on interaction with $beta_2$-adrenergic receptor sites on myometrial cell membranes. Their activity depends on the alkyl substitutions on the ethylamine side-chain

Table 33.3   Contraindications to suppression of preterm labour

Absolute contraindications
  Fetal death
  Fetal congenital anomaly incompatible with life
  Obvious clinical chorioamnionitis
  Fetal conditions requiring immediate delivery
  Maternal conditions requiring immediate delivery
Relative contraindications
  Vaginal bleeding
  Gestational hypertension
  Fetal distress
  Fetal growth retardation

and the hydroxyl groups at the 3 and 5 positions of the benzene ring. The agonist–receptor complex activates adenylate cyclase, resulting in an increase in intracellular cyclic adenosine monophosphate (cAMP; Roberts 1984). In turn this activates a protein kinase which causes both phosphorylation of membrane proteins in the sarcoplasmic reticulum responsible for reducing intracellular calcium concentrations, and an inhibition of myosin light-chain kinase activity which prevents the actin–myosin interaction necessary for smooth muscle contraction.

Safety   Maternal side effects of beta-mimetics are well documented and are described in Table 33.4. The metabolic effects are a result of beta$_2$-receptor stimulation, which promotes hepatic glycogenolysis and thus hyperglycaemia. Insulin levels rise, in part due to hyperglycaemia (Cano et al 1985) and in part due to increased pancreatic secretion via the rise in cAMP. The effect is transient, peaking at 3–6 hours after treatment starts (Young et al 1983). Transient hypokalaemia almost always occurs as a consequence of a redistribution of potassium from extracellular to intracellular compartments. Total body potassium is not changed and there are no reports of adverse effects. No replacement therapy is indicated.

Most of the concern over the use of beta-agonists centres on the severe cardiovascular side-effects. Arrhythmias are described (Merkatz et al 1980) but are usually benign. Symptomatic myocardial ischaemia, usually localized to the subendocardial region, has been described (Benedetti 1983). Most women on ritodrine develop some electrocardiographic changes (Hendricks et al 1986), with depression of the ST segment and flattening or inversion of the T wave. These most likely result from relative hypoperfusion of the subendocardial region, and as such are the normal adaptive response to the beta-agonist-induced tachycardia. These changes probably do not reflect myocardial damage. Nevertheless the findings urge extreme caution where pre-existing cardiac disease is even suspected, and alternative therapies should be explored.

Table 33.4 Maternal side-effects of beta-agonist tocolysis

Palpitations
Tremor
Restlessness
Agitation
Rash
Nausea and bloating
Elevated transaminases
Anaemia
Paralytic ileus
Glucose intolerance
Hypokalaemia
Myocardial ischaemia
Arrhythmias
Pulmonary oedema

The greatest controversy has been reserved for the risk of pulmonary oedema, which occurs in 0.3% of cases (Canadian Preterm Labour Investigators Group 1992). This does not usually occur within the first 24 hours of therapy and its aetiology is multifactorial. There is a high output state with possible capillary endothelial leaks. Stimulation of the renin–aldosterone system results in both dilutional anaemia and retention of fluid. Many of the reported severe cases, including deaths, were associated with very large volumes of crystalloid fluid. There is some evidence that the use of sodium chloride solution compared with dextrose solution is associated with an increased likelihood of fluid retention (Philipsen et al 1981). Whatever the cause, the injudicious use of beta-agonists can be lethal, and appropriate monitoring needs to be in place (see below).

Fetal side-effects are confined in practical terms to a tachycardia and hypoglycaemia. No long-term effects have been noted (Creasy 1984).

Administration   All delivery suites should have clear guidelines for the management of women on beta-agonist therapy. These should include guidance on the indications and contraindications for use, preliminary investigations, dosage schedules and frequency of increasing dose, instructions for maintainance intravenous therapy, duration of therapy, maternal and fetal monitoring required with special attention to calculation of fluid balance, and indications for abandoning therapy or adding further drugs. The maximum duration of therapy should be stated clearly, as should the chain of command for re-initiating treatment. There should be clear objectives to the therapy.

Beta-agonists should only be used where there is good evidence of preterm labour. Preliminary investigations will include a full cardiovascular history and examination, including electrocardiogram, and measurement of plasma electrolytes and haematocrit.

Beta-adrenergic agonists should be given as continuous intravenous infusions, diluted in 5% dextrose or half-strength saline solution. They should be given as high concentration solutions to utilize the minimum fluids; this may include the use of syringe pumps. They should always be given via calibrated infusion pumps and as a separate infusion. Administration schedules vary but the initial dose should be the minimum recommended. The dose should be increased every 10–20 minutes until uterine activity is less than one contraction in 15 minutes, or until maternal side-effects ensue (tachycardia greater than 140/min). The dose should then be stabilized and the infusion maintained for 12–24 hours. Gradual tapering of the dose should be encouraged after a few hours, and there is increasing evidence that doses required for maintainance of intravenous tocolysis are much less than previously expected. The major objects of tocolytic therapy are to arrange transfer to a place with appropriate neonatal facilities or to buy time for therapies which may directly influence outcome such as corticosteroids. These objects are usually achievable in 24–36 hours, and continuation of intravenous treatment beyond this period should only occur in unusual circumstances such as difficulties in finding appropriate neonatal care or where the fetus is thought previable and therapy appears partly effective. Other drugs (see below) are used where effective tocolysis for 24 hours seems unlikely or where there are contraindications to beta-agonists. Prior to their use, critical review of the suspected aetiology should be undertaken, and consideration should be given to exclusion of infection by direct examination of the amniotic fluid at this point.

Maternal monitoring is mandatory. It should include regular auscultatation of the lung bases, half-hourly to hourly vital signs, 12-hourly plasma electrolytes, strict input/output charting, and continuous pulse oximetry. In addition to standard midwifery observations, continuous cardiotocography is helpful, as much for information on the frequency of uterine activity as for fetal heart rate monitoring.

Following the tapering of intravenous treatment, some clinicians advocate the use of oral therapy (see below).

Efficacy   Randomized trials have clearly demonstrated that beta-mimetics are effective in delaying delivery in the short term (King et al 1988, Canadian Preterm Labour Investigators Group 1992). The odds of delivering within 24 hours are 0.31 (CI 0.24–0.41) and within 48 hours 0.54 (CI 0.43–0.69) (Keirse 1993b). As yet however there seems no clear improvement in outcome, although births below 37 weeks and births of infants weighing less than 2500 g are less (see Fig. 33.2).

Unfortunately, few of the existing trials referred to

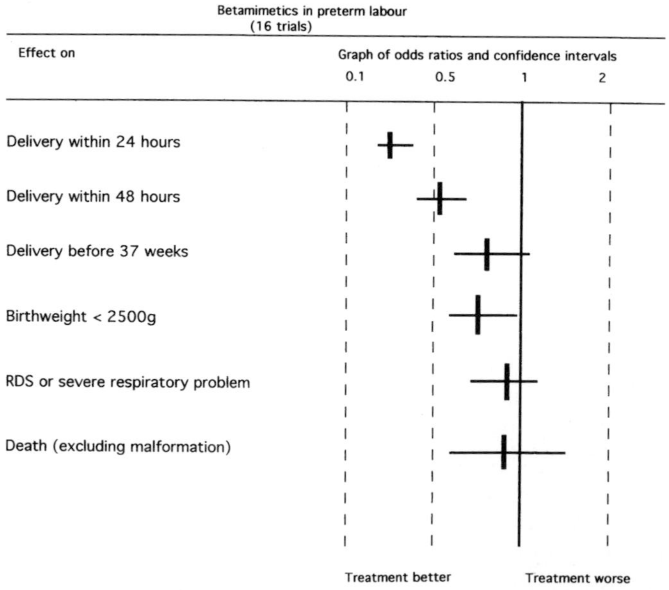

corticosteroid use, and it may well be that insufficient use of this short window of opportunity was made. Many of the trials included sizeable numbers of pregnancies beyond 34 weeks, and any effect on serious outcome may be diluted. However, the current data cannot exclude an adverse effect from the use of tocolysis, such as its use where immediate delivery was the better option. The uncertainties around the precise benefits of delaying delivery strengthen the rational approach to the management of preterm labour, with structured investigation of aetiology to identify those infants requiring urgent delivery and clear use of the time gained by tocolytics to introduce therapies with known beneficial effects on outcome, including appropriate transfer.

Prostaglandin synthetase inhibitors

Mechanism of action   Prostaglandins play a key role in both uterine activity and in facilitating cervical dilatation. Indomethacin, the only drug of this class to be studied to any extent, if given orally or rectally, has a peak action at around 2 hours, and a half-life of 2.6–11.2 hours (Duggan et al 1972). It acts by inhibiting cyclo-oxygenase, the enzyme which converts fatty acids into prostaglandin endoperoxides. Its action is reversible and enzyme activity resumes as drug levels fall. In vitro, spontaneous contractions of myometrial strips are abolished by the addition of indomethacin (Garrioch 1978). The drug passes freely to the fetus, with equivalent levels in the fetus at 5–6 hours after the maternal dose independent of gestation (Moise et al 1990).

Safety   Maternal side-effects are uncommon and usually minor (gastrointestinal disturbance, headache, vertigo, tinnitus). Postpartum haemorrhage has been reported. The classic contraindications and cautions of prostaglandin synthetase inhibitors should be recognized, namely history of duodenal ulceration, allergy to salicylates, known coagulation disorder, or known hepatic or renal dysfunction.

The main concerns regarding indomethacin, in contradistinction to ritodrine, are fetal (Table 33.5). Prostaglandins play a central role in maintaining ductal patency (Sideris et al 1983) and it is well established in animal models that prenatal ductal constriction can set in motion haemodynamic alterations which lead to persistent fetal circulation in the neonate (Tulzer et al 1991). Ductal

Betamimetics in preterm labour
(16 trials)

Effect on	Graph of odds ratios and confidence intervals

Fig. 33.2   Metanalysis of effects of beta-agonists in preterm labour.

Table 33.5   Potential fetal side-effects of indomethacin

Constriction of the ductus arteriosus
Persistent fetal circulation
Hydrops
Oligohydramnios
Bleeding disorders
Necrotizing enterocolitis/ileal perforation
Intraventricular haemorrhage

constriction with concomitant tricuspid regurgitation in human fetuses exposed to indomethacin has been demonstrated, and the duct is sensitive from as early as 27 weeks' gestation (Moise et al 1993). Despite these basic data, persistent fetal circulation has rarely been described in clinical studies.

Fetal urinary output decreases after indomethacin therapy, this being the basis for the drug's use in idiopathic polyhydramnios (Hendricks et al 1990). The precise mechanism is unclear, being a probable combination of changes in the central and peripheral effects of antidiuretic hormone and arginine vasopressin, and changes in proximal tubular absorption. It does not appear to be due to alterations in renal blood flow (Mari et al 1990).

Like all such agents, indomethacin can lead to alterations in haemostasis. These drugs can cause platelet dysfunction, inactivating cyclo-oxygenase. The effects of indomethacin are transient as the binding to the enzyme is reversible.

Experimentally there is decreased intestinal blood flow following fetal exposure to indomethacin (Meyers et al 1991) and there seems to be a specific risk to the terminal ileum. Both localized ileal perforation, often delayed and in otherwise well babies (Vanhaesebrouck et al 1988), and necrotizing enterocolitis (Major et al 1991) appear increased following the use of indomethacin tocolysis.

In newborn animals indomethacin can reduce basal brain blood flow, and attenuates hyperaemia following asphyxial injury (Leffler et al 1985). In the human fetus, ductal constriction with tricuspid regurgitation is associated with alterations in cerebral Doppler consistent with increased flow (Mari et al 1989). The most detailed study of neonatal cerebral outcome following indomethacin shows an increase in intraventricular haemorrhage, and particularly in severe haemorrhage leading to periventricular leucomalacia (Baerts et al 1990).

Despite the stated possible risks, trials using short courses of indomethacin have not demonstrated major neonatal problems. Nevertheless, caution is advised above 30 weeks' gestation, where there is existing oligohydramnios, where fetal coagulopathy is possible (e.g. alloimmunization), and in the growth-retarded fetus already at risk of necrotizing enterocolitis and severe intraventricular haemorrhage.

Administration   Prior to use fetal size and liquor volume should be established, and maternal contraindications sought. The usual daily dose is between 150 and 300 mg, and the commonest regimen in preterm labour is 100 mg rectally followed by 25 mg orally every 6 hours. It is rarely justified to continue beta-agonist therapy beyond 48 hours. Liquor volume should be assessed every 12–24 hours. If long-term use is considered, detailed echocardiography may be valuable in assessing those fetuses at risk of alterations in cerebral blood flow.

Efficacy   Prostaglandin synthetase inhibitors are highly effective in inhibiting myometrial activity, a single dose being effective in many women at term (Reiss et al 1976). The two randomized trials which compared the effects of indomethacin with placebo in delaying delivery (Niebyl et al 1980, Zuckerman et al 1984) show significant delay at 48 hours and at 7–10 days. Observational and other studies suggest that indomethacin can often rescue failed beta-agonist tocolysis but that the reverse rarely occurs. In comparative trials (Besinger et al 1991, Kurki et al 1991) with beta-agonists there appear few differences in efficacy but indomethacin is better tolerated.

The delay in delivery achieved with beta-agonists has not been translated into improvements in outcome, although the trend to reduced fetal and neonatal death is clear (odds ratio 0.61, CI 0.33–1.11). Overall prostaglandin seems an effective and well-tolerated drug but there are insufficient data regarding its fetal safety, with some studies not addressing this issue at all. For indomethacin in particular there is the fear that reductions in serious outcomes achievable by delaying delivery and use of other treatments may be countered by drug-induced morbidity.

Magnesium sulphate

Mechanism of action   In vitro studies demonstrate that magnesium can completely inhibit spontaneous contractility in gravid uterine muscle strips (Hall et al 1959). Its precise mode of action in vivo is not fully understood, but involves alterations in uptake, binding and distribution of calcium in smooth muscle cells (Altura et al 1987). Magnesium concentration is regulated by the kidney, with most of an extraneous load being excreted within 24 hours. Calcium excretion is also increased, further reducing available intracellular calcium.

Safety   The major safety concerns for the use of magnesium relate to maternal effects (Table 33.6). Flushing and perspiration occur shortly after commencement

Table 33.6   Maternal side-effects of magnesium tocolysis

Minor
  Perspiration, flushing
  Nausea
  Mild central hypothermia
  Depression tendon reflexes
Moderate
  Lethargy, sleepiness
  Diplopia, blurred vision
  Dysarthria
  Nystagmus
Severe
  Respiratory depression, cardiac arrest
  Chest pain, ECG effects
  Pulmonary oedema
  Paralysis
  Tetany
  Hypotension
  Paralytic ileus

of the loading infusion. Other side-effects occur at higher infusion rates (2.5–4 g per hour) and can be alleviated by reduction in the rate or by injection of 1 g calcium gluconate. Serious side-effects are uncommon. Chest pain may be due to myocardial ischaemia, and is usually associated with multiple therapy rather than magnesium alone. Pulmonary oedema occurs in 1% of cases (Elliot 1983), and again is more likely in complex cases involving dual therapy, prolonged therapy and medical complications. In the presence of deep tendon reflexes, there is little risk of respiratory depression, and this clinical sign is a useful marker of toxicity.

Experimentally magnesium sulphate increases uterine and placental blood flow (Thiagarajah et al 1985), and arguably may benefit certain fetuses. Long-term therapy has been linked with radiographic abnormalities of the long bones (Holcolm et al 1991). Short-term side-effects mimic those in the mother, with reduction in fetal heart rate and variability, decrease in fetal breathing, and hypotonia with poor respiratory effort at birth.

Administration Women with muscle disorders or renal impairment should not receive magnesium tocolysis.

Magnesium sulphate is commonly given as an initial loading dose of 4–6 g over 30 minutes, followed by an infusion of 2–3 g/hour for the first hour. Magnesium should be given in 5% dextrose. If uterine quiescence does not occur, then the rate can be increased by 0.5 g/hour every 30 minutes until uterine activity ceases or side-effects supervene. Once effective tocolysis is achieved, the rate is maintained at the lowest effective dose or at 2 g/hour, whichever is the lowest, for 12 hours. It is then tapered off at a rate of 0.5 g/hour. In most regimens oral beta-agonists are started at this point. As for other tocolytics, failure should trigger a more aggressive search for the cause of labour, and therapy should be continued beyond 48 hours only in exceptional circumstances.

Careful attention to fluid balance and reflexes form the key elements to maternal monitoring. Where possible, serum magnesium levels should be evaluated, especially where rates of 6–8 g/hour are thought necessary. Ineffective tocolysis at magnesium levels greater than 7 mg/dl should prompt reconsideration of infection or concealed abruption as the cause of preterm labour.

Efficacy Despite its widespread use as a tocolytic, there is little data supporting its efficacy. Two trials (Cotton et al 1984, Cox et al 1990) examined efficacy compared with a placebo, and could not demonstrate any benefit in terms of delaying delivery. Although both trials have been criticized, they are consistent in their message. Other trials have examined the efficacy of magnesium compared with beta-agonists (Keirse 1993c). The methodological quality is poor. Although better tolerated in the main than beta-agonists, these studies do not demonstrate any advantage of the use of magnesium in prolonging pregnancy or improving outcome. Outcome data are often poorly described.

At present, although magnesium may have attractive theoretical benefits, the evidence supporting its use as a primary tocolytic agent is poor. Given the proven short-term effectiveness of both ritodrine and indomethacin, its use should be confined to appropriate controlled clinical trials.

Calcium antagonists

Mechanism of action The ultimate mechanism of relaxing uterine muscle depends on reducing available calcium within myometrial cells. One group of drugs performs this function by blocking or regulating calcium entry into cells. Of the two agents commonly used as tocolytics, verapamil is the least selective and its use in preterm labour is limited by its cardiac effects. Nifedipine is a 1,4-dihydropyridine which inhibits slow voltage-dependent channels regulating calcium influx. It is absorbed rapidly from the oral mucosa and from the gastrointestinal tract, with detectable levels within minutes of administration. Its elimination half-life is around 80 minutes (Ferguson et al 1989).

Safety Adverse effects include dizziness, flushing, headache and peripheral oedema, all a consequence of vasodilatation; these occur in one in six women, and can sometimes lead to discontinuance of therapy (Talbert & Bussey 1983). Severe side-effects are extremely rare. Initial concerns over fetal welfare have been largely dispelled (Hanretty et al 1989).

Administration There is no consensus on dosage or frequency for tocolysis with nifedipine. A starting dose of 20 mg seems common, with 10–20 mg 4 to 6 hourly thereafter. Blood pressure should be monitored carefully.

Efficacy Clinical experience is limited with nifedipine. Trials to date have not been of high quality, and have not demonstrated any benefit over ritodrine in the prolongation of pregnancy (Bracero et al 1990, Ferguson et al 1990, Meyer et al 1990). It appears well tolerated, and no adverse fetal or neonatal effects have been reported. Its use should be confined to appropriate trials at present but its apparent safety justifies continuing investigation.

Antibiotics

The increasing evidence implicating infection as a major aetiological factor in preterm labour makes it logical to suppose that appropriate antibiotics might interrupt or modify the process. Antibiotics in asymptomatic bacteriuria appear to prolong pregnancy (Smaill 1993). A number of studies have been performed using ampicillin or erythromycin in preterm labour and in preterm PROM.

The data from preterm labour with intact membranes is unconvincing to date although numbers remain small.

The data on preterm PROM, however, is much more encouraging (Crowley 1993a). The odds of delivery within 7 days of membrane rupture following antibiotics is 0.53 (95% CI 0.45–0.80), although no benefit in terms of improved survival was seen. Neonatal sepsis is reduced, whether measured by blood cultures, overall infection or pneumonia (Amon et al 1988, Morales et al 1989, Johnston et al 1990). Maternal infectious morbidity is markedly reduced both before and after delivery. The failure to improve outcome given these data is puzzling, but may be due to failure to utilize corticosteroids; ruptured membranes and the fear of infection are frequently cited as contraindications for their use. It may however reflect masking of infection with associated poor outcome balancing the gains of prolongation of gestation. Further work is needed to clarify the use of antibiotics and to determine the most effective antibiotics.

Oxytocin antagonists

Much work is currently underway in developing specific antagonists to oxytocin (see Melin 1993). These may act by competing for cellular binding sites. Preliminary studies have been carried out in preterm labour using the antagonist atosiban. These demonstrate its consistent and effective reduction of uterine activity in preterm labour over 28 weeks without observable fetal or maternal side-effects (Andersen et al 1989, Goodwin et al 1994). The study of Goodwin et al (1994) had a placebo arm, and reduction in uterine activity was significantly better with atosiban. Further clinical studies are awaited.

Maintainance of tocolysis

It is often felt that tocolysis should be maintained by oral therapy after successful initial parenteral therapy. Only two drugs have been studied to any extent, beta-agonists and magnesium. For magnesium only one trial (Ricci et al 1991) has evaluated against placebo, and no advantage in terms of prolongation of pregnancy or improved outcome was demonstrated. Comparisons with oral beta-agonist therapy have not shown any advantage.

Although oral ritodrine and terbutaline are widely used, there are only four trials comparing their effect with placebo (see Keirse 1993d). The trend is towards a reduction in recurrence of preterm labour, an increase in the interval between recurrences and a reduction in preterm delivery. The evidence is not conclusive and further studies would be useful in clarifying their role. On current evidence there is some justification for their use, especially in the very preterm.

3b. Therapies to improve outcome: improving fetal lung maturity

Corticosteroids

Further argument regarding the use of corticosteroids in circumstances where preterm delivery is expected or imminent is of little value, and their use is strongly recommended in all such circumstances unless there are specific contraindications.

Mechanism of action Steroids exert their effect via enhanced production and release of pulmonary surfactant. Surfactant glycerophospholipid and protein synthesis is regulated by a number of factors including corticosteroids. At the molecular level, glucocorticoids have a complex action on transcription and post-transcriptional modification of surfactant protein A. This protein is closely involved with surfactant proteins B and C in structural change of the lamellar bodies, and in rapid formation of phospholipid surface films. Secretion of phospholipids may be in part regulated by surfactant protein A. The interaction of stimulatory and inhibitory effects are dose dependent and time dependent, and effects may differ at differing stages in development (see Mendelson et al 1993). In contrast, surfactant protein B and C expression are stimulated in a dose-dependent manner, which may be an indirect effect, mediated through other messengers.

Glucocorticoids are also implicated in lung morphogenesis, and in phospholipid synthesis itself (Gonzales et al 1986). The dependence of much of the effect of steroids on receptor-mediated gene transcription explains much of the time effect seen with therapy.

Safety Maternal concerns have centred around pulmonary oedema and infection. Cases of pulmonary oedema have been associated with tocolytic therapy, rather than therapy with corticosteroids alone. Other side-effects of corticosteroids are well documented. Given the short duration of therapy, only gastrointestinal haemorrhage remains a potential serious risk and steroids may be contraindicated where this is an issue.

There is now sufficient data to dispel the fear that, in intact membranes, there is increased maternal infectious morbidity (Crowley 1993b). Experimental studies support the lack of effect of these doses of corticosteroids on maternal resistance to infection (Cunningham & Evans 1991).

There appears no increase in neonatal infection following corticosteroid administration. Other concerns around neonatal morbidity have focused on long-term effects given the reduction in immediate morbidity and mortality demonstrated. Growth and psychomotor development have been studied in cohorts of infants from several of the trials. There is no evidence that these are impaired over 3, 6 or 10–12 years (MacArthur et al 1982, Collaborative

Group 1984, Howie 1986, Smolders-de-Has et al 1990). Available evidence in fact suggests that steroids protect against neurological abnormality. The single potential long-term adverse outcome reported to date is that of a reduction in the number of boys reaching puberty (Smolder-de-Has et al 1990). Lung growth appears normal.

Administration 24 mg of betamethasone or dexamethasone, or 2 g of hydrocortisone should be administered in 24 hours as divided doses. The most popular regimens are 8 mg 12 hourly or 12 mg 12 hourly.

Contraindications to use include history of gastrointestinal haemorrhage, overt chorioamnionitis, and other contraindications to corticosteroid use. Caution is necessary if using in hypertensive pregnancies and in diabetic pregnancies. Infants of diabetic mothers are more likely to develop hyaline membrane disease (Roberts et al 1976), and its use should be encouraged in these pregnancies. Diabetic control will require very close supervision to avoid ketoacidosis, and women may have to be managed on regimens akin to those utilized in labour.

For most women use will be combined with that of tocolysis to delay delivery to allow optimal action of steroids. For others with pregnancy complications requiring elective early delivery, consideration should be given as to whether delivery can be postponed for 24–48 hours to allow steroid administration. This will include pregnancies complicated by intrauterine growth retardation, hypertensive disease, alloimmunization and antepartum haemorrhage. Individual clinical judgement is required, but with foresight many of these deliveries can be predicted. Such prophylactic steroid use is probably insufficiently utilized.

If used in pregnancies complicated by preterm PROM, care must be taken to exclude infection. Maternal leucocyte counts will rise in response to steroid administration, and C-reactive protein estimates are helpful in determining if the rise is infectious in origin.

Efficacy The efficacy of corticosteroids is not in doubt (Crowley et al 1990, Crowley 1993a) and the key results are summarized in Figure 33.3. All groups benefit from therapy and the maximum benefit accrues if delivery occurs between 24 hours and 7 days after treatment (odds ratio 0.31). Usage rates of corticosteroids prior to preterm delivery still vary enormously, but can and perhaps should approach 75–80% (Cooke et al 1993).

Special care is required with prophylactic usage. Delivery should be delayed only until corticosteroid therapy is completed in both intrauterine growth retardation and hypertensive disease. Further delay may be the contributing factor in the increase in intrauterine deaths seen with hypertensive disease in the various trials.

Controversy remains over usage in preterm PROM. The most recent overview (Crowley 1993c), analysing 11 trials, shows a reduction in respiratory distress syndrome of the same order of magnitude as demonstrated for all

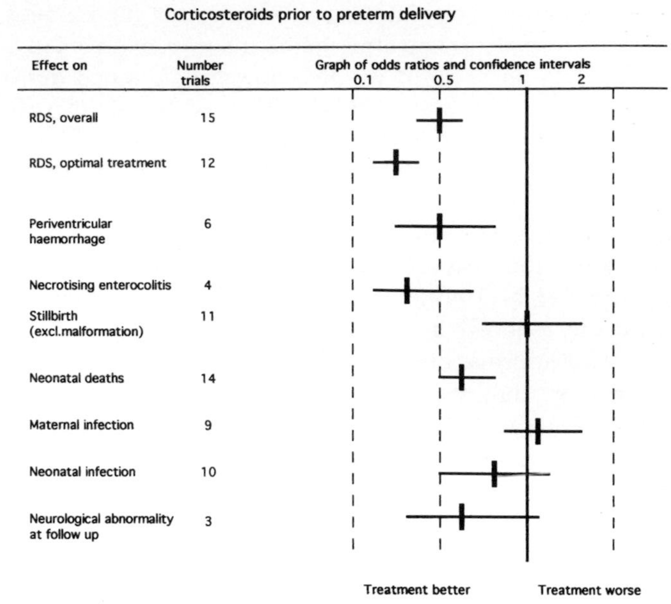

Fig. 33.3 Effects of antenatal corticosteroids.

infants (odds ratio 0.5, 95% CI 0.38–0.66) without any significant increase in neonatal infection. These data should hopefully encourage their use in this group.

Antenatal administration of corticosteroids is the most effective perinatal intervention currently available to obstetricians. Attempts should be made to administer the drug to all eligible women.

Thyroid releasing hormone

Mechanism of action Both T_4 and T_3 stimulate production of phosphatidylcholine in human lung explants (Gross et al 1980), with T_4 enhancing choline incorporation. Thyroid hormones do not appear to influence surfactant protein production (Gross 1990). The effect on phospholipid production may be synergistic with that of steroids if given together (Gonzales et al 1986) and there is a variable effect on morphological maturation. Thyroid hormone has a number of other effects, including alterations in the cardiovascular system, alterations in lung liquid flow and stimulation of prolactin secretion.

As the placenta is relatively impermeable to thyroid hormone, clinical studies have utilized either intra-amniotic injection of thyroid hormone or maternal thyroid releasing hormone (TRH). This is a tripeptide which stimulates fetal thyroid stimulating hormone (TSH) production. This stimulation occurs within 15–30 minutes, with peak levels at 30–90 minutes. Fetal T_3 levels peak at 2–4 hours.

Safety Maternal side-effects are common, with nausea, vomiting, flushing and palpitations occurring in up to one-third. Alterations in fetal physiology are seen, with changes in basal heart rate, fetal breathing activity, increases in other hormones, and neurodevelopmental alterations. Although no serious adverse effects are yet obvious, theoretical considerations with regard to brain development and oxygen consumption urge caution in its use.

Administration   TRH has to be given intravenously. Dosage regimens have not been standardized. Usually 400 µg is given, 8–12 hours apart, for 4–6 doses. There is some evidence to support 400 µg as an adequate therapeutic dose (Moya et al 1991). At 12 hours following a 400 µg dose, no elevation of thyroid hormone levels were demonstrated in cord blood, suggesting an 8-hour regimen as preferable.

Efficacy   Studies to date have concentrated on comparing the effects of TRH in addition to corticosteroids (Crowther & Grant 1993). Given the lack of effect of thyroid hormone on surfactant protein synthesis, and the known advantages of steroids, trials without steroids in these infants would likely be considered unethical.

Trials suggest promising reductions in the need for oxygen therapy (odds ratio 0.14), bronchopulmonary dysplasia (odds ratio 0.53, 95% CI 0.31–0.94) and the need for prolonged oxygen therapy (odds ratio 0.44, 95% CI 0.26–0.76). As yet no reduction in mortality or severe respiratory distress syndrome has been established. Longer-term infant outcome is not yet available, and therefore usage should be confined at present to trials. Other work needs to establish the most effective dose regimen.

3c. Therapies to improve outcome: prevention of intraventricular haemorrhage

Corticosteroids themselves have an effect on rates of periventricular haemorrhage (see Fig. 33.3). As most severe haemorrhage occurs shortly after birth, other strategies have been considered in an attempt to reduce this serious morbidity.

Antenatal vitamin K

The use of postnatal vitamin K reduces haemorrhagic disease of the newborn. Postnatal dosage takes about 4–6 hours to achieve this aim. Three small trials (Pomerance et al 1987, Morales et al 1988, Kazzi et al 1989) have examined the use of antenatally administered vitamin K. Periventricular haemorrhage was reduced in all three trials. The mechanism is unclear, given the very variable response following maternal injection, at least as gauged by cord vitamin K levels. However, the magnitude of the reduction in intraventricular haemorrhage (odds ratio 0.58) warrants consideration.

Antenatal phenobarbitone

Phenobarbitone can reduce mean arterial blood pres-

sure peaks in preterm infants. Dramatic changes in blood pressure and potentially cerebral blood flow have been implicated in the genesis of intraventricular haemorrhage. However, the drugs effects are likely to be achieved at anticonvulsant doses, and these can take up to 24 hours to obtain. Anticonvulsant levels of phenobarbitone can be obtained in cord blood within 30 minutes of maternal injection, although maternal sedation occurs. Trials of antenatal administration, now five in number (Grant & Crowther 1993), show a reduction in all and in severe intraventricular haemorrhage. The methodological quality, in terms of placebo control, postrandomization exclusions and blinding of outcome assessment, urge caution in interpretation of these encouraging results.

The most recent trial, examining the combined effect of vitamin K and phenobarbitone (Thorpe et al 1994) in a well-designed study, demonstrates only a small and not statistically significant reduction in both total intraventricular haemorrhage and in severe bleeding.

4. Intrapartum monitoring of the preterm fetus

Once labour is established or it is decided to allow labour to progress, issues regarding intrapartum monitoring of the preterm fetus must be addressed. There are three issues, namely, who should be monitored, which form of monitoring should be utilized and how should monitoring be interpreted?

There is strong evidence that metabolic acidaemia in the preterm fetus has a closer relationship with poor neurodevelopmental outcome than in the term fetus (Low et al 1981, Mires et al 1991, Gaudier et al 1992). Hypoxia and acidosis can affect lecithin production and surfactant formation. It is therefore vital that intrapartum asphyxia be avoided to improve outcome.

The issues around who should be monitored are contentious. There is an argument for only monitoring those labours where intervention would result from abnormalities of monitoring. This requires judgement on viability and ultimate prognosis, as well as the potential risks of operative intervention, including classical Caesarean section, on the mother. At gestations above 26 weeks, all labours should be monitored, unless there is good evidence of severe growth retardation with an estimated weight less than 500 g. For a normally grown fetus at 26 weeks, current survival rates are over 50%. At gestations below 22 weeks there is little realistic chance of survival at present, and monitoring would be distressing to staff and most of all to parents. Survival rates at 23–24 weeks are improving (one-third in 1992/3 in Liverpool), although handicap rates are high. All these issues should be discussed with midwifery and neonatal paediatric colleagues initially, and then with the parents, before reaching a joint decision. Difficulties in interpreting monitoring at this gestation should form part of the discussion. At

25–26 weeks, survival rates are such that intervention might now be justified for putative evidence of fetal distress, and therefore monitoring would be justified. Nevertheless, it is best to take an individual view of all the circumstances before coming to a decision with the parents.

Issues around the method of monitoring to be used follow the same pattern as for term fetuses (Neilson & Grant 1993). There remains scanty evidence to support widespread use of continuous electronic fetal heart rate monitoring in normal labours. In the preterm fetus the issue has been addressed by Luthy and colleagues (Luthy et al 1987, Shy et al 1990) in a randomized trial. They did not demonstrate any benefit of electronic fetal heart rate monitoring either in immediate neonatal outcome (Apgar scores, acidaemia, intracranial haemorrhage) or in neurological development. For uncomplicated preterm labours, it may therefore be quite appropriate to monitor using structured intermittent auscultation.

If continuous electronic fetal heart rate monitoring is used to monitor the preterm fetus, then it must be appreciated that cardiovascular physiology in the preterm fetus differs from that at term (Natale et al 1984). It is not appropriate to interpret findings as for a term fetus. Variable decelerations are extremely common, 55–75% (Ingemarrson et al 1980, Zanini et al 1980), and there is a poor correlation with pH. Variable decelerations with a late component, and those with an overshoot, seem most associated with acidosis. Tachycardia and reduced baseline variability are commonly seen in acidaemia (Westgren et al 1982), although the relationship for reduced variability has been challenged (Mires et al 1993). Late decelerations are ominous (Westgren et al 1982, Mires et al 1993). Follow-up of preterm infants with ominous continuous electronic fetal heart rate monitoring has shown a relationship with neurodevelopmental outcome, especially in the very preterm (Westgren et al 1986).

Interpretation of continuous electronic fetal heart rate monitoring is complex in the preterm, and such records need to be examined by appropriately trained medical staff, who understand the complexities of the physiology of the preterm fetus. This should allow both better recognition of ominous records and prevent unnecessary intervention based on term criteria.

5. Delivery of the preterm fetus

The preterm fetus should be delivered in a unit where appropriate neonatal care can be provided. Earlier evidence (Paneth et al 1987) that neonatal outcome is better in central units has been given support by recent comparisons of different sized neonatal units (International Neonatal Network 1993), strongly suggesting better outcome, especially in the very preterm, in the largest units.

The ideal mode of delivery will vary, dependent on the indication for delivery. For many infants of complicated pregnancies electively or semielectively delivered preterm, there may be cogent reasons for recourse to Caesarean section, both fetal and maternal. For the majority of preterm births, however, there are few data to support liberal use of abdominal delivery. Mode of delivery correlates poorly with outcome (Kitchen et al 1985). Analysis of long-term neonatal outcome in inborn infants delivering at Liverpool Maternity Hospital over the last decade similarly shows no relationship between outcome and mode of delivery. Barely 100 women have been recruited into randomized trials (Grant 1993) of elective versus selective Caesarean section, and no conclusion can be drawn from this data.

For cephalic presentations with preterm labour or preterm PROM, vaginal delivery is the preferred option. Oxytocin may be used (as in preterm PROM) but with great caution. Both prolonged labour and precipitate labour are risk factors for intracranial haemorrhage. Analgesia should be adequate. There is no necessity for routine use of epidural analgesia, although there is some evidence that outcome is better than if opiate analgesia is used. There is no evidence that forceps delivery, applied routinely, confers any fetal advantage, and as it confers maternal detriment, its use should be abandoned. All texts suggest liberal use of generous episiotomies to prevent sudden decompression of the head of the preterm infant, although the evidence for such a policy is flimsy (Lobb & Cooke 1986).

Delivery of the preterm breech generates as much controversy as for term breech delivery. There are no appropriate trials, and retrospective, prospective and cohort studies are plagued with selection bias (see Keirse 1989) making rational decision making virtually impossible. The majority of breech presentations between 28 and 34 weeks' gestation are nevertheless delivered by Caesarean section, and recent attempts to mount a randomized trial appear to have foundered on preconceived beliefs.

Caesarean section on the preterm uterus is not necessarily an easy option, and should not be seen as a way of avoiding trauma. A poorly formed lower segment in the very preterm may make classical Caesarean section, low vertical incision, J and T incisions, and trauma likely. Delivery of a fragile preterm infant through a small low transverse uterine scar in a thick lower segment is likely to be as traumatic as a well-conducted normal or vaginal breech delivery.

Summary

The overall management of preterm labour and delivery is summarized in Table 33.8. The key to successful management is a well-structured and comprehensive set of guidelines dealing with diagnosis, therapy and delivery, with early and close involvement of senior staff. Neonatal mortalities of two or less per 1000 are achievable with this closely linked and comprehensive perinatal approach.

PRETERM PREMATURE RUPTURE OF THE MEMBRANES

Many of the factors and management decisions discussed for preterm labour are relevant for preterm premature rupture of the membranes (PROM), but some issues differ.

Aetiology and risk factors

Many of the risk factors described earlier apply equally to preterm PROM. In particular, previous preterm delivery (odds ratio 2.8), early pregnancy bleeding (odds ratio 2.4 for first-trimester bleeding, odds ratio 4.4 for second-trimester bleeding) and cigarette smoking (odds ratio 2.1) emerge as important variables in women subsequently presenting with preterm PROM (Harger et al 1990).

The mechanism by which bleeding in the first half of pregnancy predisposes to preterm PROM is unclear but could include ascending infection or disruption of nutritional support to part of the membranes. The data on smoking are controversial but consistent (Meyer & Tonascia 1977) and the mechanism may be mediated through damage to decidual blood vessels.

The primary aetiological mechanism is again infection as outlined in Figure 33.1. Where organisms have been sought from amniotic fluid, positive cultures have been found in about one-third. *Chlamydia trachomatis* has been implicated (Gravett et al 1986), as has group B streptococcus (Alger et al 1988). Much recent interest has focused on the role of apparently less pathogenic organisms such as those involved in bacterial vaginosis (Gravett et al 1986, McDonald et al 1991).

Management issues in preterm PROM

There are a number of complex issues to be dealt with in the management of preterm PROM as outlined in Table 33.7. The argument between expectant versus interventional management is driven by fear of serious maternal morbidity and poor survival rates in early preterm

Table 33.7 Issues in preterm PROM

Viability
Pulmonary hypoplasia
Maternal infection
Antenatal fetal monitoring
Tocolysis
Antibiotics
Corticosteroids
Digital examination

PROM. Loss rates are clearly linked to gestation at delivery rather than infection (Newton et al 1987), but for pregnancies where labour does not ensue rapidly after rupture of the membranes the risk of infection has been overstated (Kappy et al 1979). In the absence of clear evidence of infection, most clinicians now advocate an expectant approach to 32–34 weeks. One area where this may be challenged is where group B streptococcus is isolated. The effectiveness of intrapartum antibiotics may be reduced if expectant management is pursued (Newton et al 1987).

Viability

The question of viability arises when preterm PROM occurs early. As for any cause of severe oligohydramnios prior to 20 weeks' gestation, the outcome is poor. The risk of chorioamnionitis is high, and the risk of pulmonary hypoplasia exceeds 50% (Rotschild et al 1990). In the study of Taylor & Garite (1984) with a mean gestational age at preterm PROM of 23 weeks, only 10% of pregnancies produced a neurologically normal long-term survivor. Although more recent studies have slightly better outcomes, significant proportions of survivors have serious sequelae. Given this information, it may be appropriate to raise therapeutic termination as an option. No therapy is currently available to replace or maintain successfully amniotic fluid in these circumstances, although some interesting approaches to plugging the cervix are under investigation.

The most difficult area is between 22 and 24 weeks. Neonatal survival is still poor and there is a high incidence of handicap in survivors. Other than infection, the main concern is pulmonary development. There is good evidence that the development of pulmonary hypoplasia is dependent on the gestation of membrane rupture rather than duration (Rotschild et al 1990). Prediction is difficult, but nomograms of chest circumference or lung length (Roberts & Mitchell 1990) may help.

Maternal infection

Maternal sepsis remains the most serious hazard to expectant management. Both maternal death and postpartum hysterectomy secondary to sepsis have been reported, and overall infection rates are high. Digital vaginal examination may contribute to this (Lewis et al 1991), although the data are not strong.

Monitoring for developing sepsis relies on conventional clinical surveillance. C-reactive protein estimates seem the most reliable (Fisk 1988), although cut-off values need to be modified for pregnancy. Persistent levels above 20 mg/l or single estimates above 30–40 mg/l are highly suggestive of infection. The presence of symptomatic infection is an absolute indication for delivery.

Antenatal monitoring

Preliminary assessment of the fetus in preterm PROM does not differ from that of preterm labour. If liquor is collectable from the vagina, then it is useful to have available gram staining of this fluid. If labour does not supervene, then fetal surveillance is necessary. Its use here is in the prediction of fetal sepsis.

The non-stress test alone may be helpful, with high sensitivity (Vintzileos et al 1986a) for indices of chorio-amnionitis and neonatal sepsis, although the false-positive rate remains around 40%. Amniotic fluid volume itself has been proposed as a predictor (Gonick et al 1985, Vintzileos et al 1985), with maximum pools less than 1 cm the key. It is not as sensitive or specific as the non-stress test, but may be useful.

A number of biophysical parameters have been used to predict infection. Fetal breathing activity is reduced after preterm PROM (Roberts et al 1991a) and a number of groups have documented an association between subsequent sepsis and reduced breathing (Vintzileos et al 1986b, Goldstein et al 1988). However, although very sensitive, false-positive rates are 50%. Fetal movement, total fetal activity and fetal biophysical profile scoring show similar predictive abilities (Roberts et al 1991b), with sensitivities in excess of 90%, negative predictive values around 95% but with false-positive rates of 25–40%. Given current information, the most appropriate monitoring appears to be frequent ultrasound assessment of fetal activity and breathing, with amniocentesis reserved for exclusion of false-positive non-invasive results. Despite the wealth of observational data, none of these strategies have been subjected to an appropriate trial. Whether such intensive monitoring should be hospital based is also open to debate. The only trial of hospital versus home (Carlan et al 1993), although small, demonstrated no differences.

Tocolysis

The use of parenteral tocolysis in women with preterm PROM in established or suspected labour is controversial. There is little doubt that in the presence of ruptured membranes, tocolysis is less effective. Few randomized trials have specifically addressed the issue of prolongation of pregnancy in this group. The trials of Christensen (Christensen et al 1980) and Weiner (Weiner et al 1988) did suggest some short-term gains akin to those seen in overviews of tocolytic therapy, but no improvement in outcome. Steroids were not used in either trial. Pragmatically, there seems little justification in using tocolysis beyond 28 weeks' gestation except to facilitate in utero transfer. In less mature pregnancies, there may be value in trying to gain time to administer steroids given the supportive evidence from trials of corticosteroids in PROM.

Corticosteroids and antibiotics

The issues around antibiotic usage remain to be resolved as discussed earlier, although there is clear evidence of a reduction in neonatal and maternal sepsis. Evidence now favours the use of steroids in preterm PROM (Crowley 1993c). An unresolved issue is whether steroids should be repeated in continuing pregnancies with early PROM, given the reduction in efficacy seen after 1 week. Practice varies from regular dosage until elective delivery, single dosage following admission, and repeated doses up until 28–30 weeks' gestation. No clinical studies are available, but scientific evidence might support the latter regimen.

In summary, most women with preterm PROM will progress to preterm labour within 48 hours, and their management is not different from those admitted in preterm labour. For the smaller group of women who do not labour, expectant management with surveillance of both mother and fetus for evidence of sepsis is appropriate. Strategies for both are empirical, as no trials have been conducted. Intervention should occur only if there is evidence of clinical maternal infection or evidence of fetal infection, preferably based on invasive testing of amniotic fluid rather than on non-invasive ultrasound tests with high false-positive rates. For women with very early preterm PROM, full information on outcome should be available, and discussion of termination should be considered.

PARENTS

It is important to involve parents at every stage of the management of preterm labour and delivery. The woman will require skilled midwifery and medical support, not least because most parent education does not commence until the third trimester. For primigravidae in particular, and given the sociodemographic associations of preterm delivery, labour itself, and operative delivery especially, are ordeals suddenly thrust upon them. Family support is vital and there should be no restrictions placed on companionship in labour in these circumstances.

Careful attention should be focused on explaining what tests will be performed, what drugs will be used and their effects, how the baby will be monitored, and what the expectations might be. All involved in such care should be aware of local survival rates by weight and gestation, and early involvement of neonatal paediatric colleagues is to be encouraged. Where possible, the father should visit the neonatal unit prior to delivery, and if elective preterm delivery is contemplated, the entire family should visit.

Postnatally, midwifery and medical staff need to be aware of the different potential reactions. Parents may react to the separation by infrequent visiting. There may be distress following a visit to the neonatal unit, with the baby attached to complex equipment and often not looking like a proper baby. The daunting difficulties in maintaining breast milk production under these circumstance should not be underestimated.

Neonatal intensive care units often have well-developed support systems for parents and other family members, but it is important that the obstetric and midwifery team remain involved and interested.

Follow-up is important, both from the point of view of continuinig support for the family, but also to discuss the reasons for preterm delivery and to discuss the management of future pregnancies (Table 33.8).

Table 33.8   Management of preterm labour and delivery

Clear diagnosis of preterm labour or need to deliver
Rapid investigation into aetiology of labour/PROM
Accurate assessment of fetal age, weight and condition
Appropriate and selective use of short-term tocolysis
Widespread use of corticosteroids
Consideration of fetal monitoring
Careful choice of mode of delivery
Careful choice of place of delivery
Availability of skilled paediatric assistance

REFERENCES

Agustsson P, Patel N 1987 The predictive value of fetal breathing movements in the diagnosis of preterm labour. British Journal of Obstetrics and Gynaecology 94: 860–863

Alger L S, Lovchik J C, Hebel J R et al 1988 The association of *Chlamydia trachomatis, Neisseria gonorrhoeae*, and group B streptococci with preterm premature rupture of the membranes and pregnancy outcome. American Journal of Obstetrics and Gynecology 159: 397–404

Altura B M, Altura B T, Carella A et al 1987 Mg^{2+}–Ca^{2+} interacts in contractility of smooth muscle: magnesium versus organic calcium channel blockers on myogenic tone and agonist-induced responsiveness of blood vessels. Canadian Journal of Physiology and Pharmacology 65: 729–745

Amon E, Lewis S V, Sibai B M, Villar M A, Arheart K L 1988 Ampicillin prophylaxis in preterm premature rupture of the membranes: a prospective randomised study. American Journal of Obstetrics and Gynecology 159: 539–543

Andersen L F, Lyndrup J, Akerlund M, Melin P 1989 Oxytocin receptor blockade: a new principle in the treatment of preterm labour? American Journal of Perinatology 6: 196–199

Anderson A 1977 Preterm labour: definition. In: Anderson A (ed) Proceedings of the Fifth Study Group of the Royal College of Obstetricians and Gynaecologists. RCOG, London

Baerts W, Fetter W F, Hop W J et al 1990 Cerebral lesions in preterm infants after tocolytic indomethacin. Developmental Medicine and Child Neurology 32: 910–918

Bakketeig L S, Hoffman H J 1981 Epidemiology of preterm birth: results from a longitudinal study of births in Norway. In: Elder M G, Hendricks C H (eds) Preterm labour. Butterworths, London, pp 17–46

Barros F C, Huttly S R A, Victoria C G et al 1992 Comparison of the causes and consequences of prematurity and intrauterine growth retardation: a longitudinal study in Southern Brazil. Paediatrics 90: 238–244

Bejar R, Curbelo V, Davis C, Gluck L 1981 Premature labour. Bacterial sources of phospholipase. Obstetrics and Gynecology 57: 479–482

Benedetti T J 1983 Maternal complications of parenteral betasympathomimetic therapy for premature labour. American Journal of Obstetrics and Gynecology 145: 1–6

Berkowitz G S, Kelsey J L, Holford T R et al 1982 Physical activity and the risk of spontaneous preterm labour. Journal of Reproductive Medicine 28: 581–585

Besinger R E, Niebyl J R, Keyes W G 1991 Randomised comparative trial of indomethacin and ritodrine for the long term treatment of preterm labour. American Journal of Obstetrics and Gynecology 164: 981–988

Blondel B, Le Coutour X, Kaminski M et al 1990 Prediction of preterm delivery: is it substantially improved by routine vaginal examination? American Journal of Obstetrics and Gynecology 162: 1042–1048

Boer K, Samlal R A K, Smit B J, Kreijenbroek M E, Hogerzeil H V 1993 Twenty years' drug policy in obstetric care in Amsterdam. In: Koppe J G, Eskes T K A B, van Geijn H P, Weisenhann P F, Ruys J H (eds) Care, concern and cure in perinatal medicine. Parthenon Press, Carnforth, Lancashire, pp 221–231

Bracero L A, Leikin E, Kirshenbaum N, Tejani N 1990 Comparison of nifedipine and ritodrine for the treatment of preterm labour. American Journal of Obstetrics and Gynecology 163: 77–81

Canadian Preterm Labour Investigators Group 1992 Treatment of preterm labour with beta-adrenergic agonist ritodrine. New England Journal of Medicine 327: 308–312

Cano A, Tovar I, Parilla J J 1985 Metabolic disturbances during intravenous use of ritodrine: increased insulin levels and hypokalaemia. Obstetrics and Gynecology 65: 356–360

Carlan S T 1993 Home versus hospital monitoring for preterm premature rupture of the membranes. Obstetrics and Gynecology 81: 61–64

Casey M L, Cox S M, Beutler B, Milewich L, McDonald P C 1989 Cachectin/tumour necrosis factor-alpha formation in human decidua. Potential role of cytokines in infection-induced preterm labour. Journal of Clinical Investigation 83: 430–436

Christensen K K, Ingemarsson I, Leideman T et al 1980 Effect of ritodrine on labour after premature rupture of the membranes. Obstetrics and Gynecology 55: 187–190

Collaborative Group on Antenatal Steroid Therapy 1984 Effects of antenatal dexamathasone administration in the infant; long-term follow up. Journal of Paediatrics 104: 259–267

Collaborative Group on Preterm Birth Prevention 1993 Multicenter randomised, controlled trial of a preterm birth prevention program. American Journal of Obstetrics and Gynecology 169: 352–366

Cooke R W I 1992 Annual audit of neonatal morbidity in preterm infants. Archives of Disease in Childhood 67: 1174–1176

Cooke R W I, Walkinshaw S A, Ryan S 1993 Steroids for babies. Lancet 341: 569

Cotton D B, Strassner H T, Hill L M, Schifrin B S, Paul R H 1984 Comparison of magnesium sulfate, terbutaline and a placebo for the inhibition of preterm labour. Journal of Reproductive Medicine 29: 92–97

Cox S M, Sherman M L, Leveno K J 1990 Randomised investigation of magnesium sulfate for prevention of preterm birth. American Journal of Obstetrics and Gynecology 163: 767–772

Creasy R K 1984 Preterm labor and delivery. In: Creasy R K, Resnik R (ed) Maternal-fetal medicine. Principles and practice. W B Saunders, Philadelphia, p 415

Creasy R K, Gummer B A, Liggins G C 1980 A system for predicting spontaneous preterm birth. Obstetrics and Gynecology 55: 692–695

Crenshaw C, Jones D E D, Parker R T 1973 Placenta previa: a survey of 20 years experience with improved perinatal survival by expectant therapy and cesarean delivery. Obstetrical and Gynecological Survey 28: 461–468

Crowley P 1993a Antibiotics for prelabour preterm rupture of the membranes. In: Enkin M, Keirse M J N C, Renfrew M, Neilson J P (eds) Pregnancy and childbirth module. Cochrane database of systematic reviews. Update Software, Oxford (review no 04391, vol disk issue 2)

Crowley P 1993b Corticosteroids prior to preterm delivery. In: Enkin M, Keirse M J N C, Renfrew M, Neilson J P (eds) Pregnancy and childbirth module. Cochrane database of systematic reviews. Update Software, Oxford (Review no 02955, vol disk issue 2)

Crowley P 1993c Corticosteroids after preterm prelabour rupture of the membranes. In: Enkin M, Keirse M J N C, Renfrew M, Neilson J P (eds) Pregnancy and childbirth module. Cochrane database of systematic reviews. Update Software, Oxford (review no. 04395. vol disk issue 2)

Crowley P, Chalmers I, Keirse M J N C 1990 The effects of corticosteroid administration before preterm delivery: a review of the evidence from controlled trials. British Journal of Obstetrics and Gynaecology 97: 11–25

Crowther C A, Grant A M 1993 Antenatal thyrotropin-releasing hormone (TRH) prior to preterm delivery. In: Enkin M, Keirse M J N C, Renfrew M, Neilson J P (eds) Pregnancy and childbirth module. Cochrane database of systematic reviews. Update Software, Oxford (review no 04749. vol disk issue 2)

Cunningham D S, Evans E E 1991 The effects of betamethasone on maternal cellular resistance to infection. American Journal of Obstetrics and Gynecology 165: 610–615

Deter R L, Rossavik I K, Harrist R B, Hadlock F P 1986 Mathematical modelling of fetal growth: development of individual growth curve standards. Obstetrics and Gynecology 68: 156–161

Dudley D J, Trautman M S, Edwin S S et al 1992 Biosynthesis of interleukin-6 by cultured human chorion laeve cells: regulation by cytokines. Journal of Clinical Endocrinology and Metabolism 75: 1081–1086

Duggan D E, Hoggans A F, Kwan K C et al 1972 The metabolism of indomethacin in man. Journal of Pharmacology and Experimental Therapeutics 181: 563–569

Dunlow S G, Duff P 1990 Microbiology of the lower genital tract and amniotic fluid in asymptomatic preterm patients with intact membranes and moderate to advanced degrees of cervical effacement and dilatation. American Journal of Perinatology 7: 235–238

Editorial 1991 Trends in fertility and infant and maternal health— United States, 1980–88. MMWR 40: 381–390

Egley C C, Katz V L, Herbert W N P 1988 Leukocyte esterase: a simple bedside test for the detection of bacterial colonisation of amniotic fluid. American Journal of Obstetrics and Gynecology 159: 120–122

Elliot J P 1983 Magnesium sulfate as a tocolytic agent. American Journal of Obstetrics and Gynecology 147: 277–284

Ferguson J E I, Schutz T, Pershe R, Stevenson D K, Blaschke T 1989 Nifedipine pharmacokinetics during preterm labor tocolysis. American Journal of Obstetrics and Gynecology 161: 1485–1490

Ferguson J E, Dyson D C, Schutz T, Stevenson D K 1990 A comparison with nifedipine or ritodrine. Analysis of efficacy and maternal, fetal and neonatal outcome. American Journal of Obstetrics and Gynecology 163: 105–111

Fisk N M 1988 Modification to selective conservative management in preterm premature rupture of the membranes. Obstetrical and Gynecological Survey 43: 328–334

Friedman M L, McElin T W 1969 Diagnosis of fetal ruptured membranes: clinical study and review of the literature. American Journal of Obstetrics and Gynecology 104: 544–550

Garn S M, Shaw H A, McCabe K D 1977 Effects of socioeconomic status and race on weight defined and gestational prematurity in the United States. In: Reed D M, Stanley F J (eds) The epidemiology of prematurity. Urban and Schwartzenburg, Baltimore, p 127

Garrioch D B 1978 The effect of indomethacin on spontaneous activity in the isolated human myometrium and on the response to oxytocin and prostaglandin. British Journal of Obstetrics and Gynaecology 85: 47–52

Gaudier F L, Goldenberg R L, Peralta M et al 1992 Prediction of long term neurologic handicap in very low birth weight infants. American Journal of Obstetrics and Gynecology 166: 419

Gibbs R S, Blanco J D 1982 Premature rupture of the membranes. Obstetrics and Gynecology 60: 671–679

Goldenberg R L, Davis R O, Cooper R L et al 1990 The Alabama Preterm Birth Prevention Project. Obstetrics and Gynecology 75: 933–939

Goldstein I, Romero R, Merrill S et al 1988 Fetal body and breathing movements as predictors of intra-amniotic infection in preterm premature rupture of the membranes. American Journal of Obstetrics and Gynecology 159: 363–368

Gonick B, Bottoms S F, Cotton D B 1985 Amniotic fluid volume as a risk factor in preterm premature rupture of the membranes. Obstetrics and Gynecology 65: 456–459

Gonzales L W, Ballard P L, Ertsey R et al 1986 Glucocorticoids and thyroid hormones stimulate biochemical and morphological differentiation of human fetal lung in organ culture. Journal of Clinical Endocrinology and Metabolism 62: 678–691

Goodwin T M, Paul R, Silver H et al 1994 The effect of the oxytocin antagonist atosiban on preterm uterine activity in the human. American Journal of Obstetrics and Gynecology 170: 474–478

Grant A M 1993 Elective vs selective Caesarean delivery of the small baby. In: Enkin M, Keirse M J N C, Renfrew M, Neilson J P (eds) Pregnancy and childbirth module. Cochrane database of systematic reviews. Update Software, Oxford (review no 06597 vol disk issue 2)

Grant A M, Crowther C A 1993 Phenobarbital prior to preterm delivery. In: Enkin M, Keirse M J N C, Renfrew M, Neilson J P (eds) Pregnancy and childbirth module. Cochrane database of systematic reviews. Update Software, Oxford (review no 04261, vol disk issue 2)

Gravett M G, Nelson H P, DeRouen T et al 1986 Independent association of bacterial vaginosis and chlamydia trachomatis infection with adverse pregnancy outcome. Journal of the American Medical Association 256: 1988–1993

Gross I 1990 Regulation of fetal lung maturation. American Journal of Physiology 259: L337–L344

Gross I, Wilson C M, Ingelson L D et al 1980 Fetal lung in organ culture. III. Comparison of dexamethasone, thyroxine, and methylxanthines. Journal of Applied Physiology 48: 872–877

Hadlock F P, Harrist R B, Sharman R S et al 1985 Estimation of fetal weight with the use of head, body and femur measurements—a prospective study. American Journal of Obstetrics and Gynecology 151: 333–337

Hall D G, McGaughey H S, Corey E L et al 1959 The effects of magnesium therapy on the duration of labour. American Journal of Obstetrics and Gynecology 78: 27–32

Hall M H 1985 Incidence and distribution of preterm labour. In: Beard R W, Sharp F (eds) Preterm labour and its consequences, Proceedings of the Thirteenth Study Group of the Royal College of Obstetricians and Gynaecologists. Royal College of Obstetricians and Gynaecologists, London, pp 5–13

Halliday H L 1988 Care of the preterm babies in the first hour. Care of the Critically Ill 4: 7–12

Hanretty K P, Whittle M J, Howie C A, Rubin P C 1989 Effect of nifedipine on Doppler flow Velocity waveforms in severe pre-eclampsia. British Medical Journal 299: 1205–1207

Harger J H, Hsing A W, Tuomala R E et al 1990 Risk factors for preterm premature rupture of the fetal membranes: a multicenter case-control study. American Journal of Obstetrics and Gynecology 163: 130–137

Hendricks S K, Keroes J, Katz M 1986 Electrocardiographic changes associated with ritodrine-induced maternal tachycardia and hypokalaemia. American Journal of Obstetrics and Gynecology 154: 921–923

Hendricks S K, Smith J R, Moore D E et al 1990 Oligohydramnios associated with prostaglandin synthetase inhibitors in preterm labour. British Journal of Obstetrics and Gynaecology 97: 312–316

Herron M A, Katz M, Creasy R K 1982 Evaluation of a preterm birth prevention program: a preliminary report. Obstetrics and Gynecology 59: 452–456

Hill W C, Fleming A D, Martin R W et al 1990 Home uterine activity monitoring is associated with a reduction in preterm birth. Obstetrics and Gynecology 76: 13s–18s

Hillier S L, Martius J, Krohn M, Kiviat N, Holmes K K, Eschenbach D A 1988 A case-control study of chorioamniotic infection and histologic chorioamnionitis in prematurity. New England Journal of Medicine 319: 972–978

Hoffman H J, Bakketeig L S 1984 Risk factors associated with the occurrence of preterm birth. Clinical Obstetrics and Gynecology 27: 539–552

Holbrook R H, Laros R K, Creasy R K 1989 Evaluation of a risk-scoring system for prediction of preterm labour. American Journal of Perinatology 6: 62–68

Holcolm W L, Schackelford G D, Petrie R H 1991 Magnesium

tocolysis and neonatal bone abnormalities. Obstetrics and Gynecology 78: 611–614

Howie R N 1986 Pharmacological acceleration of lung maturation. In: Villee C A, Villee D B, Zuckerman J (eds) Respiratory distress syndrome. Academic, London, pp 385–396

Iams J D, Johnson F F, O'Shaughnessy R W et al 1987 A prospective random trial of home uterine activity monitoring in pregnancies at increased risk of preterm labour. American Journal of Obstetrics and Gynecology 157: 638–643

Iams J D, Stilson R, Johnson F F, Williams R A, Rice R 1990a Symptoms that precede preterm labour and preterm premature rupture of the membranes. American Journal of Obstetrics and Gynecology 162: 486–490

Iams J D, Johnson F F, Hamer C 1990b Uterine activity and symptoms as predictors of preterm labour. Obstetrics and Gynecology 76: 42s–46s

Ingemarsson E, Ingemarrsson I, Solum T et al 1980 A one-year study of routine fetal heart rate monitoring during the first stage of labour. Acta Obstetrica et Gynaecologica Scandinavica 59: 297–300

Ingemarsson I 1976 Effect of terbutaline on premature labour: a double blind placebo controlled study. American Journal of Obstetrics and Gynecology 125: 520–524

International Neonatal Network 1993 The CRIB (Clinical risk index for babies) score: a tool for assessing initial neonatal risk and comparing performance of neonatal intensive care units. Lancet 342: 193–198

Johnston M M, Sanchez-Ramos L, Vaughn A J, Todd M W, Benrubi G I 1990 Antibiotic therapy in preterm premature rupture of membranes: a randomised, prospective, double-blind trial. American Journal of Obstetrics and Gynecology 163: 743–747

Kapatais-Zoumbos K, Chandler D K F, Barlie M F 1985 Survey of immunological A protease activity among selected species of Ureoplasmas and Mycoplasmas: specificity for host immunoglobulin. Infection and Immunity 47: 704–709

Kappy K A, Cetrulo C L, Knuppel R A 1979 Premature rupture of the membranes: a conservative approach. American Journal of Obstetrics and Gynecology 134: 655–661

Katz M, Gill P J, Newman R B 1986 Detection of preterm labour by ambulatory monitoring of uterine activity: a preliminary report. Obstetrics and Gynecology 68: 773–778

Kazzi N J, Ilagan N B, Liang K C et al 1989 Maternal administration of vitamin K does not improve the coagulation profile of preterm infants. Paediatrics 84: 1045–1050

Keirse M J N C 1989 Preterm delivery. In: Chalmers I, Enkin M, Keirse M J N C (eds) Effective care in pregnancy and childbirth. Vol 1. Pregnancy. Oxford University Press, Oxford, pp 1270–1292

Keirse M J N C 1993a Home uterine activity monitoring for preventing preterm delivery. In: Enkin M, Keirse M J N C, Renfrew M, Neilson J P (eds) Pregnancy and childbirth module. Cochrane database of systematic reviews. Update Software, Oxford (review no 06656 vol disk issue 2)

Keirse M J N C 1993b Betamimetic tocolytics in preterm labour. In: Enkin M, Keirse M J N C, Renfrew M, Neilson J P (eds) Pregnancy and childbirth module. Cochrane database of systematic reviews. Update Software, Oxford (review no 03237 vol disk issue 2)

Keirse M J N C 1993c Magnesium sulphate versus betamimetics for tocolysis in preterm labour. In: Enkin M W, Keirse M J N C, Renfrew M, Neilson J P (eds) Pregnancy and childbirth module. Cochrane database of systematic reviews. Update Software, Oxford (review no 06194 vol disk issue 2)

Keirse M J N C 1993d Oral betamimetics for maintainance after preterm labour. In: Enkin M, Keirse M J N C, Renfrew M, Neilson J P (eds) Pregnancy and childbirth module. Cochrane database of systematic reviews. Update Software, Oxford (review no 04380 vol disk issue 2)

Keirse M J N C, Rush R W, Anderson A B M, Turnbull A C 1978 Risk of preterm delivery in patients with previous preterm delivery and/or abortion. British Journal of Obstetrics and Gynaecology 85: 81–86

King J F, Grant A M, Keirse M J N C, Chalmers I 1988 Beta-mimetics in preterm labour: an overview of the randomised controlled trials. British Journal of Obstetrics and Gynaecology 95: 211–222

Kirbinen P, Joupilla P 1978 Polyhydramnios. A clinical study. Annales

Chirurgiae et Gynaecologiae Senniae 67: 117–123

Kitchen W, Ford G W, Doyle L W et al 1985 Caesarean section or vaginal delivery at 24 to 28 weeks gestation: comparison of survival and neonatal and two-year morbidity. Obstetrics and Gynecology 66: 149–157

Klebanoff M A, Shiono P H, Rhoads G G 1990 Outcomes of pregnancy in a national sample of resident physicians. New England Journal of Medicine 323: 1040–1045

Knuppel R A, Lake M F, Watson D L et al 1990 Preventing preterm birth in twin gestation: home uterine activity monitoring and perinatal nursing support. Obstetrics and Gynecology 76: 24s–27s

Kovacs L, Molnar B G, Huhn E, Bodis L 1988 Mg substitution in pregnancy: a prospective randomised double blind study. Geburtshife Frauenheilkd 48: 595–600

Kragt H, Kierse M J N C 1990 How accurate is a woman's diagnosis of threatened preterm delivery? British Journal of Obstetrics and Gynaecology 97: 317–323

Kulpa P J, White B M, Visscher R 1987 Aerobic exercise in pregnancy. American Journal of Obstetrics and Gynecology 156: 1395–1403

Kurki T, Eronen M, Lumme R et al 1991 A randomised double-dummy comparison between indomethacin and nylidrin in threatened preterm labour. Obstetrics and Gynecology 78: 1093–1097

Kurki T, Sivonen A, Renkonen O V, Savia E, Ylikorkala O 1992 Bacterial vaginosis in early pregnancy and pregnancy outcome. Obstetrics and Gynecology 80: 173–177

Lamont R F, Rose M, Elder M G 1985 Effects of bacterial products on prostaglandin E2 production by amnion cells. Lancet ii: 1131–1133

Lamont R F, Taylor-Robinson D, Wigglesworth J S, Furr P M, Evans R T, Elder M G 1987 The role of mycoplasmas, ureoplasmas, and chlamydiae in the genital tract of women presenting in spontaneously early preterm labour. Journal of Medical Microbiology 24: 253–257

Launer L J, Villar J, Kestler E et al 1990 The effect of maternal work on fetal growth and duration of pregnancy: a prospective study. British Journal of Obstetrics and Gynaecology 97: 62–70

Leffler C W, Busija C W, Fletcher A M et al 1985 Effects of indomethacin upon cerebral haemodynamics in newborn piglets. Paediatric Research 19: 1160–1164

Leveno K J, Cox K, Roark M L 1986 Cervical dilatation and prematurity revisited. Obstetrics and Gynecology 68: 434–435

Lewis D F, Major C A, Towers C V, Harding J A, Asrat T, Garite T J 1991 Effects of digital vaginal exams on latency period in preterm premature rupture of the membranes. American Journal of Obstetrics and Gynecology 164: 381

Lobb M O, Cooke R W I 1986 The influence of episiotomy on the neonatal survival and incidence of periventricular haemorrhage in the very-low-birth-weight infants. European Journal of Obstetrics, Gynaecology and Reproductive Biology 22: 17–21

Lockwood C J, Senyei A E, Dische M R et al 1991 Fetal fibronectin in cervical and vaginal secretions as a predictor of preterm delivery. New England Journal of Medicine 325: 669–674

Lockwood C J, Wein R, Lapinski R, et al 1993 The presence of cervical and vaginal fetal fibronectin predicts preterm delivery in an inner-city obstetric population. American Journal of Obstetrics and Gynecology 169: 798–804

Lopez Bernal A, Hansell D J, Khong T Y, Keeling J W, Turnbull A 1990 Placental leukotriene B4 release in early pregnancy and in term and preterm labour. Early Human Development 23: 93–99

Low J A, Karchmar J, Brockhoven L et al 1981 The probability of fetal metabolic acidosis during labour in a population at risk as determined by clinical factors. American Journal of Obstetrics and Gynecology 141: 941–951

Lumley J 1987 The epidemiology of prematurity. In: Wood E C, Yu Y H Y (eds) Prematurity. Churchill Livingstone, Edinburgh

Lumley J 1993 The epidemiology of preterm birth. Baillière's Clinical Obstetrics and Gynaecology 7: 477–498

Lumley J, Astbury J. Advice for pregnancy. In: Chalmers l, Enkin M, Keirse M J N C (eds) Effective care in pregnancy and childbirth. Vol 1. Pregnancy. Oxford University Press, Oxford, pp 237–254

Luthy D, Shy K, van Belle G et al 1987 A randomised trial of electronic fetal heart rate monitoring in preterm labour. Obstetrics and Gynecology 69: 687–695

MacArthur B A, Howie R N, Denzoete J A, Elkins J 1982 School progress and cognitive development of 6-year old children whose mothers were treated antenatally with betamethasone. Paediatrics 70: 99–105

Macfarlane A, Cole S, Johnson A, Botting B 1988 Epidemiology of birth before 28 weeks of gestation. British Medical Bulletin 44: 861–893

Main D M, Gabbe S, Richardson R et al 1985 Can preterm deliveries be prevented? American Journal of Obstetrics and Gynecology 151: 892–898

Main D M, Katz M, Chiu G et al 1988 Intermittent weekly contraction monitoring to predict preterm labour in low risk women: a blinded study. Obstetrics and Gynecology 72: 757–761

Major C A, Lewis D F, Harding J A et al 1991 Does tocolysis with indomethacin increase the incidence of necrotizing enterocolitis in the low birthweight neonate. American Journal of Obstetrics and Gynecology 164: 361

Mamelle N, Gabbe S G, Richardson D et al 1984 Prematurity and occupational activity during pregnancy. American Journal of Epidemiology 119: 309–322

Mari G, Moise K J, Deter R L et al 1989 Doppler assessment of the middle cerebral artery during constriction of the fetal ductus arteriosus after indomethacin therapy. American Journal of Obstetrics and Gynecology 161: 1528–1531

Mari G, Moise K J, Deter R L et al 1990 Doppler assessment of the renal blood flow velocity waveform during indomethacin therapy for preterm labour and polyhydramnios. Obstetrics and Gynecology 75: 199–201

McDonald H M, O'Loughlin J A, Jolley P, Vigneswaran R, McDonald P J 1991 Vaginal infection and preterm labour. British Journal of Obstetrics and Gynaecology 98: 427–435

McGregor J 1988 Prevention of preterm birth: new initiatives based on microbial–host interactions. Obstetrical and Gynecological Survey 43: 1–14

McGregor J A, Lawellin D, Franco-Buff A et al 1986 Protease production by microorganisms associated with reproductive tract infection. American Journal of Obstetrics and Gynecology 154: 109–114

McGregor J A, French J I, Lawelin D et al 1987 In vitro study of bacterial protease-induced reduction of chorioamniotic membrane strength and elasticity. Obstetrics and Gynecology 69: 167–174

McLean M, Walters W A, Smith R 1993 Prediction and early diagnosis of preterm labor: a critical review. Obstetrical and Gynecological Survey 48: 209–225

Meis P J, Ernest J M, Moore M L et al 1987 Regional program for prevention of premature birth in northwest Carolina. American Journal of Obstetrics and Gynecology 157: 550–556

Melin P 1993 Oxytocin antagonists in preterm labour and delivery. Ballière's Clinical Obstetrics and Gynaecology 7: 577–600

Mendelson C R, Alcorn J L, Gao E 1993 The pulmonary surfactant protein genes and their regulation in fetal lung. Seminars in Perinatology 17: 223–232

Mercer B M, Sklar S, Shariatmader A et al 1987 Fetal foot length as a predictor of gestational age. American Journal of Obstetrics and Gynecology 156: 350–355

Merkatz I R, Peter J B, Barden T P 1980 Ritodrine hydrochloride. A beta-mimetic agent for use in preterm labour. II. Evidence of efficacy. Obstetrics and Gynecology 56: 7–12

Meyer M 1977 Effects of maternal smoking and altitude on birth weight and gestation. In: Reed D M, Stanley F J (eds) The epidemiology of prematurity. Urban and Schwarzenberg, Baltimore, pp 81–104

Meyer M B, Tonascia J A 1977 Maternal smoking, pregnancy complications and perinatal mortality. American Journal of Obstetrics and Gynecology 128: 494–502

Meyer W R, Randall H W, Graves W L 1990 Nifedipine vs ritodrine for suppressing preterm labour. Journal of Reproductive Medicine 35: 649–653

Meyers R L, Gadalpan E, Cluman R I 1991 Patent ductus arteriosus, indomethacin and intestinal distention: effects on intestinal bloodflow and oxygen consumption. Paediatric Research 29: 569–574

Mires G J, Agustsson P, Forsyth J S, Patel N 1991 Cerebral pathology in the very low birth weight infant: predictive value of peripartum metabolic acidosis. European Journal of Obstetrics, Gynecology and Reproductive Medicine 42: 181–185

Mires G J, Owen P, Lee C P, Patel N B 1993 Electronic fetal heart rate monitoring in prematurity. In: Spencer J A D, Ward R H T (eds) Intrapartum fetal surveillance. RCOG, London, pp 95–109

Mitchell M D, Dudley D J, Edwin S S, Lundin-Schiller S 1991 Interleukin-6 stimulates prostaglandin production by human amnion and decidual cells. European Journal of Pharmacology 192: 189–191

Moise K J 1993 The effect of advancing gestational age on the frequency of fetal ductal constriction secondary to maternal indomethacin use. American Journal of Obstetrics and Gynecology 168: 1350–1353

Moise K J, Ou C-N, Kirshon B et al 1990 Placental transfer of indomethacin in the human pregnancy. American Journal of Obstetrics and Gynecology 162: 549–554

Mortensen O A, Franklin J, Lofstrand T et al 1987 Prediction of preterm birth. Acta Obstetrics Gynaecologica Scandinavica 66: 507–512

Morales W J, Angel J L, O'Brien W F, Knuppel R A, Marsalisi F 1988 The use of antenatal vitamin K in the prevention of early neonatal intraventricular haemorrhage. American Journal of Obstetrics and Gynecology 159: 774–779

Morales W J, Angel J L, O'Brien W F, Knuppel R A 1989 Use of ampicillin and corticosteroids in premature rupture of the membranes: a randomised trial. Obstetrics and Gynecology 73: 721–726

Moya F, Mena P, Foradori A et al 1991 Effect of maternal administration of thyrotropin-releasing hormone on the preterm fetal pituitary-thyroid axis. Journal of Paediatrics 119: 966–971

MRC/RCOG Working Party on Cervical Cerclage 1993 Final report of the MRC/RCOG multicentre randomised trial of cervical cerclage. British Journal of Obstetrics and Gynaecology 100: 516–523

Mueller-Heubach E, Reddick D, Barnett B et al 1989 Preterm birth prevention: evaluation of a prospective controlled randomised trial. American Journal of Obstetrics and Gynecology 160: 1172–1178

Murray J L, Bernfield M 1988 The differential effect of prenatal care on the incidence of low birth weight among Blacks and Whites in a prepaid health care plan. New England Journal of Medicine 319: 1385–1391

Nageotte M P, Casal D, Senyei A E 1994 Fetal fibronectin in patients at increased risk for premature birth. American Journal of Obstetrics and Gynecology 170: 20–25

Natale R, Nasello C, Turluik R 1984 The relationship between movement and accelerations in the fetal heart rate between 24 and 32 weeks gestation. American Journal of Obstetrics and Gynecology 148: 591–595

Neilson J P, Grant A M 1993 The randomised trials of intrapartum electronic fetal heart rate monitoring. In: Spencer J A D, Ward R H T (eds) Intrapartum fetal surveillance. RCOG, London, pp 77–93

Newton E R, Kennedy J L, Louis F et al 1987 Obstetric diagnosis and perinatal mortality. American Journal of Perinatology 4: 300–308

Niebyl J R, Blake D A, White R D, Kumor K M, Dubin N H 1980 The inhibition of labour with indomethacin. American Journal of Obstetrics and Gynecology 136: 1014–1019

Nwosu E C, Welch C R, Manasse P, Walkinshaw S A 1993 Longitudinal assessment of amniotic fluid index. British Journal of Obstetrics and Gynaecology 100: 816–819

Olsen S F, Sorensen J, Secher N J, et al 1992 Randomised controlled trial of effect of fish-oil supplementation on pregnancy duration. Lancet 339: 1003–1007

Paneth N, Kiely J L, Wallenstein S, Susser M 1987 The choice of place of delivery. Effect of hospital level on mortality in all singleton births in New York City. American Journal of Diseases of Children 141: 60–64

Papiernik E 1993 Prevention of preterm labour and delivery. Ballière's Clinical Obstetrics and Gynaecology 7: 499–522

Papiernik E, Bouyer J, Dreyfus J et al 1985 Prevention of preterm birth: a perinatal study in Haguenau, France. Paediatrics 76: 154–158

Philipsen T, Erikson P S, Lyngaard F 1981 Pulmonary edema following ritodrine-saline infusion in preterm labour. Obstetrics and Gynecology 58: 304–308

Plaut A G 1978 Microbial IgA proteases. New England Journal of Medicine 298: 1459–1462

Pomerance J J, Teal T G, Gogolok J F, Brown S, Stewart M E 1987 Maternally administered antenatal vitamin K1: effect on neonatal prothrombin activity, partial thromboplastin time, and intraventricular haemorrhage. Obstetrics and Gynecology 70: 235–241

Powell P G, Pharoah P O D, Cooke R W I 1987 How accurate are the perinatal statistics in your region? Community Medicine 9: 226–231

Prendeville W J 1993 17 Alphahydroxyprogesterone caproate in pregnancy. In: Enkin M, Keirse M J N C, Renfrew M, Neilson J P (eds) Pregnancy and childbirth module. Cochrane database of systematic reviews. Update Software, Oxford (review no 04399 vol disk issue 2)

Quatero H W P, Fry C H 1989 Placental corticotrophin releasing factor may modulate human parturition. Placenta 10: 439–445

Reece E A, Goldstein I, Pilu G, Hobbins J 1987 Fetal cerebellum growth unaffected by intrauterine growth retardation: a new parameter for prenatal diagnosis. American Journal of Obstetrics and Gynecology 157: 632–638

Reiss U, Atad J, Reuinstein I et al 1976 The effect of indomethacin in labour at term. International Journal of Obstetrics and Gynaecology 143: 369–374

Ricci J M, Hariharan S, Helfgott A, Reed K, O'Sullivan M J 1991 Oral tocolysis with magnesium chloride: a randomised controlled prospective clinical trial. American Journal of Obstetrics and Gynecology 165: 603–610

Robert M F, Neff R K, Hubell J P, Taeusch H W, Avery M E 1976 Association between maternal diabetes and respiratory distress syndrome in the newborn. New England Journal of Medicine 294: 357–360

Roberts J M 1982 Current understanding of pharmacologic mechanisms in the prevention of preterm birth. Clinical Obstetrics and Gynecology 27: 592–615

Roberts A B, Mitchell J M 1990 Direct ultrasonographic measurement of fetal lung length in normal pregnancies and pregnancies complicated by prolonged rupture of the membranes. American Journal of Obstetrics and Gynecology 163: 1560–1566

Roberts A B, Goldstein I, Romero R, Hobbins J 1991a Fetal breathing movements after preterm premature rupture of the membranes. American Journal of Obstetrics and Gynecology 164: 821–825

Roberts A B, Goldstein I, Romero R, Hobbins J C 1991b Comparison of total fetal activity measurement with the biophysical profile in predicting intra-amniotic infection in preterm premature rupture of the membranes. Ultrasound in Obstetrics and Gynecology 1: 36–39

Robson S C, Gallivan S, Walkinshaw S A, Vaughan J, Rodeck C H 1993 Ultrasonic estimation of fetal weight: use of targeted formulas in small for gestational age fetuses. Obstetrics and Gynecology 82: 359–364

Romero R, Mazor M 1988 Infection and preterm labour. Clinical Obstetrics and Gynecology 31: 553–584

Romero R, Mazor M, Wu Y K et al 1988a Infection in the pathogenesis of preterm labour. Seminars in Perinatology 12: 262–279

Romero R, Emamian M, Quintero R 1988b The value and limitations of the gram stain in the diagnosis of intraamniotic infection. American Journal of Obstetrics and Gynecology 159: 114–119

Romero R, Mazor M, Wu Y K, Avila C, Oyarzun E, Mitchell M D 1989 Bacterial endotoxin and tumour necrosis factor stimulate prostaglandin production by human decidua. Prostaglandins, Leukotrienes, and Essential Fatty Acids 37: 183–186

Romero R, Avila C, Santhanam U, Seghal P B 1990a Amniotic fluid interleukin 6 in preterm labour. Journal of Clinical Investigation 85: 1392–1400

Romero R, Jimenez C, Lohda A K 1990b Amniotic fluid glucose concentrations: a rapid and simple method for the detection of intra-amnionitis in preterm labour. American Journal of Obstetrics and Gynecology 163: 968–974

Romero R, Avila C, Brekue C A, Morotti R 1991 The role of systemic and intrauterine infection in preterm parturition. Annals of the New York Academy of Sciences 622: 355–375

Rotschild A, Ling E W, Puterman M L, Farqhuarson D 1990 Neonatal outcome after prolonged preterm rupture of the membranes. American Journal of Obstetrics and Gynecology 162: 46–52

Rush R W, Kierse M J N C, Howat P 1976 Contribution of preterm delivery to perinatal mortality. British Medical Journal 2: 965–968

Russell P 1979 Inflammatory lesions of the human placenta. I. Clinical significance of acute chorioamnionitis. American Journal of Diagnosis in Gynecology and Obstetrics 1: 127–137

Sbarra A J, Thomas G B, Cetrulo C L et al 1987 Effect of bacterial growth on the bursting pressure of fetal membranes in vitro. Obstetrics and Gynecology 70: 107–110

Schoendorf K C, Hogue C J R, Rowley D et al 1992 Mortality among infants of black as compared to white college educated parents. New England Journal of Medicine 326: 1522–1526

Shepard M J, Richards V A, Berkowitz R L et al 1982 An evaluation of two equations for predicting fetal weight by ultrasound. American Journal of Obstetrics and Gynecology 142: 47–54

Shy K, Luthy D, Bennett F et al 1990 Effects of electronic fetal heart rate monitoring as compared to periodic auscultation on neurologic development of premature infants. New England Journal of Medicine 322: 588–593

Sibai B M, Villar M A, Bray E 1989 Mg supplementation during pregnancy: a double blind randomised controlled clinical trial. American Journal of Obstetrics and Gynecology 161: 115–119

Sideris E B, Yokochi K, Van Helder T et al 1983 Effects of indomethacin and prostaglandins E2, 12 and D2 on the fetal circulation. Advances in Prostaglandin, Thromboxane Leukotriene Research 12: 477–486

Smaill F 1993 Antibiotic versus no treatment for asymptomatic bacteriuria. In: Enkin M, Keirse M J N C, Renfrew M, Neilson J P (eds) Pregnancy and childbirth module. Cochrane database of systematic reviews. Update Software, Oxford (review no 03170 vol disk issue 2)

Smolders-de-Has H, Neuvel J, Schmand B, Treffers P E, Koppe J G, Hoeks J 1990 Physical development and medical history of children who were treated antenatally with corticosteroids to prevent respiratory distress syndrome. Paediatrics 86: 65–70

Spatling L, Spatling G 1988 Mg supplementation in pregnancy: a double blind study. British Journal of Obstetrics and Gynecology 95: 120–125

Talbert R L, Bussey H I 1983 Update on calcium channel blocking agents. Clinical Pharmacology 2: 403–416

Tamura R K, Sabbagha R E 1984 Diminished growth in fetuses born preterm after spontaneous labour or rupture of the membranes. American Journal of Obstetrics and Gynecology 148: 1105–1110

Taylor J, Garite T J 1984 Premature rupture of the membranes before fetal viability. Obstetrics and Gynecology 64: 615–620

Thiagarajah S, Harbert B M, Bourgeois F J 1985 Magnesium sulfate and ritodrine hydrochloride: systemic and uterine haemodynamic effects. American Journal of Obstetrics and Gynecology 153: 666–674

Thomsen A C, Morup L, Brogaard Hansen K 1987 Antibiotic elimination of group B streptococci in urine in prevention of preterm labour. Lancet i: 591–593

Thorpe J A, Parriott J, Ferette-Smith D, Meyer B A, Cohen G R, Joynson J 1994 Antepartum vitamin K and phenobarbitol for preventing intraventricular haemorrhage in the premature newborn: a randomised double-blind, placebo controlled trial. Obstetrics and Gynecology 83: 70–76

Tulzer G, Gudmundsson S, Rotondo K M et al 1991 Acute fetal ductal occlusion in lambs. American Journal of Obstetrics and Gynecology 165: 775–778

Turnbull A C 1977 Aetiology of preterm labour. In: Anderson A (ed) Proceedings of the Fifth Study Group of the Royal College of Obstetricians and Gynaecologists. RCOG, London, pp 56–70

Tyson J, Guzick D, Rosenfield C R et al 1990 Prenatal care evaluation and cohort analyses. Paediatrics 85: 195–204

van den Berg B J, Oechsli F 1984 Prematurity. In: Bracken M B (ed) Perinatal epidemiology. Oxford University Press, Oxford, pp 69–85

Vanhaesebrouk P, Thiery M, Leroy J G et al 1988 Oligohydramnios, renal insufficiency, and ileal perforation in preterm infants after in utero exposure to indomethacin. Journal of Paediatrics 113: 738–743

Vince G S, Starkey P M, Jackson M C, Sargent I L, Redman C W 1990 Flow cytometric characterisation of cell populations in human pregnancy decidua and isolation of decidual macrophages. Journal of Immunological Methods 132: 181–189

Vintzileos A M, Campbell W A, Nochimson D J, Weinbaum P J 1985

Degree of oligohydramnios and pregnancy outcome in patients with premature rupture of the membranes. Obstetrics and Gynecology 66: 162–167

Vintzileos A M, Campbell W A, Nochimson D J, Weinbaum P J 1986a The use of the nonstress test in patients with premature preterm rupture of the membranes. American Journal of Obstetrics and Gynecology 155: 149–153

Vintzileos A M, Campbell W A, Nochimson D J, Weinbaum P J 1986b Fetal breathing as a predictor of infection in premature rupture of the membranes. Obstetrics and Gynecology 67: 813–817

Volpe J J 1992 Effect of cocaine use on the fetus. New England Journal of Medicine 327: 399–407

Walkinshaw S A, Siney C, Kidd M, Manasse P, Morrison C 1993 Outcome of pregnancy in opiate dependent women within a methadone treatment programme. In: First International Conference on Practical Obstetrics, Paris, p 156

Wang E, Smaill F 1989 Infection in pregnancy. In: Chalmers I, Enkin M, Keirse M J N C (eds) Effective care in pregnancy and childbirth. Oxford, Oxford University Press, pp 534–564

Wariyar U, Richmond S, Hey E 1989 Pregnancy outcome at 24 to 31 weeks gestation: mortality. Archives of Disease in Childhood 64: 670–677

Weiner C P, Renk K, Klugman M 1988 The therapeutic efficacy and cost-effectiveness of aggressive tocolysis for premature labor associated with premature rupture of the membranes. American Journal of Obstetrics and Gynecology 159: 216–222

Wen S W, Goldberg R L, Cutter G R, Hoffman H J, Cliver S P 1990 Intrauterine growth retardation and preterm delivery: perinatal risk factors in an indigent population. American Journal of Obstetrics and Gynecology 162: 213–218

Westgren M, Holmquist P, Svenningsen N, Ingemarsson I 1982 Intrapartum fetal monitoring in pre-term deliveries: prospective study. Obstetrics and Gynecology 60: 99–106

Westgren M, Malcus P, Svenningen N 1986 Intrauterine asphyxia and long term outcome in pre term fetuses. Obstetrics and Gynecology 67: 512–516

WHO 1977 Manual of the International Classification of Diseases, Injuries and Causes of Death, vol 1. World Health Organization, Geneva

Wilcox M A, Johnson I R, Maynard P V, Smith S J, Chilvers C E D 1993 The individualised birthweight ratio: a more logical outcome measure of pregnancy than birthweight alone. British Journal of Obstetrics and Gynaecology 100: 342–347

Young D C, Toofanian A, Leveno K J 1983 Potassium and glucose concentrations without treatment during ritodrine tocolysis. American Journal of Obstetrics and Gynecology 145: 105–106

Zanini B, Paul R H, Huey J R 1980 Intrapartum fetal heart rate: correlation with scalp pH in preterm fetuses. American Journal of Obstetrics and Gynecology 136: 43–47

Zuckerman H, Shalev E, Gilad G, Katzuni E 1984 Further study of the inhibition of premature labour by indomethacin. Part II. Double blind study. Journal of Perinatal Medicine 12: 25–29

34. Prolonged pregnancy

Linda Cardozo

Material in this chapter contains contributions from the first edition and we are grateful to the previous authors for the work done.

INTRODUCTION

Prolonged pregnancy causes anxiety and distress for many women, their families, midwives and obstetricians. The main reason for this is the risk of late intrauterine death which may occur while the baby remains in utero. Despite many trials, there is still no consensus regarding the most appropriate management of this difficult situation. Thus in many instances the decision as to whether to intervene in a prolonged pregnancy is based on tradition and emotion rather than scientific data.

DEFINITION

Terminology is confusing. A *prolonged pregnancy* exceeds 40 weeks (280 days) from known time of ovulation or conception. The expressions *postdates* and *post-term* are used synonymously to describe a pregnancy which exceeds 294 days from the last menstrual period—assuming a 28-day cycle (FIGO 1980). However, confusion exists because the term *postmaturity*, which is often used synonymously with prolonged pregnancy, actually describes the state of the baby. Postmaturity, dysmaturity and placental dysfunction all refer to an infant with clinical signs of intrauterine malnutrition which may occur at any

Table 34.1   Features of the postmaturity syndrome

Absence of vernix caseosa
Absence of lanugo hair
Abundant scalp hair
Long fingernails
Dry, cracked desquamated skin
Body length increased in relation to body weight
Alert and apprehensive facies
Meconium staining of skin and membranes

gestation (Table 34.1). Kloosterman (1979) described as postmature

every fetus that dies before or during labour or shows signs of severe fetal distress during a normal labour; whereas its development and degree of maturity would have guaranteed survival of a healthy individual, if it had been brought into the outer world at a slightly earlier date.

HISTORICAL PERSPECTIVE

As long ago as 399 BC Aristotle appreciated that the gestation period for human pregnancy varied considerably and that prolonged pregnancy was not uncommon. He wrote:

Now all other animals bring the time of pregnancy to an end in a uniform way; in other words, one single term of pregnancy is defined for each of them. But in the case of mankind alone of all animals the times are diverse for pregnancy may be of seven months duration or of eight months or of nine and still more commonly of ten (lunar) months, whilst some women go even into the eleventh month (Aristotle Works Vol II).

In 1883 a woman who was pregnant for 476 days gave birth to a boy weighing 13 lb (5.8 kg). Her last menstrual period was on 17 July 1882 with an expected date of delivery of 24 April 1883. In May 1883 she had some labour pains and these continued on and off for the next few months. In September 1883 the cervix admitted two fingers and in November 1883 she went into spontaneous labour with the forceps delivery of a male infant (Ferguson et al 1982).

Comparing prolonged human pregnancy with certain mammalian pregnancies, Mills (1970) proposed the term fetal hibernation to be applied to cases in which there was evidence of retarded fetal growth followed by resumption of normal development. This hypothesis based on clinical estimations of uterine size and duration of amenorrhoea was rejected by Campbell et al (1970) who stressed how unreliable uterine palpation is in the estimation of fetal growth, size and maturity.

NORMAL DURATION OF PREGNANCY

Not only is there dispute amongst clinicians regarding the duration of normal pregnancy but other disciplines use different starting points so care must be taken when comparisons are made. Embryologists and reproductive biologists use ovulatory age or fertilization age while clinicians calculate the estimated date of delivery from the last menstrual period.

Modern obstetricians still support Naegele's rule, which adds 280 days or 9 calender months plus 7 days to the last menstrual period (Naegele 1812). This was introduced when ovulation was thought to follow soon after menstruation; a concept which was rejected when it was realized that Orthodox Jewish women, who are barred from intercourse at this time, were extremely fertile. However, Naegele's rule is still employed although other studies have shown some variation in the mean length of gestation. (Table 34.2).

Despite the fact that more accurate methods of determining the time of ovulation and conception are now available, there still remains some debate as to the duration of normal pregnancy.

INCIDENCE

The prevalence of prolonged pregnancy is about 10% when based on the first day of the last menstrual period (Ballantyne & Brown 1922, Anderson 1972, Chalmers & Richards 1977). However, the introduction of a routine ultrasound examination in early pregnancy almost halved this to about 6% (Vorherr 1975, Grennert et al 1978, Eik-Nes et al 1984, Cardozo et al 1986). A more recent study has shown that accurate dating in early pregnancy can reduce the incidence of prolonged pregnancy to as little as 1% (Boyd et al 1988). This is important as the outcome for women whose labour is induced for *uncertain postmaturity* is significantly worse than for those with certain dates (Gibb et al 1982).

LEGAL IMPLICATIONS

A precise knowledge of gestation is important for obstetric care but also has legal implications. In such cases the plaintiff is usually the supposed father who is disputing paternity on the grounds that he had no opportunity for sexual intercourse with his wife within usually accepted limits of pregnancy duration.

In Gaskill versus Gaskill (Times Law Report 1921) the petitioner, Mr Gaskill, a soldier at the time, gave evidence that on 4 October 1918 he had sexual intercourse with his wife for the last time. He left for Salonika on 12 October 1918 and did not return to England until September 1919. On 1 September 1919 his wife gave birth to a child. The lapse of time since the husband's departure was 331 days. Dr Munroe, the doctor in charge, stated that the child weighed around 11 lb and the labour was prolonged. The only evidence of adultery was the abnormal length of pregnancy. An extract from the judgement by the Lord Chancellor summarizes the case:

No other fact or circumstance has been deduced which in the slightest degree casts any reflection upon the chastity or modesty of the respondent who has on oath denied adultery. I can only find her guilty if I come to the conclusion that it is impossible, having regard to the present state of medical knowledge and belief, that the petitioner can be the father of the child. In these circumstances I accept the evidence of the respondent and find that she has not committed adultery and accordingly dismiss the petitioner.

A more recent medicolegal trend has been observed by Freeman (Elliott & Flaherty 1984) who reported that in North America approximately 40% of cases of obstetric malpractice involved post-term pregnancies.

DIAGNOSIS OF PROLONGED PREGNANCY

In order to avoid unnecessary intervention accurate dating

Table 34.2 Average duration of pregnancy

Author	Method of assessment	Days from LMP
Naegele (1812)	LMP	280
Cary (1948)	Artificial insemination	285 (271 from conception)
Kortenoever (1950)	LMP	282
Stewart (1952)	Basal body temperature	280–284 (266–270 from conception)
Park (1968)	LMP	287–289
Guerrero & Florex (1969)	Basal body temperature	280
Nakono (1972)	LMP	278.5

LMP = last menstrual period.

Table 34.3 Methods of assessing gestational age

History	Last menstrual period
	Symptoms of pregnancy
	Nausea
	Breast tenderness
	Urinary frequency
	Vaginal discharge
	Quickening
Examination	Uterine size
	Fundal height
Investigations	Beta human chorionic gonadotrophin
	Ultrasound
	Gestational sac
	Crown–rump length
	Biparietal diameter
	Femur length
	Head circumference
	Abdominal circumference
	X-ray
	Epiphyses

is essential. The basic symptoms and signs are shown in Table 34.3.

History and examination

Anderson et al (1981a) showed that the date of a woman's last menstrual period was the best clinical predictor of the date of confinement; prediction of the actual day of delivery in women with known dates was not improved by ultrasound. In their study 71% of the women were able to recall their last menstrual period exactly; 25% could provide an approximate date and in 4% the date was completely unknown. This differs from other studies. Campbell (1974) reported a 40% incidence of suspect menstrual histories and Warsof et al (1983) a 45% incidence. Wenner & Young (1974) found that one-third of their group of women had a non-specific date of last menstrual period, and showed that in other studies between 14% and 58% of patients are uncertain of their last menstrual period. Basal body temperature charts or other symptoms and signs of ovulation, including Mittelschmerz, which has been demonstrated to be a preovulatory rather than postovulatory symptom, may also be of help (O'Herlihy et al 1980). Information on menstrual patterns, the use of ovulation-induction agents or recent discontinuation of hormonal contraception may be beneficial.

Using the last menstrual period, quickening, fetal heart tones first audible, the uterus at the level of the umbilicus and fundal height measurements, Anderson et al (1981b) developed a more comprehensive approach to the problem of gestational age (Table 34.4). In women with a known last menstrual period additional information did not improve the prediction of delivery date; however if the last menstrual period was uncertain or unknown, averaging the predicted delivery dates by several clinical

Table 34.4 Mean observed intervals to delivery date from LMP and obstetric landmarks (from 418 patients; Anderson et al 1981b)

	Mean interval to delivery (days)	SD (days)
Known LMP	284.2	14.6
Quickening	156.3	18.0
Fetal heart first audible	136.2	17.0
Uterus at umbilicus	140.8	14.9

LMP = last menstrual period.

examinations provided a prediction of delivery date as precise as if the last menstrual period had been known. This may be of particular value in late pregnancy when ultrasound is not as useful for estimating gestational age and clinical data recorded in the antenatal notes may become the main basis on which gestational age is estimated.

Quickening, defined as the date when the patient first feels fetal movements for three consecutive days, is of limited value. Traditionally quickening is said to occur some time between 16 and 20 weeks after the onset of the last menstrual period. In a prospective study of 200 patients O'Dowd & O'Dowd (1985) concluded that the range of quickening is wide, 15–22 weeks for primigravidae and 14–22 weeks for multigravidae.

Because of the wide biological variations, neither bimanual nor abdominal examination is sufficiently accurate to be useful in the estimation of gestational age. Serial estimations of fundal height with the results plotted graphically may be of benefit in the detection of intrauterine growth retardation.

Investigations

A variety of hormones have been estimated during pregnancy but the wide variation in biological norms has rendered them useless in dating a pregnancy.

Rapid enzyme immunoassay kits for the beta subunit of human chorionic gonadotrophin (hCG) are available and can detect an early pregnancy before a period has been missed. Lagrew et al (1983) measured quantitative levels of hCG in women of less than 60 days' gestation and observed only a 3.5-day mean difference between predicted and actual gestation.

Ultrasound scanning is now the best method available for dating a pregnancy. Transabdominal measurement of the gestational sac diameter was first described but was considered to be inaccurate because of inclusion of the yolk sac. Weiner (1981) showed that the definitive sonographic diagnosis of intrauterine pregnancy required the demonstration of fetal heart motion which could only be detected at 49 days' gestational age or at approximately the time of peak hCG levels (10 000–20 000 ng/ml). However, the advent of vaginal ultrasonography has enabled earlier identification of a viable pregnancy

(Timor-Tritsch et al 1988). In a series of 38 wheel-dated pregnancies these authors showed that a well-defined intrauterine gestational sac could be seen at 4 weeks and 1–4 days of menstrual age when the beta subunit of hCG was 450–750 mu/ml. They also showed that using transvaginal ultrasound, a yolk sac should be visible by 5.5 weeks and that a heart beat should be seen not later than 6.5 weeks when the crown–rump length measures 5–6 mm. Body movements appear at 8.5 weeks' gestation and discrete limb movements at 9 weeks and 2–3 days.

From around 9 weeks onwards transabdominal ultrasonic measurement of the crown–rump length can be used to predict accurately the expected date of delivery (Drumm et al 1976). At around 12 weeks the fetus develops a kyphosis and the crown–rump length measurement loses accuracy. The biparietal diameter, femur length, head circumference and abdominal circumference all become more relevant. The accuracy of pregnancy dating from 12 to 20 weeks by ultrasound is probably almost as good as that carried out earlier.

In the third trimester prediction of gestational age without prior information is more difficult. In the past radiological detection of fetal femoral and tibial epiphyses was used to confirm a clinical assessment of fetal maturity. The distal femoral epiphysis can first be detected between the 35th and 40th week and by term is present in 95% of fetuses. The proximal tibial epiphysis appears between the 37th and 42nd week and by term is present in 75% of cases.

Amniotic fluid sampling has been used to confirm fetal maturity. Measurement includes fetal fat-filled cells, amniotic creatinine, and lecithin/sphingomyelin ratios. These have fallen out of favour for not only are they invasive but also alternative methods of assessment have been developed.

AETIOLOGY

Although prolonged pregnancy is often within normal limits, several studies have attempted to identify aetiological factors.

Seasonal variation

Pronounced seasonal variations in the length of pregnancy have been demonstrated by Boe (1951); pregnancy being longer in the summer than the winter months, with an average difference of 2.5–4 days.

Improved living standards

The hypothesis that improved living standards may lead to prolonged pregnancy was raised with the knowledge that poor nutrition leads to prematurity. Boe (1951) found that since 1900 there has been a tendency for the average duration of pregnancy and size of babies to increase, but only to a minor degree. During the starvation in the Netherlands that followed the occupation the duration of pregnancy did not appreciably shorten although birthweights tended to fall (The Dutch Famine Birth Cohort Study 1993).

Hereditary and racial factors

Prolonged pregnancy tends to recur in successive pregnancies in the same woman, and the condition often runs in families. Surveys have shown a significantly shorter mean length of gestation and lower frequency of pregnancies which continue beyond 42 weeks' gestation in black than in white women (Barron & Vessey 1966, Tuck et al 1983). This difference has not been observed in Asian woman (Bissenden et al 1981, Tuck et al 1983).

Hormonal influence

Oestrogen and cortisol play a role in the initiation of labour. A defect in the pituitary–adrenal axis may be of importance in prolonged pregnancy and occurs in cases of anencephaly. However, there is little evidence of endocrinological defects in the majority of prolonged pregnancies, except in a small number of cases with placental sulphatase deficiency and congenital adrenal hyperplasia.

Placental ageing

The myth of the ageing placenta has been dispelled by Fox (1979). He demonstrated that there are no morphological features of the term or post-term placenta at either light or electron microscope level which can be considered as a manifestation of ageing. Studies have also demonstrated that total placental DNA rises in a linear fashion beyond the 40th week of gestation (Fox 1983); the placenta grows, at a decreased growth rate, during the later stages of pregnancy. The placenta is rather like the liver in that once it has reached its optimal size it shows little evidence of cell replication but retains a latent potential for growth activity. Fetal growth continues, although at a reduced velocity, after 38 weeks of pregnancy (Gruenwald 1967) and babies delivered at 42 weeks' gestation are nearly three times as likely to weigh over 4000 g compared to those delivered between 40 and 41 weeks (Boyd et al 1983).

SIGNIFICANCE OF PROLONGED PREGNANCY

Fetal implication

There is no doubt that perinatal mortality is lowest at term. It does not rise significantly until after 42 weeks' gestation and then only slightly. Clifford (1954) demonstrated the classical U-shaped curve of perinatal mortality with the nadir at 272–289 days. The perinatal mortality rate was demonstrated to be significantly increased in postmature infants but only in primigravidae and not multigravidae. Earlier, Ballantyne & Browne (1922) suggested that postmaturity was dangerous and induction of labour should be performed at or soon after term. Browne revised his position in 1957 when he studied hospital reports from 20 hospitals with a large variation in the frequency of induction of labour for prolonged pregnancy; no significant difference in mortality rates was found. Clayton (1941) noted an increase in perinatal mortality but no change occurred when analysis was restricted to babies who died for no apparent cause.

The 1958 survey of the National Birthday Trust reviewed by McClure-Browne (1963) showed significant increases in perinatal mortality after 42 completed weeks of gestation. However, the significance of oligohydramnios, intrauterine growth retardation, glucose intolerance and other causes of fetal compromise was not appreciated and antenatal tests of fetal well-being were not available. Other reports (Dawkins et al 1961) emphasized the association of hypertension in the postmature pregnancy with perinatal death; however uncomplicated postmaturity was rarely associated with death.

Butler & Bonham (1963) also analysed the National Birthday Trust study of births in Britain in 1958 and reported that the lowest perinatal mortality rate was at 40 weeks; by 44 weeks' gestation the rate had risen more than threefold. At 41 weeks the perinatal mortality was almost the same as at 40 weeks but by 42 weeks it had doubled. Performing the same calculations from the 1970 National Birthday Trust nationwide survey of births in Britain, Chamberlain et al (1970) showed the influence of postdates had changed since 1958: the perinatal mortality rate was lower at 41–42 weeks than at 39–40 weeks and at 43+ weeks was just over twice that at 39–40 weeks.

A retrospective study of perinatal mortality in term (37–41 weeks) and post-term (> 42 weeks) pregnancies delivered at the National Maternity Hospital, Dublin, between 1974 and 1981, showed that the perinatal mortality, exclusive of lethal malformations, was 5.0 per 1000 at 37–42 weeks and 9.4 per 1000 after 42 weeks (Crowley et al 1984).

The increase in perinatal mortality which may exist can be reduced by careful monitoring and selective intervention. The majority of infants born following a prolonged pregnancy have an uncomplicated perinatal course (Paterson et al 1970, Schneider et al 1978). However macrosomia may occur. Approximately 10% of all infants are born weighing more than 4000 g and 1% of infants weigh more than 4500 g (Spellacy et al 1985). The incidence of macrosomia is three- to seven-fold more frequent in prolonged pregnancy than in term deliveries. These babies are at greater risk of perinatal mortality and mor-

bidity, especially the risk of shoulder dystocia (Modanlou et al 1980).

Amniotic fluid volume deceases from approximately 37 weeks' gestation onwards (Phelan et al 1987a). During the postdates period it is estimated that there is a 33% decline in the amniotic fluid volume each week (Beischer et al 1969). Measurement of the amniotic fluid index (Phelan et al 1987b) allows the clinician to follow changes in amniotic fluid volume. Fetal heart rate patterns are affected by changes in amniotic fluid volume. Gabbe et al (1977) have shown an inverse relationship between the amniotic fluid volume and fetal heart rate decelerations. When oligohydramnios or fetal heart rate decelerations are present in postdates pregnancies there is a significantly greater likelihood of meconium-stained amniotic fluid (Rutherford et al 1987). However, in the majority of cases, meconium staining of the amniotic fluid in utero is benign (Green & Patel 1978).

Intrapartum implications

Different studies have shown a varying incidence of fetal distress in postdate infants during labour. Miller & Read (1981) and Klapholz & Friedman (1977) documented no increase in the incidence of fetal distress, whereas Freeman et al (1981) and Schneider et al (1978) demonstrated a significant increase. There is an increased incidence of meconium in post-term amniotic fluid in labour (Miller & Read 1981) which, in combination with fetal distress, may lead to a poor outcome. The incidence of meconium aspiration syndrome can be reduced by adequate suction of the respiratory tract at delivery (Carsons 1976). However, post-term fetuses may be at increased risk of meconium aspiration in utero (Freeman & Lagrew 1991). In addition prolonged pregnancy is associated with oligohydramnios which may be an indicator of poor placental reserve and may lead to cord compression and fetal compromise either antenatally or in labour.

Neonatal and childhood implications

In the past congenital malformations were increased by up to 50% in post-term pregnancies (Vorherr 1975). Infants born at term have been compared to those born post-term in a study by Field et al (1977). The post-term, postmature infants had more perinatal complications and lower motor scores at birth. At 8 months of age their daily motor scores were similar to those of control infants but their mental scores were lower. They also had more illness and feeding and sleep disturbances; however long-term follow up was not performed. An earlier study of 400 000 births found an increase in perinatal mortality, fetal distress, birth injury, meconium aspiration and congenital malformations in the postdates infant (Zwerdling 1967). Follow-up showed a continued increase in mortality among infants up to 2 years of age, although at 5 years no difference in mortality rates was noted between babies born at term and those born postdates.

The influence of prolonged pregnancy on infant development at 1 and 2 years of age following otherwise uncomplicated pregnancies, with meticulous dating, was investigated by Shime et al (1986). At 1 and 2 years the general IQ, physical milestones and intercurrent illness of normal infants and those of prolonged pregnancies were not found to be significantly different.

Maternal implications

For many women who are eagerly or anxiously awaiting the birth of their child, emotional or even psychological disturbances may be encountered if delivery does not occur at or soon after the estimated date of delivery. This may be exacerbated by poor counselling. Those women who go into spontaneous labour prior to their estimated date of delivery are fortunate as the risks to both them and their baby have been shown to increase as term progresses (Saunders & Paterson 1991); however this does not help with the management of those women whose pregnancy progresses beyond this time. Therefore the importance of accurate dating by early ultrasonic examination cannot be overstressed (Votta & Cibils 1993).

ANTENATAL MANAGEMENT

Management of prolonged pregnancy remains controversial with no right or wrong path to follow. However, postmaturity is still one of the commonest indications for induction of labour in many hospitals in the UK and USA, and has been for nearly 20 years (Chalmers & Richards 1977). Some of the dilemma is the fault of obstetricians and midwives who still give an estimated date of delivery to all women. In 1958 Wrigley wrote: 'No exact date for the onset of labour should be given and if no exact date is given then management of the condition can vary from patient to patient.'

Although induction of labour was first recommended as the best method of preventing postmaturity by Ballantyne & Brown (1922), it was not until the advent of effective methods of induction in the 1950s that induction for postmaturity became more common. The subject was hotly debated and in 1958 Gibberd wrote of 'the choice between death from postmaturity and death from induction of labour'; in 1959 Theobald replied 'the choice between death from postmaturity or prolapsed cord and life from induction of labour'.

Over thirty years ago, McClure-Browne (1963) studied 16 986 pregnancies in the National Birthday Trust Survey and demonstrated an increased fetal morbidity after 42 weeks' gestation. From these data he suggested induction of labour at 42 weeks, when the associated morbidity of

such a policy equalled that of non-intervention. Knox et al (1979), Hauth et al (1980) and Gibb et al (1982) have all shown that routine induction at 42 weeks does not improve neonatal outcome. Although several studies have shown an increase in the Caesarean section rate associated with routine induction (Vorherr 1975, Gibb et al 1982), this may be due to the technique employed for induction of labour. Studies which have employed prostaglandins in the induction process have not shown a significantly higher Caesarean section rate (Cardozo et al 1986, Papageorgiou et al 1992).

Harris et al (1983) found that in a group of well-documented 42-week pregnancies the mean cervical score was 3.6 and only 8.2% had a Bishop's score >7; they concluded that amongst patients with prolonged pregnancy the cervix tends to be unfavourable for induction. A low Bishop's score is associated with a high induction failure rate (Friedman et al 1966), which explains why routine attempts at induction when the patient has reached 42 weeks' gestation are often unsuccessful (Hauth et al 1980). It has been shown that physiological cervical ripening is a slow gradual process (Hendricks et al 1970).

Antenatal surveillance and selective induction of labour

Antenatal assessment of fetal well-being can be carried out using several methods but, unfortunately, none seems to be wholly satisfactory. The tests employed vary according to the facilities available and financial constraints. Clinical assessment based on palpation of the abdomen, symphysis–fundal height measurement and the impression of oligohydramnios give a poor prediction of fetal well-being in utero.

The recognition that reduction in maternally perceived fetal movement may precede fetal death by a day or longer (Sadousky & Yaffe 1973) led to the development of the Cardiff count to ten kick chart (Pearson & Weaver 1978). This was a popular and inexpensive method of evaluating fetal health but unfortunately it does not always predict fetal compromise in time for appropriate action to be taken, and maternal compliance may be poor. It was best used as a screening test to detect those who needed a more specific assessment of the fetal state such as antenatal cardiotocography which is still widely used to check fetal well-being in post-term pregnancy. A reactive trace can still be defined according to the criteria proposed by Everston et al (1979) as good variability (range >5 beats per minute, frequency > than 2 cycles per minute), two accelerations or fetal movements in 20 minutes and no decelerations. But a reactive trace is only a good index of fetal health at the time of the assessment. In a recent study comparing term and post-term fetal heart rate patterns using computer-assisted analysis a statistically significant decrease in the number of accelerations and a decrease in baseline variability was observed in pregnancies which had exceeded 42 weeks' gestation (Bartnicki et al 1992).

The biophysical profile as described by Manning et al (1981) is commonly employed to assess fetal well-being in utero in post-term pregnancies. The combined observations of five fetal biophysical variables (qualitative amniotic fluid volume, fetal movement, breathing, tone and limb activity) are assessed. Johnson et al (1986) reviewed 307 consecutive post-term pregnancies assessed by biophysical profile scoring. Twice-weekly scores differentiated precisely between normal fetuses and those at risk of intrauterine hypoxia. When the profile score was normal, waiting for spontaneous labour resulted in healthy neonates and a much lower Caesarean section rate (15% compared to 42% prophylactic induction). Although the biophysical profile has been shown to have a low false-negative rate (Manning et al 1990), fetal deaths do still occur within 1 week of a normal test (Watson et al 1991).

Doppler ultrasound measurements of umbilical artery flow velocity waveforms are simple to record and may differentiate between normal and high-risk pregnancies (Trudinger et al 1987). In a recent study of several biophysical measures of fetal well-being in utero, Doppler ultrasound showing absence of umbilical artery end-diastolic flow seemed to be the most sensitive predictor of the post-term fetus at risk of compromise (Pearce & McParland 1991).

Several techniques have been employed to assess amniotic fluid volume. Originally Manning et al (1980) regarded a pocket of fluid less than 1 cm in vertical diameter as abnormal. More recently the development of a four-quadrant approach to the evaluation of amniotic fluid volume has enabled oligohydramnios to be diagnosed with more precision (Phelan et al 1987a, b). By obtaining vertical diameters in each of four quadrants of the uterus, the amniotic fluid index can be calculated. An index of less than 5 cm is associated with adverse perinatal outcome (Rutherford et al 1987).

Even when fetal surveillance combines twice-weekly antenatal cardiotocography together with examination of the amniotic fluid index, fetal death occasionally unexpectedly occurs. Grubb et al (1992) studied 8038 consecutive post-term pregnancies in this way. There were nine antepartum fetal deaths and no intrapartum deaths giving a fetal mortality rate of 1.12 per 1000. A lower stillbirth rate of 0.44 per 1000 has been reported using twice-weekly biophysical profiles but an occasional death of an otherwise healthy fetus does still occur (Manning et al 1987).

Induction of labour versus serial monitoring

Even the results of prospective randomized controlled trials comparing different management regimens are at variance. There have been two such studies reported recently. Herabutya et al (1992) showed no significant difference in Caesarean section rate and perinatal mortality in a prospective randomized controlled trial of 108 women following either elective induction at 42 weeks or serial antenatal monitoring. Unfortunately greater numbers would have been required for a powerful study.

The large Canadian multicentre study (Hannah et al 1993), studied 3407 women with uncomplicated singleton pregnancies who reached 41 weeks (287 days) or more, as defined by certain dates or ultrasound scanning prior to 26 weeks' gestation. Women were assigned randomly either to induction of labour within 4 days of randomization or increased antenatal surveillance until spontaneous labour occurred (or an indication to expedite delivery arose). In this study expectant management was associated with a higher Caesarean section rate (24.5%) than induction of labour (21.2%) because of an increased incidence of fetal distress during the first stage. Unfortunately, fetal distress was undefined and may have been related to the higher incidence of meconium staining of the amniotic fluid in the non-induction group—to be expected at a later gestation. There was no difference in the incidence of meconium aspiration, one of the greatest neonatal risks of prolonged pregnancy; nor were any other differences in perinatal outcome recorded. It is interesting to note that in this large study of uncomplicated prolonged pregnancies the intervention rate (instrumental plus operative delivery) was 49% amongst those randomized to induction of labour and 51% for those who were monitored whilst awaiting spontaneous labour. In the UK this would be considered by midwives, obstetricians and mothers to be an unacceptably high level of intervention in an otherwise normal physiological process.

A recent meta-analysis of all published, randomized, controlled trials (Crowley 1991) revealed seven deaths in all reports studied, only one of which occurred in a woman in whom the intention was to induce labour. However, the author concluded that for meaningful statistics regarding perinatal mortality a study would need to recruit 30 000 women.

It is therefore impossible at present to always make absolute guidelines. Routine induction of labour at term is not appropriate; the question is when should intervention occur? Forty-three weeks' gestation has been suggested (Bergsjo et al 1989), as induction of labour at this gestation is associated with a lower incidence of failure (Augensen et al 1987). However the timing of delivery should be based on any risk factors and should be a joint decision made by the woman and her attendants. Earlier induction of labour would obviously be preferable for a 40-year-old primigravida with a long history of infertility, even following an uncomplicated pregnancy, whereas this may be inappropriate for a 25-year-old multipara.

The state of the cervix (Bishop's score) should also

be taken into account and if delivery with an unfavourable cervix is thought to be essential, in some cases it may be preferable to consider elective lower segment Caesarean section under epidural block rather than risk the need for an emergency Caesarean section under general anaesthesia in the middle of the night, as this carries a higher risk of morbidity and mortality to the mother and asphyxia to the baby. Recent data from King's College Hospital, London (Kelleher & Cardozo 1992) have revealed an unacceptable incidence of unrecognized maternal morbidity associated with Caesarean section and this may be compounded by the need for repeated operative deliveries in subsequent pregnancies. Thus we need to consider if there is anything that we can do for a woman who goes past term. It has been suggested that membrane stripping is associated with earlier spontaneous labour and no complications (McColgin et al 1990) but this is a form of intervention which many women might dislike.

In view of the controversy it is mandatory that a decision to induce or not should be shared between the woman, her partner and the obstetrician and, if possible, her views respected. Women's opinions differ. In a prospective questionnaire-based study of 500 women with uncomplicated singleton pregnancies, only 45% at 37 weeks' gestation were agreeable to expectant management after 42 weeks (Roberts & Young 1991). However, the possibility of allowing pregnancy to progress beyond 42 weeks was only raised at this late gestation in the third trimester and of course the majority of these women was expecting to deliver at 40 weeks. Thus counselling in early pregnancy, probably at the booking clinic with an explanation that pregnancy may continue well beyond the expected date of delivery, may increase the acceptance of expectant management (Choudury & Versi 1992).

There is no doubt that a certain proportion of complications associated with prolonged pregnancy can be avoided by close surveillance even if our techniques of monitoring are far from perfect.

INTRAPARTUM MANAGEMENT

Obviously the management of labour in a post-term pregnancy needs to be individualized. However, it is often difficult to tell which babies are at increased risk of hypoxia due to low fetal reserves. Lagrew & Freeman (1986) have demonstrated an increase in fetal distress in postdate pregnancies and concluded that they should all be electronically monitored from the onset of labour to delivery. In the presence of thick meconium or oligohydramnios, fetal scalp blood sampling may be indicated even with a normal fetal heart rate pattern. Oligohydramnios increases the likelihood of compression of the umbilical cord and subsequent vagal activation induces gastrointestinal peristalsis and the release of meconium. Meconium occurs in 25–43% of postdate labours

(Zwerdling 1967, Schneider et al 1978, Miller & Read 1981, Yeh & Read 1982). The management of meconium aspiration in the neonate is also contentious and has varied between chest compression at delivery; saline lavage of the airways; and prompt endotracheal suction for meconium, beyond the vocal cords, by a paediatrician immediately after delivery. None of these measures has been shown to satisfactorily avoid meconium aspiration syndrome in the neonate. Measurement of umbilical cord gases at delivery is beneficial to document neonatal condition at delivery and guide future management.

Oligohydramnios has been significantly associated with fetal distress, in part due to umbilical cord compression (Leveno et al 1984). Gabbe et al (1977) induced and then relieved cord compression by removing and then replacing amniotic fluid in Rhesus monkeys. Miyazaki & Taylor (1983) reported relief of both variable and prolonged deceleration by infusing saline solution into the uterus during labour in humans. However this technique of amnioinfusion has not gained popularity.

Two studies, both performed in Germany (Holtorff & Schmidt 1966, Schussling & Radzuweit 1968), found the prevalence of uterine inertia in labour occurring in prolonged pregnancy to be twice that reported in labour occurring at term. This has not been confirmed by Cardozo et al (1986) who found that the prevalence of abnormal labour patterns was similar in the prolonged pregnancy group to the term pregnancy group. As a total of 25% of post-term infant are born weighing more than 4 kg (Lagrew & Freeman 1986), anticipation of shoulder dystocia is important.

CONCLUSION

The occurrence of prolonged pregnancy is unfortunate and our current management is haphazard. As 66% of primigravidae deliver after the estimated date of delivery calculated from their last menstrual period, we are really providing women with inaccurate information regarding the normal timing of the birth of their child. Thus we should reconsider the need to give women an accurate expected date of delivery and perhaps it would be better to provide a range of dates covering term (from 37 completed weeks to 42 completed weeks of gestation). However, this would still mean that some women would have a prolonged pregnancy and for them and their advisers there is no clear-cut decision. As long as a baby remains in utero there is always the possibility of an occasional antenatal death of a perfectly normal fetus.

Antepartum surveillance to enable women to go into spontaneous labour requires better methods of predicting ongoing fetal well-being. It is possible that in the future Doppler blood flow measurements combined with the amniotic fluid index will prove to be a more sensitive indicator of fetal compromise. With the established tests in current use, approximately one otherwise normal fetus in 1000 prolonged pregnancies is likely to die in utero. This has to be balanced against the increased risks of intervention and especially Caesarean section in women who undergo induction of labour, especially in the pres-

ence of an unfavourable cervix. At present, the decision regarding timing of delivery in women with an otherwise uncomplicated prolonged pregnancy is still based on imperfect techniques of antenatal surveillance and techniques of induction of labour which are not always reliable.

REFERENCES

Anderson D G 1972 Postmaturity: a review. Obstetrical and Gynecological Survey 27: 65–69

Anderson H F, Johnson T R B, Barclay M L, Flora J D 1981a Gestational age assessment 1. Analysis of individual clinical observations. Obstetrics and Gynecology 139: 173–177

Anderson H F, Johnson T R B, Flora J D, Barclay M L 1981b Gestational age assessment II. Prediction from combined clinical observation. American Journal of Obstetrics and Gynecology 140: 770–774

Augensen K, Bergsjo P, Eikeland T, Askrik K, Carlgen J 1987 Randomised comparison of early versus late induction of labour in post-term pregnancy. British Medical Journal 294: 1192–1195

Ballantyne J W, Browne F J 1992 The problems of postmaturity and prolongation of pregnancy. Journal of Obstetrics and Gynaecology of the British Empire 29: 177–238

Barron S L, Vessey M P 1966 Birth weight of infants born to immigrant women. British Journal of Preventative and Social Medicine 20: 127–134

Bartnicki J, Ratanasin T, Meyenburg M, Saling E 1992 Post-term pregnancy: computer analysis of the antepartum fetal heart rate patterns. International Journal of Gynecology and Obstetrics 37: 243–246

Beischer N A, Brown J B, Towsend L 1969 Studies in prolonged pregnancy. III. Amniocentesis in prolonged pregnancy. American Journal of Obstetrics and Gynecology 103: 496–500

Bergsjo P, Gui-dan H, Su-qin Y, Zhi-zeng G, Bakketerg L S 1989 Comparison of induced versus non-induced labour in post-term pregnancy. Acta Obstetricia et Gynecologica Scandinavica 68: 683–687

Bissenden J G, Scott P H, Hallum J, Mansfield H N, Scott P, Wharton B A 1981 Racial variations in tests of fetoplacental function. British Journal of Obstetrics and Gynaecology 88: 109–114

Boe F 1951 Variations in the duration of pregnancy and in the weight of newborn infants. Acta Obstetricia et Gynecologica Scandinavica 30: 247–255

Boyd M E, Usher R H , McLean F H 1983 Fetal macrosomia: prediction, risks, proposed management. Obstetrics and Gynecology 61: 715–722

Boyd M E, Usher R H, McClem F H, Kramer M S 1988 Obstetric consequences of post maturity. American Journal of Obstetrics and Gynecology 158: 334–338

Browne F J 1957 Foetal postmaturity and prolongation of pregnancy. British Medical Journal 1: 851–855

Butler N R, Bonham D G 1963 Perinatal Mortality. The First Report of the 1958 British Perinatal Mortality Survey under the Auspices of the National Birthday Trust Fund. Livingstone, Edinburgh

Campbell S 1974 The assessment of fetal development by diagnostic ultrasound. Clinics in Perinatalogy 1: 507–519

Campbell S, Underhill R A, Beazley J M 1970 Fetal hibernation. Lancet i: 468

Cardozo L, Fysh J, Pearce J M 1986 Prolonged pregnancy: the management debate. British Medical Journal 293: 1059–1063

Carsons B S, Losey R W, Bowes W A, Simmons M A 1976 Combined obstetric and pediatric approach to prevent meconium aspiration syndrome. American Journal of Obstetrics and Gynecology 126: 712–715

Cary W H 1948 Results of artificial inseminations with an extramarital specimen (semi-adoption). American Journal of Obstetrics and Gynecology 56: 727–732

Chalmers I, Richards M 1977 Intervention and casual inference in obstetric practice. In: Chard T, Richards M (eds) Benefits and hazards of the new obstetrics. Spastics International Medical Publications, London, pp 34–61

Chamberlain G, Philipp E, Howlett K, Masters K (eds) 1970 British births 1970, vol 2, obstetric care. Heinemann Medical, London

Choudury M, Versi E 1992 Management of prolonged pregnancy—an analysis of womens attitudes before and after term. British Journal of Obstetrics and Gynaecology 99: 272

Clayton S G 1941 Foetal mortality in postmaturity. Journal of Obstetrics and Gynaecology of the British Empire 48: 450–460

Clifford S H 1954 Postmaturity with placental dysfunction. Clinical syndrome and pathological findings. Journal of Pediatrics 44: 1–13

Crowley P 1991 Elective induction at 41 weeks gestation. In: Chalmers I (ed) Oxford database of perinatal trials. Version 1.2 disk issue 5, record 4144. Oxford University Press, Oxford

Crowley P, O'Herlihy C, Boylan P 1984 The value of ultrasound measurement of amniotic fluid volume in the management of prolonged pregnancies. British Journal of Obstetrics and Gynaecology 91: 444–448

Dawkins M J R, Martin J D, Spector W G 1961 Intrapartum asphyxia. Journal of Obstetrics and Gynaecology of the British Commonweath 68: 604–610

Drumm J E, Clinch J, MacKenzie G 1976 The ultrasonic measurement of fetal crown rump length as a method of assessing gestational age. British Journal of Obstetrics and Gynaecology 83: 417–421

The Dutch Famine Birth Cohort Study 1993 Designed validation of exposure and selected characteristics of subjects after 45 years follow up. Paediatric and Perinatal Epidemiology 7: 354–367

Eik-Nes S H, Okland O, Aure J C, Ulstein M 1984 Ultrasound screening in pregnancy: a randomised controlled trial. Lancet i: 1347–1349

Elliott J P, Flaherty J F 1984 The use of breast stimulation to prevent postdate pregnancy. American Journal of Obstetrics and Gynecology 149: 628–632

Everston L R, Gauthier R J, Schifrin B S, Paul R H 1979 Antepartum fetal heart rate testing. Evolution of the non stress test. American Journal of Obstetrics and Gynecology 133: 29–33

Ferguson I L C F, Taylor R W, Watson M 1982 Records and curiosities in obstetrics and gynaecology. Baillière Tindall, London

Field T M, Dabiri C, Hallock N, Shuman H H 1977 Developmental effects of prolonged pregnancy and the postmaturity syndrome. Journal of Paediatrics 90: 836–839

FIGO 1980 International classification of diseases. International Journal of Gynaecology and Obstetrics 17: 634–640

Fox H 1979 The placenta as a model for organ ageing. In: Beaconsfield P, Villee C (eds) Placenta—a neglected experimental animal. Pergamon, Oxford, pp 351–378

Fox H 1983 Placental pathology. In: Studd J (ed) Progress in obstetrics and gynaecology, vol 3. Churchill Livingstone, Edinburgh, pp 47–56

Freeman R K, Lagrew D C 1991 Prolonged pregnancy in obstetrics. In: Gabbe S G, Niebyl J R, Sampson J I (eds) Normal and problem pregnancies, 2nd edn. Churchill Livingstone, New York, pp 945–956

Freeman R K, Garite T J, Mondanlou H, Dorchester W, Rommall C, Devaney M 1981 Post date pregnancy: utilization of contraction stress testing for primary fetal surveillance. American Journal of Obstetrics and Gynecology 140: 128–135

Friedman E A, Niswander K R, Bayonet-Rivera N P, Sachtleben M R 1966 Relations of prelabor evaluation in inducibility and the course of labor. Obstetrics and Gynecology 28: 495–501

Gabbe S G, Ettinger B B, Freeman R K, Makrhn C B 1977 Umbilical cord compression associated with amniotomy: laboratory observations. American Journal of Obstetrics and Gynecology 126: 353–355

Gibb D M F 1985 Prolonged pregnancy. In: Studd J (ed) The management of labour. Blackwell Science, Oxford, pp 108–122

Gibb D M F, Cardozo L D, Studd J W W, Cooper D J 1982 Prolonged pregnancy: is induction of labour indicated? A prospective study. British Journal of Obstetrics and Gynaecology 89: 292–925

Gibberd G F 1958 The choice between death from post-maturity and death from induction of labour. Lancet i: 64–66

Green J W, Patel R H 1978 The value of amniocentesis in prolonged pregnancy. Obstetrics and Gynecology 51: 293–298

Grennert L, Persson P H, Genuser G 1978 Benefits of ultrasonic screening of a pregnant population. Acta Obstetricia et Gynecologica Scandinavica 78(suppl): 5–14

Grubb D K, Rbello Y A, Paul R H 1992 Post-term pregnancy: fetal death rate with antepartum surveillance. Obstetrics and Gynecology 79: 1024–1026

Gruenwald P 1967 Growth of the human fetus. In: McLaren A (ed) Advances in reproductive physiology, vol 2. Logos Press, London, pp 279–309

Guerrero R, Florex P E 1969 Duration of pregnancy. Lancet ii: 268–269

Hannah M G, Hannah W J, Hellman J, Hewqson S, Milner R, Willan A 1993 Induction of labor as compared with serial antenatal monitoring in post-term pregnancy– a randomised controlled trial. New England Journal of Medicine 326: 1587–1592

Harris B A, Huddleston J F, Sutlitt G, Perlis H W 1983 The unfavourable cervix in prolonged pregnancy. Obstetrics and Gynecology 62: 171–174

Hauth J C, Goodman M T, Gilskap L C, Gilskap J E 1980 Post term pregnancy I. Obstetrics and Gynecology 56: 467–469

Hendricks C H, Brenner W E, Kraus G 1970 Normal cervical dilatation pattern in late pregnancy and labor. American Journal of Obstetrics and Gynecology 106: 1065–1082

Herabutya Y, Prasertsawat P O, Tongyai T, Isarangura N A, Ayudthya N 1992 Prolonged pregnancy: the management dilema. International Journal of Obstetrics and Gynecology 37: 253–358

Holtorff J, Schmidt H 1966 Die verlangerte Schwangerschaft und ihr Einfluss auf das Schicksal des Kindes. Zentralblatt fur Gynaekologie 88: 441–449

Johnson J M, Harman C R, Lange I R, Manning F A 1986 Biophysical profile scoring in the management of the post term pregnancy—an analysis of 307 patients. American Journal of Obstetrics and Gynecology 154: 269–273

Kelleher C, Cardozo L D 1992 Caesarean section—unrecognised morbidity. In: Proceedings of the 26th British Congress of Obstetrics and Gynaecology, Manchester

Klapholz H, Friedman E A 1977 Incidence of intrapartum fetal distress with advancing gestational age. American Journal of Obstetrics and Gynecology 127: 405–407

Kloosterman G J 1979 Epidemiology of postmaturity. In: Keirse M J N C, Anderson A B M, Bennebroek Gravenhorst J P (eds) Human parturition. Martinus Nijoff, The Hague, pp 247–261

Knox G E, Huddleston J F, Flowers C E, Eubanks A, Sutliffe G 1979 Management of prolonged pregnancy: results of a prospective randomised trial. American Journal of Obstetrics and Gynecology 134: 376–384

Kortenoever M E 1950 Pathology of pregnancy: pregnancy of long duration and post mature infant. Obstetrical and Gynecological Survey 5: 812–814

Lagrew D C, Freeman R K 1986 Management of post date pregnancy. American Journal of Obstetrics and Gynecology 154: 8–13

Lagrew D C, Wilson E A, Jawad M J 1983 Determination of gestation age by serum concentration of human chorionic gonadotrophin. Obstetrics and Gynecology 61: 37–40

Leveno K J, Quirk J G, Cunningham F G et al 1984 Prolonged pregnancy. I. Observations concerning the causes of fetal distress. American Journal of Obstetrics and Gynecology 150: 465–473

Manning F A, Platt L D, Sipoz L 1980 Antepartum fetal evaluation: development of a fetal biophysical profile. American Journal of Obstetrics and Gynecology 136: 787–790

Manning F A, Baskett T F, Morrison I, Lange I 1981 Fetal biophysical profile scoring: a prospective study in 1184 high risk patients. American Journal of Obstetrics and Gynecology 140: 289–294

Manning F, Morrison I, Harman C R, Lange I, Menticoglu S 1987 Fetal assessment based on fetal biophysical profile scoring: experience in 19 221 referred high risk pregnancies X1. An analysis of false negative fetal deaths. American Journal of Obstetrics and Gynecology 157: 880–884

Manning F, Morrison I, Herman C, Menticoglou S 1990 The abnormal biophysical profile score V. Predictive accuracy according to score composition. American Journal of Obstetrics and Gynecology 162: 918–927

McClure-Browne J C 1963 Postmaturity. American Journal of Obstetrics and Gynecology 85: 573–582

McColgin S W, Hampton H C, McCaul J F, Howard P R, Andrew M E, Morrison J C 1990 Stripping membranes at term: can it safely reduce the incidence of post-term pregnancies? Obstetrics and Gynecology 76: 678–680

Miller F C, Read J A 1981 Intrapartum assessment of the postdates fetus. American Journal of Obstetrics and Gynecology 141: 516–520

Mills W G 1970 Fetal hibernation? Lancet i: 334–336

Miyazaki F S, Taylor N A 1983 Saline amnioinfusion for relief of variable or prolonged decelerations. A preliminary report. American Journal of Obstetrics and Gynecology 126: 670

Modanlou H K, Dorchester W L, Thorosian A, Freeman R K 1980 Macrosomia: maternal, fetal and neonatal implications. Obstetrics and Gynecology 55: 420–423

Naegele F C 1812 Erfahrung und Abhandlungen des weiblichen Geslechter, Mannheim

Nakano R 1972 Post term pregnancy Acta Obstetricia et Gynecologica Scandinavica 51: 217–222

O'Dowd M J, O'Dowd T M 1985 Quickening—a re-evaluation. British Journal of Obstetrics and Gynaecology 92: 1037–1039

O'Herlihy C, Robinson H P, de Crespigny L J 1980 Mittelschmerz is a preovulatory symptom. British Medical Journal 280: 986

Papageorgiou I, Tsionou C, Minaretzis D, Michalas S, Aravatinos D 1992 Labor characteristics of uncomplicated prolonged pregnancies after induction with intracervical prostaglandin E_2 gel versus intravenous oxytocin. Gynecological and Obstetric Investigation 34: 92–96

Park G L 1968 The duration of pregnancy. Lancet ii: 1388–1389

Paterson P J, Dunstan M K, Trickey N R A, Beard R W 1970 A biochemical comparison of the mature and postmature fetus and newborn infant. Journal of Obstetrics and Gynaecology of the British Commonwealth 77: 390–397

Pearce J M, McParland P J 1991 A comparison of Doppler flow velocity wave forms, amniotic fluid columns and non-stress test as a means of monitoring post date pregnancies. Obstetrics and Gynecology 77: 204–208

Pearson J F, Weaver J B 1978 Fetal activity and fetal wellbeing: an evaluation. British Medical Journal 1: 1305–1307

Phelan J P, Ahn M O, Smith C V et al 1987a Amniotic fluid index measurements during pregnancy. Journal of Reproductive Medicine 32: 601–604

Phelan J P, Smith C V, Broussard P, Sucell M 1987b Amniotic fluid volume assessment with the four quadrant technique at 36–42 weeks gestation. Journal of Reproductive Medicine 32: 540–543

Roberts L J, Young K R 1991 The management of prolonged pregnancy—an analysis of womens attitudes before and after term. British Journal of Obstetrics and Gynaecology 98: 1102–1106

Rutherford S E, Phelan J P, Smith C V et al 1987 The four quadrant assessment of amniotic fluid volume: an adjunct to antepartum fetal heart rate testing. Obstetrics and Gynecology 70: 353–356

Sadousky E, Yaffe H 1973 Daily fetal movement recording and fetal prognosis. Obstetrics and Gynecology 41: 845–850

Saunders N, Paterson C 1991 Effect of gestational age on obstetric performance: when is 'term' over? Lancet 338: 1190–1192

Schneider J M, Olson R W, Curet L B 1978 Screening for fetal and neonatal risk in post date pregnancy. American Journal of Obstetrics and Gynecology 131: 473–478

Schussling G, Radzuweit H 1968 Ubertragung in der Schwangerschaft. Zentralblatt fur Gynaekologie 49: 143–147

Shime J, Librach C L, Gare D J, Cook C 1986 Influence of prolonged pregnancy on infant development at 1 and 2 years of age. A prospective controlled study. American Journal of Obstetrics and Gynecology 154: 341–345

Spellacy W N G, Miller M S, Winegar A et al 1985 Macrosomia: maternal characteristics and infant complications. Obstetrics and Gynecology 66: 158–161

Stewart H L 1952 Duration of pregnancy and postmaturity. Journal of the American Medical Association 148: 1079–1083

Theobald G W 1959 The choice between death from postmaturity or prolapsed cord and life from induction of labour. Lancet i: 59–66

Timor-Tritsch I E, Farine D, Rosen M G 1988 A close look at early embryonic development with the high frequency transvaginal transducer. American Journal of Obstetrics and Gynecology 159: 676–681

Times Law Reports 1921 Gaskill v Gaskill 1921, 12 August, p 977

Trudinger B J, Cook C M, Giles W B, Connelly A, Thompsom R S 1987 Umbilical artery flow velocity waveforms in high risk pregnancy. Randomised controlled trial. Lancet i: 188–190

Tuck S M, Cardozo L D, Studd J W W, Gibb D M, Cooper D J 1983 Obstetric characteristics in different racial groups. British Journal of Obstetrics and Gynaecology 90: 892–897

Vorherr H 1975 Placental insufficiency in relation to post-term pregnancy and fetal post-maturity. American Journal of Obstetrics and Gynecology 123: 67–105

Votta R A, Cibils L A 1993 Active management of prolonged pregnancy. American Journal of Obstetrics and Gynecology 168: 557–563

Warsof S L, Pearce J M, Campbell S 1983 The present place of routine ultrasound screening. Clinics in Obstetrics and Gynaecology 10: 445–458

Watson W, Katz V, Bowen W 1991 Fetal death after normal biophysical profile. American Journal of Perinatalogy 8: 94–96

Weiner C P 1981 The pseudogestation sac in ectopic pregnancy. American Journal of Obstetrics and Gynecology 139: 959–961

Wenner W, Young E B 1974 Nonspecific date of last menstrual period. An indication of poor reproductive outcome. American Journal of Obstetrics and Gynecology 120: 1071–1079

Wrigley A J 1958 Postmaturity. Lancet i: 1167–1168

Yeh S Y, Read J A 1982 Management of post term pregnancy in a large obstetric population. Obstetrics and Gynecology 60: 282–287

Zwerdling M A 1967 Factors pertaining to prolonged pregnancy and its outcome. Pediatrics 40: 202–212

35. Abnormal uterine action

Philip J. Steer

Uterine action in labour is variously considered to be abnormal if it falls into one of the following categories:

1. *Hypotonic:* too little.
2. *Hypertonic:* too much.
3. *Incoordinate:* abnormal in pattern.
4. *Inefficient:* not associated with progressive cervical dilatation.

Of these, the first, third and fourth are often associated. Incoordinate contractions (irregular in shape and timing) are probably of no significance unless they are also hypotonic (Turnbull 1957, Seitchik & Chatkoff 1977). Hypertonic uterine action is a special case and will be considered separately.

THE NORMAL LEVEL OF UTERINE ACTIVITY IN LABOUR

Uterine action cannot be categorized as hypotonic or hypertonic without knowledge of the normal levels of uterine action; there is no precise agreement about these. Variations will depend to a considerable extent on the population studied. The rate of cervical dilatation in labour is directly proportional to the level of uterine action (i.e. higher levels of uterine activity are associated with higher rates of cervical dilatation; Steer et al 1984).

Hence, the selection for study of women progressing rapidly in labour (often described arbitrarily as normal) is likely to result in a higher mean level of observed uterine activity than if a total unselected population sample is studied. The rate of cervical dilatation is also inversely proportional to the resistance to progress, a hypothetical concept which involves pelvic and fetal size, presentation, and consistency of the soft tissues and cervix (Rossavik 1978, Arulkumaran et al 1985, Steer et al 1985). For any particular level of uterine activity, the higher the resistance, the slower is the rate of cervical dilatation. Therefore, if women are short and have large babies so that their resistance to progress is high, for a particular rate of cervical dilatation they will have a higher level of uterine activity than women with a low resistance, for example, grand multiparae (Al-Shawaf et al 1987). Thus to enable true comparison of results, researchers should quote values of uterine action in relation to groups specified in terms of parity, height, birthweight and rate of cervical dilatation. Most reported studies lack this type of information and thus are difficult to compare with each other. However, despite their lack of precise comparability, a number of important conclusions can be drawn from the reported data (Fig. 35.1).

Firstly, uterine action increases by about 50% as labour progresses. Secondly, mean uterine activity levels fall somewhere between 1000 and 1500 kPas/15 min or 130–200 Montevideo units (see Ch. 29). Most studies give a similar distribution around the mean value such that the 10th percentile is about 700 kPas/15 min and the 90th percentile is about 1800 kPas/15 min. By analogy with other distributions (such as birthweight) where the 10th and 90th percentiles are used as the boundaries of normality, it seems reasonable to designate levels < 700 kPas/15 min as hypotonic and > 1800 kPas/15 min as hypertonic.

The individual components of uterine activity

The three terms used to describe the main components of a uterine contraction are basal tonus, active pressure

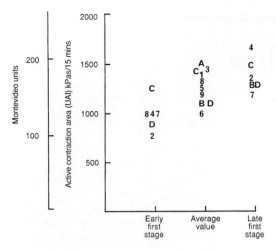

Fig. 35.1 Normal levels of uterine activity in spontaneous labour.
1 = Zambrana et al (1960); 2 = Poseiro & Noriega-Guerra (1961);
3 = Cibils & Hendricks (1965); 4 = El Sahwi et al (1967); 5 = Krapohl
et al (1970); 6 = Mendez-Bauer et al (1975); 7 = Pontonnier et al
(1975); 8 = Lindmark & Nilsson (1977); 9 = Flynn et al (1978);
A = Cowan et al (1982); B = Steer et al (1984); C = Gibb et al (1984);
D = Arulkumaran et al (1984).

(peak pressure above basal tonus) and frequency. The shape of the contraction can also be described.

The reported range of normal baseline tonus varies from 0.8 to 2.6 kPa (5–20 mmHg) depending on the measuring technique used (external pressure transducer connected to a fluid-filled intrauterine catheter or internal catheter-tipped pressure transducer) and the position of the transducer relative to the upper level of amniotic fluid within the uterus (see Ch. 29). Values greater than 3 kPa are likely to represent hypertonus and will compromise maternal blood flow into the placenta, resulting in fetal hypoxia.

The rate of cervical dilatation is more closely related to the mean active pressure of contractions than any of the other variables (Richardson et al 1978). Active pressure needs to be at least 2 kPa to produce progressive cervical dilatation and contractions are most efficient above 3.5 kPa (Caldeyro et al 1950). Mean active pressure averaged over the active phase of labour is approximately 5 kPa (SD 1.3: 40 mmHg, SD 10), rising to 6.3 kPa in the late first stage (Alvarez & Caldeyro 1950, Krapohl et al 1970, Pontonnier et al 1975, Steer et al 1984). Fetal oxygen supply, on the other hand, is related more to the frequency and duration of contractions and to basal tonus (Martin 1965, Brotanek et al 1969, Morishima et al 1975, Novy et al 1975). The mean frequency averaged over the active phase of labour is 4/10 minutes (SD 1.1), rising to a mean of about 5/10 minutes in the late first stage (Alvarez & Caldeyro 1950, Krapohl et al 1970, Pontonnier et al 1975, Steer et al 1984). The duration of contractions however is remarkably constant throughout labour in any particular individual, normally ranging between 70 and 90 seconds (Krapohl et al 1970, Pontonnier et al 1975).

HYPOTONIC UTERINE ACTIVITY

Most cases of slow progress in labour are associated with hypotonic uterine activity and are therefore likely to respond to oxytocics (Steer et al 1985). This suggests that in most cases there is not an inherent defect in the ability of the uterus to contract but that uterine contractility is at an early stage of its evolution. Such a conclusion is supported by the report of Hemminki et al (1985) who showed that 83% of women progressing slowly in labour subsequently developed normal levels of uterine activity when managed expectantly (ambulation was encouraged) rather than being given oxytocics. A similar evolution of activity was seen in women progressing slowly in labour and nursed in the lateral recumbent position with epidural anaesthetic rather than being ambulant (Bidgood & Steer 1987).

However, in a few cases, hypotonic uterine activity fails to respond to oxytocics. It has long been suggested that in some cases this is due to the suppression of uterine activity by the autonomic nervous system. Bourne & Burn noted in 1927 that 'the effect of emotion appears to be to delay the uterine contractions in labour', and since they considered one of the main effects of emotion to be the stimulation of the sympathetic nervous system, they investigated the effects of injections of adrenaline into labouring patients. They demonstrated that the intravenous injection of 5 minims of adrenaline produced complete cessation of uterine contractions for 12 minutes, following which the contractions began again. They also observed that the administration of hypnotics to the labouring mother sometimes produced a marked increase in uterine activity. They suggested that 'the augmentor action of hypnotics such as chloral may in part be due to the depression by these hypnotics of inhibitory impulses passing from the brain centres of anxious or emotional patients to the uterus by way of the sympathetic supply'.

The inhibitory effects of adrenaline on uterine activity were confirmed by Kaiser & Harris (1950). They monitored uterine activity with the Reynolds multichannel tocodynamometer. In large doses (such as to have unacceptably severe side-effects) adrenaline stimulated the uterus. However, in lower concentrations which had no demonstrable systemic effect, they found that adrenaline was 'strikingly inhibitory' to uterine activity. They also noted that 'in difficult labour there is a state of emotional stress which may well induce excessive secretion of endogenous adrenaline'. They considered that the disordered patterns of uterine activity involved in inertial labour resembled in many respects that induced by exogenous adrenaline: 'Systemic sedation and nerve-conduction blocks may in some cases shorten the length of labour by allaying apprehension'.

A similar theme was pursued by Arthur & Johnson (1952). They compared the outcome in 22 cases of prolonged labour treated with caudal anaesthesia with 26 controls. The mean duration of labour in the test group was 51 hours with a 14% Caesarean section rate, compared with 66 hours and a 50% Caesarean section rate in the controls. They attributed the difference to an improvement in uterine activity produced by the analgesia. Similar claims have been made for epidural anaesthesia (Moir & Willocks 1967).

Caldeyro-Barcia et al have claimed that an improvement in incoordinate activity can be produced by spinal anaesthesia (Caldeyro et al 1950) and also by hypnotic sleep (Caldeyro-Barcia & Alvarez 1952).

Jeffcoate (1963) recommended the use of intravenous morphine or pethidine to treat incoordinate uterine activity, and reported an example of improvement in the pattern of uterine activity and the rate of cervical dilatation following an intravenous infusion of pethidine.

An illustrative example of the apparent augmentor action of a hypnotic observed by the author is shown in Figure 35.2. A primigravida was admitted to the labour ward complaining of painful contractions, one every 3 minutes. A vaginal examination revealed ruptured membranes, and a cervix that was fully effaced but only 2 cm dilated. A further examination 4 hours later showed the cervix to be only 3 cm dilated and because of the slow progress an oxytocin infusion was commenced. Four hours later the infusion rate had reached 12 mU/min, without any obvious effect on uterine activity or cervical dilatation. External tocography showed apparently normal contractions (Fig. 35.2a). In view of the lack of progress, the oxytocin infusion rate was increased again, reaching 20 mU/min after a further 4 hours. At this point the cervix had reached only 5 cm dilatation and an intrauterine catheter was inserted. This showed the typical pattern of incoordinate uterine activity (Fig. 35.2b). Instead of a contraction wave originating at the pacemaker site (which is usually one or other uterine cornu) and propagating progressively down the uterus towards the cervix (fundal dominance; Caldeyro et al 1950), various parts of the uterus contract independently at irregular intervals (Calder et al 1950). An external tocograph placed over a particular part of the uterus may show a deflection indistinguishable from a normal contraction whenever that part contracts. However, the intrauterine pressure reflects the sum of activity in the whole uterus, and therefore shows the weak and irregular pressure rises which occur when the muscle fibres of the uterus fail to act in unison.

Because oxytocin had manifestly failed to correct the abnormal contraction pattern, a hypnotic dose of pethidine (150 mg) was administered intramuscularly. By about an

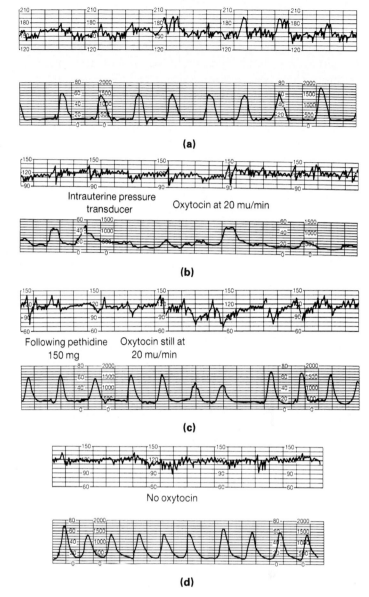

(a)

Intrauterine pressure transducer   Oxytocin at 20 mu/min

(b)

Following pethidine   Oxytocin still at
150 mg   20 mu/min

(c)

No oxytocin

(d)

Fig. 35.2 (a)–(d) An example of hypotonic incoordinate labour, resistant to oxytocin infusion but apparently responding to maternal sedation with pethidine.

hour later (Fig. 35.2c), the contractions had improved to such an extent that a fetal bradycardia developed and the oxytocin had to be turned off. Uterine activity continued at a normal level without further oxytocic stimulation (Fig. 35.2d), and a normal delivery occurred 6 hours later.

Mitrani et al (1975) hypothesized that since adrenaline exerts its suppressive effect on uterine activity via the uterine muscle beta-receptors, a beta-blocker such as propranolol could be used to treat incoordinate activity. They treated 10 primigravidae in dysfunctional labour with intravenous propranolol at the rate of 1 mg/min for 4 minutes. The authors observed a marked increase in uterine activity in all cases; in two cases there was tachysystole with hypertonus sufficient to produce fetal bradycardia. This interesting observation has never been repeated, nor have systematic studies of the effect of hypnotics on dysfunctional labour been carried out using modern techniques for recording uterine activity. This partly reflects the difficulty of studying a relatively uncommon event, and partly the current emphasis on oxytocics as the primary treatment for dysfunctional labour. This latter emphasis can largely be attributed to the work of O'Driscoll and his colleagues at the National Maternity Hospital in Dublin. For example, in 1969 O'Driscoll et al wrote:

> no distinction was made in the present series between hypotonic and hypertonic uterine activity and oxytocin proved equally effective in both circumstances. This is completely at variance with the experience of Jeffcoate, who found that oxytocin often makes matters worse when given in labour complicated by incoordinate activity. It is our experience that the correct treatment of incoordinate action is to increase the rate of oxytocin infusion and not the dose of analgesic drugs.

The resolution of this dispute awaits further study.

HYPERTONIC UTERINE ACTIVITY

Spontaneous uterine hypercontractility without placental abruption is rare, probably occurring in not more than one in 3000–4000 pregnancies. Most cases of hypoxia in labour are due to intrauterine growth retardation with consequent inability of the fetus to withstand the normal stress of labour, rather than excessive uterine activity (Lissauer & Steer 1986). Nonetheless, cases of excessive uterine activity without obvious causes are sometimes seen. There is no evidence that an unusually high active pressure of contractions (i.e. above 12 kPa) is associated with any clinical problem; an increase in any of the other three contraction variables above normal levels, however, may lead to problems with fetal oxygen supply.

Duration

Figure 35.3 illustrates a case of spontaneous labour where the duration of contractions averaged 120 seconds. Frequency and baseline tone were normal. Figure 35.3a shows small decelerations synchronous with contractions which became larger 2 hours later (Fig. 35.3b). After a further 2 hours (Fig. 35.3c) the decelerations became prolonged and a fetal blood sample showed a pH of 7.15. Delivery was effected by Caesarean section as the cervix was still only 6 cm dilated. Frequency and basal tonus remained normal throughout.

Frequency

Figure 35.4 illustrates a case of spontaneous labour

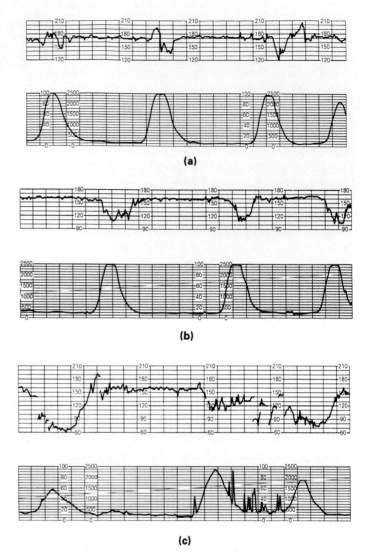

Fig. 35.3   (a)–(c) An example of spontaneous uterine hypercontractility—prolonged duration of contractions.

where contraction frequency became excessive without obvious cause (the traces illustrated form a continuous sequence). Contraction frequency was normal initially (Fig. 35.4a) but as contractions increased to six every 10 minutes, early fetal heart rate (FHR) decelerations appeared (Fig. 35.4b). As the frequency increased to seven every 10 minutes, the decelerations became larger (Fig. 35.4c). Eventually intrauterine pressure failed to return to a normal tonus between contractions and a persistent fetal bradycardia developed (Fig. 35.4d). A slow intravenous infusion of salbutamol (150 µg) was given with immediate reduction in the frequency and active pressure of contractions, and recovery of the FHR. The contractions then continued to be normal until the second stage (Fig. 35.4e), when some mild hypertonus recurred. However, a healthy infant was born after only 15 minutes in the second stage.

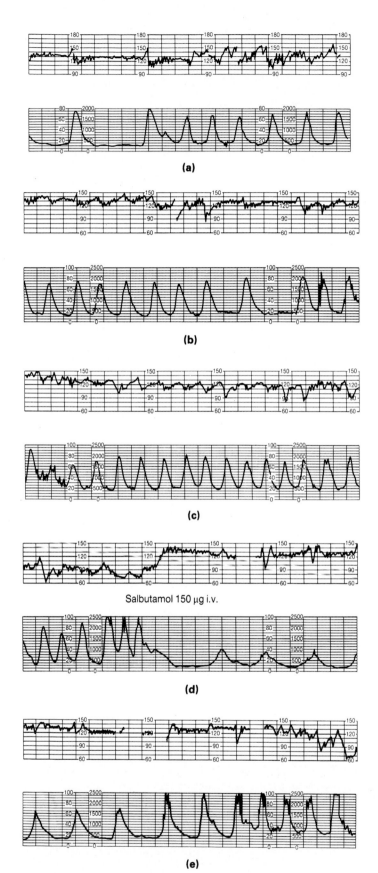

Fig. 35.4　(**a**)–(**e**) An example of spontaneous uterine hypercontractility—excessive frequency of contractions.

Salbutamol 150 μg i.v.

Hypertonic uterine action with placental abruption

Placental abruption occurs in about one in 100 pregnancies, and is severe enough to kill the fetus in one in every eight cases (Pritchard et al 1985). Death may occur due to extensive placental separation but in many cases the excessive uterine activity produced by the massive release of prostaglandins from the disrupted decidua is also a major factor. Odendaal in 1976 drew attention to the high mean frequency of contractions seen in association with abruption. Mean contraction frequency recorded in 37 studied cases was 7.9 in 10 minutes, with some occurring as often as 16 in 10 minutes.

The importance of excessive contraction frequency as a sign in the diagnosis of abruption was emphasized by Saunderson & Steer in 1978. They pointed out that the high frequency of contractions meant that associated late decelerations could be misinterpreted as increased baseline variability, or a reduced baseline rate with accelerations. Such a case is shown in Figure 35.5. The contractions were recorded with an external tocodynamometer, so true baseline tone is not shown. In the initial half of the tracing, without careful synchronization of the FHR changes with the contractions it would be easy to interpret it as showing a baseline FHR of 125 beats/min with frequent accelerations. In the latter half of the tracing, however, the reduced baseline variability and the increasing amplitude of the late decelerations make the correct diagnosis more obvious. Figure 35.6 shows a similar case with intrauterine pressure recording, using a Gaeltec catheter-tipped pressure transducer (see Ch. 29).

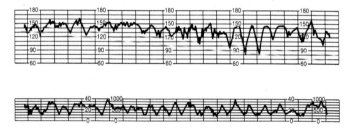

Fig. 35.5　Uterine hypercontractility associated with placental abruption, recorded with an external tocodynamometer.

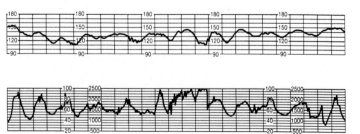

Fig. 35.6　Uterine hypercontractility associated with placental abruption, recorded with a catheter-tip pressure transducer.

The initial baseline tone is set rather high, at 25 mmHg; however, the subsequent rise of baseline tone by 25 mmHg to 50 mmHg, the abnormal contraction pattern, and the excessive frequency of contractions are all typical of abruption. The FHR is grossly abnormal, with loss of variability and late decelerations. The baby was delivered by emergency Caesarean section with a cord artery pH of 6.98; however, it made a good long-term recovery.

Hyperstimulation with oxytocics

One of the commonest causes of uterine hyperactivity in modern clinical practice is the use of oxytocics. Bourne & Burn warned against the careless use of oxytocin in 1927 and Liston & Campbell echoed their warnings in 1974. The use of oxytocin at infusion rates up to 40 mU/min is associated with a uterine hyperstimulation rate of 30–40% (Caldeyro-Barcia et al 1957, Seitchik & Castillo 1982, Arulkumaran et al 1987, Bidgood & Steer 1987, Mercer et al 1991). The more physiological school advocates measuring uterine activity by direct measurement of the pressure achieved during contractions and only giving oxytocin if there is a demonstrable deficiency in the strength of the contractions (Steer et al 1985, Bidgood & Steer 1987). Oxytocin dose rate is titrated upwards until a target value of uterine activity is reached (usually 1500–1700 kPas/15 min, or 150–200 Montevideo Units). The usual infusion rate of oxytocin required to induce this level of uterine activity at term is 2–8 mU/min, with a mean of 4 mU/min (Caldeyro-Barcia et al 1957, Steer et al 1985, Blakemore et al 1990). The American College of Obstetricians and Gynecologists now recommends that oxytocin infusion to induce or augment labour should commence at an initial dose of 0.5–1 mU/min, increasing by 1–2 mU/min every 30–60 minutes. Retrospective studies have confirmed that there is no evident advantage to using higher dosage regimens (Foster et al 1988, Brindley & Sokol 1988, Wein 1989). There is no conclusive evidence that either of these two approaches, either active or physiological, is superior one from the other. Satin et al (1992) have recently reported a prospective (although not randomized) study in which they compared a low dose regimen, 1 mU/min starting dose and 1 mU/min increments until 8 mU/min then 2 mU/min increments to a maximum of 20 mU/min, with a high dose regimen, starting dose 6 mU/min and 6 mU/min up to a maximum dose of 42 mU/min. They found a reduced duration of augmented labour with the high dose regimen, but no significant decrease in overall Caesarean section rate in either augmented or induced labour. However, in both augmented and induced labour, the high-dose regimen significantly increased the incidence of uterine hyperstimulation (by 13–15%). They commented that the use of high-dose versus low-dose regimens 'produces a risk benefit dilemma for which we

have no answer'. A leading article in the *Lancet* in 1988 commented that 'At present, low-dose oxytocin infusion with careful assessment of uterine activity is the best policy in most cases' (Leading Article 1988). However, the data sheet for Syntocinon (the synthetic oxytocin used in clinical practice) lists absolute contraindications to its use in labour as including 'hypertonic uterine inertia' (i.e. failure of the cervix to dilate despite a high level of uterine contraction), 'mechanical obstruction to delivery' (which is often only suspected when the cervix fails to dilate) and 'fetal distress'. Thus extreme caution should be exercised when giving oxytocin in the absence of intrauterine pressure measurement, and it should always be withheld or stopped if the FHR becomes in any way abnormal. Failure to observe these precautions is one of the major sources of litigation in both the USA and UK (Fuchs 1985, Taylor & Taylor 1988, M Symonds, personal communication) and is almost always indefensible. An obvious example of oxytocin-induced hypertonus is shown in Figure 35.7. However, the effects of hyperstimulation may be more subtle. Figure 35.8 shows the tracing of a woman who was having her labour induced. Oxytocin had been increased over the first 90 minutes to 12 mU/min. This dose produced satisfactory uterine activity and it was maintained at this level for the next 2.5 hours. However, as labour proceeded, the uterus became more sensitive to the oxytocin and the frequency of contractions gradually increased, until at the beginning of the tracing shown it had reached seven in 10 minutes. The FHR showed loss of variability with late decelerations, indicating fetal hypoxia. Fortunately the hyperstimulation

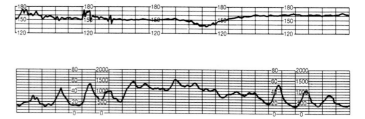

Fig. 35.7 Uterine hypercontractility associated with oxytocin infusion—acute hyperstimulation.

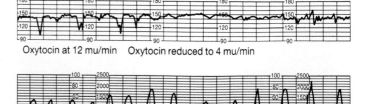

Oxytocin at 12 mu/min   Oxytocin reduced to 4 mu/min

Fig. 35.8 Uterine hypercontractility associated with oxytocin infusion—chronic hyperstimulation; restoration of normal contraction pattern with reduction in oxytocin infusion rate.

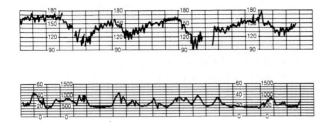

Fig. 35.9 Uterine hypercontractility associated with vaginal prostaglandin administration.

was recognized, and the infusion rate was reduced to 4 mU/min. Over the next 15 minutes the frequency subsided to a more normal five in 10 minutes and the FHR returned to normal. The tracing also illustrates the reduced active pressure associated with excessive contraction frequency; the active pressure rose from 4 kPa (30 mmHg) to 8 kPa (60 mmHg) as the frequency fell.

Prostaglandin administration is also associated with abnormal uterine action (Felmingham et al 1976, Sutton & Steer 1979, Lamb 1981). Figure 35.9 shows the excessively frequent and incoordinate contractions which occurred following the vaginal administration of a 2.5 mg prostaglandin E_2 pessary used to induce labour. Large late decelerations demonstrated the resulting fetal hypoxia and emergency delivery by Caesarean section was necessary.

INEFFICIENT UTERINE ACTIVITY

By definition, any level or type of uterine activity which does not produce progressive cervical dilatation is inefficient. Some workers prefer this term to expressions such as hypotonic, incoordinate, and hypertonic. However, the cervix may fail to dilate despite apparently normal contractions, because of cephalopelvic disproportion or cervical dystocia. Some authorities recommend the use of oxytocics in this situation, despite the risk of uterine hyperstimulation (British Medical Journal Leading Article 1972) but this is a controversial issue and more properly considered in Chapter 36. More recently some workers have noted a rise in the plasma concentrations of the metabolites of prostaglandin $F_{2\alpha}$ in labour associated with progressive cervical dilatation; this rise was not observed even in the presence of apparently normal contractions if cervical dilatation did not occur (Fuchs et al 1983, Weitz et al 1986). The significance of this observation is not yet clear. More recently, Gough et al (1990) have suggested that a major factor in inefficient uterine action is a low force generated between the fetal presenting part (usually the head) and the lower segment/cervix. They studied 31 women in slow labour, and found that once uterine activity levels had been normalized by appropriate oxytocin infusion, women who eventually needed Caesarean section for inadequate cervical dilatation rates

had poor forces (mean 16.5 g wt, range 6–31) between the presenting part and the cervix in comparison to those who achieved a vaginal delivery (mean 45 g wt, range 22–100). This was despite similar levels of uterine activity in both groups. It therefore appears that however strong the uterine contractions, if they cannot deliver an adequate force to the cervix, it will fail to dilate. Margono et al (1993) have suggested that another factor which might prevent cervical dilatation is inadequate fundal dominance, a concept introduced by Caldeyro et al (1950) and elaborated by Jeffcoate (1963). This concept suggests that in order to be effective, uterine contractions should commence at the cornua of the uterus (the designated pacemaker sites) and sweep downwards over the uterus. If the lower segment contracts at the same time, or before the upper segment, the effect may be to prevent descent of the head, and thus reduce the effective dilating force. Margono et al studied 22 women in labour, 15 of whom had active phase arrest of labour, by inserting two intra-uterine catheters, one into the lower segment area and the other up to the fundus. They showed that in the 16 women who delivered vaginally, the upper segment pressures were always higher than those in the lower segment. In the six who were delivered by Caesarean section, the pressures were higher in the lower segment. Even more recently, Olah et al (1993) have demonstrated that in the latent phase of labour almost 50% of women in labour exhibit contractions of the cervix, and have since suggested that if this persists into the active phase, such women are at increased risk of Caesarean section. In such cases, the use of oxytocin is likely to be ineffective, and may even be counterproductive.

ABNORMAL UTERINE ACTION AND POSTURE IN LABOUR

Williams (1952) was the first worker to demonstrate clearly that the supine position in labour can be associated with the development of abnormal uterine action. In the case he reported, uterine activity with the parturient in the sitting position was normal, with a contraction frequency of three in 10 minutes and an active pressure of 5.3 kPa (40 mmHg). When the woman was allowed to lie supine, the contraction frequency rose to 6.4 in 10 minutes and the active pressure fell to 2.1 kPa (16 mmHg). A similar example recorded by the author is shown in Figure 35.9. The change in pattern is abrupt and dramatic. In this case the FHR continues unaffected, but in some cases the increase in contraction frequency is associated with signs of hypoxia. Caldeyro-Barcia et al reported in 1960 that similar changes could be observed in 94% of women in spontaneous labour, and in 76% of those in oxytocin-induced labour. The mechanism by which the supine position can produce abnormal uterine action in this way is completely unknown.

THE MANAGEMENT OF ABNORMAL UTERINE ACTION

The key to appropriate management is the recognition of the category of abnormality. It is particularly important to recognize promptly hypertonic uterine activity, as it is potentially harmful to the fetus. In addition, the diagnosis of uterine hyperactivity may be the first clue to a diagnosis of placental abruption.

Placental abruption

Abruptio placentae is not only likely to have serious implications for the fetus because of interference with placental gaseous exchange, but it can also have major consequences for the mother (particularly blood loss leading to shock, and coagulopathy: see Chs 18 and 23). In severe cases, with lower abdominal pain and vaginal bleeding or the signs of shock (pallor, sweating, tachycardia and hypotension) the diagnosis may be obvious, but *in the early stages of abruption the possibility is all too easily overlooked*. For example, the lower abdominal pain and uterine irritability may be misattributed to a urinary tract infection.

In any pregnant woman, the occurrence of spontaneous uterine contractions with a frequency exceeding 1 every 2 minutes should lead one to consider the diagnosis of placental abruption.

In addition, the mother may give a history of continuous lower abdominal pain, or backache, which persists between contractions. She may give a history of bleeding per vaginam; this may be quite slight and is sometimes only elicited on direct questioning. Examination is likely to show uterine tenderness, which is often localized but in severe cases will spread to include the entire uterus.

Cardiotocography has an important place in the early diagnosis of abruption, because it facilitates recognition of tachysystolia (excessively frequent contractions). In addition, the interference with placental perfusion which occurs in abruption often causes fetal hypoxia, resulting in abnormal fetal heart rate patterns. In their early stages, these abnormalities (such as loss of variability and shallow late decelerations) are not readily detectable using the Pinard stethoscope. Because of their subtlety it is important that the cardiotocography should be performed carefully, with particular attention to the placement of the external tocodynamometer (contraction transducer). Ideally the mother should be in the semi-Fowler position, sitting up at about 60° to the horizontal, supported by pillows, with the tocodynamometer sited firmly in the midline about 12 cm below the fundus of the uterus. If the mother is lying on her side, then the tocodynamometer should be placed in a similar position but displaced about 10 cm towards the upper side. Only tachysystolia is demonstrable using an external contractions transducer, since neither baseline tone nor amplitude of contractions can be measured in absolute terms using commercially available tocodynamometers. The demonstration of raised baseline tone requires the insertion of an intrauterine catheter. Ideally this should have a catheter-tipped pressure transducer. This is because the maximum error in measurement of baseline tone using this type of catheter is about 2 kPa (15 mmHg) due to variations in hydrostatic pressure at different points within the uterus. In contrast, if a fluid-filled catheter with external pressure transducer is used, unless the transducer is placed carefully at the same level as the uterus, very large offsets in measured baseline tone can occur, making the assessment of true baseline tone unreliable.

Once the diagnosis of abruption has been made, management depends on whether the fetus remains in good condition and upon the state of the cervix. If the mother's condition is satisfactory and if the FHR remains normal then conservative management can proceed with continuing and continuous monitoring of maternal condition, uterine activity and FHR.

If the fetus is sufficiently mature and the cervix is favourable, an induction of labour by artificial rupture of the membranes is probably advisable in case there is a further and larger abruption later on. If the FHR is abnormal or if there is any concern over the mother's condition, immediate delivery is the only safe treatment. Caesarean section will often be the method of choice, particularly if the cervix is unfavourable or if the FHR abnormality is severe.

Attempts to suppress uterine activity with tocolytics such as ritodrine or salbutamol should never be made in the presence of placental abruption for raised intrauterine tone limits the inflow of blood into the uterus and if the tone is reduced, it may precipitate further catastrophic intrauterine bleeding. In addition, if the mother is developing tachycardia and hypotension, these will be exacerbated by tocolytics. This is in contrast to the situation with antepartum haemorrhage due to placenta praevia, where the bleeding is not restricted by raised intrauterine tone but instead is often provoked by uterine contractions. In this situation tocolytics can be used relatively safely and often result in the cessation of bleeding. However, the same caveats about the use of tocolytics in placenta praevia apply with respect to maternal condition; they should not be used if tachycardia and hypotension suggest haemodynamically significant blood loss.

Uncomplicated tachysystolia

If abruption can be ruled out as a cause of excessive uterine contractions, then tocolytics can be used with advantage to reduce the level of uterine action to within normal limits. They are particularly useful as an emergency measure if hypercontractility is secondary to an oxytocic such as prostaglandin E_2 whose action cannot easily be terminated. Oxytocin has a short half-life in the blood; if hyperstimulation occurs with oxytocin use, it is usually sufficient to discontinue the infusion. The effect will wear off within 5–10 minutes.

Inadequate uterine activity

This is usually diagnosed initially because of a slow rate of cervical dilatation. The rate of dilatation below which progress is designated slow varies from one obstetric unit to another but in the UK usually lies between 1 cm an hour and 1 cm every 2 hours. About 75% of slow labours are due to inadequate levels of uterine activity (Steer et al 1985) and most of these will respond effectively to intravenous oxytocin infusion at a rate between 2 and 8 mU/ min (techniques for augmentation of labour are covered fully in Ch. 37). Ideally such infusion should be monitored by intrauterine pressure measurement, particularly in women of high parity, in those with a uterine scar and in those where the fetus is known to be at particular risk (e.g. small-for-gestational-age). If intrauterine pressure monitoring is not available, then contraction frequency should not be stimulated beyond one contraction every 2 minutes, and the rate of infusion should be reduced by half as soon as there is any sign of abnormality of the FHR, and reduced further if the abnormality persists.

INCOORDINATE UTERINE ACTION

There is no need to treat incoordinate uterine action so long as the FHR and the rate of cervical dilatation remain normal. As previously mentioned, the role of oxytocin in the management of incoordinate activity where both overall levels of activity and rates of cervical dilatation are low remains controversial. The author's experience is that the cervical dilatation rate increases in parallel with any increase in uterine activity, even if that uterine activity appears incoordinate. It therefore seems appropriate to use oxytocin infusion in the first instance, and in many cases improvement in the level of uterine activity and the rate of cervical dilatation will occur. Prostaglandins are not recommended as they have an inherent tendency to produce incoordinate uterine contractions and may make the situation worse. If, however, there is a poor response to oxytocin, further measures may be tried. It must be emphasized that at the present time there are no firm scientific data to support the use of these measures.

Firstly, the posture of the woman should be adjusted; while the supine position should always be avoided any other position in which uterine activity improves should be maintained. If this is not effective then adequate analgesia must be ensured. This will usually be a regional block such as an epidural anaesthetic. This not only produces an improvement in uterine activity but also provides analgesia, which is important in prolonged labour; if the mother is comfortable and fetal condition is satisfactory, it may be possible to wait long enough so that even a slow rate of cervical dilatation will result in a vaginal delivery. Care should be taken to continue observing FHR and uterine contractions as the anaesthetic is administered, particularly if an oxytocin infusion is being given; if the uterus suddenly becomes more sensitive and there is hypertonus, fetal hypoxia may result. If there is also hypotension from the epidural (despite preloading the circulation with fluid) the effect on the fetus can be catastrophic. If there is still no improvement in the overall level of uterine activity, then sedation with 150 mg pethidine may be tried as a last resort. At the present time there is insufficient evidence on which to recommend the use of beta-blockers such as propranolol.

CONCLUSION

The main categories of abnormal uterine action are hypotonic (too little), hypertonic (too much), incoordinate (abnormal in pattern) and inefficient (not associated with progressive cervical dilatation).

The main priority in dealing with hypertonic activity is to decide whether it is due to placental abruption. If not, it may be treated with tocolytics.

None of the other abnormalities matters as long as fetal condition is satisfactory and the cervix is dilating at an adequate rate. If the cervix is dilating at less than 1 cm every 2 hours then ideally intrauterine pressure measurement should be undertaken and oxytocin infusion commenced if activity is deficient; the dose rate should be titrated against response. Persistent incoordinate action associated with poor progress should be treated initially with regional anaesthesia and subsequently with sedation if poor progress persists. If neither of these treatments is effective and delivery cannot be anticipated within a reasonable time (depending on maternal and fetal condition), then delivery by Caesarean section is indicated.

REFERENCES

Al-Shawaf T, Al-Moghvaby S, Akiel A 1987 Normal levels of uterine activity in primigravidae and women of high parity in spontaneous labour. Journal of Obstetrics and Gynaecology 8: 18–23

Alvarez H, Caldeyro R 1950 Contractility of the human uterus recorded by new methods. Surgery, Gynecology and Obstetrics 91: 1–13

American College of Obstetrics and Gynecology 1987 Induction and augmentation of labor. Technical Bulletin no 110. American College of Obstetricians and Gynecologists, Washington DC

Arthur H R, Johnson G T 1952 Continuous caudal anaesthesia in the management of cervical dystocia. Journal of Obstetrics and Gynaecology of the British Empire 59: 372–377

Arulkumaran S, Gibb D M F, Lun K C, Heng S H, Ratnam S S 1984 The effect of parity on uterine activity in labour. British Journal of Obstetrics and Gynaecology 91: 843–848

Arulkumaran S, Gibb D M F, Ratnam S S, Lun K C, Heng S H 1985 Total uterine activity in induced labour—an index of cervical and pelvic tissue resistance. British Journal of Obstetrics and Gynaecology 92: 693–697

Arulkumaran S, Michelsen J, Ingemarsson I, Ratnam S S 1987 Obstetric outcome of patients with a previous episode of spurious labor. American Journal of Obstetrics and Gynaecology 157: 17–20

Bidgood K A, Steer P J 1987 Randomised control study of oxytocin augmentation of labour. British Journal of Obstetrics and Gynaecology 94: 512–517

Blakemore K J, Nai-Geng Q, Petrie R, Paine L 1990 A prospective comparison of hourly and quarter hourly oxytocin dose increase intervals for the induction of labor at term. Obstetrics and Gynecology 75: 757–761

Bourne A, Burn J H 1927 The dosage and action of pituitary extract and the ergot alkaloids on the uterus in labour, with a note of the action of adrenaline. Journal of Obstetrics and Gynaecology of the British Empire 34: 249–272

Brindley B E, Sokol R J 1988 Induction and augmentation of labor: basis and methods for current practice. Obstetrics and Gynecology Survey 43: 730–743

British Medical Journal Leading Article 1972 Active management of labour. British Medical Journal 4: 126

Brotanek V, Hendricks C H, Yoshida T 1969 Changes in uterine blood flow during uterine contractions. American Journal of Obstetrics and Gynecology 103: 1108–1116

Caldeyro R, Alvarez H, Reynolds S R M 1950 A better understanding of uterine contractility through simultaneous recording with an internal and seven channel external method. Surgery, Gynecology and Obstetrics 91:641–650

Caldeyro-Barcia R, Alvarez H 1952 Abnormal uterine action during labour. Journal of Obstetrics and Gynaecology of the British Empire 59: 648–654

Caldeyro-Barcia R, Sica-Blanco Y, Poseiro J J et al 1957 A quantitative study of the action of synthetic oxytocin on the pregnant human uterus. Journal of Pharmacology 121: 18–31

Caldeyro-Barcia R, Noriega-Guerra L, Cibils L A et al 1960 Effect of position changes on the intensity and frequency of uterine contractions during labour. American Journal of Obstetrics and Gynecology 80: 284–290

Cibils L A, Hendricks C H 1965 Normal labour in vertex presentation. American Journal of Obstetrics and Gynecology 91: 385–395

Cowan D B, Van Middlekoop A, Philpott R H 1982 Intrauterine pressure studies in African nuiliparae: normal labour progress. Journal of Obstetrics and Gynaecology of the British Empire 89: 364–369

El-Sahwi S, Gaafar A A, Toppozada H K 1967 A new unit for evaluation of uterine activity. American Journal of Obstetrics and Gynecology 98: 900–903

Felmingham J E, Oakley M C, Atlay R D 1976 Uterine hypertonus after induction of labour with prostaglandin E_2 tablets. British Medical Journal 1: 586

Flynn A M, Kelly J, Hollins G, Lynch P F 1978 Ambulation in labour. British Medical Journal 2: 591–593

Foster T C, Jacobson J D, Valenzuela G 1988 Oxytocin augmentation of labor; a comparison of 15 and 30 minute dose increment intervals. Obstetrics and Gynecology 71: 147–149

Fuchs F 1985 Cautions on using oxytocin for inductions. Contemporary Obstetrics and Gynecology 24: 13–14

Fuchs A-R, Goeschen K, Husslein P, Rasmussen A B, Fuchs F 1983 Plasma concentrations of oxytocin and 13,14-dihydro-1,5-ketoprostaglandin $F_{2\alpha}$ in spontaneous and oxytocin-induced labour at term. American Journal of Obstetrics and Gynecology 147: 497–507

Gibb D M F, Arulkumaran S, Lun K C, Ratnam S S 1984 Characteristics of uterine activity in nulliparous labour. British Journal of Obstetrics and Gynaecology 91: 220–227

Gough G W, Randall N J, Genevier E S, Sutherland I A, Steer P J 1990 Head to cervix forces and their relationship to the outcome of labor. Obstetrics and Gynecology 75: 613–618

Hemminki E, Lenck M, Saariksoki S, Henriksson L 1985 Ambulation versus oxytocin in protracted labour: a pilot study. European Journal of Obstetrics, Gynecology and Reproductive Biology 20: 199–208

Jeffcoate T N A 1963 Physiology and mechanism of labour. In: Claye A, Bourne A (eds) British obstetric and gynaecological practice. Heinemann Medical, London, pp 145–183

Kaiser I H, Harris J S 1950 The effect of adrenalin on the pregnant human uterus. American Journal of Obstetrics and Gynecology 59: 775–784

Krapohl A J, Myers G G, Caideyro-Barcia R 1970 Uterine contractions in spontaneous labour. American Journal of Obstetrics and Gynecology 106: 378–387

Lamb M P 1981 Prostaglandins in obstetrics. British Medical Journal 282: 1398

Leading Article 1988 How actively should dystocia be treated? Lancet i: 160–160

Lindmark G, Nilsson B A 1977 A comparative study of uterine activity in labour induced with prostaglandin F2alpha or oxytocin, and in spontaneous labour. Acta Obstetrica et Gynecologica Scandinavica 56: 87–94

Lissauer T J, Steer P J 1986 The relationship between the need for neonatal resuscitation, abnormal cardiotocograms in labour and cord blood gas measurements. British Journal of Obstetrics and Gynaecology 93: 1060–1066

Liston W A, Campbell A J 1974 Dangers of oxytocin induced labour to fetuses. British Medical Journal 3: 606–607

Margono F, Minkoff H, Chan E 1993 Intrauterine pressure wave characteristics of the upper and lower uterine segments in parturients with active phase arrest. Obstetrics and Gynecology 81: 481–485

Martin C B 1965 Uterine blood flow and placental circulation. Anesthesiology 26: 447–459

Mendez-Bauer C, Arroyo J, Garcia Ramos C et al 1975 Effects of standing position on spontaneous uterine contractility and other aspects of labour. Journal of Perinatal Medicine 3: 89–100

Mercer B, Pilgrim P, Sibai B 1991 Labor induction with continuous low dose oxytocin infusion: a randomized trial. Obstetrics and Gynecology 77: 659–663

Mitrani A, Bettinger M, Abinader E G, Sharf M, Klein A 1975 Use of propranolol in dysfunctional labour. British Journal of Obstetrics and Gynaecology 82: 651–655

Moir D D, Willocks J 1967 Management of incoordinate uterine action under continuous epidural anaesthesia. British Medical Journal 3: 396–400

Morishima H O, Daniel S S, Richards R T, James L S 1975 The effect of increased maternal Pao_2 upon the fetus during labour. American Journal of Obstetrics and Gynecology 123: 257–264

Novy M J, Thomas C L, Lees M H 1975 Uterine contractility and regional blood flow responses to oxytocin and prostaglandin E_2 in pregnant rhesus monkeys. American Journal of Obstetrics and Gynecology 122: 419–433

Odendaal H J 1976 The frequency of uterine contractions in abruptio placentas. South African Medical Journal 50: 2129–2131

O'Driscoll K, Jackson R J A, Gallagher J T 1969 Prevention of prolonged labour. British Medical Journal 2: 447–480

Olah K S, Gee H, Brown J S 1993 Cervical contractions: the response of the cervix to oxytocic stimulation in the latent phase of labour. British Journal of Obstetrics and Gynaecology 100: 635–640

Pontonnier G, Puech F, Granjean H, Rolland M 1975 Some physical and biochemical parameters during normal labour. Biology of the Neonate 26: 159–173

Poseiro J J, Noriega-Guerra L 1961 Dose response relationships in uterine effects of oxytocin infusions. In: Caldeyro-Barcia R, Heller H (eds) Oxytocin. Pergamon, Oxford

Pritchard J A, MacDonald P C, Gant N F 1985 Placental abruption. In: Williams obstetrics. Appleton-Century-Crofts, Norwalk, Connecticut, pp 395–407

Richardson J A, Sutherland I A, Allen D W 1978 A cervimeter for conunuous measurement of cervical dilatation in labour—preliminary results. British Journal of Obstetrics and Gynaecology 85: 178–184

Rossavik I K 1978 Relation between total uterine impulse, method of delivery and 1 minute Apgar score. British Journal of Obstetrics and Gynaecology 85: 847–851

Satin A J, Leveno K J, Sherman M L, Brewster D S, Cunningham F G 1992 High versus low dose oxytocin for labor stimulation. Obstetrics and Gynecology 80: 111–116

Saunderson P R, Steer P J 1978 The value of cardiotocography in abruptio placentae. British Journal of Obstetrics and Gynaecology 85: 796–797

Seitchik J, Castillo M 1982 Oxytocin augmentation of dysfunctional labour. American Journal of Obstetrics and Gynecology 144: 899–905

Seitchik J, Chatkoff M L 1977 Intrauterine pressure waveform characteristics of successful and failed first stage labour. Gynecological Investigation 8: 246–253

Steer P J, Carter M C, Beard R W 1984 Normal levels of active contraction area in spontaneous labour. British Journal of Obstetrics and Gynaecology 91: 211–219

Steer P J, Carter M C, Beard R W 1985 The effect of oxytocin infusion on uterine activity levels in slow labour. British Journal of Obstetrics and Gynaecology 92: 1120–1126

Sutton M, Steer P J 1979 Induction of labour. British Medical Journal 3: 671

Taylor R W, Taylor M 1988 Misuse of oxytocin in labour. Lancet i: 352

Turnbull A C 1957 Uterine contractions in normal and abnormal labour. Journal of Obstetrics and Gynaecology of the British Empire 64: 321–333

Wein P 1989 Efficacy of different starting doses of oxytocin for induction of labor. Obstetrics and Gynecology 74: 863–868

Weitz C M, Ghodgaonker R B, Dubin N H, Niebyl J R 1986 Prostaglandin F metabolite concentration as a prognostic factor in preterm labour. Obstetrics and Gynecology 67: 496–499

Williams E A 1952 Abnormal uterine action during labour. Journal of Obstetrics and Gynaecology of the British Empire 59: 635–641

Zambrana M A, Gonzalez-Panizza V H, Santiso-Gaivez R et al 1960 Relacion de la contractilidad espontanea del utero con el progreso del parto. In: Third Uruguayan Congress of Obstetrics and Gynecology 3: 354. Cited in: Greenhill J P (ed) Obstetrics, 3rd edn. WB Saunders, Philadelphia, pp 281, 304

36. Abnormal fetal presentations and cephalopelvic disproportion

John Malvern

Material in this chapter contains contributions from the first edition, which may take the form of personal experience and opinion. We are grateful to the previous authors for the work done.

The commonest presentation of the fetus in the late pregnancy is cephalic. This is not because of the shape of the pelvis or the fetal head, but because of the pyriform-shaped cavity of the uterus (particularly in primigravidae), which allows more room for lower limb activity in the fundal region thus necessitating the other pole to occupy the cervical region. With increasing gravidity the uterine wall becomes more lax and the cavity more apple-shaped, thus allowing a higher incidence of malpresentation and malposition of the presenting fetal pole, and an increased likelihood of an unstable lie. Similarly, when fetal movement is restricted by obstructions within the uterus such as septae, uterine fibroids or another fetus then there is greater likelihood of malpresentation. When the pelvic cavity has become occupied by some soft tissue swelling either within the uterus in the form of placenta praevia or uterine fibroids or from without by ovarian tumours in the pouch of Douglas, the presenting part is unable to enter the pelvic brim and the fetal lie stands a greater chance of being unstable.

During the early stages of labour a favourable presentation and position is one where the baby's head is entering the mother's pelvis with the occiput directed towards the side wall or some point between it and the symphysis pubis. The subsequent labour and delivery should be a normal physiological function requiring no obstetric intervention. Unfortunately, in some women either the presentation or the position is not normal and this may lead to complications requiring special management and occasionally operative treatment.

A considerable amount of difficulty arises from the shape of the human birth canal. When eye contact became a most important tool for the developing hominid as she descended from the trees (Morgan 1972), she started to walk with an upright stance. The subsequent development of the gluteal and thigh muscles led to thickening and strengthening of the bones of the pelvis and forward curvature of the lower half of the sacrum. Eye contact during intercourse required a forward facing procreation tract so that the vagina gradually turned at a right angle to the brim of the pelvis and to the uterus itself. Delivery of a child came to mean not only pushing it through a rigid bony canal, the entrance to which was wider from side to side while the exit was larger from front to back, but negotiation of a right-angled bend half way down the canal followed by traversing strong perineal muscles designed more for keeping things in than letting them out (Stewart 1984a; Fig. 36.1).

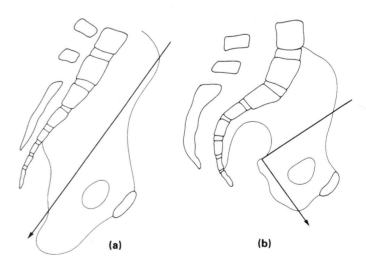

Fig. 36.1 (a) Gorilla pelvis showing straight birth canal. (b) Human pelvis showing birth canal with right-angle turn.

657

These changes were accompanied by an increase in the size of the human brain required to develop and utilize the skills which humans need to remain the dominant animal (Moore 1970), so that as the pelvis was becoming less suitable for delivery the most important part of the infant increasingly came to have more difficulty fitting through it.

These disadvantages are normally overcome by what are known as the mechanics of labour. The bigger parts of the baby, such as the head, shoulders, and breech, enter the pelvis with their largest diameters running transversely. They rotate as they descend so that the same diameters leave the pelvis in an anterior–posterior direction. Because the spine is inserted into the back of the skull, pressure directed along it will make the head flex (Fig. 36.2). Thus, before labour commences or in its early stages the occipito-frontal diameter of the head is in the transverse diameter of the pelvis. As it descends it quickly flexes so that the occipito-frontal diameter becomes the suboccipito-bregmatic, identical in length with the biparietal diameter at 9.5 cm. These form a circle to apply pressure equally all round the cervix, resulting in a reflex arc which stimulates fundal contractility and subsequently more downward pressure. When the head reaches the gutter formed by the levator muscles deep in the pelvis, the occiput, which is larger than the sinciput, is funnelled forwards to present at the vulval opening. With further downward pressure it can emerge from the larger of the two diameters at the pelvic outlet, finally extending as it does so.

Subsequent restitution and external rotation of the

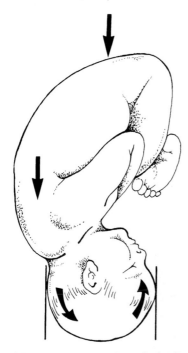

Fig. 36.2 Fundal pressure directed down fetal spine promotes flexion rather than extension of head.

head are merely reflections of the remainder of the baby coming through the pelvis but are not important as the largest part of it has by now delivered.

Using these mechanics most babies negotiate the pelvis safely. However, in a small number of cases the presentation is not cephalic or if it is, it rotates the wrong way in midpelvis, extending instead of flexing and these mechanisms cannot apply. Such problems form the basis of this chapter. It is written from a western European perspective where it is tempting to manage them by delivering the baby abdominally. This solution is not always available in the less well developed areas of the world and even in more advanced countries the tendency to treat every complication by Caesarean section has been criticized because, however straightforward for the baby, it is a major procedure for the mother (Chalmers 1984, Gilstrap et al 1984, Yudkin & Redman 1986).

The first page of this chapter concentrates on the function of the mother delivering her baby and does not dwell on the different pelvic shapes. Fetal size in utero is related to the height of the mother. Thus, tall women should have large pelves and be capable of delivering large babies while smaller women with smaller pelves should have correspondingly lighter infants. Antenatal X-rays of the pelvis may label a small woman as having a contracted pelvis and lead to unnecessary interference. Radiology should be restricted to those with breech presentation or after delivery in patients who have had an unexpectedly difficult birth for no obvious reason (O'Brien & Cefalo 1982, Floberg et al 1987, Krishnamurthy et al 1991).

DEFINITIONS

The definitions used in this chapter are as follows.

The *attitude* of the fetus describes the relationship between the fetal head and limbs to the trunk. Usually this is one of flexion.

The *lie* of the fetus is its relationship to the long axis of the uterus. This can be longitudinal, oblique or transverse.

The *presentation* is that part of the fetus presenting in the lower pole of the uterus or at the pelvic brim.

The *presenting part* is that part of the presentation which lies immediately inside the internal os.

The *position* defines the relationship of the presentation or the presenting part to the maternal pelvis.

The *denominator* is that part of the presentation or the presenting part which denotes the position. For a cephalic presentation with the vertex as the presenting part, the denominator is the occiput. With a face as the presenting part it is the chin and for a breech it is the sacrum.

It is important to distinguish between presentation and presenting part. For example, a patient can have a cephalic presentation with the brow or the face as a presenting part: it is incorrect to refer to these as brow or face presentations.

It is also incorrect to write vertex as the presentation on abdominal palpation. It is the presenting part at the commencement of most labours before the head has flexed.

OCCIPITO-POSTERIOR POSITIONS OF THE HEAD

Occipito-posterior position means that the occiput, the denominator for the position of the head, points posteriorly in the pelvis, either directly at the sacrum (direct occipito-posterior) or to one side of it in the region of the sacroiliac joints (oblique occipito-posterior). This may be the case during the antenatal period, or at any time in labour right up to delivery. Because the head rotates during labour, discussion about these positions has to include women in whom the occiput points sideways (occipito-lateral, occipito-transverse). It is accepted that 10–20% of cephalic presentations enter labour with the occiput directed posteriorly (Myerscough 1982). Some rotate to occipito-anterior so that by the time of delivery, only 5% remain occipito-posterior or have arrested in the occipito-lateral position while attempting to turn towards the front.

This position of the fetal head is one of the commonest causes of a high head at term, and can be recognized by the difficulty in locating the fetal back, the scaphoid concave area between the pubic symphysis and umbilicus and the prominence of the fetal limbs anteriorly. The fetal heart may be also more difficult to locate, as it can either head directly anteriorly or out in the flanks.

There are several possible causes for the abnormal position. Braxton Hicks contractions may not be strong enough to push the head into the brim and make it flex prior to the onset of labour (Fig. 36.3a). Conversely the fact that the head is extended presents a rectangular-shaped outline to the lower segment so that the stimulus to fundal contractility may be irregular and incomplete (Fig. 36.3b). In late pregnancy, attempts by the uterus to turn the baby's head and shoulders may be impeded by the latter catching on to the mother's lower lumbar spine and sacral promontory. Hypertonus in the fetus can prevent the normal flexed attitude in utero.

The babies of women with either anthropoid or android pelves are more likely to be occipito-posterior. The former is very uncommon but is usually large; the baby presents directly occipito-posterior for the whole labour and delivers easily in that position. Viewed from above, the more commonly found android pelvis is triangular in shape with the apex at the symphysis pubis so that the larger part of the fetal head finds more room in the back of the pelvis and turns into the sacral curve as it descends (Holmberg et al 1977, Stewart 1984b).

Whatever the precise aetiology, the fact that the baby's spine is juxtaposed to the mother's means that downward pressure along the spine is more likely to extend the head than flex it, thus increasing the diameters presented to the pelvic brim. In addition, since the head is rarely directly occipito-posterior, the biparietal, its largest transverse diameter, will be trying to squeeze through the space between the sacral promontory and the pectineal line while the smaller bitemporal measurement will have all the space available from the sacroiliac joint to the back of the symphysis pubis (Fig. 36.4). Uterine contractility is adversely affected because the cervix is not stimulated correctly by the rectangular surface presented by the

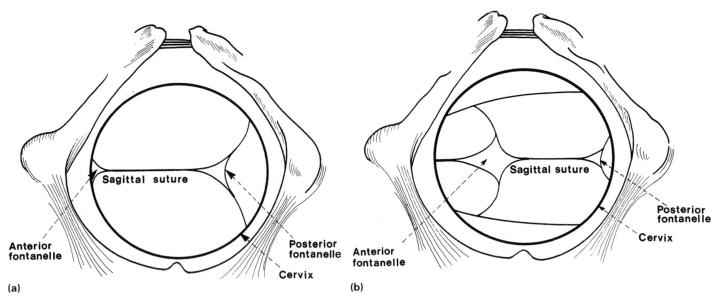

Fig. 36.3   **(a)** Flexed head presenting as a circle to the cervix. Biparietal diameter 9.5 cm; suboccipito-bregmatic diameter also 9.5 cm. **(b)** Deflexed head presenting a rectangular surface to the cervix. Biparietal diameter 9.5 cm; occipito-frontal diameter 11.5 cm.

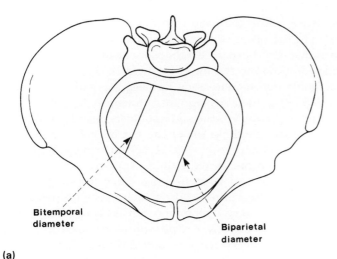

Bitemporal diameter   **Biparietal diameter**

(a)

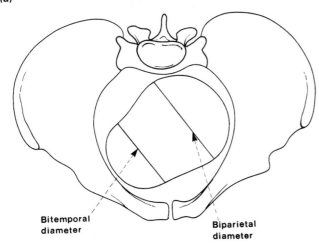

Bitemporal diameter   **Biparietal diameter**

(b)

Fig. 36.4 **(a)** Left occipito-anterior position. Biparietal diameter (9.5 cm) lying between the sacroiliac joint and the summit of the symphysis pubis. Bitemporal diameter (8.5 cm) occupies the smaller sacrocotyloid dimension. **(b)** Left occipito-posterior position. Biparietal diameter squeezed into the sacrocotyloid while the bitemporal has excess space.

Table 36.1 Mode of vaginal delivery of 482 babies presenting as occipito-posterior or with deep transverse arrest at full dilatation at Grady Memorial Hospital in 1971.

Mode of delivery	Percentage
Spontaneous	33.8
Forceps occipito-posterior	39.8
Manual rotation/forceps	16.7
Kiellands forceps	14.4
Vacuum extraction	2.0

as it descends in the pelvis. In a small number of cases this extension continues so that first the baby's brow and then its face becomes the presenting part.

The resultant trend towards prolonged labour possibly with operative delivery increases morbidity for both mother and child. Phillips & Freeman (1974) in a retrospective review of 1082 cases which were born vaginally reported an operative delivery rate of 66% with 22% requiring rotation. There was more puerperal pyrexia and so many episiotomies extended posteriorly that the authors recommended never using a midline technique. Friedman et al (1977) examined 656 children aged between 3 and 4 years and found that a history of prolonged labour and mid-forceps either together or independently had an adverse effect on subsequent intelligence.

The diagnosis of an occipito-posterior position can be suspected antenatally on abdominal palpation. With the baby lying on its back when the mother is examined, its flexed legs mean that the maximum protrusion of the maternal abdomen viewed from the side is well above the umbilicus with a sharp fall down to the xyphi sternum and a gentle slope towards the symphysis pubis (Fig. 36.5). The head will feel smaller because the sinciput is anterior and the back may be difficult to palpate clearly.

Management of the occipito-posterior position

There is no point in attempting to alter the position during the antenatal period as many correct themselves once labour starts; most cases are not diagnosed until labour is well established and some may have arisen only in its early stages. However, it is important to emphasize that because the condition may be associated with incoordinate uterine action, the cervix is most unlikely to be ripe if induction is being considered.

Once labour is underway some cases of occipito-posterior position progress quickly and either rotate to occipito-anterior spontaneously or deliver as face to pubes before the malposition has been diagnosed. These cause no problem apart from a tendency towards perineal damage. Most cases come to light because of failure to progress in labour and in units where active management is practised

extended head (Fig. 36.3b). When the occiput eventually meets the pelvic floor it may fail to rotate to the front partly because of the long way it has to travel, through three-eighths of a circle, and partly because the posterior shoulder remains caught on the wrong side of the mother's sacral promontory. In many cases the head rotates through 45° and can go no further, eventually ending up as deep transverse arrest. Some turn the same distance but posteriorly and become persistent occipito-posterior positions. Neither delivers or can be delivered as easily as a well-flexed head in the normal occipito-anterior position. Thus, progress of labour is marred by misapplication of the head to the cervix, the largest transverse diameter of the head trying to pass through the smallest diameter of the pelvic brim and the tendency of the head to deflex and present bigger and bigger diameters

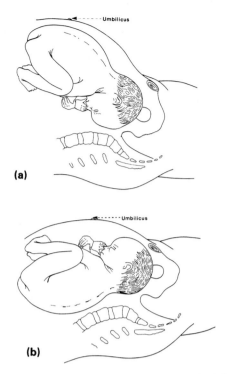

Fig. 36.5 Lateral view of abdomen near term. **(a)** Occipito-anterior position: maternal umbilicus at summit of abdominal swelling. **(b)** Occipito-posterior with umbilicus inferior to summit.

a vaginal examination quickly reveals the abnormal position. It is essential that such examinations are thorough and produce as much information as possible. Abnormal positions often develop moulding and caput formation as labour progresses and it is easier to define the suture lines on the fetal skull in the early stages.

The degree of deflexion of the fetal head is also noted and not only should the bony pelvis be assessed but the thickness and elasticity of the maternal soft tissues may be relevant to subsequent attempts at operative delivery. Application of the cervix to the presenting part is assessed, especially during a contraction. If it is not well applied, then uterine contractility is inadequate, however much discomfort the patient is having. Observations as to the colour of the amniotic fluid and whether the cord can be palpated are also important. A vaginal examination which merely states the dilatation of the cervix and the station of the head is not sufficient for the management of complicated cases and has no place in a good unit. Such limited information could have been obtained by rectal examination, which is much quicker.

Having made the diagnosis of occipito-posterior it is important to remember that while the position of the head may slow its descent down the birth canal there is no reason why the cervix should not become fully dilated provided the labour is managed actively. A rate of 1 cm/hour (as in patients with an occipito-anterior position)

must be anticipated; Syntocinon should be administered in sufficient doses if this does not occur spontaneously. There is considerable doubt as to how much of the drug may be necessary. Gibb et al (1984) found that Chinese primigravidae in Singapore required much higher intra-uterine pressures to achieve progress than was found by either Seitchik & Castillo (1983) or Steer and his colleagues (1985a), who felt that intrauterine pressures above 1500 kPa/15 min caused uterine hyperstimulation and fetal distress. Steer et al (1985b) also recommended the use of a closed loop system which Gibb et al (1985) found not to be as effective as manually controlled infusion. Arulkumaran and his co-workers (1985), writing about induction of labour, again used higher doses, stressing the importance of maternal soft tissue resistance.

For labour wards which do not have the benefit of catheter-tipped transducers and for the sake of simplicity it seems that the quantity of oxytocic required is that which is sufficient to dilate the cervix without causing more than four contractions in 10 minutes or fetal distress. Since it takes 40 minutes for the level of plasma oxytocin to peak, there is no point in increasing the infusion rate more quickly (Seitchik et al 1984). Both oxytocin and glucose can cause neonatal and maternal hyponatraemia so normal saline should be used as an infusion base (Singhi et al 1985). The fetus must be continuously monitored and the mother is an ideal candidate for an epidural, although a labouring woman does not always appreciate the analgesia provided (Morgan et al 1982). There is no need to give glucose intravenously to combat ketosis if the labour appears slow (Dumoulin & Foulkes 1984). Maternal dehydration can be dealt with by intravenous saline (Morton et al 1985). Indeed, if dehydration occurs the obstetrician in charge must question the preceding management of the case and make certain that labour advances more quickly.

With this approach every cervix should become fully dilated. In some, the head will have descended to the pelvic floor and deliver spontaneously either with the occiput anterior or in the direct occiput posterior position. The latter may require a large enough episiotomy to prevent excess tearing of the perineum. Provided that some progress is being made and the baby's heart rate and pH remain normal, patience and care will result in a spontaneous delivery for many women. However, if the head remains high a full reassessment of the case is essential. If the pelvis appears smaller than was first thought; if the antenatal records imply that the baby always felt large; if the mother is small or even if the father is tall (Pritchard et al 1983), then there may be a degree of disproportion even without an abnormal position. There is no point in doing pelvimetry as even with a large pelvis, failure of the head to descend to a level where forceps or vacuum extraction can be safely applied will result in abdominal delivery (Bottoms et al 1987). In such instances the operator must not feel in any way that labour has been wasted.

If none of these applies, an increase in the amount of oxytocin may effect further descent or rotation of the head. This is especially so if an epidural is in situ. Goodfellow et al (1983) have shown that the oxytocin surge stimulated by dilatation of the upper vagina is suppressed by conduction analgesia. Allowing the epidural to wear off neither shortens the second stage nor reduces the incidence of forceps delivery (Phillips & Thomas 1983), but instituting an infusion (Kirwan 1983) or increasing the dose (Bates et al 1985) may improve progress. Despite the finding of Smith et al (1982) that delayed pushing in the second stage did not lessen the need for instrumental delivery, Maresh et al (1983) reported exactly the opposite. They also stated that the resultant prolongation of the second stage had no adverse effect on mother or child, which concurred with Cohen's view (1977) that there was no point in having time limits for the second stage. Nevertheless, most obstetricians would agree with Kadar et al (1986) that the prospect of a normal delivery after 3 hours in the second stage is most unlikely.

For some women a change of position may be helpful. Despite the inconsistent findings of many workers, most of whom have concentrated on the effects of ambulation in the first stage of labour—Dunn (1978), Flynn et al (1978) and Lupe & Gross (1986) feel an upright posture helps while McManus & Calder (1978a,b), Williams et al (1980), Calvert et al (1982) and Stewart & Calder (1984) all feel it makes no difference—squatting, semi-squatting, lying on the side or sitting in a birth chair may enable the woman who feels the urge to push to do so more effectively than lying on her back even when propped up with pillows. Failure of any of these measures will lead to operative vaginal delivery.

Operative vaginal delivery

This must start with careful palpation of the abdomen. If any part of the head can be felt above the symphysis pubis its station in the pelvis is higher than may have appeared to be the case on vaginal examination, usually because of moulding or caput or both. While such a finding is not an absolute contraindication to vaginal delivery it acts as a warning not to persist if the first attempt is unsuccessful.

The woman is put into the lithotomy position with both buttocks slightly over the edge of the bed. If vaginal examination shows the head to be directly occipito-posterior and low in the pelvis, a direct application of a Neville Barnes-type forceps with the aid of a suitable episiotomy and gentle traction should deliver the baby. However, if the head fails to descend it will be necessary to rotate it manually, with straight forceps or by means of a vacuum extractor. This will also be the case if the head is in the oblique occipito-posterior position or is arrested at mid-cavity in the deep transverse position.

The lower birth canal must be suitably anaesthetized. Depending on the procedure undertaken, pudendal block may be adequate but in many who do not already have an epidural in place, a single-shot caudal may be inserted quickly, making certain that a wedge is placed under one of the patient's buttocks when she is returned to the lithotomy position.

Manual rotation of the head

This involves the operator's hand grasping the sinciput and rotating it towards the sacrum. An alternative method is to insert the hand alongside the head, turning the head with pressure from the palmar surface of the fingers. Placing the fingertips in the suture lines may help, as does an abdominal hand pulling the anterior shoulder of the baby in the appropriate direction.

It is simpler if the operator uses the right hand for rotation so that once the head has been turned the first blade of the forceps can be applied immediately. The left hand is then inserted quickly along the right side of the pelvic wall in an effort to hold the head in its new position while the right blade is put in place. Correct application means that the handles will close easily with the operator rechecking the suture lines before using any traction. Non-closure demands that the blades should be removed and the vaginal assessment repeated.

Insertion of a hand alongside the baby's head leaves even less room in the pelvis, so to effect rotation it may be necessary to push the head into the upper pelvis or even out of the pelvis, which will turn a low- or mid-cavity forceps into a high-forceps and this is not recommended. Ideally, the operator should have slim fingers which can fit around the head without displacing it upwards: unfortunately, this attribute often goes with weak hands so that those best shaped for the manoeuvre are not always strong enough to carry it out. For these reasons manual rotation should be restricted to cases where the head is obliquely posterior low in the pelvis and easily turned to direct occipito-posterior for delivery in that position.

Forceps rotation

Forceps have the advantage that the blades are thinner than human fingers so that the operator keeps the head low when applying them. In the direct or oblique occipito-posterior position the blades of a Keillands-type of instrument can be applied directly. Rotation is then performed with one hand while the index finger of the other is kept on the sagittal suture to make certain it is turning with the forceps. Rotation may be helped by either pulling down or pushing up the head a centimetre or two and since there is no pelvic curve the handles of the forceps must always be directed more posteriorly than with axis traction forceps. In the direct occipito-posterior position, rotation can be either clockwise or anticlockwise, usually towards the side on which the back has been palpated abdominally. With an obliquely posterior head the rotation is towards the side on which the occiput already is. In both cases it is important to remember that if rotation in one direction is unsuccessful it is worth trying to turn the forceps the other way.

As soon as the occipito-anterior position is attained the same forceps are used to effect delivery. Removing them and reapplying ordinary traction forceps not only risks increased trauma to the maternal tissues but the head may turn back in the process.

For those who feel that the head in deep transverse arrest is better allowed to rotate at its own level than at one chosen by the operator, Barton's forceps may be more suitable (see Ch. 38). A sharp angle makes the posterior blade easier to apply than Keillands and rotation occurs spontaneously as traction is applied (Parry-Jones 1968).

Vacuum extractor

This instrument has the advantage that it occupies no space to the side of the baby's head. When properly applied, it actually flexes the baby's head, reducing one of the diameters presenting to the pelvic outlet from the occipito-frontal to the smaller suboccipito-bregmatic. In addition, with traction the head can rotate to whichever position enables it to be delivered most easily. Details on this subject are given in Chapter 38.

Two further points should be emphasized in connection with operative delivery for abnormal cephalic positions—relating to episiotomy and failed forceps delivery.

Episiotomy

Because the head is extended the episiotomy may need to be larger than for an occipito-anterior position. With instrumental delivery there is a temptation to do the episiotomy prior to inserting either the forceps or the vacuum in order to make the application easier. This should be avoided: failure to effect the delivery and subsequent Caesarean section means the patient will have an unnecessary wound in her perineum. In addition, until one knows which way the head will rotate it is impossible to be sure whether the episiotomy is better done on the right or the left side. If the head is right occipito-transverse and rotation forceps are applied with the aid of a right mediolateral episiotomy (Fig. 36.6), clockwise rotation will drag the posterior blade across the episiotomy site with the risk of extending it and causing severe

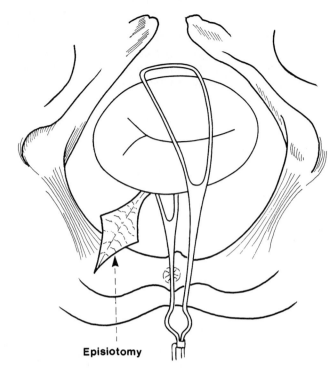

Fig. 36.6 Rotation forceps. With clockwise rotation the posterior blade will pass through the episiotomy, risking extension. In this case the incision should have been made on the left side of the perineum.

trauma. The operator should aim to reserve the incision until vaginal delivery is certain, by which stage even a midline incision may be adequate.

Episiotomy discomfort worries many puerperal women more than anything else (Reading et al 1982) and great care should be taken in its performance and repair. Midline incisions are easier to suture but unfortunately are not less painful than mediolateral ones (Coats et al 1980). A subcuticular repair (Isager-Sally et al 1986) with polyglycolic suture material (Roberts & McKay Hart 1983, Grant 1986) is better than other techniques.

Failed forceps delivery

No surgeon likes a procedure to fail but it is important to remember that a forceps delivery which requires a strong pull is occasionally followed by shoulder dystocia. Benedetti & Gabbe (1978), along with Acker and his colleagues (1985, 1986), have shown that secondary arrest or a prolonged second stage with mid-cavity forceps is a warning sign for this complication. While in theory it can be overcome by a variety of manoeuvres (Harris 1984, Carter 1986, Gross et al 1987), including replacement of the head and later Caesarean section (Sandberg 1985), in practice fetal mortality and morbidity are high.

If rotation cannot be achieved, if a large vacuum cup properly applied comes off, or if firm one-handed traction with forceps applied to a head in the direct occipito-anterior position fails to deliver the baby, Caesarean section must be undertaken. Lowe (1987) reported in the years 1981–1985 at St. Mary's Hospital, Portsmouth, that out of 25 872 deliveries, 225 women with selected criteria had delay in the second stage. Among these, 42 had an operative delivery for fetal distress; 122 went for trial of forceps of which 75 (62%) were successful and the remainder had a Caesarean section. The remaining 61 had a failed operative vaginal delivery.

With foresight, operative deliveries which look as though they may be difficult can be done in an operating theatre with everything prepared to proceed to Caesarean section, but any maternity unit which never has a failed operative delivery is under-reporting its cases or doing traumatic vaginal deliveries.

FACE AND BROW PRESENTING PARTS

These two abnormal presenting parts may be considered together as they are similar in many respects. Cruikshank & Cruikshank (1981) quote an incidence of one in 500 for the face and one in 1500 for the brow as presenting parts. The chin is the denominator when the face is presenting but traditionally there is no such marker for a brow; it is thought that the large occipito-mental diameter can never pass through a pelvis and therefore no mechanism is necessary. The diameters of a face are the normal biparietal (9.5 cm) and the submento-bregmatic, which is the same as the occipito-frontal of a deflexed vertex (11.5 cm). However, labour can be more difficult than with an extended head because the facial bones do not mould as satisfactorily as parietal ones; if the chin rotates posteriorly, then the large area of skull comprising the vertex and the occiput cannot follow the face out under the symphysis. Both conditions are due to hyperextension of the fetal neck, usually cases of occipito-posterior position which extend first into a brow and then into a face either before labour but usually as labour is progressing. Abnormalities such as anencephaly or tumours of the fetal neck may also be associated.

The principal complication for the mother is that of operative delivery, often Caesarean section. For the baby there exists the danger of the presenting part attempting to mould adequately enough to fit through the pelvis and therefore straining the intracranial membranes with resultant intracranial haemorrhage. The excess oedema of eyelids, nose, lips and cheeks found when the face presents looks spectacular but resolves quickly. Vaginal operative delivery must be done by someone experienced to avoid causing damage to these organs.

Diagnosis is suspected on palpation when the head will be high or will feel larger than normal with a sharp angulation between the fetal back and the occiput. Often an ultrasound scan or X-ray is done to exclude abnormality and shows the unusual presenting part. Most cases appear for the first time in labour, when vaginal examination will demonstrate the root of the nose and the two orbital ridges of a brow, or the nose, the mouth and the two orbital hollows of a face. Confirmation by a senior colleague is often of value: these cases are rare and occasionally the mouth can be mistaken for the anal orifice.

Management of face and brow

There is no point in attempting to correct the abnormality prior to the onset of labour, the advent of which will hopefully lead to the head flexing and the vertex becoming the presenting part. If there is an over-riding requirement to deliver the baby, elective Caesarean section is usually a wiser choice than inducing labour with the high presenting part, even if the cervix is suitable.

Once labour starts it should be managed in the normal fashion until full dilatation. Seeds & Cefalo (1982) pointed out that many brows convert to a vertex or a face and most faces are mento-anterior. The cervix should be expected to dilate at 1 cm/hour and Syntocinon may be used to achieve this, remembering that many of these patients are multiparous and the abnormal presenting part can lead to obstructed labour and rupture the uterus. Thus if after 1 hour of contractions which have been considered adequate there is no increase in dilatation of the cervix or alteration in the presenting part, such as a brow turning to a face or a face descending in the pelvis, it is safer to deliver the baby by Caesarean section. At full dilatation, management will be determined by the size of the pelvis. If it is small, the presenting part will remain high and Caesarean section will be needed. If large, as is often the case, the presenting part will descend below the spines and may come to vaginal delivery.

Face presentation may be encouraged to deliver spontaneously provided that the chin is already anterior or is rotating forwards. Should it be mento-posterior, it is usually high in the pelvis and although rotation forceps can be successfully applied, most operators will opt for Caesarean section as the wiser choice. However, Cruikshank & Cruikshank (1981) report a section rate of only 15% in a review of 2373 faces with 72% requiring low-forceps and only 12% needing mid-forceps.

Manipulations such as Thorn's manoeuvre for turning a brow into a vertex do work but the complication is so rare that few people have much experience of their use. Provided the head is engaged, it is possible to treat a forward-facing brow as an exaggerated occipito-posterior position. It can be flexed with a vacuum cup or by applying a Neville Barnes forceps with the handles held very posteriorly at first and then brought forwards.

Most experienced obstetricians and midwives have seen babies delivered brow first with no untoward effects but there are no references in the literature to this being an acceptable procedure. The author has personally applied a 4-cm vacuum cup to a brow which delivered with one gentle pull. The baby was subsequently found to weigh 3750 g.

TRANSVERSE LIE

A transverse lie involves the long axis of the fetus lying at right angles to the uterus. The incidence is 2% early in the third trimester but only 0.3% at term. Most cases have no obvious aetiology and are presumably due to laxity of the abdominal musculature in a multiparous patient. However, this must not be assumed until pelvic tumours such as placenta praevia, fibroids and ovarian cysts have been excluded, along with fetal malformations, including twins. Rarely the cause is an abnormal uterus with the baby fixed in a transverse lie, its back pointing towards the lower segment. Antenatal diagnosis is usually easy with two poles of the fetus felt on either side of the abdomen. Ultrasound must be done to exclude the various abnormalities already mentioned. Vaginal examination is contraindicated for fear of disturbing a possibly low-lying placenta.

Once labour starts the diagnosis is made in the same manner but vaginal examination can confirm the lie by feeling a shoulder or the baby's ribs. The shoulder can feel like the breech, hence the importance of having the facility to do ultrasound scans in the delivery suite.

Management

Provided the gestational age has been confirmed, a persistently transverse or unstable lie should be managed conservatively until 37 weeks' gestation. At that stage external cephalic version may be done and repeated at each antenatal visit until the presentation is cephalic. This is easier to perform if the baby is facing downwards (Fig. 36.7a) than if it is facing upwards (Fig. 36.7b) but should always be attempted. As the volume of amniotic fluid diminishes nearer term the uterus may close down on the fetus and hold it in a longitudinal lie. The mother must be given strict instructions to come into hospital if there is any sign of labour and many units will feel happier if they can admit her 2 or 3 weeks before term for daily observation.

There are three methods of managing these cases after 37 weeks—conservative, stabilizing induction, and elective Caesarean section.

The conservative approach involves keeping the mother in hospital in the hope that the lie will straighten either before labour or when it starts. This is expensive and disruptive to the patient's family life; there is no guarantee that the membranes will not rupture spontaneously with cord prolapse and death of the baby before an emergency Caesarean section can be undertaken.

Stabilizing induction is done by first converting the lie to a cephalic presentation, starting an oxytocin infusion

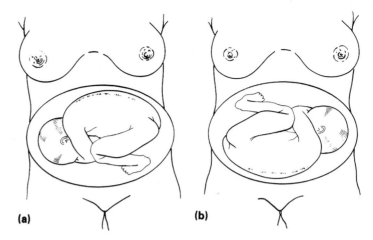

Fig. 36.7 Transverse lie. **(a)** Baby facing pelvis: pushing down the head produces flexion and makes version easy. **(b)** Baby facing maternal diaphragm: pushing down the head extends the fetal spine and makes version difficult.

and having a midwife sitting with the patient and checking the lie frequently. Once the head enters the pelvic brim the membranes are ruptured and the infusion continued. Edwards & Nicholson (1969) produced excellent results with this approach but while it works well with patients of low parity, in the grand multipara the tendency is for the membranes to rupture spontaneously before the head enters the brim and the lie then becomes oblique or reverts to transverse as the amniotic fluid drains out. Elective Caesarean section is the safest route for the baby provided it is mature. For the mother it is a major procedure but may be safer than the emergency operation necessary if either of the other modes of management is unsuccessful.

If the transverse lie is first diagnosed in labour, placenta praevia and fetal abnormality must be excluded by ultrasound, which can also sometimes demonstrate a cord in the lower segment (Lange et al 1985). Provided these other complications are not present, external version to a longitudinal lie may be attempted between contractions. The bladder is kept empty with an indwelling catheter and if the fetus remains longitudinal a normal labour is anticipated. Vaginal examination is done when the membranes rupture to exclude cord prolapse; cord prolapse or failure of the fetus to stabilize will demand immediate Caesarean section. If the diagnosis is not suspected until after the membranes have ruptured the uterus will be wrapped tightly around the baby, making abdominal palpation more difficult. Careful vaginal examination will reveal an arm, a shoulder or some ribs, all of which can be mistaken for a breech presentation. Immediate Caesarean section is essential to prevent ruptured uterus in all cases where the baby is alive and in most where it is dead.

Internal version is contraindicated even with a live fetus and intact membranes, because while the cervix may appear fully dilated, once the procedure ruptures the membranes the uterus will clamp down on the baby and the cervix will then be found to be only 6 or 7 cm dilated with subsequent entrapment of the aftercoming head.

Transverse lie in labour is most commonly found with a second twin. This differs from a singleton pregnancy in that the cervix has already been fully dilated and will not start to close down for 20 or 30 minutes. The fetal lie is checked or corrected abdominally and with rupture of the membranes, maternal effort and possibly an oxytocin infusion will push the presenting part into the pelvis and the baby will deliver. With any signs of fetal distress, internal version and then breech extraction are permissible. Helped by suitable analgesia and occasionally general anaesthesia a hand pushes up the membranes, grasps a foot and pulls it down through the membranes, tearing them as it emerges. It is important not to release amniotic fluid before grasping the foot as the uterus clamps down on the baby and by the time the foot is located attempts to turn the baby can harm it and rupture the uterus.

A compound presentation is uncommon, and is diagnosed in labour by vaginal examination. Most cases have a limb beside the fetal head. Provided the latter is descending with contractions the head usually pushes its way past the limb and labour continues normally. A high unstable presentation should be managed as for transverse lie, with repeated vaginal examinations to exclude cord prolapse and monitor alterations in the presentation.

BREECH PRESENTATION

The incidence of breech presentation varies with fetal maturity. Scheer & Newbar (1976) report a 16% incidence at 32 weeks, falling to 7% at 38 weeks and 5% at 40 weeks. Thus it should not be considered abnormal until late in pregnancy and causes no problems unless premature labour intervenes. Nearer term a breech presentation is due to something preventing spontaneous version. Fianu & Vaclavinkova (1978) stated that 78% of breech babies had cornual implantations of the placenta, compared with 4% of cephalic presentations, although Luterkort et al (1984) contested this. Where there is no such obvious pathology the lesion would appear to lie in the infant's inability to kick itself around. Thus any baby born after a breech delivery must be suspected of having some neurological impairment of its lower limbs until proved otherwise.

Faber-Nijolt and his colleagues (1983) felt that the mild neurological dysfunction found after breech birth was not always due to the vaginal delivery while O'Connell & Keane (1985) have described several inherent differences in breech babies. Torgrim & Bakke (1986) reported that breech babies have shorter cords than cephalic-presenting babies, but whether this is due to their lack of mobility or whether the short cord actually prevents them turning in utero is not clear.

The mechanism of breech labour involves the bitrochanteric diameter (9.25 cm) entering the pelvis in the transverse plane, rotating in mid-cavity and presenting at the pelvic outlet in the anterior–posterior diameter. The buttocks deliver in this position and then the whole body rotates to allow the shoulders to do exactly the same. Delivery of the anterior shoulder occurs as the head enters the pelvis in the transverse diameter, hopefully flexed as much as possible. Internal rotation then occurs so that the chin appears at the perineum, followed by the face, and then flexion allows the remainder of the skull to leave the pelvis. Thus there are no difficulties about the mechanics: the problem of a vaginal delivery is that the largest and least compressable part of the baby comes out last.

Because of the irregular outline of the breech, spontaneous rupture of the membranes may be followed by cord prolapse. This is not always as serious as in a cephalic presentation because the soft breech is less likely to compress the cord, although the cord may still go into spasm and cause acute fetal hypoxia. The ill-fitting breech can also be associated with slower labour but this appears to happen only in multiparous women (Clinch & Matthews 1985). The classical complication at the end of labour is that caused by the bitrochanteric diameter being smaller than the biparietal, so that the breech and the lower limbs can fit through a cervix or pelvis which is not sufficiently large for the after-coming head.

The small baby is unlikely to have bony problems but as the head is relatively larger than in the mature baby it may be caught in a partially dilated cervix, causing acute asphyxia. This can happen to the larger baby, especially if a foot pressing on the maternal rectum causes the mother to push before full dilatation.

In both premature and mature babies the skull does not have sufficient time to mould when passing through the pelvis; Wigglesworth & Husemeyer (1977) have shown the danger of damage to the occipital bone which increases the possibility of intracranial haemorrhage. Nevertheless, most premature breeches suffer more from the complications of immaturity than the actual mode of delivery and good management in labour rarely allows a mature breech to get into trouble.

Diagnosis in the antenatal period should be made by abdominal palpation and if the presentation persists, ultrasound to exclude fetal abnormality and demonstrate the placental site will confirm it. Occasionally, vaginal examination in labour reveals a previously unsuspected case.

Management of breech presentation has traditionally distinguished between primigravid and multigravid mothers. While this is correct in virtually every other type of obstetric complication, it is of little value in breech because most cases are really side-effects of premature labour. Small breeches suffer from immaturity as well as from the mode of delivery and should therefore be considered separately from larger babies. A dividing line of 37 weeks is convenient to take because until that gestation no active measures are needed on account of the presentation.

Management of the preterm breech in labour

The incidence of breech presentation in babies born before 37 weeks is approximately 15%. They are not a cohesive group. Some mothers arrive with ruptured membranes or a small antepartum haemorrhage but few contractions, and yet are found a few hours later with the cervix fully dilated and a bearing-down sensation, having had no obvious labour. Others labour, but at 6 or 7 cm push the small limbs and body through the cervix, which remains insufficiently stretched to allow passage of the aftercoming head.

On admission to the delivery suite the mother's chart should be checked to see that fetal abnormality has been ruled out. Even if this is the case ultrasound must be employed to confirm it, to exclude a low-lying placenta, to make an estimate of fetal weight, and possibly to assess the presence or absence of fetal breathing which may give some indication of whether labour is likely to proceed (Besinger et al 1987). Anderson (1981) reported that in up to 80% of cases where the mother thinks she is in premature labour contractions cease spontaneously and the pregnancy continues. Therefore immediate vaginal examination is contraindicated: it may introduce infection leading to chorioamnionitis or premature rupture of the membranes if these are still intact (Iams et al 1987, Sbarra et al 1987).

Nevertheless, the baby must be monitored by external techniques as in some cases the cord will be in the lower segment of the uterus and virtually prolapsed. Should contractions persist or the membranes rupture, vaginal examination may be undertaken in the expectation that the baby is going to be delivered. To prevent the mother pushing before full dilatation an epidural or caudal block should always be utilized (David & Rosen 1976, Crawford 1985). This will also relax the pelvic floor, reducing pressure on the fetal head when it passes through as well as facilitating any vaginal manoeuvre which may become necessary.

The actual delivery is the same as for a mature breech but there is some evidence that a caul delivery is better for the baby than rupturing the membranes (Goldenberg & Nelson 1984). The infant must be handled particularly gently, with a paediatrician present for the birth. Should the cervix clamp down on the head, rapid infusion of a tocolytic may relax it somewhat but this is not always available so the head should be flexed with one hand abdominally and the middle finger of the vaginal hand in the baby's mouth. Turning the baby into the transverse diameter may make it easier to deliver through the cervix.

If this is unsuccessful, scissors with the intracervical blade guarded by a finger are used to incise the cervix at 4 and 8 o'clock. The previously described manoeuvre should then deliver the head. The edges of the cervical incisions are grasped with sponge-holding forceps and are usually easy to suture as the cervix hangs down into the vagina.

Caesarean section for preterm breech

Whether preterm vaginal breech delivery has any place was first questioned by Ingemarsson and his colleagues in 1978. They showed that babies delivered by Caesarean section between 1975 and 1977 had a better outlook than those born vaginally between 1971 and 1974. Other writers concurred (Duenhoelter et al 1979, Weaver 1980, Kauppila et al 1981) but Crowley and Hawkins (1980), in a review of 11 papers, indicated that while babies weighing between 1000 and 1500 g did better, the prognosis for smaller ones was not improved by an abdominal approach. Further confirmation of this soon appeared (Lamont et al 1983, Main et al 1983, Yu et al 1984, Morales & Koerten 1986). On the other hand, Cox et al (1982) found that increasing the use of Caesarean section, whatever the fetal size, carried no advantage. Olshan and his colleagues (1984) agreed, partly because their series included babies weighing 700–1500 g. Kitchen and co-workers had stated in 1982 that abdominal delivery for very small breech babies did not reduce long-term handicap and in 1985, describing infants born between 24 and 28 weeks' gestation, showed no statistical difference between the two modes of delivery. Both Rayburn et al (1983) and Effer et al in the same year came to the conclusion that the side-effects of immaturity were far more important than the mode of delivery, while Myers & Gleicher (1987) in a review of the critical factors involved in breech delivery concluded that a clearcut case had not yet been made for elective Caesarean section in any particular group of premature breech babies.

However, Canadian workers (Bodmer et al 1986) felt that since head entrapment killed seven out of 55 premature breech babies born between 25 and 28 weeks's gestation, perhaps Caesarean section should be undertaken for all babies weighing less than 1000 g. Karp and his colleagues (1979) had already tried to distinguish between the various types of presenting part and felt that small footling breeches should always be delivered by Caesarean section, but that those with extended legs could be allowed a trial of labour.

At present it would seem sensible to consider Caesarean section in babies thought to weigh between 1000 and 1500 g, allowing the others to progress in labour and always remembering how difficult it can be to assess fully a premature breech baby in early labour.

Reporting from a hospital where the policy is to utilize abdominal delivery, Westgren et al (1985a) remarked that many cases advanced so quickly that it was not possible to estimate the baby's weight before delivery was imminent. Admitting that the study was retrospective, they had difficulty in showing that Caesarean section produced a statistically better result but reported that 25% of the deaths in the vaginally delivered group were due to head entrapment.

Management of the mature breech baby

If by 37 weeks the malpresentation persists, external cephalic version should be attempted. There is no point in considering the procedure before this gestation in view of the possibility of spontaneous version occurring. Kasule and his colleagues (1985) showed that version at various stages after 30 weeks produced no significant difference in the ultimate vaginal breech delivery, Caesarean section or perinatal mortality rates between those in whom version was attempted and controls. On the other hand several groups of workers have shown that version in the last 3 weeks of pregnancy results in a lower incidence of Caesarean section (Van Dorsten et al 1981, Hofmeyer 1983, Brocks et al 1984, Phelan et al 1985, Morrison et al 1986). All of these employed tocolytics. Dyson et al (1986) give details of dosage and point out that either ritodrine or terbutaline can be used.

The same factors which are thought to prevent spontaneous version also make external cephalic version more difficult. These are primigravidity, extended legs and firm abdominal muscles (Westgren et al 1985b) but even so, after the 37th week spontaneous version will result in only one-third of the number of cephalic presentations at term which will follow use of the external cephalic procedure (Hofmeyer et al 1986). Ferguson & Dyson (1985) even use version with tocolysis after labour has commenced. Their paper describes 22 term breeches in labour. Attempted version failed in seven with ruptured membranes, but succeeded in 11 of the remaining cases, of whom 10 had spontaneous vaginal deliveries.

In an extensive review Savona-Ventura (1986) agrees with the concept of attempting version late in pregnancy. He reminds the reader that many authors have reported transient fetal heart irregularities after the procedure but points out that if more serious complications arise the baby is mature enough to be delivered immediately. He also points out that while there is no significant fall in perinatal mortality as a result of version, it does lower neonatal morbidity and reduces the maternal morbidity associated with Caesarean section.

An active policy of version with tocolysis cannot yet be justified in women with a history of antepartum haemorrhage, hypertension or previous Caesarean section, but there is nothing to stop them using Elkins' manoeuvre. Elkins (1982) describes 71 women with confirmed breech presentation after the 37th week of gestation. All were instructed to adopt the knee–chest position for 15 minutes every 2 hours of waking time for 5 days. A total of 65 babies underwent spontaneous version and all had normal vaginal deliveries. Of the six who failed to turn, two had low-lying placentas, two had unusually short cords and one mother had a bicornuate uterus. All six underwent Caesarean section: there were no perinatal deaths in either group and no evidence of side-effects or complications from the manoeuvre.

After the baby has been turned, patients who are rhesus-negative will need anti-D immunoglobulin. All mothers must then be seen weekly to ascertain that the cephalic presentation persists. If it does not, it must be accepted that the baby is unable to tolerate being head-down and is best left as a breech. Whatever happens it is important to monitor the baby in labour, as doing the version may well have wrapped the cord around its neck or body, which can subsequently cause problems.

Management of the persistent breech presentation

Failure of version means that a decision must be made as to whether a breech presentation should be delivered by elective Caesarean section or allowed to go into labour. During the 1970s Caesarean section was being used increasingly: in the U.S., it rose for breeches from 11.6% in 1970 to 79.1% in 1985 (Croughan-Minilane 1990). Cheng and Hannah in 1993 pointed out that a percentage of mothers sectioned for breech experienced significant morbidity. In 1982 Green et al reported that a Caesarean section rate increase from 22% to 94% produced no significant improvement for breech babies either in the short or long term. A review by Russell (1982) lamented the increased Caesarean section rate without giving concrete alternatives. Gimovsky et al (1983), in a preliminary report of a randomized study, recommended that the section rate should not exceed 50%, while a year late Watson and Benson produced an overall abdominal delivery rate of 36%. Despite this trend towards vaginal delivery, Flanagan and colleagues (1987) found it necessary to perform elective Caesarean section on 68% of 623 term breeches. To resolve such conflicting views it is suggested that the practising clinician should assess every mature breech in a series of simple steps, as described below.

Abdominal palpation, done by an experienced obstetrician, may occasionally indicate that the infant is so large that elective Caesarean section is justified. Ultrasound, after excluding abnormality, should be used to estimate the fetal weight. If this is more than 4000 g, again a Caesarean section may be indicated. The fetal attitude is also important and even with a small baby, extension of the head is an unfavourable finding. Westgren et al (1981) reported an incidence of 7.4% neck extension in a series of breeches. There was a 22% incidence of neurological problems in these babies if delivered vaginally, but none after Caesarean section. They advocated abdominal delivery if the neck was extended to any degree.

X-ray pelvimetry should be used in patients not so far chosen for elective section, even if they have had a previous vaginal delivery of a good-sized baby. Ridley et al (1982) have shown that neonates whose mothers underwent a radiological assessment of their pelvis were fitter than those in whom this was not done, whatever the eventual route of delivery.

The simplest method is a standing lateral X-ray of the pelvis; Gimovsky et al (1985), along with Adam and his co-workers (1985), have shown that digital radiography is more accurate than conventional techniques and, like computerized tomography, results in less fetal and maternal irradiation (Kopelman et al 1986). Computational tomography (CAT scans) and magnetic resonance imaging will be used in the future; pelvic dimensions will probably be slightly larger if the patient is lying down.

Whatever method is used it is essential that a picture should be seen by the obstetrician in charge. While the radiologist will give accurate measurements, the shape of the pelvis must be taken into consideration. A well-curved sacrum supplies a large pelvic cavity but if the upper anterior surface is flat, any part of the baby negotiating the brim has to pass down a tunnel, as opposed to slipping between two narrow points. On occasion, the anterior surfaces of the first and second sacral vertebrae are so prominent that they actually produce funnelling in the upper pelvis (Fig. 36.8). To a lesser extent, the size of the sacrosciatic notch will indicate pelvic adequacy, the digital assessment of the subpubic angle helps in evaluating the size of the pelvic outlet and the presence of a potential

dead space. Should any of these unfavourable features be present or if the anterior–posterior diameter of either the inlet or the outlet is less than 11.5 cm, Caesarean section may be indicated.

Thus it is safe to allow a trial of labour in term breeches provided it is competently supervised, and that the unit in which it takes place is adequately equipped and staffed so that if it fails, the fact that the subsequent section is undertaken on an emergency rather than an elective basis is unlikely to increase maternal morbidity or mortality (Bingham & Lilford 1987).

Inducing labour prematurely in an attempt to achieve a smaller baby would have to be done so early in the pregnancy that the chances of successful induction would be much reduced. Induction for other reasons is not totally contraindicated but most obstetricians would regard two pregnancy complications as a reason for Caesarean section.

Management of labour in the mature breech

Once labour commences cervical dilatation and descent of the breech should be plotted on a partogram, as with a cephalic presentation. Vaginal examination is done to exclude cord prolapse and to confirm whether the breech is flexed or extended, while a monitoring clip is attached to the buttock. Rupture of the membranes along with an oxytocin infusion is permissible in a fully assessed patient, provided the procedures are used to accelerate a dilatory labour in its early stages rather than to drive an over-sized breech through the pelvis (Beazley et al 1975). As with premature breeches, epidural anaesthesia both relieves pain and prevents the mother pushing involuntarily before full dilatation. Failure of the cervix to dilate at a standard rate or of the breech to descend should be accepted as indicating that the baby is larger (or the pelvis smaller) than the prelabour assessment had implied, and Caesarean section will be required. There is no need to encourage maternal efforts immediately the cervix is fully dilated but once she does start pushing, failure of the breech to descend should lead to section rather than breech extraction. The bitrochanteric diameter is usually a little smaller than the biparietal; if the former does not pass easily through the pelvis, neither will the latter.

Provided labour progresses satisfactorily preparation should be made for an assisted breech delivery. This involves a standard forceps trolley on which there is also a sterile razor and a scalpel with a no. 1 blade. The mother is in the lithotomy position with a wedge under one side of the buttocks if she has an epidural. If not, it will be necessary to infiltrate the perineum and preferably do a pudendal block once the breech has descended on to it. Episiotomy is essential but is reserved until the fetal anus has appeared at the vulva. Once done, maternal

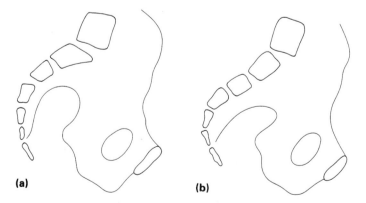

(a)   **(b)**

Fig. 36.8 Lateral view of pelves with identical inlet measurements. However, (**a**) has a good sacral curve so that once the brim is negotiated there is adequate space, while (**b**) has a straight sacrum so the head has to travel to mid-cavity before there is extra space.

effort should deliver the baby's buttocks and, with flexed legs, the lower limbs. With extended legs the operator will have to flex each knee joint separately, pushing it to the side of the baby so that the foot pops out.

The mother is encouraged to bear down until the trunk up to the scapula becomes visible. Cord pulsation is checked and a small loop pulled down to prevent a tight cord impeding further progress. The mother is asked to push again and the shoulders should deliver one at a time, along with the arms folded over the chest.

Failure of the shoulders to deliver is dealt with by lifting up the baby's legs and trunk, which enables a finger to reach an elbow joint; flexing it, and delivering it across the chest. This is repeated for the other side. Gentle rotation of the fetal trunk at the same time will assist this manoeuvre. Rarely, the baby's abdomen is facing the operator: if so, the trunk is turned and as the mother pushes, one shoulder will deliver under the symphysis with further rotation producing the other. With extended arms it is necessary to slide an index finger along the baby's scapula over the shoulder and down into the antecubital fossa to deliver the elbow between the body and the side of the vulva. These manoeuvres virtually always deliver the shoulders.

If case selection has been good, at this stage the baby's head may start to appear without any further effort on the operator's part. He or she should attempt to apply forceps to control the speed of delivery but if this is not possible the legs may be swung out and up in a Burns Marshall manoeuvre, keeping the vulva completely covered with the other hand. It is essential that the baby's legs should be kept vertically in the air and the weight taken off the cervical spine. Hyperextension of the neck with the body being held over the mother's abdomen will occlude the vertebral arteries and can lead to necrosis of the cervical cord. Excess weight on the cervical spine will either have the same effect or dislocate the baby's neck. The operator's vulval hand can then be opened slowly to allow first the baby's face and then the remainder of the head to deliver. The latter should be supported while the operator sits down with the baby across his or her knee.

Should maternal effort not push down the head, more assistance is needed as the occiput must be low enough in the pelvis to hinge around the back of the symphysis and not be caught above it. Simply permitting the baby to hang may delay progress: the manoeuvre can cause extension rather than flexion of the head as the head swivels on an axis through the biparietal eminences (Fig. 36.9). Therefore, while the baby is hanging feet down, the operator must insert two fingers behind the symphysis pubis to push up an anterior lip of cervix which is often dragged down by the occiput and will slow its final descent (Fig. 36.10). This will also tend to flex the head, an action which can be further assisted either by

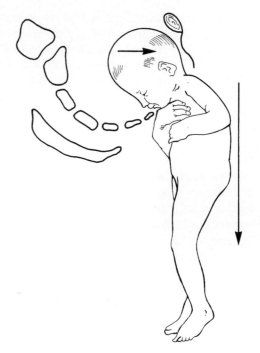

Fig. 36.9 Trunk of breech allowed to hang. Traction on fetal spine would extend not flex the head. Contrast this with Figure 36.2.

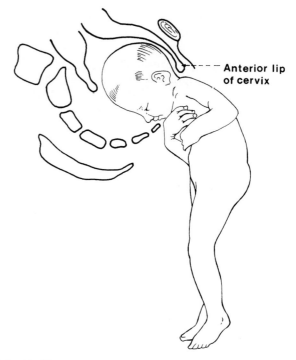

Fig. 36.10 Hanging breech. Anterior lip of cervix pulled down by occiput must be pushed up before forceps can be applied.

some suprapubic pressure or by renewed maternal effort or by both. Once the hair line is visible the head is delivered. The baby's feet are grasped and, using as much traction as required to keep the body straight and take weight off its neck, they are swung outwards and upwards to be held by an assistant, using a towel to make certain they do not slip. The operator then applies a Neville Barnes forceps and delivers the head slowly, sucking out the mouth as soon as it can be seen and remembering that the final part of the head only appears as the face flexes on to the chest.

Problems

Shoulder dystocia rarely occurs without extended arms; this has usually been caused by traction on the fetus early in the delivery. The body is pulled down leaving the arms behind rather than the uterus pushing down the whole fetus in a flexed attitude. Often the arms can be brought down as already described but lack of success means that Lovset's manoeuvre will be required. The classical procedure comprises three rotations but the fewer done the better, as each involves traction and rotation of the whole body. The baby must be held by the thighs—never by the trunk—and the operator must wrap the legs in a towel so that they do not slip when gripped.

Should the head not enter the pelvis after the shoulders have delivered, the baby's body must be turned sideways and suprapubic pressure used to flex the head and push it into the pelvis. This may be helped on occasions by the vaginal hand inserting a finger into the baby's mouth to flex it. Both these actions also make the head descend if it has entered the pelvis but is still not low enough to apply forceps.

Continued failure of the head to engage is the sole indication for symphysiotomy. The technique is described by Hartfield (1973), Philpott (1980) and Gebbie (1982), although the latter points out that in a mature baby, if the head is not going to fit through the pelvis the buttocks too should be obstructed. With proper predelivery assessment the technique will never be necessary, nor should such bizarre measures as replacing the body of the baby and proceeding to Caesarean section, as described by Iffy et al (1986), although their case probably succeeded only because the uterus was still distended by the second twin. Such potential disasters emphasize the importance of delivery suites having the facilities available to make rapid assessment in unbooked or unsuspected breech deliveries (Davis & Brunfield 1984).

The Mauriceau Smellie Veit manoeuvre is favoured by some obstetricians for routine delivery of the head. While a finger in the mouth may cause flexion, traction on the cervical spine will do the opposite. Combined, they can draw the base of the skull away from the vault, stretching the falx cerebri and producing a perfect way of tearing the tentorium cerebelli as well as causing brachial plexus injuries. The manoeuvre is best avoided. On the other hand, inexperienced operators can forget that unlike a conventional forceps application, a breech delivery means that the smallest part of the baby's skull appears at the vulva first with the large parietal area at the back of the pelvis. Thus, if the forceps handle is straightened out too soon after insertion of the blade, the distal part of the blade will dig into the side of the baby's head and it will not be possible to lock the handles. The tip must be kept pointed at the sacrum for as long as possible, which means that the guiding hand has to be inserted well into the vagina until the tip has passed round the occiput. Properly trained obstetricians can manage this: those taught simply to open the labia will find the correct application virtually impossible.

UMBILICAL CORD PRESENTATION AND PROLAPSE

This malpresentation occurs about once in every 300 deliveries. Cord presentation is said to take place when the cord lies below the level of the presenting part and is said to have prolapsed following rupture of the membranes and its release into the vagina.

Sometimes a malpresentation of the cord can be identified on ultrasound scan, but more often it is found on vaginal examination when, if the fetus is alive, it becomes an obstetric emergency.

This malpresentation is often associated with the condition in which the presenting part of the fetus is incompletely filling the pelvis, thus allowing room for the umbilical cord to pass between it and the pelvic wall. Thus this condition should be suspected with a high head, polyhydramnios, a footling or flexed breech, transverse lie and a small fetus, either premature or a member of a multiple pregnancy.

Diagnosis

This is usually made on vaginal examination following rupture of the membranes. If the fetus has not already died it is in imminent danger of doing so by either spasm of the vessels in the cord exposed to the air or more likely due to compression of the cord against the pelvic wall. On the rare occasions the diagnosis is made in the second stage then a forceps delivery is indicated. In all other cases the mother should be placed in a head down position so as to dislodge the presenting pole from the pelvis to avoid cord compression. The hand of the examiner should be kept in the vagina to prevent further prolapse of the cord and its compression, and arrangements should be made as quickly as possibly by others in the department for immediate Caesarean section.

The essence of good management is anticipation. Prophylactic measures such as the admission of patients to hospital with unstable and transverse lie in the last 3 weeks of pregnancy, and the avoidance of artificially rupturing the membranes before the fetal pole has become deeply engaged in the pelvis, and the early vaginal examination following spontaneous rupture of the membranes will all help to reduce the mortality and morbidity for the fetus.

CAESAREAN SECTION FOR ABNORMAL POSITIONS AND PRESENTATIONS

Abdominal delivery for fetal malposition or malpresentation often takes place at the end of a long labour and may technically be more difficult than with a normal presentation. Although there is no need to use any of the more complicated extraperitoneal approaches which are occasionally suggested (Wallace et al 1984), there should always be someone experienced scrubbed up in theatre; the operating table must be tilted laterally or a simple wedge inserted under the mother's right buttock (Endler & Donath 1985) and a paediatrician skilled in neonatal resuscitation should be present. Several other points are worth emphasizing.

Occipito-posterior positions

However high the head feels on vaginal examination, at Caesarean section it can be difficult to extricate from the pelvis and an assistant must be scrubbed up ready to push it up vaginally. It must be assumed that the lower segment of the uterus will be thin and may tear readily. Therefore the surgeon should make the uterine incision fairly high in the lower segment so that if it does extend downwards the subsequent repair will be easier. He or she should aim to insert a hand around the side of the baby's head and deliver it slowly out of the pelvis before bringing it anteriorly through the wound. In this way the head is flexed, with the chin going on to the baby's chest. Tears arise because the chin catches on the upper edge of the wound and as the face, followed by the brow, the vertex, and finally the occiput deliver, the lower edge is stretched to allow passage of these large diameters and often splits. Such lacerations are never easy to repair and occasionally involve the base of the bladder. The same comments apply to face and brow presenting parts, where the diameters may be even larger and, especially with the brow, the labour may have become obstructed, leading to excess thinning of the lower segment and occasionally a constriction ring.

Transverse lie

With intact membranes the operator has the choice of looking for the baby's head and steering it quickly into the incision as the uterus clamps down when the amniotic fluid rushes out. In practice, a limb appears in the incision: usually this is an arm. It should be replaced quickly, a leg grasped and the baby extracted as a breech. Many operators choose a breech delivery as a first option, pushing the membranes in front of the operating hand, finding a limb, palpating its lower end to make certain it is a foot and withdrawing it through the incision just as the amniotic fluid starts to escape.

With a transverse lie and already ruptured membranes the lower segment of the uterus will be so narrow that a conventional incision would not be large enough for any baby. The anaesthetist should be asked to give a rapid dose of a uterine relaxant for 2 or 3 minutes (Akamatsu 1975, Maduska 1981). Jovanovic (1985) has made the point that if the uterine incision is enlarged by cutting rather than tearing, with the extremes of the incision pointing upwards rather than laterally, then not only will the aperture be larger but any extension will go upwards rather than downwards and be easier to repair. Should these measures not be successful the operator has no choice but to proceed to enlarge the incision vertically from its middle point, making an inverted T incision. To avoid the possibility of this, many obstetricians regard transverse lie with ruptured membranes as almost the sole remaining indication for the classical operation. Here, the bladder should be pushed down and the incision brought as far as possible into the lower segment and only extended upwards as needed.

In all cases the inside of the uterus must be inspected to exclude an abnormality such as a small septum or a fibroid which might have caused the transverse lie. This is carefully noted in the patient's chart for future reference, along with inspection of the ovaries and tubes, to rule out other tumours which may have had the same effect.

Premature breech

If the baby is very small the lower segment may not have formed. Although Haesslein & Goodlin (1979) proposed solving this problem by using a classical incision, most other workers do not agree with them. Westgren et al (1982) advocated a bolus of uterine relaxant, probably terbutaline, just before opening the uterus, although Westgren later modified this when writing with Paul in 1985, suggesting that the lower segment should be carefully examined and in some cases a vertical incision performed. Hobel & Oakes (1980) thought that halothane at the induction of anaesthesia was best for all small section babies. Schutterman & Grimes (1983), reviewing 416 breeches of all gestations allocated randomly to transverse or low vertical incisions, found no advantages for low vertical incisions.

It would appear that the normal lower segment transverse incision, with an added uterine relaxant in some cases, is satisfactory for breech section. Whatever incision is used the baby must be delivered as gently as with the vaginal approach: forceps are essential for the aftercoming head. In order that no part of the baby is caught in the abdominal wound the incision should be sufficiently big to take the beak of a large, not just a small, Doyen retractor.

Mature breech

Section for mature breech should produce no technical difficulties but forceps should be available for controlling delivery of the aftercoming head. The ideas about not hyperextending or placing too much weight on the cervical spine apply equally forcibly.

An analysis in the management for mature breech deliveries in North West Thames (Thorpe-Beeston et al 1992), the incidence of intrapartum and neonatal death was shown to be higher in association with vaginal birth (0.83%) compared with Caesarean section (0.03%). However, this analysis of 3447 breech deliveries was not conducted as a randomized control trial, and there was no detailed information, whether or not the loss of the eight fetuses by vaginal delivery was in any way associated with the mechanism of breech delivery nor was the criteria in each centre for allowing vaginal delivery outlined.

THE NEWBORN BABY

All babies born after abnormal presentations or positions require a thorough paediatric examination even if the delivery was spontaneous and however well they may appear at the time. The unusual moulding due to the abnormal position of the head or the speed of this moulding may cause intracranial lesions. Some will have had operative vaginal deliveries which, however easy they may seem to the attendant, are more traumatic for the fetus. Above all, there is always the suspicion that the malpresentation or the malposition has been due to some abnormality in the fetus. This is especially so in the case of the breech baby. Many of these will be premature and paediatric assessment will be routine in any case.

In the mature breech, it should be assumed until proved otherwise that some inherent defect in the baby prevented it from turning a somersault in utero; one looks forward to studies assessing whether those in whom external version has been successful suffer from the same disabilities.

Above all, it is important to be aware that not all neonatal deficiencies are due to the mode of delivery or to incorrect obstetrical management in labour. Illingworth (1985) stressed that most cases of cerebral palsy or mental subnormality follow a normal pregnancy and delivery: to ascribe brain damage solely to events occurring during labour is too simplistic.

Abnormal presentations and positions will continue to arise in obstetrical practice. It is essential that labour ward routines should be constantly updated to counteract the adverse effects of abnormal presentations on both mother and child. Fetal assessment by cardiotocography and pH estimations is accepted, but Modanlou and his coworkers (1982) feel that it is important to establish the relationship between the whole baby and the maternal pelvis. The authors point out that the average fetal size is increasing and that more effort should be made to diagnose macrosomia at term. Knowledge of the chest circumference and its ratio to head size should reduce the incidence of shoulder dystocia and contribute to a fall in the number of difficult vaginal deliveries. Each labour is a trial: one looks forward to the day when the result can be forecast accurately in every labouring woman.

CEPHALOPELVIC DISPROPORTION

Cephalopelvic dystocia has been recognized as a grave complication of human parturition since earliest times. Its more serious consequences—a uterine rupture, vesicovaginal fistula, maternal and fetal death, birth injury—still exact a steady toll of suffering in the developing world. The prevalence of cephalopelvic dystocia in the human species is related to the unique size of the human brain and cranium at the time of birth in the newborn, and to the erect posture, which influences the mother's pelvic shape and size.

Most, if not all, the disasters which may result from unrecognized or unrelieved cephalopelvic dystocia can be prevented through timely and appropriate intervention. It was, therefore, an important milestone in obstetric care when the concept of cephalopelvic disproportion was first propounded in the late 19th century. The idea embodied in the concept of disproportion was that disparity in size between the head and the pelvis could be assessed and identified before labour, or early in labour before serious dystocia occurred.

In this way, the attendants are alerted to the anticipated risk of difficult labour, and delivery can be planned with appropriate skilled supervision. In historical perspective, the concept of cephalopelvic disproportion was one of the first elements in the development of preventive prenatal care.

Initially, disproportion was diagnosed through the use of relatively crude clinical assessments of the fetal head fitting in the pelvic brim. The prevalence of disproportion tended to be overestimated, and its importance was sometimes exaggerated. For many years it was a generally accepted dogma that if in a primigravida engagement of the head failed to occur by the 36th week of pregnancy, cephalopelvic disproportion should be suspected. This teaching was subsequently shown by Weekes & Flynn (1975) and by Sharma & Soni (1978) to be quite erroneous. The modal interval between engagement and the onset of labour is, in fact, less than 7 days.

Later, during the second quarter of this century,

radiological methods of pelvic measurement were developed; some obstetric radiologists claimed remarkable accuracy for their predictions of the degree of mechanical difficulty which would occur in labour. Since the heyday of radiological prediction in the 1950s, the pendulum has swung back towards a more empirical outlook. This chapter will seek to present a balanced contemporary view of cephalopelvic assessment and of the management of disproportion. First it is necessary to consider the major factors influencing pelvic size and shape, so that the epidemiology of pelvic contraction can be better understood.

Factors influencing pelvic morphology

The girdle of bone which bounds the birth canal has an important weight-bearing function throughout life. Among pronograde animals, weight-bearing is shared by all four limbs, but in the erect human posture the lower limbs, through the pelvic girdle, support the whole weight of the rest of the body.

In an infant the developing component parts of the bony pelvis are still separated by wide margins of osteogenic cartilage, and the pelvic cavity has a long oval (dolichopellic) shape. The formation and consolidation of bone depends on an adequate intake of mineral—calcium, phosphorus—and of vitamin D, which promotes mineral absorption (Table 36.2).

During normal growth, the rate of increase in the density and strength of the bones matches the progressive increase in the child's body weight at every stage. If, however, the requirement for mineral and vitamin D is not fully met during the years of growth, particularly during the growth spurts of infancy and adolescence, nutritional disease of bone is likely to develop and overall growth may be stunted. The impaired strength of the affected bone will permit distortion by the stresses of weight-bearing. Obesity in childhood will increase these distorting forces so that the knock-kneed overfed child of an affluent family is only too commonly seen. Excessive

load-carrying in childhood can be expected to have a similar influence.

Florid rickets and osteomalacia are now rarities in Britain but there is clear evidence from biochemical studies and measurements of bone density that nutritional bone disease occurs in less overt forms in the neonate (Lancet Editorial 1986), the infant (Amiel & Crosbie 1963), the adolescent (Ford et al 1976) and the adult (British Medical Journal Editorial 1979).

The delicacy of the balance normally maintained between weight-bearing stress and bone strength during growth is also demonstrated if the growing child suffers from disease or injury affecting one lower limb, and has an impairing gait over a period of time. Even a modest extra share of weight-bearing carried by the good leg is usually sufficient to distort the side wall of the pelvis on the healthy side, because of the extra pressure on the acetabular floor, despite normal consolidation of bone. When the condition affects the infant before he or she can stand or walk, the body weight in the sitting position is transmitted through the imperfectly ossified pelvic girdle to the ischial tuberosities, which tend to splay apart, widening the pubic arch and the transverse diameters of the lower pelvis. The upper part of the sacrum is pushed forward, but the lower sacrum rotates backwards, pivoting on the sacroiliac joints.

When, however, nutritional bone disease develops during the later growth spurt of adolescence (11–13 years old in females) the pelvis in its lower part is subjected to different compressive forces through the acetabula. The bony structure of the lower and anterior parts of the pelvis is much lighter than the dense posterior arch, and ossification is completed later; these parts are pushed medially. As a consequence, the brim of the pelvis loses its rounded contour anteriorly, the pubic arch may be narrowed, and the side walls of the mid and lower pelvis are approximated, with funnelling of the birth canal (Fig. 36.11).

In rare instances of severe adult osteomalacia, the softened pelvic bones are grossly distorted into a triradiate form (Fig. 36.12), clearly illustrating the nature and direction of the main weight-bearing stresses on the pelvic girdle. However, milder forms of adult osteomalacia occur, as has been documented, for example, in Arab and Bedouin women by Fahmy (1973), Toppozada (1964) and by Chaim et al (1981). In these milder forms of nutritional bone disease in the adult, the commonest deformity is a progressive protrusion of the upper sacrum, reducing the conjugate diameter of the pelvic brim. Even a modest reduction in pelvic capacity of this nature can have disastrous obstetric consequences in a multiparous woman.

The pattern of pelvic contraction in a community, therefore, reflects the nutritional experience of the females concerned from their infant years. In Britain and similar

Table 36.2 Nutritional/metabolic bone disease: factors influencing vitamin D metabolism

Source	Form of vitamin D	Interfering factors
Diet	Ergocalciferol Vitamin D_2	Poor nutrition Phytates
Skin	7-Dehydrocholesterol	
UV light	Cholecalciferol Vitamin D_3	Lack of sunlight
Liver	25-OHD$_3$	Liver disease Anticonvulsants
Kidney	1,25-(OH)$_2$D$_3$ Calcitriol	Vitamin D dependent rickets Renal osteodystrophy Renal tubular disorders

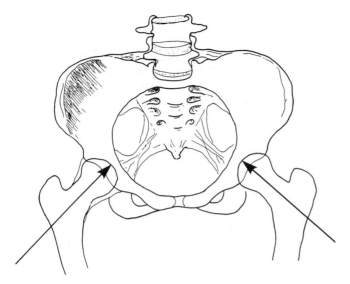

Fig. 36.11 Pelvis illustrating the almost transverse compression effect of weight-bearing. This could lead to funnelling of the lower pelvis if the compressive forces acted in the presence of nutritional bone disease.

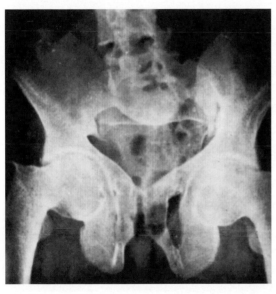

Fig. 36.12 X-ray of pelvis showing osteomalacia. Reproduced with permission from Myerscough (1982).

developed countries, such bone changes in the infant have been virtually eliminated by ensuring an adequate intake of vitamin D, and are only liable to develop in the infant of very low birthweight. A surprising amount of nutritional bone disease, much of it overt, has been discovered among adolescents, mainly in immigrant Asian communities. Causal factors in these subjects include a diet rich in phytate (chapatti flour), and limited exposure of the skin to sunlight. Similarly, evidence of osteomalacia in multiparous immigrant women during pregnancy and lactation can be demonstrated. Prophylaxis with vitamin D (500 u/day) is indicated, but compliance is often poor.

In an overall view, the nutritional factors described are found to be the dominant influence on pelvic size and shape. Genetic variations certainly exist, but in practical terms are of secondary importance.

Among the tallest, best nourished women, therefore, the brim of the pelvis commonly retains a long oval (dolichopellic) shape, and all the pelvic diameters are adequate for parturition, as Greulich & Thoms first demonstrated (1939). This pelvic shape is the truly gynaecoid pelvis, if that word is to be used.

Among women of near-average stature and nutrition, the pelvic brim is rounded, and although the conjugate diameter is often less than the transverse diameter, no serious flattening has occurred during growth. Shorter women with a less favourable nutritional background include more frequent examples of brim-flattening amounting to significant deformation, which is liable to result in cephalopelvic disproportion.

Convergent funnelling of the pelvic side walls was recognized many years ago by Whitridge Williams (1941) to be a relatively common (perhaps the commonest) form of pelvic deformation then encountered in American women. This may well also be true of Britain at the present time. The configuration of this type of pelvic deformation and its associated features are consistent with the view that it results from less severe nutritional bone disease in the adolescent, often with excessive weight-bearing stress due to obesity. By the time of the adolescent growth spurt, the posterior arch of dense bone between the acetabula, formed by the thick lower part of the ilium and the ala of the sacrum, is relatively resistant to deformation, but the strut-like form of the anterior and lower pelvis renders it more malleable.

The specific deformations which may result include slight flattening of the posterior segment of the brim, beaking of the anterior segment of the brim, and convergent funnelling of the side walls in the lower parts of the pelvis. The angle of the pubic arch may thus be reduced.

Summarizing in simple outline, therefore, it is evident that more severe nutritional bone disease in infancy is liable to result in deformation maximal at the pelvic brim, with reduction in the anteroposterior diameter, while less severe forms of the condition in the older child may cause deformation mainly of the lower pelvis, reducing the transverse diameters towards the outlet. Because this latter type of deformity is the one most likely to be encountered in Britain and other developed countries, the traditional view that a lateral pelvic X-ray delineates the most important pelvic dimensions may need to be revised.

Recognition of cephalopelvic disproportion

Failure to recognize or to be able to provide obstetric care in patients with severe disproportion and obstructive labour has disastrous consequences characterized by uterine rupture (particularly with increasing parity), avascular necrosis of the pelvic floor leading to vesicovaginal and rectovaginal fistulae, and intrauterine death from asphyxia. Therefore careful observation by the obstetrician and midwife to the possibility of disproportion long before progress in labour becomes arrested is essential.

The size of the fetus

Dystocia may arise in the presence of a normal size and shaped pelvis because the fetus is excessively large. Macrosomia (>4000 g) is often hereditary, related to the size of one or both the parents, more frequently found in increasing parity and in patients with undiagnosed or poorly controlled gestational diabetes. It is also often associated with prolonged pregnancy and maternal obesity and high weight gain in pregnancy.

Gross abnormality of the fetus such as hydrocephalus, abdominal ascites, excessive enlargement of the fetal bladder and organ tumours may also lead to dystocia and obstructive labour. Fortunately all these excessive growth abnormalities are easily measured with ultrasound and avoiding steps can then be taken.

General features

The relationship between stature and pelvic size has been recognized for many years. It derives from the stunting of growth which accompanies impaired nutrition in infancy and early childhood. The degree of brim-flattening is thus likely to be reflected in the degree of growth-stunting. Contraction of the outlet, however, originating at a later stage in growth, is less closely associated with restriction of stature.

Primigravidae of less than 155 cm (5′ 1″) should, therefore, be carefully assessed at or shortly before the onset of labour. Women whose height is 165 cm (5′ 5″) or greater will rarely manifest disproportion. Those women with a limp or a history of pelvic fracture will also all require careful earlier review. These guidelines are relevant to British practice. However, in the developing world, where malnutrition is rife, almost every primigravida must be regarded as having a pelvis of uncertain capacity.

Among parous patients a history of previous dystocia is always relevant, but its absence provides no firm assurance that disproportion will not develop. Birthweight tends to increase as parity advances and, besides, insidious flattening of the brim may develop in the multipara with osteomalacia.

Prelabour assessment

This is of some value as a screening procedure in primigravidae of small stature. The modal interval between engagement of the head and the onset of labour in primigravidae is less than 7 days, and in 80% of cases the interval is less than 14 days (Weekes & Flynn 1975). Non-engagement of the head is therefore unlikely to be of importance before the 39th week, but is of greater prognostic significance at the time of onset of labour.

In such cases a rough clinical assessment of possible brim-flattening can be attempted by estimating the diagonal conjugate. If the anterior surface of the first (or second) piece of the sacrum can be reached with the tip of the examining fingers, the anteroposterior dimensions of the upper pelvis are less than adequate. At the same time, the level of the head should be carefully assessed, and expressed as the amount of head (in fifths) still palpable in the abdomen (see Fig. 36.13). This simple and reproducible assessment provides a more reliable and objective guide to possible disproportion than do tests of head-brim fitting. If after the 39th week the head remains four-fifths palpable, cephalopelvic disproportion must be suspected.

A clinical assessment of the capacity of the pelvic outlet is also possible before or during labour. The angle of divergence of the pelvic rami (subpubic angle) can be felt anteriorly, and the anteroposterior diameter to the tip of the sacrum assessed with the extended fingers, in a manner similar to the diagonal conjugate estimate. However, the transverse dimensions of the lower pelvis are most significant, so that both the interischial spinous and the intertuberous diameters should be assessed. The prominence of the spine is felt vaginally; the intertuberous width can be roughly gauged with a closed fist externally. But clinical outlet assessment is of very limited accuracy as a screening test. Floberg et al (1986) screened a large group of primigravidae both clinically and radiologically. One-half of the patients with contracted outlets were not identified by clinical assessment. If the evidence from this prelabour assessment—taking into account short stature, high head, and unfavourable clinical pelvimetry—points towards possible disproportion, X-ray pelvimetry is usually of value.

Radiological pelvimetry

If as a result of clinical assessment before or during labour cephalopelvic disproportion is suspected, the wise course is to obtain accurate information about the pelvic dimensions by radiological pelvimetry. The newer imaging techniques of computational tomography (CAT scan) and magnetic resonance imaging are useful in depicting pelvic morphology, and may replace radiological methods.

In most of the Western world, two films provide adequate information for pelvic assessment. These are a frontal view using the semi-orthodiagraphic (tube-shift) method to define the transverse diameters at both brim and outlet and a lateral view depicting the anteroposterior diameters (Borell & Radberg 1964). The techniques of

X-ray pelvimetry have been refined over the years to minimize fetal exposure to radiation which, with the method described, is about 2 mGy. To reduce exposure to radiation even further, it is possible to use one film alone as the initial screening procedure. In developed countries it is logical, for the reasons outlined earlier in the chapter, to use the transverse pelvimetry film for screening. The radiation exposure involved is only a small fraction of that resulting from a lateral film. If the transverse diameters are adequate, no lateral film is required.

When both exposures are performed, the information they provide about the anteroposterior and transverse diameters at brim and outlet levels can be combined to calculate the approximate cross-sectional area of the birth canal at these levels. The area estimate (π r_1 r_2), as Allan (1947) demonstrated, correlates more closely with the incidence of cephalopelvic dystocia than does any single diameter. In the lower pelvis, where the axis of the birth canal is more sharply curved and the level of the different diameters does not coincide, Borell & Fernstrom (1960) advocated the combining of three diameters—the interspinous, intertuberous and sagittal—into a single index, the sum of the outlet. This should measure more than 32 cm.

The role of pelvimetry   The value of pelvimetry lies in:

1. Identifying those patients, few in our community, whose pelvic contraction, combined with other unfavourable features, justifies elective Caesarean section. Section in labour, despite the protective use of antibiotics, still carries a maternal risk which is about three times greater than elective abdominal delivery.
2. Forewarning the obstetrician about borderline disproportion. He or she is then guided in the conduct of trial labour not only by observation of the progress of descent and dilatation, but also by knowledge of the degree of mechanical difficulty which the head would encounter at lower levels in the pelvis.
3. Influencing the mode of delivery in outlet dystocia, the most common type of disproportion in the developed world, and one which is easily overlooked. The fine judgement required in deciding between abdominal or vaginal intervention is reinforced if objective pelvic measurements are known.

It must be acknowledged that, in the past, pelvimetry has often been employed inappropriately and sometimes with indiscriminate zeal. This has led to scepticism about its value, though this is counterbalanced by medicolegal concern about the consequences of ignoring pelvimetry. A panel convened jointly by the American Colleges of Obstetrics and Gynecology and of Radiology suggested guidelines for the use of pelvimetry, which would restrict the method to about 3% of parturients in the American population (United States Department of Health Education and Welfare 1980).

Interpretation of pelvimetry findings   As with most biological measurements, it is not helpful or appropriate to attempt to define absolute limits of normality. Disproportion must take account not only of the size of the pelvis, but also of the size of the head. Formerly X-ray cephalometry was attempted, and Moir (1947) developed methods of incorporating head size in his system of pelvic assessment as he sought to refine its predictive value. Sonar cephalometry now provides a much more accurate and safe method of measuring head size, which has yet to be applied systematically in the assessment of disproportion.

Table 36.3 sets out for various pelvic parameters the borderline zone between pelvic adequacy and absolute disproportion.

Cephalopelvic disproportion in primigravidae

First stage of labour

The alerting features in this situation include:

1. The head remains three- or four-fifths palpable abdominally.
2. The latent phase may be prolonged.
3. The active phase of dilatation is retarded. Eventually the progress of dilatation may cease, often between 7 and 9 cm.
4. The cervix may be poorly applied to the head, and in neglected cases may become oedematous.
5. As the progress of dilatation ceases, excessive head moulding is likely to become apparent and fetal heart rate decelerations during contractions tend to occur. Initially this is the result of head compression only, but ultimately it is also due to hypoxia.

Second stage of labour

When cephalopelvic dystocia only becomes evident at this late stage in labour, it is usually because the pelvis is contracted in its lower part. Although the first stage of labour may not have been unduly prolonged, often there will have been some premonitory sign of impending difficulty. Typically the partogram indicates that the rate of cervical dilatation in its later stages has slowed down,

Table 36.3   Borderline zone between pelvic adequacy and absolute disproportion

Variable	Measurement (cm)
Brim area	90^2–110^2
Obstetrical conjugate	9.0–11.5
Outlet area	80^2–100^2
Sum of outlet	31.0–33.5

and one- or two-fifths of the head remains palpable abdominally. On vaginal examination, the arrest of descent of the head may be masked by an increasingly large caput and head moulding is pronounced. The impaction of the head prevents anterior rotation of the occiput, so a persistent occipito-posterior or occipito-transverse position may be found.

Head moulding in cephalopelvic dystocia

Philpott & Stewart (1974) described a simple system of scoring to assess the degree of head moulding quantitatively. Moulding is assessed in at least two locations, i.e. lambdoidal suture, sagittal suture and, if possible, coronal suture. It is scored in three degrees:

+   indicates closing of the suture line
++   indicates reducible overlap
+++ indicates irreducible overlap of the cranial bones.

When the sum of the moulding scores at two of the sites is five or six pluses, serious disproportion is present and safe vaginal delivery will rarely be possible.

Fetal distress due to cephalopelvic dystocia

Two factors are responsible for the fetal distress which may arise during mechanically difficult labour:

1. Fetal head compression slows the fetal heart rate due to the rise in intracranial pressure accompanying contractions in the presence of marked head moulding. The decelerations synchronize with the contractions and are particularly likely to occur as the head, having moulded into a contracted pelvic inlet, then begins to descend more rapidly into the pelvic cavity.
2. When the progress of descent and dilatation is arrested, and labour is prolonged, fetal hypoxia is likely to develop. This causes late decelerations of the fetal heart rate typical of fetal asphyxia.

In cases of serious disproportion, both these effects may be seen together; the decelerations begin early during the contractions but reach a delayed nadir and recover slowly. This combined variable deceleration pattern is typical of the fetal distress caused by major cephalopelvic dystocia.

Management of cephalopelvic disproportion in primigravidae

It is necessary to consider primigravidae and parous women separately, because the pattern of their labours in the presence of cephalopelvic disproportion is quite different; this applies particularly to the risk of uterine rupture. The uterus of the primigravida reacts to mechanical difficulty with reduced contractility, though the myometrium may not relax normally between contractions. The undamaged primigravid uterus, therefore, can be relied on not to rupture spontaneously.

Elective Caesarean section

In the absence of other unfavourable features, elective Caesarean section is only indicated if the degree of pelvic contraction is severe, and particularly if the diameters are seriously reduced at more than one level. In other instances, complications such as malpresentation, advanced age, infertility, or diabetes will justify an elective operation, even when the pelvis is only moderately contracted. Although the maternal risk from abdominal delivery is small, it should not be forgotten that, despite antibiotic cover, section in labour carries a risk more than twice as great as an elective procedure. It also prejudices the management of future deliveries.

Trial of labour

In cases of minor or moderate cephalopelvic disproportion, which make up the great majority in this country, a trial of labour is the appropriate management. The term implies that the outcome of labour is uncertain because of mechanical difficulty, and that particularly vigilant monitoring of progress and of fetal well-being are required.

In some instances the trial will be relatively tentative, and will only be allowed to continue if there is progressive advance. But in the case of a young primigravida, where the pelvic contraction affects only one principal diameter, there should be greater persistence to achieve vaginal delivery, and augmentation of the uterine action with oxytocin infusion may be indicated if spontaneous uterine activity is not adequate.

Duration of trial of labour It is not helpful to specify some arbitrary time limit for a trial of labour. If oxytocin augmentation of labour is utilized to maintain good uterine action, it should become clear within 12–18 hours at the most whether safe vaginal delivery will be possible. If during the active phase there is arrest of dilatation and descent over a period of 3–4 hours with good contractions, abdominal delivery is indicated. To secure adequate but not excessive uterine activity in the presence of disproportion it may be helpful to monitor intrauterine pressure with a catheter manometer, as a guide to oxytocin dosage.

Monitoring fetal well-being Continuous electronic fetal heart rate recording should be utilized during trial of labour. External transducers can often provide an adequate signal, failing which a scalp electrode should be used. The deceleration patterns encountered during cephalopelvic dystocia have already been described.

Intermittent scalp-blood sampling to check fetal pH may be necessary if the fetal heart rate tracing is of uncertain interpretation.

Monitoring the progress of labour   Regular accurate clinical observations on the partogram are essential to the proper conduct of a trial of labour. The successive observations of cervical dilatation and descent of the head should usually be made at intervals of 3–4 hours. It is important that the level of the head should be assessed both by vaginal and abdominal palpation. The abdominal findings are, in this situation, generally the more significant.

Methods of assessment of head level   The earliest clinical techniques of palpation of the head focused on head-brim fitting, and the question addressed was: 'Is the head engaged?' or 'Has the widest diameter entered the brim?' The lateral contours of the accessible portion of the head were therefore explored by deep palpation in the iliac fossae, to gain an impression whether the fingertips could feel beyond the widest part of the head.

Later, the concept of vaginal station of the head was promulgated in the USA. The level of the head was defined by a vaginal assessment, using the ischial spines as a reference level, and relating the lowest part of the head (vertex) to this level, in estimated centimetres of vertical distance. Thus a station of −2 indicated that the vertex was still 2 cm above the ischial spine level. Such an assessment of vaginal station may not correlate exactly with the findings on abdominal palpation because of the elongation of the head produced by moulding and variations in the pelvic depth.

In terms of the basic mechanics of disproportion, it is the amount of head remaining above the pelvic brim which provides the most significant indicator of difficulty yet to be overcome. This principle was recognized by the South African obstetricians Crichton (1952), Notelelowitz (1973), Lasbery (1963) and Philpott & Castle (1972) and a system of assessment was devised which defined the head level in terms of the amount—in fifths—of the head palpable abdominally (Fig. 36.13).

To define the level of the head accurately in this way, a different pattern of palpation should be adopted,

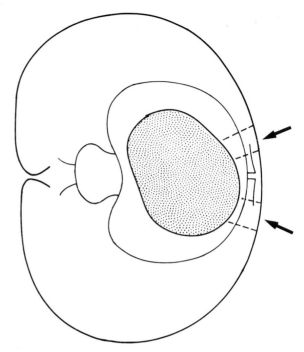

Fig. 36.14   Cross-section at level of fetal head. The head is most accessible to palpation near the midline.

aiming to define the level of the highest part of the head felt in or near the midline. The distance between this level and the top of the symphysis can be expressed as finger-breadths of an average adult hand, which in turn represents the number of fifths of the head above the brim. Figure 36.14, depicting a cross-sectional view through the mother's body at the level of the head, illustrates how close to the abdominal surface the head lies near the midline. The technique is, therefore, more definitive and less uncomfortable for the patient.

By using both vaginal examination and the method of abdominal palpation described for assessment of the descent of the head much greater accuracy will be achieved. If there appears to be a discrepancy between the two findings, it is the amount of head remaining palpable in the abdomen which has the greater significance, for the reasons already described.

Disproportion at the pelvic brim is relatively easy to diagnose, assess and manage in labour, but disproportion at lower levels in the pelvis is more common in Britain, and is often unsuspected. It is therefore, in the writer's experience, the more dangerous condition, calling for skill, patience, and fine judgement in its management.

Pain relief   During a trial of labour analgesia can with advantage be secured by epidural nerve block, though other forms of pain relief are not excluded.

Outcome of a trial of labour   A trial of labour should usually be terminated if, despite active management, there is failure to progress over a period of 3–4 hours, or if a major degree of fetal distress is diagnosed. Stewart

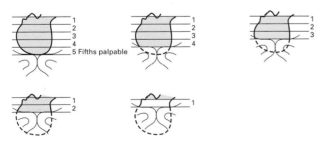

Fig. 36.13   Fifths of a head; a concept for translating clinical findings from abdominal palpation of the fetal head into degrees of descent through the mother's pelvis.

Table 36.5   Scheme for selecting mode of delivery

Amount of head palpable (fifths)	Mode of delivery
0/5	Ventouse or forceps
1/5	Trial ventouse
	If fetal distress, Caesarean section
2/5	Caesarean section or symphysiotomy
3/5+	Caesarean section

& Philpott (1980) proposed a systematic outline plan for selecting the safest mode of delivery in the presence of disproportion. Their scheme, based on a study of African women, needs to be modified for application in Britain. A simplified plan of action is shown in Table 36.5. It should be noted that:

1. In the presence of disproportion, the ventouse provides a safer method of assisted delivery than the forceps.
2. Potentially difficult vaginal delivery should never be attempted in the presence of fetal distress.
3. Symphysiotomy has been shown in many parts of the world to provide a safer alternative than a Caesarean section for appropriately selected cases.

Cephalopelvic disproportion in parous women

For several important reasons, disproportion in parous women presents different and much more dangerous problems than in primiparae. The patient's history of uneventful delivery may falsely reassure the obstetrician, as well as the woman herself. But in a subsequent labour, the infant is likely to be bigger, or the presentation may be abnormal, or the pelvis, in some instances, smaller! Surprise dystocia may therefore occur.

The tempo of labour will be more rapid in a parous woman, and the character of uterine action in the presence of disproportion, unlike that of primigravidae, is likely to be vigorously reactive, culminating in neglected cases in tonic contraction of the uterus and uterine rupture. The pattern of progress of cervical dilatation on the partogram (Soglow & Friedman 1967) is not invariably retarded, so that an important warning sign which is present in primigravidae cannot be relied on. Diagnosis of mechanical difficulty rests on other features of the labour—delay in descent of the head, exaggerated moulding, and sometimes unremitting uterine activity.

If the presence of disproportion is undetected and labour is augmented with oxytocin, the danger of uterine rupture is very real but insidious. The classical signs of impending spontaneous rupture of an unscarred uterus—frequent, violent uterine contractions and possibly an exaggerated retraction ring (Bandl's ring)—do not usually appear prior to rupture during oxytocin infusion in parous women. Often the only warning sign of impending iatrogenic rupture may be the failure of the uterus to relax between apparently normal contractions. For these reasons, labour should not be augmented in parous women where disproportion is thought to be present.

The management of disproportion in parous women therefore requires particular vigilance; careful assessment of progress, including vaginal examination, may be required at intervals of as little as 1–2 hours during the active phase of the first stage of labour. In grand multiparae, disproportion presents formidable risks, and such labours should always be supervised by an experienced obstetrician.

Conclusions

The shape and size of the bony pelvis are principally determined by nutritional factors, operating particularly during the years of growth. If progressive consolidation of the bones is not adequate to sustain the stresses of weight-bearing, distortion of the pelvis occurs.

Major degrees of pelvic contraction and serious cephalopelvic dystocia have therefore become much less common as the nutritional status of British women has improved, and their mean stature increased. In particular, marked brim-flattening is now rarely seen in the UK, but pelvic funnelling may be encountered and outlet dystocia may develop with little advance warning. The ability to anticipate difficulty and to assess accurately the degree of disproportion is all-important if correct decisions about the safe mode of delivery are to be ensured.

Cephalopelvic disproportion occurring for the first time in multigravidae can be due to either an increase in fetal size or a reduction in pelvic capacity, or both. The risk of uterine rupture in these circumstances is appreciable, and is magnified if uterine action is augmented with oxytocin.

REFERENCES

Acker D B, Sachs B P, Friedman E A 1985 Risk factors for shoulder dystocia. Obstetrics and Gynecology 66: 762–768

Acker D B, Sachs B P, Friedman E A 1986 Risk factors for shoulder dystocia in the average-weight infant. Obstetrics and Gynecology 67: 614–618

Adam P, Alberge Y, Castellano S, Kassab M, Escude V 1985 Pelvimetry by digital radiography. Clinical Radiology 36: 327–330

Akamatsu T J 1975 Anaesthesia for Caesarean section. Clinics in Obstetrics and Gynaecology 2: 647–659

Allan E P 1947 Standardised radiological pelvimetry. British Journal of Radiology 20: 108, 164, 205, 451

Anderson A B M 1981 Second thoughts on stopping labour. In: Studd J (ed) Progress in obstetrics and gynaecology, vol I. Churchill Livingstone, Edinburgh, pp 125–138

Arniel G C, Crosbie J C 1963 Infantile rickets returns to Glasgow. Lancet ii: 423

Arulkumaran S, Gibb D M F, Ratnam S S, Lun K C, Heng S H 1985 Total uterine activity in induced labour—an index of cervical and pelvic tissue resistance. British Journal of Obstetrics and Gynaecology 92: 693–697

Bates R G, Helm C W, Duncan A, Edmonds D K 1985 Uterine activity in the second stage of labour and the effect of epidural analgesia. British Journal of Obstetrics and Gynaecology 92: 1246–1250

Beazley J M, Banovic I, Feld M S 1975 Maintenance of labour. British Medical Journal 2: 248–250

Benedetti T J, Gabbe S G 1978 Shoulder dystocia. A complication of fetal macrosomia and prolonged second stage of labor with midpelvic delivery. Obstetrics and Gynecology 52: 526–529

Berkus M D, Ramamurthy R S, O'Connor P S, Brown K, Hayashi R H 1985 Cohort study of silastic obstetric vacuum cup deliveries: I. Safety of the instrument. Obstetrics and Gynecology 66: 503–509

Berkus M D, Ramamurthy R S, O'Connor P S, Brown K J, Hayashi R H 1986 Cohort study of silastic obstetric vacuum cup deliveries. II. Unsuccessful vacuum extraction. Obstetrics and Gynecology 68: 662–666

Besinger R, Compton A, Hayashi R 1987 The presence of fetal breathing movements as a predictor of outcome in preterm labour. American Journal of Obstetrics and Gynecology 157: 753–757

Bingham P, Lilford R J 1987 Management of the selected term breech presentation: assessment of the risks of selected vaginal delivery versus caesarean section for all cases. Obstetrics and Gynecology 69: 965–977

Bodmer B, Benjamin A, McLean F H, Usher R H 1986 Has caesarean section reduced the risks of delivery in the preterm breech presentation? American Journal of Obstetrics and Gynecology 154: 244–250

Borell U, Fernstrom I 1960 Radiologic pelvimetry. Acta Radiologica suppl 191

Borell U, Radberg C 1964 Orthodiagraphic pelvimetry with special references to capacity of distal part of pelvis and pelvic outlet. Acta Radiologica (Diagnostica) 2: 273

Bottoms S F, Hirsch V J, Sokol R J 1987 Medical management of arrest disorders of labor: a current overview. American Journal of Obstetrics and Gynecology 156: 935–939

British Medical Journal Editorial 1979 Rickets in Asian immigrants. British Medical Journal 1: 1744

Brocks V, Philipsen T, Secher N J 1984 A randomized trial of external cephalic version with tocolysis in late pregnancy. British Journal of Obstetrics and Gynaecology 91: 653–656

Calvert J P, Newcombe R G, Hibbard R M 1982 An assessment of radiotelemetry in the monitoring of labour. British Journal of Obstetrics and Gynaecology 89: 285–291

Cardozo L D, Gibb D M F, Studd J W W, Cooper D J 1983 Should we abandon Kielland's forceps? British Medical Journal 287: 315–317

Carter V 1986 Another technique for resolution of shoulder dystocia. American Journal of Obstetrics and Gynecology 154: 964

Chaim W, Alroi A, Leiberman J R, Cohen A 1981 Severe contracted pelvis appearing after normal deliveries. Acta Obstetricia et Gynecologica Scandinavica 60: 131

Chalmers I 1984 Trends and variations in the use of caesarean delivery. In: Clinch J, Matthews T (eds) Perinatal medicine. MTP Press, Lancaster, p 145

Chalmers J A 1968 The management of malrotation of the occiput. Journal of Obstetrics and Gynaecology of the British Commonwealth 75: 889–891

Cheng M, Hannah M 1993 Breech delivery at term. Obstetrics and Gynecology 82: 605–618

Chiswick M L 1980 Forceps delivery—neonatal outcome. In: Beard R W, Paintin D B (eds) Outcome of obstetric intervention in Britain. RCOG, London, pp 33–41

Chiswick M L, James D K 1979 Kielland's forceps: association with neonatal morbidity and mortality. British Medical Journal 1: 7–9

Coats P M, Chan K K, Wilkins M, Beard R J 1980 A comparison between midline and mediolateral episiotomies. British Journal of Obstetrics and Gynaecology 87: 408–412

Cohen W R 1977 Influence of the duration of second stage labor on perinatal outcome and puerperal morbidity. Obstetrics and Gynecology 49: 266–269

Collea J V, Rabin S C, Weghorst G R, Quilligan E J 1978 The randomized management of term frank breech presentation: vaginal delivery versus cesarean section. American Journal of Obstetrics and Gynecology 131: 186–195

Cox C, Kendall A C, Hommers M 1982 Changed prognosis of breech-presenting low birthweight infants. British Journal of Obstetrics and Gynaecology 89: 881–886

Crawford J S 1985 Lumbar epidural analgesia for labour and delivery: a personal view. In: Studd J (ed) The management of labour. Blackwell Scientific Publications, Oxford, pp 226–234

Crichton D 1952 The accuracy of X-ray cephalometry in utero. Proceedings of the Royal Society of Medicine 45: 535

Croughan-Minilane M, Petite D, Gordis L, Golditch I 1990 Obstetrics and Gynecology 75: 821–825

Crowley P, Hawkins D F 1980 Review: premature breech delivery—the caesarean section debate. Journal of Obstetrics and Gynaecology 1: 2–6

Cruikshank D P, Cruikshank J E 1981 Face and brow presentation: a review. Clinical Obstetrics and Gynecology 24: 333–351

Cyr R M, Usher R H, McLean F H 1984 Changing patterns of birth asphyxia and trauma over 20 years. American Journal of Obstetrics and Gynecology 148: 490–498

David H, Rosen M 1976 Perinatal mortality after epidural analgesia. Anaesthesia 31: 1054–1059

Davis R O, Brunfield C G 1984 The use of real-time ultrasound in the management of obstetric emergencies. Clinical Obstetrics and Gynecology 27: 68–77

Dierker L J, Rosen M G, Thompson K, Lynn P 1986 Midforceps deliveries: long-term outcome of infants. American Journal of Obstetrics and Gynecology 154: 764–766

Drife J O 1983 Kielland or Caesar? British Medical Journal 287: 309–310

Duenhoelter J H, Wells E, Reich J S, Santos-Ramos R, Jimenez J M 1979 A paired controlled study of vaginal and abdominal delivery of low birth weight breech fetus. Obstetrics and Gynecology 54: 310–313

Dumoulin J G, Foulkes J E 1984 Ketonuria during labour. British Journal of Obstetrics and Gynaecology 91: 97–98

Dunn P M 1978 Posture in labour. Lancet i: 496–497

Dyack C 1980 Rotational forceps in midforceps delivery. Obstetrics and Gynecology 56: 123–126

Dyson D C, Ferguson J E, Hensleigh P 1986 Antepartum external version under tocolysis. Obstetrics and Gynecology 67: 63–68

Edwards R L, Nicholson H O 1969 The management of the unstable lie in late pregnancy. Journal of Obstetrics and Gynaecology of the British Commonwealth 76: 713–718

Effer S B, Saigal S, Rand C et al 1983 Effect of delivery method on outcomes in the very low-birth weight breech infant: is the improved survival related to cesarean section or other perinatal care maneuvers? American Journal of Obstetrics and Gynecology 145: 123–128

Elkins V H 1982 Procedure for turning breech. In: Enkin M, Chalmers I (eds) Effectiveness and satisfaction in antenatal care. Spastic International Medical Publishers, London, p 216

Endler G C, Donath R W 1985 Inflation device to prevent aortocaval compression during pregnancy. Anesthesia and Analgesia 64: 1015–1016

Faber-Nijholt R, Huisjes H J, Touwen B C L, Fidler V J 1983 Neurological follow-up of 281 children born in breech presentation: a controlled study. British Medical Journal 286: 9–12

Fahmy K 1973 Disproportion in multiparae. Journal of the Kuwait Medical Association 7: 119

Ferguson J E, Dyson D C 1985 Intrapartum external cephalic version. American Journal of Obstetrics and Gynecology 152: 297–298

Fianu S, Vaclavinkova V 1978 The site of placental attachment as a factor in the aetiology of breech presentation. Acta Obstetricia et Gynecologica Scandinavica 57: 371–372

Flanagan T A, Mulchahey K M, Korenbrot C C, Green J R, Laros R K 1987 Management of term breech presentation. American Journal of Obstetrics and Gynecology 156: 1492–1502

Floberg J, Belfrage P, Carlsson M, Ohlsen H 1986. The pelvic outlet.

A comparison between clinical evaluation and radiologic pelvimetry. Acta Obstetricia et Gynecologica Scandinavica 65: 321

Floberg J, Belfrage P, Ohlsen H 1987 Influence of pelvic outlet capacity on labor. A prospective pelvimetry study of 1429 selected primiparae. Acta Obstetricia et Gynecologica Scandinavica 66: 121–126

Flynn A M, Kelly J, Hollins G, Lynch P F 1978 Ambulation in labour. British Medical Journal 2: 591–593

Ford J A, McIntosh W B, Butterfield R 1976 Clinical and subclinical vitamin D deficiency in Bradford children. Archives of Disease in Childhood 51: 939

Friedman E A, Sachtleben M R, Bresky P A 1977 Dysfunctional labor. American Journal of Obstetrics and Gynecology 127: 779–783

Gebbie D 1982 Symphysiotomy. Clinics in Obstetrics and Gynaecology 9: 663–683

Gibb D M F, Arulkumaran S, Lun K C, Ratnam S S 1984 Characteristics of uterine activity in nulliparous labour. British Journal of Obstetrics and Gynaecology 91: 220–227

Gibb D M F, Arulkumaran S, Ratnam S S 1985 A comparative study of methods of oxytocin administration for induction of labour. British Journal of Obstetrics and Gynaecology 92: 688–692

Gilstrap L C, Hauth J C, Toussaint S 1984 Cesarean section: changing incidence and indications. Obstetrics and Gynecology 63: 205–208

Gimovsky M L, Wallace R L, Schifrin B S, Paul R H 1983 Randomised management of non frank breech presentation at term: a preliminary report. American Journal of Obstetrics and Gynecology 146: 34–40

Gimovsky M L, Willard K, Neglio M, Howard T, Zerne S 1985 X-ray pelvimetry in a breech protocol: a comparison of digital radiography and conventional methods. American Journal of Obstetrics and Gynecology 153: 887–888

Goldenberg R L, Nelson K G 1984 The unanticipated breech presentation in labor. Clinical Obstetrics and Gynecology 27: 95–105

Goodfellow C F, Hull M G R, Swaab D F, Dogterom J, Buijs R M 1983 Oxytocin deficiency at delivery with epidural analgesia. British Journal of Obstetrics and Gynaecology 90: 214–219

Goodlin R C 1986 Modified manual rotation in midpelvic delivery. Obstetrics and Gynecology 67: 128–130

Grant A 1986 Repair of episiotomies and perineal tears. British Journal of Obstetrics and Gynaecology 93: 417–419

Green J F, McLean F, Smith L P, Usher R 1982 Has an increased cesarean section rate for term breech delivery reduced the incidence of birth asphyxia, trauma, and death? American Journal of Obstetrics and Gynecology 142: 643–648

Greis J B, Bierniarz J, Scommegna A 1981 Comparison of maternal and fetal effects of vacuum extraction with forceps or cesarean deliveries. Obstetrics and Gynecology 57: 571–577

Greulich W W, Thoms H 1939 A study of pelvis type and its relationship to body build in white women. Journal of the American Medical Association 112: 485

Gross S J, Shime J, Farin D 1987 Shoulder dystocia: predictors and outcome. American Journal of Obstetrics and Gynecology 156: 334–336

Haesslein H C, Goodlin R C 1979 Delivery of the tiny newborn. American Journal of Obstetrics and Gynecology 134: 192–197

Halme J, Ekbladh L 1982 The vacuum extractor for obstetric delivery. Clinical Obstetrics and Gynecology 25: 167–175

Harris B A 1984 Shoulder dystocia. Clinical Obstetrics and Gynecology 27: 106–111

Hartfield V J 1973 A comparison of the early and late effects of subcutaneous symphysiotomy and of lower segment caesarean section. Journal of Obstetrics and Gynaecology of the British Commonwealth 80: 508–514

Healy D L, Quinn M A, Pepperell R J 1982 Rotational delivery of the fetus: Kielland's forceps and two other methods compared. British Journal of Obstetrics and Gynaecology 89: 501–506

Hobel C J, Oakes G K 1980 Special considerations in the management of preterm labor. Clinical Obstetrics and Gynecology 23: 147–164

Hofmeyr G J 1983 Effect of external cephalic version in late pregnancy on breech presentation and caesarean section rate: a controlled trial. British Journal of Obstetrics and Gynaecology 90: 392–399

Hofmeyr G J, Sadan O, Myer I G, Galal K C, Simko G 1986 External cephalic version and spontaneous version rates: ethnic and other determinants. British Journal of Obstetrics and Gynaecology 93: 13–16

Holmberg N G, Lilieqvist B, Magnusson S, Segerbrand E 1977 The influence of the bony pelvis in persistent occiput posterior position. Acta Obstetricia et Gynecologica Scandinavica 66: (suppl) 49–54

Iams J D, Clapp D H, Contos D A, Whitehurst R, Ayers L, O'Shaughnessy R W 1987 Does extra-amniotic infection cause preterm labor? Gas–liquid chromatography studies of amniotic fluid in amnionitis, preterm labour, and normal controls. Obstetrics and Gynecology 70: 365–368

Iffy L, Apuzzio J J, Cohen-Addad N, Zwolska-Demczuk B, Francis-Lane M, Olenczak J 1986 Abdominal rescue after entrapment of the aftercoming head. American Journal of Obstetrics and Gynecology 154: 623–624

Illingworth R S 1985 A paediatrician asks—why is it called birth injury? British Journal of Obstetrics and Gynaecology 92: 122–130

Ingemarsson I, Westgren M, Svenningsen N W 1978 Long-term follow-up of preterm infants in breech presentation delivered by caesarean section. Lancet ii: 172–175

Isager-Sally L, Legarth J, Jacobsen B, Bostofte E 1986 Episiotomy repair—immediate and long-term sequelae. A prospective randomised study of three different methods of repair. British Journal of Obstetrics and Gynaecology 93: 420–425

Jovanovic R 1985 Incisions of the pregnant uterus and delivery of low-birth weight infants. American Journal of Obstetrics and Gynecology 152: 971–974

Kadar N, Romero R 1983 Prognosis for future childbearing after midcavity instrumental deliveries in primigravidas. Obstetrics and Gynecology 62: 166–170

Kadar N, Cruddas M, Campbell S 1986 Estimating the probability of spontaneous delivery conditional on time spent in the second stage. British Journal of Obstetrics and Gynaecology 93: 568–576

Karp L E, Doney J R, McCarthy T, Meis P J, Hall M 1979 The premature breech: trial of labor or Cesarean section? Obstetrics and Gynecology 53: 88–92

Kasby C B, Poll K 1982 The breech head and its ultrasound significance. British Journal of Obstetrics and Gynaecology 89: 106–110

Kasule J, Chimbira T H K, Brown I McL 1985 Controlled trial of external cephalic version. British Journal of Obstetrics and Gynaecology 92: 14–18

Kauppila O, Gronroos M, Aro P, Aittoniemi P, Kuoppala M 1981 Management of low birth-weight breech delivery: should Cesarean section be routine? Obstetrics and Gynecology 57: 289–294

Kirwan P 1983 Oxytocin and the second stage of labour. Irish Journal of Medical Science 152: 201–202

Kitchen W H, Yu V Y H, Orgill A A et al 1982 Infants born before 29 weeks' gestation: survival and morbidity at 2 years of age. British Journal of Obstetrics and Gynaecology 89: 887–891

Kitchen W, Ford G W, Doyle L W et al 1985 Cesarean section or vaginal delivery at 24 to 28 weeks' gestation: comparison of survival and neonatal and 2-year morbidity. Obstetrics and Gynecology 66: 149–157

Kopleman J N, Duff P, Karl R T, Schipul A H, Read J A 1986 Computed tomographic pelvimetry in the evaluation of breech presentation. Obstetrics and Gynecology 68: 455–458

Krishnamurthy S, Fairlie F, Cameron A, Walker I, Mackenzie J 1991 The role of postnatal x-ray pelvimetry. British Journal of Obstetrics and Gynaecology 98: 716–718

Lamont R F, Dunlop P D M, Crowley P, Elder M G 1983 Spontaneous preterm labour and delivery at under 34 weeks' gestation. British Medical Journal 286: 454–457

Lancet Editorial 1986 Metabolic bone disease of prematurity. Lancet i: 200

Lange I R, Manning F A, Morrison I, Chamberlain P F, Harman C R 1985 Cord prolapse: is antenatal diagnosis possible? American Journal of Obstetrics and Gynecology 151: 1083–1085

Lasbery A H 1963 The symptomatic sequelae of symphysiotomy. A follow-up study of 100 patients subjected to symphysiotomy. South African Medical Journal 37: 231

Lowe B 1987 Fear of failure: a place for the trial of instrumental delivery. British Journal of Obstetrics and Gynaecology 94: 60–66

Lupe P J, Gross T L 1986 Maternal upright posture and mobility in labor—a review. Obstetrics and Gynecology 67: 727–734

Luterkort M, Persson P, Weldner B 1984 Maternal and fetal factors in breech presentation. Obstetrics and Gynecology 64: 55–59

Maduska A L 1981 Inhalation analgesia and general anesthesia. Clinical Obstetrics and Gynecology 24: 619–633

Main D M, Main E K, Maurer M M 1983 Cesarean section versus vaginal delivery for the breech fetus weighing less than 1500 grams. American Journal of Obstetrics and Gynecology 146: 580–584

Maresh M, Choong K H, Beard R W 1983 Delayed pushing with lumbar epidural analgesia in labour. British Journal of Obstetrics and Gynaecology 90: 623–627

McManus T J, Calder A A 1978a Upright posture and the efficiency of labour. Lancet i: 72–74

McManus T J, Calder A A 1978b Posture in labour. Lancet i: 1041

Modanlou H D, Komatsu G, Dorchester W, Freeman R K, Bosu S K 1982 Large-for-gestational-age neonates: anthropometric reasons for shoulder dystocia. Obstetrics and Gynecology 60: 417–423

Moir J C 1947 The use of radiology in predicting difficult labour. Journal of Obstetrics and Gynaecology of the British Empire 54: 20

Moolgaoker A S, Ahamed S O S, Payne P R 1979 A comparison of different methods of instrumental delivery based on electronic measurements of compression and traction. Obstetrics and Gynecology 54: 299–309

Moore R 1970 Evolution. Life Nature Library. Time–Life International (Nederland), NV, p 165

Morales W J, Koerten J 1986 Obstetric management and intraventricular hemorrhage in very-low-birth-weight infants. Obstetrics and Gynecology 68: 35–40

Morgan B 1972 The descent of woman. Souvenir Press, London, pp 21–42

Morgan B M, Bulpitt C J, Clifton P, Lewis P J 1982 Occasional survey: analgesia and satisfaction in childbirth (the Queen Charlotte's 1000 mother survey). Lancet ii: 808–811

Morrison J C, Myatt R E, Martin J N et al 1986 External cephalic version of the breech presentation under tocolysis. American Journal of Obstetrics and Gynecology 154: 900–903

Morton K E, Jackson M C, Gillmer M D G 1985 A comparison of the effects of four intravenous solutions for the treatment of ketonuria during labour. British Journal of Obstetrics and Gynaecology 92: 473–479

Myers S A, Gleicher N 1987 Breech delivery: why the dilemma? American Journal of Obstetrics and Gynecology 156: 6–10

Myerscough P R 1982a Occipitoposterior positions of the vertex. In: Munro Kerr's operative obstetrics, 10th edn. Baillière Tindall, London, pp 50–60

Myerscough P R 1982b Munro Kerr's operative obstetrics. Baillière Tindall, London, p 139

Notelowitz M 1973 Beware the weeping womb. South African Journal of Obstetrics and Gynaecology 47(3): 1653–1655

O'Brien F, Cefalo R C 1982 Evaluation of X-ray pelvimetry and abnormal labor. Clinical Obstetrics and Gynecology 25: 157–164

O'Connell P, Keane A 1985 The term breech: subsequent growth and development. In: Clinch J, Matthews T (eds) Perinatal medicine. MTP Press, Lancaster, p 219

O'Driscoll K, Meagher D, MacDonald D, Geoghegan F 1981 Traumatic intracranial haemorrhage in firstborn infants and delivery with obstetric forceps. British Journal of Obstetrics and Gynaecology 88: 577–581

Olshan A F, Shy K K, Luthy D A, Hickok D, Weiss N S, Daling J R 1984 Cesarean birth and neonatal mortality in very low birth weight infants. Obstetrics and Gynecology 64: 267–270

O'Neil A G B, Skull E, Michael C 1981 A new method of traction for the vacuum cup. Australian and New Zealand Journal of Obstetrics and Gynaecology 21: 24–25

Paintin D B 1982 Mid-cavity forceps delivery. British Journal of Obstetrics and Gynaecology 89: 495–500

Parry-Jones E 1968 Barton's forceps: its use in transverse position of the fetal head. Journal of Obstetrics and Gynaecology of the British Commonwealth 75: 892–901

Phelan J P, Stine L E, Edwards N B, Clark S L, Horenstein J 1985 The role of external version in the intrapartum management of the transverse lie presentation. American Journal of Obstetrics and Gynecology 151: 724–726

Phillips K C, Thomas T A 1983 Second stage of labour with or without extradural analgesia. Anaesthesia 38: 972–976

Phillips R D, Freeman M 1974 The management of the persistent occiput posterior position. Obstetrics and Gynecology 43: 171–177

Philpott R H 1980 Obstructed labour. Clinics in Obstetrics and Gynaecology 7: 601–619

Philpott R, Castle W M 1972 Journal of Obstetrics and Gynaecology of the British Commonwealth 79: 592, 599

Philpott R H, Stewart K S 1974 Intensive care of the high-risk fetus in Africa. Clinics in Obstetrics and Gynaecology 1: 241

Pritchard C W, Sutherland H W, Carr-Hill R A 1983 Birthweight and paternal height. British Journal of Obstetrics and Gynaecology 90: 156–161

Rayburn W F, Donn S M, Kolin M G, Schork M A 1983 Obstetric care and intraventricular hemorrhage in the low birth weight infant. Obstetrics and Gynecology 62: 408–413

Reading A E, Sledmere C M, Cox D N, Campbell S 1982 How women view postepisiotomy pain. British Medical Journal 284: 243–246

Ridley W J, Jackson P, Stewart J H, Boyle P 1982 Role of antenatal radiography in the management of breech deliveries. British Journal of Obstetrics and Gynaecology 89: 342–347

Roberts A D G, McKay Hart D 1983 Polyglycolic acid and catgut sutures, with and without oral proteolytic enzymes, in the healing episiotomies. British Journal of Obstetrics and Gynaecology 90: 650–653

Russell J K 1982 Breech: vaginal delivery or caesarean section. British Medical Journal 285: 830–831

Sandberg E C 1985 The Zavanelli maneuver: a potentially revolutionary method for the resolution of shoulder dystocia. American Journal of Obstetrics and Gynecology 152: 479–484

Savona-Ventura C 1986 The role of external cephalic version in modern obstetrics. Obstetrical and Gynecological Survey 41: 393–400

Sbarra A J, Thomas G B, Cetrulo C L, Shakr C, Chaudhury A, Paul B 1987 Effect of bacterial growth on the bursting pressure of fetal membranes in vitro. Obstetrics and Gynecology 70: 107–110

Scheer K, Nubar J 1976 Variation of fetal presentation with gestational age. American Journal of Obstetrics and Gynecology 125: 269–270

Schutterman E B, Grimes D A 1983 Comparative safety of the low transverse versus the low vertical uterine incision for cesarean delivery of breech infants. Obstetrics and Gynecology 61: 593–597

Seeds J W, Ccfalo R C 1982 Malpresentations. Clinical Obstetrics and Gynecology 25: 145–156

Seitchik J, Castillo M 1983 Oxytocin augmentation of dysfunctional labor. American Journal of Obstetrics and Gynecology 145: 526–529

Seitchik J, Amico J, Robinson A G, Castillo M 1984 Oxytocin augmentation of dysfunctional labor. American Journal of Obstetrics and Gynecology 150: 225–228

Sharma S, Soni I K 1978 The time of engagement of the fetal head. Journal of Obstetrics and Gynaecology of India 28: 410

Singhi S, Chookang E, Hall J St E, Kalghatgi S 1985 Iatrogenic neonatal and maternal hyponatraemia following oxytocin and aqueous glucose infusion during labour. British Journal of Obstetrics and Gynaecology 92: 356–363

Smith A R B, James D K, Faragher E B, Gilfillan S 1982 Continuous lumbar epidural analgesia in labour—does delaying 'pushing' in the second stage reduce the incidence of instrumental delivery? Journal of Obstetrics and Gynaecology 2: 170–172

Soglow S R, Friedman E A 1967 Feto-pelvic disproportion in multiparae. Obstetrics and Gynecology 29: 848

Steer P J, Carter M C, Beard R W 1985a The effect of oxytocin infusion on uterine activity levels in slow labour. British Journal of Obstetrics and Gynaecology 92: 1120–1126

Steer P J, Carter M C, Choong K, Hanson M, Gordon A J, Pradhan P 1985b A multicentre prospective randomised controlled trial of induction of labour with an automatic closed-loop feedback controlled oxytocin infusion system. British Journal of Obstetrics and Gynaecology 92: 1127–1133

Stewart D B 1984a The pelvis as a passageway. I. Evolution and adaptations. British Journal of Obstetrics and Gynaecology 91: 611–617

Stewart D B 1984b The pelvis as a passageway. II. The modern human pelvis. British Journal of Obstetrics and Gynaecology 91: 618–623

Stewart P, Calder A A 1984 Posture in labour: patients' choice and its effect on performance. British Journal of Obstetrics and Gynaecology 91: 1091–1095

Stewart K S, Philpott R H 1980 Fetal response to cephalopelvic disproportion. British Journal of Obstetrics and Gynaecology 87: 641

Thorpe Beeston J G, Banfield P J, Saunders N J St G 1992 Outcome of breech delivery at term. British Medical Journal 305: 746–747

Toppozada H K 1964 Clinical pelvimetry I. Alexandria Medical Journal 10: 287

Torgrim S, Bakke T 1986 The length of the human umbilical cord in vertex and breech presentations. American Journal of Obstetrics and Gynecology 154: 1086–1087

Traub A I, Morrow R J, Ritchie J W K, Dornan K J 1984 A continuing use for Kielland's forceps? British Journal of Obstetrics and Gynaecology 91: 894–898

United States Department of Health Education and Welfare Public Health Service Food and Drugs Administration 1980 The selection of patients for X-ray examination. Brown R F et al (eds)

Vacca A, Grant A, Wyatt G, Chalmers I 1983 Portsmouth operative delivery trial: a comparison of vacuum extraction and forceps delivery. British Journal of Obstetrics and Gynaecology 90: 1107–1112

Van Dorsten J P, Schifrin B S, Wallace R L 1981 Randomized control trial of external cephalic version with tocolysis in late pregnancy. American Journal of Obstetrics and Gynecology 141: 417–424

Wallace R L, Eglinton G S, Yonekura M L, Wallace T M 1984 Extraperitoneal cesarean section: a surgical form of infection prophylaxis? American Journal of Obstetrics and Gynecology 148: 172–177

Watson W J, Benson W L 1984 Vaginal delivery for the selected frank breech infant at term. Obstetrics and Gynecology 64: 638–640

Weaver J B 1980 Breech delivery—obstetric outcome. In: Beard R W, Paintin D B (eds) Outcomes of obstetric intervention in Britain. RCOG, London, pp 47–62

Weekes A R L, Flynn M J 1975 Engagement of the fetal head in primigravidae and its relationship to duration of gestation and time of onset of labour. British Journal of Obstetrics and Gynaecology 82: 7

Westgren M, Paul R H 1985 Delivery of the low birthweight infant by cesarean section. Clinical Obstetrics and Gynecology 28: 752–762

Westgren M, Grundsell H, Ingemarsson I, Muhlow A, Svenningsen N W 1981 Hyperextension of the fetal head in breech presentation: a study with long-term follow-up. British Journal of Obstetrics and Gynaecology 88: 101–104

Westgren M, Ingemarsson I, Ahlstrom H, Lindroth N, Svenningsen N W 1982 Delivery and long-term outcome of very low birthweight infants. Acta Obstetricia et Gynecologica Scandinavica 61: 25–30

Westgren L M R, Songster G, Paul R H 1985a Preterm breech delivery: another retrospective study. Obstetrics and Gynecology 66: 481–484

Westgren M, Edvall H, Nordstrom L, Svalenius E, Ranstam J 1985b Spontaneous cephalic version of breech presentation in the last trimester. British Journal of Obstetrics and Gynaecology 92: 19–22

Wigglesworth J S, Husemeyer R P 1977 Intracranial birth trauma in vaginal breech delivery: the continued importance of injury to the occipital bone. British Journal of Obstetrics and Gynaecology 84: 684–691

Williams R M, Thom M H, Studd J W W 1980 A study of the benefits and acceptability of ambulation in spontaneous labour. British Journal of Obstetrics and Gynaecology 87: 122–126

Williams W 1941 Obstetrics. Appleton-Century, New York

Yu V Y H, Bajuk B, Cutting D, Orgill A A, Astbury J 1984 Effect of mode of delivery on outcome of very-low-birthweight infants. British Journal of Obstetrics and Gynaecology 91: 633–639

Yudkin P L, Redman C W G 1986 Caesarean section dissected, 1978–1983. British Journal of Obstetrics and Gynaecology 93: 135–144

37. Induction and augmentation of labour

Andrew A. Calder

INTRODUCTION

Labour is an inevitable consequence of pregnancy. Only two events can prevent the onset of labour once pregnancy has become well established—the death of the undelivered mother or surgical removal of the fetus. The timing of the onset of labour may vary widely, but it will happen, sooner or later.

INDUCTION

Induction of labour is an obstetric procedure designed to pre-empt the natural process of labour by initiating its onset artificially before this occurs spontaneously. Many women whose labours are induced today would, left alone, labour tomorrow while for others, induction advances the process by many days or even weeks. The decision to advance the labour is taken to serve some interest—usually that of the offspring; less often it is that of the mother and rarely it is that of the obstetrician or the clinical service.

Few medical issues have generated so much controversy in the past 20 years as have the use and abuse of labour induction. In the early 1970s the media mounted a public challenge to the speciality on this issue, the impact of which can still be felt today. At the time, many obstetricians rightly felt that the presentation of the arguments by the media was dishonest and distorted. Many felt bitter that their professional judgement and competence were subjected to such public challenge, but few would now deny that the long-term effects have been beneficial. Obstetricians were made aware of the need to re-examine their motives, to be more accountable and, most of all, to explain more fully and discuss their views with the person most intimately and immediately concerned—the prospective mother.

Authoritarianism is cosy and simple, while informed discussion is time-consuming and bothersome. Nevertheless, induction of labour represents such a profound interference with natural laws that the clinician must be prepared to justify it to his or her patients, to the wider public and to him- or herself.

The obstetrician must be conscious of a feeling of power. Among a profession often accused of trying to usurp the authority of the Almighty, obstetricians may be at risk from the temptation to exercise God-like power. They have few more potent clinical weapons at their disposal and it therefore behoves them to use this power wisely and only for reasons which can be amply justified.

Putting aside the largely contentious question of intervention for the benefit of the obstetric services or of the clinical staff (which is hard to defend on purely medical grounds, but might in certain circumstances be justified on the basis of the best deployment of resources), labour induction must be seen to benefit the mother or the offspring or both. The particular challenge of obstetrics which lies in the need to care for two parties simultaneously is seen in its sharpest focus when the interests of the mother and those of the fetus may appear to be in conflict. The last few years have seen an increase in the number of mothers who yearn for what has come to be called natural childbirth and who eschew obstetric interference in any form. To such women, the induction of labour may be particularly abhorrent; often it seems that such mothers believe that if they are sufficiently determined in their mental approach they will achieve a normal and trouble-free pregnancy, labour and delivery.

There is as yet no evidence that yearning for natural childbirth is an effective protection against antepartum haemorrhage, gestational diabetes, placental insufficiency and such disorders. In consequence, it may often be necessary to insist that some mothers subordinate their aspirations for a fulfilling birth experience to the more pressing interests of their offspring. This may seem an obvious course, but few obstetricians have not had the experience of trying to convince what appears to be an infuriatingly stubborn mother that she has her priorities wrong. Happily, most mothers see the well-being of their offspring as paramount, but this emphasizes the need for the obstetrician to be on the firmest ground in giving advice and not to recommend induction lightly.

Many of the difficulties we now face date from the era when enthusiasm for our new-found ability to induce labour outstripped sound clinical judgement. It is easy to employ emotional blackmail in persuading a mother of our case for induction by suggesting that her failure to agree may put her baby at risk. We must therefore constantly strive for intellectual and clinical honesty in the advice we offer.

Indications for induction of labour

The essence of the indications for induction of labour lies in our assessment of the components which contribute to the obstetric balance (Calder 1983; Fig. 37.1). Intervention is only appropriate when its risks are judged to be fewer than those associated with non-intervention.

Fetal indications

Labour induction for fetal indications assumes that the welfare of the offspring is better served by being delivered than by remaining in utero. Certain obstetric complications are well known to carry clear-cut fetal risks (e.g. rhesus disease, diabetes, severe pre-eclampsia); in others

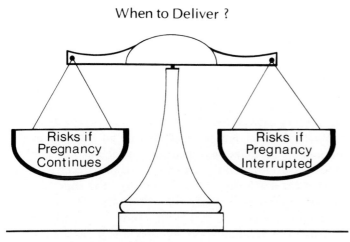

When to Deliver ?

Fig. 37.1 The obstetric balance.

the risks are less consistent. These latter may be described as epidemiological indications in conditions such as prolonged pregnancy, mild and moderate pre-eclampsia or increased maternal age. It is these latter categories which have contributed most to the widely varying rates of labour induction and to the consequent controversy. The firmer indications account for fewer than 10% of confinements in most populations (Studd & Cardozo 1985), whereas marginal indications may be identified in anything from 10% to 50% of the remainder. It is the interpretation of the significance and weight of such indications that determines the frequency with which induction is applied in any given obstetric service.

Essentially the obstetrician must assess the relative risks for the fetus of continuing in utero or being delivered. The inaccessibility of the fetus to clinical examination and assessment makes the risks in utero difficult to quantify but the risks after delivery may be no more precise. The increasing willingness of obstetricians to confer with their neonatal colleagues is greatly welcomed but ultimately the decision is a matter of judgement based on the assessment of several uncertainties. Birthweight, estimated by clinical methods or by ultrasound and gestational age are important factors in predicting neonatal problems but other factors, especially those complications which are under consideration, may have a crucial bearing on whether or not the neonate has a stormy introduction to extrauterine life.

The past two decades have witnessed increased sophistication in the methods of assessment of both types of risk. Diagnostic ultrasound has allowed more precise measurement of fetal growth and well-being. Cardiotocography may give valuable information about the fetal condition. The assessment of the fetal biophysical profile (Manning et al 1980) is gaining in popularity.

Such measures are also useful in predicting neonatal difficulties so that the value of amniocentesis to allow measurement of liquor phospholipids (Gluck & Kulovich 1973) in order that the fetal lung maturity can be determined now plays a smaller part than it once did.

A further factor concerns the skills and facilities available for the care of the newborn. Clearly the availability of the highest level of neonatal intensive care will put a very different complexion on the prospect of delivery. In the absence of such facilities there is little merit in delivering a grossly immature infant with little prospect of survival.

It is a matter of balance. In most pregnancies the balance (Fig. 37.1) remains firmly tipped against interference and remains so until the spontaneous onset of labour at term. In some instances the risks in utero may be seen to be gradually rising and delivery may be contemplated at an appropriate moment. The radical obstetrician favours early intervention in the belief that it is better to deliver the offspring before it has been seriously compromised. A conservative colleague will favour delaying intervention until evidence of fetal compromise is clearly seen, which may never happen.

Rhesus disease Maternal rhesus isoimmunization illustrates many of the matters considered above. The risks of this complication are almost all directed towards the fetus. Haemolysis of fetal red blood cells may lead to progressive anaemia, cardiac failure and eventually to hydrops fetalis. The earlier these complications appear the greater is the likelihood that intervention will be required to prevent fetal death in utero. Such intervention may be labour induction if it is judged that the fetus is sufficiently mature; otherwise blood transfusion of the fetus in utero is required.

Hitherto the methods of assessing these factors have been fairly imprecise. The maternal antibody pattern is no more than a general pointer, while liquor bilirubin assessment is only a crude index of fetal haemoglobin levels. Methods of direct fetal blood sampling may now bring greater precision to the management of this condition and measurement of liquor phospholipids remains a useful procedure in this condition (Whitfield 1982).

The outcome of each case depends on the race between declining haemoglobin concentration and advancing fetal maturation. When it is judged that the fetus is sufficiently mature, delivery is indicated, perhaps by labour induction.

Diabetes Maternal diabetes confers major hazards on the offspring. Poor control of the maternal blood glucose level increases the risks of fetal and maternal complications, leading to increased rates of perinatal death and morbidity. Sudden fetal demise in utero during the last weeks of gestation is less common nowadays because of improvements in diabetic control but induction of labour remains an important weapon in the battle to achieve a successful outcome to these pregnancies.

Severe pre-eclampsia This condition may be associated with impaired placental function leading to growth retardation or even death of the fetus in utero. Timely induction of labour may be appropriate in the fetal interest.

Maternal indications

It is rare nowadays to have to consider labour induction purely in the maternal interest. Nevertheless some maternal diseases such as valvular disorders of the heart, hypertension, renal disease, liver disease and certain autoimmune disorders may, especially if deteriorating, require consideration to be given to delivery in the maternal interest. Malignant conditions present a particularly taxing challenge.

Few maternal diseases are actually improved during pregnancy; in general the extra burden of pregnancy hastens their progression. The existence of such conditions is often recognized before pregnancy but commonly may only come to light or indeed may arise de novo during the course of pregnancy.

The process of ending the pregnancy may in itself pose an added risk but as a general if not invariable rule, when a mother's life is becoming threatened by such a disease during pregnancy, it is to her benefit to have the pregnancy removed from the clinical picture. In the past, women with serious medical conditions were often strongly counselled not to embark on pregnancy at all or if they did conceive therapeutic abortion was immediately advised. This is now less common for two reasons. First, the likely course of the disease states concerned and the effects of pregnancy on them are better understood. Secondly, the methods of pregnancy interruption have been steadily improved.

It remains true that the earlier a pregnancy is terminated, the safer it will be for the mother concerned but it is now more possible to intervene at any stage of gestation if the need to do so becomes apparent. Whereas formerly for the pregnancy to stand a good chance of success it had to continue for at least 36 weeks, nowadays, thanks to the advances in neonatal care, it may have a good chance of a successful outcome in many good neonatal units after only 28 weeks. In addition, in years gone by the dangers from methods of interruption rose steeply after the first trimester and did not begin to decline until the natural course of pregnancy was almost complete. Thus there was a window, or perhaps more aptly a closed door, between 12 and 36 weeks during which interruption carried greater hazards and this encouraged the view that early abortion might be best.

The advent of prostaglandins has brought the ability to induce labour throughout gestation. Thus a mother with a serious disease may now more often be allowed to embark on a pregnancy on the understanding that if her condition deteriorates dangerously as it advances the pregnancy may need to be interrupted. It may however have advanced far enough to be successful. The desire for parenthood is so strong that such women should not be forbidden the chance to reproduce on the grounds of uncertain deleterious effects. We can now more often put the question to the test without incurring unacceptable risks.

The decision to intervene

The foregoing may help to explain the reasons why induction of labour has been such a controversial procedure in recent times. Obstetricians have argued bitterly about the appropriate use of induction. The rates of induction in different hospitals and between different clinicians, differing widely, have been the subject of pride or the object of criticism. Many of these arguments have been sterile because the populations of mothers concerned have differed greatly in the risks they face.

Nevertheless, with the advance of obstetrics as a clinical science we are steadily moving away from the days of induction of labour for vague theoretical or epidemiological risks to more enlightened times where the indications are based on risks more precisely identified within the individual mother or fetus. Increased capacity for studying the condition and behaviour of the fetus in utero, although far from perfect, is assisting this process. Closer contact with the neonatologist and careful obstetric and neonatal audit allow more accurate prediction of the outlook for a particular neonate. Thus the various components in the obstetric balance can be measured with greater precision and the decision that labour induction is required reaches a sounder footing.

AUGMENTATION OF LABOUR

The need to intervene to augment labour implies two things: firstly, that labour has already begun, and secondly that its quality or progress is unsatisfactory. An additional category of indication can be included under this heading, namely, the situation in which the fetal membranes have ruptured but labour has not become established. This latter situation is conventionally described as premature rupture of the membranes, an unsatisfactory description because the term prematurity implies that the fetus is immature. Nevertheless, for want of a better description, the term premature rupture of the membranes will be used to refer to this clinical problem.

In deciding on the clinical need for augmentation of labour, two difficulties arise. First of all, the diagnosis of labour is itself far from easy. Many mothers are admitted to maternity units in what may be described as false or hesitant labour and, left alone, many of these will not progress to establish in labour. It is a moot point whether in such circumstances at term it is better to apply conservative or active policies. Many obstetricians, fearing that such false or hesitant labours may be associated with unrecognized fetal compromise, may favour intervention. Others, however, are more inclined simply to observe and await the definite onset of labour.

Where the membranes have ruptured but labour has not immediately followed, there is a general belief that delivery is desirable in a relatively short period. In most such instances a conservative approach will be followed by spontaneous labour in the majority of instances within a day or two. The sword of Damocles which hangs over all such clinical situations is, however, intrauterine infection. For this reason, most obstetricians will favour stimulation of uterine contractility, if this does not itself become established within a certain number of hours.

When labour has been diagnosed, it should proceed to delivery within certain accepted time limits. In the past it was conventional to define upper time limits for the normal durations of first- and second-stage labour. Much more profitable is the application of the principle of partography, which owes its origins to the work of Friedman (1967) in the USA and Philpott (1972) in Southern Africa. Thus, the progress of labour may be plotted graphically and deviations from the normal pattern may be recognized early. Various different partograms have been described, but all share the ability to define a labour which has deviated from the normal pattern of progress and where this is slow, augmentation may be indicated (see Ch. 29).

It must, however, be remembered that there are a number of causes for unsatisfactory progress in labour and poor uterine contractility is but one of these. Feto-pelvic disproportion may also be responsible for poor cervimetric progress, especially in the latter phase of cervical dilatation, and while augmentation of uterine contractility may represent a useful clinical step in reaching the diagnosis, the dangers associated with obstructed labour and augmented uterine contractility (uterine rupture and fetal demise) must never be forgotten.

Active management of labour

One of the most radical contributions to obstetric care in the latter half of the present century has been the philosophy which has emanated from the National Maternity Hospital in Dublin known as active management of labour (O'Driscoll & Stronge 1975). This doctrine, which applies to primiparous labours with cephalic presentations only, has as its articles of faith the need to optimize the prospects of a successful first labour by:

1. Ensuring an accurate diagnosis that labour has indeed begun.
2. Ensuring that thereafter cervical dilatation progresses at a rate no slower than 1 cm per hour.
3. Avoiding confounding the prospects of success by resort to unnecessary maternal analgesia.

These objectives are pursued by a policy of endeavouring to provide continuous support in labour from the same midwife and by the aggressive administration of oxytocin if the criteria for progress in labour are not met.

This approach has been pursued with religious zeal in Dublin with remarkable success and while it has not been exported to other parts of Europe with comparable results, it has undoubtedly led to a greater clarity of thinking in the management of labour in general.

METHODS OF INDUCTION AND AUGMENTATION OF LABOUR

Although for practical reasons it will be necessary to consider induction and augmentation separately and to regard them as different types of obstetric intervention, the only important distinction between the two lies in the extent to which the process of spontaneous labour has already begun. Just as we regard the ovarian cycle as consisting of a number of phases (follicular–ovulatory–luteal–menstrual), it is important to regard each birth cycle as a continuum from pregnancy to delivery through the sequence pregnancy–prelabour–latent labour–active labour–delivery.

In physiological terms the onset of human labour is not the sudden event it often appears, but rather a culmination of a gradual process evolving over a period of several weeks. This period is well described as prelabour and it sees the critical conversion of the myometrium from a state of inhibition to one of stimulation. Less obvious than the change in the myometrium is the radical modification which takes place in the tissues of the uterine cervix to allow delivery to take place.

Uterine contractility

At no stage in its life history is the human uterus entirely at rest. In the non-pregnant state it shows episodic contractility with peaks at the time of ovulation and menstruation. In pregnancy, the pattern of contractility which was so carefully studied and beautifully described by Caldeyro-Barcia (1958) is shown in Figure 37.2. This shows the uterine contractility throughout pregnancy, parturition and the early puerperium and demonstrates that the quiescent myometrium of pregnancy begins a build-up of activity about 4–5 weeks before the onset of labour proper. This steadily evolves throughout the phase of prelabour until labour becomes fully expressed.

Cervical ripening

Just as the powerful contractions of clinical labour are

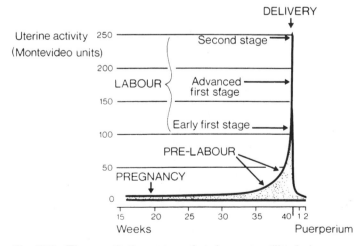

Fig. 37.2 The quantitative pattern of uterine contractility during pregnancy, pre-labour and labour (from Caldeyro-Barcia 1958).

preceded by a period of gradual evolution, so are the dramatic changes of effacement and dilatation which the cervix undergoes during labour. A number of careful studies (Bishop 1964, Anderson & Turnbull 1969, Hendricks et al 1970) have demonstrated that the rapid change in the shape of the cervix during labour begins imperceptibly during prelabour. Moreover, the change in the physical properties of the connective tissue which forms the main mass of the cervical stroma and which allows the shape change to take place probably begins even earlier. The non-pregnant and early-pregnant cervix has a firm and unyielding character attributed to the collagen fibres which it possesses in abundance. These undergo radical modification to afford the massive increase in compliance in the tissue which is essential to allow the stretching and dilatation during labour necessary for delivery.

In spite of extensive studies of the nature of these modifications, the exact mechanisms are not fully elucidated. The proteoglycans of the cervical ground substance appear to undergo changes which in turn alter the physical properties of the tissue. Since these molecules are mostly responsible for the binding of the collagen fibres it seems likely that a change in such binding might contribute to the altered physical properties of the cervix. There may, however, be a more fundamental modification of the collagen consisting of a quantitative reduction or indeed a qualitative change in type.

Muscle is relatively sparse in cervical tissue and is thought to contribute little to these processes. The principal cellular element, the fibroblast, was formerly regarded as the orchestrator of most of these tissue changes, since it seemed to be the source of both collagen and proteoglycan synthesis and also of the lytic enzymes responsible for their removal from the tissue (Liggins 1978, Calder 1979). More recently, greater interest has focused on the possible role of inflammatory cells, notably neutrophils, infiltrating the tissue of the cervix during the ripening process and modifying the cervical stroma by degranulating and releasing their lytic enzymes such as collagenase and elastase (Liggins 1981, Calder & Greer 1992, Barclay et al 1993).

The normal physiological control of the transition from pregnancy to labour thus requires the development not only of uterine contractility, but of a maturing process in the cervix which lowers its resistance to dilatation. Throughout pregnancy, the cervix functions as a closed sphincter, but as delivery approaches it must be capable of rapid opening. A normal coordinated and successful labour and delivery requires that the corpus and cervix of the uterus must act in synchrony, altering their roles from those required to maintain the pregnancy to those necessary to allow its culmination with delivery. This synchronous relationship between the two components of the uterus is illustrated in Figure 37.3.

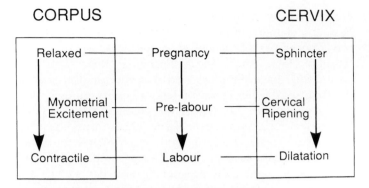

Fig. 37.3 The inter-related changes in the corpus uteri and cervix uteri during pregnancy, pre-labour and labour.

HORMONAL CONTROL OF LABOUR

The endocrine control of parturition represents a jigsaw in which many of the pieces of scientific knowledge are still missing. This has been carefully reviewed in Chapter 29. Many of the agents which have been shown to influence uterine contractility have been explored as possible agents for induction or inhibition of human labour. The list of candidates is extensive, including arginine vasopressin, corticotrophin, corticosteroids, catecholamines, oxytocin, oestrogens, progesterone, adenyl cyclase, relaxin and prostaglandins. Of these, only oxytocin and prostaglandins have been used extensively in clinical practice, although many of the others have been the subject of experimental studies.

It seems likely that the final event responsible for the onset of labour contractions in the human is an increased synthesis of prostaglandins of the E and F series within the uterine compartment, from the decidua and fetal membranes (Keirse 1979). Once this synthesis has been initiated, labour is likely to become established. Csapo & Pulkinnen (1979) described the prostaglandins as 'the ultimate uterine stimulant' and clearly their production within the uterine compartment is subject to higher endocrine control in which the placental steroids, oestrogen and progesterone, appear to play a crucial role. The role of relaxin in human parturition is as yet far from clear, but represents an exciting prospect for further study.

The uterus only becomes fully sensitive to exogenous oxytocin in late pregnancy (Fuchs 1973). The early pregnant uterus is insensitive to oxytocin, but becomes sensitive if prostaglandin E_2 or prostaglandin $F_{2\alpha}$ is administered. This favours the conclusion that the rise of prostaglandin activity in prelabour sensitizes the myometrium to the action of oxytocin.

As far as cervical ripening is concerned there is little evidence to support an important role for oxytocin. On the other hand, the prostaglandins (especially prostaglandin E_2) appear to be centrally concerned in this process and again this may be under the control of steroid hormones (Lerner 1980) and possibly relaxin (Steinetz et al 1980).

Thus, it seems likely, and perhaps not surprising, that similar endocrine control mechanisms operate for both the activation of myometrial contractility and for the induction of cervical ripening.

Practical aspects

We have considered the reasons why it may be necessary to recommend induction or augmentation of labour and the physiological background against which we must consider how to intervene. Beazley (1975) argued that all labour induction should more properly be called augmentation or acceleration of labour since, as has been stated earlier, it simply brings forward an inevitable future prospect. Clearly the physiological status of the individual mother, and in particular the position she occupies on the spectrum illustrated in Figure 37.4, will determine whether her management requires to fall into the category of induction of labour or that of augmentation. In practical terms, if she has not passed from the phase of prelabour into the phase of latent labour, we must regard intervention as induction, whereas if she has already begun latent labour, albeit unsatisfactorily, the intervention should be classified as augmentation.

It has been shown that prelabour occupies several weeks in late pregnancy and it is important to emphasize that the point occupied by the mother within that evolutionary phase has a crucial bearing on her response to labour induction. Thus, if she is still in very early prelabour she has a very different induction prospect from someone in late prelabour. In simple terms, the closer the onset of spontaneous labour, the easier and more successful will labour induction prove. The converse is even more important. Labour induction undertaken when spontaneous labour is a distant prospect is fraught with much more difficulty and many more complications.

This would be of little consequence if there was no way of judging the mother's situation within prelabour,

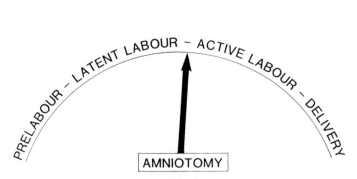

Fig. 37.4 Spectrum of phases in the transition from pregnancy to delivery. The membranes may rupture spontaneously or be ruptured artificially at any point in this spectrum.

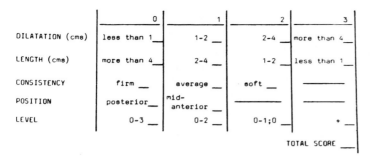

	0	1	2	3
DILATATION (cms)	less than 1	1-2	2-4	more than 4
LENGTH (cms)	more than 4	2-4	1-2	less than 1
CONSISTENCY	firm	average	soft	
POSITION	posterior	mid-anterior		
LEVEL	0-3	0-2	0-1;0	+

TOTAL SCORE __

Fig. 37.5 Modified Bishop's score (Calder et al 1974).

but because cervical ripening is a central event during this phase, an assessment of the degree to which this has developed provides a helpful guide.

Assessment of cervical ripening is based on the scoring system devised by Bishop (1964); indeed, in Bishop's original study, he showed that there was a clear inverse relationship between the cervical score and the time programmed for spontaneous onset of labour. Stated simply, a high Bishop score indicates that spontaneous labour is imminent, while a low Bishop score denotes that it is a distant prospect. More importantly, a high Bishop score predicts a good response to labour induction, while a low score presages difficulties.

Clinical assessment of cervical state is an essential element in the process of considering and implementing a decision to induce labour. For this purpose we employ a slight modification of Bishop's original scoring system (Calder et al 1974) which has proved easier to apply in practice (Fig. 37.5).

Techniques of induction and augmentation

A historical review of labour induction (Donald 1972) describes a wide variety of mechanical and chemical assaults, many of them bizarre, and embraces a wide spectrum of success and failure. Such success as was achieved by mechanical interference (such as bougies or balloons passed through the cervix) was probably because they stimulated the release of endogenous prostaglandins within the uterine compartment (Keirse 1979). The only mechanical method which has stood the test of time is amniotomy.

Many chemical substances possess the ability—in varying degrees—to stimulate the myometrium, but most of these are unsatisfactory for labour induction or augmentation. Thus, ergometrine, although a potent myometrial stimulant and a valuable agent in the prevention and treatment of postpartum haemorrhage, has no place before delivery on account of its unpredictable effect and the danger of inducing myometrial spasm. Sparteine sulphate was popular for a time, but never gained an established place in clinical practice. Castor oil, an agent with a well-recognized capacity to stimulate gastrointestinal smooth

muscle, was widely employed until about 20 years ago, but its effects on the myometrium were uncertain and it fell from grace.

Oxytocin

The chemical substance most widely used for labour induction has been the posterior pituitary polypeptide, oxytocin. Controversy has abounded throughout the 80 years since it was discovered by Sir Henry Dale (Dale 1906) and since its first clinical application by William Blair Bell (Bell 1909). The first preparations were crude pituitary extracts of widely varying potency. Unpredictable absorption from intramuscular injection sometimes led to catastrophes from violent and uncontrolled uterine stimulation. In a famous public lecture before the Second World War, the eminent American clinician Joseph Bolivar DeLee roundly condemned oxytocin and illustrated his point by holding up in one hand a ruptured uterus and in the other a dead fetus. Quoting from holy scripture (Proverbs chapter 23 verse 32) he declared: 'It biteth like a serpent and stingeth like an adder.' His dramatic declaration emphasized the dangers of inappropriate use of this powerful agent.

In spite of this, oxytocin has evolved into a safe therapeutic weapon. The three main developments which have allowed this have been firstly, the isolation of pure oxytocin, its chemical characterization (DuVigneaud et al 1953) and its subsequent commercial synthesis (Boissonas et al 1955); secondly, the acceptance that intravenous administration using controlled infusion apparatus was the safest and most reliable means of administration (supplanting intranasal, sublingual and buccal oxytocin); and thirdly, the recognition that the oxytocin sensitivity of the pregnant uterus varies widely between individuals and at differing stages of pregnancy. From this last development evolved the principle of oxytocin titration against uterine response (Turnbull & Anderson 1968).

Prostaglandins

This important group of bioactive compounds has roles in almost all body functions. Unlike oxytocin, they are not circulating hormones, but are synthesized and released at, or very close to, their target organ. Because of this and because of the rapidity with which circulating prostaglandins are inactivated, systemic administration of these agents requires large doses and is likely to provoke troublesome side-effects. Consequently, in clinical obstetric practice, local routes of administration within the genital tract have gained wider acceptance because of a greater degree of specificity, the need for a lower dosage, and consequently the virtual elimination of unwanted side-effects. Prostaglandin $F_{2\alpha}$ and prostaglandin E_2 are the two prostaglandins which have been used extensively in labour induction, and of these prostaglandin E_2 has been found to be the agent of choice.

A SCHEMATIC APPROACH TO LABOUR INDUCTION AND AUGMENTATION

In present-day obstetric practice, the clinician has at his or her disposal a triad of weapons. The three prongs of the attack are as follows:

1. Amniotomy (introduced by Thomas Denman of the Middlesex Hospital more than 200 years ago).
2. Oxytocin (introduced by Blair Bell 85 years ago).
3. Prostaglandins (introduced for labour induction within the past 25 years).

The art of labour induction and augmentation depends on a rational combination of these three weapons.

As a general rule, the prostaglandins have their greatest effect in the prelabour and latent labour phase before amniotomy. Oxytocin, in contrast, is of little value before amniotomy, but flourishes thereafter, especially in active labour. Amniotomy is the cornerstone of successful induction and its timing is paramount in relation to both the progression of the natural physiological processes and the employment or otherwise of prostaglandins and/or oxytocin (Fig. 37.6). Some clinical situations may demand the use of none of the three weapons (as in spontaneous labour, spontaneous membrane rupture and efficient progression to delivery), while others may require all three. Between these extremes lies a spectrum of situations. Some may need amniotomy alone; some prostaglandins and then amniotomy; some amniotomy and then oxytocin. The particular requirement depends on the clinical condition of the individual patient.

Assessment of the patient

The appropriate technique for labour induction or augmentation therefore depends on the point which has been reached along the physiological progression from pregnancy to delivery. In theory, it should be possible to determine whether uterine contractility is absent or present, but since the uterus is never entirely quiescent and since it is not always possible to diagnose established labour, even in the presence of apparently strong uterine contractions, this is more difficult in practice.

The most convincing evidence of progress in labour is descent of the presenting part within the birth canal. Abdominal examination allows assessment of the level of the presenting part, but in practice this is no more than a rough guide to the progress of labour.

The clinical history and abdominal examination are not in themselves sufficient. The best source of information is vaginal examination and assessment of the cervical score (Fig. 37.5). This also allows determination of whether the membranes are intact or not, if this issue is in doubt.

The place of prostaglandins

Prostaglandin E_2 is the prostaglandin which is best suited for labour induction. It is more potent and less likely to provoke side-effects than prostaglandin $F_{2\alpha}$ and achieves its best results when given locally within the genital tract. It is indicated where the cervix is unripe, with a low cervical score, especially in primigravidae (Calder 1979).

The unripe genital tract offers the choice of three routes of prostaglandin administration—extra-amniotic, endocervical or vaginal. The first two routes are effective for cervical ripening with relatively low doses, of the order of 0.5 mg prostaglandin E_2, but are more invasive than the simpler vaginal route, which requires a larger dose. Vaginal administration of prostaglandin in pessaries or gel formulations, repeated if necessary, is effective in ripening the cervix and increasing the cervical score (Calder 1986). Side-effects are rare, although care must be taken to avoid uterine hyperstimulation, and a careful watch should be kept for this complication.

Vaginal prostaglandin E_2 is also valuable for labour induction when the cervix is already ripe. A single dose of 1–2 mg prostaglandin E_2 gel is generally effective in establishing latent labour and if this is reinforced by amniotomy, the majority proceed to active labour and delivery without further stimulation (Kennedy et al 1982). Local prostaglandins may also be used for induction of labour following amniotomy or for augmentation, but in this regard their advantages over oxytocin are less clear.

Other routes of prostaglandin administration have been largely abandoned, although some clinicians continue to favour oral administration of tablets containing 0.5 mg prostaglandin E_2. These require to be given more frequently, perhaps as often as every hour, but are effective both for induction in favourable cases and for augmentation.

The main advantages of the use of prostaglandins

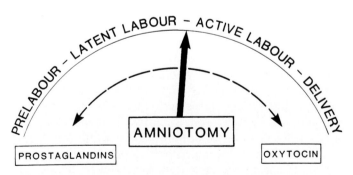

Fig. 37.6 A scheme for labour induction. Prostaglandins may be used to greatest advantage in prelabour and latent labour prior to amniotomy. Oxytocin is most effective following amniotomy. The best timing for amniotomy is after latent labour has begun.

appear to lie in their ability to reproduce many of the features of spontaneous labour. From the woman's viewpoint they are less disagreeable than the use of intravenous oxytocin, which requires complicated infusion apparatus and limits her mobility. In the case of the unfavourable induction, especially the primigravada with a low cervical score, prostaglandins result in a lower incidence of maternal and fetal complications during labour, and in particular a reduction in the Caesarean section rate compared to the rate associated with amniotomy and intravenous oxytocin. In addition, from the fetal point of view the incidence of birth asphyxia and neonatal jaundice appear to be reduced. Finally, postpartum haemorrhage is less common.

The place of amniotomy

Intact fetal membranes have been described as the biggest single hindrance to progress in labour and clearly amniotomy has a potent labour-promoting effect. Amniotomy has a central place in labour induction and augmentation, but it should not be employed until the cervix is ripe. The optimal timing of amniotomy in labour whether it be spontaneous or induced is when uterine contractility is well established and the cervix has completed the process of effacement and is 3 or 4 cm dilated. This corresponds with the point of transition from latent to active labour (Fig. 37.6).

The place of oxytocin

As has already been stated, oxytocin is of little clinical value prior to amniotomy. Amniotomy stimulates the release of endogenous prostaglandins within the uterine compartment, notably from the amnion and the decidua, and this appears to sensitize the myometrium to the action of oxytocin. It is best given by intravenous infusion and should be controlled by a mechanical infusion pump, since reliance on gravity-feed can result in dangerously wild fluctuations in dose rate.

Oxytocin can be employed immediately after either spontaneous or artificial membrane rupture or its use may be delayed until the response to membrane rupture is assessed. Some clinicians prefer to wait before administering intravenous oxytocin, but most feel there is little to be gained by this and prefer to proceed without delay.

The solution of oxytocin should not be too dilute (ideally 20 iu/l) and administration should begin at the rate of 1 mu/min and increased, preferably on a logarithmic scale to a maximum of around 32 mu/min. It should rarely be necessary to go above this maximum dose. Administration of oxytocin should be controlled carefully using an infusion pump with electronic control. A paediatric infusion set ensures precise regulation. When higher doses of oxytocin are used, it is wise to record the amniotic fluid pressure by means of an intrauterine catheter connected to a pressure recorder.

Hazards of induction of labour

As was emphasized at the start of this chapter, labour induction is a potentially hazardous step. There may be hazards inherent in the fact of interruption, or in the method employed. If the fetus is immature it faces a number of dangers and may perish as a direct result of immaturity.

Amniotomy carries two particular hazards: firstly, in the absence of a well fitting presenting part, the umbilical cord may prolapse during amniotomy. Secondly, pathogenic bacteria may be introduced at the time of amniotomy, and if delivery is delayed thereafter this is likely to lead to intrauterine infection of serious clinical import for mother or offspring, or both.

There are specific hazards associated with oxytocic agents, the most obvious of which is uterine hyperstimulation and consequent fetal hypoxia.

Prostaglandins

Apart from uterine hyperstimulation, prostaglandins are relatively free of hazards, although they may be the cause of irksome side-effects. These are largely minimized by the use of local routes of administration.

Oxytocin

Oxytocin has been shown to be associated with a number of dangers, some of which may be serious. The antidiuretic action of this hormone can lead to water intoxication of the mother, and this has on occasion been fatal. There has also been an association with neonatal jaundice, although this is usually mild. There may be an increased tendency towards atonic postpartum haemorrhage, even if, as is recommended, the infusion of oxytocin is continued for 30–60 minutes after delivery.

Although these hazards are potentially very dangerous, careful adherence to appropriate guidelines in respect of induction of labour should result in their being rare.

FUTURE PROSPECTS

Further improvements in methods of induction and augmentation of labour will undoubtedly accrue from our ever-increasing understanding of the physiological control of parturition. In addition, pharmacological control is also likely to improve with the emergence of new therapies and more sophisticated delivery vehicles, especially for prostaglandins. The antiprogesterone drugs have already had a major impact in interruption of early pregnancy (Roger & Baird 1987, 1990) and the first of these, Mifepristone, has already been explored as a potential agent for cervical ripening in the context of labour induction at term (Frydman et al 1991).

CONCLUSIONS

Labour should not be induced or augmented unless there are clear clinical indications to do so. An understanding of the physiology of labour is crucial to good clinical practice.

The method chosen to accomplish delivery should be tailored to the obstetric features of each individual patient. If delivery is indicated when the cervix is unripe, the choice must lie between elective Caesarean section and therapeutic cervical ripening. If cervical ripening is chosen, this is best achieved by local prostaglandin E_2 therapy.

Amniotomy, the cornerstone of induction, should not be performed before the cervix is ripe. Oxytocin comes into its own following membrane rupture, whether artificial or spontaneous. The dose should be titrated against the uterine response.

REFERENCES

Anderson A B M, Turnbull A C 1969 Relationship between length of gestation and cervical dilatation, uterine contractility and other factors during pregnancy. American Journal of Obstetrics and Gynecology 105: 1207–1214

Barclay C B, Brennand J E, Kelly R W, Calder A A 1993 Interleukin-8 production by the human cervix: another factor in cervical ripening. American Journal of Obstetrics and Gynecology 169: 625–632

Beard R W 1968 The effect of fetal blood sampling on caesarean sections for fetal distress. British Journal of Obstetrics and Gynaecology 75: 1291–1295

Beazley J M 1975 In: Beard R, Brudenell M, Dunn P, Fairweather D (eds) The management of labour. Royal College of Obstetricians and Gynaecologists, London, pp 25–26

Bell W B 1909 The pituitary body and the therapeutic value of infundibular extract in shock, uterine atony and intestinal paresis. British Medical Journal 2: 1609–1613

Bishop E H 1964 Pelvic scoring for elective induction. Obstetrics and Gynecology 24: 266–268

Boissonas R A, Guttmann S, Jaquenand P A, Waller T P 1955 A new synthesis of oxytocin. Helvetica Chimica Acta 38: 1491–1495

Calder A A 1979 Management of the unripe cervix. In: Keirse M J N C, Anderson A B M (eds) Human parturition. Leiden University Press, Leiden, pp 201 217

Calder A A 1983 Methods of induction of labour. In: Studd J (ed) Progress in obstetrics and gynaecology, vol 3. Churchill Livingstone, Edinburgh, pp 86–100

Calder A A 1986 Cervical ripening. In: Bygdeman M, Berger G S, Keith L G (eds) Prostaglandins and their inhibitors in clinical obstetrics and gynaecology. MTP Press, Lancaster, pp 145–264

Calder A A, Greer I A 1992 Cervical physiology and induction of labour. Ballière's Clinical Obstetrics and Gynaecology 6: 771–786

Calder A A, Embrey M P, Hillier K 1974 Extra-amniotic prostaglandin E_2 for the induction of labour at term. Journal of Obstetrics and Gynaecology of the Commonwealth 81: 39–46

Caldeyro-Barcia R 1958 Uterine contractility in obstetrics. Proceedings of the Second International Congress of Gynaecology and Obstetrics, Montreal, vol 1, pp 65–78

Csapo A I, Pulkinnen 1979 The mechanisms of prostaglandin action on the pregnant human uterus. Prostaglandins 17: 283–299

Dale H H 1906 On some physiological aspects of ergot. Journal of Physiology 34: 163

Donald I 1972 A review of procedures in induction of labour. The case of prostaglandin E_2 and $F_{2\alpha}$. In obstetrics and gynaecology. Symposia Specialists, Miami, pp 5–11

DuVigneaud V, Ressler C, Trippet S 1953 The sequence of amino acid in oxytocin with a proposal for the structure of oxytocin. Journal of Biological Chemistry 205: 949–955

Friedman E A 1967 Labor. Clinical evaluation and management. Meredith, New York

Frydman R et al 1991 Mifepristone for induction of labour. Lancet 337: 488–489

Fuch F 1973 Initiation of labour. In: Klopper A, Gardner J (eds) Endocrine factors in labour. Cambridge University Press, Cambridge, pp 1–24

Gluck L, Kulovich M V 1973 Lecithin/sphingomyelin ratios in amniotic fluid in normal and abnormal pregnancies. American Journal of Obstetrics and Gynecology 115: 539–546

Hendricks C H, Brenner W E, Kvans G 1970 Normal cervical dilatation pattern in late pregnancy and labor. American Journal of Obstetrics and Gynecology 106: 1065–1082

Keirse M J N C 1979 Endogenous prostaglandins in human parturition. In: Keirse M J N C, Anderson A, Bennebroek Gravenhorst J (eds) Human parturition. Leiden University Press, Leiden, pp 101–142

Kennedy J H, Stewart P, Barlow D H, Hillan E, Calder A A 1982 Induction of labour: a comparison of a single prostaglandin E_2 vaginal tablet with amniotomy and intravenous oxytocin. British Journal of Obstetrics and Gynaecology 89: 704–707

Lerner U 1980 The uterine cervix and the initiation of labor: action of estradiol-17β. In: Naftolin F, Stubblefield P G (eds) Dilatation of the uterine cervix. Raven Press, New York, pp 301–316

Liggins G C 1978 Ripening of the cervix. Seminars in Perinatology 2: 261–271

Liggins G C 1981 Cervical ripening as an inflammatory reaction. In: Ellwood D A, Anderson A B M (eds) The cervix in pregnancy and labour: clinical and biochemical investigations. Edinburgh, Churchill Livingstone, pp 1–9

Manning F A, Platt L D, Sipos 1980 Antepartum fetal evaluation. Development of a fetal biophysical profile score. American Journal of Obstetrics and Gynecology 136: 787–795

O'Driscoll K, Stronge J M 1975 The active management of labour. Clinical Obstetrics and Gynaecology 2: 3–17

Philpott R H 1972 Graphic records in labour. British Medical Journal 4: 163–165

Rodger M W, Baird D T 1987 Induction of therapeutic abortion in early pregnancy with meiepristone in combination with prostaglandin pessary. Lancet ii, 1415–1418

Roger M W, Baird D T 1990 Pretreatment with mifepristone (RU486) reduces interval between prostaglandin administration and expulsion in second trimester abortion. British Journal of Obstetrics and Gynaecology 97: 41–45

Steinetz B G, O'Byrne E M, Kroc R L 1980 The role of relaxin in cervical softening during pregnancy in mammals. In: Naftolin F, Stubblefield P G (eds) Dilatation of the uterine cervix. Raven Press, New York, pp 157–177

Studd J W W, Cardozo L 1985 Evaluation of induction of labour. In: Studd J (ed) The management of labour. Blackwell, Oxford, pp 123–132

Turnbull A C, Anderson A B M 1968 Induction of labour; results with amniotomy and oxytocin titration. Journal of Obstetrics and Gynaecology of the British Commonwealth 75: 32–41

Whitfield C R 1982 Future challenges in the management of rhesus disease. Progress in Obstetrics and Gynaecology 2: 48–61

38. Operative vaginal delivery*

Geoffrey Chamberlain

Material in this chapter contains contributions from the first edition and we are grateful to the previous author for the work done.

FORCEPS DELIVERY

Historical background

Until the 17th century, many instruments had been devised to bring forth the tardy child. Midwives commonly used a variety of household utensils including pot hooks and ladles whilst the man-midwives used purpose-designed hooks, knives and tongs, none of which were intended to deliver a live baby.

With the advent of the obstetric forceps, live births from obstructed labour became a practical possibility and it is not surprising that their inventors tried to keep the instruments a closely guarded Chamberlen family secret; this they succeeded in doing for three generations. The forceps were probably devised by Peter, who delivered Queen Anne. Dr Peter's son Hugh tried to sell the secret to Mauriceau in Paris in 1670 but failed to accomplish the test which Mauriceau set him—the delivery of a rhachitic dwarf. Hugh, physician to King Charles the Second, fell out of favour and in 1690 left the country for Amsterdam where he sold the secret to Roger van Roonhuyze. In fact it seems that Hugh had sold him but one of the pair of blades. Evidently the secret leaked out or was unravelled in several places in the first half of the 18th century. These mechanical aids to delivery were so successful that they gained ground in an atmosphere and philosophy of medicine which was antimechanical. The addition of a pelvic curve to the blades was first advocated by Smellie in 1762, a concept which was also described by Johnson (1769) in Edinburgh and Levret (1751) in France.

To improve the mechanical advantage of the forceps when delivering a high head, modifications of the shank and handles were made which facilitated traction in the correct axis of the birth canal. The most successful axis traction rods were devised by Neville of Dublin in 1886 as an attachment which could be combined with various types of long forceps then in use. In particular they became wedded to the Barnes forceps and the virtually indestructible Neville–Barnes instruments are, a century later, still in use (albeit without the traction rods) in many units without thought for the original design and purpose of the instrument.

Variations

In 1929 Das catalogued over 600 different obstetric forceps and more have been described since then. His classic work and that of Laufe (1968), together with the references previously cited, provide stimulating and thought-provoking reading for the modern obstetrician.

Choice of instrument in modern practice

Different instruments work better in different hands. The only essential rules in the choice of forceps are that they should be appropriate to the task and that the operator should be experienced in their use. It is possible to undertake all forceps deliveries using two, or at most three, instruments. For outlet forceps delivery a short-shanked light forceps of the Wrigley type is the most suitable (Fig. 38.1). For mid-cavity forceps when the sagittal suture is in the anteroposterior diameter, an instrument with a longer shank is needed (Fig. 38.1); it should be as light in weight as possible and should have dimensions appropriate to modern practice. For forceps rotation, if such manoeuvres are undertaken, Kielland's forceps are most widely used. For delivery of the aftercoming head in breech presentation the conventional long-shanked forceps are suitable but the Piper forceps, in which the pelvic curve is set behind the long axis, is widely used.

---

*In a previous edition, this chapter was in two parts, the former on forceps by Professor Bryan Hibbard and the latter on vacuum extraction by Professor Geoffrey Chamberlain. In this edition, both have been condensed and brought into one chapter by the Editor; he gratefully acknowledges the larger amounts of material in the first half which are so good that he continued to use parts of Professor Hibbard's contribution.

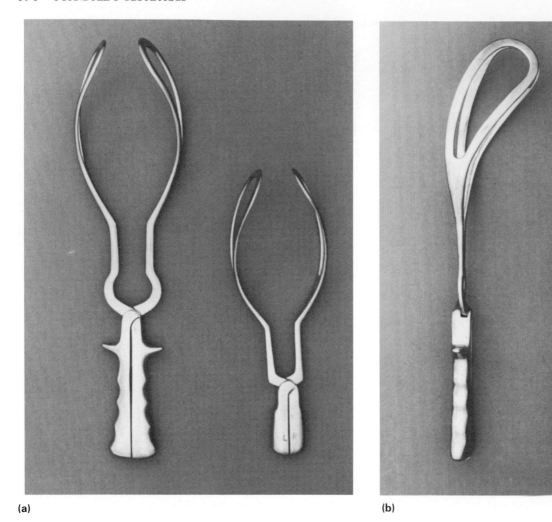

Fig. 38.1 Anderson's long forceps (left) and Wrigley's forceps (right) compared. (**a**) Plan; (**b**) elevation. From Hibbard (1988) with permission.

Terminology

The definitions of certain terms used to describe forceps deliveries vary greatly from author to author; this makes comparison of data difficult.

A *high-forceps* delivery is one in which the fetal head is not engaged and on vaginal examination the vertex is well above the level of the ischial spines. The hazards of such a procedure are so great that it should hardly ever be comtemplated in modern obstetric practice, except in surroundings where a Caesarean section cannot be performed and where the operator is highly experienced in vaginal operative delivery. The former situation is now getting rarer while the latter are also becoming extinct.

A *mid-forceps* delivery is performed when the head is in the mid pelvic cavity with the vertex at or near the level of the ischial spines. Internal rotation of the head is often incomplete and will need to be corrected before traction can be applied. The management of such cases is one of the most controversial current issues.

A *low-forceps* delivery usually refers to those cases in which the head is at or near the pelvic floor or even visible at the introitus, although perineal distension does not occur with contractions.

Outlet forceps refer to when the vertex has reached the pelvic floor, the sagittal suture is in the anteroposterior diameter and only maternal soft tissues are impeding the delivery of the head.

It is unfortunate that the terms outlet and low are used more or less synonymously and indiscriminately by many obstetricians, because according to the definitions given, low-forceps delivery may be necessitated by some degree of cephalopelvic disproportion and the problems and hazards are more akin to those of mid-forceps delivery, although of lesser degree. Until general agreement is reached it is incumbent on units or individuals to define their use of these terms clearly.

Indications for forceps delivery

The need to expedite vaginal delivery may arise because

of poor progress or because of some maternal or fetal emergency, the latter often being consequent on the former.

Delay in the second stage

It used to be customary to apply arbitrary time limits for the duration of the second stage of labour, commonly 2 hours in nulliparae and 1 hour in multiparae. These are not particularly useful, especially as it is usually uncertain when the second stage actually began. Of far more importance is the progress, judged by serial assessment of the descent of the presenting part, and the position and attitude of the head. Expulsive forces may be insufficient to maintain progressive labour because they are inherently weak or because there is undue resistance to descent of the head caused by cephalopelvic disproportion or by soft-tissue obstruction. Disproportion is a relative concept which may be due to a relatively large head, a relatively small or misshapen pelvis, or to positional disproportion caused by malpresentation so that a larger fetal head diameter presented.

There are no absolute criteria for intervention when progress is unduly slow, providing there are no other acute complicating factors. Too early interference may involve the operator in an unnecessarily difficult operative delivery, perhaps with the need for rotation of the head. With a little more patience some further progress could have been achieved, followed by an easier forceps delivery. On the other hand unnecessary waiting increases the physical and mental discomfort for the mother and the risk of hypoxia and trauma for the baby.

An outlet forceps delivery carries no significant risk for the mother or baby and is freely employed when there is delay due to relative rigidity of the maternal soft tissues or when maternal expulsive efforts are inadequate because of exhaustion, non-co-operation, or lack of the bearing-down reflex associated with epidural anaesthesia.

Specific maternal and fetal indications

Although there are certain clearcut conditions which in themselves indicate the need for urgent delivery, more commonly intelligent anticipation of maternal or fetal deterioration, particularly in cases of prolonged labour, leads to obstetric intervention.

Maternal compromise *Maternal obstetric indications* include eclampsia, severe pre-eclampsia and intrapartum haemorrhage. *Intercurrent illness,* such as severe cardiac or pulmonary disease, may be an indication for early recourse to forceps delivery if progress is not rapid, to minimize physical strain.

Maternal distress to former generations of obstetricians meant a mother exhausted physically and mentally, dehydrated and ketotic, with a raised pulse rate and often mildly pyrexial. To allow such a situation to develop in modern obstetric practice is indefensible. However the term is still used and refers to circumstances where progress is slow and further encouragement of the mother is to no avail.

Fetal compromise There are some clearly recognized and defined complications in the second stage, such as umbilical cord prolapse and premature separation of the placenta, in which early delivery, usually by forceps, is imperative.

More commonly, there is gradually accumulating evidence of fetal distress—a clinical concept implying progressive fetal hypoxia and acidaemia—for which no specific cause is identified although in many cases there are defined risk factors, such as maternal age, hypertension, prolonged pregnancy and intrauterine growth retardation. Other alerting factors include the passage of meconium-stained amniotic fluid, fetal bradycardia and late deceleration patterns on a cardiotocograph. However, as in the first stage of labour, action based on fetal heart rate patterns alone will lead to many unnecessary interventions and unless the pattern is truly alarming, or delivery is likely to be achieved quickly and easily by episiotomy and outlet forceps delivery, fetal blood sampling may be performed before deciding on the need for, and mode of, delivery.

Alternative methods of management

Since indications for forceps delivery are rarely, if ever, absolute, other options need to be considered.

Wait

When the head is in the mid-cavity and incompletely rotated, temporizing may result in some further progress and avoid the need for rotation as well as bringing the head lower in the pelvis. There is of course no case for waiting if there is arrest of progress.

Encourage stronger uterine action

This may be done by administration of oxytocin, as advocated by O'Driscoll & Meagher (1980), at least in primigravidae. The authors distinguish two phases in the second stage of labour. In phase 1 the head is high in the pelvis and the occiput is usually lateral. It is a natural extension of the first stage of labour and there is no maternal desire to push. Phase 2 begins when the head reaches the pelvic floor and the mother has a compulsive desire to push. O'Driscoll & Meagher take the extreme view that vaginal delivery with forceps should never be attempted in phase 1, when a need for urgent delivery is met by Caesarean section. If there is no urgency, adequate uterine activity can be restored by oxytocin infusion, replacing traction by propulsion. Although there may be an eventual need for forceps delivery it is likely to be easier. The other side of the coin is that oxytocin may result in further impaction and if Caesarean section is ultimately needed, displacement and delivery of the head may be more difficult. Clearly careful selection of cases for such a form of management is vital if trauma is to be avoided.

Caesarean section

Abandonment of mid-forceps operations, especially those involving rotation of the fetal head, has gained favour in recent years, not only because of the attitudes expressed by O'Driscoll & Meagher (1980) but because of increasing concern with defensive obstetrics occasioned by attitudes to litigation in the event of misfortune. The risks of Caesarean section are clear and relatively well quantified. The risks of forceps delivery from the mid-cavity are not and, in spite of an extensive literature, judgement continues to be based on common sense rather than statistical analyses of often dubious validity. From the published literature, including the review by Cohen & Friedman (1983), it is evident that judgement is confounded by many factors, including the following: there have been no prospective or controlled trials; varying definitions have been used; indications for forceps delivery vary and series may or may not include rotations performed by various means; management policies include varying degrees of conservatism; it is difficult to be certain whether many fetal complications and condition at birth are propter hoc or post hoc, cause or effect; distinction is not made between operations performed by skilled and unskilled obstetricians; the availability of senior assistance or facilities for immediate Caesarean section in case of undue difficulty is a relevant factor. Many of these problems are highlighted by the provocative papers of Cardozo et al (1982) and Chiswick & James (1979) and the extensive correspondence which followed them.

On the basis of available evidence there does not appear to be a case for absolute abandonment of mid-cavity forceps delivery, even if it involves rotation, in favour of Caesarean section but the following general guidelines should ensure that these potentially dangerous operations can be relatively safe for mother and baby and the longer-term sequelae of Caesarean section can be minimized:

1. Caesarean section should generally be carried out if there is confirmed evidence of fetal asphyxia and the head has not reached the pelvic floor, so that there is only soft-tissue resistance to be overcome. Reassessment in the operating theatre immediately prior to section is often advisable as the situation may have changed in the interim.
2. Caesarean section is indicated in mid-cavity arrest in multigravidae, with or without malpresentation as this

nearly always indicates disproportion of a degree which would make vaginal delivery dangerous.
3. If mid-forceps delivery is contemplated, senior staff should always be directly involved in assessment and supervision of the delivery. If for any reason senior assistance is not immediately available or advice is available only by telephone, Caesarean section is likely to be a preferable option.
4. If the preceding labour pattern suggests the possibility of disproportion, such as a long 7–10 cm cervical dilatation interval (Davidson et al 1976; Fig. 38.2), assessment in the operating theatre with facilities immediately available for Caesarean section is required before attempting forceps application.
5. Adequate anaesthesia must be established. This usually means epidural or spinal anaesthesia—pudendal nerve block and local infiltration are inadequate.

Ventouse

The advantages and disadvantages of the ventouse are discussed on page 713. Forceps and ventouse, rather than rivalling each other, should be regarded as complementary in varying circumstances and their use kept for the appropriate occasion.

Prerequisites for forceps delivery

There are certain fundamental rules which must be fulfilled before forceps delivery is attempted, irrespective of an apparent urgency to deliver the baby. Indeed an emergency situation is just the time when discipline and adherence to well established principles are most required.

1. The cervix must be fully dilated.
2. The membranes must be ruptured.

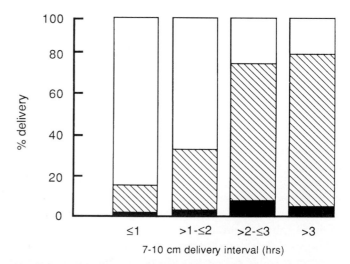

Fig. 38.2 Facility of forceps delivery related to the 7–10 cm cervical dilatation period (occipito-anterior presentations). ■ = difficult; ▨ = moderate; □ = easy. After Davidson et al (1976).

3. The position and station of the head must be identified with certainty and the head must be in a suitable position for delivery, with prior rotation if necessary.
4. There must be no major cephalopelvic disproportion.
5. There must be adequate facilities for neonatal resuscitation and special care.

In addition it is usually recommended that the bladder should be empty. This is arguable, as the bladder is an abdominal organ at this stage and is not likely to contribute to mechanical difficulty. Neither is bladder trauma more likely if there is urine in it—indeed it might even be protective. A possible exception is when forceps rotation is being performed and it is of some importance to know that there is no pre-existing bladder injury indicated by haematuria. Hence a catheter is passed before delivery for the same reason.

Technique

Occipito-anterior forceps delivery

The first essential for safe delivery of the baby is that the forceps blades should lie in correct relationship to the fetal head. To this end careful reassessment and rehearsal of the position of the blades are a desirable preliminary. The blades are designated left and right. The left blade is that which is applied on the left side of the mother's pelvis and is held in the operator's left hand. It fits comfortably into the slightly cupped right hand of the operator (Fig. 38.3).

The patient should be on an obstetric bed capable of head-down tilt or on an operating table. Most obstetricians favour the lithotomy position but necessary precautions are a wedge under one buttock to avoid aortocaval compression and minimal flexion and abduction of the thighs compatible with access.

There are three phases to the operation—application of the blades, adjustment and articulation, and traction.

Application of the blades The left blade is selected and the handle is held between the finger and thumb of the left hand. The blade rests in the cupped right hand and the handle is approximately parallel with the right inguinal ligament (Fig. 38.4). Only two fingers of the right hand need to be inserted into the vagina to guide the tip of the blade into position alongside the fetal head as the handle is swept round in an arc. Only minimal force should be necessary and grasping the handle of the forceps like a joystick is quite unnecessary. If application and manipulation are not possible with a finger and thumb grasp something is wrong and the situation should be reassessed. The right blade is applied in like manner.

Adjustment and articulation With proper application and positioning the forceps blades should come together and lock easily but some minor adjustments

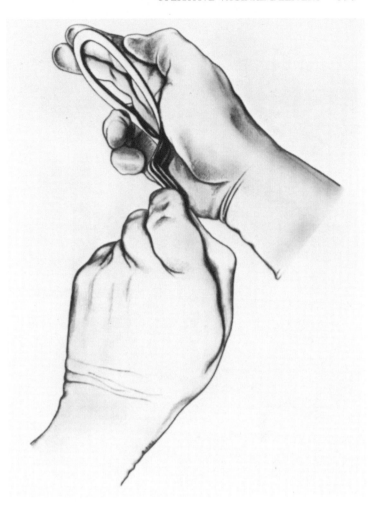

Fig. 38.3 Identification of the left blade of the forceps. The blade fits comfortably into the right hand and the fingers guard the tip. From Hibbard (1988) with permission.

may be necessary. Optimally the blades should ultimately grasp the head at right angles to the submentovertical diameter. If the head is not quite directly in the antero-posterior diameter of the pelvis, the forceps should be applied in correct relationship to the head rather than the pelvis.

The positioning is checked by feeling the lambdoid suture 2 cm from the shank of the forceps and the symmetry of the forceps in relation to the suture lines and fontanelles.

If the blades do not lock easily, undue manipulation is likely to be traumatic to mother and baby. Removal and reassessment are indicated.

Traction Traction is best applied by the fingers placed between the shanks of the forceps (Fig. 38.5). This imposes some limit to the degree of traction force which can be applied, gives a better feel of the direction of traction and avoids any risk of head compression from gripping the handles. The traction force is also limited if the forearm is kept in a flexed position.

The aim of traction is to augment the natural forces. The direction of traction should be in the axis of the birth

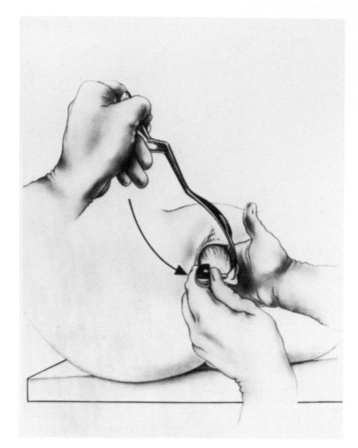

Fig. 38.4 Insertion of the left blade. The handle starts parallel with the inguinal ligament on the opposite side. From Hibbard (1988) with permission.

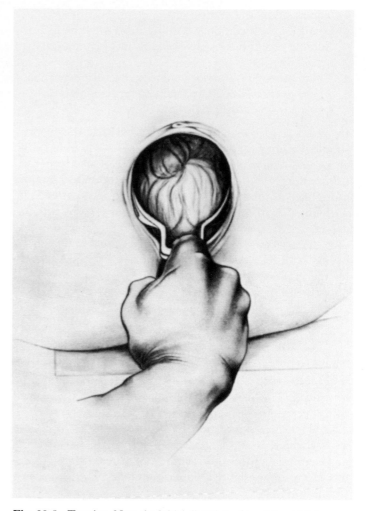

Fig. 38.5 Traction. Note the initial direction of traction which is related to the station of the head in the birth canal. The traction force is applied via the index finger between the shanks of the forceps. From Hibbard (1988) with permission.

canal, altering the angle as the head descends (Fig. 38.6). Traction is applied intermittently and synchronously with uterine contractions. There should always be some descent of the head during traction, even though it retreats in the intervening period. Lack of descent suggests a degree of disproportion incompatible with safe vaginal delivery. When the head is distending the perineum and the biparietal diameter is at the level of the ischial tuberosities an episiotomy is performed. Crowning and delivery of the head are achieved in a controlled manner by swinging the handles of the forceps upwards so that the head extends (Fig. 38.7). The blades are removed and delivery is completed in the normal manner, followed by inspection of the birth canal for lacerations and repair of the episiotomy.

Forceps delivery for cephalic malpresentations

The clinical features and general management of occipitoposterior and transverse positions are discussed elsewhere (see Ch. 36). In summary, with delay associated with these malpositions the options are:

1. Caesarean section.
2. Manual rotation and forceps delivery.

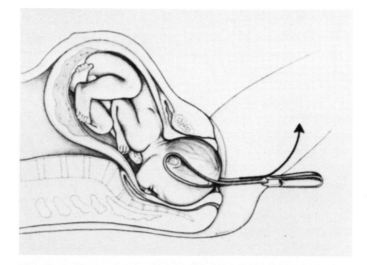

Fig. 38.6 The direction of traction follows the axis of the birth canal, reproducing the normal mechanism of labour. From Hibbard (1988) with permission.

hazardous, and increasing difficulty is related to, for example, the duration of the 7–10 cm dilatation interval (Davidson et al 1976; Fig. 38.2). Therefore such procedures must always be undertaken or supervised by the most senior person available and are often best carried out as a trial of forceps in the operating theatre with facilities immediately available for Caesarean section if conditions prove unfavourable.

Preliminaries to forceps rotation

Essential preliminaries are:

1. Assemble the full team, including anaesthetist and paediatrician.
2. Ascertain that conditions are as previously assessed and that a traumatic vaginal delivery is potentially feasible.
3. Decide on the place of delivery, i.e. delivery room or operating theatre.
4. Decide on the method of pain relief with the patient and anaesthetist.

Manual rotation

This is the least popular option and may lead to unexpected and unwanted problems.

To facilitate rotation it is usually necessary to disimpact the head by pushing it upward. This increases the risk of cord prolapse and may leave the head at a higher level after rotation, so making forceps application more difficult and more hazardous. Undue displacement may even result in the head being above the pelvic brim. Further, to have the occiput anterior when the head is high in the pelvic cavity is unanatomical and is contrary to the normal mechanism of labour. One of the basic rules of assisted delivery is to endeavour to mimic the normal mechanism of labour as closely as possible.

In general, if displacement is necessary to rotate the head, Caesarean section is a better option.

Forceps rotation and delivery

Although there is an experienced body of opinion which believes that forceps rotation of an occipito-posterior presentation should never be undertaken (O'Driscoll & Meagher 1980), the majority identify a place for forceps rotation in carefully selected cases. However, it is clear that in some units where there is ready and early recourse to forceps delivery the number of rotational forceps is unnecessarily high, and that with a little more time natural rotation often occurs which can be followed by an easier and straightforward forceps application.

Forceps of the conventional long type have been used for rotation after correct cephalic application but, because of the pelvic curve of the blades, to maintain the correct

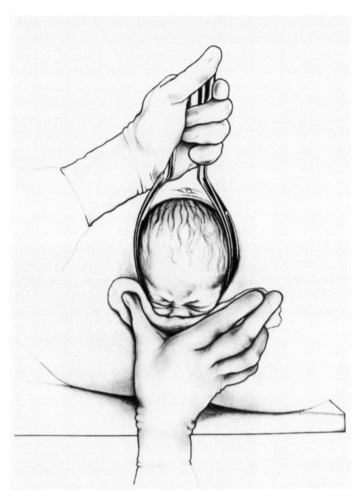

Fig. 38.7 Completion of delivery of the head by extension. The handles of the forceps are almost vertical. From Hibbard (1988) with permission.

3. Forceps rotation and delivery.
4. With occipito-posterior position, delivery as an occipito-posterior.
5. Ventouse delivery.

When delivering from the transverse position it is important to distinguish between *true deep transverse arrest*, where pelvic contraction is likely, rotation must be assisted and delivery may be difficult, and *transverse position without arrest*, when delivery may be required because of fetal compromise but the pelvis is of normal configuration. In the latter case the head is still in mid-cavity, but has not had time to rotate from the transverse position in which it engaged in the pelvis. In such cases traction, either by ventouse or forceps, is associated with autorotation as the head descends to the pelvic outlet. This was the desirable objective emphasized by Kielland in 1916.

The choice of operative procedure is dependent not only on the clinical conditions, but on the skills and training of the operator. All such deliveries are potentially axis of the blades during rotation the handles must be swept round in a wide arc (the Scanzoni manoeuvre) which is difficult to judge accurately. It can lead to a dangerous degree of rotatory force, with risk of intracranial damage as well as trauma to the birth canal. This type of manipulation has no place in modern practice.

Kielland's forceps

Of the many types of forceps designed for rotation of the head only two have found wide favour over a long period. Kielland's forceps have been particularly popular in Europe, whilst Barton's forceps have had most support in America. The use of the former will be described. Those readers who wish to make a detailed study of Barton's forceps and their modifications are referred particularly to the monograph by Parry Jones (1972).

Kielland first described his forceps in 1916 although he had publicly demonstrated them in 1910. Thus his description of their use was based on his considerable experience at the time of writing and is worthy of reconsideration. The forceps were designed primarily for extraction of the incompletely rotated head, using a correct cephalic application (oblique application had previously been a common practice). Contrary to what is often believed, Kielland condemned the use of forceps when the head was above the pelvic brim. He reiterated the observations of the previous generation who had developed axis traction forceps that: 'the extraordinary force necessary . . . lay principally in the misdirected traction . . . resulting from the pelvic curve'. Kielland's design might be regarded as the simplest form of axis traction because 'the bayonet-like shape permits the axis of the blade to lie parallel to the axis of the handle . . . traction can therefore follow the direction of the handles' (Fig. 38.8). One potential disadvantage is that the initial direction of traction is through the perineum, so that a large and early episiotomy is required.

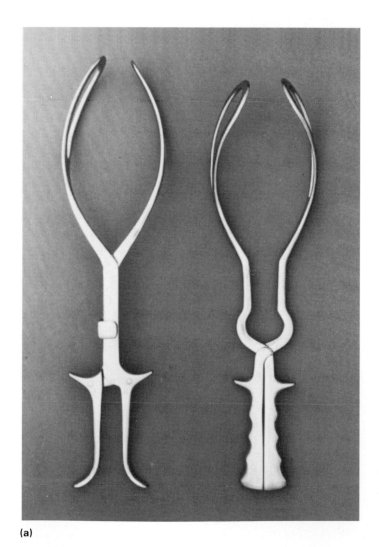

(a)

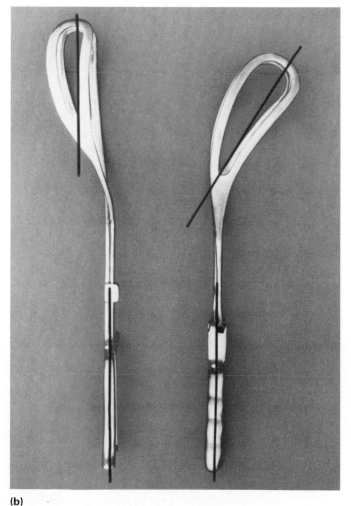

(b)

Fig. 38.8 Kielland's forceps (left) and Anderson's forceps (right) compared. (**a**) Plan; (**b**) elevation. Note that in the Kielland's forceps the axes of the blades and handles are parallel. From Hibbard (1988) with permission.

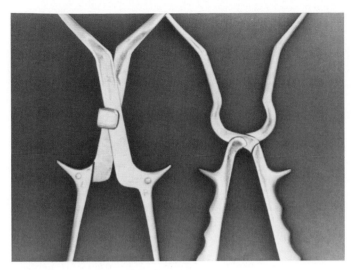

Fig. 38.9 The locks of Kielland's (left) and conventional forceps (right) compared. The sliding lock of the Kielland's forceps facilitates application when there is asymmetric moulding of the head. From Hibbard (1988) with permission.

The other outstanding feature of the instrument is the sliding lock (Fig. 38.9) which permits satisfactory cephalic application even in cases of gross asynclitism, although in modern practice such a condition is rarely encountered, as intervention has usually taken place at an earlier stage.

Other minor details of design are important, especially in relation to the method of application of the blades. For a detailed discussion the reader is referred to the classic monograph by Parry Jones (1952). Parry Jones defined ideal criteria for forceps which are almost fulfilled by the Kielland instrument:

1. Simple in construction.
2. Suitable for all positions of the head.
3. Require only a single application with minimal manipulation.
4. Permit true axis traction.
5. Satisfactory for rotation of the fetal head without applying excessive stressing forces.

Nevertheless, in inappropriate, unskilled hands Kielland's forceps are potentially dangerous and specialist training and continuing practice are required for their safe use. Hence there has been a growing tendency to abandon mid-cavity rotation in favour of Caesarean section. In some working circumstances ventouse delivery may be a satisfactory or even desirable alternative, with less risk of trauma but more risk of failure. Also, the ventouse does not reduce the already limited available pelvic space.

Application of Kielland's forceps It is helpful to rehearse the application of the blades once the station of the head and position of the occiput have been identified, remembering that the aim is to obtain a correct cephalic application with the concavity of the pelvic curve of the forceps directed towards the occiput. To aid orientation

there is a raised knob on the upper surface of each finger lug and these should point in the direction of the occiput.

The anterior (superior) blade is always applied first— i.e. the left blade for a right occipito-lateral position and the right blade for a left occipito-lateral position.

Three methods of application of the anterior blade are described and the relative merits have long been debated. The most controversial is the classic method recommended by Kielland himself. He was aware of criticism of what many regarded as a dangerous technique but put the counter arguments very convincingly in his original paper (1916).

Classic application The superior blade is selected and inserted with the cephalic concavity directed anteriorly (Fig. 38.10), i.e. upside down in relation to the fetal head. The index and middle fingers of one hand are used to guide the tip of the blade and protect the fetal and maternal soft tissues. The other hand grasps the forceps 'with a full grip (like a sword, not a pen)' (Kielland 1916). The handle is initially kept nearly horizontal but when the tip of the blade encounters the fetal head the handle is depressed and the blade should then slide easily into the cavity of the uterus. Failure to recognize this can lead to damage to the lower uterine segment.

The blade is introduced until the shank impinges on the posterior vaginal wall and the narrow bevelled section between the base of the blade and the shank is between the head and the symphysis pubis. The blade is then rotated, maintaining the axis, so that it slides into correct position in relation to the head. The direction of rotation is important, as will be seen if the procedure is rehearsed. The arc which the blade describes is minimized if the concavity of the pelvic curve fits the convexity of the head,

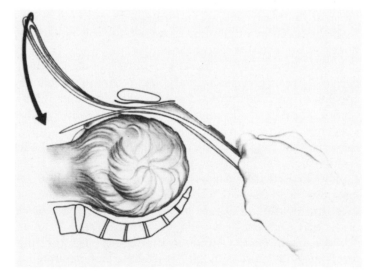

Fig. 38.10 Classic method of application of the anterior blade of Kielland's forceps. Note the position of the shank between the head and the symphysis pubis. From Hibbard (1988) with permission.

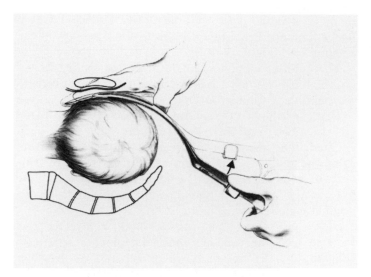

Fig. 38.11   Direct application of the anterior blade. Note the use of the operator's fingers to avoid injury to the birth canal by the tip of the forceps. From Hibbard (1988) with permission.

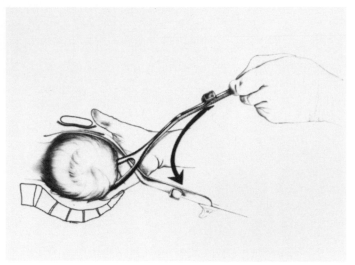

Fig. 38.12   Wandering method of application of the anterior blade. Insertion is started as with a conventional forceps application, swinging the blade round to a correct cephalic application as insertion proceeds. From Hibbard (1988) with permission.

so the correct direction of rotation is always towards the concave rim of the blade. The knobs on the handles act as a guide—rotation is carried out to the side on which the knob is felt.

The available space between the head and the symphysis may not be sufficient to carry out this manoeuvre safely, particularly if the head is well down in the pelvic cavity.

Direct application   This apparently simple option is only feasible when the head is low in the pelvis because the initial position of the handle is such that it may be hampered by the perineum or the end of the operating table (Fig. 38.11).

The main force used during introduction is elevation of the handle and, as with the classic method, advancement of the blade follows naturally, with minimal effort. Again protection of the soft tissues with the operator's fingers is an essential feature.

Wandering method   This is the most popular option, perhaps because it is closer to the technique used for application of conventional forceps. The ultimate anterior blade, whether it be right or left, is inserted in the standard manner along the side wall of the pelvis and is then wandered by swinging it round to a correct cephalic relationship as insertion proceeds (Fig. 38.12). It is usually advised that it is easier to wander the blade from insertion over the forehead and this has the advantage that during the early part of insertion the pelvic curve of the blade matches the curve of the birth canal.

The posterior blade   Although it might appear from the foregoing that more difficulty is likely to be encountered with the anterior rather than the posterior blade the opposite is often the case—a point again emphasized by Kielland (1916)—because of obstruction by the sacral promontory (Fig. 38.13).

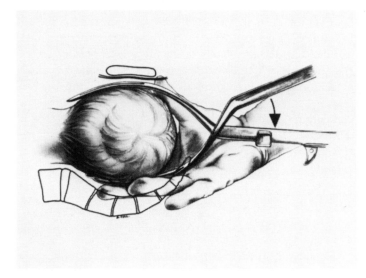

Fig. 38.13   Direct application of the posterior blade. From Hibbard (1988) with permission.

Half of the right hand is introduced into the hollow of the sacrum and is used to facilitate direct application of the blade, which often drops into position with minimal pressure. If the sacral promontory is a problem it is important for any manipulation to be carried out gently whilst the soft tissues are guarded by the operator's fingers. Sometimes in cases of difficulty a slightly oblique introduction and wandering application may be helpful.

Traction and rotation   Accepting that the desirable objective is to mimic the normal mechanism of labour as closely as possible, traction force in the exact direction of the handles should be applied first and if there is advancement of the head this can be continued without any external rotating force; the head should rotate spontaneously as it descends through the birth canal.

It must be recognized that, because of the design of the forceps, the direction of traction is more posteriorly than with conventional forceps and an early generous episiotomy is required. Also, if the patient is in the lithotomy position effective traction is difficult with the operator in a standing position or sitting on a normal operating stool. Although Kielland advocated tilting the bed to facilitate traction a better alternative is for the operator to kneel or sit on a low footstool.

Delivery is completed in the conventional manner, avoiding compression of the handles and using only the finger lugs to exert traction force (Fig. 38.14).

If the head does not descend readily during the initial traction attempt the situation should be reappraised, with the alternative options of rotation in the mid-cavity or Caesarean section.

Mid-cavity rotation must be carried out with gentleness and sensitivity. Slight upward dislodgement of the head, especially with a funnel-shaped pelvis, may facilitate rotation. Only the finger lugs should be used for applying rotational pressure. Traction and rotational forces should not be applied at the same time.

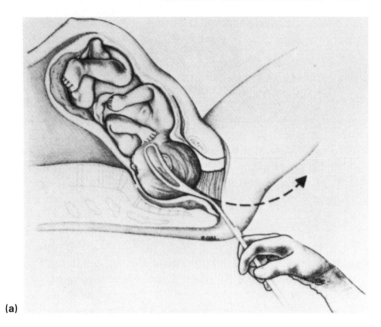

(a)

Forceps delivery as an occipito-posterior

The second stage of labour is likely to be prolonged with an occipito-posterior position even if spontaneous delivery eventually occurs. Generally delay which is sufficient to warrant intervention suggests the need to correct the malpresentation before applying traction, but in some cases forceps delivery as an occipito-posterior may be justified and preferable. Particular circumstances in which this option should be considered include a satisfactory bony pelvic outlet, as with an anthropoid pelvis (which favours occipito-posterior positions) and delay due to soft-tissue obstruction. The head must be below the level of the ischial spines and the position must be directly occipito-posterior (occipito-sacral).

The forceps are applied in the conventional manner, with correct pelvic application, taking care not to place the blades too far anteriorly in relation to the head as they may then slip off. A generous episiotomy is usually required and traction is directed posteriorly until the glabella is under the apex of the pubic arch. The handles of the forceps are then swung upwards so that the head is delivered by flexion.

Complications

Most complications of forceps delivery result from errors of judgement and inexperience. When labour has been prolonged and difficult there is an added element of maternal tissue bruising, devitalization and risk of sepsis

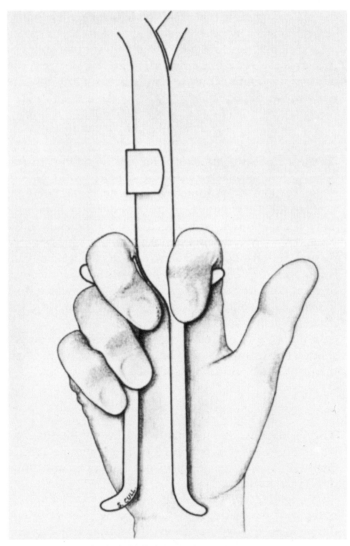

(b)

Fig. 38.14 (a) The direction of traction with Kielland's forceps. (b) The traction force is applied via the finger lugs and not by grasping the handles. From Hibbard (1988) with permission.

which is likely to increase the problems arising from any operative trauma.

The perineum and vagina

There is a risk of extension of the episiotomy and additional vaginal lacerations occurring during application of the blades and during traction, particularly if forceps of unsuitable design are used. Any additional trauma makes suturing more difficult and increases the risk of painful scars and dyspareunia.

The cervix

The cervix is particularly susceptible to damage during rotational deliveries, either during the application of the blades or during the rotation. Lateral lacerations may extend upwards in the lower uterine segment, with rupture of the uterine artery or main branches. Damage anteriorly can involve the bladder, with production of a vesicocervical vesicovaginal fistula. Traumatic haemorrhage may be severe and in any cases of doubt concerning trauma full exploration in operating theatre conditions is obligatory. Attempts at semi-blind suturing in the delivery room without adequate exposure and assistance are only likely to compound the problem.

Urinary complications

These include retention of urine and infection. In particular a careful watch should be kept to avoid retention with overflow if epidural analgesia has been used. Any difficult delivery should be followed by catheterization and if haematuria is revealed special precautions are necessary. Gross haematuria suggests the possibility of tearing and fistula formation, and detailed examination is required. Lesser degrees of haematuria are indicative of bruising and devitalization. This may be associated with tissue necrosis and the risk of late fistula formation when tissue breakdown occurs.

In all cases of haematuria continuous bladder drainage should be instituted and continued for some days after the urine has been macroscopically clear of blood.

Pelvic sepsis

This is usually due primarily to the conditions which led to the need for operative delivery but the risks are greatly increased by unskilled manipulations and trauma during the delivery.

The patient will be predisposed to *back strain* and nerve root or sciatic plexus damage by poor positioning during delivery, with excessive flexion and abduction of the hips, or from the use of excessive traction force.

Anaesthetic complications are discussed in Chapter 32.

Fetal injury

The infant is at particular risk of intracranial trauma and haemorrhage if forceps are abused, particularly if they are misapplied, so that there is not a true cephalic fit. Forceps of unsatisfactory design may lead to undue compression or may slip, causing facial abrasion.

Compression distortion injuries result in tears of the tentorium and rupture of the bridging veins. Rupture of the great vein of Galen leads to bleeding into the posterior fossa with compression of the brain stem, but supratentorial haemorrhages are more common.

Skull fractures are usually linear and not of lasting consequence. Depressed fractures, which may follow forceps delivery, are very uncommon but can result in subdural or subarachnoid haemorrhage.

Cephalhaematomas are seen most commonly over the parietal bone.

Facial nerve palsy is caused by pressure at the point where the nerve emerges from the stylomastoid foramen or as it passes over the mandibular ramus. The lesion is of lower motor neurone type, with paresis of the whole of the affected side of the face. Uncommonly, temporal bone fracture results in seventh nerve injury, the lesion being of upper motor neurone type and involving the lower two-thirds of the face.

Failed forceps delivery

This term implies that a forceps delivery was initiated in the delivery room in the belief that it could be completed successfully but that it had to be abandoned in favour of Caesarean section. It would be more appropriate to include cases in which vaginal delivery had been achieved, but only after a second attempt by a more experienced operator, and cases in which there is undue morbidity or even mortality.

Most cases of failed forceps arise from disobeying the ground rules, inexperience and lack of discipline. The commonest contributory factors are unrecognized malpresentation, incomplete dilatation of the cervix and congenital malformations causing obstruction.

A trial of forceps which is not successful might also be regarded as failed forceps but if the trial is conducted according to defined rules—by a skilled operator, in the operating theatre, with adequate anaesthesia, and with the team and equipment ready for immediate Caesarean section—there should be no significantly increased risk of morbidity.

THE VACUUM EXTRACTOR

The vacuum extractor has virtually replaced the forceps in many countries of northern Europe and Africa. Its use however is much more limited in Britain and the

Commonwealth while in the USA it is hardly used at all. Inertia is one of the hardest barriers to overcome. What one always has done is attractive, to change is difficult; probably because of this mental inertia the vacuum extractor has not been taken up more widely in the Western world. It is interesting to speculate that the underemployment of this useful instrument may be associated with the skills of forceps delivery learnt traditionally over the years and which people are loath to release from their grasp.

The definitive instrument is the one described by Malmstrom with a few modifications which have since been added. He first described his instrument in 1954 and in 1957 this was superseded by the instrument we all know now with the well-known circumferential bulge, which allows a chignon of scalp to be sucked into it. The narrower ring of the edge of the extractor means a better grip is obtained on the fetal head by this cap than with any other previous instrument. It was Malmstrom's equipment and the modifications made by Bird (1969) that are now incorporated into the instruments used in the Western world. Soft caps were introduced in an effort to reduce fetal trauma (O'Neil et al 1981) and several studies have shown they are significantly less likely to injure the scalp than metal ones. The results are best summarized in a meta-analysis by Chenoy & Johnson (1992).

Indications

The vacuum extractor has often been described as a replacement for forceps. Its use should be considered as complementary to the forceps for, although there are common indications, each instrument has its own individual criteria for use. Attempts at forceps delivery are usually contraindicated when the cervix is not yet fully dilated (see Ch. 38); one of the uses of the vacuum extractor in skilled hands used to be to bring the head down on to the cervix when there was delay in labour and so cause full dilation from 7 or 8 cm.

Because a vacuum extractor usually takes longer to assemble, apply and use properly, it is of less use when there is acute fetal distress in the second stage of labour; most skilled obstetricians can deliver a baby in the second stage more swiftly with forceps than they can with a vacuum extractor. However, many indications for operative vaginal delivery are not for acute fetal distress but relate to slow progress at the end of the first stage or in the second stage of labour; for these, the vacuum extractor is ideal.

First stage

In the first stage of labour the major indication for the vacuum extractor is lack of advance and delay at the end of the first stage. There should be no obvious cephalopelvic disproportion and the operator should reasonably expect to delivery the baby per vaginam. Occasionally, there may be a place for a trial of vacuum extraction, performed in an operating theatre with all facilities ready for Caesarean section.

At the latter part of the first stage, if fetal distress or a prolapsed cord occurs, delivery is usually by Caesarean section. However, if the operator is skilled in vacuum extraction and the woman is multiparous, it is likely that he could deliver the baby vaginally safely and much more swiftly than the time it takes to get an operating theatre ready and perform a Caesarean section (Bird 1982).

Second stage

In the second stage of labour, the vacuum extractor is of major use when there has been delay. If, in the absence of overt cephalopelvic disproportion, there is no descent of the fetal head after 20 minutes of active contractions assisted by maternal effort, it is probable that the pelvic floor is holding up the fetal head. Sometimes, particularly after epidural analgesia, the head does not rotate fully and so descent is hindered; then a vacuum extractor will complete delivery very easily.

The use of the vacuum extractor for fetal distress in the second stage depends upon the degree of distress and the skill of the operator. Often a forceps delivery will be swifter but with a skilled operator and a less serious degree of fetal hypoxia, the vacuum extractor may be preferred. The skill of the operator is stressed here since an unskilled operator takes a long time to assemble the equipment of the vacuum extractor and then to raise the requisite negative pressure. All this must be done before the active process of extraction can be commenced and could take 10–15 minutes, whereas the application of the forceps blades takes a minute or so.

Another useful function of the vacuum extractor is to help the woman whom the obstetrician does not wish to have a long or fatiguing second stage, such as a mother with heart disease or raised blood pressure. Here the efforts of the second stage can be shortened very readily with a vacuum extractor. The obstetrician will be pulling with the woman's own contractions so that she can be making some small effort and does have the satisfaction of delivering her baby vaginally, although the real effort is by the obstetrician.

The vacuum extractor is used occasionally in other instances. For instance, it is a very good instrument for the delivery of a second twin when the fetal head is high and the cervix appears not to be completely dilated despite the birth of the first twin. It is an ideal instrument in these circumstances but this is rare and few operators are skilled in this procedure. It is of great use in occipito-lateral and occipito-posterior positions.

In some parts of the world a Caesarean section could lead to difficult sequelae in the woman's subsequent social and reproductive life. In parts of Central Africa, for example, a Caesarean section is considered a shameful thing and the woman's future place in the family may be jeopardized. Here the use of symphysiotomy combined with vacuum extraction has proved a boon and the literature in this specific area is well documented (Lancet Leading Article 1974).

Contraindications

The vacuum extractor is contraindicated for any presentation other than a cephalic one, preferably reasonably flexed. Hence it should not be used on a face or brow presentation, a breech or a transverse lie. If the fetus is immature (under 32 weeks' gestation), the likelihood of cephalohaematoma with the vacuum extractor rises sharply so that many would not wish to use the instrument on such small infants. Should the obstetrician think that any reasonable degree of cephalopelvic disproportion is present, the vacuum extractor must not be used to try to overcome a mechanical block.

The apparatus

Many obstetricians in the Western world use Malmstrom's equipment (1957) or its major modifications put forward by Bird (1969). Some prefer to use a soft cap made from pliable silicone or plastic.

Metal caps are usually provided of three diameters—40, 50 or 60 mm. Although there is one of 30 mm, most hospitals do not possess this. The caps are of toughened steel, chromium-plated and shaped like a flattened hemisphere. The edge is curved in so that the rim has a smaller diameter than the cavity of the hemisphere a little higher up. Thus, if it is placed against the fetal scalp and air is evacuated from the cavity, the scalp is sucked in to fill the space of the hemisphere; the chignon, so produced, has a greater diameter above the rim than the rim itself, so that traction can be applied to the overhang (Fig. 38.15).

The soft caps are mostly 60 mm in diameter. The silastic model is a trumpet-shaped cap of silicone elastomer (Fig. 38.16); a plastic cup (Mityvac) comes with its own hand pump as a kit for action. The Silc cup of silicone rubber is said to have improved adherence to the fetal scalp (Fig. 38.17). A new version comes with a cord traction system. The CMI cap, made of malleable plastic, comes with its own reusable pistol grip hand pump and is said to produce less trauma to the fetal head (Fig. 38.18).

Air is evacuated from the cap through a thick-walled rubber tube. In the original equipment, this evacuation was from the centre of the cap and through this vacuum tube ran the traction equipment. Bird (1969) suggested

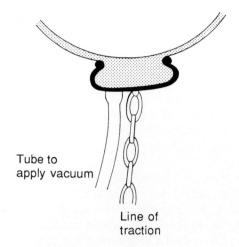

Tube to
apply vacuum

Line of
traction

Fig. 38.15   The chignon produced on the scalp.

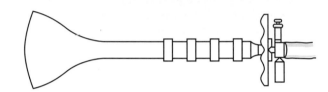

Fig. 38.16   A silastic cup.

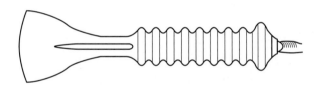

Fig. 38.17   A Silc cup.

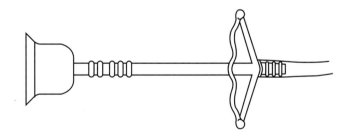

Fig. 38.18   A CMI cup.

that the vacuum outlet should be to one side and independent of the traction (Fig. 38.19). This makes the cap more manoeuvrable with better application to a badly flexed head, since it can be slipped nearer to the bregma. There are also vacuum extractor caps with the tube on the side wall of the cap—an extension of the same principle. This is known as the posterior cap and was also designed by Bird (1976). Carmody et al (1996) were

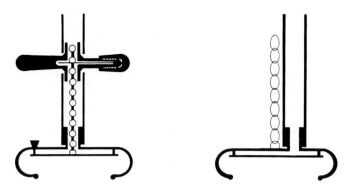

Fig. 38.19 The commonly used vacuum extraction caps. **Left:** cross-section of Malmstrom's (1957) apparatus with a central vacuum vent and the traction system through the vacuum tube. **Right:** Bird's (1969) modification showing the lateral vacuum vent and the traction chain separate.

unable to show any great benefit for the use of this cap in a randomized controlled trial of 123 women.

If the traction chain passes down the centre of the evacuation tube, the traction handle has to be incorporated into the vacuum system. This means assembling the equipment at the time it is going to be used; this can be a fiddly business, and extremely exasperating when one wants to get on with the work in hand of delivering the baby. It is here that the experience of the operator counts since he knows that assembly has to be done in a careful and methodical way. The chain used for this type of vacuum traction usually has finer links than Bird's modification. The holding pin can be bent and links of the chain may be deformed, leading to difficulties in passing the chain down the tube. Bird's modification has a shorter, stronger chain and its shortness makes angled traction less likely.

A vacuum can be achieved by hand or mechanically; the former makes use of a small hand pump, a reverse of a bicycle pump with the valves placed the other way; hence, instead of blowing things up, each stroke removes air. The hand pump can be worked by an unskilled and unscrubbed assistant. Electrical pumps have been developed which can be controlled by a foot pedal by the operator. The more sophisticated mechanical pumps allow for small gas leakages in the equipment and automatically maintain an even negative pressure which can be preset. This is of great importance for if the operator does not notice any loss of the vacuum, he will be working with inefficient equipment; this can lead to damage of the scalp. The hand pumps are cheap and easily portable but if a vacuum extractor is to be used to any extent on a hospital unit, it is worth acquiring the larger electrical pump.

The equipment is completed by a vacuum bottle through which the air from the extractor passes before going on to the pump. This is essential for a certain amount of blood, amniotic fluid and mucus is drawn into the system and this must not be allowed to enter the pump system. The bottle must be cleaned out carefully after each delivery and sterilized with one of the liquid chemical antiseptic agents. The level of vacuum is measured from this bottle with a simple aneroid barometer, graduated from 0 to $-1.0\,kg/cm^2$. This is probably the most sensitive part of the whole apparatus and the part most likely to be damaged. It does not need sterilization because it is outside the sterile field but the rough life in the labour ward often damages it. This can lead to an under-representation of the reading which might be dangerous (Chamberlain 1965).

After use, the operators themselves should disassemble the equipment and clean it, taking it to pieces and washing all the parts exposed to blood before it is sent off for sterilization. Only then will they be sure that it is going to come back after sterilization ready for use on the next occasion. If they leave it to others, however well meaning, the equipment may be sent for sterilization in an assembled condition prepared for the last delivery; the rubber evacuation tubes are still attached to the vent lugs on the cap. When during sterilization this is heated, the metal of the lug expands and the rubber will be stretched under heat. The tube may then lose some of its elasticity and when the equipment cools, the rubber stays in an expanded position so that it is inefficient to maintain a vacuum. The equipment is robust but needs thoughtful handling and is best looked after by the operator.

Use of the ventouse

The equipment is unpacked and assembled by the scrubbed-up operator. A cap of the most appropriate size is chosen. Generally this should be one of the larger caps (50 or 60 mm diameter) for with a larger size of chignon, less negative pressure will be applied per cm^2 over the skin, hence this will be less traumatic to the fetal scalp. If the cervix is not dilated, a 40 mm cap may be required; it is most unusual to apply a vacuum extractor these days to a woman who is less than 7 cm dilated and so the 30 mm cap is very rarely required.

No antiseptic creams should be used on the skin or at the vaginal preparation of the woman. Aqueous sterilizing solutions only should be used since cream causes too great an increased lubrication which might allow the cap to slip. This is most important.

The cap is then applied to the fetal head under sterile conditions, placing it as far back as possible. Ideally it should be over the posterior fontanelle, in the midline of the fetal head (Fig. 38.20). The further forward it is from this, the more it is likely to deflect the head as tension is put on the chain. Further, if the cap is not placed in the midline, when traction occurs it causes asynclitism so that larger head diameters than necessary have to engage in the maternal pelvis (Figs 38.21–38.23). These

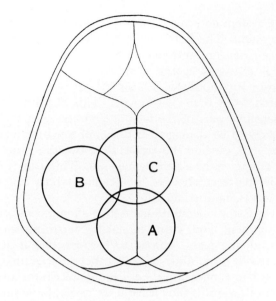

Fig. 38.20   The cap should ideally be as far back as possible over the bregma (A). If it is off the midline (B) it allows an asymmetrical pull and so larger diameters of the fetal head engage. If it is further forward than the bregma (C) the head is deflexed.

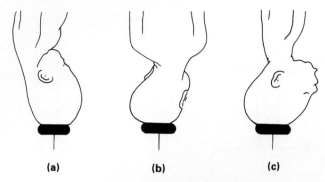

Fig. 38.21   The consequences of applications shown in Figure 57.3 are: (**a**) good application—good flexion; (**b**) off the midline—asynclitism; (**c**) too far forward—deflexion.

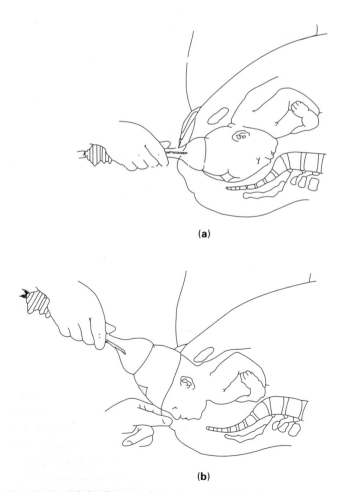

Fig. 38.22   (**a**) Application of silastic cap. (**b**) Delivering the head; note change of angle of traction.

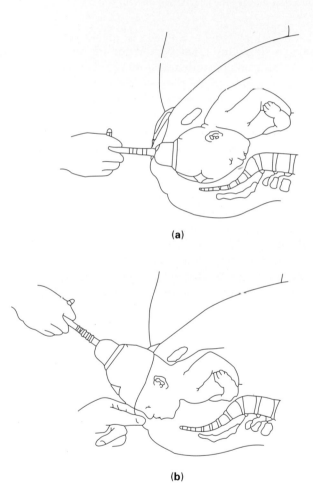

Fig. 38.23   (**a**) Application of CMI cap. (**b**) Delivering the head; note change of angle of traction.

points are important and should be checked when the cap is first placed on the head.

Negative pressure is now applied. When done with the hand pump it is conventional to do this in stages, lowering the pressure by $-0.2\,\text{kg/cm}^2$ on each occasion, but if the operator is happy that the cup is correctly positioned, there is no need to pause between each bout of pumping.

With an electrical pump, evacuation of air can be done continuously and thus the rate of induction of vacuum is quicker.

Once the cap has been attached to the scalp by the first phase of vacuum, its position must be carefully checked. It is also important that the operator runs a finger round the whole perimeter of the cap to ensure that there is no maternal tissue caught. There may be a fold of redundant vaginal wall, particularly posteriorly, which gets sucked into the cap; if a first-stage vacuum extraction is performed, part of the cervix can get caught. This step is most important and circumferential digital examination should be repeated between each bout of hand-pumping or at intervals if the continuous electrical pump is used. If this is not done, the operator will inadvertently pull down on both maternal and fetal tissues. Either the vacuum will not work since air will enter so that the cap comes off or, worse, the cap may compress the maternal tissues sufficiently to allow delivery to take place but a tear of the vagina or cervix follows as part of the delivery. Both can be avoided by checking several times that there has been no entrapment of maternal tissue.

After a vacuum of -0.8 kg/cm^2 has been achieved and before traction, the operator should assess the line of pull which will be most effective. If the head is in mid-cavity or just above it, then the pull would have to be very posterior, so much so that occasionally a preliminary episiotomy must be performed to allow the line of traction to be correct. This is most important for if the operator merely pulls at right angles to the vulva, then the actual traction on the cap will be oblique and cause it to skid on the head, producing lacerations of the scalp or eventually detachment with failure of the method.

Traction is usually applied with the operator's right hand on the handle, but the function of the left hand is very important. The index finger of the left hand should be placed on the cap near the periphery if a central vent model is used, or on the opposite side from the vent if a lateral vent cap is used. This ensures that the cap does not rock or become pulled obliquely. The middle fingertip rests on the fetal head to give a guide about real descent with traction. If the uterus is contracting, then traction on the vacuum extractor is best done synchronously with these and, if the cervix is fully dilated, the mother is encouraged to bear down with each contraction in the usual way. If there are no contractions, then the operator makes his own rhythm pulling for about 30–40 seconds every 2 minutes.

Care must be taken not to dislodge the cap. If it is felt to move laterally by the index finger of the left hand, or if a sucking noise of air entering the equipment is heard, traction should stop and the position of the cap should be reassessed. It may be too lateral or more likely, too far forward on the head. There might be unsuspected cephalopelvic disproportion and the head is not going to come down; this should be considered by the operator. If these points are evaluated and it is considered that vacuum extractor delivery should continue, the negative pressure should be restored to -0.8 kg/cm^2 and another attempt should be made. It is unwise to have more than one attempt at re-application of the cap and it may be that a larger size of cap should be used the second time. The method should be considered to have failed if the cap comes off twice and another method of delivery should then be used.

During traction, the operator must concentrate on thinking about the level of the head in the pelvis and apply traction at right angles to the cap surface wherever it is pointing. This means that the traction will be very posterior at first, towards the mother's anus when the head is high, gradually curving round so that as the head finally enters the lower pelvis, traction is almost at right angles to the vulva (Fig. 38.24). No attempt should be made to try to rotate the fetus into an occipito-anterior position. The traction force is a linear one and the fetal head will then rotate in its own way so that its diameters engage advantageously in the various diameters of the maternal pelvis. This is the vacuum extractor's great advantage, that the head can follow its own pattern of rotation. As the head crowns, the negative pressure should be released, either by the foot pump or by the operator's assistant; the cap can then be easily detached when the

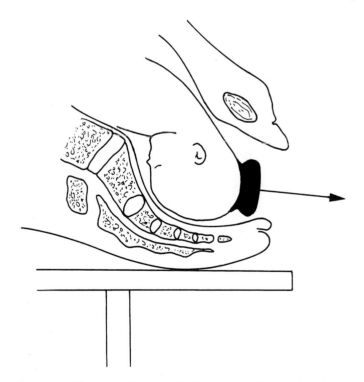

Fig. 38.24 The cap has been applied far back; the head is well flexed and progress is good. The head is now just below mid-cavity and so traction can be less posterior than when the head was higher.

negative pressure is released. There is always a chignon and there may even be a little abrasion of skin.

The operator should be on guard for shoulder dystocia which seems to be a little commoner amongst babies born by vacuum extraction. This is probably associated with the slight difficulty the woman had at delivering the head and the size of the baby in relation to the pelvis (McFarland et al 1986). In consequence, it is wise not to give Syntometrine until the anterior shoulder has actually appeared under the symphysis pubis.

The baby is resuscitated in the usual fashion. It is a sensible precaution before handing the baby to the parents to warn them that there will be a little bump on the head and to tell them that it will go down within 48 hours. Many operators actually swathe the baby in a sterile cloth and tactfully cover the top of the head with that cloth, claiming it is there to reduce heat loss. It is actually there to stop the parents seeing the chignon on their first view of their offspring. After the placenta is delivered and any episiotomy has been repaired, the operator will examine the baby fully with the parents; he can then show the diminishing chignon to them, explaining its significance and its rapid rate of disappearance.

Failed vacuum extraction

Failure rates are not often published, except by people who have performed large series of vacuum extractions. Hence, they are the failure rates of those who are interested and most experienced. A good example is Bird (1982) who had a failure rate of 3.2% among 1334 women when the Malmstrom classical cap was used and 0.5% among 2452 women when he used his modified cap. Bratt (1965) reported a failure rate of 2.3% among 1135 women. The failure rates are overall higher when soft caps are used. An average failure rate of 14% is reported by Vacca in 1992 in a cumulative series of 1074 cases by nine authors. This he compares with a failure of 4.5% among 16 authors on 4741 mothers using rigid caps. In a randomized controlled trial, Chenoy & Johanson (1992) found the overall success rate to be similar—85% for the silastic cap and 87% for the metal cap. Fewer babies had significant scalp trauma with the silastic cap but it was more likely to fail if there was an excessive caput.

Failure rates decrease with increased experience. The commonest reason for non-delivery is that the operator applies traction to the cap in an oblique fashion and not in the axis of the birth canal at the station where the fetal head is. In the first few cases, the operator may not pull hard enough and this will result in no delivery; occasionally he may pull too hard. There is a skill about vacuum extraction which tests the mind and the hands of the operator in a finer way than do forceps deliveries for this is the gentleman's way of delivering a baby. It is

wise for all operators to practise vacuum extraction on easy cases first—on outlet presentations for the first few times, graduating to vacuum extraction required for mid-cavity deliveries.

In addition, the equipment can go wrong. There may be loose rubber-to-air vent connections due to ageing of the rubber following improper sterilization. The pump may be inefficient because the valve flange is not properly lubricated (a few drops of paraffin applied soon puts this right). It is essential that all equipment should be maintained properly, preferably by those who use it.

The operator may have chosen the wrong case on which to try vacuum extraction. There may actually be some cephalopelvic disproportion or a greater degree of deflection of the fetal head than the operator had first imagined, such as a brow presentation. Sometimes after a long labour when a large oedematous caput has formed, the vacuum cap does not grip so well and comes off with a more limited tractive effort.

In essence, failed vacuum extraction is due to one of three causes:

1. The cap is not gripping the scalp properly because maternal tissue is trapped or there is inefficient equipment. The management is to re-apply the cap, excluding the maternal tissues, or to correct the leaks in the apparatus.
2. There is detachment of the cap following incorrect traction technique. There may alternately be a caput succedaneum, or the cap may have been put on the wrong part of the fetal head. The reports by Vacca (1992) referred to previously showed detachment of metal caps in 14% and soft caps in 34%.
3. Although the cap will accept strong traction, the head will not descend; the commonest reason is cephalopelvic disproportion or a misapplication of the cap so that it is too far forward or off the midline.

The operator should ensure that the fetal head is descending with each tractive effort and that it is not just the scalp which comes down. Generally speaking, the operator should consider another method of delivery if, after correct application of the cap, the head is not brought into the position of crowning within three or four proper bouts of traction. If the cap comes off, it should not be re-applied more than once.

Side-effects

The major problem that vacuum extraction might pose for the mother is that a fold of her vagina or cervix is sucked in between the cap and the fetal head; it may then be damaged, leading to haemorrhage.

The fetus is not usually seriously affected by vacuum extraction. Any attempt to correlate fetal hypoxia with the use of the vacuum extractor is confounded by the indications for the use of the instrument. Generally, if the vacuum extraction is used for an easy, uncomplicated delivery and not more than three or four episodes of traction are required, there is no hypoxia.

Scalp injuries are moderately common. Abrasions to the scalp and skin occur; these relate to the rotation or moving of the cap on the skin which in turn is associated with a badly placed cap. If the cap is detached suddenly, this too can cause skin damage.

Cephalohaematomata can occur if a skin vein is damaged by chance; more rarely subgaleal haemorrhages have been reported (Robinson & Rossiter 1968). Again, this is probably associated with prolonged and strenuous traction which may be associated with a long and difficult labour.

Intracranial haemorrhage relates to the duration and strength of the pulling of the vacuum extractor. Plauché (1979) recorded a range of intracranial injury up to 8%. The upper end of this came from the more difficult vacuum extractions following the more difficult labours. The neurological and behavioural sequelae of such deliveries have been examined by Leijon (1980). He found that neonatal depression with later lower auditory and visual responses could occur but could often be explained by the abnormal presentations and the long labour, in addition to the long vacuum extraction. Naske et al (1976) found that there was a greater incidence of brain damage in babies born by vacuum cap delivery compared with those delivered spontaneously; there was no difference between those born with a vacuum cap as opposed to those born by forceps. Again it is hard to sort out the propter hoc from the post hoc—was the damage caused by the indication for using a vacuum extractor or its use? Generally, most workers find little adverse effect on neurological or intellectual development.

Campbell et al (1975) found an increased incidence of neonatal jaundice in mature infants born by vacuum extraction compared with those born by forceps. This is rarely a serious problem and light therapy was not often required. Jaundice follows even without apparent bruising of the infant's scalp and the workers assumed this was due to breakdown of blood in the chignon.

In the longer term, rare reports of alopecia have appeared. The author has seen two such children aged over 1 year with a distinct cleancut circle of hair loss which would have corresponded to the position and size of the vacuum cap used at their birth. However, one sees well rounded patches of alopecia occurring spontaneously.

Comparison of vacuum extraction with the use of forceps

Vacuum extraction is simple to use and, generally speaking, can be practised by less skilled people than can forceps delivery. In many parts of the underdeveloped world,

midwives are perfectly competent with vacuum deliveries whereas they have not been appropriately trained to be able to use forceps. The application of forceps requires a greater knowledge of fetal and pelvic anatomy and a greater familiarity with pelvic examinations.

The vacuum extractor occupies less space at the side wall of the pelvis than do the forceps and so does not add to any potential disproportion. When traction is applied with the vacuum extractor, this is a linear pull and the head can follow its own mechanisms in the pelvis for rotation. Using a pair of forceps, the head is gripped in four places and rotation is in the control of the operator. This may be appropriate with the skilled obstetrician who has performed many forceps deliveries but with the less well trained, perhaps nature knows best and the head can be allowed to follow its own course.

The disadvantages of the vacuum extractor compared with forceps are that the equipment is more complex and so more likely to go wrong and that it requires maintenance whereas little can happen to two blades of a pair of forceps. The vacuum extractor is also less portable than forceps.

Vacuum extraction can be performed with the help of little extra pain relief. Often it can be done without any additional analgesia since the application of the cap is not much more painful for the woman than is a vaginal examination. Putting on forceps is a more difficult art, particularly if the head is in mid-cavity. Then, a more extensive regional block is required than for a vacuum extraction. In a study of mothers randomly allocated to forecps delivery or vacuum extraction, Garcia et al (1985) found that women required less analgesia for vacuum extraction but had more worries about their babies because of the jaundice.

Forceps delivery can be done more swiftly than vacuum extraction by most operators, provided the head is in a reasonable position in the pelvis and the cervix is fully dilated. Thus, if the baby shows signs of fetal distress in the second stage of labour—one of the major indications for operative vaginal delivery—forceps are to be preferred. However, the other major indication for accelerated delivery is delay in the second stage; for this, the vacuum extractor is an excellent instrument.

The baby nearly always has a chignon for 24–48 hours after a vacuum extraction and there is a higher prevalence of jaundice. After a forceps delivery, particularly with rotation, there are transient forceps marks on the cheeks.

It is interesting to observe how the spread of any new technique occurs in medicine. There are at first case reports from the enthusiasts; thence the technique is taken up eagerly by those who wish to try innovations. They too usually find it useful and report on it enthusiastically. After this follows a series of reports on the side-effects and complications that have occurred during the first enthusiasm of usage but have not been reported immediately; only after some years does the proper use of the technique stabilize. To some extent usage depends on the phase in the propagation of practice when an operator starts to use equipment. He may join it in the first enthusiasms or later at the complications stage. As the operator then becomes a practical teacher, he advises others what he thinks is right and teaches the wider use of what he believes in.

These mechanisms probably account for the patchy use of the vacuum extractor in the world. Earlier reports, such as by Snoeck in 1960, were that the forceps had been virtually abandoned in his hospital and vacuum extraction had taken over. Similarly, there are many Scandinavian and German hospitals where forceps are rarely used. In a large part of the Middle East where there is influence of teachers from the European area, there is also a relatively low use of forceps and a higher employment of the vacuum extractor. The incidence of operative vaginal deliveries has increased in most countries but in England and the USA these deliveries are still mostly by forceps rather than vacuum extraction.

A few comparative trials have been performed of these instruments. Greis et al (1981) compared vacuum extraction births with those by forceps delivery. Results showed that the forceps deliveries were associated with a threefold increased incidence of birth canal trauma, while anaesthesia requirements and perinatal morbidity were much less than those with vacuum extraction. Schenker & Serr (1967) compared 300 women delivered by vacuum extraction with 300 retrospectively examined forceps deliveries. Maternal complications were halved in the vacuum extraction group while the rate of fetal complications was the same in both groups; the incidence of fetal problems increased considerably when the traction time with the ventouse was longer than 15 minutes and when the cervix was not fully dilated.

A randomized controlled trial was performed in Ports-mouth by Vacca et al (1983) when 304 women requiring operative delivery in the second stage of labour were randomly allocated to vacuum extraction or forceps groups. Maternal trauma, use of analgesia and blood loss at delivery were significantly less after vacuum extraction. The authors found that mild neonatal jaundice was increased in this group; more serious neonatal problems were rare in both the forceps and vacuum extraction groups. With this number of women, statistically significant conclusions could not be drawn but this is an important study and the subject deserves a wider randomized controlled trial.

More recently, Johanson et al (1993) reported a multi-centre randomized controlled trial of 607 women divided into vacuum extraction or forceps assisted delivery. There was less maternal trauma with vacuum extraction. Although there were more with cephalohaemotomas in the vacuum group, the babies had fewer facial injuries. The incidence of retinal haemorrhages was the same but suckling difficulties were more frequent in the forceps group.

Conclusions

When further research has been properly evaluated, it may well be that the vacuum extractor will be able to take its proper place. In the opinion of those who are experienced in its use, the vacuum extractor is probably most appropriate when delivering a woman, particularly multiparous, who has been shown not to have cephalo-pelvic disproportion but who develops delay at the end of the first stage or in the second stage of labour. The vacuum extractor should be used in parallel with forceps rather than in competition. Skills in the management of delivery with both sets of equipment should be gained in training and kept bright by constant repetition in practice.

REFERENCES

Bird G C 1969 Modifications of Malmstrom's vacuum extractor. British Medical Journal 111: 526

Bird G C 1976 The importance of flexion in vacuum extraction delivery. British Journal of Obstetrics and Gynaecology 83: 194–200

Bird G C 1982 The use of the vacuum extractor. Clinical Obstetrics and Gynecology 9: 641–661

Bratt T 1965 Indications for and results of the use of the ventouse. Journal of Obstetrics and Gynaecology of the British Commonwealth 72: 883–888

Campbell N, Harvey D, Norman A P 1975 Increased frequence of neonatal jaundice. British Medical Journal 11: 548–552

Cardoza L D, Gibb D, Studd J W W et al 1982 Predictive value of cervimetric labour patterns in primigravidae. British Journal of Obstetrics and Gynaecology 89: 33–38

Carmody F, Grant A, Somchiwang M 1986 Vacuum extraction: a randomised controlled comparison of the new generation cup with the original Bird cup. Journal of Perinatal Medicine 14: 95–100

Chalmers J A 1971 The ventouse. Year Book Medical Publishers, Chicago, p 116

Chamberlain G 1965 Vacuum extractor—a possible danger. Lancet i: 632

Chenoy R, Johanson R et al 1992 A randomized prospective study comparing delivery with metal and silicone rubber vacuum extraction caps. British Journal of Obstetrics and Gynaecology 99: 360–364

Chiswick M L, James D K 1979 Kielland's forceps: association with neonatal morbidity and mortality. British Medical Journal 1: 7–9

Cohen W R, Friedman E A 1983 Management of labor. University Park Press, Baltimore

Das K 1929 The obstetric forceps: its history and evolution. The Art Press, Calcutta

Davidson A C, Weaver J B, Davies P, Pearson J F 1976 The relation between ease of forceps delivery and speed of cervical dilatation. British Journal of Obstetrics and Gynaecology 83: 279–283

Garcia J, Anderson J, Vacca A, Elbourne D, Grant A, Chalmers I 1985 Views of women about instrumental delivery using vacuum extraction and forceps. Journal of Psychosomatic Obstetrics and Gynaecology 4: 1–9

Giffard W 1734 Cases in midwifery. E Hody, London

Greis J B, Biermanz J, Scommegna A 1981 Comparison of maternal and fetal effects of vacuum extraction with forceps and Caesarean deliveries. Obstetrics and Gynecology 57: 571–577

Hibbard B M 1988 Principles of Obstetrics. Butterworths, London

Johanson R et al 1993 ARCT comparing a vacuum extractor policy with forceps delivery. British Journal of Obstetrics and Gynaecology 100: 524–530

Johnson R W 1769 A new system of midwifery founded on practical observations, London

Kadar N, Romero R 1983 Prognosis for future childbearing after mid-cavity instrumental deliveries in primigravidae. Obstetrics and Gynecology 62: 166

Kielland C 1916 The application of forceps to the unrotated head. Monatsschrift für Geburtshilffe und Gynakologie 43: 48–78

Lancet Leading Article 1974 Symphysiotomy and vacuum extraction. Lancet i: 396–397

Laufe L E 1968 Obstetric forceps. Harper & Row, New York

Leijon I 1980 Neurology and behaviour of the newborn infants delivered by vacuum extraction. Acta Paediatrica Scandinavica 69: 625–631

Levret A 1751 Suite des observations sur les causes et les accidens de plusieurs accouchemens laboreux. Delaguette, Paris

Malmstrom T 1954 Vacuum extraction. Acta Obstetricia et Gynecologica Scandinavica 33 (suppl 4): 3

Malmstrom T 1957 The vacuum extractor. An obstetrical instrument. Acta Obstetricia et Gynecologica Scandinavica 5: 153–156

McFarland L, Raskin M, Darling J, Benedetti 1982 Erb/Duchenne's palsy. Obstetrics and Gynecology 68: 784–788

Naske R V, Poustka F, Presslich J 1976 Zusammenhange zwischen operativer Geburtsbundigung und Zerebralschadigung des Kinder. Wiener Klinische Wochenschrift 88: 319–324

O'Driscoll K, Meagher D 1980 Active management of labour. Saunders, London

O'Neil A G, Skull E, Michael E 1981 A new method of traction for the vacuum cup. Australian and New Zealand Journal of Obstetrics and Gynaecology 21: 24–25

Parry Jones E 1952 Kielland's forceps. Butterworths, London

Parry Jones E 1972 Barton's forceps. Sector, London

Plauché W C 1979 Fetal cranial injuries related to delivery with the Malmstrom vacuum extractor. Obstetrics and Gynecology 53: 750–757

Robinson R J, Rossiter M A 1968 Massive subaponeurotic haemorrhage in babies of African origin. Archives of Disease in Childhood 43: 684–687

Ryden G 1986 Vacuum extraction or forceps? British Medical Journal 292: 75–76

Schenker J C, Serr D M 1967 Comparative study of delivery by vacuum extraction and forceps. American Journal of Obstetrics and Gynecology 98: 32–35

Snoeck J 1960 The vacuum extractor (ventouse)—an alternative to the obstetric forceps. Proceedings of the Royal Society of Medicine 53: 749

Speert H 1958 Obstetric and gynecologic milestones: essays in eponymy. Macmillan, New York

Tarnier E 1877 Description de deux nouveaux forceps. Martinet, Paris

Vacca A, Grant A, Wyatt G, Chalmers I 1983 A comparison of vacuum extraction and forceps delivery. British Journal of Obstetrics and Gynaecology 90: 1107–1112

Vacca A 1992 Handbook of extraction in obstetric practice. Edward Arnold, London, p 63

Willughby P 1972 Observations in midwifery. Edited from the original manuscript by Henry Blenkinsop (1863) with a new introduction by John L. Thornton, S R Publishers, Wakefield

39. Caesarean section*

G. Justus Hofmeyr

Material in this chapter contains contributions from the first edition and we are grateful to the previous author for the work done.

The evolution of Caesarean section during this century as a relatively safe procedure, largely due to improved anaesthetic techniques and antiseptic procedures, has revolutionized obstetric practice. Many vaginal procedures such as internal version, destructive operations and symphysiotomy have become rare or obsolete. The spectre of obstructed labour leading to fetal death and maternal mutilation or death, still prevalent in many parts of the world, has been eliminated for women with access to medical facilities.

In recent years, however, the use of Caesarean section has become increasingly controversial. Uncertainty exists about the relative risks and benefits of the operation (Chamberlain 1993) as the indications are progressively widened, and concern is expressed among health professionals and consumers about its increasing use. Increases have varied considerably between centres and countries (Stephenson et al 1993). A large increase in Caesarean sections in the USA after 1965 appeared to be justified by improved perinatal mortality rates, yet similar perinatal improvements occurred in Dublin with minimal increase in Caesarean sections (Fig. 39.1).

Detailed accounts of the indications for Caesarean section will be found in the chapters dealing with the relevant complications of pregnancy. This chapter will deal in principle with the process of decision making preceding Caesarean section, discuss the indications with an emphasis on those relative indications which may account for differences in Caesarean section rates, and describe the operation itself.

THE DECISION PROCESS PRIOR TO CAESAREAN SECTION

The choice between vaginal and abdominal delivery is often complex, involving several factors:

1. The relative risks to the mother, both physical and emotional, immediate and remote. Despite remarkable improvements in safety, Caesarean section does increase the risk of maternal death, probably by a factor of 2–5. Puerperal complications such as sepsis are increased (see Ch. 43), and Caesarean section may be associated with postnatal emotional morbidity (Boyce & Todd 1992, Hannah et al 1992, Salmon & Drew 1992), and complicates the management of subsequent pregnancies (Enkin 1989). Special attention needs to be given to the potential long-term risks of Caesarean section in women who may not have access to or seek medical care in subsequent pregnancies.
2. The likelihood of successful vaginal delivery. Because the risk to the mother of intrapartum emergency Caesarean section may be as much as twice that of elective Caesarean section, when the likelihood of successful vaginal delivery is small, elective Caesarean section may be a safer option than trial of labour with respect to the immediate risks to the mother (Lilford et al 1990).
3. The relative risks to the fetus. Caesarean section is in general considered a safe option for the fetus. Possible adverse effects such as lack of the preparation for adaptation to extrauterine life which occurs during labour, including the outpouring of catecholamines, and early separation from the mother with reduced chance of successful breastfeeding, are at present poorly understood, but need to be considered.

---

*This chapter is dedicated by the author to the memory of Dr Antony Barker who, in 1971, taught a fourth year medical student posted to the Charles Johnson Memorial Hospital in Zululand to perform Caesarean sections under local infiltration analgesia and encouraged his trembling attempts with the words: 'better a shaky hand than a shaky mind'.

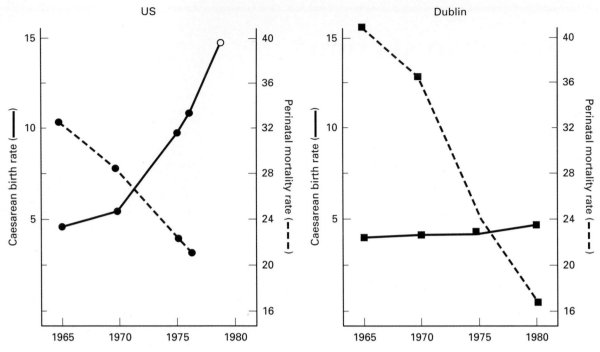

Fig. 39.1 Caesarean birth rates per 100 deliveries (solid lines) and perinatal mortality rates per 1000 deliveries (dashed lines) in the USA, according to Bottoms et al (1980) and in the National Maternity Hospital, Dublin. (See p. 874.)

Iatrogenic prematurity, though greatly reduced for women with access to early pregnancy ultrasound examination, has not been eliminated.

4. The urgency of the need for delivery.
5. When a choice exists between Caesarean section and induction of labour, the ripeness of the uterine cervix may influence the decision.
6. The preference of the mother.

The decision is often complicated by the fact that the interests of the mother and fetus are contradictory, and value-judgements of relative priorities need to be made. Many of the recent increases in Caesarean section rates are accounted for by indications such as suspected fetal distress and breech presentation for which the overall benefit to the fetus is uncertain while the increased risk to the mother is certain.

The following principles may help to give structure to the decision-making process:

1. It is important not to opt for Caesarean section as an easy option on the basis of a vague notion that several features of the pregnancy are suboptimal. Rather evaluate each potential indication critically, and choose Caesarean section only if a clearly defined indication is present. It is often useful to break down the decision into stages: Is this the optimal time for delivery? Is Caesarean section preferable for the mother? Is Caesarean section preferable for the fetus?

2. Valid information about relative risks and benefits in specific circumstances is often scarce. Wherever possible, rely upon objective information such as that from randomized trials rather than subjective impressions; try to assess the risk of the individual woman against a trial population into which she would fit, e.g. First World approaches may not be appropriate in a Third World situation.

3. Every effort should be made to guard against the understandable tendency to choose the option least likely to result in litigation (Savage & Francome 1993) rather than the one most likely to be in the true interests of mother and baby.

4. Some decisions will inevitably in retrospect appear to have been wrong. It is important to acknowledge to ourselves and to the parents that our knowledge is incomplete and we are not able to predict every eventuality. We should not promise perfection. Having made the best possible decision in the light of available information, we and the parents must accept the consequences of the decision.

Indications for Caesarean section

These may be divided into maternal, fetal and combined indications. Many are relative or controversial. Indications which account for large differences in Caesarean section rates between centres with differing policies will be discussed in more detail.

Maternal indications

Maternal indications include situations in which prompt delivery is needed to safeguard the mother's health, vaginal delivery is impossible or contraindicated, or labour is contraindicated:

Life-threatening uterine haemorrhage Whatever the cause of the haemorrhage, prompt delivery may be needed to limit blood loss.

Eclampsia or imminent eclampsia Caesarean section may be needed unless rapid vaginal delivery is feasible.

Previous classical Caesarean section Classical Caesarean section must be followed by Caesarean section in subsequent pregnancies, preferably before the onset of labour, because of the relatively high risk and serious nature of upper uterine segment scar dehiscences. In a recent UK survey, 95% of consultants responded that they would not allow trial of scar following a classical Caesarean section (Roberts et al 1994). Whether midline lower segment incisions which encroach on the upper segment, and transverse incisions which strictly are placed in the upper segment because of a poorly formed lower segment should be managed as classical incisions is not clear.

Previous lower segment Caesarean section Repeat Caesarean section is a major contributor to Caesarean section incidences (Yudkin & Redman 1986). Attempts to predict successful delivery after Caesarean section and the likelihood of scar dehiscence on the basis of the indication for the previous operation, the number of previous Caesarean sections, and assessment of pelvic size (Krishnamurthy 1991) have been unsuccessful (Enkin 1989, Hofmeyr 1989). For example, previous Caesarean section for failure to progress in labour or cephalopelvic disproportion is associated with an only slightly lower rate of successful vaginal delivery than when the previous Caesarean section was for other indications. Interestingly the risk of scar dehiscence is considerably lower, probably because the original uterine incision was usually placed in a well-formed lower segment following prolonged labour (Enkin 1989, Hofmeyr 1989). The reported results for trials of labour following more than one Caesarean section are similar to those reported for one previous Caesarean section.

Overall, scar dehiscence occurs unpredictably in 0.5–2% of cases allowed a trial of labour. Of greater importance than the incidence is the fact that in a maternity unit with ready recourse to Caesarean section, these dehiscences are seldom associated with serious sequelae for mother or infant. The relative risks and benefits of elective repeat Caesarean section compared with trial of labour in women without current indications for Caesarean section have not been determined by randomized studies. The evidence from prospective cohort studies and decision analysis studies, though obviously subject to bias, are in favour of trial of labour (Enkin 1989). Maternal and fetal condition and the progress of labour should be monitored closely, and prompt Caesarean section performed if deterioration of any of these parameters occurs.

Uterine rupture This will vary in severity from dehiscence of a uterine scar with a live fetus within the uterine cavity and minimal bleeding, to expulsion of the fetus and placenta into the peritoneal cavity, particularly in the case of a previously unscarred uterus. In the latter circumstance, hysterectomy is often required.

Placenta praevia Major placenta praevia is an absolute indication for Caesarean section. The place of Caesarean section for minor placenta praevia is controversial.

Pelvic space-occupying lesions These include entrapped ovarian tumours and low-lying uterine fibromyomas.

Gross pelvic contraction The use of X-ray pelvimetry to predict cephalopelvic disproportion has been shown to be insufficiently accurate to be useful (Hofmeyr 1989). This is not surprising as pelvic size is only one of several factors determining successful delivery. In all but the most extreme cases of pelvic contracture, the presence or absence of cephalopelvic disproportion should be diagnosed by trial of labour using a partogram. Imaging pelvimetry by X-ray or CT scan should be reserved for cases in which specific pelvic inadequacy is suspected.

Previous surgical correction of urinary incontinence Vaginal delivery is considered to constitute a risk to the integrity of such repairs.

Extrauterine pregnancy This is a rare and surprisingly difficult condition to diagnose. Even ultrasound examination may be misleading, as omentum stretched over the gestational sac may have the appearance of uterine wall. Suspect extrauterine pregnancy if the fetal lie is bizarre and if attempts at induction of labour are unsuccessful. Lateral abdominal X-ray typically shows fetal parts overlying the mother's spine. The fetus is delivered by laparotomy. The placenta is often attached to bowel and the broad ligament, and attempted removal may cause major blood loss. If removal of the placenta does not appear straightforward, ligature and cut the cord at the placental insertion, and leave the placenta in situ.

Cervical carcinoma Vaginal delivery is considered to constitute a risk for haemorrhage or dissemination of invasive cervical carcinoma. Classical Caesarean section has been recommended, followed by radical hysterectomy if appropriate. Premalignant conditions of the cervix tend to regress after vaginal delivery and are not an indication for Caesarean section.

Serious medical illness In cases of serious maternal compromise such as severe cardiac, respiratory, musculoskeletal or neurological illness, the relative risks of labour compared with surgery need to be weighed up in the light of the specific circumstances of each case.

Bearing-down efforts contraindicated In situations such as severe hypertension or cerebral aneurysm, it is usually preferable to avoid bearing-down efforts by the use of effective regional analgesia and assisted delivery rather than Caesarean section.

Maternal preference The reason for Caesarean section request may vary from a morbid fear of labour to simple convenience. It may be argued that the mother has the right to informed choice of the method of delivery, including the right to accept the increased risks to herself of Caesarean section. Labour and vaginal delivery may have benefits for the fetus, and what some may consider an unnecessary Caesarean section may be seen as an infringement of the rights of the fetus, particularly when Caesarean section is requested before full term for convenience. In the absence of information from clinical trials on which to base decisions, the author's practice is to strongly discourage Caesarean section by choice, explaining the increased risk to the mother and possible adverse effects for the fetus, but having done so to respect the mother's right to an informed choice, provided that the possibility of iatrogenic prematurity is excluded. This question is discussed further by Chamberlain (1993).

Fetal indications

Fetal indications for Caesarean section include the need for prompt delivery, the need to avoid labour and the need to avoid vaginal delivery:

Suspected fetal distress Randomized trials of electronic fetal heart rate (FHR) monitoring during labour compared with intermittent auscultation have shown a doubling of Caesarean sections for fetal distress when FHR monitoring was complemented by selective fetal blood sampling, and a four times increase when it was not (Grant 1989, Neilson 1993). The only discernible improvement in neonatal outcome was a reduction in neonatal convulsions in certain trials (MacDanold et al 1985). These occurred only in labours which were prolonged or stimulated with oxytocics, and the long-term outcomes were good. Thus there is no evidence that electronic FHR monitoring during uncomplicated labour improves neonatal outcome. There is also little or no evidence that the large increase in Caesarean sections for suspected fetal distress in recent years has had any effect on the incidence of cerebral palsy (Stanley & Blair 1991). In a randomized comparison, the rate of Caesarean section for fetal distress in labours with FHR monitoring alone was twice that which occurred when FHR monitoring was supplemented with fetal electrocardiogram (ECG) waveform analysis (Westgate et al 1992).

FHR monitoring is inherently imprecise, particularly with respect to the overdiagnosis of fetal distress. Before labour, non-reactive FHR patterns may be associated with fetal distress, but more often are not. During labour, early and variable FHR decelerations usually reflect an appropriate vagal response to fetal head compression or umbilical cord compression. Even late decelerations may reflect an appropriate fetal response to no more than mild hypoxia during uterine contractions. Thus many FHR patterns create diagnostic uncertainty, and the understandable tendency is to expedite delivery in case fetal distress is indeed present.

The rate of Caesarean sections not really needed for suspected fetal distress during labour may be reduced by several methods: fetal scalp blood pH measurement, or newer techniques such as fetal ECG waveform analysis may be used to confirm the diagnosis. Intrauterine resuscitation may be used. The mother is placed in the lateral position, oxygen is administered by facemask, and excessive uterine contractions are inhibited by reducing oxytocic administration or administering a beta-adrenergic agent. Early or variable decelerations can be abolished in the majority of cases by saline amnioinfusion, with significant reduction in the rate of Caesarean section (Hofmeyr 1992a). Meconium staining of the amniotic fluid is sometimes associated with fetal distress, but the association is too weak to justify Caesarean section.

Presentation or prolapse of the umbilical cord Caesarean section is needed unless prompt vaginal delivery is feasible, or the baby is dead. Palpation of the cord for pulsation is an unreliable indicator of whether the fetus is alive, and may aggravate spasm of the cord vessels. Auscultate for the fetal heart beat, and confirm with Doppler detection or ultrasound if unsure. Methods described to reduce compression of the cord between the presenting part and the pelvis while preparing for Caesarean section include the Sims' or knee–elbow position, filling the bladder with 500 ml normal saline, stopping oxytocic administration, tocolysis and digital elevation of the presenting part per vaginam. With appropriate management, it is unusual for fetal death to occur after the diagnosis has been made.

Brow or face presentation For brow presentation, a short trial of labour is worthwhile as delivery may occasionally occur when the baby is small, the pelvis is unusually large, or conversion to vertex or mento-anterior face presentation occurs during labour. In most cases Caesarean section is needed. Mento-posterior face presentation can deliver vaginally only if long anterior rotation takes place.

Transverse or oblique lie Transverse or oblique lie may be corrected in the majority of cases by external version during labour or immediately prior to the induction of labour, provided that the membranes are intact (Hofmeyr 1993). For persistent non-longitudinal lie in labour there is no option other than Caesarean section.

Breech presentation There is convincing evidence that the chance of breech presentation at delivery and Caesarean section may be reduced by external cephalic version at term (Hofmeyr 1991, 1993).

The method of delivery for persistent breech presentation

remains problematical. Neonatal outcome is worse after breech than cephalic delivery, but this discrepancy may be due to pre-existing fetal problems which have resulted in breech presentation rather than harm during breech delivery (Hytten 1982). Randomized trials of vaginal versus Caesarean delivery for frank (Collea et al 1980) and non-frank (Gimovsky et al 1983) breech presentations have failed to show any difference in perinatal outcome. However, large retrospective studies have suggested a poorer perinatal outcome following vaginal rather than abdominal breech delivery, and the authors have argued in favour of routine Caesarean section for breech presentation at term (Thorpe-Beeston et al 1992). The policy in our department is to allow vaginal delivery for breech presentation provided that the fetus is estimated to weigh between 1500 and 3750 g, is a frank or complete breech presentation (the combined diameters of thighs and trunk are likely to exceed those of the aftercoming head), does not have an extended neck or cord completely encircling the neck on ultrasound examination, is well grown and without evidence of distress, and most importantly that labour progresses favourably as assessed with the partogram. The breech should descend readily into the pelvis, reaching the level of the ischial spines by the time that the cervix is 6 cm dilated, and the pelvic floor when the cervix is fully dilated.

The policy of routine Caesarean section for breech presentation increases the risk of delivery for the mother without evidence of improved neonatal outcome. In the long term, such a policy results in self-perpetuating inexperience when the need for emergency breech delivery arises unavoidably.

Several recent reports have appeared of successful management of obstruction to delivery of the aftercoming head of the breech by tocolysis, replacement of the infant in the uterus and Caesarean section (Hofmeyr 1992b). The author prefers to use symphysiotomy and forceps delivery of the aftercoming head. Rapid delivery can be effected provided that a symphysiotomy set is routinely kept at hand during breech deliveries.

Prematurity   The use of Caesarean section for breech presentations estimated to weigh below 1500 g is controversial (Crowley & Hawkins 1980), particularly when viability is uncertain. Evidence from randomized trials to guide management is lacking. In a recent survey of consultants in England and Wales, 76% of respondents reported routinely using Caesarean section for uncomplicated preterm breech delivery, 35% considered that there is sufficient evidence to support this policy, and overall 71% reported that their management was affected by medicolegal considerations (Penn & Steer 1991). Preterm vertex delivery is not an indication for Caesarean section.

Multiple pregnancy   Caesarean section is indicated in multiple pregnancy when adverse factors are present such as extreme prematurity (estimated fetal weight below 1500 g), discordant fetal growth, single amniotic sac, conjoined twins and higher order multiple pregnancies than twins.

Macrosomia   It has been suggested that the risk of shoulder dystocia can be reduced by the use of elective Caesarean section when the fetus is estimated to weigh more than 4500 g, or in diabetic women more than 4000 g. Such a policy would however result in an unacceptably high rate of Caesarean sections, and most cases of shoulder dystocia would be missed (Hofmeyr 1992b). The only feasible way of addressing the problem of shoulder dystocia is by ensuring that all birth attendants are skilled in its management, particularly the early use of the McRobert's manoeuvre. Several reports have recently appeared, mainly in the North American literature, of successful management of absolute shoulder dystocia by the Zavanelli manoeuvre—replacement of the head into the uterus using tocolysis, and Caesarean section (Hofmeyr 1992b).

Fetal anomaly   Fetal anomaly is not an indication for Caesarean section unless the nature of the anomaly is such that vaginal delivery may cause fetal injury or impair the chance of surgical correction. A difficult ethical dilemma is gross hydrocephaly. The choice lies between Caesarean section with a large uterine incision which may have to be a classical incision, or cephalocentesis to permit vaginal delivery.

Fetal thrombocytopenia   Autoimmune thrombocytopenia is associated with an unpredictable risk of fetal thrombocytopenia. Suggested management policies include routine Caesarean section or selective Caesarean section when the fetal platelet count from scalp blood sampling or cordocentesis is below 25 000 per ml.

Infections which may be acquired during delivery   Active genital herpes simplex infection carries a significant risk of serious neonatal infection which may be reduced by Caesarean section if performed before rupture of the membranes. Group B haemolytic streptococcal infection of the vagina is common (Van Oppen & Feldman 1993) and the incidence of serious neonatal infection is considered too low to justify Caesarean section. Six-hourly douching with chlorhexidine in water during labour may reduce the risk of infection. Similarly, the risk of neonatal laryngeal papillomas is considered too small to justify Caesarean section for maternal human papillomavirus infection.

The possibility that Caesarean section may reduce the risk of vertical infection with hepatitis virus or human immunodeficiency virus has not been established (European Collaborative Study 1992). The avoidance of penetrating scalp electrodes and scalp blood sampling is recommended.

Fetomaternal indications

Fetomaternal indications for Caesarean section are related to disproportion.

Arrested progress in labour The term cephalo-pelvic disproportion is best avoided as an indication for Caesarean section, for two reasons. First, it is often difficult to distinguish between true cephalopelvic disproportion and inefficient uterine action as the cause of arrested progress in labour. Secondly, the term cephalo-pelvic disproportion suggests an absolute obstruction, and may bias the mother and caregiver against trial of vaginal delivery in a subsequent pregnancy as discussed in 'Previous lower segment Caesarean section' above. In a recent study, Caesarean section for fetal distress as well as for dystocia was significantly more frequent in women randomly allocated to receive epidural analgesia during labour (Thorp et al 1993).

How to avoid unnecessary Caesarean sections

In summary, the rate of Caesarean sections may be reduced by:

1. Operating only when a clear-cut indication exists.
2. Performing external cephalic version at term for breech presentation and prior to induction or in early labour for transverse or oblique lie.
3. Having a policy of vaginal breech delivery in selected cases.
4. Allowing carefully monitored trial of previous Caesarean section scar whenever no clear contraindication exists.
5. Diagnosing cephalopelvic disproportion only after adequate trial of labour with partographic monitoring, ruptured membranes and, when indicated, oxytocin stimulation and intrauterine pressure monitoring.
6. Avoiding electronic FHR monitoring in uncomplicated labours.
7. Confirming suspected fetal distress with fetal blood sampling or other diagnostic measures.
8. Managing suspected fetal distress initially with intrauterine resuscitative measures.
9. Managing variable or early FHR decelerations with amnioinfusion.
10. Reducing the use of epidural analgesia during labour.

THE CAESAREAN SECTION OPERATION

Caesarean sections were performed in several ancient civilizations, usually when the mother was moribund or dead. Isolated reports of maternal survival have appeared since the 16th century. Of historical interest was a successful Caesarean section in 1826 by Dr James Barry, the British Army Medical Officer at the Cape of Good Hope (Sandler 1967). However, up to the last quarter of the 19th century, maternal mortality was excessively high. In 1878 Lapage reported that no women operated upon in Paris between 1799 and 1877 survived. The uterine wound was usually left unsutured. In 1876 Porro described a technique of amputating the uterine body and removing the ovaries, which reduced the maternal mortality. In 1882 Sanger described a satisfactory technique of suturing the classical uterine incision, using two rows of sutures. This, together with the introduction of general anaesthesia and antiseptic techniques, contributed to declining maternal mortality. The first recorded transverse lower uterine segment Caesarean section (TLUSCS) has been credited to F.A. Kehrer in 1882. The lower segment operation was championed in the UK by Munro Kerr, who first used it in 1911.

Many variations of the Caesarean section operation have been described, and each surgeon eventually settles on a technique which suits him- or herself. The description which follows includes practical hints and techniques which the author has found useful, in the knowledge that many effective alternatives exist.

Fetal maturity

For non-urgent Caesarean sections, fetal maturity should be confirmed. If doubt exists, particularly if ultrasound assessment of gestational age has not been performed before 20 weeks, it is preferable to await the spontaneous onset of labour. Ultrasound has largely replaced the confirmation of fetal lung maturity by amniocentesis using the alcohol shake test or measurement of the lecithin-sphingomyelin ratio or phosphatidyl glycerol level.

In general, planning elective Caesarean section to be performed when labour commences has the advantages of reducing the risk of iatrogenic immaturity, allowing time for potentially self-correcting indications such as fetal malpresentation to resolve, and ensuring a well-formed lower uterine segment with possible reduction of the risk of dehiscence in subsequent pregnancies. The disadvantage is the need to operate at an unscheduled time.

Preoperative counselling

Counsel the parents carefully about the details and implications of the operation. Many women regard giving birth as an important life event and view Caesarean section as a personal failure. Stress the positive aspects of the woman's part in the pregnancy and subsequent care of her child. Discuss anaesthetic options and find out whether the parents have any special requests regarding the birth. Enquire about the mother's attitude to donor blood transfusion. The option of sterilization should have been discussed routinely during the antenatal period. If not, it should be made clear that a last-minute decision is not essential, as sterilization can be performed at a later date. If uncertainty exists the decision should be postponed.

Written consent to the operation is signed by the mother. Informed consent implies the discussion of possible complications of the surgery such as haemorrhage requiring hysterectomy, and anaesthetic complications. A difficult issue is the problem of anxiety created by the detailed description of potential complications as part of the informed consent process.

Preparation for surgery

The woman's fitness for surgery should be ascertained, including appropriate special investigations. If undue haemorrhage is anticipated, donor blood should be available in the operating theatre.

Neither starvation nor any of several medications commonly used is effective in achieving an empty, non-acidic stomach during pregnancy (Johnson et al 1989). Particulate antacids are probably contraindicated. The use of antacids or gastroprokinetic agents should not create a false sense of security. The risk of gastric content aspiration should be minimized by the application of effective cricoid pressure by a competent assistant from the time of induction of general anaesthesia until the correct placement of the endotracheal tube has been confirmed and the cuff inflated.

Pubic hair shaving causes skin abrasion which may promote infection. Non-abrasive clipping of pubic hair in the proposed line of incision is preferable. Effective emptying of the urinary bladder should be ensured prior to surgery, usually by means of an indwelling urinary catheter.

The paediatrician should be advised of any anticipated neonatal problem.

Prophylactic antibiotics and heparin

There is unequivocal evidence from a large number of randomized trials that the use of prophylactic antibiotics is associated with a clinically important reduction in infectious morbidity after both emergency and elective Caesarean section (Smaill 1993). The added benefit of prophylactic antibiotic therapy for longer than 1 day is uncertain. Details of antibiotic prophylaxis are given in Chapter 43 on puerperal sepsis.

The use of prophylactic low-dose heparin in other surgical disciplines has been shown to reduce the risk of pulmonary embolism (Collins et al 1988). Its use does not appear to be associated with increased blood loss at Caesarean section (Hill et al 1988). The evidence available is thus in favour of the use of heparin prophylaxis, probably routinely but certainly for those with risk factors. Calcium heparin may be used, 5000 units subcutaneously 8 hourly, commencing 2 hours before the operation (see Ch. 44).

Choice of anaesthesia

General anaesthesia carries certain specific risks, particularly gastric content aspiration and failed intubation. Attempts to minimize the depressant effect of anaesthetic agents on the neonate have resulted in the risk of the mother being paralysed but aware of the operation in the early stages. Regional and general anaesthesia for Caesarean section are considered in Chapter 32.

Preparation in theatre

Ensure that any drugs which may be needed, such as oxytocin, ergometrine, prostaglandin F2 alpha and a beta-adrenergic agent such as hexoprenaline (Ipradol) are available in theatre. Position the mother on the table with 15 degrees of left lateral tilt. There is clear evidence that the fetal condition is improved by this simple manoeuvre (Pearson & Rees 1989). The use of 5 degrees of reverse Trendellenburg's position has been shown to reduce the incidence of venous air emboli diagnosed with precordial Doppler monitoring. Oxygen should be administered to the mother at 100% concentration until the delivery of the infant.

The author uses the mnemonic SHIP as a final checklist before scrubbing up:

1. Has the question of Sterilization been finalized?
2. Is the fetal Heart still audible? Particularly when Caesarean section is performed for fetal distress, fetal death may occur before the operation is commenced.
3. Is the Indication still valid? For example, if the Caesarean section is for failure to progress in labour, a vaginal examination should be performed as unexpected progress may have taken place; breech presentation should be reconfirmed by palpation as spontaneous version may occur even during labour.
4. Palpate the Position of the fetus. It is important to know the orientation of the occiput so that it can be rotated anteriorly during delivery.

When regional analgesia is used, ask the mother whether she wishes to hold and put the baby to breast immediately after delivery, and arrange her gown and sterile drapes appropriately.

The abdominal incision

Transverse incisions

Compared with vertical incisions, the Pfannenstiel (low transverse) skin incision is somewhat slower to perform, more liable to haematoma formation and cannot easily be enlarged if extended access is required. These limitations are generally accepted in view of its excellent cosmetic and functional results. The first two drawbacks may be reduced by use of the Cohen incision (described in Pearsen & Rees 1989).

Vertical incisions

If operative complications such as extensive intra-abdominal adhesions or excessive haemorrhage are anticipated, a midline or paramedian incision is preferable. For classical Caesarean sections, a paramedian incision is preferable because of the ease of extension above the umbilicus.

The parietal peritoneum

Open the parietal peritoneum as high up as possible, taking care not to injure an unexpectedly high bladder, particularly in cases of obstructed labour or previous Caesarean section.

Various techniques of extraperitoneal approach to the uterus (Wallace et al 1984) or of suturing parietal to visceral peritoneum, thus closing off the peritoneal cavity before opening the uterus, have been described. These methods designed to reduce the spread of infection to the peritoneal cavity are seldom used in current obstetric practice.

Uterine incisions

The transverse lower uterine segment incision

Ensure that the lower segment is wide enough to allow an adequate transverse incision to accommodate the baby without lateral extension into the uterine vessels. Ensure that a fetal pole is present in or can be made to enter the lower segment, failing which a constriction between the upper and lower uterine segments may prevent the presenting part being brought down to a lower segment incision. If either of the above conditions is not met, use a midline incision. Correct any rotation of the uterus. Open the loosely adherent visceral peritoneum covering the lower uterine segment transversely, separate the peritoneum digitally from the lower segment, and displace it inferiorly, together with the bladder, using a Doyen's retractor.

Incise the myometrium of the lower uterine segment with a scalpel transversely in the midline, 1–2 cm below the junction with the upper segment, using gentle strokes of the scalpel. If membranes are intact and liquor volume normal, the shiny fetal membranes are seen to bulge outward. If possible, complete the myometrial incision without rupturing the membranes. Extend the incision

laterally with slight upward curvature, using curved scissors. Protect the baby with a finger deep to the blade of the scissors, and cut first towards and then away from yourself. Alternatively use the index finger of each hand to tear the myometrium laterally. Once the membranes rupture, the uterus begins to contract down, and the baby should be delivered without undue delay. Remove the Doyen's retractor before delivering the baby.

The midline (De Lee) lower uterine segment incision

Open the visceral peritoneum transversely as for the transverse incision, and reflect the bladder off the lower segment down to the level of the cervix. Incise the uterus vertically in the midline just below the upper segment. Insert the index finger of the left hand down the lower segment in the midline, extra-amniotically if the membranes remain intact, until the cervix is identified. Open the lower segment vertically with dissecting scissors as far as a point 2 cm above the identified cervix. If the incision is still not long enough, extend it upwards as far as necessary into the upper uterine segment. For the purposes of subsequent pregnancies, an incision which encroaches significantly on the upper segment should be regarded as at increased risk of dehiscence (Hauth et al 1992).

Closure of the uterus may be by means of two layers of continuous sutures. The author prefers a single-layer interrupted suture closure as for the transverse incision. It is important to ensure that the first suture secures the lowest extent of the incision, using the technique described below for securing the lateral angles of the transverse incision.

The classical uterine incision

If the placenta is anterior, map its borders with ultrasound preoperatively, as described for a lower segment incision with placenta praevia. Ensure adequate access to the upper uterine segment by means of a paramedian abdominal incision. Correct any rotation of the uterus and incise the upper segment vertically in the midline, attempting to avoid rupturing the membranes. Extend the incision sufficiently for delivery of the fetus, using a scalpel or large pair of scissors. Separate any overlying placenta in the direction of its nearest margin. Deliver the fetus by the legs or head, whichever presents, taking care not to allow an arm to prolapse. Manage the third stage of labour as described below.

A feature of the classical incision is marked retraction of the superficial layers of the myometrium, which may be difficult to approximate. Most texts describe two or more layers of interrupted or continuous sutures, sometimes with a series of full thickness tension sutures as well.

Delivery of the baby

When using the transverse lower segment incision, careless technique for delivery of the head is a common cause of tearing of the lower uterine segment. To avoid this it is essential to elevate the position of the head in the uterus to above the level of the uterine incision and to rotate the occiput anteriorly before any attempt is made to deliver the head through the uterine incision. If operating from the patient's right side, insert four fingers of the left hand between the lower uterine segment and the fetal head. Gently elevate the head from the mother's pelvis, taking care to pull upwards with the whole arm rather than using a levering movement of the wrist, which may cause tearing of the lower uterine segment. Resistance to elevation of the head is often the result of contraction of the uterus about the fetus, particularly in the presence of obstructed labour or ruptured membranes. Avoid the use of force. The resistance is usually easily overcome by intravenous administration of a beta-adrenergic agent. Occasionally a deeply engaged head may need to be disengaged by means of a vaginal examination by an assistant.

As the head is elevated, lift the fingers nearest the fetal occiput ahead of the other fingers, thus rotating the occiput anteriorly. Once the head is above the level of the uterine incision and the occiput anterior, use four fingertips of the right hand, palm upward, to displace the lower edge of the uterine incision posteriorly, then remove the left hand to apply fundal pressure while guiding the head through the incision with the fingertips of the right hand, which remain outside the uterus. The uterine incision is thus minimally distended by the head alone in a well-flexed occipito-anterior position. If meconium is present, use suction on the baby's airways immediately. Continue fundal pressure and carefully guide the shoulders through the uterine incision. If regional analgesia is being used, dry and hand the baby to the mother as soon as possible and put to the breast if requested, care being taken to avoid cooling.

Some surgeons prefer to use curved obstetric forceps to deliver the head, and the use of the soft vacuum extractor cup has also been described.

Delivery for malpresentation

If one foot or both feet are presenting, take a firm hold preferably of the posterior foot, if that cannot be done, grasp both feet, and gently extract the leg or legs followed by the breech. Make quite sure that a hand is not delivered in error. For frank breech presentation, use the technique described above for cephalic presentation. For transverse lie, correction to a longitudinal lie may be possible before opening the uterus. If not, insert a hand after opening the uterus and bring either the head or more likely one or both feet, whichever is most accessible, down to the incision and proceed as described already. Tocolysis is advisable if any manipulation of the fetal position is required.

When delivering the aftercoming head of a breech, it is important to maintain flexion of the head using the Mauriceau–Smellie–Veit manoeuvre or obstetric forceps.

Placenta praevia

If the diagnosis is at all in doubt, confirm by careful vaginal examination under anaesthesia immediately prior to surgery. Careful preoperative localization of the placental margin with ultrasound is helpful in planning the approach to the uterine cavity. A classical incision is seldom justified.

If the placenta covers the lower uterine segment anteriorly, the uterine wall will be very vascular and the delivery should be completed quickly and efficiently to minimize blood loss. Keeping in mind the relationship of the nearest placental margin to the proposed incision, open the myometrium as usual without incising the placenta. Separate the placenta from the uterine wall in the direction of the nearest margin, move the placental edge out of the way, and deliver the baby. Occasionally it may be necessary to cut through the placenta to reach the baby. Clamp the umbilical cord immediately in case fetal placental vessels have been divided.

Place as many broad Green-Armytage haemostatic clamps around the uterine wound edge as needed to obtain haemostasis. After removal of the placenta, take particular care to ensure that the lower segment placental site is not bleeding actively, undersewing bleeding points if necessary, before closing the uterus.

The use of tocolysis during Caesarean section

Contraction of the uterus, either following prolonged labour or in response to the uterine incision and escape of liquor, may make the delivery of the baby difficult and result in unnecessary trauma to the baby, particularly if premature, and the uterus. Effective relaxation of the uterus can be achieved within 30 seconds by administering a beta-adrenergic agent such as hexoprenaline (Ipradol) 5 µg intravenously. An alternative is to use halothane, which causes uterine relaxation in high doses. Over the past 15 years the author has developed the following approach:

1. Always have a beta-adrenergic agent available in theatre.
2. For significant prematurity, malpresentation and multiple pregnancy, give the tocolytic routinely 1 minute before incising the myometrium.
3. For advanced or prolonged labour, ask the

anaesthetist to have the tocolytic drawn up and ready to administer. If the baby's head cannot be lifted from the pelvis with ease, administer the tocolytic, wait 30 seconds, then proceed with the delivery.

4. For any unanticipated difficulty with delivery, consider prompt tocolysis.

The possibility that tocolysis may inhibit third-stage contraction of the uterus has not been systematically studied. In practice the author has not been aware of any noticeable difference in the response of the uterus to oxytocin infusion following tocolysis in the dosage described.

Glyceryl trinitrate sublingual spray has also been described as an effective tocolytic to facilitate intrauterine manipulations during delivery (Greenspoon & Kovacic 1991).

Delivery of the placenta and membranes

Once the anterior shoulder has been delivered, administer oxytocin by slow intravenous injection or infusion. Avoid routine manual removal of the placenta, which is associated with an increased risk of postoperative endometritis (McCurdy et al 1992) and increased blood loss. While awaiting placental separation, secure the midpoint of the lower edge of the uterine incision with a broad haemostatic Green-Armytage forceps. Reinsert the Doyen's retractor only after identifying the lower edge of the uterine incision, as the retractor may cover it and the posterior uterine wall be mistaken for the wound edge. Control any actively bleeding points of the uterine wound with similar forceps.

Deliver the placenta and membranes with cord traction once the uterus has contracted firmly. Remove and replace any forceps in place on the uterine wound edge as the membranes are peeled off the underlying uterine wall. Explore the uterine cavity manually to exclude retained placental tissue. If labour had not commenced, wear an extra glove on the left hand which can be discarded once the cervix has digitally been checked to be sufficiently dilated to allow free drainage of blood.

Excessive haemorrhage

If bleeding from the uterine cavity is excessive, avoid closing the uterus before the bleeding has been controlled, usually by undersewing bleeding points with figure-of-eight 2/0 chromic catgut sutures. Control bleeding from severed branches of the uterine artery at the angles of the incision by means of full thickness myometrial sutures placed parallel to and above and below the incision. If uterine contraction is inadequate, administer ergometrine and commence an infusion of oxytocin 20 units in 1000 ml normal saline. If this is not effective, consider administering prostaglandin F2 alpha 1 mg diluted to 10 ml slowly directly into the myometrium taking care to avoid intravascular injection, which would cause serious maternal complications. If bleeding continues, ligate one or both internal ileac arteries close to the bifurcations of the common ileac arteries, after displacing the ureters medially (van Gelderen 1975). If all else fails, do not delay in resorting to hysterectomy as a life-saving procedure.

Closure of the transverse lower uterine incision

Externalization of the uterus reduces blood loss somewhat, but increases the risk of postoperative endometritis and causes discomfort, nausea and vomiting during operation with regional analgesia. Movement of the Doyen's retractor from side to side by the assistant, taking care not to damage the bladder, provides adequate exposure for closure of the non-exteriorized uterus.

Most texts describe closure with two layers of continuous sutures. Secure both angles of the incision with full thickness sutures. The first continuous layer should include the inner two-thirds of the myometrium and exclude the decidua. The outer layer should invert the wound edges. A recent randomized trial found a single layer of continuous locking sutures to be quicker and require fewer haemostatic sutures than a double layer (Hauth et al 1992).

The author uses a single layer of interrupted figure-of-eight sutures. To obtain apposition of the full thickness of myometrium including the outer edges, the sutures (excluding the angle sutures) are placed obliquely through the myometrium and crossed inside the uterus. Number 1 chromic catgut is preferred to polyglycolic acid suture material because of its greater elasticity and lesser tendency to cut through tissues.

Sterilization

Sterilization at the time of Caesarean section may be associated with an increased failure rate. A possible explanation is that during pregnancy the Fallopian tubes are oedematous and more friable. The use of clips or ligation techniques developed for use in the non-pregnant state may cut into the tube with proximal sinus formation. In an attempt to minimize this risk, the author uses a ligation and separation technique.

Pass 0 chromic catgut through a clear area in the mesosalpinx. Ligate the tube twice medially and once laterally, and divide it about 1.5 cm from the uterus between the ligatures, ensuring that the medial stump is able to reach the uterine insertion of the round ligament without tension. Hold the tip of each stump with artery forceps. Pass another 0 chromic catgut suture through the base of the round ligament from front to back, taking about two-thirds of the thickness of the ligament. Loop the suture around the medial stump of the tube from below to above and pass it back through the round ligament from back to front, 0.5 cm lateral to the first passage. Pull the suture ends to tuck the medial stump of the tube in behind the round ligament. Pass the lateral stump of the tube in front of the round ligament between the two ends of the suture and tie the suture over it.

Abdominal closure

Check the adnexa and major abdominal organs for disease before closure. When using regional analgesia, the questionable benefit of palpating upper abdominal organs in asymptomatic women needs to be weighed against the discomfort this may cause. Ensure good haemostasis. If any doubt exists about the effectiveness of haemostasis, drain the relevant area.

Doubt has been cast on the value of peritoneal closure, as spontaneous reperitonization has been shown to occur when the peritoneum is left unsutured. Secure closure of the sheath is important. If a continuous suture is used, tie a knot after the first and again after the second stitch to avoid the possibility of unravelling as tension is placed on the continuous suture. Number 1 polyglycolic acid is usually adequate, but a non-absorbable suture such as nylon should be used for vertical abdominal incisions in the presence of obesity or maternal conditions associated with poor wound healing. Nylon 2/0 mattress sutures may be used for the skin, or continuous subcuticular for transverse incisions. The author infiltrates the subcutaneous tissues with 0.5% bupivacaine to reduce postoperative pain, although the effectiveness of this technique has been questioned.

Postoperative care

Adequate analgesia and routine observations including vaginal blood loss should be ensured. Women who have undergone Caesarean section need extra help and encouragement to manage their babies and establish breastfeeding, and hospital routines should be established which minimize the separation of mothers and babies except at the mother's request. Early mobilization of the mother should be actively encouraged.

During a straightforward Caesarean section the bowel is scarcely exposed, particularly if the uterus is not externalized, and paralytic ileus is rarely a problem. The author's policy is therefore not to limit oral fluids after Caesarean section unless there is a particular reason to do so. Once oral fluids are being well tolerated and the woman's condition is stable, the intravenous infusion is discontinued and food gradually introduced. On one occasion a woman being operated upon with regional analgesia who was desperately thirsty was given a cup of tea during closure of the abdominal wall with no ill effect and much enjoyment. A recent small study has shown no significant difference in gastrointestinal function between women allowed to drink immediately postoperatively and those starved for 24 hours (Guedj et al 1991).

Postoperative care should include careful temperature monitoring, as puerperal sepsis is considerably more common following Caesarean section than following vaginal delivery (see Ch. 43).

CONCLUSION

Caesarean section has become a prominent feature of obstetric practice. Careful attention must be paid to the indications for the operation, anaesthetic and operative technique, and the special needs of women delivered with this method.

Acknowledgements

Caesarean section is an operation learned by apprenticeship. I acknowledge my teachers, particularly Derek Merrell, Adelaide Kock and Ernst Sonnendecker; and the University of the Witwatersrand for support to complete this chapter.

REFERENCES

Bottoms S F, Rosen M G, Sokol R J 1980 The increase in the cesarean birth rate. New England Journal of Medicine 302: 559
Boyce P M, Todd A L 1992 Increased risk of postnatal depression after emergency caesarean section. Medical Journal of Australia 156: 172–174
Chamberlain G 1993 What is the correct caesarean section rate? British Journal of Obstetrics and Gynaecology 100: 403–404
Collea J, Chein C, Quilligan E 1980 The randomized management of term frank breech presentation: a study of 208 cases. American Journal of Obstetrics and Gynecology 137: 235–244
Collins R, Scrimgeour A, Yusuf S, Peto R 1988 Reduction in fatal pulmonary embolism and venous thrombosis by perioperative administration of subcutaneous heparin: overview of results of randomized trials in general, orthopedic and urologic surgery. New England Journal of Medicine 318: 1162–1173
Crowley P, Hawkins D S 1980 Premature breech delivery—the Caesarean section debate. Journal of Obstetrics and Gynaecology 1: 2–6

Enkin M 1989 Labour and delivery following previous caesarean section. In: Chalmers I, Enkin M, Keirse M J N C (eds) Effective care in pregnancy and childbirth. Oxford University Press, Oxford, pp 1196–1215
European Collaborative Study 1992 Risk factors for mother-to-child transmission of HIV-1. Lancet 339: 1007–1012
Gimovsky M, Wallace R, Schifrin B, Paul R 1983 Randomized management of the non-frank breech presentation at term: a preliminary report. American Journal of Obstetrics and Gynecology 146: 34–40
Grant A 1989 Monitoring of the fetus during labour. In: Chalmers I, Enkin M, Keirse M J N C (eds) Effective care in pregnancy and childbirth. Oxford University Press, Oxford, pp 846–882
Greenspoon J S, Kovacic A 1991 Breech extraction facilitated by glyceryl trinitrate sublingual spray. Lancet 338: 124–125
Guedj P, Eldor J, Stark M 1991 Immediate postoperative oral hydration after caesarean section. Asia Oceanea Journal of Obstetrics and Gynaecology 17: 125–129

Hannah P, Adams D, Lee A, Glover V, Sandler M 1992 Links between early post-partum mood and post-natal depression. British Journal of Psychiatry 160: 777–780

Hauth J C, Owen J, Davis R O 1992 Transverse uterine incision closure: one versus two layers. American Journal of Obstetrics and Gynecology 167: 1108–1111

Hill N C W, Hill J G, Sargent J M, Taylor C G, Bush P V 1988 Effect of low dose heparin on blood loss at caesarean section. British Medical Journal 296: 1505–1506

Hofmeyr G J 1989 Suspected fetopelvic disproportion. In: Chalmers I, Enkin M, Keirse M J N C (eds) Effective care in pregnancy and childbirth. Oxford University Press, Oxford, pp 493–498

Hofmeyr G J 1991 External cephalic version at term: how high are the stakes? British Journal of Obstetrics and Gynaecology 98: 8–13

Hofmeyr G J 1992a Amnioinfusion: a question of benefits and risks. (Commentary). British Journal of Obstetrics and Gynaecology 99: 449–451

Hofmeyr G J 1992b Breech presentation and shoulder dystocia in childbirth. Current Opinion in Obstetrics and Gynecology 4: 807–812

Hofmeyr G J 1993 External cephalic version at term. Fetal and Maternal Medicine Review 5: 213–222

Howell C J 1993 Spinal vs epidural block for caesarean section. In: Enkin M W, Keirse M J N C, Renfrew M J, Neilson J P (eds) Pregnancy and childbirth module. Cochrane database of systematic reviews: review no 07057. Update Software, Oxford

Hytten F 1982 Breech presentation: is it a bad omen? British Journal of Obstetrics and Gynaecology 89: 879–880

Johnson C, Keirse M J N C, Enkin M, Chalmers I 1989 Nutrition and hydration in labour. In: Chalmers I, Enkin M, Keirse M J N C (eds) Effective care in pregnancy and childbirth. Oxford University Press, Oxford, pp 827–832

Krishnamurthy S, Fairlie F, Cameron A D, Walker J J, Mackenzie J R 1991 The role of postnatal x-ray pelvimetry after caesarean section in the management of subsequent delivery. British Journal of Obstetrics and Gynaecology 98: 716–718

Lilford R J, Van Coeverden De Groot H A, Moore P J, Bingham P 1990 The relative risks of caesarean section (intrapartum and elective) and vaginal delivery: a detailed analysis to exclude the effects of medical disorders and other acute pre-existing physiological disturbances. British Journal of Obstetrics and Gynaecology 97: 883–892

McCurdy C M, Magann E F, McCurdy C J, Saltzman A K 1992 The effect of placental management at cesarean delivery on operative blood loss. American Journal of Obstetrics and Gynecology 167: 1363–1366

MacDonald D, Grant A, Sheridan-Pereira M, Boylan P, Chalmers I 1985 The Dublin randomised trial of intrapartum fetal heart monitoring. American Journal of Obstetrics and Gynecology 152: 524–539

Neilson J P 1993 Cardiotocography during labour. British Medical Journal 1: 528–529

Pearson J, Rees G 1989 Technique of caesarean section. In: Chalmers I, Enkin M, Keirse M J N C (eds) Effective care in pregnancy and childbirth. Oxford University Press, Oxford, pp 1234–1245

Penn Z J, Steer P J 1991 How obstetricians manage the problem of preterm delivery with special reference to the preterm breech. British Journal of Obstetrics and Gynaecology 98: 531–534

Ranney B, Stanage W F 1975 Advantages of local anaesthesia for caesarean section. Obstetrics and Gynecology 45: 163–167

Roberts L J, Beardsworth S A, Trew G 1994 Labour following caesarean section: current practice in the United Kingdom. British Journal of Obstetrics and Gynaecology 101: 153–155

Salmon P, Drew N C 1992 Multidimensional assessment of women's experience of childbirth: relationship to obstetric procedures, antenatal preparation and obstetric history. Journal of Psychosomatic Research 36: 317–327

Sandler E M 1967 The first caesarean section at the Cape of Good Hope. South African Medical Journal 41: 20–21

Savage W, Francome C 1993 British caesarean section rates: have we reached a plateau? British Journal of Obstetrics and Gynaecology 100: 493–496

Smaill F 1993 Prophylactic antibiotics in caesarean section (all trials), review no 03690; prophylactic antibiotics for elective caesarean section, review no 03775; 1-day vs 3–5 day courses of antibiotics for caesarean section, review no 03250. In: Enkin M W, Keirse M J N C, Renfrew M J, Neilson J P (eds) Pregnancy and childbirth module. Cochrane database of systematic reviews. Update Software, Oxford

Stanley F J, Blair E 1991 Why have we failed to reduce the frequency of cerebral palsy? Medical Journal of Australia 154: 623–626

Stephenson P A, Bakoula C, Hemminiki E et al 1993 Patterns of use of obstetrical interventions in 12 countries. Paediatric Perinatal Epidemiology 7: 45–56

Thorp J A, Hu D, Albin R et al 1993 The effect of intrapartum epidural analgesia on nulliparous labor: a randomized controlled trial. American Journal of Obstetrics and Gynecology 168: 319

Thorpe-Beeston J, Banfield P, Saunders N 1992 Outcome of breech delivery at term. British Medical Journal 305: 746–747

Van Gelderen C J 1975 Internal iliac artery ligation in obstetrics and gynaecology. South African Medical Journal 49: 1997–2000

Van Oppen C, Feldman R 1993 Antibiotic prophylaxis of neonatal group B streptococcal infections. British Medical Journal 1: 531–532

Wallace R L, Eglinton G S, Yonekura M L, Wallace T M 1984 Extraperitoneal caesarean section: a surgical form of infection prophylaxis? American Journal of Obstetrics and Gynecology 148: 172–177

Westgate J, Harris M, Curnow J S H, Greene K R 1992 Randomised trial of cardiotocography alone or with ST waveform analysis for intrapartum fetal heart rate monitoring. Lancet 340: 194–198

Westmore M D 1990 Epidural opioids in obstetrics—a review. Anaesthetic Intensive Care 18: 292–300

Yudkin P L, Redman C W G 1986 Caesarean sections dissected 1978–1983. British Journal of Obstetrics and Gynaecology 93: 135–144

40. Postpartum haemorrhage and abnormalities of the third stage of labour

Frank Loeffler

Material in this chapter contains contributions from the first edition and we are grateful to the previous author for the work done.

PRIMARY POSTPARTUM HAEMORRHAGE

Conventional definition

Primary postpartum haemorrhage is conventionally defined as a blood loss of 500 ml or more occurring within 24 hours of delivery of the baby. Using the conventional definition, its incidence is around 5% of deliveries.

Limitations of conventional definition

Estimation of blood loss

The assumption underlying the above definition is that birth attendants can measure revealed postpartum blood loss with reasonable accuracy. Unfortunately that is not generally so, underestimates being much more common than overestimates. Various authors (DeLeeuw et al 1962, Pritchard et al 1962, Newton 1966) using spectrophotometric measurement of haematin in fluid lost and also that eluted from relevant pads and bed linen, estimated that the blood loss in the third stage of labour and the succeeding 24 hours is normally in the region of 600 ml.

Variable response to blood loss

The effect of any volume of blood loss postpartum on the pulse, blood pressure and general condition of any parturient depends on her initial blood volume, haematocrit and haemoglobin concentration. Thus some women can lose up to 1 litre of blood without any systemic effect while others develop hypotension, tachycardia, faintness and air hunger after losing only 300 ml of blood. Rigid volumetric definitions of blood loss thus have their limitations.

Failure to appreciate concealed postpartum blood loss

Concentration on the measurement of revealed blood loss can distract attention from the fact that many serious postpartum haemorrhages are associated with concealed bleeding. Such bleeding may be concealed in the uterine cavity (as retained clot), in the broad ligament, the peritoneal cavity (both after uterine rupture) or in the paravaginal or vulval tissue spaces.

Early and delayed bleeding

Most primary postpartum haemorrhage occurs within the first 4 hours after delivery of the baby, at which time parturients are usually under close supervision by midwives or doctors. Bleeding which is delayed and may occur when the birth attendants are no longer with a patient may go unrecognized and thus has its own particular danger. It is thus wise to recommend regular observation of general condition, blood pressure, pulse rate, abdominal signs, the size and consistency of the uterus and the amount of vaginal loss in the first 12–24 hours postpartum. Equally, it is of great importance to look for paravaginal or vulval haematoma formation in any woman who complains of excessive pain after delivery.

Postpartum haemorrhage and maternal mortality

Confidential enquiries into maternal deaths have been conducted in England and Wales since 1952 and have been published 3 yearly. Northern Ireland began similar enquiries and reports in 1956 and Scotland did the same from 1965 onwards. 1991 saw publication of the first report which dealt with the entire UK and it covered the 3-year period 1985 to 1987 inclusive (Report on Confidential Enquiries into Maternal Deaths in the United Kingdom, 1985–87 1991).

There were nearly 2.3 million births in 1985–87 and 139 direct maternal deaths (i.e. deaths directly attributable to pregnancy complications), making a rate of 61 per million births or one in about 38 000. Of these 139 direct maternal deaths, only six (4.3%) were due to postpartum haemorrhage and in four out of the six deaths due to postpartum haemorrhage care was thought to be substandard.

Results pooled from 11 population-based studies from eight developing countries (Maine et al 1987) suggested that postpartum haemorrhage accounted for 28% of maternal deaths. Thus postpartum haemorrhage must still be regarded as making a major contribution to maternal mortality and proper facilities for and methods of treatment become a matter of paramount importance.

Causes of primary postpartum haemorrhage

The following are the main causes of primary postpartum haemorrhage:

1. Uterine atony (in about 90%).
2. Genital tract trauma (in about 7%).
3. Coagulation disorders.
4. Large placenta.
5. Abnormal placental site.
6. Increased vascularity of the uterus.

Each of the items listed merits brief consideration.

Uterine atony

Uterine atony is when the contraction and retraction of the uterus, so vital for haemostasis after delivery, fails to occur. Uterine atony may be secondary to poor management of the third stage of labour (described later). It may also occur in a uterus whose contractile and retractile function is impaired by placental abruption which is often associated with diffuse bleeding into, and consequent damage of, the uterine musculature. Further associations are previous overdistension by twins or polyhydramnios, fibroids or a very full bladder.

Genital tract trauma

Lacerations of the vagina and cervix, or rupture of the uterus may all be the cause of postpartum haemorrhage.

Coagulation disorders

Coagulation disorders may occur with amniotic fluid embolism or after diffuse intravascular coagulation associated with placental abruption or severe pre-eclampsia. Only rarely do we see patients known to have coagulation disorders due to liver disease, autoimmune disease, or inherited vascular, platelet or coagulation factor deficiencies. Occasionally a patient comes to delivery who is anticoagulanted for medical reasons, usually with heparin.

A large placenta

Large babies, twins and grossly hydropic babies, particularly those affected by rhesus isoimmunization, can have a very large placenta attached to a large placental site and this disposes to postpartum haemorrhage.

Abnormal placental site

Major degrees of placenta praevia mean that most of the placental site is in the lower uterine segment which does not contract or retract after delivery. Severe postpartum haemorrhage may thus complicate Caesarean section for placenta praevia and the obstetrician must be alert to this possibility.

Increased vascularity of the uterus

Grande multiparae are at increased risk of postpartum haemorrhage. This may well be because they can have a very vascular uterus with large dilated pelvic vessels which bleed much more readily and heavily with any degree of uterine atony than does the uterus with normal vasculature.

Prevention of primary postpartum haemorrhage

Prophylactic use of oxytocic drugs at the onset of the third stage of labour

There is little doubt that the prophylactic use of oxytocic drugs reduces the risk of postpartum haemorrhage by something like 30–40%. This point has been proven in nine trials involving over 4000 women (see Enkin et al 1989). It is therefore difficult to understand why it is that some women will not consent to this form of prophylactic treatment.

The drug most commonly used in the UK is Syntometrine (5 units of Syntocinon and 0.5 mg of ergometrine maleate in 1 ml of fluid) and it is given by deep intramuscular injection either when the baby's head is crowning or just after the baby is delivered. The risk of entrapment of an undiagnosed second twin is a theoretical risk in circumstances where routine ultrasound scanning is not practised. An additional problem with Syntometrine is its tendency to induce vomiting and occasionally a rise in blood pressure, particularly in hypertensive patients. This effect is probably caused by ergometrine which is therefore contraindicated in patients with hypertension. Past histories of asthma and cardiac disease are also regarded as relative contraindications to the use of Syntometrine. In those circumstances an intramuscular injection of 10 units of Syntocinon may be given, although Syntocinon is not as quick acting as Syntometrine and therefore not as effective in reducing the incidence of primary postpartum haemorrhage.

Active management of the third stage of labour

Active management of the third stage implies early clamping of the umbilical cord and delivery of the afterbirth by controlled cord traction as soon as the uterus contracts and there are signs of placental separation (bleeding) and descent (lengthening of the cord). Again it is evidence obtained from controlled trials in around 1200 women of active versus physiological management (no oxytocics, no cord clamping, maternal effort instead of cord traction) which leads to the advocacy of active management (Enkin et al 1989).

Avoidance of genital tract trauma

Clearly, reducing genital tract trauma must reduce the incidence of postpartum haemorrhage. The genital tract trauma associated with instrumental delivery can be minimized by ensuring that only people with appropriate competence and training conduct or supervise such deliveries. As forceps delivery, particularly with the Kielland's instrument, is more likely to be associated with injury to the genital tract than is vacuum extraction, every obstetric unit should be taking steps to introduce vacuum extraction using up-to-date and well-maintained equipment whenever assistance with this method is appropriate.

At this point it would be relevant to refer to Caesarean section. On most occasions good technique makes the procedure simple and safe. However there are circumstances (as with major degrees of placenta praevia, or when the uterus is torn during attempts to extract a large baby or an impacted head) in which blood loss may be heavy and rapid and the skill of an experienced operator is required. Easy access to such expertise can prevent disaster.

Circumstances which increase the danger of primary postpartum haemorrhage

Anaemia

An anaemic woman has low reserves of blood volume and haemoglobin and even moderate loss may cause problems. Hence checking haemoglobin levels antenatally to ensure that they remain above 10 g/dl and prescribing haematinics (iron and folic acid) either prophylactically or whenever indicated, constitutes good practice. It is also necessary to investigate any anaemia which is refractory to treatment.

Inadequate access to clinical and laboratory support

Postpartum haemorrhage occurring in inadequately staffed maternity units or in units without good access to resuscitation facilities and haematology laboratories or opinions are particularly dangerous. Postpartum haemorrhage usually occurs unexpectedly and must be a great worry to anyone involved in home confinement where immediate access to medical aid is anything but easy, despite Flying Squads and paramedical teams. This applies particularly when midwives or doctors are working single-handed. Delays in instituting resuscitation and treatment can convert a manageable bleed into a life-threatening complication.

Treatment of primary postpartum haemorrhage

There are three clinical scenarios which merit separate consideration:

1. Postpartum haemorrhage before delivery of the placenta.
2. Postpartum haemorrhage occurring after delivery of the afterbirth.
3. Massive postpartum haemorrhage.

Postpartum haemorrhage before delivery of the placenta

An attempt should be made to stop the bleeding by making the uterus contract by massaging it and administering an oxytocic drug intravenously; Syntocinon 10 units or an ampoule of Syntometrine should be used.

Venous access should be obtained with an intravenous infusion, blood being taken at the same time for grouping and cross-matching. Intravenous fluids, either plasma volume expanders like Haemaccel or cross-matched blood, may need to be given and Syntocinon may be added to the infusion fluid. If acute hypotension occurs in circumstances where no intravenous fluids are available (e.g. during home confinement), the patient should be laid flat and the foot of her bed or legs elevated.

The placenta will need to be delivered either by controlled cord traction or manual removal of the placenta under suitable analgesia or general anaesthesia. Credé's manoeuvre (attempting to squeeze the placenta out of the uterus like a stone out of a plum) and fundal pressure should not be used in these circumstances for delivery of the placenta and membranes.

If bleeding continues thereafter, the steps outlined in the next section will need to be followed.

Postpartum haemorrhage after delivery of the placenta and membranes

Once again, the uterus should be massaged into a firm contraction and all clot should be expressed from the uterine cavity. Intravenous oxytocic drugs should also be administered and venous access should be obtained so that resuscitation with appropriate fluids can be instituted if necessary. Blood should be obtained for grouping and cross-matching. It is prudent to catheterize the bladder to make sure it is empty.

The placenta should be inspected to ensure that no placental cotyledons or membranes are missing. If there is doubt about completeness of either, the uterus may have to be explored under analgesia or general anaesthesia.

If bleeding continues after the uterine cavity is apparently empty and the uterus is firmly contracted, genital tract trauma should be suspected. As soon as the patient is in a satisfactory condition, she should be taken to the operating theatre for examination under general anaesthesia. A good light, suction, assistants, a large vaginal speculum, and a plentiful supply of sponge holders with which to grasp the cervix so that it can be adequately inspected will greatly facilitate the identification of genital tract trauma. When it is located, suturing will usually control the bleeding.

Massive postpartum haemorrhage

This is fortunately a rare complication, but when it occurs requires very active multidisciplinary management. It is dealt with further in Chapter 41. The role of each member of the team is considered here.

Having gone through the manoeuvres already described, it would now be wise to assemble a team—an extra experienced obstetrician, an extra midwife, an anaesthetist and a haematologist—to help the doctor and midwife who will have looked after the patient so far.

The *haematologist* should be asked to advise on what investigations are appropriate; a prothrombin time, partial thromboplastin time, thrombin time, fibrinogen titre, a platelet count and measurement of fibrin degradation products may be needed for precise identification of a coagulation defect. The haematologist should also alert the laboratory about the emergency and indicate that generous supplies of blood may be required. Guidance should be sought about the administration of platelets and various blood products and also about measures which might have to be taken to counter the biochemical effects of massive transfusion of blood.

The *anaesthetist* should be given charge of resuscitation which may require a further intravenous line and a central venous pressure line to monitor the administration of intravenous fluids. Undertransfusion rather than overtransfusion is the tendency in patients with massive haemorrhage. Foley catheterization of the bladder for strict measurement of hourly urine output is essential.

The extra *midwife* summoned to the scene should be given full responsibility for keeping accurate charts of pulse, blood pressure, fluid balance, central venous pressure, temperature, respiratory rate and the results of any investigations that may be done.

If the bleeding continues and there is no lower genital tract trauma, consideration will have to be given to desperate measures which may include:

1. The administration of one or several doses of 250 mg (1.0 ml) of Hemabate (carboprost promethamine) by deep intramuscular injection.
2. Bimanual compression of the uterus between a fist in the vagina and an abdominal hand on the uterine fundus: this is a most exhausting manoeuvre. Packing of the uterus is not a reliable means of arresting uterine haemorrhage.
3. Laparotomy for suture of a ruptured uterus, internal iliac artery ligation or hysterectomy. Extremely experienced clinicians are needed to make decisions about and undertake these procedures.

Patients who have massive haemorrhage may develop renal, liver or pituitary failure and may require transfer to renal or intensive care units.

OTHER CAUSES OF COLLAPSE WITHIN 24 HOURS OF DELIVERY

Not all postpartum collapse or apparent shock with hypotension is due to haemorrhage. There are a number of other causes which may produce a similar clinical picture and these include:

1. amniotic fluid embolism
2. pulmonary embolism
3. acute cardiac failure due to decompensation in patients with valvular disease of the heart or a cardiomyopathy
4. pneumonitis due to inhalation of gastric contents
5. pneumothorax
6. a cerebrovascular accident
7. eclampsia
8. hypoglycaemia
9. septicaemia.

The foregoing conditions are only mentioned because they require specific therapeutic measures, and resuscitation involving the intravenous infusion of large volumes of fluid could seriously harm patients with these conditions.

ABNORMALITIES OF THE THIRD STAGE OF LABOUR

Retained placenta

Physiologically, the uterus should contract soon after the delivery of the baby. The placenta will then separate from the uterine wall and is spontaneously expelled. Oxytocin has been used to hasten this process which may take up to half an hour or more. Despite the routine use of oxytocics the third stage may be delayed. Possible explanations for this delay are inadequate uterine contraction and retraction and, rarely, a morbidly adhered placenta.

The management of the retained placenta has varied considerably from time to time but in modern practice, manual removal of the placenta is employed if there is failure to deliver the placenta half an hour after the delivery of the baby. This may be performed earlier if the patient is bleeding and the placenta has failed to separate completely. Ready resort to this procedure has been facilitated by the advent of antibiotics, the availability of blood transfusion and the safety of modern anaesthetic techniques.

Technique

The patient who has a retained placenta is often shocked, having had postpartum haemorrhage. Adequate resuscitation is mandatory before attempting manual removal. This should include giving blood if the patient is bleeding and the administration of a second dose of the oxytocic to encourage uterine contraction and placental separation. Failure to deliver the placenta despite these measures indicates transfer of the patient to the operating theatre and the administration of a general anaesthetic.

The patient is placed in the lithotomy position. One hand is placed on the abdomen to encourage the uterus to contract and a last attempt is made with the Brandt–Andrews' method of controlled cord traction. If this fails, the abdominal hand should steady the uterus, pressing it down on to the vaginal hand. The vaginal hand should be insinuated through the cervical os and the retraction ring, if one is present, to the upper segment of the uterus, following the cord to its placental insertion. The lower edge of the placenta is then located and, with a sawing motion, the operator proceeds to detach the placenta from the uterus. When there is total separation of the placenta, it is removed and an intravenous oxytocic—preferably Syntometrine, unless contraindicated—administered to promote uterine contraction. The patient is given a course of antibiotics to prevent infection following intrauterine manipulation. Uterine perforation is a rare complication of this procedure.

Placenta accreta

The morbid adherence of the placenta to the uterus is termed placenta accreta. The penetration of the placenta up to the myometrium is termed placenta increta; when it penetrates the myometrium to the serosa, the term placenta percreta is used. The diagnosis of the latter two conditions is retrospective and is only found when laparotomy and hysterectomy are performed.

The morbidly adherent placenta is commonly associated with placenta praevia, or a previous Caesarean section scar or uterine perforation.

Placenta accreta is diagnosed when difficulty is encountered during delivery of the placenta and manual removal has to be performed. When part of the placenta is morbidly adherent and not removed, there are two possible outcomes: the bleeding may be minimal or the patient may continue bleeding. When bleeding is minimal, the patient should be observed and warned of the possibility of secondary postpartum haemorrhage, which usually occurs 10–14 days after delivery. However, if bleeding continues and the patient is desirous of having more children, conservative treatment with oxytocics or prostaglandins should be tried first; internal iliac ligation or hysterectomy are the last resort. When the subject has completed her family, a hysterectomy may be considered as the method of choice.

Acute uterine inversion

This is an uncommon complication of the third stage of labour. There are three degrees of inversion.

1. The inverted fundus reaches the cervical os.
2. The whole body is inverted up to the cervical os.
3. The uterus, cervix and vagina are completely inverted.

Acute inversion may be spontaneous or the result of mismanagement of the third stage of labour. Spontaneous inversion is often associated with a fundal placental site. Other associated factors are uterine atony, an arcuate or unicornuate uterus. In patients with uterine atony, the inversion may occur following a cough, sneeze or any other act causing an increase in intra-abdominal pressure.

Mismanagement of the third stage of labour may result in uterine inversion. This occurs when traction on the cord is attempted before uterine contraction and placental separation are established. However, the most common cause is resort to Credé's method of expelling the placenta when the uterus is relaxed. Rarely, it may follow a manual removal of the placenta when the abdominal hand is firmly pressed on the uterus and the vaginal hand is withdrawn too quickly. This results in the creation of a negative pressure and the uterus inverts.

The most dramatic presentation is the complaint of severe lower abdominal pain and the feeling of prolapse followed by collapse and haemorrhage. In milder degrees of inversion the patient may complain of pain and haemorrhage. When only indentation of the fundus occurs, symptoms are minimal and it usually corrects spontaneously. The shock produced by a uterine inversion is commonly neurogenic in origin as considerable traction is placed on the infundibulopelvic and round ligaments. Haemorrhagic shock may further complicate the situation since uterine atony and partial placental separation may have occurred.

When called to see such a patient, the obstetrician should always exclude a submucous fibroid protruding from the os. The diagnosis is easy enough as the uterine body and fundus are palpable in the abdomen in this situation.

Prevention is the mainstay of management of acute uterine inversion. One should never exert traction on the cord when the uterus is still relaxed, and countertraction should be applied when the uterus finally contracts, when delivery of the placenta should be attempted. Credé's manoeuvre should not be employed.

If the inversion occurs at the time of delivery, with the obstetrician in attendance, it is probably best to replace the uterus immediately, and follow with an intravenous bolus dose of an oxytocic to initiate uterine contraction. The patient should then be sent to the operating theatre for manual removal of the placenta. If the inversion is only detected some time after the event, and the woman is in shock, it is best to resuscitate her with intravenous fluids and blood. Pain is alleviated by packing the vagina to relieve the tension on the infundibulopelvic ligaments. The patient should then be transferred to the operating theatre and a general anaesthetic administered.

Hydrostatic replacement, as described by O'Sullivan (1945), has made correction of an inversion simple. This involves infusing warm saline from a container held about 1 m above the patient via a rubber tube into the vagina. To minimize the leak of saline, an assistant will be required to use his or her hands at the vaginal orifice to block it. The hydrostatic pressure would correct the inversion quite dramatically as the uterus pops back into place. However, a considerable amount of saline may be required to replace the uterus. If the placenta is still attached to the uterus it should be removed manually and then an oxytocic should be administered to ensure uterine contraction. For obvious reasons it is most important to exclude any uterine rupture before employing O'Sullivan's technique.

SECONDARY POSTPARTUM HAEMORRHAGE

Secondary postpartum haemorrhage is defined as any sudden loss of fresh blood (regardless of volume) from the genital tract occurring after the first 24 hours and within 6 weeks of delivery of the baby. Most secondary postpartum haemorrhage is due to retained and often infected products of conception. Sometimes the bleeding may be due to slough separating from a blood vessel in a lower genital tract laceration. On the rarest of occasions the bleeding may be due to a choriocarcinoma.

Most women with secondary postpartum haemorrhage have not lost sufficient blood to become shocked. Such patients should be examined clinally; those with retained and infected products may be febrile and have a tender, subinvoluted uterus with offensive lochia. Such patients should have a high vaginal swab taken for culture and should be treated with antibiotics which are effective against aerobic and anaerobic organisms. Evacuation of the uterus should be undertaken. The procedure requires care as the postpartum uterus is soft and relatively easy to perforate; any tissue obtained should be sent for histological examination. At the end of the procedure, the lower genital tract should always be inspected for bleeding points. Oxytocic drugs are usually given during the procedure and may be continued for 12–24 hours afterwards.

Even if the clinical signs do not suggest retained and infected products of conception, an ultrasound scan to check the contents of the uterus should be done. If the uterine cavity is empty and there is no evidence of infection, conservative management as an outpatient may be indicated.

On rare occasions secondary postpartum haemorrhage may be severe and cause shock. Heavy bleeding is sometimes seen with secondary haemorrhage after a Caesarean section. Such patients may not respond to the treatment already outlined and may require large blood transfusions, intensive care, and even some of the heroic measures outlined in the preceding section on massive haemorrhage.

REFERENCES

De Leeuw N K M, Lowenstein L, Tucker E C, Dayal S 1968 Correlation of red cell loss at delivery with changes in red cell mass. American Journal of Obstetrics and Gynecology 100: 1092–1011

Enkin M, Keirse J N C, Chalmers I 1989 A guide to effective care in pregnancy and childbirth. Oxford, Oxford University Press, pp 235, 237

Maine D, Rosenfeld A, Wallis M et al 1987 Prevention of maternal deaths in developing countries. The Centre for Population and Family Health, University of Colombia, New York

Newton M 1966 Postpartum haemorrhage. American Journal of Obstetrics and Gynecology 94: 711–717

O'Sullivan J V 1945 A simple method of correcting puerperal uterine inversion. British Medical Journal 2: 282

Pritchard J A, Baldwin R M, Dickey J C, Wiggins K M 1962 Blood volume changes in pregnancy and the puerperium. American Journal of Obstetrics and Gynecology 84: 859

Report on Confidential Enquiries into Maternal Death in the United Kingdom, 1985–87 1991 HMSO, London

41. Massive blood loss in obstetrics

H. F. Seeley

INTRODUCTION AND HISTORY

Blood has always held a special significance for the human race. Sacrifice and the ritual shedding of blood have played an important role in many ceremonies, both sacred and secular. The life-sustaining properties of blood were certainly known to the Romans who used haemorrhage as a relatively painless means of committing suicide.

A brief, but entertaining, history of blood transfusion is given by Marshall & Bird (1983).

The first human blood transfusion may have taken place in 1492. More than 100 years before Harvey first described the circulation, Pope Innocent VII was given blood from three young men, thus ensuring the death of all four involved. Denis of Montpellier seems to have been the first to transfuse blood from an animal to man in 1667, an experiment repeated by Lower in England in the same year. Others followed their example so it was not surprising that 3 years later blood transfusions were forbidden by law in both countries (James 1982). During the 18th century the medical profession became more interested in blood-letting than blood transfusion as a therapeutic manoeuvre, and bleeding became a common treatment even for the severely injured.

During the early 19th century Blundell showed that blood of different species was incompatible. He and Cline reintroduced the practice of human blood transfusion, mainly to treat those who had suffered major haemorrhage during childbirth. Though only small volumes were transfused the procedure seems to have had some success.

Three factors were responsible for major advances in the early 20th century. First, the American surgeon Crile showed that infusions of warm saline could reduce mortality in experimental haemorrhage. Second was the discovery by Landsteiner of the ABO groups in human blood. Third was the development of an anticoagulant that could be infused safely. These advances were refined during the treatment of casualties from the First World War; armed conflict provided, as Hippocrates noted it always does, a chance to improve the treatment of the severely injured.

Once the scientific foundations of the treatment of severe haemorrhage had been established the concept of irreversible shock developed. If resuscitation was inadequate or subject to excessive delay then death ensued despite subsequent restoration of circulating volume. It seemed that prolonged hypotension could lead to a state of hypoxic tissue damage that was irretrievable. With modern techniques for the support of failing lungs, heart and kidneys the distinction between reversible and irreversible shock has become blurred. However, these techniques are expensive, time-consuming and not always successful so that early recognition and competent treatment of massive haemorrhage are essential.

Massive blood loss is usually obvious in obstetric patients. Covert haemorrhage is more insidious as almost the entire blood volume can be sequestered internally with a normal haemoglobin concentration in what little blood remains in the circulation. Though every first-aid manual lists the classic signs and symptoms of haemorrhagic shock, the diagnosis is often missed if bleeding is not obvious and the classic signs are absent or misinterpreted. A loss of 25% of blood volume may prove fatal yet in the early stages of shock the arterial pressure can remain unaltered. This illustrates how the concept of shock has changed. Shock is now defined in terms of a circulation which cannot meet the overall metabolic requirements of the cells; it should not be defined in terms of specific values of pulse or blood pressure.

MASSIVE BLOOD LOSS IN OBSTETRICS

During the period 1985–87, 10 maternal deaths in the UK were directly attributed to antepartum and postpartum haemorrhage (Department of Health, Welsh Office, Scottish Home and Health Department, Department of Health and Social Services, Northern Ireland 1991). In seven of these care was considered substandard. In another 12 cases bleeding contributed to a fatal outcome. Thus excessive blood loss played a part in 16% of all direct deaths during this period.

Confidential Enquiries for the triennium 1979–81 (Department of Health and Social Security 1986) drew attention to three factors which were important in deaths from haemorrhage:

1. Failure to anticipate the high risk associated with operative delivery for placenta praevia in women with previous Caesarean section.
2. Failure to deal efficiently with massive blood loss. This included underestimation of blood loss and subsequent under-transfusion of blood, and, conversely, excessive infusion of crystalloid solutions leading to pulmonary oedema.
3. Failure to anticipate, detect at an early stage, or deal efficiently with coagulation failure.

Enquiries for the period 1985–87 (Department of Health, Welsh Office, Scottish Home and Health Department, Department of Health and Social Services, Northern Ireland 1991) identified additional factors:

1. Deficiencies in antenatal care reflected in anaemic patients coming into labour, women at high risk of bleeding being booked for delivery in inappropriate units, and failure to anticipate problems in women who refuse blood transfusion on religious grounds.
2. Treatment of severely shocked patients by anaesthetic and obstetric staff with inadequate experience.
3. Failure to resort to heroic surgery such as internal iliac artery ligation or even hysterectomy at a sufficiently early stage.

The Enquiries also reported that cumulative figures for the period 1970–84 show that risk of death from haemorrhage increases with age. Women having their second babies are at lower risk than primigravidae, but subsequently risk increases with parity.

Though the Confidential Enquiries reports are a laudable exercise in clinical audit, maternal mortality is an insensitive index of medical competence (Reynolds 1986). The victims of massive blood loss may survive more by luck than by good management. Failure to recognize and adequately to treat major blood loss remains an important cause of morbidity and mortality in obstetrics. National data on the incidence of heavy bleeding in obstetrics are not collected statutorily. Probably the best documented blood loss is postpartum haemorrhage, and in those hospitals which publish reports the rate seems to vary between 2% and 6% (Chamberlain 1992).

Massive blood loss is a phrase used in many accounts of the physiopathology and treatment of haemorrhage. However, like Lewis Carroll's Humpty Dumpty, authors understand massive to mean just what they choose it to mean—neither more nor less. One useful definition is an acute haemorrhage in which at least half the initial blood volume is lost (Horsey 1982). In obstetric practice the threat of massive blood loss should be considered once the patient has lost 1000–1500 ml.

PHYSIOPATHOLOGY OF MASSIVE BLOOD LOSS

Physiological background

Body fluid compartments

In the average adult intravascular or blood volume is about 5 litres. Blood consists of 2 litres of cellular elements suspended in plasma. Extracellular fluid consists of two components, the plasma and the interstitial space: the latter has a fluid volume of about 11 litres. The cellular elements of blood are part of the intracellular space which has a total volume of about 28 litres (Schultze 1982).

Capillary exchange takes place between plasma and the interstitial space (Ross 1982b). The barrier to exchange consists of the endothelial cells, the junctions between them and the basement membrane on which the cells lie. The exact structure of this barrier in any tissue determines the ease with which larger molecules gain access to the interstitial space. In the liver, molecules the size of albumin can cross with ease; in the central nervous system the barrier is so tight that even small molecules may have difficulty in crossing.

Lipid-soluble molecules such as oxygen and carbon dioxide will diffuse rapidly across the whole surface of the capillary wall. Water, water-soluble substances and ions pass more slowly through fenestrations and intercellular clefts. Large molecules will pass only through fenestrations, though on occasions they may be transported actively through endothelial cells. Thus the transfer of respiratory gases between plasma and the interstitial space will be very rapid; that of water, ions and small molecules rather less so, and the transfer of larger molecules such as albumin will be much slower.

Fluid is kept in the intravascular compartment by the oncotic pressure of the plasma proteins; the most important in this respect is albumin. The concentration of albumin in interstitial fluid is much lower than that in plasma, though the extravascular mass of albumin slightly exceeds that in the intravascular compartment (Marshall & Bird 1983). Though formulated some 90 years ago, Starling's hypothesis which explains capillary exchange remains fundamentally unchallenged (Guyton 1986a). At the arterial end of the capillary, hydrostatic pressure exceeds oncotic pressure and the net filtration pressure favours loss of fluid from the capillary to the interstitial space. At the venous end of the capillary the situation is reversed and the fluid moves back into the circulation. Overall, slightly more fluid leaves the circulation than enters, the surplus being returned to the intravascular compartment via the lymphatic system.

Control of arterial blood pressure

The prime function of the circulation is to provide the tissues with oxygen and nutrients and to remove metabolic waste. Thus the tissues constitute the master, with the heart and various control systems of the circulation acting as the servant (Cutfield 1983). Depending on specific activities, different tissues will have differing demands: thus blood flow to skeletal muscle will increase during exercise while that to the gut increases after a meal. All tissues have the ability to regulate blood flow in response to changing demand; this illustrates the master–servant relationship with the circulation. However, the speed with which flow and demand are matched, the process of autoregulation, varies from organ to organ.

For individual tissues blood flow is more important than blood pressure. However, circulatory control relies on maintaining a constant pressure reservoir from which organs can draw blood according to their varying needs. Blood flow is regulated by changing arteriolar tone and by opening and closing precapillary sphincters. These changes result from local build-up of metabolites; the exact metabolites which effect these changes vary from tissue to tissue.

It is a paradox that the physiological monitoring of the circulation is based largely on pressure measurement whilst the function of the system is to deliver flow (George & Winter 1985). Two suggestions have been made to explain this paradox. First, circulatory control must protect the arterial system from the destructive effects of excessive hydrostatic pressure. Second, pressure is much more easily sensed than flow.

Control of the circulation is governed by the equation:

mean arterial pressure = cardiac output × systemic vascular resistance.

Arterial pressure is sensed by high-pressure receptors, the baroreceptors of the carotid sinuses and aortic arch. Information on arterial pressure is passed to integrating centres in the brainstem via the glossopharyngeal and vagus nerves (Ross 1982a).

Cardiac output is the product of heart rate and stroke volume. Heart rate is controlled by the opposing actions of the sympathetic and vagus nerves on the sinoatrial node. Stroke volume is controlled by changes in venous tone which determines right atrial filling pressure, and by changes in myocardial contractility; both these changes are mediated by the sympathetic nervous system.

Systemic vascular resistance is controlled by variations in arteriolar vasoconstriction; these, too, are mediated by the sympathetic nervous system. The maintenance of systemic vascular resistance may be regarded as a perpetual contest between local tissue demands which tend to reduce regional resistance, and a parsimonious central control whose tendency to vasoconstrict maintains, in conjunction with changes in cardiac output, the required value of arterial pressure.

Control of blood volume

Under normal conditions blood volume is maintained within narrow limits in spite of wide variation in fluid intake. Intravascular fluid volume is sensed by low-pressure (stretch) receptors in the atria: the response to changes in blood volume is both neural and hormonal (Ross 1982a).

Information from the atrial stretch receptors travels via the vagus nerves and is integrated within the central nervous system. Renal sympathetic tone is modified accordingly, leading to changes in urine output. An additional mechanism, which acts through nervous pathways involving the hypothalamus–pituitary axis, is the adjustment of the secretion rate of antidiuretic hormone.

Aldosterone, a hormone promoting reabsorption of water and sodium by the kidney, is also involved in the control of blood volume. One of the factors controlling the secretion of aldosterone is renin, a hormone released from the kidney in response to sympathetic stimulation and to changes in the composition of glomerular filtrate. Adrenocorticotrophic hormone and similar substances released from the pituitary may also by involved in the control of aldosterone secretion (Sawin 1982).

Other hormones participate in the control of blood volume. Atrial natriuretic peptide is released from the atria in response to stretch; this hormone promotes an increased loss of water and sodium in the urine (Kaye & Camm 1985). Further third factors which promote diuresis may also be involved (de Wardener & MacGregor 1983).

Thus blood volume is controlled by neural and hormonal mechanisms which match circulating volume to urine output. A decrease in blood volume results in a fall in urine output; an increase promotes a diuresis.

Homeostatic response to massive blood loss

The homeostatic response to massive blood loss can be discussed under three headings:

1. Physiological control systems which regulate arterial pressure and blood volume.
2. Emergency systems which come into operation when physiological controls are stretched beyond their normal operating limits.
3. Inappropriate responses which may actually jeopardize the patient's survival.

Response of physiological systems

Following massive blood loss the arterial pressure control system attempts to sustain blood pressure by intense sympathetic activity. Increases in heart rate and myocardial contractility try to maintain cardiac output; venoconstriction aims to maintain right heart filling pressure and reduce the functional volume of the circulation. Arteriolar constriction overrules local autoregulatory mechanisms which match blood flow to demand, so increasing systemic vascular resistance. However, this vasoconstriction is not uniformly distributed; it occurs mainly in the splanchnic area, kidney, skeletal muscle and skin. Flow to the brain and myocardium is preserved.

The effects of intense sympathetic nervous activity are augmented by adrenaline released from the adrenal medulla. Circulating adrenaline constricts metarterioles which, though responsive to catecholamines, are not sympathetically innervated.

As blood volume falls renal sympathetic vasoconstriction and increased levels of circulating antidiuretic hormone and aldosterone cause a marked fall in urine output. Levels of atrial natriuretic peptide and other third factors promoting diuresis are presumed to fall, although this has not yet been established.

Emergency systems

As arterial pressure and blood volume fall precipitously emergency systems come into operation. Peripheral arterial chemoreceptors are stimulated, resulting in an augmented sympathetic response and increased rate and depth of respiration. This stimulation occurs before hypoxaemia and acidaemia develop in arterial blood and results from a reduction in blood flow to the chemoreceptors. On the basis of flow per unit mass of tissue, blood supply to these organs is massive: the reduction in flow which occurs during hypovolaemia is interpreted as a fall in arterial Po_2 and pH.

During hypotension, activation of the renal baroreceptor causes release of increasing amounts of renin into the circulation. Acting through the renin cascade this hormone causes increased production of angiotensin II. Angiotensin has many actions (Miller 1981): it is an extremely powerful vasoconstrictor acting mainly on the arterioles of the skin, kidney and splanchnic area; it promotes retention of water and sodium by the kidney, both by direct action and through release of aldosterone; it facilitates sympathetic neurotransmission and promotes thirst (Guyton 1986b). The story of Sir Philip Sidney, who suffered great thirst after injury and loss of blood, is a reminder that thirst may be the overwhelming symptom of haemorrhage.

After massive blood loss antidiuretic hormone is released in large quantities from the posterior pituitary. In high dose, antidiuretic hormone increases still further the splanchnic vasoconstriction induced by sympathetic stimulation, circulating catecholamines and angiotensin. This property is used in the treatment of bleeding oesophageal varices.

Fluid moves into the circulation from the interstitial space. Intense arteriolar constriction leads to a fall in hydrostatic pressure at the arterial end of the capillary. The normal Starling equilibrium is disturbed and there is a net inward flux of fluid from the interstitial space into the capillary. In severe haemorrhage refill rates of 1000 ml/hour can be achieved (Marshall & Bird 1983). Albumin also moves into the circulation from the interstitial space, although at a slower rate.

Severe haemorrhage induces a number of metabolic changes. Increased release of adrenocorticotrophic hormone causes a rise in plasma cortisol; high levels of cortisol may be necessary for the normal homeostatic response to haemorrhage. Catecholamines stimulate glucagon secretion, resulting in hyperglycaemia and increased levels of glycerol and free fatty acids in blood. In the longer term the negative nitrogen balance associated with the stress response develops.

Inappropriate responses

Fear, pain and anxiety markedly increase sympathetic activity. Thus, the response of the severely injured casualty or the obstetric patient with postpartum haemorrhage is more dramatic than that of a volunteer bled during a physiology experiment. Blood pressure and central venous pressure may be above normal in the early stages of haemorrhagic shock in spite of significant loss of circulating volume (Marshall & Bird 1983).

Bradycardia develops in some patients rendered hypotensive as a result of haemorrhage. This response, apparently inappropriate, may be due to increased vagal tone (Sander-Jensen et al 1986).

Inappropriately high blood pressures and central venous pressures, and inappropriately slow pulse rates may obscure the diagnosis, especially if haemorrhage is concealed.

The endogenous opiate, beta-endorphin, may be released with adrenocorticotrophic hormone after massive blood loss. Though endorphin may have the laudable effect of increasing pain threshold after injury, it may exacerbate arterial hypotension and even jeopardize survival (Faden & Holaday 1979).

Summary of homeostatic response to massive blood loss

The homeostatic response attempts to maintain arterial pressure and effective blood volume. Intense sympathetic activity causes venoconstriction, tachycardia and increased myocardial contractility, all of which aim to limit falls in cardiac output. Sympathetic activity also increases systemic vascular resistance; however, the arteriolar constriction is not uniformly distributed and occurs mainly in skin, skeletal muscle, the kidney and the splanchnic area. Splanchnic ischaemia is intense as sympathetic vasoconstriction is augmented by the actions of adrenaline, antidiuretic hormone and angiotensin in the circulation. The fact that blood pressure is maintained rather than overall flow means that arterial pressure is a poor guide to cardiac output (George & Winter 1985). Pulse pressure is a much better indicator since diastolic pressure depends on systemic vascular resistance and systolic pressure depends on stroke volume (George & Tinker 1983).

Blood volume is maintained by venoconstriction, which reduces the volume of the intravascular compartment, and by neural and hormonal actions on the kidney which reduce urine output. Fluid intake is promoted by thirst. Blood is diverted from regions where vasoconstriction is marked and fluid from the interstitial space is drawn into the circulation.

Investigation into the haemodynamic and neuroendocrine responses to haemorrhage is beset with problems. The responses differ depending on the species studied and whether the animal is conscious or anaesthetized. There are ethical limits to the induction or simulation of severe haemorrhage in human subjects.

Recently there has been renewed interest in a phenomenon noted during experiments conducted during the Second World War, namely that the response to haemorrhage in conscious humans is biphasic (Barcroft et al 1944). A modern account of this response is given by Schadt & Ludbrook (1991). Initially, arterial pressure is maintained solely by sympathetic and renin-mediated selective vasoconstriction. After about 30% of blood volume has been lost, a sympathoinhibitory phase develops abruptly with bradycardia, vasodilatation and a profound fall in arterial pressure. However, levels of circulating adrenaline, angiotensin and vasopressin rise. The central nervous pathways initiating the inhibitory phase probably involve endogenous opioids, serotonin and vasopressin.

Adverse consequences of the homeostatic response

The homeostatic response to massive blood loss involves intense splanchnic vasoconstriction. The profound ischaemia which results is exacerbated by the reduced oxygen-carrying capacity which follows loss of red cell mass.

Cells vary in their ability to withstand hypoxia; the astrocytes of the central nervous system are notoriously susceptible whilst skeletal muscle and liver cells are relatively resistant. Survival after hypoxia does not, however, imply normal cell function during the time of ischaemia. The splanchnic area can withstand a period of greatly reduced blood flow but if this is prolonged then adverse consequences are inevitable.

The pathological changes during haemorrhagic shock have been the subject of intense study. Most of the present understanding has come from animal experiments in which conditions can be carefully controlled. The brief survey which follows encompasses one written before; it is reproduced here by kind permission of the publishers (Seeley 1987). For more detailed accounts the reader should consult reviews by George & Tinker (1983), Runciman & Skowronski (1984) and Ledingham & Ramsay (1986).

The adverse consequences of massive bleeding can be considered under two headings: changes at the cellular and microcirculatory level, and effects on organ function.

Effects on cells and microcirculation

Three main disturbances of cell function can be discerned—alterations in regulation of cell volume, alterations in energy metabolism and the disruption of lysosomes (Ledingham & Ramsay 1986). Cell membrane function is disturbed with an influx of sodium, calcium and water and a loss of potassium and magnesium. The cells swell as do the mitochondria. Calcium flux within the cell is disturbed. As blood flow becomes sluggish, oxygen extraction increases so that venous oxygen content falls; ultimately metabolism becomes anaerobic with the production of large quantities of lactic acid. Lysosomal enzymes, found in particular abundance in the liver, spleen and pancreas, leak into other cell structures. These enzymes, together with peptide fragments and cellular debris, also pass into the circulation and may produce adverse effects in more distant parts of the body.

Proteolytic enzymes act on precursors present in plasma to form kinins. Kinins cause vasodilatation and increase capillary permeability, so antagonizing sympathetic vasoconstriction and promoting loss of fluid from the circulation into the interstitial space. Kinins also depress myocardial contractility and initiate disseminated intravascular coagulation (DIC). Histamine released from damaged cells further increases vasodilatation and capillary permeability. Serotonin (5-HT) released from platelets may contribute to the pulmonary hypertension which occurs.

The precise role of prostaglandins and leukotrienes in shock is not established. Different prostaglandins may have opposing actions, some promoting and others inhibiting platelet aggregation, some causing vasodilatation and others vasoconstriction.

Hypoxic damage to endothelial cells, exposure of collagen fibres, failure of production of prostacyclin, sludging of red cells and aggregation of platelets are other factors which may initiate DIC. The obstetric patient is already at increased risk as pre-eclampsia, abruptio placentae and amniotic fluid embolism may be complicated by DIC.

Although sympathetic discharge causes intense precapillary vasoconstriction in the initial stages, build-up of local metabolites, together with kinins, histamine and other vasoactive products, ultimately overcomes the centrally mediated forces and leads to vasodilatation and increased capillary permeability. The postcapillary venules appear more resistant to these local forces than the pre-capillary vessels so that hydrostatic pressure within the capillary rises and fluid moves into the interstitial space. Increased tissue pressure within the interstitial space compresses the capillaries, reducing still further blood flow in the microcirculation.

Effects on organ function

In the gastrointestinal tract the ischaemia is most marked in the mucosal layer. The integrity of the mucosal barrier is lost and the body is invaded by intestinal bacteria and their toxins. Although in the past there has been great emphasis on the role of absorbed endotoxin, the toxins of Gram-positive bacteria may be just as important (George & Tinker 1983). Mucosal damage is most marked in the stomach where superficial erosions and petechial bleeding may contribute to further blood loss. The large intestine appears to be much more resistant (Runciman & Skowronski 1984) although ischaemic necrosis of the right colon has been reported after haemorrhagic shock (Flynn et al 1983).

The liver suffers a reduction in blood flow from both hepatic artery and portal vein, the latter normally supplying some 60% of the liver's oxygen requirements. The hepatic reticuloendothelial system fails, allowing bacteria absorbed from the gut to gain access to the circulation. Bacterial toxins have adverse effects on cell function and vascular control, and activate the coagulation and complement cascades.

During severe haemorrhage blood flow to the pancreas may be reduced by 85%. Pancreatic lysosomes seem particularly susceptible to hypoxic disruption and at least nine myocardial depressant polypeptides of pancreatic origin have been identified during shock. Myocardial depressant factor is one such polypeptide which also impairs reticuloendothelial function.

A further myocardial depressant, passive transferable lethal factor, is released from the reticuloendothelial system during shock. Fibronectin, a serum opsonin essential for the normal functioning of the reticuloendothelial system, is depleted during haemorrhagic shock (Singer & Goldstone 1985).

During acute hypotension renal blood flow is reduced as a result of sympathetic stimulation. The kidney contributes to the homeostatic response to haemorrhage by reducing urine output. Hypotension may be followed by acute renal failure. It is likely that many factors are involved in the initiation, maintenance and recovery phases of acute renal failure: among the suggested mechanisms are afferent arteriolar vasoconstriction due to angiotensin, catecholamines and prostaglandins; altera-tion in the distribution of renal blood flow, and post-ischaemic tubular dysfunction.

As described above, intense vasoconstriction in certain regions allows cellular debris and active substances, collectively known as mediators, to enter the circulation. These products have deleterious effects on more distant organs.

The lung is involved in haemorrhagic shock. In the early stages hyperventilation occurs, probably due to the actions of catecholamines on the central nervous system, the effect of vasoactive substances on lung receptors and stimulation of the chemoreceptors. Prolonged un-corrected hypovolaemia may lead to adult respiratory distress syndrome (ARDS). A product of the complement cascade, activated complement fraction 5 (C5a), has been shown to cause leucocyte aggregation in the lung. D-antigen, a product of fibrin degradation, may play a similar role.

These leucocyte aggregates release free oxygen radicals and proteases which destroy cellular and structural elements in the lung. These changes themselves stimulate further leucocyte aggregation and activate the complement and clotting cascades. Circulating catecholamines, serotonin, histamine and prostaglandins contribute to the pulmonary hypertension observed during haemorrhagic shock. The ventilation/perfusion (V/Q) abnormalities caused by vasoactive substances lead to arterial hypoxaemia which is exacerbated by the shunting of mixed venous blood of low oxygen content.

Increases in rate and myocardial contractility are part of the normal sympathetic response of the heart to haemorrhage. However, if severe hypovolaemia persists, myocardial function is impaired by lactic acidosis and by circulating myocardial depressants such as kinins, myocardial depressant factor and passive transferable lethal factor. Myocardial oxygenation is jeopardized by tachycardia, rising ventricular end-diastolic pressure and falling arterial diastolic pressure. The subendocardial region is at particular risk.

The brain is essential for co-ordinating the autonomic response to haemorrhage. The cerebral circulation shows remarkable powers of autoregulation, matching flow to requirements within seconds over a wide range of perfusing pressures. It is surprising therefore that restlessness and clouding of consciousness may be seen at values of arterial pressure that are well tolerated in the postoperative recovery room. One explanation is that sympathetic stimulation shifts the autoregulation curve to the right; autoregulation is therefore lost at higher pressures than usual and cerebral ischaemia occurs even during mild hypotension (Lassen & Christensen 1976).

The physiopathology of massive blood loss: summary

The body's initial response to massive blood loss is remarkably effective. Blood flow to the heart and brain is maintained whilst that to regions more tolerant of ischaemia, such as skeletal muscle and the splanchnic area, is greatly reduced.

However, the response cannot be sustained indefinitely. Prolonged ischaemia in the splanchnic area leads to invasion of the portal system by bacteria and their toxins; these gain access to the systemic circulation because the liver fails to filter them. These invaders, together with products released from hypoxic cells, initiate the coagulation and immune cascades which proceed in an uncontrolled fashion. Mediators are formed which overcome all aspects of the homeostatic response by promoting vasodilatation and loss of fluid into the interstitial space, and by depressing myocardial contractility. Many factors conspire to initiate DIC, which further impairs flow in the microcirculation whilst promoting increased bleeding from wounds. Thus a vicious circle is set up which leads to collapse of homeostatic compensation. Even if resuscitation succeeds in saving the victim's life, the running-amok of systems which have a local protective function may cause prolonged damage to kidneys and lungs.

The signs and symptoms of progressive blood loss are shown in Table 41.1.

TREATMENT OF MASSIVE BLOOD LOSS

The physiopathology of massive blood loss has been the subject of intense study. Animal experiments have identified many adverse metabolic consequences of haemorrhagic shock and as a result therapeutic regimens have been suggested which might prevent or at least modify these untoward effects. These include the administration of steroids, adrenergic agonists and antagonists, prostaglandins and prostaglandin inhibitors, clotting factors and anticoagulants, and infusions of various cocktails containing energy-rich compounds involved in cellular metabolism. Though they have shown promise in animal experiments none is yet of proven value in man.

Successful resuscitation must therefore rely on the principles succinctly stated by Ledingham & Ramsay (1986):

The objective of treatment is to restore adequate oxygen availability for the metabolic requirements of the tissues. The immediate aims are to augment intravascular volume, optimise cardiac output and its distribution, and ensure adequate pulmonary gas exchange. These aims are achieved by minimising further fluid loss and replacing estimated loss with either colloid or crystalloid solutions and transfusion with concentrated red cells to a haematocrit of 30–35%; by the judicious use of pharmacological agents; and by the administration of oxygen together with mechanical ventilation when indicated.

Fluids available for restoring blood volume

In view of the availability of blood for transfusion in the UK it might at first seem surprising that there should be any discussion about the best fluid for the treatment of massive haemorrhage. However, blood has obvious disadvantages for immediate treatment in an emergency:

1. Bloods of donor and recipient must be tested for compatibility before transfusion. Unless blood has been previously cross-matched, delay will be inevitable.
2. Blood has a limited shelf-life (currently 35 days) and must be stored in a suitable refrigerator.
3. Functional changes occur during storage. Banked blood does not have the same properties as freshly drawn blood.

For these reasons other fluids are also used during resuscitation. The properties of all available fluids will now be discussed.

Stored blood and red cell concentrates

The changes which take place during storage of blood have been listed by Marshall & Bird (1983). A certain percentage of red cells die, initially because of the effects of transfer from the donor and subsequently through natural ageing. Levels of 2,3-diphosphoglycerate (2,3-DPG) within the red cells fall, shifting the oxygen–haemoglobin dissociation curve to the left: haemoglobin becomes more avid for oxygen and less ready to release it when required. Platelets and neutrophils lose their function and the labile clotting factors (V, VIII, IX and X) disappear. The pH falls to 6.7, the Pco$_2$ rises to over 14 kPa and the potassium to 20 mmol/l. The functional elements in stored blood are therefore red cells, whose haemoglobin

Table 41.1 Classification of haemorrhagic shock in relation to clinical criteria and percentage of total blood volume lost (from Hanson 1978 with permission)

Classification	Blood loss as a percentage of total blood volume	Blood pressure (mmHg)	Symptoms and signs
Compensated preshock	10–15	Normal	Palpitations Dizziness Tachycardia
Mild	15–30	Slight fall	Palpitations Thirst Tachycardia Weakness Sweating
Moderate	30–35	70–80	Restlessness Pallor Oliguria
Severe	35–40	50–70	Pallor Cyanosis Collapse
Profound	40–50	50	Collapse Air hunger Anuria

has an increased affinity for oxygen, and albumin, much of which may already have been removed by the transfusion service. The accompanying fluid will be rich in potassium, citrate, lactic acid and ammonia.

It follows that during massive blood transfusion other elements found in fresh blood may be required. If the transfused blood has been in the form of red cell concentrate, then albumin (usually as 4.5% human albumin solution) or plasma substitutes will be needed. The logical way to assess the need for colloid is to measure plasma oncotic pressure but this technique is not widely available. The Confidential Enquiries (Department of Health and Social Security 1986) protocol for managing major haemorrhage recommends infusion of colloid if more than 3 units of red cell concentrate have been given.

Massive transfusion demands replacement of labile clotting factors in the form of fresh frozen plasma (FFP) and cryoprecipitate. Recommended doses differ; some suggest 1 unit of FFP as routine after 4 units of blood, while others recommend 1 unit after as many as 10 units of blood (Marshall & Bird 1983). More FFP and cryoprecipitate will be needed if DIC occurs. In all cases of massive transfusion the help of a haematologist is required and labile factors can be given on the basis of clotting studies.

Dilutional thrombocytopenia may be a problem during massive blood replacement but bleeding from this cause is more likely to appear 8–12 hours after transfusion (Marshall & Bird 1983). Platelet transfusion should be given on the advice of a haematologist; such expert help is of particular importance in the management of DIC.

Platelets, FFP and cryoprecipitate are scarce and costly materials. Cheaper fluids should be used to restore circulating volume until major haemorrhage has been stopped, if necessary by immediate surgery.

There is renewed interest in the particular properties of fresh blood (Isbister 1992). The platelets of whole blood less than about 48 hours old have not yet developed a storage lesion and there is some evidence for the efficacy of fresh blood in the treatment of massive haemorrhage. However, fresh blood is rarely available in an emergency.

The importance of 2,3-DPG and changes in oxygen affinity during transfusion have been reviewed by MacDonald (1977). There are theoretical reasons for believing that changes in oxygen affinity would be important in obstetric patients under two circumstances: first, if massive transfusion was required before delivery; second, during transfusion in patients with sickle cell anaemia. In such cases the use of fresh blood, or blood preserved in a medium which maintains normal levels of 2,3-DPG, might be considered if circumstances permit. However, the risks of inadequate circulating haemoglobin, whatever its oxygen affinity, far outweigh those associated with shifts in the dissociation curve.

In dire emergency, when it is considered that lack of oxygen-carrying capacity (rather than hypovolaemia) represents an immediate danger to the patient's life, group O Rh-negative blood can be given. If the patient's blood group and antibody screen are known, ABO-compatible uncross-matched blood is preferable. A patient's blood group can now be established within minutes and a satisfactory cross-match can be made in about half an hour (Singer & Goldstone 1985). It must be emphasized that these are times from arrival at the laboratory; rapid and reliable transport between labour ward or operating theatre and the laboratory is essential.

Crystalloids and colloids

These solutions have many attractions for the restoration of circulating volume. The problems of blood-grouping and incompatibility are absent, shelf-life is measured in years, and storage requirements are much less stringent than those for blood.

Crystalloids are isotonic solutions of small ions. When given intravenously equilibration between circulation and interstitial space is rapid. Hartmann's solution is probably the most popular crystalloid: its composition closely resembles that of extracellular fluid except that bicarbonate is given in the form of lactate. After infusion the liver converts the lactate ion to bicarbonate. Fears that any existing lactate acidosis might be aggravated by this solution have proved groundless (Ledingham & Ramsay 1986). Enthusiasm for the use of Hartmann's solution dates from studies of the loss of extracellular fluid during surgery by Shires and his colleagues (1961).

Colloids are solutions of large molecules whose molecular weight is sufficient to exert significant oncotic pressure. In practice this implies a molecular weight of 30 000 or above; the molecular weight of albumin is about 70 000. All colloids will increase circulating volume; those whose oncotic pressure exceeds that of plasma (for example, 25% albumin and 10% pentastarch) will draw additional fluid from the interstitial space into the circulation.

Albumin, usually given in the form of 4.5% human albumin solution (HAS), is regarded as the gold standard colloid. Following infusion of albumin there is a small but significant frequency of severe reactions of about 0.003% (Twigley & Hillman 1985). The main objections to HAS are cost and limited availability. During its preparation HAS is heat-treated to inactivate hepatitis B virus (Marshall & Bird 1983); this process has been shown also to inactivate HIV (Hilfenhaus et al 1986).

Several plasma substitutes are available which will maintain intravascular volume. They are readily obtainable and all are cheaper than HAS. However, severe reactions are three to 10 times more common, depending on the study quoted and the particular colloid. As with all rare side-effects, any quoted frequency should be interpreted with caution.

Three types of colloid are available for use as plasma substitutes: dextran 70, modified gelatins and hydroxy-ethyl starches. The properties of these colloids have been the subject of reviews (Singer & Goldstone 1985, Twigley & Hillman 1985, Mythen et al 1993).

Dextran 70 is a cheap and effective colloid for replacement of minor to moderate blood loss. However, adverse effects on haemostasis limit its use to a maximum of about 1 litre per day in the average adult. It is therefore not the colloid of choice after massive haemorrhage.

Modified gelatins are also cheap colloids. In hypovolaemia their half-life in the circulation is between 5 and 7 hours. Two preparations are available, a succinylated gelatin (Gelofusine) and a urea-linked gelatin (Haemaccel). The formulations of these two gelatins differ considerably; the high calcium and potassium content of Haemaccel should be noted. Gelatins do not affect haemostasis, nor do they interfere with cross-matching; however, a urea-linked gelatin has been shown to cause a fall in plasma fibronectin, although the clinical effects of this change have not been established (Brodin et al 1984).

Hetastarch (Hespan) has been available for some time in Europe and the USA but has only recently been introduced into the UK. It can claim to be a true plasma substitute as increases in oncotic pressure persist for several days after infusion (Haupt & Rackow 1982). Fears of a specific interference with blood clotting have not been substantiated (Diehl et al 1982). It is the most expensive plasma substitute, though considerably cheaper than HAS. Pentastarch has a shorter duration of action and its effects persist for some 12 hours.

Fluids used for resuscitation

Restoring red cell mass

Although Olympic athletes have been known to use red cell infusions to improve their performance, most humans carry 25% more haemoglobin than they actually need (Doenicke et al 1977). Although it is tempting to try to restore haemoglobin levels to normal during resuscitation, a haematocrit of 30–35% represents the best compromise between oxygen-carrying capacity and blood viscosity (Hanson 1978, Ledingham & Ramsay 1986). Despite the recommendation that haematocrit should not be allowed to fall below 25% (Singer & Goldstone 1985), recent experience with patients who refuse blood transfusion, either for religious reasons or through fear of contracting AIDS, suggests that low levels of haemoglobin are better tolerated than was believed 10 or 15 years ago.

If more than half the circulating volume has been lost (about 2500 ml in the average adult) blood with normal haemoglobin–oxygen affinity (relatively fresh blood, or blood with special preservatives) should be given if available. If red cell concentrates are infused additional HAS or plasma substitutes will be needed to maintain oncotic pressure.

Additional fluids: colloid and crystalloid

Whilst there is general agreement on the criterion for maintaining red cell mass there is surprising dissension over the best fluids for restoring plasma volume; the arguments about the colloid/crystalloid controversy have been summarized by Ledingham & Ramsay (1986). Many clinicians use both types of fluid during resuscitation from massive haemorrhage and there is evidence from animal experiments to support this compromise (Smith & Norman 1982). The detailed arguments of the colloid/crystalloid controversy may seem somewhat arcane to the obstetrician faced with the problem of treating massive blood loss, and the following recommendations are based on those of Marshall & Bird (1983); a more detailed protocol is given by Hanson (1978).

Suggested procedure—initial resuscitation

The fluids used during initial resuscitation depend on clinical circumstances. Two groups of patients can be distinguished:

1. If resuscitation has been delayed and there has been a period of prolonged hypovolaemia (more than 30 minutes) fluid will have been lost from both circulation and interstitial space. The first fluid should be crystalloid, either Hartmann's solution or isotonic saline. The circulation should show improvement after infusion of 1–2 litres, after which 2 units of cross-matched blood are given. If blood is still not available 1 litre of colloid, either modified gelatin or hetastarch, can be given pending its arrival. Whole blood is preferable but if only red cell concentrates are available additional colloid is necessary to replace removed albumin: hetastarch is the logical plasma substitute under these circumstances.

   An alternative strategy for resuscitation of patients with prolonged hypovolaemia is undergoing trials at present (Rocha e Silva & Velasco 1992). This involves infusion of small volumes of hypertonic solutions in the early phase of resuscitation.

2. If sudden severe haemorrhage occurs in hospital there is no excuse for any delay in resuscitation. The main fluid loss will be from the circulation and significant shift of fluid from the interstitial space will not yet have occurred. The first fluid should be blood or colloid. In torrential haemorrhage uncross-matched blood may be life-saving. After 1–1.5 litres has been infused the situation can be reassessed.

Suggested procedure—subsequent fluids

Once the initial resuscitation has been completed, further blood, colloid, crystalloid and clotting factors will be needed. Subsequent fluid therapy can be based on the following measurements:

1. Central venous pressure.
2. Arterial pressure.
3. Heart rate (from electrocardiogram).
4. Haemoglobin and haematocrit.
5. Urine output.
6. Core–peripheral temperature difference.
7. Serum potassium, acid–base state, clotting studies.

Frequent measurements are needed to assess the reversal of the homeostatic response and the redistribution of fluids into various compartments and damaged tissues.

As normovolaemia (judged by central venous pressure and core–peripheral temperature difference) is approached, the haematocrit should be used to guide further red cell transfusion. Blood loss is often overestimated and patients can end up with raised haemoglobin levels (Marshall & Bird 1983). The advantages of a lowered haematocrit have already been described.

The need for colloid is more difficult to assess unless oncotic pressure can be measured. However, a ratio of infused colloid : crystalloid of 2 : 1 represents a useful guide.

Clotting factors and platelets should be given on the advice of a haematologist.

Oxygen administration should be routine and artificial ventilation will be needed if adequate pulmonary gas exchange cannot otherwise be maintained.

If hypotension persists despite adequate restoration of circulating volume, myocardial depression is present due to factors such as sepsis or persistence of myocardial depressant factor. Inotropic support may be required. Although rare in obstetric resuscitation, the possibility of cardiac tamponade or tension pneumothorax must always be considered.

Practical aspects

Venous access

Two intravenous lines should be set up using 14- or 16-gauge cannulae. Percutaneous cannulation can be very difficult in the hypovolaemic patient and a peripheral cut-down or insertion of internal jugular or subclavian lines may be required.

Blood-warmer

A warming device is essential whenever blood or other refrigerated fluid is infused rapidly. It is desirable even when fluid at room temperature is given in large quantity.

Infusors

Blood is a viscous fluid and pressure bag infusors are needed to maintain adequate flow. Martin's pumps and hand-pumped giving sets are clumsy and cause haemolysis; they should be considered obsolete.

Microfiltration

The need for microfiltration of stored blood during massive transfusion is being questioned (Derrington 1985). It was hoped that removal of microaggregates from stored blood would reduce the incidence of ARDS: evidence for the success of microfiltration in this respect is sparse. These filters may help to prevent post-transfusion reactions by trapping granulocytes; however, they may activate complement and promote formation of new microaggregates. Microfilters should not be used when transfusing fresh blood or platelets; they must be discarded whenever they impede flow during transfusion.

Central venous pressure and arterial line

Central venous pressure measurement is mandatory for correct management. Intra-arterial pressure monitoring is very helpful in the management of hypotensive patients; the arterial cannula also allows easy and frequent measurement of blood gases and acid–base state.

Metabolic effects

Stored blood is acid and rich in potassium and citrate. However, the classical problem of potassium intoxication is rare now that warming is routine during massive transfusion (Marshall & Bird 1983). Calcium and potassium are physiological antagonists. If there is electrocardiographic evidence of hyperkalaemia, calcium is given intravenously; otherwise it is rarely required. Citrate intoxication is unlikely unless the patient is hypothermic or has hepatic or renal disease (Doenicke et al 1977). Although a metabolic acidosis may be seen immediately after massive transfusion, the metabolism of citrate to bicarbonate results later in an alkalosis; there is therefore no case for the routine administration of bicarbonate (Horsey 1982).

Protocol for dealing with massive blood loss

The successful management of massive obstetric haemorrhage demands speed, skill and experience. The Confidential Enquiries for 1979–81 (Department of Health and Social Security 1986) recommend that every obstetric unit should have its own agreed procedure which is well known to medical and nursing staff. Although the exact details of the procedure will vary with local circumstances, the following principles should be kept in mind during its formulation:

1. The procedure should be agreed in consultation with obstetricians, anaesthetists, haematologists, nursing staff and porters.
2. The importance of recognizing the mother at high risk cannot be overemphasized. All women attending the antenatal clinic should have their blood grouped and screened for antibodies. High-risk mothers should have blood cross-matched before delivery.
3. Once massive haemorrhage has occurred a general alert should be broadcast at the earliest opportunity. Experienced staff can be assembled and if necessary an operating theatre can be put on stand-by; elective surgery may need to be postponed.
4. The clinical management must be specified in detail, indicating the necessary equipment and the fluids to

be infused. The volumes of blood samples for cross-matching and clotting studies and the type of specimen tubes required must be specified exactly. Inadequate volumes of sample delivered to the laboratory in inappropriate tubes can only introduce unacceptable delay.

The Confidential Enquiries for 1985–87 (Department of Health, Welsh Office, Scottish Home and Health Department, Department of Health and Social Services, Northern Ireland 1991) give guidelines for the management of massive haemorrhage which can form the basis of an individual contingency plan.

Acknowledgements

The author wishes to thank two colleagues at St George's Hospital for their help and advice—Dr J Parker-Williams, consultant haematologist, and Dr I Findley, consultant anaesthetist in charge of obstetric anaesthesia and analgesia.

REFERENCES

Barcroft H, McMichael J, Edholm O G, Sharpey-Shafer E P 1944 Posthaemorrhagic fainting. Study by cardiac output and forearm flow. Lancet i: 489–491

Brodin B, Hesselvik F, von Schenk H 1984 Decrease of plasma fibronectin concentration following infusion of a gelatin-based plasma substitute in man. Scandinavian Journal of Clinical and Laboratory Investigation 44: 529–533

Chamberlain G V P 1992 The clinical aspects of massive haemorrhage. In: Patel N (ed) Maternal mortality—the way forward. RCOG, London, pp 54–62

Cutfield G R 1983 The systemic and pulmonary circulations. In: Tinker J, Rapin M (eds) Care of the critically ill patient. Springer-Verlag, Berlin, pp 19–36

Department of Health and Social Security 1986 Report on Confidential Enquiries into Maternal Deaths in England and Wales 1979–1981. Report on Health and Social Subjects 29. HMSO, London

Department of Health, Welsh Office, Scottish Home and Health Department, Department of Health and Social Services, Northern Ireland 1991 Report on Confidential Enquiries into Maternal Deaths in the United Kingdom 1985–87. HMSO, London

Derrington M C 1985 The present status of blood filtration. Anaesthesia 40: 334–347

de Wardener H E, MacGregor G A 1983 The relation of a circulating sodium transport inhibitor (the natriuretic hormone?) to hypertension. Medicine 62: 310–326

Diehl J T, Lester III J L, Cosgrove D M 1982 Clinical comparison of hetastarch and albumin in postoperative cardiac patients. Annals of Thoracic Surgery 34: 674–679

Doenicke A, Grote B, Lorenz W 1977 Blood and blood substitutes. British Journal of Anaesthesia 49: 681–688

Faden A I, Holaday J W 1979 Opiate antagonists: a role in the treatment of hypovolaemic shock. Science 205: 317–318

Flynn T C, Rowlands B J, Gilliland M, Ward R E, Fischer R P 1983 Hypotension-induced post-traumatic necrosis of the right colon. American Journal of Surgery 146: 715–718

George R J D, Tinker J 1983 The pathophysiology of shock. In: Tinker J, Rapin M (eds) Care of the critically ill patients. Springer-Verlag, Berlin, pp 163–187

George R J D, Winter R J D 1985 The clinical value of measuring cardiac output. British Journal of Hospital Medicine 34: 89–95

Guyton A C 1986a Capillary dynamics and exchange of fluid between the blood and intestitial fluid. In: Textbook of medical physiology, 7th edn. W B Saunders, Philadelphia, pp 348–360

Guyton A C 1986b Regulation of blood volume, extracellular fluid volume, and extracellular fluid composition by the kidneys and by the thirst mechanism. In: Textbook of medical physiology, 7th edn. W B Saunders, Philadelphia, pp 425–437

Hanson G C 1978 The management of the patient suffering from severe trauma. In: Hanson G C, Wright P L (eds) Medical management of the critically ill. Academic Press, London, pp 333–354

Haupt M T, Rackow E C 1982 Colloid osmotic pressure and fluid resuscitation with hetastarch, albumin, and saline solutions. Critical Care Medicine 10: 159–162

Hilfenhaus J, Herrman A, Mauler R, Prince A M 1986 Inactivation of the AIDS-causing retrovirus and other human viruses in antihemophilic plasma protein preparations by pasteurization. Vox Sanguinis 50: 208–211

Horsey P J 1982 Blood transfusion. In: Atkinson R S, Langton-Hewer C (eds) Recent advances in anaesthesia and analgesia, vol 14. Churchill Livingstone, Edinburgh, pp 89–103

Isbister J P 1992 Blood transfusion, blood products and autologous transfusion. Current Opinion in Anaesthesiology 5: 263–271

James D C O 1982 Blood transfusion and notes on related aspects of blood clotting. In: Scurr C, Feldman S A (eds) Scientific foundations of anaesthesia, 3rd edn. Heinemann Medical, London, pp 375–389

Kaye G, Camm A J 1985 The role of the atria in fluid volume control. British Journal of Hospital Medicine 34: 82–88

Lassen N A, Christensen M S 1976 Physiology of cerebral blood flow. British Journal of Anaesthesia 48: 719–734

Ledingham I McA, Ramsay G 1986 Hypovolaemic shock. British Journal of Anaesthesia 58: 169–189

MacDonald R 1977 Red cell 2,3-diphosphoglycerate and oxygen affinity. Anaesthesia 32: 544–553

Marshall M, Bird T 1983 Blood loss and replacement. Edward Arnold, London

Miller E D 1981 The role of the renin–angiotensin–aldosterone system in circulatory control and in hypertension. British Journal of Anaesthesia 53: 711–718

Mythen M G, Salmon J B, Webb A R 1993 The rational administration of colloids. Blood Reviews 7: 223–228

Reynolds F 1986 Obstetric anaesthetic services. British Medical Journal 293: 403–404

Rocha e Silva M, Velasco I T 1992 Hemorrhagic shock: new experimental models and prehospital care. Current Opinion in Anaesthesiology 5: 258–262

Ross G 1982a The arteries and arterial pressure. In: Ross G (ed) Essentials of human physiology, 2nd edn. Year Book Medical Publishers, Chicago, pp 203–218

Ross G 1982b The microcirculation and the veins. In: Ross G (ed) Essentials of human physiology, 2nd edn. Year Book Medical Publishers, Chicago, pp 219–229

Runciman W B, Skowronski G A 1984 Pathophysiology of haemorrhagic shock. Anaesthesia and Intensive Care 12: 193–205

Sander-Jensen K, Secher N H, Bie P, Warberg J, Schwartz T W 1986 Vagal slowing of the heart during haemorrhage: observations from 20 consecutive patients. British Medical Journal 292: 364–366

Sawin C T 1982 The adrenal gland. In: Ross G (ed) Essentials of human physiology, 2nd edn. Year Book Medical Publishers, Chicago, pp 626–637

Schadt J S, Ludbrook J 1991 Hemodynamic and neurohumoral responses to acute hypovolemia in conscious mammals. American Journal of Physiology 260: H305–H318

Schultze R G 1982 Renal function and body fluids. In: Ross G (ed) Essentials of human physiology, 2nd edn. Year Book Medical Publishers, Chicago, pp 361–381

Seeley H F 1987 Pathophysiology of haemorrhagic shock. British Journal of Hospital Medicine 37: 14–20

Shires T, Williams J, Brown F 1961 Acute change in extracellular fluids associated with major surgical procedures. Annals of Surgery 154: 803–810

Singer C R J, Goldstone A H 1985 Recent advances in blood transfusion and blood products. In: Kaufman L (ed) Anaesthesia review, vol 3. Churchill Livingstone, Edinburgh, pp 156–182

Smith J A R, Norman J N 1982 The fluid of choice for resuscitation of severe shock. British Journal of Surgery 69: 702–705

Twigley A J, Hillman K M 1985 The end of the crystalloid era? Anaesthesia 40: 860–871

The puerperium

42. The physiology of the puerperium and lactation

P. W. Howie

INTRODUCTION

The puerperium is a time of major physiological, psychological and social adjustment for a new mother and her family. The care which a mother receives during the postnatal period influences greatly her attitude to the maternity services and the House of Commons Health Committee has called for a reappraisal of current ways of delivering postnatal care (House of Commons Health Committee 1992). There is evidence that postnatal care has been given insufficient attention and that good research is required to define the needs of postnatal mothers and to evolve effective strategies to meet them.

Good postnatal care is based upon a sound understanding of the physiological changes in the puerperium. The dominant physiological event is lactation, which will be discussed later in the chapter, but other profound physiological changes occur soon after delivery of the child.

PHYSIOLOGY OF THE PUERPERIUM

It takes 38 weeks for the maternal organism to respond to the structural and functional demands of pregnancy. In the newly delivered woman, all the pregnancy adaptations, except those related to lactation, return to the non-pregnant state during the puerperium. It has been traditionally taken to last 6 weeks and, in fact, most of the changes are completed within this period. These restorative processes, many of which are of considerable magnitude, take place at varying, though quite rapid, speeds.

Structural changes in the genital tract

Involution of the uterus

Immediately after the delivery of the placenta the uterus weighs approximately 900 g. The fundus, if the bladder is empty, is palpable 11–12 cm above the upper margin of the pubic symphysis. In an opened uterus, the rough area of the placental site, uncovered by epithelium, is clearly distinguishable. The cavity of the uterus is in direct continuity with the vagina and the cervix hangs as a circular curtain from the body of the uterus into the vagina. The vessels formerly supplying and draining the placenta are compressed by continuing uterine retraction and also contribute to haemostasis by contraction of the vessel wall. The uterine contractions of labour continue and, for some reason not as yet understood, are sometimes felt as afterpains mostly in women who have previously borne children.

Systematic studies of human uterine involution (Montford & Perez-Tamayo 1961) have shown the rapid decrease in tissue mass, with total weight reduced by about 50% within 7 days of parturition. Total uterine weight, water, muscular protein, collagen and hexosamine were all shown to decrease in the same proportions. The exact mechanisms involved in uterine involution are the subject of debate but are probably caused by the rapid withdrawal of placental hormones. Electron-microscope studies in postpartum guinea-pigs (Dessouky 1971) suggest that smooth muscle cells, macrophages and the endothelial cells of myometrial vessels may all participate in involution. There is autodigestion of cytoplasmic organelles, thus reducing the contents of the cytoplasm, and degradation of extracellular collagen and ground substance. These processes seem to be carried out by an increase in the number of lysosomes and in the activity of their hydrolytic enzymes.

By the end of 6 weeks the uterus has shrunk almost to its prepregnancy size and now weighs less than 100 g. Its content of fibrous tissue is greater than that of the prepregnant uterus and increases progressively with recurring pregnancies.

Within 3 days of parturition, the superficial layer of the decidua becomes necrotic and is shed in the lochia. The deeper layers of the decidua, containing the base of the glands, are retained. Proliferation of epithelial cells from the glandular remnants and growth of the adjacent stroma are rapid, resulting in the reformation of an intact endometrial surface within 7–10 days of parturition, except over the former placental site. The restoration of an endometrial covering over the latter takes approximately 3 weeks. It is derived by ingrowth from the edge of the site and also from luteal islands of glandular remnants.

The full repair of the former placental site takes up to 6 weeks. The contracted blood vessels become thrombosed and later organized by fibrous tissue; in some, recanalization eventually occurs.

The cervix is usually torn to some extent in normal parturition, hence the difference in the shape of the external os in the parous and nulliparous cervix. The cervix is open and readily admits two fingers for a few days following parturition but in the absence of infection has narrowed by the end of the first week, making it difficult to introduce even one finger.

The lochia

This is the normal discharge from the genital tract in the puerperium. For up to 3 days it is red in colour (lochia rubra) and contains a variable amount of fresh blood as well as decidual debris. It then becomes pink in colour (lochia serosa) containing still some red cells, but predominantly leucocytes and necrotic decidua. By the end of the first week it is yellowish-white in colour (lochia alba), consisting now principally of serous fluid and leucocytes. It has a characteristic sweetish odour and gradually diminishes in amount over the following 3–6 weeks.

The characteristics of the lochia may be influenced by retained products within the uterus. In a study of 100 women, Lipinski & Adam (1981) found evidence of retained tissue in 32 at 24 hours after delivery; in 22 scans, sonolucent areas were seen suggesting blood or clot which nearly always resolved spontaneously; in 10 women with echo-dense areas suggesting retained tissue, four passed tissue spontaneously and the remaining six developed symptoms which required uterine evacuation.

Other structural changes

The abdominal wall may remain soft and flabby for some weeks. The striae gravidarum gradually become paler in colour over 6–9 months. Permanent laxity of the abdominal wall, possibly with separation or divarication of the rectus abdominus muscle, tends to occur in a woman who has experienced excessive abdominal stretching during pregnancy, for example, by twins.

In the first few days of the puerperium the vaginal walls are smooth, soft and oedematous. The distension which has resulted from labour remains for a few days but the return of normal elasticity and hence normal capacity is

quick thereafter. If the woman is breastfeeding, the vaginal epithelium remains thinner than in the prepregnant state for several weeks or months, reflecting presumably the lower levels of circulating oestrogens. Episiotomies and tears of the vagina and perineum should heal well and quickly, provided adequate suturing has been undertaken. These high incidences of postnatal pain are not significantly altered by restricted, compared to liberal, policies of performing episiotomies (Sleep 1991). Randomized trials, however, have shown less pain after perineal repair with polyglycolic acid sutures (such as Dexon or Vicryl, compared with conventional catgut or silk) (Glazener et al 1993). There is no evidence that perineal pain is aided by the addition of salt or Savlon to bath water or by the local application of praxomine/hydrocortizone as a combination. Recent information, however, shows that 42% of women have perineal pain after spontaneous delivery, with 8% having pain persisting beyond 2 months; the corresponding figures after assisted vaginal delivery are 84% and 30% respectively (Glazener et al 1993). Problems are particularly likely to occur if healing is complicated by infection or haematoma and the wound, after breaking down, heals by granulation and fibrosis. A small number of women may complain of dyspareunia for up to 3 years after delivery.

From these figures, it is clear that perineal care is an important aspect of postnatal management and that effective analgesia should be given when necessary. Paracetamol and ibuprofen are superior to placebo and mefenamic acid is better than paracetamol (see Glazener et al 1993).

Hormonal changes

Sex steroids

In late pregnancy, maternal serum levels and urinary output of sex steroids represent primarily the production of the fetoplacental unit, though the corpus luteum and the remaining ovarian tissue have been shown to produce progesterone and oestradiol respectively in late pregnancy (Acar et al 1981). Daily measurements in the puerperium have shown that mean serum levels of progesterone and oestradiol fall to non-pregnant levels by 72 hours and urinary excretion of oestrone and oestradiol by the fourth day (West & McNeilly 1979, Gray et al 1987).

The return of ovarian activity and potential fertility is dependent upon whether the mother breastfeeds or not. The physiological events determining the return of fertility are discussed later in this chapter.

Pituitary hormones

Follicle-stimulating hormone (FSH) and luteinizing hormone (LH) levels remain at their low late-pregnancy levels for the first 10 days of the puerperium (Marrs et al 1981). The capability of the adenohypophysis to release FSH returns faster than for LH, and FSH levels rise to normal non-pregnant levels within 3 weeks of delivery (Rolland & Schellekens 1975). If high doses of bromocriptine are administered for 4–7 days to suppress prolactin secretion and lactation, both FSH levels and the FSH response to a bolus injection of gonadotrophic hormone-releasing hormone (GnHRH) are readily measurable during the second puerperal week (Nader et al 1975). Of the neurohypophyseal hormones, oxytocin is considered in connection with lactation. Vasopressin, unlike oxytocin, is not secreted in rapid pulses. Basal levels of 1–5 pg/ml have been described in the non-pregnant female, at the end of labour and in the puerperium (Dawood 1983). The levels increase only in response to changes in circulating blood volume and plasma renin activity.

Thyroid function

Following delivery, concentrations of thyroid-binding globulin (TBG) slowly fall back to normal over 6 weeks (Man et al 1969). For this reason, the elevated total thyroid hormone level (T4) of late pregnancy also declines to normal over the same period. Total triiodothyronine (T3), being much less bound to TBG, shows an appreciable decline by the end of the first postpartum week, though not to non-pregnant levels (Rastogi et al 1974). At this time the radioactive iodine uptake is still elevated, but not at 6 weeks after delivery. By 6 weeks the renal clearance of iodine and the absolute iodine uptake have returned to normal but the thyroid clearance rate does not reach control values until the 12th week postpartum (Aboul-Khair et al 1964).

The suprarenal cortex

Immediately after parturition there is a short-lived rise in the urinary excretion of 17-ketosteroids (Appleby & Norymberski 1957) which may be due to the stress of labour. Plasma cortisol levels, raised during pregnancy and even higher during labour, fall to normal within a week of parturition (Bayliss et al 1955). The raised plasma levels of testosterone and androstenedione decline to normal within a few days of delivery (Mizuno et al 1968).

In late pregnancy the plasma levels of renin, angiotensin II and aldosterone are elevated and this is a reflection of both increased secretion and excretion. Frequent sampling following delivery shows a significant fall in plasma renin activity and concentration and in angiotensin II levels at 2 hours, but 2 hours later the levels increase to those characteristic of late pregnancy and subsequently fall very slowly to reach non-pregnant levels by 6 weeks (Broughton-Pipkin et al 1978).

Insulin and glucose tolerance

In the early puerperium, there is a puzzling discrepancy between the response of plasma insulin and of plasma glucose to an oral glucose load. In healthy women in late pregnancy, an oral glucose challenge evokes an enhanced insulin response but in spite of this plasma glucose levels 1 and 2 hours later are higher than in the non-pregnant state. Two days postpartum, the fasting plasma insulin and insulin response curve have returned to non-pregnant values. In contrast, at this time the glucose response curve is no different from that in late pregnancy. Both insulin and glucose responses have returned to non-pregnant values by 8–10 weeks postpartum (Lind & Harris 1976).

Haemodynamic changes

Pregnancy is associated with increases in maternal heart rate, stroke volume and cardiac output. Immediately following delivery cardiac output is increased, mainly because of the relief of inferior vena caval compression and reduced venous pooling in the uterus. Thereafter, the haemodynamic changes reverse rapidly. The recent availability of non-invasive ultrasonic measurements and Doppler frequency shifts has allowed serial measurements of cardiac output to be made in the same subject (Robson et al 1987). These have shown that, 48 hours after delivery, resting cardiac output is still elevated to the same levels as at 38 weeks' gestation. Follow-up measurements at 14 days show a mean fall in cardiac output of 16%, suggesting that the return to non-pregnant values takes a considerable time. Since the pulse rate in the early puerperium quickly falls by about 10 beats/minute in the absence of infection and abnormally heavy blood loss, the persistent elevation in cardiac output must be due to a rise in stroke volume. Direct measurements have confirmed this. This slow return to non-pregnant cardiac output contrasts with the change in circulating blood volume which returns to non-pregnant levels by the 10th day of the puerperium.

The structural changes in the heart which occur during pregnancy reverse steadily during the puerperium. After an increase during the first 48 hours after delivery, left atrial dimensions return to normal within 2 weeks as does the left ventricular end-diastolic dimension. The increases in myocardial contractility which occur in pregnancy have also returned to normal by the end of the second week (Dunlop 1989).

The study of the resting blood pressure in the puerperium reflects the problems of definition. For example, some women remain normotensive during pregnancy and labour but show a rise in blood pressure in the early puerperium. Is this a manifestation of pathology and therefore outside the physiological range or is it a physiological variant? It is well known that in women developing pregnancy-induced hypertension without significant proteinuria, the blood pressure may remain elevated for 2–3 weeks postpartum and its return to normal non-pregnant levels by the 28th or 42nd day of the puerperium is used in definitions and classifications of various types of pregnancy-induced hypertensive disorders.

It is clear that the early puerperium can be associated with increased arterial blood pressure and total peripheral vascular resistance. Thus the early puerperium is a time which requires close surveillance in any women at risk of cardiac compromise from conditions such as rheumatic heart disease and there can be risks from overenthusiastic volume expansion in patients who have severe puerperal hypertension.

Body weight changes and water elimination

The average primigravida, eating to appetite, gains about 12.5 kg in weight during pregnancy. A number of measurements made during early labour and just after delivery have shown a weight loss due to labour (water loss) and parturition (products of conception) of on average 6 kg. This leaves a surplus of approximately 6.5 kg at the start of the puerperium.

When puerperal women are weighed daily under standard conditions, body weight usually remains steady or even rises for 3–4 days. It then begins to fall (Dennis & Blytheway 1965). In cases where oedema is present in late pregnancy (about 40% of the total; Dennis & Blytheway 1965), progressive weight loss from delivery is more common, though in these women daily weight loss is less in the first 3 than in the subsequent 7 days of the puerperium (Fig. 42.1). The early puerperal weight gain is more marked in multiparous women.

Body weight tends to stabilize about 10 weeks after delivery (Fig. 42.2). At this time there is still a positive balance of about 2.25 kg compared with the assumed prepregnancy weight. This positive balance is on average 0.7 kg less in women whose lactation is continuing than in those who have not lactated.

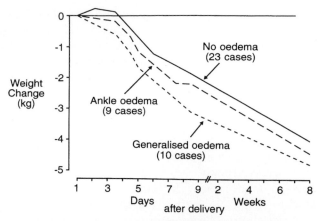

Fig. 42.2 Body weight changes from delivery until 8 weeks later in a group of 42 normal primiparae by the presence and type of clinical oedema in late pregnancy.

It has long been assumed that a diuresis commences immediately after parturition and continues for 1–2 weeks until all the additional water stored during pregnancy has been eliminated. This pattern of water shedding does indeed occur in women with clinically demonstrable oedema in late pregnancy. In the 60% who are not oedematous, however, diuresis is usually delayed until the third or fourth day of the puerperium. This means that the steady or rising body weight of the early puerperium is associated with continuing or increasing water retention at this time. The exact mechanism is not known, but it is probable that the rapid elimination of progesterone after delivery of the placenta leaves temporarily unbalanced the activity of the aldosterone–renin–angiotensin axis which reduces more slowly than progesterone. This leads to temporary retention of sodium and water. Thereafter, the increased diuresis during the early puerperium may be related to increased concentrations of atrial naturetic peptide at this time which decline thereafter as do the plasma concentrations of other vasoactive hormones (Dunlop 1989).

Haematological changes

Daily estimations of the haemoglobin concentration in peripheral venous blood show on average an initial rise on the first day of the puerperium compared with a late pregnancy measurement in the same woman. This is followed by a sharp fall to a minimum level on the fourth and fifth days. Thereafter, the haemoglobin level rises again and by the ninth day has reached about the same value as on the first day. Eight weeks postpartum there was no further change. Serial daily haematocrit measurements show parallel changes. In consequence, the mean corpuscular haemoglobin concentration remains relatively constant (Fig. 42.3). These changes occurred in women whose third-stage blood loss was within normal limits

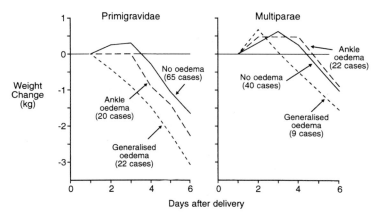

Fig. 42.1 Body weight changes in the first 6 days of the puerperium related to the presence and type of clinical oedema in late pregnancy.

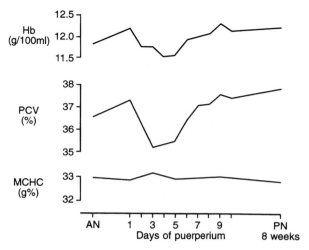

Fig. 42.3 Mean levels of haemoglobin (Hb), haematocrit (PCV) and mean corpuscular haemoglobin concentration (MCHC) in peripheral venous blood in late pregnancy and in the puerperium in 42 normal primiparae. None of the subjects showed clinical oedema in late pregnancy.

and who were given no haematinic therapy. The results suggest that the substantial fall in haemoglobin concentration and peripheral venous haematocrit in the early puerperium is due to temporary haemodilution, occurring at a time when water is being retained and when body weight is either steady or rising. In the absence of postpartum haemorrhage haemoglobin levels should therefore be measured on the first day of the puerperium rather than on the third day if a misleading diagnosis of anaemia is to be avoided (Dennis 1976).

Serial measurements of plasma volume, using the Evans Blue dilution technique, corroborate these findings. During the first 3 days of the puerperium the plasma volume in non-oedematous women either remains static or rises slightly, whereas the total red cell volume falls slightly, possibly from fresh blood loss in the lochia rubra. After the third day, plasma volume falls, reaching non-pregnant values by the ninth day. Total red cell mass remains stationary.

During pregnancy there is a steadily increasing leucocytosis; the mean leucocyte count rises from 7210/μl to approximately 10 350/μl in the third trimester (Efrati et al 1964). During and immediately after labour there is a sharp further increase to between 10 000 and 40 000/μl, made up predominantly of granulocytes. The count returns to non-pregnant levels by the sixth day postpartum (Gibson 1937, Polishuk et al 1970).

Plasma protein levels (other than fibrinogen and alpha-globulin) fall for the first 3 days of the puerperium but then rise steadily to return to non-pregnant values by the 10th day. Plasma osmolality, which in late pregnancy is 10 mosmol/kg below the non-pregnant value, rises after delivery and on average reaches the non-pregnant level of 290 mosmol/kg water by the fifth day.

Haemostasis and fibrinolysis

The blood coagulation and fibrinolytic systems are discussed in detail in Chapter 23 on coagulation disorders in pregnancy but during the puerperium some of the clotting factors, especially fibrinogen, show a rise during the first few days. By contrast, the fibrinolytic enzyme system which is depressed in pregnancy rapidly returns to normal after delivery (Bonnar 1975). To these factors must be added the initiating role of platelets, especially in injury to small vessels.

Platelet counts decrease slightly but significantly during pregnancy, but it is not known whether this is from haemodilution or increased platelet consumption. The decrease is more marked in women developing pregnancy-induced hypertension and antedates the rise in blood pressure (Bonnar 1975). Although the average fall in normotensive women is around 20%, most women at the onset of labour have a platelet count greater than 100 000/mm³. During the first 2 days postpartum the platelet count falls. There is then an outpouring into the circulation of fresh platelets with increased adhesiveness and a rapid rise in platelet count which remains elevated until the 50th day postpartum. The state of puerperal hypercoagulability therefore lasts about 7 weeks. This has obvious implications when planning prophylactic anticoagulant regimens for women at risk from thromboembolic disease.

Management of the puerperium

Although we cannot remove the patient immediately after delivery into another climate, we can qualify the air, so as to keep it in a moderate and salutary temper, by rendering it warm or cold, moist or dry, according to the circumstances of the occasion. With regard to diet women . . . even till the ninth day after delivery, ought to eat little solid food (Smellie 1752).

Smellie, the father of modern obstetrics, in his treatise merely codified the prevalent midwifery practices of his age. He accepted that the management of the puerperium has for thousands of years been the preserve of midwives in most cultures. It can justifiably be argued that, until well into the 20th century, midwives and obstetricians have done more harm than good in their advice to puerperal women. Their interference has often increased early puerperal blood loss; they have caused virulent cross-infections of the genital tract, which have probably unwittingly encouraged venous thrombosis and pulmonary embolism. Possibly the first prospective controlled trial in the puerperium was proposed 60 years ago by Baird (personal communication), working as an assistant obstetrician in Glasgow. His chief managed the puerperium by insisting that his patients should have their legs tied together for 14 days. Baird questioned the rationale of this regimen and proposed that he might try, on alternate cases, not tying the legs and see what happened. Unfortunately, we do not know the results of Baird's proposals.

This section deals with the management of the normal puerperium and also includes the observations needed to detect abnormalities at the earliest stage of their development. The establishment of lactation and the management of successful breastfeeding are discussed later in this chapter.

The first few hours

Even in women who have just gone through an uncomplicated labour and delivery, an experienced obstetrician or midwife should remain in constant attendance for at least 1 hour. Occasionally uterine atony occurs and continuous bleeding may be seen from the vulva or may result in the gradual distension of the uterus with blood and clot. If this is diagnosed early, the hypovolaemia corrected and the haemorrhage controlled, all is well, but if such continuous bleeding is missed until the woman is in hypovolaemic shock, she is at risk of losing her life. The experienced attendant should therefore palpate the uterus through the abdominal wall at frequent intervals after the delivery of the placenta, checking the vulva to ensure that no more than slight bleeding is occurring. At the end of the first hour, or sooner if there is untoward bleeding, the pulse rate, blood pressure and temperature are recorded.

If the uterus becomes soft during this time a contraction should be stimulated by massaging it through the abdominal wall. If necessary an oxytocic drug such as ergometrine 0.5 mg or Syntocinon 5 units or both, can be administered parenterally. If this results in the expulsion of more than 200 ml of blood and clot, an intravenous line should be established and a sample of blood taken with a request to the laboratory to cross-match 2 units of blood. In such a situation the patient will have to be observed carefully for several hours until the obstetrician is certain that no further uterine bleeding and relaxation will occur. An account of massive postpartum bleeding is given in Chapter 41.

Bladder function

The commonest management error occurring in the first 48 hours postpartum is failure to diagnose, and therefore to treat, bladder distension. The rate of renal urinary secretion after delivery is very variable, ranging from the oliguria of the patient with severe pre-eclampsia or eclampsia to the marked diuresis of the normotensive woman who has accumulated massive generalized oedema in late pregnancy. In addition, in many women intravenous fluids are infused during labour. If the infusion contains oxytocin in moderate or high dosage the antidiuretic effect produces additional fluid retention. When after delivery the oxytocin is discontinued, the retained fluid is usually quickly eliminated, contributing to a rapid filling of the bladder. Moreover, both the sensation and the detrusor function of the bladder may be reduced by the residual effect of epidural anaesthesia (Weil et al 1983), although the effects of epidural may be difficult to separate from those of painful lesions in the genital tract such as episiotomy, extensive lacerations and haematoma formation (Crawford 1972). Pain from abdominal incisions or prolapsing haemorrhoids are other common causes of inability to void urine completely.

It is not surprising, therefore, that urinary distension with overflow of the bladder is a frequent complication of the early puerperium. Once overdistension has been allowed to occur, bladder sensation and detrusor muscle function are further impaired and a chronic reduction of detrusor contractility can occur with collagen being laid down in between the smooth muscle fibres (Hinman 1976). When this state is reached the patient may take several weeks or even longer to recover. Throughout this time the stagnant pool of urine in the bladder predisposes to bacterial invasion and multiplication and to ascending infection of the urinary tract.

Prevention of overdistension demands close observation of the bladder after delivery to make sure that it does not overfill. The commonest finding on abdominal palpation is the upward displacement of the contracted body of the uterus and the bladder can be felt as a boggy cystic swelling. The main differential diagnosis, especially after abdominal delivery, is a haematoma in the broad ligament or below the uterovesical pouch. In cases of doubtful diagnosis an ultrasound examination can readily distinguish between the distended bladder and any other cause of suprapubic swelling.

If the woman has not voided within 6 hours of delivery, it is likely that her bladder is in danger of overdistension. Conservative measures that should be tried at this stage include walking to a commode or toilet or the administration by mouth or parenterally of an analgesic to control pain. If these measures fail to restore adequate micturition, the bladder should be catheterized. If overdistension of the bladder has been permitted the catheter should be left in situ or repeat catheterization may be required. If residual bladder volume exceeds 200 ml, an indwelling catheter should be left in the bladder for 48–72 hours, though this will increase the chance of urinary tract infection. This risk can be reduced by inserting a fine plastic suprapubic, rather than a urethral, catheter which can be safely removed when the volume of residual urine is less than 100 ml.

Care of the vulva

Shortly after the completion of the third stage of labour and perineal repair, the drapings and soiled linen are removed provided there is no excessive bleeding or other reason to keep the mother in the lithotomy position on the delivery table. The external genitalia and buttocks are washed with a warm detergent antiseptic solution or soapy water in such a way that all the liquid drains from the vulva and perineum down over the anus rather than in the reverse direction. A sterile vulval pad is then applied over the genitalia and replaced by a clean pad as necessary. After each bowel movement and before any local treatment or examination, the external genitalia should be similarly cleansed.

During the early puerperium, mothers should be discouraged from using immersion baths but instead should use bidets and showers. In hospitals, toilet seats and the rims of bidets should be wiped with a swab soaked in methylated spirit or alcohol immediately prior to use (Report of the Royal College of Obstetricians and Gynaecologists 1987).

Other standard observations

Occasionally pregnancy-induced or pregnancy-associated hypertension occurs for the first time in the early puerperium. For this reason, the pulse rate and blood pressure should be checked at least four times during the first 24 hours. If these measurements show normal values, daily recordings for the first 10 days then suffice. The same frequency of measurement is adequate for body temperature in the absence of any cause which makes an elevation more likely, e.g. tender breasts, shivering, dysuria or urinary retention. A rise in body temperature above 37°C may be taken as physiological provided it occurs only in the first 24 hours and never exceeds 38°C. Subsequent or more serious pyrexia requires investigation.

The lochia should be observed daily for colour, volume, odour and the presence of clots. The passage of clots after the first 24 hours, the prolongation of red lochia beyond the third day or the development of an offensive odour all require further investigation, especially if associated with pyrexia, tachycardia or abdominal or vulvar tenderness.

The measurement of urinary output has already been discussed in relation to bladder function. It is important to measure total 24-hour output for at least 2 days in all cases where hypertension or ante- or postpartum haemorrhage has been a complication but this accurate measurement of urinary production is not otherwise necessary.

The daily measurement of uterine fundal height above the pubic symphysis was formerly a requirement of adequate midwifery care. It is certainly valueless unless steps are taken to ensure that the bladder is empty. Whether the measurements are recorded or not, the midwife should note her opinion of uterine involution from day to day and the presence of any uterine or vulvar pain or tenderness. The condition of any abdominal or vulvar wounds should also be assessed.

Immunizations

The rhesus-negative woman who is not isoimmunized and whose baby is rhesus-positive with a negative direct Coombs' test is given 500 iu anti-D globulin within 72 hours of delivery (see Ch. 20).

Women whose early-pregnancy test showed them to be non-immune to rubella should be offered immunization in the early puerperium. This injection should however be postponed until the postnatal examination in those women who require the anti-D injection.

Diet

As mentioned above, it was formerly customary to restrict the diet of the puerperal woman who had been delivered vaginally. Such restrictions have now been removed. Following delivery, if it is unlikely that there will be any complications which may require the administration of an anaesthetic, the woman should be given something to drink if she is thirsty, or something to eat if she is hungry. A celebratory glass of champagne may, however, cause unwelcome vomiting in those unaccustomed to fizzy drinks.

The diet of the lactating mother is normally governed by local custom but should be well balanced to provide necessary nutrients. There is no evidence that the manipulation of food or fluid intake during the early puerperium has any effect on the quantity or quality of breast milk production or composition, although the nutritional status of the mother prior to and during pregnancy can in extreme deprivation have a significant effect. In spite of this, it is still common practice to attempt to manipulate solid and fluid intake in the first month after delivery. Such manipulations should be abandoned.

Women who have been delivered vaginally and who have not suffered a recognized postpartum haemorrhage should have their blood haemoglobin concentration or haematocrit checked within the first 36 hours of parturition, before the early haemodilution of the puerperium causes false low values. To avoid the side-effects of unnecessary iron supplementation only those with low values at this time should be treated. Following Caesarean section oral iron should be prescribed after 3 or 4 days since the blood loss is usually underestimated by the operator. When measured, it is rarely less than 400 ml and more commonly amounts to almost a litre (Pritchard et al 1962).

Postnatal pain

The pain following Caesarean section, its causes, management and the management of postoperative ileus are discussed in Chapter 39. During the first few days after vaginal delivery, the mother often experiences pain or discomfort from a variety of sources. These include perineal oedema or haematoma associated with tears and episiotomy, after pains from uterine contractions and breast engorgement. Less commonly, problems occur from superficial thrombophlebitis, prolapsed haemorrhoids or occasionally, postspinal headache. Often what is bearable discomfort by day becomes disturbing pain at night and causes sleeplessness. There should therefore be no hesitation in administering simple analgesics such as soluble aspirin 0.6 g or paracetamol 0.5–1.0 g as frequently as every 3 hours, if necessary and mefenamic acid for more severe pain. Although these drugs appear in breast milk, the quantity is so small that the parents can be safely reassured (Catz & Giacoia 1972, Briggs et al 1983).

For the relief of episiotomy paint a heat lamp has been a standard remedy, but in a hot environment it may produce more discomfort than relief. An ice bag, applied early frequently, and intermittently thereafter, tends to reduce swelling and allay discomfort and is equally useful for prolapsed, congested or thrombosed haemorrhoids. Local anaesthetic ointments are helpful at times to reduce the pain of haemorrhoids. Severe or persistent perineal pain is an indication for a careful examination of the area with a good light, since such pain is often due to a large vulvar, paravaginal or ischiorectal haematoma or abscess.

Constipation is still a common problem for some mothers in spite of early ambulation. Strong purgative drugs should be avoided but the mother should be encouraged to increase the roughage content of her diet and bran may be sprinkled over her cereals or vegetables. If this is inadequate, bulk-forming drugs should be prescribed such as ispaghula husk (e.g. Fybogel, Isogel, Regulan) or methylcellulose (e.g. Celevac, Colgel). When there is associated abdominal discomfort from gaseous distension, a low-volume modern enema can give much relief.

It was formerly believed that the use of abdominal binders helped involution of the uterus and the restoration of the mother's figure. They are no longer used. If the abdomen is unusually flabby or pendulous, an ordinary girdle is more satisfactory. Exercises to help restore tone to the abdominal wall muscles may be started at any time after vaginal delivery and as soon as the abdominal soreness diminishes after Caesarean section.

Psychosocial aspects of puerperal care

The great majority of babies are now delivered in hospital. This may be a large unit, staffed by specialist obstetricians, anaesthetists, paediatricians with full supporting services, or a small general practitioner hospital, but in both, midwives will normally be responsible for puerperal care of the majority of mothers.

A plan should be agreed antenatally for each mother's care to ensure that she has the support she needs both during her stay in hospital and after her return home, and that the advice she receives is consistent and that she gains confidence in her role as a parent. To ensure the plan is carried out effectively, there should be close liaison between the hospital, general practitioner, midwife and the community support services.

During her postnatal stay in hospital, whether this is for a few hours or few days, each mother should normally have her baby at her bedside and take responsibility for his or her care as soon as she is fit to do so. The baby should not be moved elsewhere unless it is at the mother's wish or unless there are over-riding medical reasons.

All mothers, especially those having their first baby, should be encouraged to discuss with staff anything that is worrying them and staff should find time to answer any questions. It is during the postnatal period that parental attitudes to their responsibilities for the maintenance of their health and that of their children and their expectations of professional aid may be influenced and established. Thus the relationships which are portrayed by the attitudes and actions of midwives, health visitors and doctors are of crucial importance. Openness should be encouraged to facilitate dialogue, to ensure that criticism and comment are helpful and to help parents gain confidence in caring for their family. (From Munro 1985, with permission of the Controller of Her Majesty's Stationery Office).

Many problems in the psychosocial field can be prevented or alleviated by education and planning in the antenatal period, reinforced by support and reassurance postpartum. Pregnant women should be forewarned about the mild depression and tearfulness which afflicts 50% of mothers during the first week, and reassured that it is likely to last only a few days at most. They should also be forewarned that, on the rare occasions when it does last for more than 4 days, they should seek medical help. One study has shown that 10–13% of puerperal women suffer from a more prolonged depression (Cox 1986). This often does not start till 3 or 4 weeks postpartum and may last for several weeks. Prominent factors in the genesis of both the early transient and the later and more prolonged depressive episodes include the emotional swing away from the elation immediately following delivery; the discomforts of the early puerperium; fatigue from lack of sleep during labour and postpartum in most hospital settings; the mother's anxiety over her ability to establish breastfeeding in the early days and her capability for caring for her infant in general after leaving hospital; and fears that she has become permanently less attractive to her husband.

The modern nuclear family often means that support from relations and neighbours during the later type of depressive phase is not available. It is the midwife, health visitor or family doctor who must be vigilant and offer support and reassurance. The prescription of mild hypnotic drugs to allow adequate sleep is often necessary and sometimes the use of tricyclic antidepressants for several weeks allows the mother to recover. If taken at night, they also promote sleep.

Sexual interest and libido may tend to take several

weeks to return and it is important that couples should be given advice antenatally that it is quite normal for a mother, especially if she is breastfeeding, not to recover her previous sex drive for sometimes as long as 9 months (Falicov 1973, Kenny 1973). The failure of couples to realize that it is quite normal for a new mother to be temporarily asexual often causes the husband at first to be bewildered and later disappointed; if the couple for any reason cannot discuss this problem with each other, the sexual aspect of their relationship may sustain permanent damage.

How long a mother and her baby should stay in hospital after delivery should be agreed antenatally as far as possible. The decision should take into account the parents' wishes, the adequacy of the physical home environment and the amount of help likely to be available to the mother from husband or partner, nearby relatives and friends and neighbours. Where the hospital environment is pleasant and not rushed, mothers elect to stay for more than 2–3 days for their first baby and even for subsequent babies provided the mother is confident that the care of her other children is satisfactory, although the current trend is for early return to the home environment.

Postnatal examination

A tradition has evolved that around 6 weeks' postpartum a formal postnatal examination is undertaken and, in most cases, the general practitioner is well placed to undertake this task. The actual physical examination is nowadays less important than the opportunity afforded to review the recent pregnancy and labour and the subsequent progress of the mother and baby. By this time the involution of the genital tract should be complete, all wounds should have healed, medical complications exacerbated by pregnancy (e.g. hypertension, diabetes) should have regressed, and menstruation may have recommenced in non-lactating mothers.

Where there have been any difficulties or complications during pregnancy, labour or the early puerperium, a full explanatory discussion is held with the mother, her questions are answered, and the likely course of the next pregnancy is explored in as much detail as seems appropriate. If there has been a perinatal death, or the birth of a low birthweight or deformed child, counselling techniques should include the reduction of parental guilt feelings as an important objective.

The method of family spacing or limitation should have been discussed antenatally and agreed in the early puerperium. This should now be reviewed and, if necessary, adjusted or revised. If the original decision was that an intrauterine device should be fitted, this is often a good opportunity for its insertion. Where desired, arrangements are made for later sterilization of husband or wife.

If it was not possible to give rubella vaccine in the early puerperium, a non-immune woman should be offered the appropriate injection.

PHYSIOLOGY OF LACTATION

Lactation is a physiological process which is common to all mammals; there is strong evidence of its evolutionary importance. Despite its central place in the natural reproductive cycle, many women find breastfeeding a difficult skill to learn and the human species is the only one in which lactation has been widely replaced by artificial feeding. Indeed, this change from breast- to bottlefeeding has been described as 'the largest uncontrolled in vivo experiment in human history' (Minchen 1985). An understanding of the physiology of lactation is necessary to understand the reasons for and the consequences of this widespread change from natural to artificial infant feeding.

Anatomy of the breast

The breast extends from the second to the sixth rib and from the sternum to the mid-axillary line with a tail extending into the axilla. It overlies the pectoralis major, serratus anterior and external oblique muscles. The main constituents of the breast are the glandular cells with their associated ducts, a very variable quantity of adipose tissue, connective tissue, blood vessels, nerves and lymphatics (Fig. 42.4). The gland lies in the superficial fascia of the thorax under its overlying skin. The lactiferous ducts lead to the nipple and dilate to form sinuses

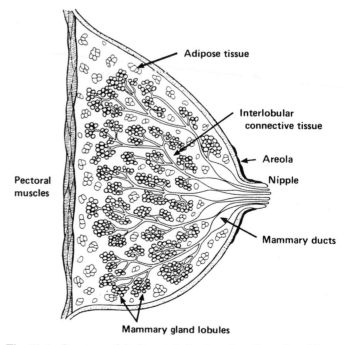

Fig. 42.4 Structure of the breast during lactation. Reproduced from Gardner & Dodds (1976) with permission.

immediately below the surface of the areola. The nipple is surrounded by the areola, a pigmented area of varying size which darkens during pregnancy. The areola contains sebaceous glands which hypertrophy and become prominent during pregnancy and are called Montgomery's tubercles. The areola is richly supplied with sensory nerves which are important during suckling (for a fuller description of the functional anatomy see Gould 1983). Throughout pregnancy the areola is said to be relatively insensitive to touch but this increases greatly immediately after delivery (Robinson & Short 1977). This change ensures that the suckling of the infant sends a stream of afferent neural impulses to the hypothalamus to control not only the process of lactation itself but also other important maternal adaptations which are discussed later.

The glandular tissue of the breast is derived from the ectoderm and is arranged in 15–20 ductal–lobular–alveolar systems (Fig. 42.4). The alveolar or secreting cells are grouped in grape-like bunches around the ductules which join to form the main ducts leading to the nipple. The alveolar cells are cuboidal cells in the resting breast which develop full secretory features during lactation. The alveolar cells are surrounded by oxytocin-sensitive contractile myoepithelial cells which play an important part in milk ejection. The ducts are lined by contractile longitudinal cells which, during the milk-ejection reflex, open the ducts widely to assist milk flow (McNeilly 1977).

Mammary growth and development

In the adult breast, four phases of mammary growth and development can be recognized. These are the resting phase, the development phase during pregnancy, the milk-secreting phase during lactation and the involutionary phase.

The human species is unusual in that a major degree of breast development occurs at puberty prior to pregnancy.

It seems likely that the reason for this is that the erotic significance of the female breast plays an important part in the attraction of male to female which is essential for human reproduction. At puberty, the milk ducts leading from the nipple branch and sprout and form a modest degree of alveolar development. The control of human breast development is not fully understood and current concepts come mainly from animal experiments in which ovaries, pituitary and adrenal are removed, followed by the replacement of hormones both individually and in combination (Cowie & Tindall 1961). These experiments suggest that mammary growth and development are under the control of multiple hormones and the exact role of each has not been precisely determined. At present it seems likely that proliferation of the ducts is primarily dependent upon oestrogen in conjunction with glucocorticoids and growth hormone (Fig. 42.5). On the other

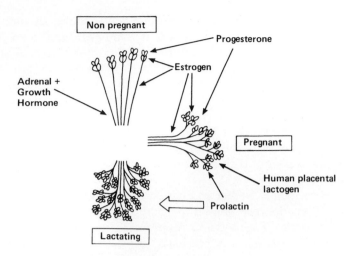

Fig. 42.5 Endocrine requirements for breast development and lactogenesis in the human. Lobulo-alveolar and ductal development appear to be steroid dependent with an undetermined role of prolactin or placental lactogen during pregnancy. Prolactin is essential for lactogenesis. Reproduced from McNeilly (1977) with permission.

hand, alveolar growth is stimulated by progesterone in the oestrogen-primed breast but may also require prolactin and prednisolone (Neville & Neifert 1983).

Once the adult breast has developed it requires only minimal stimulation by the appropriate hormones to begin milk secretion. As little as 14 days' exposure to the conjugated oestrogens followed by stimulation of prolactin secretion leads to the establishment of milk production. This sensitivity to endocrine stimuli has been used to encourage lactation in women who wish to suckle adopted infants (Auerbach & Avery 1981).

During early pregnancy there is a sharp increase in both ductal and alveolar elements of the mammary gland due to hyperplasia (Gould 1983), while during later pregnancy there is alveolar cell hypertrophy and the initiation of secretory activity. These changes during pregnancy are probably dependent upon the lactogenic hormones, prolactin and human placental lactogen, with placental oestrogens and progesterone playing an important modulatory role (Gould 1983). During human pregnancy, full milk production is inhibited by the high concentrations of progesterone (and possibly oestrogen) from the placenta and the copious milk production of established lactation does not occur until after parturition (McNeilly 1977).

Initiation and maintenance of lactation

Lactogenesis

Following parturition, there is a progressive rise in the volume of milk secreted by the breast and this is maintained in mothers who suckle their infants. During the first 30 hours after parturition, the early milk or colostrum has high concentrations of protein relative to the concentration of lactose (Fig. 42.6). During the next 3 days,

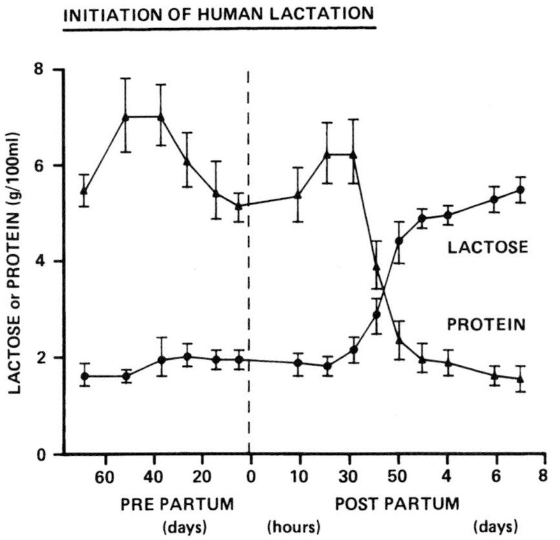

INITIATION OF HUMAN LACTATION

Fig. 42.6 Changes in lactose and protein concentrations in mammary secretions during the postpartum period, showing the sharp rise in lactose and the fall in protein concentration due to dilution. Reproduced from Kulski & Hartmann (1981) with permission.

the concentrations of lactose increase sharply under the influence of prolactin stimulation and, in order to maintain ionic equilibrium, water is drawn into the breast causing an increase in milk volume (Kulski & Hartmann 1981). At the same time, the concentrations of milk proteins fall due to a dilution effect, although the absolute amounts of the individual proteins remain constant or rise slowly (Hartmann et al 1984). After this phase of transitional milk formation, a relatively stable phase of mature milk production is reached at about day 5, after which there is a slow but steady increase in milk volume to a peak around 3 weeks' postpartum.

Galactopoiesis

Mothers who do not suckle their infants secrete some milk and this may persist for 3–4 weeks postpartum. The suckling stimulus, which releases both prolactin and oxytocin, is essential for the maintenance of lactation and these reflexes are discussed below. Provided that the breast is emptied regularly by sucking, lactation can be maintained for long periods and in some traditional communities will continue for 2 years or more (Buchanan 1975).

Most studies have estimated that after lactation is established, the average daily volume of milk production in a healthy, well-nourished mother is of the order of 750–800 ml/day (Whitehead et al 1980). More recently, studies in Australian women (Hartmann et al 1984) calculated a daily milk output of about 122 ml/day, which was in keeping with estimates made by Nims et al in the 1930s (Nims et al 1932). Differences between estimates of milk volume may also reflect the suckling practices

of the populations studied, because feeding regimens involving greater mother–infant contact may increase milk production. Mothers who are feeding twins produce twice as much milk as mothers feeding singletons (Hartmann et al 1984), strongly suggesting that suckling, which is doubled in the case of twins, is the key to milk production.

The influence of maternal diet on milk production has not been clearly defined and only small differences have been observed between Swedish and Ethiopian mothers and British and Gambian mothers (Whitehead et al 1980). It may be that babies of poorly nourished mothers have to suckle more intensively and for longer to achieve an adequate milk supply (Lunn 1985).

Prolactin and milk production

Prolactin is a long-chain polypeptide hormone which is secreted from the anterior pituitary gland in response to suckling and is essential for successful lactation.

The mechanism by which prolactin secretion is controlled is a topic of much research; current knowledge is summarized in Figure 42.7. The suckling stimulus of the baby sends afferent impulses to the hypothalamus, leading to a surge of prolactin release. Prolactin release is controlled by prolactin inhibitory factors secreted into the pituitary portal blood system; dopamine is generally considered to be the most important. The suckling-induced burst of prolactin secretion from the pituitary may be induced by the inhibition of dopamine release

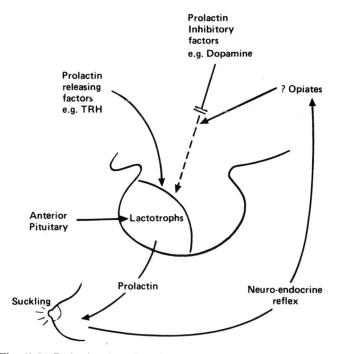

Fig. 42.7 Prolactin release is mainly under the control of prolactin inhibitory factors (dopamine) but can also be stimulated by prolactin-releasing factors (TRH-Hyrotropin-releasing hormone). Suckling may release prolactin by an opiate-mediated inhibitor of dopamine.

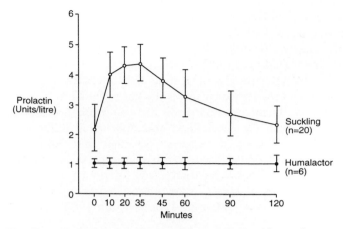

Fig. 42.8 Prolactin release in response to normal suckling and Humalactor. The Humalactor does not stimulate the nipple directly and fails to achieve effective prolactin release. Adapted from Howie et al (1980).

from the hypothalamus, although the mechanisms for control of dopamine release are not fully understood.

In response to suckling, prolactin levels rise quickly to reach a peak about 30 minutes after the baby is put to the breast and then progressively decline to reach presuckling levels after about 120 minutes (Howie et al 1980). Areolar stimulation is essential for prolactin release because the Humalactor, a breast pump which empties the breast by negative pressure, does not stimulate the nipple to release prolactin (Fig. 42.8). Basal prolactin levels are high in the immediate postpartum period and progressively decline after the sixth postpartum week at a rate which is dependent upon suckling frequency and duration (Delvoye et al 1977, Howie et al 1981a). The peak levels of prolactin achieved in response to suckling also decline progressively over time (Glasier et al 1984b).

Prolactin has a diurnal variation, being higher during hours of sleep, and it has been shown that prolactin responses to suckling are higher in the evening hours compared with those achieved earlier in the same day (Glasier et al 1984b). These considerations suggest that prolactin production is increased by frequent suckling at regular intervals throughout the 24 hours, including the night time, and that feeding practices which encourage such suckling patterns will produce optimal milk volumes. The relationship between prolactin and milk volume is complex.

The action of prolactin is to bind to receptors on the alveolar milk-secreting cells of the breast. Prolactin appears to act at multiple sites to stimulate the synthesis of several milk components, including casein, lactalbumin (which may regulate lactose synthesis), fatty acids and other constituents. It appears that prolactin interaction with the plasma membrane of the alveolar cells sets in motion a series of intracellular events which lead to the synthesis and secretion of all milk components (Neville & Berga 1983).

The importance of prolactin to lactogenesis can be demonstrated clinically because the administration in the early puerperium of bromocriptine, a dopamine agonist, rapidly reduces prolactin levels and abolishes milk production (Rolland & Schellekens 1973). There is conflicting evidence about the exact quantitative relationship between prolactin levels and milk production. On the one hand there is no correlation between prolactin levels and milk production in the early puerperium (Howie et al 1980) and mothers who have had pituitary surgery can breastfeed successfully despite having prolactin levels just above the non-pregnant range (Franks et al 1977). On the other hand dopamine receptor-blocking drugs, such as metoclopramide and sulpride, raise prolactin levels and appear to improve milk production, especially in mothers with failing lactation (Aono et al 1979, Ylikorkala et al 1982). It seems that at least basal levels of prolactin are required for milk production but that above a certain threshold the absolute levels of prolactin do not by themselves dictate the volume of milk produced.

Oxytocin and the milk-ejection reflex

The milk-ejection reflex is responsible for transferring milk from the secreting glands of the breast to the baby. The milk-ejection reflex mimics the prolactin reflex in some respects, insofar as both are initiated by suckling and mediated by afferent neural impulses from the areola to the hypothalamus. They are, however, quite separate physiologically and have important differences.

The milk-ejection reflex is mediated by the hormone oxytocin, an octapeptide synthesized in specialized magnocellular neurones in the supraoptic and paraventricular nuclei of the hypothalamus. The neuroendocrine reflex leading to oxytocin release can be initiated not just by the suckling of the infant, but also by the mother handling the baby, hearing its cry or even just thinking of feeding. In one mother who was feeding twins, McNeilly & McNeilly (1978) noted that regular spontaneous let-down could occur even in the absence of suckling. At 2 weeks' postpartum, let-down occurred at 30-minute intervals, increasing to 4-hourly intervals at 4 months' postpartum. It is of interest that the frequency of these let-down reflexes has close parallels with the observed nursing frequency in traditional hunter-gathering communities such as the !Kung in the Kalahari desert (Konner & Worthman 1980). Frequent suckling may have been the true norm for the human species until relatively recent times.

In animal studies, a burst of electrical activity in oxytocic neurones can be measured 10–15 seconds prior to milk ejection, indicating that nerve depolarization is the stimulus for oxytocin release (Poulain et al 1977). In contrast to prolactin, oxytocin is released in short bursts lasting less than a minute and frequently the largest release of oxytocin occurs in response to the cry of the baby before feeding begins (McNeilly et al 1983; Fig. 42.9).

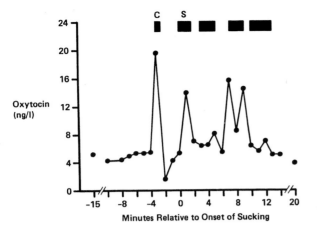

Fig. 42.9 Release of oxytocin in response to an infant's cry (C) and to suckling episodes (S), showing the importance of the presuckling stimuli in stimulating the let-down reflex. Reproduced from McNeilly et al (1983) with permission.

This understanding of the prefeeding release of oxytocin may explain, at least in part, why rooming-in of mother and baby is associated with successful breastfeeding (Cruse et al 1978).

The action of oxytocin is to bind to specific receptors on the myoepithelial cells of the breast, thereby causing them to contract. These myoepithelial cells are placed around the milk-secreting cells of the mammary gland and longitudinally in the walls of milk ducts. When the milk-ejection reflex occurs, the contraction of the myoepithelial cells around the alveoli expels the milk into the ducts (McNeilly 1977). The flow of milk to the nipple is facilitated by the wide opening of the ducts which is induced by contraction of the longitudinal oxytocin-sensitive cells in the duct walls. When the milk-ejection reflex is well established, a mother may be aware of milk being spontaneously ejected from one breast while she suckles her baby on the other.

The milk-ejection reflex is very sensitive to emotional stress (Newton & Newton 1950) and the adverse effects of threatening or discouraging remarks to the nursing mother may act in this way. Inhibition of oxytocin release may occur but catecholamines released by stress may cause constriction of the mammary vessels and prevent oxytocin access to the myoepithelial cells.

It is clear that the milk-ejection reflex is complementary to the prolactin reflex and both pathways are required for successful lactation. Various studies have suggested that pharmacological stimulation of both the oxytocin (Huntingford 1961) and the prolactin (Aono et al 1979, Ylikorkala et al 1982) pathways can improve lactation, although more work is required to define their place in clinical practice.

Infant sucking and milk transfer

In addition to milk secretion and ejection by the mother,

effective sucking by the infant is also an important part of successful breastfeeding. It is now clear that effective stripping of the milk during sucking is a very important stimulus for the maintenance of milk production (Woolridge et al 1990). In contrast to bottlefeeding, where the baby obtains the milk by negative pressure, breastfeeding involves milking of the cisterns of the breast which lie deep to the nipple. To do this, the baby must take the whole nipple into its mouth and place its tongue under the adjacent areola. A baby properly fixed in this way will milk the cisterns with its tongue and, aided by the milk-ejection reflex, will establish a good milk flow. One of the most important aspects in the clinical management of breastfeeding is to ensure that the baby is properly fixed. This can be assisted by encouraging the rooting reflex of the baby with the smell and feel of the nipple around its mouth. This makes the baby open its mouth widely and fix properly on the breast.

Detailed observation of babies during breastfeeding have shown two distinct sucking patterns which have been described as nutritive and non-nutritive sucking. Nutritive sucking is characterized by a continuous stream of strong, slow sucks while non-nutritive sucking shows an alternation of rapid shallow bursts of sucking with rests (Drewett & Woolridge 1979). Nutritive sucking occurs predominantly at the beginning of the feed and is increasingly replaced by non-nutritive sucking as the feed progresses. As a result of the changing sucking pattern, the greatest proportion of milk transfer occurs in the early part of the feed (Lucas et al 1979). In one study, over 75% of milk transfer occurred in the first 10 minutes of a 20-minute feed, although considerable variation was observed among different mothers (Howie et al 1981b). The varying patterns of sucking and milk transfer indicate that it is inappropriate to manage breastfeeding on the basis of arbitrary time schedules and the duration of a feed should be determined by the infant's response.

The physiological function of non-nutritive sucking is not clearly understood. It may be that the baby derives comfort from the close mother–infant contact but the additional sucking may also be responsible for additional prolactin release and the regulation of maternal fertility and energy balance, which are discussed later.

Mechanisms of milk secretion

A number of separate pathways are involved in the synthesis and secretion of milk products by the mammary alveolar cells. These are summarized below; a more detailed description has been given by Neville et al (1983).

Exocytosis

Many of the major components of milk, including lactose, proteins, calcium and phosphate, are packaged into secretory vesicles and secreted by exocytosis. The amino acid sequences of the milk proteins are coded in the nuclear DNA and transcribed into messenger RNA (mRNA) which moves into the cytoplasm. Under the influence of mRNA, protein synthesis occurs and the protein molecules are transferred to the Golgi system for further processing into secretory vesicles. These vesicles subsequently move to the apex of the cell and are discharged by the process of exocytosis into the alveolar lumina.

Secretion of ions and water

According to one hypothesis the major milk sugar, lactose, is synthesized when the membrane-bound enzyme, galactosyltransferase, interacts with the protein alpha-lactalbumin within the Golgi system. The Golgi system is impermeable to lactose so that an osmotic gradient is set up which attracts water into the alveolar cell. Electrolytes follow the water according to their electrochemical gradients. Chloride, however, is out of equilibrium with its concentration in the cytoplasm and it is postulated that there must be an active transport mechanism to move chloride back into the cell.

Lipid secretion

Lipid secretion is controlled by a different mechanism from the one responsible for lactose and protein synthesis. The lipids in breast milk are mainly triglycerides and are synthesized in the cytoplasm and smooth endoplasmic reticulum of the alveolar cells. The triglycerides coalesce to form fat droplets which migrate to the apex of the cell and are secreted by a mechanism which does not involve the Golgi apparatus.

Secretion of immunoglobulins

Immunoglobulin A is the principal immune protein in milk and with some other proteins can combine with specific receptors on the alveolar basement membrane before being internalized in a secretory vesicle and transported to the apex of the cell for secretion into the lumen.

Paracellular pathway

Some substances may pass between the gaps in the alveolar cells into the milk and this may be the pathway by which leucocytes and other cells enter the milk. During pregnancy and involution of the breasts, these gaps are relatively leaky but during full lactation the junctions between alveolar cells are much tighter and less permeable.

Constituents of breast milk

The composition of milk varies greatly among species, suggesting that evolution has developed specific milks suited to the needs of the young of each species (Hartmann et al 1984). Studies of human milk composition show that the concentrations of the various constituents are not constant; the constituents vary from one mother to another and in any one mother the milk content varies between one feed to another on the same day and even between the beginning and the end of the same feed. Probably the most important variable is the length of time postpartum, suggesting that the milk content adapts to meet the needs of the infant at any particular stage of development.

These considerations suggest that mother's milk is adapted to meet the needs of the young in a sensitive way which cannot be matched by artificial feeds. It also means that any statements about milk composition merely reflect an average value, around which there is considerable individual variation.

The composition of mature human milk is used as a guide for the preparation of artificial feeds; the recommended figures for some of the major constituents are shown in Table 42.1.

Carbohydrates

Human milk contains one of the highest concentrations of carbohydrate of any mammal, mainly in the form of lactose. The dramatic rise in the synthesis of lactose in the first few days after delivery is one of the main features of the transition from colostrum to mature milk. The intestinal enzyme lactase, which is responsible for the hydrolysis and subsequent absorption of lactose, develops late in fetal life so that any intestinal inflammation which interferes with lactase function will lead to lactose intolerance and diarrhoea. When lactose is digested it yields a mixture of galactose and glucose so that lactose is not considered to be an essential sugar. The reason for the high lactose content in human milk is not clear but may be important in controlling stool acidity and the characteristics of the intestinal flora.

Protein

Compared with cows' milk, the total protein content of

Table 42.1 Approximate composition of various constituents in human milk and cows' milk (from Jelliffe B & Jelliffe P 1978)

	Human milk	Cows' milk
Energy (kcal/ml)	75	66
Protein (g/100 ml)	1.1	3.5
Casein (%)	40	82
Whey proteins (%)	60	18
Lactose (g/100 ml)	6.8	4.9
Fat (g/100 ml)	4.5	3.7
Sodium (mEq)	7	20
Chloride (mEq)	11	29

human milk is much less and about 40% is in the form of casein. This means that the curds formed in human milk are much softer, more flocculent and more easily digestible for the intestinal tract. The remaining proteins are called whey proteins; they represent a mixture of soluble proteins left after the casein curd has formed. Many of these soluble proteins, such as the immunoglobulins, lactoferrin and lysozyme, are important for the anti-infective qualities of human milk and these are discussed below.

Human milk contains high concentrations of alpha-lactalbumin and, although it has been proposed as a regulator of lactose synthesis, a direct correlation between lactose and alpha-lactalbumin levels has yet to be established (Kulski & Hartmann 1981).

Fat

Lipid, which appears mainly as triglycerides, is the most variable constituent of human milk, the highest concentrations appearing in the hind-milk as milk fat globules. Fat is the major source of energy in human milk so that the estimated calorific value of 75 kcal/100 ml is at best only an approximation. The fat content of human milk is also important as the carrier of the fat-soluble vitamins A, D, E and K and of the essential fatty acids. Deficiency of vitamin D can lead to rickets, while that of vitamin K may lead to haemorrhagic disease of the newborn. The fatty acid composition of the triglycerides can vary according to the maternal diet; the influence of these dietary variations during infancy on subsequent vascular disease is a topic of interest and controversy (Hartmann et al 1984).

Minerals

Compared with cows' milk, human milk has low concentrations of sodium, chloride, iron and some other minerals. The low levels of sodium and chloride are advantageous in infants with diarrhoea because milks with a high solute load can aggravate dehydration. The concentration of iron is low (0.5 μmol/ml) in human milk and many clinicians advise iron supplements in breastfed babies. There is however a much higher absorption of iron from breast milk (> 75%) compared with cows' milk (30%) or iron-supplemented infant formula (10%; Saarinen & Siimes 1979) and although the reason for the greater bioavailability of iron from breast milk is not known, its binding to lactoferrin in human milk may be responsible.

Nutritional adequacy of breast milk

The nutritional adequacy of breast milk is a matter of controversy. Most authorities recommend that breast milk alone is sufficient to meet infants' nutritional needs until between 4 and 6 months of age. In practice most UK mothers introduce supplementary foods before this and a World Health Organization (WHO) Survey (1981) involving 27 different socioeconomic groups throughout the world showed that this was generally true. On the other hand, two studies of well-nourished mothers from the USA (Ahn & McLean 1980) and Australia (Hartmann & Prosser 1984) have shown that some mothers can adequately sustain their babies on breast milk alone for longer than this. By 8 months, however, faltering in growth will occur on breast milk alone and supplements are needed. In Western Australia, 12% of nursing mothers were giving breast milk as the sole form of fluid at 1 year with additional solids, indicating that breast milk can make a major contribution to infant nutrition well into infancy. The nutritional adequacy of breast milk is very variable, depending upon the success of milk production; clinical decisions must be made for individuals on the basis of the infant's progress.

Mammary function during weaning

During the process of weaning there is a loss of secretory activity by the mammary gland (Prosser et al 1984). When weaning is abrupt the concentrations of potassium, glucose and lactose decrease while those of sodium, chloride and protein increase. During gradual weaning the changes are similar but occur over a longer period of time. If conception occurs during lactation the rising levels of placental steroids inhibit milk secretion and this overrides the positive stimulus of the infants' suckling.

Following the cessation of regular suckling the mammary gland quickly ceases secretory activity and enters a phase of regression. The milk in the ducts and alveoli is resorbed and although there is a decrease in parenchymal elements, the breast does not return to its prenatal state as many alveoli persist.

Anti-infective properties of breast milk

Breast milk contains a number of proteins with anti-microbial activity. The anti-infective properties of breast milk are an important protection for the suckling infant, especially in areas with infected water supplies, and the antimicrobial proteins may also protect the breasts against infection and abscess formation (Hartmann et al 1984).

Lactoferrin

Lactoferrin is an iron-binding glycoprotein which inhibits bacterial growth non-specifically. *Escherichia coli* have a high requirement for free iron; lactoferrin, with its high affinity for iron, may restrict the growth of pathogenic iron-dependent bacteria. The action of lactoferrin may be low in the stomach as little iron is protein bound in an acidic environment. In the proximal duodenum, however, bicarbonate secretion will favour the binding of iron to lactoferrin and enhance its bacteriostatic action in the intestinal tract.

Lysozyme

Lysozyme is a cationic protein which is present in concentrations of 30–40 mg/100 ml of human milk. Its bactericidal activity is mediated by its ability to cleave proteoglycans in the cell walls of a number of Gram-positive and Gram-negative bacteria. The activity is promoted by other milk components, especially IgA. Lysozyme is stable in the gut because active material is present in the faeces of breastfed babies.

Immunoglobulins

The major immunoglobulin in breast milk is IgA, with smaller amounts of IgM and IgG. The concentration of IgA is particularly high in colostrum and, although the concentration of IgA falls to about 2 mg/ml in mature milk, the daily yield remains relatively constant. The IgA in breast milk is poorly absorbed and persists in the infant's gastrointestinal tract to protect against infection. The high concentration of IgA in colostrum enables it to enter the proteoglycan lining of the gastrointestinal tract and may provide initial surface protection (Watson 1980).

Specific IgA antibodies, mostly against gastrointestinal pathogens, are also present in human milk (Bezkorovainy 1979). The mechanism of their formation is illustrated in Figure 42.10. It is suggested that if the mother meets

a potential pathogen in her own gastrointestinal tract, the antigen is taken up by the gut-associated lymphoid tissue in the Peyer's patches of her terminal ileum. Plasma cells are formed which migrate to the breast where specific IgA is secreted into the breast milk. In this way, the mother is able to give her specific protection against endemic pathogens in her environment. This remarkable interaction between mother and baby is, of course, a mechanism which cannot be replicated by artificial feeds.

Other anti-infective factors

Human milk contains a growth factor for *Lactobacillus bifidus* which facilitates colonization with this organism, which competes with intestinal pathogens. Breast milk also contains cells in the form of macrophages and leucocytes, small amounts of complement and lactoperoxidases; their importance as anti-infective agents in vivo has not been defined.

Breastfeeding and infant infection

Numerous studies have demonstrated a major protective effect of breastfeeding against childhood infective illnesses, particularly gastrointestinal disease, in developing countries (Plank & Milanesi 1973, Habicht et al 1986). This protection amounts to a two-fold reduction in infant mortality and substantial improvements in morbidity.

Recent studies from developed countries, which have taken careful account of potential confounding factors, have shown that breastfeeding also protects infants against gastrointestinal disease in developed countries (Fergusson et al 1981, Kovar et al 1984). This effect, which depends upon breastfeeding being maintained for 13 weeks (Fig. 42.11), will reduce the incidence of infants' hospital admission and is maintained during the first year of life even after breastfeeding has stopped (Howie et al 1990).

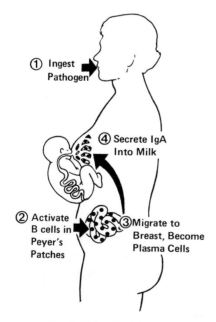

Fig. 42.10 Pathways involved in the secretion of IgA in breast milk by the enteromammary circulation Figure kindly provided by Professor R.V.Short, Monash University, Australia.

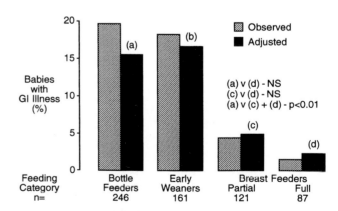

Fig. 42.11 Rates of gastrointestinal illness during the first 13 weeks of life (▨ = observed rates; ■ = rates adjusted for confounding variables) according to infant feeding method (bottle fed from birth; early weaning before 13 weeks; partial and full breast feeding for 13 weeks). Adapted from Howie et al (1990).

Maternal adaptations during lactation

During lactation, two physiological maternal adaptations take place, both of which have important practical implications. These are, first, the natural inhibition of the mother's fertility and, second, changes in maternal energy utilization which enable her to use her calories more efficiently.

Fertility after childbirth

Because of the importance of breast milk to the suckling infant, it is not surprising that maternal fertility is suppressed during lactation. In this way the baby is not prematurely displaced from the breast by a new sibling, because breast milk tends to decline during pregnancy. There is also good evidence that both maternal and child health are improved by adequate birth intervals (Morley 1977). It is therefore important to understand and maximize the natural interbirth intervals induced by breastfeeding.

Postpartum fertility in bottle- and breastfeeding mothers
Mothers who do not breastfeed have an early resumption of menstruation, ovulation and the potential for fertility. On the basis of basal body temperature rises, the earliest that ovulation has been observed after delivery is 4 weeks (Udesky 1950), although it is unusual before 5 weeks and more commonly delayed until 8–10 weeks postpartum (Howie et al 1982). Most non-lactating mothers will have resumed ovulation and menstruation by 15 weeks' postpartum. The first postpartum cycle in bottlefeeding mothers is frequently anovular (80%) or associated with an inadequate luteal phase (McNeilly et al 1982b). By the third cycle normal ovulation and luteal activity have been restored. In non-lactating women who use no contraception, 50% will have conceived by about 6–7 months postpartum (Potter et al 1965, Berman et al 1972). In contrast, breastfeeding women experience a period of lactational amenorrhoea and reduced fertility. The duration of lactational amenorrhoea varies greatly among different populations and among women within the same population. In many developing countries, lactational amenorrhoea may last for 2 years or more, whereas in developed countries menstruation and fertility may be delayed only for a few weeks (Howie & McNeilly 1982, Gross & Eastman 1985). During the greatest part of lactational amenorrhoea, ovulation is suppressed and conception cannot occur. In the 4 weeks prior to the end of lactational amenorrhoea, ovarian activity will return and 30–70% of these cycles will be ovulatory (Udesky 1950, Perez et al 1972). The longer the period of lactational amenorrhoea, the greater the chance of ovulation in the cycle prior to first menstruation (Howie et al 1982). The number of women conceiving during lactational amenorrhoea has been reported as between 1% and 10%

(Buchanan 1975), but may well be lower than this (Kennedy & Visness 1992). After the return of menstrual cycles during lactation, the potential for fertility increases but does not return to normal because many of the cycles are either anovular or associated with inadequate luteal function (McNeilly et al 1982b). On a global scale, lactational amenorrhoea is of great importance for fertility rates in countries where contraceptive usage is low. It has been estimated that in developing countries breastfeeding prevents more pregnancies than all other methods of family planning combined (Rosa 1975).

Endocrine changes after delivery

The normal endocrine control of ovarian function and how it may be modified by suckling are summarized in Figure 42.12. In response to the pulse generator in the hypothalamus, GnRH is released into the hypophyseal portal blood system. This provokes a pulsatile release of LH from the pituitary which, in combination with FSH, stimulates follicle development and oestradiol secretion in the ovary. The oestradiol promotes further follicle growth and by positive feedback stimulates the preovulatory LH surge and ovulation (McNeilly et al 1985).

During pregnancy, the high levels of placental steroids suppress the pituitary secretion of both LH and FSH to about 1% of normal (McNeilly 1979). After delivery, oestrogen and progesterone levels fall and in bottlefeeding mothers, plasma FSH and LH rise to early follicular phase levels by about 3 weeks' postpartum to stimulate ovarian activity (Glasier et al 1983).

The mechanisms which lead to the suppression of ovarian activity during lactation are not fully understood but inhibition may occur in two ways (for review see McNeilly et al 1993). In the first place, suckling induces changes in the sensitivity of the hypothalamic–pituitary axis to oestrogen, making it more sensitive to the negative feedback effects of ovarian steroids and less sensitive to positive feedback (Baird et al 1979). As a result, there is inhibition of GnRH, leading to diminished or inappropriate secretion of LH (Glasier et al 1983). When there is sufficient gonadotrophin to stimulate a small follicle during lactation, oestrogens inhibit further pulsatile LH release from the pituitary because of the changed sensitivity to feedback and prevent further follicle development (Glasier et al 1984a). As the suckling stimulus declines there is progressive recovery of gonadotrophin levels and menstrual cycles may return during lactation. Many of the cycles remain abnormal, being either anovular or having inadequate luteal phases, and these may be due to suboptimal gonadotrophin stimulation (McNeilly et al 1985).

In the second place, the prolactin which is released during suckling may contribute to ovarian inhibition during lactation. Prolactin may have a direct inhibitory

ENDOCRINE CONTROL. I

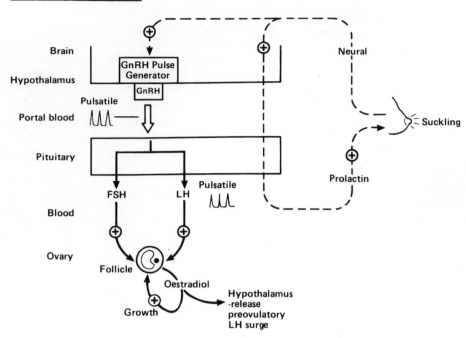

Fig. 42.12 Schematic diagram of the hypothalamic control of gonadotrophin secretion. Gonadotrophin releasing hormone (GnRH) pulses from the hypothalamus induce luteinizing hormone (LH) pulses from the pituitary which control follicle development and ovulation. Suckling, either through a direct neural input or by increased prolactin secretion, alters LH pulse secretion through an action on the GnRH pulse generator. Reproduced FSH = follicle stimulating hormone from McNeilly et al (1985) with permission.

effect on the ovary or may, through a short-loop feedback effect, contribute to the reduced gonadotrophin secretion from the pituitary (McNeilly et al 1982a). At present there is no direct evidence that prolactin plays a part in ovarian inhibition during lactation and its exact role has yet to be defined.

In countries where contraceptive usage is low, breastfeeding makes an important contribution to birth spacing and completed family size. It is clearly important not to change breastfeeding practices in countries with low contraceptive usage without fully appreciating their implications for fertility. In Africa, Asia and Latin America, contraceptive usage would have to increase sharply to keep fertility rates at their present levels if the average duration of lactational amenorrhoea was to fall (Howie 1992).

Breastfeeding, although having an important influence on fertility at a population level, is often regarded as an unreliable method of contraception for individual women. In 1988, an interdisciplinary group met in Bellagio, Italy and produced a consensus on how breastfeeding could serve as a safe and effective family planning method (Kennedy et al 1989). The guidelines (Fig. 42.13) depend upon the evidence that a mother who is still amenorrhoeic and fully breastfeeding has more than 98% protection from pregnancy during the first 6 months' postpartum.

Studies which have looked at the validity of the method of lactational amenorrhoea have shown that the continuation of lactational amenorrhoea is the most important index of continuing protection against returning fertility (Kennedy & Visness 1992). Although it does not give complete protection against conception, lactational amenorrhoea is a method of spacing pregnancies which can be valuable for many individual couples.

Maternal energy requirements during lactation

For lactating mothers the daily calorie intake recommended by WHO is 2700 kcal for the first 6 months and 2950 kcal from 6 months onwards (FAO Nutritional Studies 1950). This figure is reached by the arithmetic calculation of 2200 kcal for normal non-lactating non-pregnancy requirements plus an additional 500 kcal for the overall energy cost of the milk. Assuming an average milk volume, the average calorie value of breast milk is 750 kcal/day, which is supplemented from the maternal fat stores laid down during pregnancy to the tune of 250 kcal/day. At the end of 6 months it is assumed that the available fat stores will have been used up and an additional dietary supplement of 250 kcal/day will be required.

Observational studies on healthy lactating women in developed countries have shown that their actual calorie

Ask the mother:

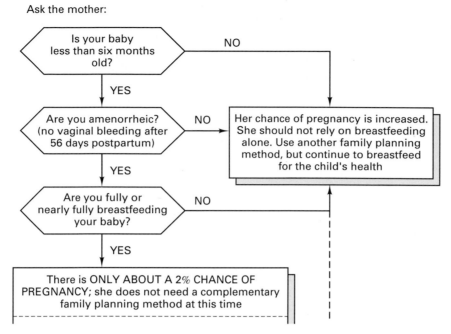

Fig. 42.13 Diagrammatic representation of the application of the lactational amenorrhoea method of fertility control for breastfeeding mothers.

intakes based on measured portions of food do not reach the theoretical recommendations. For example, Whitehead et al (1981) reported 2300 kcal/day and Butte et al (1984) reported 2170 kcal/day in mothers who had no limitation on food availability and successfully breastfed their babies. In developing countries the gap between theoretical and actual food intake is even greater. Prentice et al (1981) found that Gambian mothers took 1773 kcal/day in the dry season and 1474 kcal/day in the less plentiful wet season and, despite the calorie shortfall, breastfed their babies successfully for prolonged periods.

One possible reason for this discrepancy between the theoretical and actual energy requirements of nursing mothers is an increase in energy efficiency during lactation. Animal studies have shown that lactation is associated with an inhibition of non-shivering thermogenesis, leading to storage of all available dietary calories to be used in milk formation. In the mouse this is achieved by physiological inhibition of brown-fat cells which, in the non-lactating state, can burn off excess calories (Trayhurn et al 1982). In this way the lactating animal becomes energy efficient. Recent studies have shown that a similar adaptation takes place in nursing mothers (Illingworth et al 1986), although the biological mechanism in the human probably does not occur through brown fat. Compared with the bottlefeeding mother, the lactating mother shows an increased sensitivity to insulin (Illingworth et al 1986) and although the biological mechanisms have not been fully defined, it is clear that nursing itself harbours maternal energy resources for the benefit of the sucking infant.

This concept of maternal energy adaptation during lactation has two potential implications. First, it means that a mother who eats according to the WHO recommendations may fail to lose weight in the postpartum period. Secondly, mothers who bottlefeed in developing countries will lose the energy-sparing effect and society will have to provide more calories to meet the needs of the mother–infant pair. Further research is required to define the biological mechanism and practical implications of this physiological adaptation in nursing mothers.

Health advantages of breastfeeding

In recent years, research has identified a number of important benefits of breastfeeding particularly for preterm babies. In particular, breast milk can reduce the incidence of neonatal necrotizing enterocolitis in preterm babies with an estimated potential saving of 100 lives per year in the UK (Lucas & Cole 1990). In addition, there is some evidence that the feeding of breast milk to preterm babies may be associated with higher subsequent intelligence quotients (Lucas et al 1992). It is a pity that the problems of quarantine for breast milk due to the HIV epidemic have greatly undermined the availability of banked breast milk for preterm babies but, wherever possible, mothers should be encouraged to provide their own milk for preterm infants.

Other advantages for breastfeeding, for which there is now published evidence, include reduced levels of childhood diabetes (Borch-Johnson et al 1984, Mayer et al 1988) and childhood cancer, especially lymphoma (Davis et al 1988), and protection against premenopausal breast cancer (McTiernan & Thomas 1986, United Kingdom National Case-Control Study Group 1993). These reports require to be confirmed by further research but suggest that the benefits of breastfeeding have not yet been fully defined.

Management of breastfeeding

Despite the many advantages of breastfeeding there is evidence of its decline in many countries although this is not universal (WHO 1993).

WHO/UNICEF made a joint statement outlining 'Ten steps to successful breast feeding'. Six of these are relevant to the development of personnel supporting new mothers.

1. Have a written breastfeeding policy.
2. Train all staff.
3. Inform all pregnant women about the benefits and management of breasfeeding.
4. Help mothers to initiate breastfeeding within half an hour of birth.
5. Show mothers how to breastfeed.
6. Foster the establishment of breastfeeding support groups.

Two of the steps relate to rooming-in and are:

7. Practise 24-hour rooming-in.
8. Encourage breastfeeding on demand.

The final two relate to alternative sucking and are:

9. Give newborn infants no other food or drink, unless medically indicated.
10. Use no artificial teats.

A major complaint from many mothers is the conflicting advice which they receive from health professionals. The details of how to manage breastfeeding are beyond the scope of this chapter but there are now several texts on best practice (Royal College of Midwives 1988, Renfrew et al 1990). It is essential that all who are involved in the care of new mothers should understand the mechanisms and management of successful breastfeeding.

Conclusion

Lactation is an important part of natural human reproduction. Efforts by modern civilization to replace lactation by artificial substitutes do not detract from its physiological relevance or its practical importance in developing countries. The primary function of lactation is to nourish the infant and human milk is the ideal food for the human baby. Important secondary features of breastfeeding are the anti-infective, contraceptive and energy-sparing effects. Policies relating to the initiation and maintenance of breastfeeding, the appropriate use of supplements, contraceptive advice for nursing mothers and maternal diet must all be based on a sound understanding of the physiology of lactation.

REFERENCES

Acar B, Fleming R, Macnaughton M C, Coutts J R 1981 Ovarian function in women immediately post-partum. Obstetrics and Gynaecology 57: 468–472
Ahn C H, MacLean W C 1980 Growth of the exclusively breast fed infant. American Journal of Clinical Nutrition 33: 183–192
Aono T, Shioji T, Aki T, Hirota K, Nomura K, Kurachi K 1979 Augmentation of puerperal lactation by sulpiride. Journal of Clinical Endocrinology and Metabolism 48: 478–482
Appleby J I. Norymberski J K 1957 The urinary excretion of 17-hydroxy-corticosteroids in human pregnancy. Journal of Endocrinology 15: 310–319
Auerbach K G, Avery J L 1981 Induced lactation; a study of adoptive nursing by 240 women. American Journal of Diseases of Children 135: 340–343
Baird D T, McNeilly A S, Sawers R S, Sharpe R M 1979 Failure of estrogen-induced discharge of luteinising hormone in lactating women. Journal of Clinical Endocrinology and Metabolism 49: 500–506
Bayliss R I S, Browne J C McC, Round B P, Steinbeck A W 1955 Plasma 17-hydroxycorticosteroids in pregnancy. Lancet i: 62–64
Berman M L, Hanson K, Hillman I L 1972 Effect of breast feeding on post-partum menstruation, ovulation and pregnancy in Alaskan Eskimos. American Journal of Obstetrics and Gynecology 114: 524–534
Bezkorovainy A 1979 Breast-feeding — aid to infant health and fertility control. Population Reports Series J 4: 49–66
Borch-Johnsen K, Joner G, Mandrup-Poulsen T et al 1984 Relation between breast-feeding and incidence rates of insulin-dependent diabetes mellitus. Lancet ii: 1083–1086

Bonnar J 1975 The blood coagulation and fibrinolytic systems during pregnancy. Clinics in Obstetrics and Gynaecology 2: 321
Briggs C G, Bodendorfer T W, Freeman R K 1983 Drugs in pregnancy and lactation. A reference guide to neonatal risk. Williams & Wilkins, Baltimore
Broughton-Pipkin F B, Oats J J, Symonds E M 1978 Sequential changes in the human renin–angiotensin system following delivery. British Journal of Obstetrics and Gynaecology 85: 821
Buchanan R 1975 Breast-feeding-aid to infant health and fertility control. Population Reports Series J 4: 49–66
Butte N F, Garza C, Stuff J E, Smith E O, Nichols B J 1984 Effect of maternal diet and body composition on lactational performance. American Journal of Clinical Nutrition 39: 296–306
Catz C S, Giacoia G P 1972 Drugs in breast milk. Pediatric Clinics of North America 19: 151–166
Cowie A T, Tindall J S 1961 The maintenance of lactation in the goat after hypophysectomy. Journal of Endocrinology 23: 79–96
Cox J L 1986 Postnatal depression. Churchill Livingstone, Edinburgh
Crawford J S 1972 Lumbar epidural block in labour: a clinical analysis. British Journal of Anaesthesia 44: 66–74
Cruse P, Yudkin P, Baum J D 1978 Establishing demand feeding in hospital. Archives of Disease in Childhood 53: 76–78
Davis M K, Savitz D A, Graubard B I 1988 Infant feeding and childhood cancer. Lancet ii: 365–368
Dawood M Y 1983 Neurohypophyseal hormones. In: Fuchs F, Klopper A (eds) Endocrinology of pregnancy. Harper & Row, Philadelphia, p 204
Delvoye P, Demaegd M, Delogne-Desnoeck J 1977 The influence of the frequency of nursing and of previous lactation experience on

serum prolactin in lactating mothers. Journal of Biosocial Science 9: 447–451

Dennis K J 1976 The puerperium. In: Walker J, MacGillivray I, MacNaughton M C (eds) Combined textbook of obstetrics and gynaecology, 9th edn. Churchill Livingstone, Edinburgh, p 397

Dennis K J, Blytheway W R 1965 Changes in body weight after delivery. Journal of Obstetrics and Gynaecology of the British Commonwealth 72: 94–102

Dessouky A D 197 1 Myometrial changes in postpartum uterine involution. American Journal of Obstetrics and Gynaecology 110: 318

Drewett R F, Woolridge M 1979 Sucking patterns of human babies on the beast. Early Human Development 3/4: 315–320–329

Dunlop W 1989 The puerperium. Fetal Medicine Review 1: 43–60

Efrati P, Presentey B, MargaCith M, Rozenszajn L 1964 Leukocytes of normal pregnant women. Obstetrics and Gynaecology 23: 429–423

FAO Nutritional Studies no 5 1950 Calorie requirements. Report of the Committee on Calorie Requirements, FAO, Washington

Falicov C J 1973 Sexual adjustment during first pregnancy and postpartum. American Journal of Obstetrics and Gynaecology 117: 991–1000

Fergusson D M, Horwood J L, Shannon F T, Taylor B 1981 Breastfeeding, gastrointestinal and lower respiratory illness in the first two years of life. Australian Journal of Paediatrics 17: 191–195

Franks S, Kiwi R, Nabarro J D N 1977 Pregnancy and lactation after pituitary surgery. British Medical Journal 1: 882

Gardner D L, Dodds T C 1976 Human histology. Churchill Livingstone, Edinburgh.

Gibson A 1937 On leucocyte changes during labour and the puerperium. Journal of Obstetrics and Gynaecology of the British Empire 44: 500–509

Glasier A, McNeilly A S, Howie P W 1983 Fertility after childbirth: changes in serum gonadotrophin levels in bottle and breast feeding women. Clinical Endocrinology 19: 493–501

Glasier A, McNeilly A S, Howie P W 1984a Pulsatile secretion of LH in relation to the resumption of ovarian activity postpartum. Clinical Endocrinology 20: 415–426

Glasier A, McNeilly A S, Howie P W 1984b The prolactin response to suckling. Clinical Endocrinology 21: 109–116

Glazener C M A, MacArthur C, Garcia J 1993. Postnatal care: time for a change. Contemporary Reviews in Obstetrics and Gynaecology 5: 130–136

Gould S F 1983 Anatomy of the breast. In: Neville M C, Neifert M R (eds) Lactation, physiology, nutrition and breast-feeding. Plenum Press, New York, p 23

Gray R H, Campbell O M, Zacur H A, Labbok M H, Macrae S L 1987 Postpartum return of ovarian activity in non-breastfeeding women monitored by urinary assays. Journal of Clinical Endocrinology and Metabolism 64: 645

Gross B A, Eastman C J 1985 Prolactin and the return of ovulation in breast-feeding women. Journal of Biosocial Science (suppl 9): 25–42

Habicht J-P, Davanzo J, Butz W B 1986 Does breast feeding really save lives, or are benefits due to biases? American Journal of Epidemiology 123: 299–290

Hartmann P E, Prosser C G 1984 Physiological basis of longitudinal changes in human milk yield and composition. Federation Proceedings 43: 2448–2453

Hartmann P E, Rattigan S, Prosser C G, Saint L, Arthur D G 1984 Human lactation: back to nature. Symposium of Zoological Society of London 51: 337–368

Hinman F 1976 Postoperative overdistension of the bladder. Surgery, Gynecology and Obstetrics 142: 901–902

House of Commons Health Committee Second Report 1992 Maternity Services, vol 1. HMSO, London

Howie P W 1992 Natural family planning. British Medical Bulletin 49: 182–199

Howie P W, McNeilly A S 1982 Effect of breast feeding patterns on human birth intervals. Journal of Reproduction and Fertility 65: 545–557

Howie P W, McNeilly A S, McArdle T, Smart L, Houston M 1980 The relationship between suckling induced prolactin response and lactogenesis. Journal of Clinical Endocrinology and Metabolism 50: 670–673

Howie P W, McNeilly A S, Houston M J, Cook A, Boyle H 1981a Effect of supplementary food on suckling patterns and ovarian activity during lactation. British Medical Journal 283: 757–763

Howie P W, McNeilly A S, Houston M J et al 1981b How long should a breast feed last? Early Human Development 5: 71–77

Howie P W, McNeilly A S, Houston M J, Cook A, Boyle H 1982 Fertility after childbirth: post-partum ovulation and menstruation in bottle and breast feeding mothers. Clinical Endocrinology 17: 323–332

Howie P W, Forsyth J S, Ogston S A, Clark A, Florey C D 1990 Protective effect of breast feeding against infection. British Medical Journal 300: 11–16

Huntingford P J 1961 Intranasal use of synthetic oxytocin in management of breast feeding. British Medical Journal 1: 709–711

Illingworth P J, Jung R T, Howie P W, Lesle P, Isles T E 1986 Diminution in energy expenditure during lactation. British Medical Journal 292: 437–441

Jelliffe D B, Jelliffe E F P 1978 Human milk in the modern world. Oxford University Press, Oxford

Kennedy K I, Visness C M 1992 Contraceptive efficiency of lactational amenorrhoea. Lancet 339: 227–230

Kennedy K I, Rivera R, McNeilly A S 1989 Consensus statement on the use of breastfeeding as a family planning method. Contraception 39: 477–496

Kenny J A 1973 Sexuality of pregnant and breast-feeding women. Archives of Sexual Behaviour 2: 215

Konner. M, Worthman C 1980 Nursing frequency, gonadal function and birth spacing among !Kung hunter gatherers. Science 207: 788 –791

Kovar M G, Serdula M K, Marks J S, Fraser D W 1984 Review of the epidemiologic evidence for an association between infant feeding and infant health. Pediatrics 71 (suppl): 615–638

Kulski J K, Hartmann P E 1981 Changes in human milk composition during the initiation of lactation. Australian Journal of Experimental Biology and Medical Science 59: 101–114

Lind T, Harris V G 1976 Changes in the oral glucose tolerance test in the puerperium. British Journal of Obstetrics and Gynaecology 83: 460–463

Lipinski J K, Adam A H 1981 Ultrasonic prediction of complications following normal vaginal delivery. Journal of Clinical Ultrasound 9: 17–19

Lucas A, Cole T J 1990 Breast milk and neonatal necrotising enterocolitis. Lancet 336: 1519–1523

Lucas A, Lucas P J, Caum J D 1979 Pattern of milk flow in breast-fed infants. Lancet ii: 57–58

Lucas A, Morally R, Cole T J, Lister G, Leeson-Payne C 1992 Breast milk and subsequent intelligence quotient in children born preterm. Lancet 339: 261–264

Lunn P G 1985 Maternal nutrition and lactational infertility: the baby in the driving seat. In: Dobbing J (ed) Maternal nutrition and lactational infertility. Nestle Nutrition Workshop Series, vol 9. Raven, New York, p 41

McNeilly A S 1977 Physiology of lactation. Journal of Biosocial Science (suppl 4): 5–21

McNeilly A S 1979 Effects of lactation on fertility. British Medical Bulletin 35: 151–154

McNeilly A S, McNeilly J R 1978 Spontaneous milk ejection during lactation and its possible relevance to success of breast-feeding. British Medical Journal 2: 466–468

McNeilly A S, Glasier A, Jonassen J, Howie P W 1982a Evidence for direct inhibition of ovarian function by prolactin. Journal of Reproduction and Fertility 65: 559–569

McNeilly A S, Howie P W, Houston M J, Cook A, Boyle H 1982b Fertility after childbirth: adequacy of post-partum luteal phases. Clinical Endocrinology 17: 609–615

McNeilly A S, Robinson I C, Houston M J, Howie P W 1983 Release of oxytocin and prolactin in response to suckling. British Medical Journal 286: 257–259

McNeilly A S, Glasier A, Howie P W 1985 Endocrine control of lactational infertility 1. In: Dobbing J (ed) Maternal nutrition and lactational infertility. Nestle Nutrition Workshop Series, vol 9. Raven, New York, p 1

McNeilly A S, Tay C C K, Glasier A 1993 Physiological mechanisms underlying lactational amenorrhoea. Annals New York Academy of Sciences (in press)

McTiernan A, Thomas D B 1986 Evidence for a protective effect of lactation on risk of breast cancer in young women. American Journal of Epidemiology 124, 3: 353–358

Man E B, Reid W A, Hellegers A E, Jones W S 1969 Thyroid function in human pregnancy. III Serum thyroxine binding prealbumin and thyroxine binding globulin of pregnant women aged 14 through 43 years. American Journal of Obstetrics and Gynecology 103: 338–347

Marrs R P, Kletzky O A, Mishell D R 1981 Functional capacity of the gonadotrophs during pregnancy and the puerperium. American Journal of Obstetrics and Gynecology 141: 658–661

Minchen M (ed) 1985 Breast feeding matters. Alma, Allen and Unwin, Sydney

Mizuno M, Labotsky J, Lloyd C W, Kobayashi T, Murasawa Y 1968 Plasma androstenedione and testosterone during pregnancy and in the newborn. Journal of Clinical Endocrinology and Metabolism 28: 1133–1142

Montford I, Perez-Tamayo R 1961 Studies on uterine collagen during pregnancy and the puerperium. Laboratory Investigation 10: 1240–1258

Morley D 1977 Biosocial advantages of an adequate birth interval. Journal of Biosocial Science (suppl 4): 49–81

Munro A 1985 Maternity care in action. Part III. Care of the mother and baby, 2.3. HMSO, London

Nader S, Kjeld J M, Blair C M, Tooley M, Gordon H, Fraser T R 1975 A study of the effect of bromocriptine on serum oestradiol, prolactin and follicle stimulating hormone levels in puerperal women. British Journal of Obstetrics and Gynaecology 82: 750–754

Neville M C, Berga S E 1983 Cellular and molecular aspects of the hormonal control of mammary control. In: Neville M C, Neifert M R (eds) Physiology, nutrition and breast feeding. Plenum, New York, p 141

Neville M C, Neifert M R 1983 An introduction to lactation and breast-feeding. In: Neville M C, Neifert M R (eds) Physiology, nutrition and breast-feeding. Plenum, New York, p 3

Neville M C, Allen J C, Watters C 1983 The mechanisms of milk secretion. In: Neville M C, Neifert M R (eds) Physiology, nutrition and breast-feeding. Plenum, New York, p 49

Newton N, Newton M 1950 Relation of the let-down reflex to the ability to breast feed. Pediatrics 5: 726–733

Nims B, Macy I G, Hunscher H A, Brown M 1932 Human milk studies. Daily and monthly variations in milk components as observed in two successive lactation periods. American Journal of Diseases of Children 43: 1062–1077

Perez A, Vela P, Masnick G S, Potter R G 1972 First ovulation after childbirth: the effect of breast-feeding. American Journal of Obstetrics and Gynecology 114: 1041–1047

Plank S J, Milanesi M L 1973 Infant feeding and infant mortality in rural Chile. Bulletin of the World Health Organization 48: 203–210

Polishuk W Z, Diamant Y Z, Zuckerman H, Sadovsky A 1970 Leukocyte alkaline phosphatase in pregnancy and the puerperium. American Journal of Obstetrics and Gynecology 107: 604–609

Potter R G, New M L, Wyon J B, Gordon J E 1965 Applications of field studies to research on physiology of human reproduction: lactation and its effects upon birth intervals in 11 Punjab villages, India. Journal of Chronic Diseases 18: 1125–1140

Poulain D A, Wakerley J B, Dyball R E J 1977 Electrophysiological differentiation of oxytocin and vasopressin-secreting neurons. Proceedings of the Royal Society of London (series B) 196: 367–384

Prentice A M, Whitehead R G, Roberts S B, Paul A A 1981 Long-term energy balance in child-bearing Gambian women. American Journal of Clinical Nutrition 34: 2790–2799

Pritchard J A, Baldwin R M, Dickey J C, Wigins K M 1962 Blood volume changes in pregnancy and the puerperium. II Red blood cell loss and changes in apparent blood volume during and following vaginal delivery, caesarean section and caesarean section plus total hysterectomy. Americal Journal of Obstetrics and Gynecology 84: 1271–1282

Prosser C G, Saint L, Hartmann P E 1984 Mammary gland function during gradual weaning and early gestation in women. Australian Journal of Experimental Biology and Medical Science 62: 215–228

Rastogi G K, Sawhney R C, Sinha M K, Thomas Z, Devi P K 1974 Serum and urinary levels of thyroid hormones in normal pregnancy. Obstetrics and Gynecology 44: 176–180

Renfrew M, Fisher C, Arms S (eds) 1990 Best feeding. Celestial Arts, Berkeley, California

Report of the Royal College of Obstetricians and Gynaecologists' Sub-committee on Problems Associated with AIDS in Relation to Obstetrics and Gynaecology 1987. Royal College of Obstetricians and Gynaecologists, London

Robinson J, Short R V 1977 Changes in human breast sensitivity at puberty, during the menstrual cycle and at parturition. British Medical Journal 2: 1188–1191

Robson S C, Dunlop W, Hunter S 1987 Haemodydnamic changes during the early puerperium. British Medical Journal 294: 1065

Rolland R, Schellekens L A 1973 A new approach to the inhibition of puerperal lactation. Journal of Obstetrics and Gynaecology of the British Commonwealth 80: 945–951

Rosa F W 1975 The role of breast feeding in family planning. WHO Protein Advisory Group Bulletin 5(3): 5–10

Royal College of Midwives 1988 Successful breastfeeding: A practical guide. Royal College of Midwives, London

Saarinen U M, Siimes M A 1979 Iron absorption from breast milk, cow's milk and iron-supplemented formula: an opportunistic use of changes in total body iron determined by hemoglobin ferritin and body weight in 132 infants. Pediatric Research 13: 143–147

Sleep J 1991 Perinatal care: a series of five randomised controlled trials. In: Robinson S, Thomson AM (eds) Midwives, research and childbirth, vol II. Chapman and Hall, London, ch 8

Smellie W 1752 A treatise on the theory and practice of midwifery. D Wilson, London

Trayhurn P, Douglas J B, McGuckin M M 1982 Brown adipose tissue thermogenesis is 'suppressed' during lactation in mice. Nature 298: 59–60

Udesky I C 1950 Ovulation in lactating women. American Journal of Obstetrics and Gynecology 59: 843–849

United Kingdom National Case-Control Study Group 1993 Breast feeding and risk of breast cancer in young women. British Medical Journal 307: 17–20

Watson D L 1980 Immunological functions of the mammary gland and its secretion — comparative review. Australian Journal of Biological Science 33: 403–422

Weil A, Reyes H, Rottenberg R D, Beguin F, Herrman W L 1983 Effect of lumbar epidural analgesia on lower urinary tract function in the immediate postpartum period. British Journal of Obstetrics and Gynaecology 90: 428–432

West C P, McNeilly A S 1979 Hormonal profiles in lactating and non-lactating women immediately after delivery and their relationship to breast engorgement. British Journal of Obstetrics and Gynaecology 86: 501–506

Whitehead R G, Paul A A, Rowland M G M 1980 Lactation in Cambridge and the Gambia. Topics in Paediatrics 2: 22–23

Whitehead R G, Paul A A, Black A E, Wiles S J 1981 Recommended dietary amounts of energy for pregnancy and lactation in the United Kingdom. In: Torun B, Young V R, Rand W M (eds) Protein energy requirements of developing countries: evaluation of new data. United Nations University, Tokyo, pp 259–265

Woolridge M N, Ingram J C, Baum J D 1990 Do changes in pattern of breast usage affect the baby's nutrient intake? Lancet 336: 395–397

World Health Organization 1981 Contemporary patterns of breast-feeding. Report on the WHO collaborative study on breast feeding. WHO, Geneva

World Health Organization 1993. In: Saachen R J (ed) Breast feeding: the technical basis and recommendations for action. WHO, Geneva

Ylikorkala O, Kaupilla A, Kivinen S, Viinikka L 1982 Sulpiride improves inadequate lactation. British Medical Journal 285: 249–251

43. Puerperal sepsis

C. J. van Gelderen

Material in this chapter contains contributions from the first edition and we are grateful to the previous authors for the work done.

Ah, my little son, thou hast murdered thy mother! And therefore I suppose thou that art a murderer so young, thou art full likely to be a manly man in thine age . . . . when he is christened let call him Tristram, that is as much to say as a sorrowful birth. (Sir Thomas Malory, *Le Morte D'Arthur*, bk viii, ch 1)

Mary Wollstonecraft was perhaps the first and probably one of the most talented of the feminists, publishing *The Rights of Woman* in 1790. She was delivered of her second child on 30 August 1797, and required to have the placenta 'brought away in pieces' by Dr Poignaud, man-midwife to the Westminster lying-in hospital. After 4 days of illness, Mary developed shaking chills, a feature of childbed fever, and her condition deteriorated steadily. There was no effective treatment available, and she died 12 days after delivery.

The child, named Mary after her mother, at the age of 16 eloped with the poet Shelley, and 3 years later gave evidence of her inherited genius with the publication of her classic, *Frankenstein* (Kaiser 1976).

For several hundreds of years, infection after childbirth has been one of the chief hazards to the parturient woman, and one of the prime causes of maternal death. Ever present in sporadic nature, there have been major epidemics of puerperal sepsis which left scarcely any survivors. Such an epidemic was described by Peu in Paris in 1664, and in Lombardy, 1772 was a year in which not one woman survived childbirth (Graham 1950).

The epidemic nature of the disease in the 18th and 19th centuries was a direct result of the establishment of lying-in hospitals, with consequent overcrowding, and, more significantly, the attendance on labouring women by medical men—the so-called man-midwives.

It was perhaps natural, although in retrospect indefensible, that the medical profession was reluctant to accept this. That measures so logical, so geared toward the promotion of a favourable outcome, should in fact lead to unprecedented carnage among parturients, was beyond the comprehension of most of the physicians of the time. Indeed, for over a century, innumerable maternal deaths must have resulted from the stubborn refusal of the medical profession to recognize their own aetiological role in the spread of puerperal sepsis. Between the publication by Alexander Gordon in 1795 of a report suggesting that puerperal fever was contagious, and the eventual acceptance of the necessary preventive measures as proposed by Oliver Wendell Holmes in the USA in 1843 and Ignaz Philip Semmelweiss in Vienna in 1861, proponents of the theory of the infectious nature of the disease were scorned and scoffed at, and in many cases hounded out of office.

DEFINITIONS

Puerperal sepsis refers to infection of the genital tract after delivery. The term is synonymous with the older expressions of puerperal fever and childbed fever. Although infection of the abdominal wound following Caesarean section is more correctly termed a wound infection, such cases are commonly regarded as variants of puerperal sepsis and will be discussed in this chapter.

Puerperal morbidity is a term used to encompass all cases of significant pyrexia in the puerperium, and would include patients with puerperal sepsis, as well as those with other causes of pyrexia. The latter conditions form part of the differential diagnosis in a case of puerperal pyrexia.

Significant pyrexia in the puerperium has been defined as a temperature of 38°C (100.4°F) or higher, (measured orally by a standard technique, at least four times daily) on any 2 of the first 10 days postpartum, exclusive of the first 24 hours. Although this definition has some value in terms of alerting the attendants to the presence of illness, and for epidemiological purposes, it almost certainly leads to an underestimation of the incidence of puerperal sepsis. The early use of antibiotics may prevent the development of significant pyrexia even in the presence of meaningful disease. Neither puerperal morbidity nor significant pyrexia indicate the site of the pathology, and puerperal sepsis may occur, and be severe, without producing significant pyrexia. Sweet & Ledger (1973) suggested, with a good deal of justification, that a measure of the use of antibiotics in postpartum patients would provide a more accurate reflection of the incidence of puerperal infection. A further confounding factor is the present practice of early discharge of postpartum women. Very few women are retained in hospital for 10 days, and episodes of mild puerperal infection may well go unnoticed (Eschenbach & Wager 1980).

THE INCIDENCE OF PUERPERAL SEPSIS

Because of the difficulty in defining the condition, the incidence as reported from different centres is variable, and may range from 1% to 8% (Gibbs & Weinstein 1976). Holbrook et al (1991), in a questionnaire-based survey of 19 650 mothers, found an incidence of reported postpartum infections of 4% in all women who had delivered. However the reply rate to the questionnaire was only 36%, and of the infections reported, only 7.6% were located in the genital tract. The point is nevertheless well taken, that most studies will seriously underestimate the incidence of puerperal morbidity. Still, there is no doubt that the disease is less common, and less severe than it used to be 40–50 years ago, and studies of puerperal sepsis have been sparse in recent years.

All authors report a marked disparity in incidence between women delivered vaginally, and those delivered by Caesarean section, in whom puerperal morbidity occurs between seven and 30 times more frequently. The incidence in the latter group will also depend upon whether or not routine prophylactic antibiotics are administered to patients undergoing surgery, and upon the relative proportions of elective and emergency surgery, with the latter having a four to 10 times greater frequency of infection (Yonekura 1988).

The incidence of significant genital tract sepsis, including post Caesarean section sepsis, endomyometritis after vaginal delivery and septic perineal wounds at Baragwanath Hospital in Johannesburg, South Africa, is at present between 2% and 3% of all deliveries. The

Table 43.1 Puerperal infectious disease: Baragwanath Hospital, April 1991 to March 1992 (deliveries = 18 593, infectious disease (all types) = 542)

Condition	No.	Proportion of total (%)	Proportion of infectious disease (%)
Septic Caesarean section	203	1.1	37.5
Sepsis after vaginal delivery	101	0.5	18.6
Septic episiotomy	65	0.3	12.0
HIV positive	48	0.3	8.9
Vulval lesions (mainly condylomas)	28	0.2	5.2
Skin and cellulitis	19	0.1	3.5
Gastrointestinal	16	0.1	3.0
Pulmonary TB	16	0.1	3.0
Abscess (including breast)	13	0.1	2.4

Other infectious diseases which occurred less frequently but were nevertheless of importance because of their seriousness included malaria, typhoid, meningitis and viral infections, particularly chickenpox and hepatitis.

population served by the hospital is generally underprivileged, and we would expect the sepsis rate to be higher than that reported from more sophisticated populations; however, this does not appear to be the case. Serious infectious puerperal diseases in this hospital are listed in Table 43.1.

PATHOGENESIS

The placental site is equivalent to an open wound immediately after parturition. There are almost always lacerations of greater or lesser magnitude in the epithelium of the vagina, cervix and lower uterine segment. Iatrogenic injuries, such as Caesarean section or episiotomy incisions, provide additional breaches in the integrity of the genital tract, and local diminution in the normal defense mechanisms. The inevitable presence of blood clot and retained necrotic portions of placenta or membranes also provides an ideal culture medium for the microorganisms which inhabit the female genital tract, but which do not normally cause disease. The flora is mixed, with both aerobic and anaerobic bacteria present, including numerous species which are potentially pathogenic, such as group B haemolytic streptococci, *Bacteroides* species, *Staphylococcus aureus*, *Mycoplasma hominis* and *Escherichia coli* (Hurley 1987).

If in addition the attendant during and after labour introduces organisms to which the parturient may have no innate resistance, it is not unexpected that puerperal infection does occur. It is surprising that it does not occur more frequently.

The initial site of infection may be anywhere in the genital tract, from perineum to Fallopian tubes, but the uterus is involved in almost all cases of more than minor severity.

METHODS OF SPREAD

1. Puerperal sepsis is generally an ascending infection, proceeding along the lumen of the genital tract. The placental site is almost always involved, and the extraplacental decidua also offers very little resistance to the spread of infection, being at this time very thin, traumatized and infiltrated with blood. Translumenal spread may extend beyond the uterus, into and through the Fallopian tubes, and thence to the pelvic peritoneum where abscess formation may occur. A generalized peritonitis may ensue. The full thickness of the uterine wall, from decidua to peritoneum, is almost always involved.
2. Infection of local lacerations in the vagina and cervix may provide a portal of entry for infections which may spread along tissue planes rather than along epithelial surfaces. Extension of the process into and through the myometrium and into the parametrial tissues may be accounted for by this mechanism, which results in pelvic cellulitis, also known as parametritis. Abscess formation and peritonitis may be a sequel to extrauterine spread by this mechanism as well.
3. Spread along lymphatics may also occur, and account for extension of infection beyond the pelvis (Barnes & Bender 1955).
4. Blood-borne spread of infection from the primary site of microorganism invasion may account for septicaemia or for septic thrombophlebitis. Spread is along venous channels, commencing in the placental site vessels, and thence to the ovarian veins, the uterine and iliac vessels, and ultimately the inferior vena cava.

SEVERITY OF INFECTION AND DEGREE OF SPREAD

The severity of the infection, and the degree of spread which will occur will depend on a number of parasite- and host-related factors which must be considered when treatment is undertaken.

Parasite-related factors

The specific microorganism involved

A particular species of bacterium will have its specific method of spread and multiplication. The group A beta-haemolytic streptococcus for example will spread rapidly along tissue planes, while *Staph. aureus* tends to propagate locally to promote abscess formation.

The virulence of the specific microorganism

The virulence of a microorganism is dependent on a number of factors, such as its ability to produce toxins or enzymes, and its innate invasiveness. While different pathogenic bacteria possess these attributes in different degree (Jawetz et al 1982), it is also apparent that a particular species may exhibit variable virulence at different times. Nowhere is this more evident than in the case of the group A beta-haemolytic streptococcus (Hurley 1987), which has become a rare cause of puerperal infection, although sporadic outbreaks have occurred. Ogden & Amstey (1978) described a cluster of five cases occurring in a 9-day period at the Highland Hospital, Rochester, New York, and Silver et al (1992) described two patients with life-threatening puerperal infection due to this organism relatively recently. Separate outbreaks traced to an obstetrician who was a carrier of the organism were described in 1991 (Viglionese et al 1991).

McGregor et al (1991) have proposed phospholipase C activity as a possible virulence factor produced by microorganisms involved in reproductive tract infections.

Bacterial resistance to antibiotics

The development of bacterial resistance to antibiotic agents is a well-known phenomenon of adaptation of the organism to its environment. This property is transmitted by plasmid-borne genes (as is the degree of virulence) and confers upon its possessor the ability to survive and multiply in circumstances rendered hostile by the presence of antibiotic agents (Jawetz et al 1982). It is particularly likely to occur under hospital conditions, as a resistant native flora has often been selected out by the use of multiple antimicrobial agents over a period of time.

The magnitude of the inoculum

It stands to reason that a genital tract afflicted with a massive contamination will be more likely to develop infection than one that is lightly contaminated. This has been the basis for one of the medical profession's foremost objections to home deliveries in the past, and is still applicable where home conditions are likely to be poor.

Host-related factors

General health

The better the general health of the parturient woman, the better she will be able to withstand bacterial invasion of the genital tract. It is thus important to ensure that health is optimum at the time of labour. Attention to details such as haemoglobin level, and the treatment of intercurrent infections during the antenatal period, may minimize the chances of severe disease after delivery. Gibbs & Weinstein (1976) in their review of puerperal infection in the antibiotic era, discussed predisposing factors to the condition which were referable to poor general health, including anaemia, low socioeconomic status, and poor prenatal care. Rehu & Nilsson (1980), in contrast, could demonstrate no significant difference in the incidence of puerperal sepsis between patients with a haemoglobin concentration above 11.0 g/dl and those with a lower level. Another factor related to nutrition is that of obesity, which, when present, appears to be an important risk factor for wound infection after Caesarean section (Pelle et al 1986). Systemic disorders such as diabetes mellitus also increase the liability to infection, and dictate specific precautions.

Immune status

There is no longer any question but that the normal pregnant woman is immunologically competent, and all tests of immunological integrity reveal normal responses. Essentially, systemic cell-mediated and humoral immune mechanisms remain effective (Coulam et al 1983, Glassman et al 1985, Cunningham & Evans 1991), and although it has been suggested that suppression of cell-mediated immunity is essential for fetal survival, there is no convincing evidence that this occurs. The pregnant woman is able to withstand infection, with the possible exception of some viral diseases such as poliomyelitis and hepatitis (Feinberg & Gonik 1991), as efficiently as her non-pregnant sister. Malaria also exhibits increased virulence in pregnancy (Glassman et al 1985). Despodova et al (1989) did find lowered values of active T lymphocytes in those parturients with inflammatory complications, but these were isolated findings and further investigation is required to confirm their conclusions.

The presence in the patient of defective immunity, whether of congenital or acquired origin such as in cases of infection with the human immunodeficiency virus (HIV), would of course confer upon her a heightened susceptibility to puerperal infection.

Risk factors related to the pregnancy

Many factors related to the antecedent pregnancy and labour have been connected to the subsequent development of puerperal sepsis. The majority of these have not withstood the scrutiny of randomized controlled trials, but their possible roles in predisposing to genital tract infection merit discussion.

Route of delivery Caesarean section delivery strikingly increases the incidence of puerperal infection. All studies, from that of Gibbs & Weinstein (1976) to the more recent one of Newton et al (1990), have shown a markedly raised relative risk of sepsis (12.8 in the contemporary investigation) in patients undergoing Caesarean section. The use of prophylactic antibiotics reduces this risk, but does not eliminate it. Caesarean section remains the single unequivocal factor which confers upon the parturient a significantly increased chance of developing puerperal sepsis.

Duration of labour Although many studies have shown a correlation between prolongation of labour and puerperal morbidity (Soper et al 1989), many confounding elements come into play. Thus a prolonged labour is related to the complication resulting in the prolongation, and also to the probability of an increase in the number and invasiveness of examinations. These may have their own influence on the incidence of infection (Cox & Gilstrap 1989, Ozumba & Uchegbu 1991). Cohen (1977) found no connection between the length of the second stage and puerperal morbidity, but Saunders et al (1992) did relate this factor to early maternal morbidity.

Invasive examinations in labour This is difficult to distinguish from other factors which may be operative. If a labour is prolonged, or complicated, more frequent pelvic examinations are the rule, and additional confounding factors such as internal monitoring will also be applied more frequently. Gibbs & Weinstein (1976) could find no evidence that an increase in the number of vaginal examinations led to an increase in morbidity. Soper et al (1989) found a progressive increase in amniotic fluid infection with increasing numbers of vaginal examinations, but did not explore any relationship to puerperal morbidity. In patients going on to Caesarean section, Rehu & Nilsson (1980) found a significant increase in the rate of endometritis after one vaginal examination. This rate was not increased by further examinations. In this study, rectal examinations were also associated with an increase in morbidity rates, and that increase was related to the number of examinations.

The question of internal fetal and amniotic pressure monitoring must also be considered here. Rehu & Nilsson (1980) were not able to demonstrate any effect of internal monitoring on the incidence of sepsis over and above the effect already exerted by the pelvic examination. Newton et al (1990) found that although univariate analysis had shown significant associations between postpartum endometritis and variables such as duration of labour, rupture of membranes and internal monitoring, these were not confirmed on multivariate analysis. In general, therefore, complications of labour which lead to prolongation, or to invasive intervention, are likely to increase the risk of puerperal sepsis, particularly in patients proceeding to Caesarean section, but not to any great extent. It behoves us to keep the number of invasive examinations in labour to the minimum necessary for good obstetric care.

Rupture of the membranes and preterm labour Prolonged rupture of the membranes has traditionally been associated with an increased incidence of puerperal infection. Indeed, more argument has centred around whether infection precedes or follows the event, than around whether sepsis is predisposed to or not. Gibbs & Weinstein (1976) in their review noted a two- to four-fold increase in morbidity in the presence of prolonged rupture of membranes. Most recent studies have been concerned with the predisposition to infection in patients proceeding to Caesarean section, and most are agreed that the incidence of morbidity is increased with increasing duration of ruptured membranes. Gilstrap & Cunningham (1979) showed that the amniotic fluid was colonized by bacteria in all of 56 women who had had ruptured membranes for longer than 6 hours prior to Caesarean section, and that postoperative myometritis developed in 95% of them. Okonofua et al (1991) found a slightly increased febrile morbidity in patients of low socioeconomic status with preterm premature rupture of the membranes who were treated conservatively, and who therefore had a longer duration of ruptured membranes. The increase in morbidity was not sufficient to suggest that conservative management should be abandoned. Seo et al (1992) found more postpartum endometritis in patients with preterm premature rupture of membranes than in those in whom it had occurred at term.

Whether the infection precedes or follows the rupture of the membranes, there seems little doubt that prolonged drainage of amniotic fluid is a risk factor for the development of puerperal morbidity, particularly if the patient should require a Caesarean section. There is no convincing evidence that routine antibiotic therapy, or manoeuvres such as amnioinfusion, have an appreciable effect on the incidence of puerperal sepsis in this condition (Keirse et al 1989).

Preterm labour unassociated with premature rupture of membranes also confers upon the patient an added risk of puerperal morbidity (Seo et al 1992). Again, it is difficult to be certain which is cause and which is effect. Current opinion seems to be that the infective process precedes and is causative of the preterm labour (McGregor et al 1990, McGregor & French 1991).

Prenatal bacterial colonization of the genital tract
It stands to reason that if the genital tract is colonized with pathogenic microorganisms before the onset of labour, the chances of postpartum infection will be increased. This is not the entire explanation, as we have seen that there are numerous potentially pathogenic bacteria normally resident in the vagina, and they cause problems only in a minority of cases.

Several workers have described, however, a significant rise in the incidence of puerperal febrile morbidity when such bacterial colonization has been demonstrated. McGregor & French (1991) found an increase in post Caesarean and postpartum maternal infections when *Chlamydia trachomatis* was present in the vagina. Wager et al (1980) found an increased risk for early postpartum fever after Caesarean section, as well for postpartum fever

and endometritis following vaginal delivery, in women with a positive cervical culture for *C. trachomatis*. Harrison et al (1983) were unable to show a statistically significant relationship between *C. trachomatis* infection and puerperal endometritis, but did relate the presence of *Mycoplasma hominis* to subsequent endometritis or fever, as did Jacqui & Sedallion (1992). Newton et al (1990) were also able to predict endometritis when *M. hominis* was present in patients who subsequently underwent Caesarean section. In this study, the presence of 'bacterial vaginosis organisms' was strongly predictive of endometritis in women who went on to vaginal delivery. Similar findings were reported by Watts et al (1990). The presence of group B streptococcus in the vagina prior to labour has long been considered a risk factor for both maternal and neonatal infection. Although eradication of the organism is recommended (Wessels & Kasper 1993), the effectiveness of this approach has not been conclusively established.

Vaginal Enterobacteriaceae have not been incriminated, but Monif (1991) reported a small series of women in whom these organisms had caused bacteriuria, and 30% developed postpartum endometritis after vaginal delivery. The same Enterobacteriaceae that had been present in the urine cultures were recovered from the endometrium.

It seems reasonable to conclude that the presence of the above pathogens in the genital tract before labour is likely to predispose to infection during or after delivery. What is not certain is whether an attempt to eradicate them will have any beneficial effect.

Other determinants
Certain other factors have been incriminated as catalysts of risk for puerperal infection.

Adolescents had a significantly higher post Caesarean endometritis rate than did adults (Berenson et al 1990). Cervical cerclage has been found at least to double the rate of puerperal pyrexia, by both Rush et al (1984) and the MRC/RCOG Working Party on Cervical Cerclage (1988).

There have been numerous attempts to relate factors such as sexual intercourse during pregnancy and the size or sex of the fetus to ensuing puerperal morbidity. Proof of the relationships is not convincing.

The majority of the elements which may be considered to foster the risk of puerperal sepsis are either beyond our control or not amenable to therapy. Indeed, in some instances we find it necessary to assume the heightened risk of sepsis in order to diminish hazards of a more immediate or more severe nature. We should note the risk factors, treat those responsive to therapy and take such precautions as are available to us.

THE MICROBIOLOGY OF ESTABLISHED PUERPERAL SEPSIS

Puerperal sepsis in the modern era is commonly a polymicrobial infection (Gilstrap & Cunningham 1979). The organisms most frequently isolated are those that normally inhabit the lower genital and gastrointestinal tracts. Unusual pathogenicity is conferred upon them by the local circumstances produced by parturition. It should also be remembered that in the majority of cases, confirmation of the identity of the offending bacteria is not sought. Routine empirical therapy is applied and is generally successful, and we never really know which of the many possible microorganisms was the true culprit. It is only in cases where treatment is not attaining success, or in clinical trials or investigations, that specimens for culture are taken. In addition, many of the earlier studies seeking to identify the causative organisms in puerperal sepsis were flawed by a number of factors:

1. Cultures were taken from or adulterated in the vagina or lower cervix. It is currently required that bacteriological specimens from the female genital tract not be contaminated by vaginal or cervical flora. This entails obtaining specimens directly from the peritoneal surface through a laparoscope or by culdocentesis, or transcervically using a protected method of sampling, such as the triple-lumen aspirator described by Eschenbach et al (1986), or a double-lumen technique as recommended by Duff et al (1983).
2. Cultures for anaerobic bacteria and organisms such as *C. trachomatis* and *M. hominis* were difficult and not generally available.

For useful results to be obtained, specimens for bacteriological investigation must be taken from the endometrial cavity by a method which precludes vaginal or cervical contamination. Direct sampling of fluid collections may be performed with ultrasound control. Specimens obtained must be sent for both aerobic and anaerobic culture. Very specific sampling and laboratory methods are required to culture *C. trachomatis* and *M. hominis*, and the regional laboratory should be consulted as to how they would prefer the specimens to be processed.

Present-day investigation may be hampered by the fact that antibiotic agents are readily administered to many patients very early in the course of almost any illness, as well as for purposes of prophylaxis in patients at risk of developing infection.

Bearing these caveats in mind, the bacteria listed in Table 43.2 have been linked most frequently to cases of puerperal genital tract infection.

The finding of a single responsible microorganism is today the exception rather than the rule. Rosene et al (1986) found that in patients with endometritis, particularly in the first 48 hours after delivery, two or more species were present in more than 60% of cases. Bacteria coexisting with genital mycoplasmas were most frequently recovered. Facultative Gram-positive bacteria were present in 40% of endometrial isolates, with group B streptococci being the most common. Gram-negative aerobic

Table 43.2 Bacteria linked most frequently to cases of puerperal genital tract infection

1. **Aerobic bacteria**
   a. Gram positive
      Beta-haemolytic streptococcus, Groups B, D and A
      Staphylococcus epidermidis, rarely *St. aureus*
   b. Gram negative
      Escherichia coli
      Enterobacteriaceae including *Klebsiella pneumoniae*, *Enterobacter*, *Proteus mirabilis*, *Citrobacter*, *Pseudomonas aeruginosa*
      Haemophilus influenzae
   c. Gram variable
      Gardnerella vaginalis
2. **Anaerobic bacteria**
   Peptostreptococcus sp.
   Peptococcus sp.
   Bacteroides bivius, *B. fragilis*, *B. disiens*
   Clostridium ramosum, rarely *Cl. perfringens*
   Fusobacterium
3. **Unclassified**
   Mycoplasma hominis
   Chlamydia trachomatis

organisms were found in 22%, and anaerobic bacteria in 38% of endometrial cultures (Yonekura 1988). Rusin et al (1991) found *H. influenzae* to be an important cause of severe disease.

The group B streptococcus or *Streptococcus agalactiae* is an important infecting organism. Three cases of puerperal sepsis reported by Fry (1938) provided the first intimation that this organism could cause severe disease. By the mid 1970s, group B streptococci were recognized as an important cause of peripartum infection, both maternal and neonatal. The organism appears to be becoming more virulent, and there have been recommendations that prophylactic antibiotic therapy should be administered to proven carriers (Wessels & Kasper 1993). Work on the development of a vaccine is also proceeding (Baker et al 1988).

There have been numerous recent reports of serious puerperal sepsis, often of fatal or near fatal degree, resulting from infection with *H. influenzae* (Rusin et al 1991), *C. trachomatis* (McGregor & French 1991) and *M. hominis* (Young & Cox 1990).

The microbiology may well be different in dissimilar groups of patients. Berenson et al (1990) found isolation rates of *C. trachomatis* and that of *Gardnerella vaginalis* to be at least three times as common in adolescents compared with adults.

Puerperal sepsis is thus most commonly polymicrobial in nature, the usual offending organisms being a combination of those normally found in the lower genital tract and bowel. Any and all of these bacteria, singly or in combination, may lead to severe and life-threatening illness.

CLINICAL FEATURES

The clinical features of puerperal sepsis will depend on

the nature of the infecting organism, the site of primary infection and the rapidity and extent of spread.

In all cases a history of the antecedent pregnancy and the circumstances and course of labour should be sought. Possible risk factors should be noted as they will have a bearing on the organisms which can be anticipated to be involved. The nature of any prior administration of antibiotics must be established as this will dictate the type of both the investigation and treatment.

Examination must be directed at detecting the source and location of the infection, as well as the exclusion of any other cause for the pyrexia. Physical examination of the pyrexial postpartum woman must therefore always include the following:

1. *Head, neck and spine.* Look for evidence of anaemia, jaundice, lymphadenopathy and throat infection. Neck stiffness should also be checked for, especially if a spinal or epidural anaesthetic has been administered.
2. *Breasts.* Look for engorgement and inflammatory changes, and possible abscess formation.
3. *Heart and lungs.* Look for evidence of valvular disease in the former, and of pneumonia or collapse in the latter. This is especially important if the patient has been given an inhalational anaesthetic.
4. *Abdomen.* The abdomen must be generally examined, noting the presence of free fluid, enlargement of liver and spleen, and any abnormal masses. Particular note must be taken of uterine size and tenderness, renal angle tenderness and the presence or absence of signs of peritonitis. The presence or absence of bowel sounds should be recorded.
5. *Pelvis.* A pelvic examination must be performed in all cases. The lochia should be checked for colour, consistency and unpleasant odour. The external genitalia must be inspected, and infected lacerations sought in the lower tract. Bimanual palpation of the uterus and parametrial tissues must be done. The size of the uterus and the degree of tenderness should be noted. The pouch of Douglas must be carefully examined as this is a common site for abscess formation.
6. *Limbs.* The legs should be checked carefully for evidence of thrombosis or thrombophlebitis. The clinical signs are both misleading and non-specific. If there is any suspicion of thrombosis or embolism, specific investigations such as venography or Doppler flow studies must be instituted immediately.

Signs and symptoms will depend on whether the infection has remained localized or has spread.

Localized disease

Perineum, vulva, vagina and cervix

Infections in the perineum and vagina as a rule are sec-

ondary to lacerations or to episiotomy. They tend to remain confined to the immediate region, and to cause little in the way of general disturbance although there may be a mild degree of pyrexia. Local symptoms consist of discomfort, pain and discharge. A common predisposing element is the delayed suturing of perineal lacerations and wounds. Wounds which have for any reason not been sutured within 2–4 hours should be left to heal by second intention, which they do remarkably well. Cervical infections rarely cause problems if they remain localized.

On examination the wounds will appear reddened and oedematous. Sutures will have cut through the tissues, and there will be a disagreeable discharge. Local suppuration may occur and give rise to an ischio-rectal abscess, palpable as a fluctuant mass through the lateral vaginal fornix.

Uterus

Infection confined to the uterus may present with either local or systemic signs and symptoms. Pyrexia of significant degree is frequent in either case, and may be associated with tachycardia and rigors. General complaints such as headache, malaise, nausea and feverishness are common. Complaints of abdominal pain are usual.

The uterus is tender to palpation, and softer and larger than normal, with delay in the process of involution. There may be evidence of localized peritoneal irritation. Vaginal examination may reveal traumatic damage to the cervix or even to the lower uterine segment. There may be evidence, palpable on bimanual examination, of extra-uterine spread of infection. The lochia may be profuse and malodorous, or less commonly, scanty and inoffensive. If the cervix is open, the uterine cavity should be palpated for evidence of trauma, and for retained portions of placenta and membranes. However, ultrasound examination of the uterine cavity has the advantages that it is painless, more sensitive and specific, and not limited by inaccessibility. If it is available, it should be used as a routine.

Even localized infections may on occasion be extremely intense and should not be considered lightly. There may be extensive local tissue destruction often related to *C. perfringens* infection which may result in uterine necrosis (Patchell 1976).

Wound infections

Wound infection may complicate perineal incisions or lacerations, or the abdominal wound of a Caesarean section. If the infection has remained localized, there will be little in the way of systemic upset, and the clinical signs will be those of local inflammation, and failure to heal by first intention. If the condition is truly local, complications are rare, but often an infected Caesarean section wound is part of a more extensive process. This must be borne in mind, and regional or systemic disease must be actively sought.

Regional disease

Pelvic cellulitis

Spread of the infection to the parametrial tissue may occur at any time but tends to happen in the second week of the puerperium. If antibiotics have been administered in inadequate type or dosage, spread may occur even later, and the signs and symptoms may be partially masked. This results in a prolongation of the pyrexia, and without adequate treatment may go on to abscess formation, although slow resolution is the rule. Pain and tenderness persist, and the findings on vaginal examination are of a hard thickening tethering the uterus to the pelvic sidewall or surrounding the rectum. There may be bilateral involvement. Pelvic cellulitis is much more common after Caesarean section than after vaginal delivery. Response to intensive antibiotic therapy is usually good. On occasion surgical drainage of an abscess may be necessary (Fig. 43.1).

Adnexitis

Involvement of the tubes and ovaries may be part of a pelvic peritonitis and spread to this region is often along lymphatics and tissue planes rather than translumenal, in which case the tubal endothelium is less liable to be severely affected. If infertility results, it is therefore more

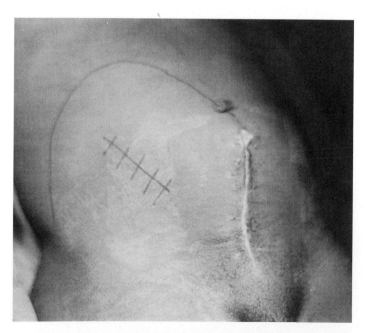

Fig. 43.1 A large parametrial abscess which was drained extraperitoneally at the site indicated. Resolution occurred rapidly thereafter. Note the absence of wound sepsis.

likely to be amenable to treatment than that resulting from a sexually transmitted infection. The signs and symptoms form a continuum with those of uterine and pelvic connective tissue infection, and treatment does not require any additional elements.

Pelvic peritonitis

This is an extension of cellulitis and adnexitis, and the diagnosis is suggested by signs of peritoneal irritation, such as guarding or rebound tenderness, in the lower abdomen. While not necessarily indicative of a more severe infection, the development of pelvic peritonitis should raise the suspicion that local defense mechanisms are not coping with the disease.

On occasion pelvic abscess formation occurs. This complication should be diagnosed early in its course when it may still respond to antibiotic therapy. At a later stage surgical drainage may be necessary. Early diagnosis is favoured by routine vaginal examination in all cases of puerperal morbidity, so that the initial stages of abscess formation are not missed, although routine ultrasound examination, if available, would be as effective. Adequate treatment of the original infection should prevent this complication, and should be sufficient therapy if it does occur.

Systemic disease

Generalized peritonitis

Once spread to the general peritoneal cavity has occurred, the disease has become severe. The diagnosis may not be as straightforward as one might think, as some of the classical signs tend to be masked by the postpartum state. Thus rigidity is often absent, although rebound tenderness is almost always found. Pyrexia tends to be high and sustained, vomiting is frequent and pain is constant. General signs of dehydration and toxicity are present. Abdominal distension with absent bowel sounds is very often an ominous sign in the puerperium, indicating peritonitis. Even after Caesarean section, distension should not be dismissed as a normal sequel of surgery. Prolonged intestinal ileus is not a feature of an uncomplicated post Caesarean section course.

Antibiotics administered for the endometritis will usually be effective for the peritonitis as well, but may need to be given in higher dosage and for a longer period of time. Surgery for intraperitoneal abscesses may become necessary.

Septic thrombophlebitis

The classic presentation of this complication is that of a patient with puerperal sepsis who does not respond to adequate doses of an appropriate antibiotic (Gibbs 1976). Signs and symptoms of pelvic and abdominal disease improve, but pyrexia remains, characterized by severe peaks every several days. The patient is often intensively investigated for obscure causes of pyrexia of unknown origin (PUO), such as typhoid fever or malaria. Pulmonary signs or symptoms offer a clue to the nature of the pathology, as septic emboli to the lungs may occur. The diagnosis is frequently made as a result of a response to a therapeutic trial of heparin therapy (Gibbs 1976). Management entails continuation of antibiotic treatment, with the addition of anticoagulant therapy. Intravenous heparin would be the most rapid and effective medication to employ. Surgical interruption of the inferior vena cava may become necessary.

Bacteraemia and septicaemia

Blanco et al (1981) found the incidence of bacteraemia to be 7.5 per 1000 obstetric admissions. There were 123 patients with puerperal endoparametritis, of whom 99 (80.5%) had delivered by Caesarean section. Bacteraemia had occurred in 3% of patients who had had a Caesarean section as opposed to 0.1% of those who had delivered vaginally. None of the patients in this study developed septic shock or died, and most responded to the initial antibiotic therapy (penicillin and an aminoglycoside).

Thus although bacteraemia is not rare in patients with puerperal sepsis, with prompt treatment the prognosis appears to be good in this group of relatively young and healthy people who constitute the obstetric population.

The picture is different when the bacteraemia is associated with hypotension, and the condition is characterized as septic shock.

Septic shock is fortunately infrequent. When it does occur in obstetric patients, the majority arise in the puerperium (Lee et al 1988), and it is much more common after Caesarean section than after vaginal delivery.

Septic shock, endotoxic shock and bacterial shock are synonyms for the same condition—inadequate tissue perfusion related to inappropriate vasodilation and circulatory maldistribution secondary to the release of vasoactive mediators. The classic causative organism was *Escherichia coli* and other members of the Gram-negative Enterobacteraciae, including the *Klebsiella–Enterobacter–Serratio* group, *Proteus mirabilis* and *Pseudomonas aeruginosa* (Duff & Gibbs 1983), but septic shock has occurred in association with streptococci (groups D, B and A) and *Staph. aureus* (Lee et al 1988). Anaerobic streptococci and *Bacteroides* species have also been incriminated. The condition is a response to the release of a lipopolysaccharide endotoxin (lipid A) after lysis of the bacterial cell wall. The endotoxin results in enhanced coagulation and fibrinolysis, and the release of inflammatory mediators such as hydrogen peroxide and free radicals (Duff &

Gibbs 1983). Practically all systems in the body suffer some degree of damage.

Clinical features are primarily those of infection associated with hypotension and (usually) oliguria, not attributable to hypovolaemia. A history of a prior operative procedure should increase suspicion of the condition. The complications include pulmonary oedema, adult respiratory distress syndrome, disseminated intravascular coagulation, renal failure and thromboembolism.

Management is complex, and is best undertaken in an intensive care facility. Aspects that will require therapy include:

Fluid balance The fluid balance must be corrected rapidly but such correction requires the control afforded by knowledge of the pulmonary capillary wedge pressure, or at the minimum, of the central venous pressure. The urine output must also always be recorded. Blood is used to replace blood loss, and thereafter crystalloid solutions are administered (Duff & Gibbs 1983).

Respiratory support The lungs are almost always involved, sometimes severely. A considerable proportion of these patients will require mechanical ventilation. This becomes essential if the arterial blood P_{CO_2} exceeds 8.0 kPa or the P_{O_2} is less than 8.0 kPa.

Circulatory support If the response to fluid replacement is not satisfactory, inotropic agents such as dopamine or dobutamine will have to be used, as obstetric patients with septic shock tend to have depressed myocardial function (Lee et al 1988).

Renal failure Kidney function must be monitored, and haemodialysis resorted to sooner rather than later.

Infection control There is no hope of saving the patient unless the infection is eradicated. Intensive antibiotic therapy must continue, and surgical removal of septic foci may be called for, including, on occasion, hysterectomy and even oophorectomy.

Corticosteroids The value of corticosteroid administration has not been established after many years and innumerable trials. Most intensive therapists do recommend their use.

Less common life-threatening puerperal infections

Necrotizing fasciitis This is a rare, rapidly progressing infection of fascia, subcutaneous tissue and skin. Characteristically muscle is spared (Janevicius et al 1982). It is associated with severe systemic disturbance and has a mortality rate of around 40%. Presenting signs include those of systemic upset such as tachycardia and leucocytosis, and local features of necrosis, cellulitis, oedema and crepitus (Pessa & Howard 1985). Golde & Ledger (1977) described four cases occurring in the puerperium, three following perineal injury, and one after Caesarean section. Two of the former group died and the remaining two had a very protracted and complicated hospital stay. It is now thought that the condition is of polymicrobial origin. Survival depends on early diagnosis, the use of broad-spectrum antibiotics and early and aggressive surgical debridement of the affected area (Patino & Castro 1991).

Tetanus Fortunately we do not see this condition in our hospital any more, but Yadav et al (1991) writing from Chandigarh in India described 50 cases with a 52% mortality. Death was most often due to respiratory complications. Prevention is much easier than treatment, and immunization during pregnancy should be recommended to patients who have not been immunized previously (Amstey 1976). Treatment involves supportive therapy including mechanical ventilation until the disease has run its course.

INVESTIGATION

Puerperal sepsis is a clinical entity, with the diagnosis based upon deduction and arrived at after thorough history and physical examination. Clinical diagnoses are necessarily uncertain and we use special investigations to eliminate imprecision as far as possible. Puerperal sepsis is reasonably well defined, and special investigations are seldom required to confirm the diagnosis, but certain basic tests are necessary and should be performed in all cases. They are simple and inexpensive, and may easily eliminate such doubts as there may be. They may be of value in cases refractory to standardized treatment and they can be useful in excluding other sources of pyrexia, or in elucidating the nature of complications of the primary condition.

The recommended tests include the following:

Blood count

The haemoglobin level will indicate whether or not the patient is anaemic. If so, she may require haematinic or even transfusion therapy to enable her to muster the best possible defense against the infection. The leucocyte count will give an indication as to the efficacy of the immune response, and the trend of repeated counts will map the progress of the infection. A low platelet count may be the first intimation of complications such as septicaemia or disseminated intravascular coagulation.

Urine culture

A clean-catch (mid-stream) specimen of urine should always be subjected to microscopy and culture. Urinary tract infection may mimic puerperal sepsis closely, and in any event may coincide with the latter condition. It is important to be aware of its presence, as urinary infection may require different treatment from puerperal sepsis as regards both the agent to administer and the duration of treatment.

Pelvic ultrasound

Pelvic ultrasound, preferably using both a vaginal probe and an abdominal sector-scanning probe, is of great value in locating collections of pus, in affording guidance in the sampling of fluid collections and in confirming the presence or absence of retained products of conception within the uterus. If it is available, the colour-flow Doppler scanner will also enable a precise diagnosis and localization of venous thrombosis to be made.

Blood urea and electrolyte estimation

It is a good idea to have an initial measurement of these indices, as renal failure may ensue later in the course of the disease, and a basis for comparison is then available.

Chest X-ray

Lung pathology, such as infection or collapse, is always a possibility (Fig. 43.2), particularly after inhalational anaesthesia, and may be the primary cause for the pyrexia. Lung complications, the result of septic or non-septic embolism, may also complicate puerperal sepsis. The early signs of adult respiratory distress syndrome may be noted in cases of septicaemia.

Microbiology

It is not our policy to request microbiological investigations on all cases of puerperal sepsis, and certainly it would be incorrect to await the results before commencing treatment. We are not alone in this practice (Filler et al 1992). Wisdom would appear to dictate that an initial bacteriological diagnosis would be beneficial in case an infelicitous choice of antibiotic has been made, but this occurs so

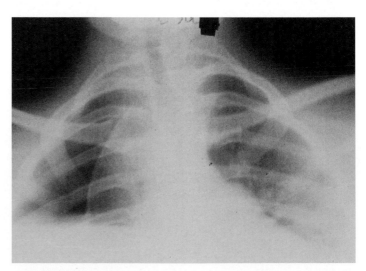

Fig. 43.2 X-ray photograph of the chest (postero-anterior) showing collapse of the right lung after a Caesarean section.

seldom these days that the costs outweigh the benefits. Certainly specimens for culture should be taken if the response to therapy is anything short of what is anticipated. If specimens for culture are taken, whether at the onset of therapy or during its course, care must be taken to avoid contamination in the lower genital tract, as outlined above.

If complications ensue, then it is mandatory that culture and sensitivity tests be performed on all fluid collections and abscesses. Blood culture is necessary if bacteraemia or septicaemia is suspected.

Other investigations have been recommended. Nikonov et al (1991) found that measurement of the lochial pH, P_{CO_2} and P_{O_2} revealed that acidosis in this fluid was diagnostic of endometritis. Abdominal X-rays showing gas in the uterus have long been taken to indicate infection with a gas-forming organism (Fig. 43.3), and to have grave implications. Wachsberg & Kurtz (1992), however, found that the detection, by means of ultrasound, of gas in the endometrial cavity was a normal finding after vaginal delivery. The presence of gas within the myometrial tissue is always significant.

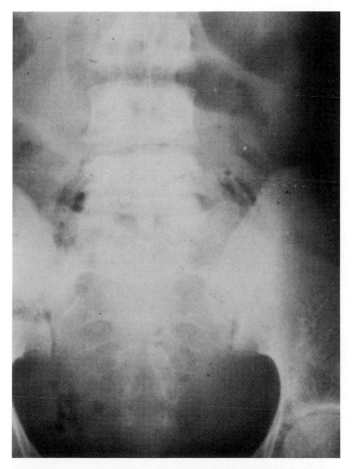

Fig. 43.3 X-ray photograph of the abdomen in a case of puerperal sepsis, showing gas shadows within the uterine cavity, and possibly in the myometrium as well. *Clostridium perfringens* was cultured from the surgical specimen.

Computerized tomography has been tried by a number of investigators (Brown et al 1986, 1991, Apter et al 1992). There was no real indication from these authors that the investigation made a helpful contribution to the management of their patients. It was nevertheless possible to make a more certain diagnosis of venous thrombosis using this imaging method, and the procedure was of value in those instances. The use of this expensive investigation cannot be recommended in cases of puerperal sepsis unless the clinician is at a loss as to how to proceed with diagnosis and treatment.

PREVENTION OF PUERPERAL SEPSIS

Basic principles

Since the days of Semmelweiss, cleanliness has been the primary weapon against puerperal infection. We are aware that we ourselves are the leading vectors of the disease, and we have learnt to take the necessary precautions against its spread. For decades each obstetric textbook would devote a considerable portion of its text to measures aimed at controlling the spread of infection. Instructions on protective clothing, hand washing and specific aseptic techniques, occupied a good many pages (Barnes & Bender 1955), and with good reason.

A good deal of this appeared to go by the board with the advent of effective antibiotic agents. Chalmers et al (1989) report that by 1984, 43% of English consultant maternity units never wore masks in the labour wards, and 90% never wore special shoes. This was partly in an endeavour to make the labour ward more user-friendly for the patient, but largely because the dropping of these measures was not seen as harmful. A reversal of this trend is now visible, but the motivation is very different. The advent of the HIV epidemic has led to a reintroduction of many of the earlier precautions, directed, however, at the protection of the attendant; perhaps the patient may also derive some benefit out of this development. It must be admitted, nonetheless, that the rate of puerperal infection did not rise when the caps and masks were abandoned, as the basic principles of cleanliness including hand scrubbing, sterile equipment, and antiseptic solutions and creams were still used (Crowther et al 1989).

These measures probably suffice for the prevention of puerperal sepsis in patients destined to deliver vaginally, as the disease is no longer as common nor as severe as it was in the days of Semmelweiss and Holmes.

The case of emergency Caesarean section

There can be no question but that the risk of puerperal infection is unacceptably high in patients undergoing non-elective Caesarean section, and the need has long been seen for some method of diminishing the incidence of a condition which was associated with a not inconsiderable mortality. Three approaches to this problem have been followed, and are discussed below:

Technical aspects of the operation

It is clear that technical skill will play a part in the prevention of intraoperative colonization of the wound. Factors which have been considered important include the duration of surgery which should not be protracted, although rushing through the operation in an attempt to beat the clock may be even more harmful.

Haemostasis should be as complete as is possible so that a collection of blood is not available to provide a culture medium for any stray bacteria.

McCurdy et al (1992) found that manual delivery of the placenta at Caesarean section resulted in a seven-fold greater incidence of endometritis than when the placenta was allowed to deliver spontaneously.

Antiseptic washes and douches

As the microbiology of post Caesarean sepsis implies that the bulk of the infecting microorganisms come from the vagina, there have been many attempts to sterilize the vagina prior to surgery, usually with scant success. Weidinger et al (1991) used an hexetidine suppository intravaginally and produced a marked reduction in the vaginal flora, but a 5-day course was necessary, and patients going on to emergency Caesarean section were not assessed. Chlorhexidine douches administered 6 hourly during labour have been noted to reduce the incidence of neonatal infections (Burman et al 1992), but the effect on maternal infection is not known. Methods such as this do merit further investigation.

Owen et al (1990) found that patients undergoing saline amnioinfusion for a variety of reasons had a significantly decreased incidence of postpartum endometritis. This technique too may repay future study.

Prophylactic antibiotics

In 1943 Richards discussed the use of sulphonamide applied locally in the prevention of postoperative sepsis in, among other operations, Caesarean section. There was sporadic interest in the topic until 1968 when Miller & Crichton published the first controlled trial, using ampicillin, and showing positive results. Since then, the number of trials has mushroomed, and in 1989 Enkin et al published a review of the results of more than 90 controlled trials. More are published each year.

The medical profession has never accepted the use of prophylactic antibiotics unreservedly. This has been based to a large extent on the perceived and anticipated ill-effects that antibiotic agents may have. These embrace drug effects on the fetus and neonate, and side-effects on the mother, which may include severe allergic reactions.

Concern has also been expressed about the effects such therapy may have on the bacterial flora, both that of the individual patient, and that of the environment. The particular fear is of promoting the emergence of new and resistant strains of bacteria.

The principal argument that can be mustered in favour of the use of prophylactic antibiotics for Caesarean section is that it unequivocally works (Smaill 1993). Enkin et al (1989) in their review reported that prophylaxis significantly reduced the rate of serious infection after Caesarean section, as well as that of postoperative febrile morbidity. Indeed, the overwhelming majority of current publications on the subject do not address the subject of whether or not prophylactic antibiotic ought to be used, but of which agent, and which route of administration to employ. There is still no certainty of the benefit-to-cost merit of this therapy in non-emergency Caesarean section where the incidence of sepsis is much lower than in the emergency case, although current trials are showing a distinct reduction in the sepsis rate in these patients as well (Smaill 1993).

At Baragwanath Hospital in January 1991, we were reluctantly persuaded to adopt a policy of using a single-dose prophylactic injection of cefoxitin administered with the premedication, and a comparison of sepsis rates before and after the institution of this policy is seen in Table 43.3. It is important to assess results from the applied policy in a unit, as opposed to those obtained under trial conditions. In the former situation there is the potential for mistakes such as omission of the treatment, and the case cannot be removed from the results. It will be noted that the sepsis rate was reduced by almost 50% after the new policy was inaugurated.

Almost all antibiotics have been used for the purpose. Most of the recent trials have employed cephalosporins of varying generations with little difference in results (Faro et al 1990, Peterson et al 1990). It is certain that each new antibiotic that is developed will be tried for the purpose of prophylaxis in cases of Caesarean section. In practice, each obstetric unit will have to decide for itself which antibiotic is appropriate for its own prophylactic use, bearing in mind such factors as cost and the spectrum of bacterial flora with which they have to cope.

Table 43.3 The effect of prophylactic antibiotic administration: Baragwanath Hospital, Johannesburg, April 1989 to March 1990 versus April 1991 to March 1992

	1989–90	1991–92
Total deliveries	19 278	18 593
Total CS (Rate)	3766 (19.5%)	3578 (19.2%)
Septic CS	394	203
Septic CS as proportion of total CS	10.5%	5.7%
Septic CS as proportion of total sepsis	58.3%	37.5%

The routine use of prophylactic antibiotics for patients undergoing emergency Caesarean section was instituted in January 1991.
CS = Caesarean section.

The route of administration has also been a point of discussion. Systemic use has been most popular, but there is a case to be made for local application in the form of irrigation of the operative field. The main advantage of the latter is that it is the surgeon's responsibility to administer the therapy, and other members of staff do not have to be depended upon. Wu (1992) found no difference between systemic and local administration, and both were better than placebo. Lewis et al (1990) also found irrigation to be effective.

Most practitioners prefer to administer the first dose after the clamping of the cord, in order to avoid any ill-effects on the fetus, and this policy makes good sense, even if it results in a marginal diminution in the effectiveness of the regimen.

The trend is towards shorter and shorter courses of antibiotic, although Enkin et al (1989) concluded from their review that short courses of antibiotics were less effective than longer courses, and single-dose regimens than multiple-dose regimens. Perhaps the development of longer-acting agents such as ceftriaxone will resolve this problem.

THE MANAGEMENT OF PUERPERAL SEPSIS

Epidemiological considerations

Notification of puerperal sepsis is no longer required, as the disease has to a large extent lost its epidemic nature, and it is seldom necessary to trace contacts and close hospitals in an effort to contain spread.

Many maternity hospitals still have separate wards for patients with postpartum infection, but the practice of isolation is tending to disappear. Provided they are not understaffed, and have the facilities for coping with serious illness, isolation wards do provide a satisfactory method of dealing with puerperal infection. It is not a bad thing for patients with wound sepsis to be segregated from others with clean wounds, provided they are not made to feel that their dismissal from the company of their peers is because of some deficiency on their part. If *Streptococcus pyogenes* group A is cultured, then isolation is mandatory.

General care

As in any illness, the general care of the patient is important. Adequate fluid and caloric intake must be ensured, by intravenous infusion if necessary. Anaemia if present should be corrected, and repeated checks of haemoglobin, leucocyte and platelet counts should be requested.

Pain must be treated with adequate dosage of analgesic agents, and sources of distress such as a distended urinary bladder or distended bowel must be attended to. Urinary retention is a frequent concomitant to pelvic infection, especially if there has been abscess formation, and the placing of an indwelling catheter will not only relieve the discomfort, but also provide the means of accurate measurement of the urinary output.

The question of breastfeeding is vexed. Our policy is to continue to encourage breastfeeding unless the patient is in too much physical distress to cope with it. If the woman is to continue with breastfeeding, there may need to be modification of the medication that is prescribed, bearing in mind that most substances are excreted into the breast milk in varying concentration.

Local therapy

Local treatment of infected wounds follows the standard principles normally employed in such cases. Drainage must be promoted, and it is usually necessary to remove a variable number of the more superficial sutures.

Treatment of an abdominal wound afflicted with severe suppuration and large amounts of slough usually involves irrigation and the application of local medication. Irrigation with solutions such as hydrogen peroxide, Eusol or dilute Savlon (cetrimide + chlorhexidine) is usual, and local applications used may be Debrisan (dextranomer) or Aserbine (a mixture of propylene glycol with benzoic, malic and salicylic acids). Secondary suturing is almost always required.

For perineal sepsis, local cleansing with dilute Savlon is recommended, and healing is almost always excellent.

Antibiotics

Antibiotic therapy is the mainstay of treatment for puerperal sepsis, and has revolutionized the outcome of this formerly dreaded disease. There are probably as many regimens of therapy as there are maternity units, and there is not much to choose between them in terms of results. It can be predicted with confidence that each newly developed antibiotic agent will be put up in trial in cases of puerperal morbidity against one of the older effective formulations.

The principles of antibiotic therapy for puerperal sepsis remain inviolate, however, and they include the following:

1. The disease is polymicrobial in origin, and treatment must therefore cover Gram-positive and -negative, aerobic and anaerobic microorganisms.
2. Multiple-agent therapy is acceptable and perhaps to be preferred.
3. Parenteral, preferably intravenous administration is advisable in the first instance. The change to oral administration may be made when the patient is recovering, intestinal ileus is no longer present and there is certainty concerning gastrointestinal absorption capacity. The antibiotic agent should therefore be capable of administration by both parenteral and oral routes (although Dinsmoor et al

(1991) found that there was no difference between patients followed up with oral therapy compared to those given placebo after successful intravenous treatment of postpartum endometritis).

4. The common pathogens in a particular geographical area should be known, and their probable susceptability to the planned therapy borne in mind.

Our own preferred antibiotic regimen at the present time consists of a combination of:

Ampicillin 500 mg to 1 g 6 hourly by intravenous injection
Amikacin 500 mg 12 hourly by intravenous injection
Metronidazole 1 g suppository 8 hourly per rectum.

Intravenous metronidazole, 500 mg 6 hourly by intravenous infusion is preferred to the rectal suppository in very ill patients, or those with lower bowel complications. In the event of poor or absent response, the initial reaction is to substitute clindamycin, 600 mg 6 hourly by intravenous infusion, for both the ampicillin and the metronidazole.

Bacteriological specimens for culture are then taken, and any further change in therapy will be directed by the microbiologist's report.

Cefoxitin, having been commenced as a prophylactic, will be continued in the puerperium in those cases where macroscopic infection is detected at Caesarean section.

There are many other regimens which have been established to be effective. In the USA the most frequently used initial therapy is a combination of clindamycin and gentamicin (Ledger 1990) but almost all the cephalosporins and the broad-spectrum synthetic penicillins have been used, alone or in combination, and usually with success. The most recent trials have been directed at establishing single-agent therapy which will cover all the potential pathogens and the results appear to be satisfactory.

Some of the antibiotics being tried as single-agent therapy are listed in Table 43.4.

In a recent review, Pastorek & Sanders (1991) expressed

Table 43.4 Antibiotics tried as single-agent therapy

Cephalosporins and cephamycins
Cefoxitin (Martens et al 1990a)
Cefamandole (Peterson et al 1990)
Moxalactam
Cefotaxime (Dinsmoor & Gibbs 1988)
Ceftazidime (Dinsmoor & Gibbs 1988)
Ceftriaxone

Penicillins with or without beta-lactamase inhibitor
Pipericillin
Ticarcillin (+ clavulanic acid) (Faro et al 1991)
Ampicillin (+ sulbactam) (Martens et al 1990b)
Amoxycillin (+ potassium clavulanate)

Fluoroquinolones
Norfloxacin
Ciprofloxacin (Maccato et al 1991)

some enthusiasm for the use of single-agent beta-lactam antibiotics for post Caesarean endomyometritis, and welcomed the addition of the beta-lactamase inhibitors to these drugs.

The present situation seems to be that any number of antibiotics or combinations of antibiotics are effective. The choice is going to depend on affordability and availability as well as effectiveness.

Surgery

Traditionally surgery has not played a leading role in the management of puerperal sepsis. The response to antibiotics is usually excellent, and surgery is reserved for those cases with complications, or which deteriorate in spite of appropriate treatment.

Operative treatment may be called for if the presence of retained portions of placenta or membrane in the uterus is strongly suspected or confirmed. These devitalized tissues form a perfect bed for the seeding of microorganisms, and the anaerobes particularly will flourish. Gentle curettage of the uterine cavity, by preference utilizing the suction curette, should be performed.

Abscesses that do not respond to antibiotic therapy need to be evacuated. First attempts may be made at emptying the cavity by needle under ultrasound guidance. If the abscess reaccumulates surgical drainage is required. The approach will depend on the situation of the abscess, and may be by colpotomy through the posterior vaginal fornix, extraperitoneally through the abdominal wall (Fig. 43.1) or by means of laparotomy. The latter is the most frequent approach employed in practice (Ledger 1990). If laparotomy is performed for any reason, it is advisable to wash the peritoneal cavity thoroughly with warm normal saline. If any appreciable amount of pus is found in the peritoneal cavity, it has become standard practice to plan on performing at least one second-look laparotomy to clear any remaining areas of suppuration, and to rewash the abdomen. This may be repeated on several occasions although, not surprisingly, the prognosis deteriorates with each successive procedure. If a second-look procedure is anticipated, it is helpful to leave the wound open, external to the rectus sheath. This will also facilitate management of local wound sepsis, which is an invariable accompaniment.

On occasion, hysterectomy is required. When the response is poor, and the patient's condition is deteriorating despite appropriate antibiotic being given in adequate dosage, removal of the septic focus may be the only course available. This is particularly likely in case of uterine necrosis as caused by *C. perfringens* infection, and may also be necessitated in patients with septic shock and its complications. Our natural reluctance to sterilize a young and fertile woman often leads us to delay in deciding to perform this operation although it may be life-saving.

We make the decision as a last resort, and sometimes, we decide too late.

Once in a while surgery is necessitated by the development of a complication of the original condition. Thus it may become necessary to operate to relieve a bowel obstruction which may have arisen as a consequence of adhesion of the intestine to the inflamed pelvic organs. Bowel may also have been damaged at the original Caesarean section. In cases of pelvic vein thrombophlebitis

with septic embolization it may become necessary to occlude, at least partially, the inferior vena cava.

Surgery is never the first-line therapy for puerperal sepsis. When it is necessary, however, the decision to proceed must not be delayed while antibiotics are chopped and changed, but rather the planned procedure should be expedited.

We should do as little as possible but as much as is necessary.

REFERENCES

Amstey M S 1976 Immunization in pregnancy. Clinical Obstetrics and Gynecology 19: 47–60

Apter S, Shamann S, Ben-Baruch G, Rubinstein Z J, Barkai G, Hertz M 1992 CT of pelvic infection after cesarean section. Clinical and Experimental Obstetrics and Gynecology (Padova) 19: 156–160

Baker C J, Rench M A, Edwards M S, Carpenter R J, Hays B M, Kasper D L 1988 Immunization of pregnant women with a polysaccharide vaccine of group B streptococcus. New England Journal of Medicine 319: 1180–1185

Barnes J, Bender S 1955 The abnormal puerperium. In: Holland Sir E (ed) British obstetric and gynaecological practice: obstetrics. Heinemann, London, pp 821–850

Berenson A B, Hammill H A, Martens M G, Faro S 1990 Bacteriologic findings of post-cesarean endometritis in adolescents. Obstetrics and Gynecology 75: 627–629

Blanco J D, Gibbs R S, Castaneda Y S 1981 Bacteraemia in obstetrics: clinical course. Obstetrics and Gynecology 58: 621–625

Brown C E L, Lowe T W, Cunningham F G, Weinreb J C 1986 Puerperal pelvic thrombophlebitis: impact on diagnosis and treatment using X-ray computed tomography and magnetic resonance imaging. Obstetrics and Gynecology 68: 789–794

Brown C E L, Dunn D H, Harrell R, Setiawan H, Cunningham F G 1991 Computed tomography for evaluation of puerperal infections. Surgery, Gynecology and Obstetrics 172: 285–289

Burman L G, Christensen P, Christensen K et al 1992 Prevention of excess neonatal morbidity associated with group B streptococci by vaginal chlorhexidine disinfection during labour. Lancet 340: 65–69

Chalmers I, Garcia J, Post S 1989 Hospital policies for labour and delivery. In: Chalmers I, Enkin M, Keirse M J N C (eds) Effective care in pregnancy and childbirth. Vol 2: Childbirth. Oxford University Press, Oxford, pp 815–819

Cohen W R 1977 Influence of the duration of second stage labor on perinatal outcome and puerperal morbidity. Obstetrics and Gynecology 49: 266–269

Coulam C B, Silverfield J C, Kazmar R E, Fathman C G 1983 T lymphocyte subsets during pregnancy and the menstrual cycle. American Journal of Reproductive Immunology 4: 88–90

Cox S M, Gilstrap L C III 1989 Postpartum endometritis. Obstetrics and Gynecology Clinics of North America 16: 363–371

Crowther C, Enkin M, Keurse M J N C, Brown I 1989 Monitoring the progress of labour. In: Chalmers I, Enkin M, Keirse M J N C (eds) Effective care in pregnancy and childbirth. Vol 2: Childbirth. Oxford University Press, Oxford, pp 833–845

Cunningham D S, Evans E E 1991 The effects of betamethasone on maternal cellular resistance to infection. American Journal of Obstetrics and Gynecology 165: 610–615

Despodova T S, Rusev R, Barov D 1989 Changes in specific and nonspecific immune reactivity in women with a complicated obstetrico-gynecologic status. Akusherstvo I Ginekologiia (Sofiia) 28: 6–10

Dinsmoor M J, Gibbs R S 1988 The role of the newer antimicrobial agents in obstetrics and gynecology. Clinical Obstetrics and Gynecology 31: 423–433

Dinsmoor M J, Newton E R, Gibbs R S 1991 A randomized, double-blind, placebo-controlled trial of oral antibiotic therapy following intravenous antibiotic therapy for postpartum endometritis. Obstetrics and Gynecology 77: 60–62

Duff P, Gibbs R S 1983 Maternal sepsis. In: Berkowitz R L (ed) Critical care of the obstetric patient. Churchill Livingstone, New York, pp 189–217

Duff P, Gibbs R S, Blanco J D, St Clair P J 1983 Endometrial culture techniques in puerperal patients. Obstetrics and Gynecology 61: 217–222

Enkin M, Enkin E, Chalmers I, Hemminki E 1989 Prophylactic antibiotics in association with caesarean section. In: Chalmers I, Enkin M, Keirse M J N C (eds) Effective care in pregnancy and childbirth. Vol 2: Childbirth. Oxford University Press, Oxford, pp 1246–1269

Eschenbach D A, Wager G P 1980 Puerperal infections. Clinical Obstetrics and Gynecology 23: 1003–1035

Eschenbach D A, Rosene K, Tompkins L S, Watkins H, Gravett M G 1986 Endometrial cultures obtained by a triple-lumen method from afebrile and febrile postpartum women. Journal of Infectious Diseases 153: 1038–1045

Faro S, Martens M G, Hammill H A, Riddle G, Tortolero G 1990 Antibiotic prophylaxis: is there a difference? American Journal of Obstetrics and Gynecology 162: 900–907

Faro S, Hammill H A, Maccato M, Martens M 1991 Ticarcillin/clavulanate for treatment of postpartum endometritis. Reviews of Infectious Diseases 13: S758–S762

Feinberg B B, Gonik B 1991 General precepts of the immunology of pregnancy. Clinical Obstetrics and Gynecology 34: 3–16

Filler L, Shipley C F IIIrd, Dennis E J IIIrd 1992 Postcaesarean endometritis: a brief review and comparison of three antibiotic regimens. Journal of the South Carolina Medical Association 88: 291–295

Fry R M 1938 Fatal infections by haemolytic streptococcus group B. Lancet i: 199–201

Gibbs R S 1976 Treatment of refractory postpartum fever. Clinical Obstetrics and Gynecology 19: 83–95

Gibbs R S, Weinstein A J 1976 Puerperal infection in the antibiotic era. American Journal of Obstetrics and Gynecology 124: 769–785

Gilstrap L C III, Cunningham F G 1979 The bacterial pathogenesis of infection following cesarean section. Obstetrics and Gynecology 53: 545–549

Glassman A B, Bennett C E, Christopher J B, Self S 1985 Immunity during pregnancy: lymphocyte subpopulations and mitogen responsiveness. Annals of Clinical and Laboratory Science 15: 357–362

Graham H (pseud) 1950 Eternal Eve. Heinemann, London

Golde S, Ledger W J 1977 Necrotizing fasciitis in postpartum patients. A report of four cases. Obstetrics and Gynecology 50: 670–673

Gordon A 1795 A treatise on the epidemic puerperal fever of Aberdeen. Robinson, London

Harrison R H, Alexander E R, Weinstein L, Lewis M, Nash M, Sim D A 1983 Cervical Chlamydia trachomatis and mycoplasmal infections in pregnancy. Journal of the American Medical Association 250: 1721–1728

Holbrook K F, Nottebart V F, Hameed S R, Platt R 1991 Automated postdischarge surveillance for postpartum and neonatal nosocomial infections. American Journal of Medicine 91: 125S–130S

Holmes O W 1843 The contagiousness of puerperal fever. New England Quarterly Journal of Medicine and Surgery 1: 503–520

Hurley R 1987 Microbiology. In: Philipp E, Barnes J, Newton M (eds) Scientific foundations of obstetrics and gynaecology, 3rd (international) edn. Heinemann, London

Jacqui P, Sedallion A 1992 Role of mycoplasmas in the last month of pregnancy and postpartum pathology. Prospective study of 577 pregnancies. Revue Francais de Gynecologie et d'Obstetrique 87: 134–144

Janevicius R V, Hann S-E, Batt M D 1982 Necrotizing fasciitis. Surgery, Gynecology and Obstetrics 154: 97–102

Jawetz E, Melnick J L, Adelberg E A (eds) 1982 Microbial genetics. In: Review of medical microbiology. Lange, Los Altos, ch 4, p 51

Kaiser I H 1976 The obstetric death of Mary Wollstonecroft. American Journal of Obstetrics and Gynecology 125: 1–2

Keirse M J N C, Ohlsson A, Treffers P E, Kanhai H H H 1989 Prelabour rupture of the membranes preterm. In: Chalmers I, Enkin M, Keirse M J N C (eds) Effective care in pregnancy and childbirth. Vol 1: Pregnancy. Oxford University Press, Oxford, pp 666–693

Ledger W J 1990 Infections of the female pelvis. In: Mandell G, Douglas R G Jr, Bennet J E (eds) Principles and practice of infectious diseases. Churchill Livingstone, New York, pp 965–970

Lee W, Clark S L, Cotton D B et al 1988 Septic shock during pregnancy. American Journal of Obstetrics and Gynecology 159: 410–416

Lewis D F, Otterson W N, Dunnihoo D R 1990 Antibiotic prophylactic uterine lavage in caesarean section: a double-blind comparison of saline, ticarcillin and cefoxitin irrigation in indigent patients. Southern Medical Journal 83: 274–276

Maccato M L, Faro S, Martens M G, Hammill H A 1991 Ciprofloxacin versus gentamycin/clindamycin for postpartum endometritis. Journal of Reproductive Medicine 36: 857–861

Martens M, Faro S, Hammill H, Maccato M 1990a Treatment of postpartum endometritis. Hospital Practice (Office edition) 25 (suppl 4): 13–19

Martens M G, Faro S, Hammill H A, Smith D, Riddle G, Maccato M 1990b Ampicillin/sulbactam versus clindamycin in the treatment of postpartum endomyometritis. Southern Medical Journal 83: 408–413

McCurdy C M, Magann E F, McCurdy C J, Saltzman A K 1992 The effect of placental management at cesarean delivery on operative blood loss. American Journal of Obstetrics and Gynecology 167: 1363–1366

McGregor J A, French J I 1991 Chlamydia trachomatis infection during pregnancy. American Journal of Obstetrics and Gynecology 164: 1782–1789

McGregor J A, French J L, Richter R et al 1990 Antenatal microbiologic and maternal risk factors associated with prematurity. American Journal of Obstetrics and Gynecology 163: 1465–1473

McGregor J A, Lawellin D, Franco-Buff A, Todd J K 1991 Phospholipase C activity in microorganisms associated with reproductive tract infection. American Journal of Obstetrics and Gynecology 164: 682–686

Miller R D, Crichton D 1968 Ampicillin prophylaxis in caesarean section. South African Journal of Obstetrics and Gynaecology 6: 69–70

Monif G R 1991 Intrapartum bacteriuria and postpartum endometritis. Obstetrics and Gynecology 78: 245–248

MRC/RCOG Working Party on Cervical Cerclage 1988 Interim Report of the Medical Research Council/Royal College of Obstetricians and Gynaecologists Multicentre Randomised Trial of Cervical Cerclage. British Journal of Obstetrics and Gynaecology 95: 437–445

Newton E R, Prihoda T J, Gibbs R S 1990 A clinical and microbiological analysis of risk factors for puerperal endometritis. Obstetrics and Gynecology 75: 402–406

Nikonov A P, Burlev V A, Ankirskaia A S, Sergeev M V, Lutfullaeva N A 1991 Diagnostic value of lochial pH, P_{CO_2} and P_{O_2} in puerperal endometritis. Akusherstvo I Ginekologiia (Moskva) 6: 42–44

Ogden E, Amstey M S 1977 Puerperal infection due to group A beta hemolytic streptococcus. Obstetrics and Gynecology 52: 53–55

Okonofua F E, Onwudwiegu U, Odunsi O A 1991 Preterm premature rupture of fetal membranes in a low socioeconomic population: results of conservative management. International Journal of Obstetrics and Gynecology 34: 35–39

Owen J, Henson B V, Hauth J C 1990 A prospective randomized study of saline solution amnioinfusion. American Journal of Obstetrics and Gynecology 162: 1146–1149

Ozumba B C, Uchegbu H 1991 Incidence and management of obstructed labour in eastern Nigeria. Australian and New Zealand Journal of Obstetrics and Gynaecology 31: 213–216

Pastorek J G II, Sanders C V Jr 1991 Antibiotic therapy for postcesarean endomyometritis. Reviews of Infectious Diseases 13: 752S–757S

Patchell R D 1976 Clostridial myonecrosis of the postpartum uterus with radiologic diagnosis. Obstetrics and Gynecology 51: 14S–15S

Patino F P, Castro D 1991 Necrotizing lesions of soft tissues. World Journal of Surgery 15: 235–239

Pelle H, Jepson O B, Larsen S O et al 1986 Wound infection after caesarean section. Infection Control and Hospital Epidemiology 7: 456–461

Pessa M E, Howard R J 1985 Necrotizing fasciitis. Surgery, Gynecology and Obstetrics 161: 357–361

Peterson C M, Medchill M, Gordon D S, Chard H L 1990 Cesarean prophylaxis: a comparison of cefamandole and cefazolin by both intravenous and lavage routes, and risk factors associated with endometritis. Obstetrics and Gynecology 75: 179–182

Rehu M, Nilsson C G 1980 Risk factors for febrile morbidity associated with cesarean section. Obstetrics and Gynecology 56: 269–273

Richards W R 1943 An evaluation of the local use of sulfonamide drugs in certain gynecological operations. American Journal of Obstetrics and Gynecology 46: 541–545

Rosene K, Eschenbach D A, Tompkins L S, Kenny G E, Watkins H 1986 Polymicrobial early postpartum endometritis with facultative and anaerobic bacteria, genital mycoplasmas and Chlamydia trachomatis: treatment with piperacillin or cefoxitin. Journal of Infectious Diseases 153: 1028–1036

Rush R W, Isaacs S, McPherson K, Jones L, Chalmers I, Grant A 1984 A randomized controlled trial of cervical cerclage in women at high risk of preterm delivery. British Journal of Obstetrics and Gynaecology 91: 724–730

Rusin P, Adam R D, Peterson E A, Ryan K J, Sinclair N A, Weinstein L 1991 Haemophilus influenzae: an important cause of maternal and neonatal infections. Obstetrics and Gynecology 77: 92–96

Saunders N S, Paterson C M, Wadsworth J 1992 Neonatal and maternal morbidity in relation to the length of the second stage of labour. British Journal of Obstetrics and Gynaecology 99: 381–385

Semmelweiss I P 1861 Die aetiologie, der begriff und die prophylaxis des kindbettfiebers. Pest Vienna and Leipzig

Seo K, McGregor J A, French J I 1992 Preterm birth is associated with increased risk of maternal and neonatal infection. Obstetrics and Gynecology 79: 75–80

Silver R M, Heddleston L N, McGregor J A, Gibbs R S 1992 Life-threatening puerperal infection due to group A streptococci. Obstetrics and Gynecology 79: 894–896

Smaill F 1993 Prophylactic antibiotics in caesarean section (all trials). In: Enkin M W, Keirse M J N C, Renfrew M J, Neilson J P (eds) Pregnancy and childbirth module. Cochrane database of systematic reviews: review no 03690, 18 December 1992. Cochrane Updates on Disk, Update Software, Oxford

Soper D E, Mayhall C G, Dalton H P 1989 Risk factors for intraamniotic infection: a prospective epidemiologic study. American Journal of Obstetrics and Gynecology 161: 562–568

Sweet R L, Ledger W J 1973 Puerperal infectious morbidity: a two-year review. American Journal of Obstetrics and Gynecology 117: 1093–1100

Viglionese A, Nottebart V F, Bodman H A, Platt R 1991 Recurrent group A streptococcal carriage in a health care worker associated with widely separated nosocomial outbreaks. American Journal of Medicine 91: 329S–333S

Wachsberg R H, Kurtz A B 1992 Gas within the endometrial cavity at postpartum US: a normal finding after spontaneous vaginal delivery. Radiology 183: 431–433

Wager G P, Martin D H, Koutsky L et al 1980 Puerperal infectious morbidity: relationship to route of delivery and to antepartum Chlamydia trachomatis infection. American Journal of Obstetrics and Gynecology 138: 1028–1033

Watts D H, Krohn M A, Hillier S L, Eschenbach D A 1990 Bacterial vaginosis as a risk factor for post-cesarean endometritis. Obstetrics and Gynecology 75: 52–58

Weidinger H, Passloer H J, Kovacs L, Berle B 1991 The advantage of preventive vaginal antisepsis with hexetedine in obstetrics and gynecology. Geburtshilfe und Frauenheilkunde 51: 929–935

Wessels M R, Kasper 1993 The changing spectrum of group B streptococcal disease. New England Journal of Medicine 328: 1843–1844

Wu Y 1992 Prevention of post-operative infection by using antibiotics in 217 cases of cesarean section. Chung-Hua Fu Chan Ko Tsa Chih (Peking) 27: 73–75

Yadav Y R, Yadav S, Kala P C 1991 Puerperal tetanus. Journal of the Indian Medical Association 89: 336–337

Yonekura M L 1988 Treatment of postcesarean endomyometritis. Clinical Obstetrics and Gynecology 31: 488–500

Young M J, Cox R A 1990 Near fatal puerperal fever due to *Mycoplasma hominis*. Postgraduate Medical Journal 66: 147–149

44. Venous thrombosis and pulmonary embolism

John Bonnar

INTRODUCTION

Thrombosis is the process by which liquid blood flowing through the vascular system turns into a solid mass of platelets, cells and fibrin within the blood vessel. The most serious vascular complication that can arise during pregnancy or the puerperium is venous thrombosis with pulmonary embolism. As maternal deaths from haemorrhage, eclampsia and sepsis have decreased over the last 30 years, pulmonary embolism has become a leading cause of maternal mortality in many obstetric services. Since 1952, the Confidential Enquiries into Maternal Deaths in England and Wales recorded almost 1000 maternal deaths from pulmonary embolism. From 1970, pulmonary embolism has ranked as the first or second most important cause of maternal death (Department of Health and Social Security 1994).

Since the majority of patients with pulmonary embolism die within 1 hour without diagnosis and treatment, the number of deaths will not be greatly reduced by improvements in treatment of the established condition. Deaths from pulmonary embolism can be reduced by more attention to predisposing factors and to selective use of effective prophylactic measures in high-risk patients, especially in late pregnancy and the early puerperium.

The accurate diagnosis of venous thrombosis and pulmonary embolism is of vital importance in pregnancy. Besides the immediate threat to the mother and the possible hazards to the fetus of treatment, the diagnosis of thrombosis has long-term implications for the woman—the wisdom of having any further pregnancies and the need for prophylaxis therein, the use of the combined pill, oestrogen replacement at and after the menopause and the increased risks of future surgery.

The diagnostic problem usually arises when the symptoms and clinical signs are minimal. It is less common to find classic presentation of iliofemoral thrombosis with a white leg (phlegmasia alba dolens) and the extreme form with intense swelling of the leg, deep cyanosis and diminished arterial pulses, with or without impending gangrene (phlegmasia caerulea dolens). The reduction of incidence of these conditions is most likely a result of the improvement in the general health of pregnant women, younger mothers and lower parity, recognition of the dangers of bedrest during pregnancy and especially after delivery, the use of prophylactic measures and the early diagnosis and treatment of the disease. Thromboembolic disease is best decribed by the term venous thrombosis, specifying the segments of the venous system involved and with pulmonary embolism as its major complication.

PATHOGENESIS OF VENOUS THROMBOSIS IN PREGNANCY

The basis for much of our understanding of the genesis of venous thrombosis was described in the mid 19th century by Virchow (1860). He postulated a triad of factors which predisposed to thrombosis:

1. Impaired blood flow resulting in venous stasis.
2. Changes in the blood coagulability.
3. Alteration or damage to the intima of the vein.

Changes in the vessel wall are now recognized as crucial to the understanding of arterial thrombosis but are less relevant for venous thrombogenesis. Vessel wall damage appears to be a poor stimulus to fibrin formation and has never been convincingly demonstrated as a significant aetiological factor in venous thrombosis (Thomas 1987). The only known additional factor that can rapidly transform static blood into a venous thrombosis is the generation of thrombin. If thrombin is present in areas of retarded blood flow, platelets aggregate and fibrinogen is converted to fibrin which provides the basic structure of a venous thrombus (Fig. 44.1). The degree of local fibrinolytic activity in the blood influences the extent to which fibrin will be deposited on an initial platelet nidus and whether a platelet fibrin nidus will be propagated or disappear.

Certain physiological changes of pregnancy predispose to thrombosis. The blood coagulation system undergoes major changes during pregnancy with marked increases in several of the plasma proteins concerned with clotting. In particular, the levels of fibrinogen, factors VII, VIII and X show a substantial rise. The natural inhibitors of blood coagulation, protein C and protein S, have been shown to alter in pregnancy with protein C increasing and protein S decreasing. Inherited deficiency of these inhibitors will predispose to venous thrombosis in pregnancy. In late pregnancy an increased ability to neutralize heparin is also present; this disappears following delivery (Bonnar

1976). This heparin resistance is probably due to the local activation of coagulation in the uteroplacental circulation. Fibrinolytic activity in plasma decreases progressively from early pregnancy and the amount of plasminogen activator which can be released from the venous endothelium is also reduced. These changes in fibrinolysis during pregnancy may be due to the progressive increase of the level of fast-acting tissue-type plasminogen activator inhibitor (Aznar et al 1986).

In late pregnancy, the velocity of venous blood flow in the lower limbs is reduced by about 50% and this is accompanied by a rise in venous pressure by about 10 mmHg. This is due to increased venous distensibility as well as the pressure of the gravid uterus which impedes venous return. The substantial increase of venous blood flow from the gravid uterus along the internal iliac veins will also cause back pressure on the venous return in the external iliac veins draining the lower limbs.

The pathogenesis of thrombosis in pregnancy is therefore most likely to be a product of the increased tendency to venous stasis in the lower limbs, combined with a shift in the balance between coagulation and fibrinolysis towards enhanced coagulation and diminished fibrinolysis, which will encourage thrombus growth.

Incidence in pregnancy

The incidence of thromboembolic complications in pregnancy is probably greatly underestimated and in published reports varies between two and five per 1000 deliveries (Aaro & Juergens 1974, Coon 1977). In a population study in the USA, approximately one-half of all venous thromboembolic events occurring in women below the age of 40 were related to pregnancy or the puerperium (Coon et al 1973). The Confidential Enquiries into Maternal Deaths reported 24 deaths from pulmonary embolism in 1988–90, similar to 25 deaths in the previous triennia (Department of Health and Social Security 1994). Deaths in 1988–90 included 13 deaths during pregnancy, and 11 after delivery. Of the latter, eight followed Caesarean section and three vaginal delivery. Table 44.1 shows the number of deaths from pulmonary embolism from 1952 to 1990. The number of deaths following all forms of vaginal delivery has fallen steadily since 1955, but those following Caesarean section have not decreased at the same rate. Since 1979 about half of the deaths have occurred during the antenatal period and these have been distributed throughout pregnancy.

Table 44.2 shows the interval between delivery and fatal pulmonary embolism following vaginal delivery and Caesarean section during the years 1970–87. Deaths from postpartum pulmonary embolism can occur at any time, whatever the mode of delivery. The most dangerous period is the first 7 days, followed by the second week, after which the risk decreases. About 15% of the deaths

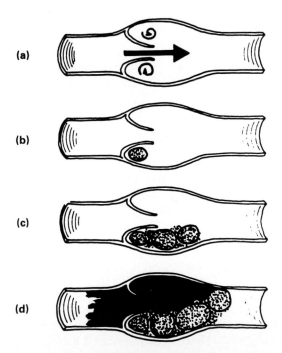

Fig. 44.1 Stages in the development of a thrombus in the valve pocket. (**a**) Vortex flow in the venous valve pocket results in an area of maximum stasis with local accumulation of activated clotting factors, platelets, leucocytes and red blood cells. (**b**) Following thrombin generation a platelet fibrin nidus forms, consisting of successive alternate layers of aggregated platelets and fibrin. (**c**) Platelet–fibrin aggregates develop on the propagating head of the thrombus and lead to thrombus growth. (**d**) Retrograde extension of the thrombus occurs when the forward propagating thrombus grows to occlude the vein. From Thomas (1987).

Table 44.1 Maternal death due to pulmonary embolism in England and Wales from 1952 to 1990

	After abortion or during pregnancy	After vaginal delivery	After Caesarean section	Total
1952–54	4	104	30	138
1955–57	24	114	26	164
1958–60	36	80	22	138
1961–63	47	66	27	140
1964–66	27	43	25	95
1967–69	28	36	18	82
1970–72	24	23	15	62
1973–75	17	13	6	36
1976–78	16	20	9	45
1979–81	17	4	7	28
1982–84	13	4	12	29
1985–87	17	5	3	25
1988–90	13	3	8	24

From Department of Health and Social Security (1994).

Table 44.2 Interval between delivery and pulmonary embolism following vaginal delivery and Caesarean section (1970–87)

	Vaginal delivery	Caesarean sections
1–7 days	27 (40%)	19 (37%)
8–14 days	14 (20%)	12 (23%)
15–42 days	27 (40%)	21 (40%)
Total	68 (100%)	52 (100%)

From Department of Health and Social Security (1991).

following vaginal delivery and following Caesarean section occurred within 24 hours. This indicates that prophylactic measures against thromboembolism in high-risk patients should cover the period of labour and Caesarean section.

Specific aetiological factors in obstetric patients

The Confidential Enquiries indicate that where thromboembolism results in a maternal death, the following factors are important:

1. *Method of delivery:* the increased risk of thromboembolism after Caesarean section is clearly shown in Table 44.1. The frequency of fatal pulmonary embolism during these years was on average more than 10 times greater after Caesarean section than after vaginal delivery.
2. *Age and parity:* the risk of fatal pulmonary embolism increases more sharply with advancing age—particularly in those aged 35 years or more—than with increasing parity.
3. *Excessive obesity (exceeding 76 kg or 12 stone):* obesity is generally accepted as an important factor in the development of thromboembolism. Approximately one in five women dying of pulmonary embolism are in this category.
4. *Hospitalization and restricted activity:* women admitted to hospital on account of obstetric complications such

as hypertension and placenta praevia are at increased risk, probably because of the restricted activity.
5. *Suppression, of lactation by oestrogens:* oestrogen administration has been shown to predispose to thromboembolism in several clinical situations. The association between suppression of lactation with stilboestrol and thromboembolism was first suggested by Daniel et al (1967). These authors showed a 10-fold increase in non-fatal thromboembolism in low-parity women of 25 years and over who were not lactating compared to those who were. For this reason it seems unwise to introduce combined oestrogen—progestogen oral contraception in the immediate puerperium.
6. *History of deep vein thrombosis of pulmonary embolism in association with pregnancy, surgery or the contraceptive pill:* women with a previous proven deep vein thrombosis or pulmonary embolism must be regarded as especially at risk during pregnancy. Likewise, women undergoing a surgical operation during pregnancy are at greater risk.
7. *Lupus anticoagulant-associated thrombotic disease:* the presence of lupus anticoagulant is associated with an increased thrombotic tendency and recurrent abortions.
8. *Hereditary thrombotic disease:* women with any of the known hereditary thrombotic disorders must be considered at increased risk of thromboembolic complications during pregnancy, e.g. hereditary antithrombin III deficiency, protein C and protein S deficiency.

THE DIAGNOSIS OF DEEP VEIN THROMBOSIS AND PULMONARY EMBOLISM DURING PREGNANCY

Clinical features

Deep vein thrombosis

The normal discomforts of pregnancy can often mimic the symptoms of leg vein thrombosis. Leg cramps, swelling of the ankles, slight cyanosis of the legs and on standing an increased prominence of the superficial veins are often seen, especially in late pregnancy. Venous thrombosis when present will almost invariably cause more symptoms in one leg than the other and predominantly in the left leg. The diagnosis of deep vein thrombosis is almost certain when physical signs such as definite tenderness and induration of the calf muscles, unilateral oedema and increased skin temperature of the leg are present. The diagnostic problem lies in the patient in whom the clinical signs are either absent or equivocal. Examination of the lower limbs should include comparison of the minimum circumference at the calf and thighs. A difference of 2 cm or more at identical sites on the legs should be regarded as significant. In the early stages, even extensive thrombi are often asymptomatic and their presence may first be suspected with the occurrence of pulmonary embolism. Autopsy studies have shown that in almost half the patients there are no clinical signs or symptoms referable to the limbs and fatal embolism may be the first indication of thrombosis.

Unlike early or localized thrombosis, the clinical diagnosis of extensive femoral or iliofemoral thrombosis is much more accurate, as the majority of propagating venous thrombi completely occlude the lumen, causing obstruction of the venous return. The patient usually presents with pain in the calf or thigh and swelling of the leg. The onset is usually rapid but there is often a history of previous pain in the calf muscles.

Examination of the affected limb will usually show swelling and oedema with dilatation of the superficial veins. The increase in skin temperature of the affected limb is because most of the venous return is taking place through the superficial veins. The distal part of the limb may however be pale or cyanosed with absent or reduced pedal pulses. This is the result of secondary arterial spasm which often accompanies massive iliofemoral thrombosis. When thrombosis extends into the iliofemoral segment, tenderness is usually present along the course of the femoral vein.

Prospective studies using radioactive fibrinogen tests and phlebography have shown that only half the patients with early deep vein thrombosis have demonstrable clinical symptoms or signs. The reverse is also true: some 25–50% of patients with clinical signs of thrombosis have no demonstrable venous thrombi. Therefore the treatment of patients based purely on clinical signs will result in a significant proportion receiving unnecessary treatment with its attendant hazards.

Whenever possible objective diagnostic methods should be used to confirm the presence of suspected deep vein thrombosis.

Pulmonary embolism

The symptoms and signs of pulmonary embolism are predominantly associated with the cardiovascular and respiratory systems. The immediate effects vary from clinically silent to sudden death and depend on the size of the embolus and the preceding health of the patient. In the author's experience, pregnant women with iliofemoral thrombosis frequently show evidence on lung scanning of small symptomless pulmonary emboli. These small emboli are probably cleared from the pulmonary circulation within a few days by the potent fibrinolytic activity in the lung vasculature.

When pulmonary infarction occurs it is usually accompanied by the sudden onset of dyspnoea, pleural pain, haemoptysis or cough and a pleural friction rub may be detected. The classic symptoms of massive pulmonary embolism are severe chest pain, air hunger, extreme apprehension and sudden collapse. Predominant clinical signs are cyanosis, rapid breathing and jugular vein distension. Syncope is primarily a finding of massive pulmonary embolism and depends upon the degree of pulmonary vascular obstruction with the resulting decrease in cerebral blood flow.

Where pulmonary embolism occurs suddenly and unexpectedly, acute severe myocardial infarction is the principal differential diagnosis. Distended neck veins which reflect the abnormally elevated pressure of the strained right ventricle are a useful sign of massive embolism; the neck veins are usually not engorged when syncope occurs in association with severe myocardial infarction.

Where pulmonary embolism is suspected, chest X-ray, electrocardiogram (ECG) and lung scanning should be carried out. The two most common plain chest X-ray findings are the presence of a consolidation or infiltration and an elevated hemidiaphragm on the affected side. ECG changes occur in 85% of patients with pulmonary embolism. The changes include rhythm disturbances, QRS abnormalities and ST–T wave alterations. An ECG is not specific in diagnosing pulmonary embolism but is useful in excluding acute myocardial infarction, which may be confused with massive pulmonary embolism. If facilities are available, a combination of perfusion and ventilation lung scanning is a highly specific and accurate method of diagnosing or excluding pulmonary embolism in a previously healthy patient. Pulmonary angiography is also a definitive method but carries some risk.

The clinical diagnosis of both venous thrombosis and pulmonary embolism in pregnancy is so subject to error that wherever possible an objective diagnostic technique should be used. Indeed there are few situations in which diagnostic certainty is more important. An erroneous diagnosis and institution of potent but unnecessary anticoagulant therapy in pregnancy will carry significant hazards for both mother and fetus. This may not be appreciated by physicians who may be less aware of the hazard of bleeding complications in the fetus and the risk of severe haemorrhage from the placental site before, during and after delivery.

Investigations

Ascending phlebography

When carried out by a skilled radiologist, phlebography will provide the most accurate and precise diagnosis of leg vein thrombosis, giving information not only about the presence of a thrombus but also its exact position, size and whether it is loose or adherent to the vein wall. Modern X-ray diagnostic equipment, including the image intensifier and television monitor screen, has enabled

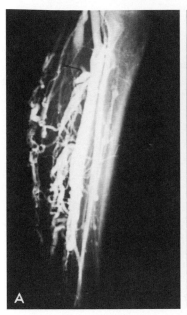
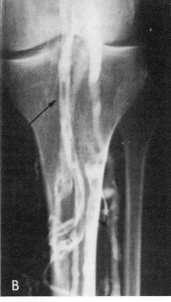

Fig. 44.2 (**A**) Phlebogram of the veins of the calf. The small thrombi in the soleal veins are usually of no clinical significance. (**B**) Thrombi in the deep veins of the calf seen as filling defects (arrow) extending up into the popliteal vein.

venographic techniques to become a reliable method for demonstrating most venous thrombi of clinical interest. Phlebography in expert hands detects at least 95% of peripheral thrombi (Browse 1978). Satisfactory demonstration of the external and common iliac veins is achieved in approximately 90% of patients. The low-viscosity contrast medium is injected into a vein on the dorsum of the foot and the whole venous system of the leg is examined up to the external and common iliac veins (Figs 44.2, 44.3). Lateral views of the calf are required to detect thrombi

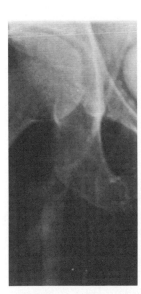
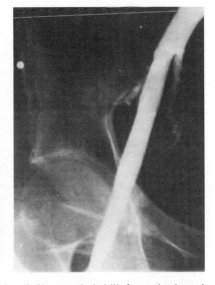

Fig. 44.3 Phlebogram showing (**left**) an occluded iliofemoral vein and (**right**) the normal appearance of the femoral, external, internal and common iliac veins.

in the soleal veins. Partially occluding thrombi are seen as well defined translucent areas with a rim of contrast medium surrounding them. A sudden and sharp obstruction to the column of contrast medium and spread of the flow into a network of collateral vessels indicates obstruction of the major venous channel.

Complications of phlebography include extravasation of contrast medium at the injection site and superficial thrombophlebitis. It has also been claimed that pulmonary embolism may occur as a result of dislodgement of a thrombus during the examination. Kakkar (1987) did not observe this complication in nearly 1500 patients in whom phlebography was performed in the presence of established extensive thrombosis.

Postphlebography deep vein thrombosis has also been claimed as a complication of ascending phlebography. This complication has an incidence of less than 1% if small amounts of contrast medium are used and the deep veins are flushed out with 100 ml of isotonic saline containing 2500 units of heparin.

Contrast phlebography has often been withheld during pregnancy because of fear of the radiation hazard to the fetus. While this may apply in the first trimester, venograms can be used in the second and third trimester. A large measure of protection to the pregnant uterus and fetus can be provided by shielding the mother's abdomen with a lead apron. Since 25–50% of patients in whom venous thrombosis is suspected from symptoms and signs do not have thrombosis, phlebography with minimum radiation will usually be indicated unless facilities are available for isotope venography. Certainly, the risk of unnecessary anticoagulant therapy to the mother and the fetus must greatly exceed any radiation risk to the fetus. Most studies show no increase in teratogenicity following in utero exposure to low doses of radiation (Ginsberg et al 1989).

Radionuclide venography and lung scanning

Radionuclide venography was introduced by Webber et al (1969), who showed that the injection of a suitable lung scanning agent into the venous system of the foot could be used for investigating the presence not only of thrombi in the deep veins of the lower limb but also for locating pulmonary emboli. Macroaggregates of albumin (MAA) or microspheres labelled with ^{99m}Tc (technetium) have been investigated and appear to be a safe and accurate method of diagnosing thromboembolic disease during pregnancy (Johnson et al 1974, Ennis & Dowsett 1983, Lisbona et al 1987).

The technique of radionuclide venography is simple to perform but accuracy depends on meticulous attention to detail. The optimal imaging technique uses a moving scanning bed and gamma camera system to perform the venography and subsequent lung scan. A 21 gauge butterfly needle with a two-way tap is inserted into the dorsal veins of both feet. An activity of 2 mCi ^{99m}Tc–MAA is made in 5 ml of saline for each limb and injected simultaneously by hand. A tourniquet above the malleoli allows the deep veins to be filled with the radionuclide. The popliteal and femoral veins are clearly defined as wide bands of activity uniting via the iliac veins to form the vena cava. MAA have an affinity for fresh clot and adhere to its surface, resulting in a hot spot. Hot spots or increased radionuclide activity can result from causes other than thrombosis and accurate interpretation requires correlation with other scintigraphic signs. Venous obstruction with demonstration of collateral vessels is usually better demonstrated with scintigraphic techniques than with contrast venography. In late pregnancy this can occur with the vena cava because of the pressure from the uterus.

Properly carried out, radionuclide venography is reported to have a correlation with contrast phlebography of greater than 90% (Ennis & Dowsett 1983). In the iliofemoral segment, the correlation is greater than 95%. Malone (1983) has shown that the dose to the fetus is as low as 3 mrad where there is complete tagging of the isotope and macroaggregates. Radionuclide venography is less invasive than phlebography and the radiation hazard is very much smaller. Prior administration of potassium perchlorate is an obvious precaution when using ^{99m}Tc compounds in order to block the maternal and fetal thyroid.

The excretion of radiopharmaceuticals in human breast milk has been studied; discontinuation of breast-feeding following administration of a radiopharmaceutical is strongly recommended. Since about 2% of injected activity is secreted in breast milk, the technique is best avoided in lactating mothers (Malone 1983).

The main disadvantages of radionuclide venography are that the patient has to be examined by a gamma camera in an isotope department and such cameras are not readily available in maternity hospitals. The chief advantage of isotope venography combined with lung scanning is that the major venous channels and the lung fields can be examined at the same time.

Ultrasonic scanning

Doppler ultrasonic examination provides a useful screening method for the diagnosis of deep vein venous thrombosis in pregnancy. The apparatus is usually readily available in obstetric units. The ultrasonic probe is placed over the femoral vein which is located immediately medial to the femoral artery. The blood flow sounds in the femoral vein may be absent if the vein is completely obstructed, and the characteristic rushing sounds due to the sudden increase in blood flow which follows gentle compression of the relaxed calf will not be heard. Because of the presence of collateral venous channels in the calf, ultrasound will not detect minor calf vein thrombosis.

Ultrasonic examination has the benefit of being non-invasive. Real-time ultrasound scanning can be used to visualize the deep veins directly. Compression ultrasonography, where the vein is compressed under ultrasound vision, can detect proximal vein thrombosis with accuracy. Studies comparing ultrasound with phlebography report an accuracy of 90–95% for the diagnosis of femoral or iliac vein thrombosis and a 15–20% sensitivity to calf vein thrombosis (Browse 1978). Compression ultrasonography has been developed recently and is highly sensitive and specific for thrombi in the femoral and popliteal veins but less sensitive for iliac vein thrombosis. Greer et al (1990) have shown real-time ultrasound to be sensitive and specific in pregnancy.

Radioactive-labelled fibrinogen

The use of ^{125}I (iodide) fibrinogen has proved a most reliable technique for the early detection of leg vein thrombosis and provides an accurate method for assessing the efficacy of various methods of prophylaxis. The amount of radiation exposure following the injection of 100 μCi ^{125}I-labelled fibrinogen is calculated to be approximately 200 mrem delivered to blood, 20 mrem to tissues and 5 mrem to the kidneys. This is less than the acceptable annual total body absorbed radiation dose (550 mrem/year) recommended for the general population by the British National Council on Radiation Protection (Kakkar 1987). Studies carried out in antepartum and postpartum patients showed no evidence of ^{125}I-labelled fibrinogen crossing the placenta, although free ^{125}I was present in small quantities (Friend & Kakkar 1972). In the puerperium, ^{125}I-fibrinogen would also result in radioactive iodine being excreted in breast milk. For these reasons ^{125}I-fibrinogen has rarely been used in pregnancy or the puerperium. With careful precautions, the method could be used in the puerperium in non-lactating high-risk patients for the early detection of leg vein thrombosis. In postpartum women, Friend & Kakkar (1970) reported an incidence of 3% of calf vein thrombi.

Limb impedance plethysmography

The non-invasive technique of plethysmography has been used for the diagnosis of deep vein thrombosis in the non-pregnant patient. The method involves filling the calf veins under resting conditions with a pressure cuff and measuring the rate of emptying of the calf, after releasing the cuff, to detect obstruction to the venous flow. The tests will not detect most calf vein thrombi since they do not obstruct the main outflow tract. Similarly, small non-occlusive thrombi in the popliteal and femoral veins may also be missed. We have studied the method during pregnancy and found the technique to be unreliable during the second half of pregnancy. The impedance test cannot distinguish between thrombotic and non-thrombotic venous obstruction; the pressure of the gravid uterus and the raised venous pressure of the lower limbs is a probable explanation of the false positive results. If plethysmography is negative in the first half of pregnancy serial testing over 7–14 days is recommended. If the test remains normal clinically important venous thrombosis is highly unlikely.

Lung scanning

Pulmonary embolism disturbs the regional perfusion of the lungs and the use of radioactive tracer techniques allows a rapid and simple study of the perfusion pattern. Lung scanning is recommended in all patients with suspected pulmonary embolism. The exception would be the patient with massive pulmonary embolism with hypotension, when pulmonary angiography should be performed if pulmonary embolectomy is contemplated.

When a perfusion scan with multiple views is normal, the probability of pulmonary embolism is so low that clinically significant pulmonary embolism can be excluded. When the perfusion pattern or regional distribution of blood flow is abnormal, a ventilation scan should also be carried out, particularly if there is any history of other cardiopulmonary disease. Patients with pulmonary embolism show multiple lesions which have vascular configurations. An abnormal perfusion scan with a normal ventilation scan of the affected area is characteristic of pulmonary embolism. In patients with lung disease, a matched perfusion and ventilation abnormality will usually, but not always, exclude thromboembolism. A ventilation-perfusion isotope lung scan can be used during pregnancy as the radiation dose to the fetus is low—about 0.2 mGy (Department of Health and Social Security 1994).

Pulmonary angiography

Selective pulmonary angiography remains the only definitive method of identifying pulmonary embolism during life. A positive diagnosis of pulmonary embolism can be made by angiography if one of two findings is present: an intravascular filling defect or a pulmonary arterial vessel cut-off (Sasahara 1987). The technique is most helpful in patients with underlying heart and lung disease who are suspected of having pulmonary embolism. These patients may present with non-specific symptoms and signs and may have an abnormal scan with doubtful lesions or matched ventilation–perfusion defects. In addition to demonstrating emboli, the pressures in the right side of the heart and pulmonary circulation can be measured. Such measurements can yield valuable information relating to severity which may influence treatment and prognosis. Many hospitals, however, do not have adequate angiographic facilities or a trained team capable of performing studies of good quality with safety. In pregnancy fetal radiation exposure should be minimized by using the brachial approach when possible.

Laboratory investigations

Laboratory investigation should include full blood count and platelet count, blood film, coagulation screen and if possible functional assays of antithrombin III, protein C and protein S, lupus inhibitors and other antiphospholipid antibodies.

Especially if there is a history or a family history of repeated venous thrombosis, the level of antithrombin III in plasma should be investigated. Congenital deficiencies or defects of antithrombin III occur in about one in 5000 of the population and are usually but not always associated with a serious thrombotic tendency. Purified preparations of antithrombin III are available and their use should be considered when a pregnant woman with congenitally deficient antithrombin III experiences a thrombotic event, or prophylactically to cover the time of maximum risk during labour and the first 2 weeks after delivery. The frequency of protein C and protein S deficiency among women with thromboembolism in pregnancy is unknown.

Diagnostic requirements for treatment

Since all hospitals do not have the same facilities and expertise, it is unrealistic to insist that all patients with venous thrombosis or suspected pulmonary embolism should be investigated in an identical manner. In dealing with a particular patient two factors should be considered: the urgency of diagnosis and the availability of the diagnostic procedures.

For the pregnant woman, a clinical diagnosis of venous thrombosis or pulmonary embolism should be confirmed by an objective test such as venography and lung scanning or ultrasound. Contrast ascending phlebography protecting the gravid uterus with a lead apron is recommended. If available, Doppler ultrasound examination should be used but the interpretation of results is highly dependent on the experience of the examiner.

Since diagnostic evaluation may be time-consuming, an intravenous bolus of 5000 units of heparin should be given if there is strong clinical suspicion of extensive thrombosis involving the iliofemoral segment or evidence of pulmonary embolism. The patient should be continued on a heparin infusion at an hourly rate of 15–25 µ/kg per hour, the rate being adjusted to keep the activated partial thromboplastin time (APTT) about 1.5 to 2 times the control value, and if the diagnosis is confirmed, treatment continued. If the diagnosis is not confirmed heparin can be stopped. The only exception to administering heparin would be in patients with bleeding from placenta praevia, or in patients with suspected massive pulmonary embolism and hypotension in whom pulmonary embolectomy was contemplated.

TREATMENT OF THROMBOSIS DURING PREGNANCY

Before discussing specific antithrombotic therapy to be used in pregnancy, the general aspects of management are worth emphasizing. The pregnant woman lying on her back in late pregnancy is likely to aggravate venous stasis in the legs due to the compression of the vena cava. She should therefore be advised to rest on one side and not to lie on her back. Venous return from the lower limbs is encouraged by elevation of the foot off the bed by 15–20 cm. Exercise of the affected leg should be restricted only by pain. Mobilization and leg exercises are of vital importance in opening up collateral venous channels and are likely to be major factors in preventing long-term venous insufficiency. When effective antithrombotic treatment is instituted, active mobilization to reduce venous stasis is no longer regarded as increasing the risk of thromboembolism. The leg should be kept firmly bandaged until acute swelling has subsided and progressive ambulation should be commenced as soon as leg symptoms allow.

In several reviews of the management of thromboembolic disease during pregnancy and the puerperium, there is now general agreement on specific treatment (Bonnar 1981, Weiner 1982, 1985, Letsky & de Swiet 1984, Letsky 1985, Astedt 1989, Haemostasis and Thrombosis Task Force 1993). Patients with venous thrombosis should be heparinized by continuous intravenous administration until the acute symptoms have subsided, followed by intermittent subcutaneous heparin in the long term. Warfarin should be avoided in pregnancy. Prophylactic subcutaneous heparin should be used in hereditary thrombotic disorders and in women with previous major thromboembolic complications. Fibrinolytic agents would not normally be used during pregnancy.

Anticoagulant therapy in pregnancy

The aim of specific treatment in deep vein thrombosis with or without pulmonary embolism is to prevent propagation and embolization. The choice of anticoagulant therapy lies with heparin alone or heparin in combination with oral anticoagulants.

Heparin therapy

Heparin is a sulphated polysaccharide with important anticoagulant and thrombotic properties; it is known to inhibit a number of activated clotting factors including factors XIIa, XIa, IXa, Xa and thrombin. Heparin exhibits its effect by complexing with the antithrombin III molecule, changing the latter's molecular configuration. The inhibitory activity of antithrombin III is greatly increased and its ability to neutralize activated clotting factors is enhanced. Thrombin, once formed, requires relatively large amounts of heparin to inhibit its effect; in contrast, factor Xa is inhibited by very small amounts of heparin. The inhibition of factor Xa can prevent the conversion of prothrombin to thrombin and is the basis of thrombosis prophylaxis using low-dosage heparin. Once a thrombus has developed and thrombin is present, much larger amounts of heparin are required. Other effects of heparin include potentiation of heparin co-factor II and inhibition of platelet function (Hirsh 1986).

Commercial heparin preparations for the treatment of thrombosis are prepared from bovine lungs or porcine intestines. These heterogeneous compounds have a molecular weight which varies between 3000 and 40 000 daltons. The unfractionated forms can be partially purified by depolymerization methods and show diverse functions depending upon their molecular size and binding to antithrombin III. Clinical trials of low molecular weight heparin (4000–9000 daltons) have shown that it is as good as unfractionated heparin with less bleeding complications (Kakkar et al 1993) in the prevention of deep vein thrombosis. Neither unfractionated mucosal heparin nor the low molecular weight heparins cross the placenta to the fetus (Bonnar 1976, Forestier et al 1984, Andrew et al 1985, Melissari et al 1992). Low molecular weight heparin requires once-daily administration and may have a lower risk of both thrombocytopenia and heparin-induced osteoporosis. Dahlman (1993) reported osteoporotic fractures in 2.2% of pregnant women receiving long-term subcutaneous unfractionated heparin.

Oral anticoagulants (coumarin derivatives)

Oral anticoagulants have a molecular weight of approximately 1000 and readily cross the placenta. The elevated levels of coagulation factors in the pregnant woman contrast sharply with the situation in the fetus and newborn in whom the levels of factors II, VII, IX and X are low. Although warfarin and other oral anticoagulants may be safe for the mother when she is within the therapeutic range, the fetus is likely to be considerably overdosed because of immature liver enzyme systems and the low levels of vitamin K-dependent clotting factors.

Reports in the literature indicate that in pregnant women taking oral anticoagulants, fetal mortality is around 15–30%. Tejani (1973) reported 32 pregnant women with a heart valve prosthesis who received oral anticoagulant therapy at some stage of their pregnancy. In this group 11 fetal or neonatal deaths occurred and three infants had major congenital abnormalities. In a review of world literature between 1945 and 1978, Hall et al (1980) found 418 cases which had received coumarin derivatives. Overall one-third of these pregnancies had abnormal fetal outcome. The abnormalities were mainly due to haemorrhage, warfarin embryopathy, central nervous system effects and spontaneous abortion. The critical period of exposure for warfarin embryopathy appears to be between 6 and 9 weeks of gestation. The main features are: saddle nose, nasal and mid-face hypoplasia, frontal bossing and short stature with stippled epiphyses and short extremities, calcification of thyroid cartilage, cardiac defects, low-set ears, mental retardation and blindness (Stevenson et al 1980). The severity of the syndrome is variable and follow-up studies indicate that most survivors have a good outcome; one-half have no severe disability.

Exposure of the pregnant woman to coumarin derivatives in the second and third trimesters may be associated with an increased incidence of central nervous system abnormalities resulting in mental retardation and blindness. Intracranial bleeding in the fetus in the second and third trimester may also lead to secondary central nervous system deformities. The overall risk of central nervous system effects appears to be about 3%.

The retrospective analysis of Hall et al (1980) estimated that with the use of coumarin derivatives one-sixth of pregnancies end in abortion or stillbirth; one-sixth result in abnormal liveborn infants and about two-thirds have a relatively normal outcome. Given that the literature is biased towards reporting complicated cases, it is likely that these retrospective estimates are the worst possible and that in practice the risks are probably much less.

In an earlier review of the use of oral anticoagulants in pregnancy, Hirsh and colleagues (1970) suggested that the risk to the fetus occurred mainly at term and was related to fetal trauma arising during childbirth. In 14 patients in whom oral anticoagulants were withdrawn after the 37th week of gestation no fetal or neonatal complications were reported. Hirsh et al concluded that the main hazard of oral anticoagulant drugs resulted from their use during the first trimester or in late pregnancy prior to delivery. Although the risk to the fetus can be reduced by discontinuing oral anticoagulant therapy at the 37th week of pregnancy, premature labour and delivery are not predictable. A preterm infant delivered under the influence of oral anticoagulants is at increased risk of cerebral haemorrhage.

Oral anticoagulant therapy should be avoided if at all possible during pregnancy; if a woman conceives while taking oral anticoagulants, she should be advised to discontinue them as early as 6 weeks of gestation. If anticoagulant therapy is essential during the first trimester, heparin can be used, as described later.

Neutralizing warfarin therapy

In some situations anticoagulant therapy may have to be neutralized because of bleeding. Impaired renal function and concurrent administration of drugs which inhibit platelet function increase the risk of bleeding complications with anticoagulants. If the anticoagulant effect of warfarin has to be reversed immediately, an infusion of 1–2 units of fresh plasma should be given. Aqueous vitamin K preparations reverse the effect of warfarin within 24 hours. The dosage of vitamin K given orally or intravenously depends on the clinical situation. Where there is serious haemorrhage and a firm decision is taken not to re-introduce anticoagulants, a dose of 25–50 mg should be given. This will render the patient resistant to further anticoagulant treatment for about 2 weeks. Where there is frank haemorrhage but it is intended to continue therapy, 15 mg should be given to reduce the drug effect without cancelling it. Where the routine coagulation test shows an excessive effect but the patient is not bleeding, a dose of 5 mg can be prescribed.

Fibrinolytic agents

Recent surgery or delivery is considered a contraindication to thrombolytic therapy. If streptokinase or urokinase is used when delivery is imminent or within 1 week of childbirth, severe haemorrhage from the placental site is to be expected. Likewise, extensive bleeding will occur from any genital tract lacerations or episiotomy wounds. The risk of bleeding will be greatest at the time of delivery and in the early puerperium.

THERAPY OF VENOUS THROMBOEMBOLISM

Pregnant women who develop venous thrombosis should be heparinized according to the protocol shown in Table 44.3 (Hathaway & Bonnar 1987). In late pregnancy a greater amount of heparin is required for adequate anticoagulation than in the non-pregnant state (Bonnar 1976, Whitfield et al 1983). For acute heparinization 50–75

Table 44.3 Protocol for heparin therapy of thromboembolism in pregnancy

Baseline diagnostic studies
1. Venogram by ascending contrast, by radionuclide venography or by Doppler ultrasound
2. Perfusion ventilation scanning
3. Coagulation studies: platelet count activated partial thromboplastin time (APTT); prothrombin time; activated whole blood clotting time (ACT); hereditary disorder screening tests as indicated

Acute heparinization
Sodium heparin 50–75 u/kg i.v. bolus injection followed by 15–25 u/kg/h by continuous infusion or pump to prolong the APTT or ACT to 1.5–2 times normal; continue therapy for 5–7 days

Long-term prophylaxis
Administer 5000–10 000 units of sodium heparin subcutaneously every 12 hours. Monitor with heparin level (0.5–0.3 u/ml plasma) or APPT, ACT (1.5 times normal) at 2–4 hours postinjection and adjust dose accordingly. When a dosage of 20 000 u or greater per 24 hours is required, an 8-hourly regimen is preferable

units of sodium heparin per kg should be given as an intravenous bolus injection, followed by 15–25 u/kg/h by continuous infusion to prolong the partial thromboplastin time to 1.5–2 times the baseline or mean control value. For adequate anticoagulation and avoidance of bleeding complications, strict attention to detail is essential. Intermittent bolus injections should not be used because of the increased risk of bleeding. Continuous intravenous heparin by infusion or pump should be given initially for 5–10 days. The precise duration of the initial treatment must be tailored to the individual but the objective is to maintain full anticoagulation until active thrombosis has been arrested, thrombi in the leg veins have been firmly attached to the vessel wall and the process of organization has begun. Where intravenous therapy for this period proves impossible, treatment can be given by subcutaneous injection into the flank of the anterior abdominal wall. Dosage of subcutaneous heparin of 10 000 units at 8-hourly intervals will usually provide adequate anticoagulation.

If the woman is in the puerperium, treatment with oral anticoagulants such as warfarin can be commenced and the heparin discontinued once the effect of the oral anticoagulant has been established. During pregnancy oral anticoagulants are best avoided and subcutaneous heparin can be given as an alternative. Subcutaneous prophylactic heparin is an effective substitute for warfarin and can be used alone in the prevention of recurrent thrombosis both in the non-pregnant and pregnant woman (Bonnar 1976, Hellgren & Nygards 1982, Hull et al 1982). Long-term prophylaxis can be provided with sodium heparin in a dosage of 5000–10 000 units 8–12 hourly to prolong the partial thromboplastin time to 1.5 times normal at 2–4 hours following the subcutaneous injection. Low molecular weight heparin administered once a day may also have a role in long-term treatment.

Subcutaneous heparin

Particular care is required in instruction of medical and nursing staff and patients in the use of subcutaneous heparin. A concentrated aqueous solution of 25 000 iu of heparin in 1 ml is used. Preloaded syringes with 5000 and 10 000 units of heparin are available; these are particularly useful for self-administration in pregnancy.

A fold of skin is gently raised on the lateral aspect of the anterior abdominal wall in the flank. This is facilitated by the patient bending forwards. The skin is cleansed and the 25 or 26 gauge needle 1.5 cm in length inserted to its full depth at right angles to the skin. The hub of the needle is held firmly between the thumb and index finger as the exact dose of heparin is injected. The needle is slowly removed at the same angle as it was inserted, taking care to avoid any damage to the skin and subcutaneous fat at the injection site. The injection site should not be rubbed or massaged. Subcutaneous heparin is best avoided in the arms and legs. Apart from being more painful and causing bruising in these areas, limb movements may accelerate the rate of absorption of the heparin.

For safe and effective long-term therapy with subcutaneous heparin, two weekly measurements of the plasma heparin level or the heparin effect on plasma are advisable to ensure that adequate heparin is being given, especially during the third trimester. Increased heparin neutralization occurs in the second half of pregnancy due to the enhanced coagulation and platelet activity in the uteroplacental circulation. Ideally the heparin level or partial thromboplastin time should be checked 2–4 hours after the subcutaneous injection as this is the time of the peak levels. The platelet count should also be measured, since some patients develop thrombocytopenia during heparin therapy. In view of the greater bioavailability of sodium heparin than calcium heparin, we prefer a 12-hourly regimen with sodium heparin during pregnancy (Bonnar & Ma 1979).

Wide individual variation is found in the levels of plasma heparin after subcutaneous injection; in late pregnancy some women require 10 000 units of heparin 8 hourly to produce an adequate level. When a dosage of 10 000 units subcutaneously is used, the plasma heparin levels should be monitored at weekly intervals. Our experience indicates that a plasma level of 0.1–0.3 u/ml provides effective protection against thrombosis in pregnancy without causing bleeding problems.

At the onset of labour, heparin therapy can be temporarily discontinued. If the woman wishes epidural anaesthesia the APTT should be checked with the platelet count and if normal epidural anaesthesia should be safe. The relative benefits and risks should be considered in discussion with the patient and the anaesthetist (Greer & de Swiet 1993). The relative heparin resistance present in late pregnancy and labour disappears immediately after delivery. In the puerperium a dosage of 5000 units of sodium heparin 12 hourly is usually sufficient and warfarin can be commenced soon after delivery. Heparin therapy should be continued until warfarin is effective. Warfarin is best continued for 3 months after delivery if the patient has suffered a pulmonary embolism during the pregnancy or following a previous pregnancy; breastfeeding should be encouraged.

When a woman has had a previous thrombotic complication, prophylactic treatment during labour and in the puerperium is advisable. If a thromboembolic complication has occurred in the antenatal period of a previous pregnancy, the choice lies between clinical surveillance with ultrasonic examination to detect DVT or prophylactic treatment from at least 4–6 weeks before the gestation time when the previous episode occurred. Lao and colleagues (1985) used no prophylactic treatment antenatally in 26 pregnant women with a previous history of thromboembolism and used treatment only at delivery with dextran 70 and for 6 weeks in the puerperium with heparin or warfarin. Of the 26, only six of the patients had had their original episode of thromboembolism in association with pregnancy. Using this regimen, one patient (4%) had a suspected pulmonary embolism and another patient who had had deep vein thrombosis at 38 weeks' gestation was given subcutaneous heparin from 37 weeks of pregnancy onwards.

De Sweit et al (1987) reported an extension of this study to 59 pregnancies 25 of whom had had their previous thromboembolism in pregnancy. He reported no further cases of antenatal thromboembolism and no cases postnatally using the regimen of dextran 70 infusion during labour and prophylaxis for 6 weeks postpartum with heparin or dextran. Dextran infusion during labour is no longer given for the reasons given below.

In the individual patient with a previous thromboembolism, the risk of a recurrence during pregnancy has to be weighed against the possible effects of subcutaneous heparin causing bone demineralization. Since approximately one-half of the maternal deaths due to pulmonary embolism now occur during pregnancy, it would seem advisable to provide well-controlled prophylactic treatment during pregnancy with subcutaneous heparin where a patient has suffered a serious thromboembolic complication during her previous pregnancy. A large multicentre trial is required to resolve the question of the need for prophylaxis during pregnancy for a patient with a single episode of previous deep vien thrombosis. Possibly in the future, low molecular weight heparin may be an alternative but as yet it remains to be evaluated for use in pregnancy.

Complications of heparin therapy

Complications associated with heparin therapy include hypersensitivity reactions, osteoporosis, thrombocytopenia and bleeding. Hypersensitivity may be manifest as urticaria and in rare situations as anaphylaxis. Osteoporosis after long-term use of heparin has been reported in pregnancy (Hall et al 1980, de Swiet et al 1983). Heparin causes demineralization of bone but this is seldom apparent unless heparin is given for more than 5 months in doses of 20 000 units daily (Hirsh 1991). Heparin-induced thrombocytopenia and bleeding or intravascular coagulation are rare effects of bovine lung heparin; porcine mucosal heparin, which is used mainly within the British Isles, rarely causes any significant thrombocytopenia.

Bleeding is the most important of the heparin complications and occurs in about 5–10% of patients on full-dose intravenous heparin. The risk of bleeding is particularly high in patients who have been exposed to recent surgery or trauma with bolus intravenous injections of heparin; in patients who have taken additional drug therapy such as aspirin, and in the presence of renal disease or pre-eclampsia. Partial thromboplastin times more than 2.5 times control, or plasma heparin levels over 0.5 iu/ml predispose to haemorrhage (Bonnar 1977). If bleeding occurs, stopping the heparin infusion for 8–12 hours usually allows haemostasis to recover. Where rapid reversal of the heparin effect is required, protamine sulphate can be given. For every estimated 100 units of heparin in the circulation, administer 1 mg protamine sulphate intravenously. The partial thromboplastin time or heparin assay should be repeated soon after the protamine injection; again, after 3 hours, further protamine may be required as it is eliminated faster than the heparin.

PROPHYLAXIS OF THROMBOEMBOLISM WITH DEXTRAN 70

The efficacy of dextran 70 in preventing venous thrombosis after pelvic surgery was shown in double-blind controlled studies (Bonnar & Walsh 1972, Bonnar 1975). Dextran 70 (Lomodex) infusion was commenced after the induction of anaesthesia and 500 ml was given during the operation; a further 500 ml was started usually before the patient left the operating theatre and infused over the next 3–6 hours. Kline and colleagues (1975) used the same regimen in surgical patients in a randomized controlled study; these authors showed a significant reduction in fatal pulmonary embolism but not in deep vein thrombosis. Browse (1977) also found a significant reduction in pulmonary emboli as detected by ventilation–perfusion scanning in patients receiving 1l dextran 70.

Recently, acute fetal distress associated with Dextran anaphylactoid reaction has been reported in mothers given Dextran 70 during epidural anaesthesia or during Caesarean section. Dextran-induced anaphylactoid reactions may be associated with uterine hypertonus within minutes of starting the infusion with subsequent severe fetal bradycardia. The uterine hypertonus may cause fetal death or neurological sequelae. In a recent survey in France, 32 cases of maternal anaphylactoid reaction associated with acute fetal distress were reported (Barbier et al 1992). These reactions have also occurred in pregnant women despite the use of immunoprophylaxis with Dextran hapten (Berg et al 1991). The risk of severe anaphylactoid reactions with Dextran 70 has been estimated at one in 821 (Paull 1987).

The risk of Dextran 70 treatment in a pregnant woman will usually exceed the risk of thromboembolism. In view of the risk to the fetus, Dextran 70 should be avoided during pregnancy. During labour or Caesarean section Dextran 70 should be withheld until after delivery of the baby (Royal College of Obstetricians & Gynaecologists 1995).

SPECIAL PROBLEMS DURING PREGNANCY

Massive pulmonary embolism

The use of cardiopulmonary bypass has improved the

results of the surgical approach to massive thrombo-embolism. Surgical intervention may be indicated where the acute resuscitation measures have failed, severe hypo-tension persists and angiography shows that peripheral pulmonary perfusion is reduced by 75%.

A decision must be based upon the clinical and haemo-dynamic state of the patient as well as the ready avail-ability of the surgical team and required facilities. If the patient survives long enough to be put on cardiopulmo-nary bypass, embolectomy is likely to be successful.

Vena caval occlusion

The vena cava may be completely ligated or partially interrupted with a variety of teflon clips. Such measures are rarely indicated and should be considered only if the mother's life is threatened by recurrent thromboemboli and lower limb venography demonstrates loose thrombi. The introduction of the inferior vena cava umbrella filter, which can be positioned under fluoroscopy with local anaesthesia, has minimized the hazards of inferior vena cava interruption. This technique seems preferable in the rare situations where interruption of the vena cava is indicated.

Cerebral thrombosis

The acute onset of headaches and neurological deficits such as hemiparesis or dysphasia, focal seizures, fever and sinus tachycardia in a pregnant or postpartum patient may be the result of cerebral venous thrombosis. Com-puterized tomography may suggest the diagnosis but often carotid angiography is required to demonstrate the occluded vessels. Three reports emphasize the safety and efficacy of heparin treatment in this rare but serious disorder (Srinivasan 1983, Halpern et al 1984, Bousser et al 1985). Cerebral arterial thrombosis can present in pregnancy as a typical stroke (Wiebers & Whisnant 1985). The use of systemic anticoagulation is controversial in these cases but can usually be treated safely if com-puterized tomography shows only an ischaemic pattern without haemorrhage. The Report on Maternal Deaths for 1988–90 included nine cases of cerebral thromboses (Department of Health and Social Security 1994).

Septic pelvic vein thrombophlebitis and ovarian vein thrombosis

These thrombotic complications may present with pyrexia and non-specific signs of inflammation but accurate diagnosis is difficult. Septic pelvic vein thrombophlebitis can arise as a complication of puerperal sepsis and may lead to pulmonary embolism. Heparinization and anti-biotic therapy are indicated (Weiner 1985). Acute ovarian vein thrombosis may present as severe adnexal pain and fever in the postpartum period. The condition is usually diagnosed at laparoscopy and the clot may extend into the vena cava and renal veins (Bahnson et al 1985). Heparinization is indicated for 10–14 days.

Hereditary thrombotic disorders

The incidence of thromboembolic complications during pregnancy in women with hereditary antithrombin III deficiency has been estimated at around 70% (Hellgren et al 1982). Full therapeutic doses of heparin are recom-mended throughout pregnancy (Brandt & Stenbjerg 1979). Antithrombin III levels should be checked periodically. At delivery marked falls in antithrombin III and thrombo-cytopenia may develop even on heparin (Brandt 1981). In this situation antithrombin III concentrates or fresh frozen plasma should be given and repeated every second day during the first postpartum week.

Cardiac prosthetic valves

Women on long-term anticoagulants with cardiac pros-thetic valves require careful counselling about pregnancy and the fetal risks. The optimal anticoagulation regimen for prophylaxis against thromboembolic complications in pregnant women with cardiac prosthetic valves remains controversial. In many previous reports, combinations of heparin and warfarin have been studied. The use of warfarin in the first trimester is associated with congenital anomalies and spontaneous abortion (O'Neill et al 1982). Subcutaneous low-dose heparin alone has been associated with major embolic events using a dose of 5000 units of heparin twice daily (Bennett & Oakley 1968, Wang et al 1983); this would be an inadequate dose in a pregnant woman. In 18 pregnancies treated by heparin therapy, adjusted to keep the thromboplastin time at 1.5 times control during the first and third trimester, with warfarin used between the 13th and the 36th week, no maternal thromboembolic complications or congenital malforma-tions occurred but early abortions attributable to warfarin therapy were seen (Lee et al 1986). In view of the fetal hazards of warfarin the following recommendations would seem reasonable (Hathaway & Bonnar 1987):

1. Pregnancy is contraindicated in women with prosthetic heart valves who have had previous thromboembolic complications and who require continuous anticoagulation with warfarin. In such patients the risk of further thrombotic episodes and fetal complications is very high.
2. In patients with cardiac valve prostheses who are at lower risk for thrombosis, warfarin should be discontinued or replaced by therapeutic heparinization prior to conception because of the high incidence of abortion in warfarin-treated patients.

3. Patients should be given subcutaneous heparin throughout pregnancy in a dosage adjusted to prolong the partial thromboplastin time to 1.5 times normal.

4. Heparin therapy should be continued for at least 1 week after delivery until the patient is re-established on warfarin. Breastfeeding is not contraindicated.

5. If a patient continues with warfarin during pregnancy careful planning of her delivery is important. Every effort should be made to change to heparin 2–3 weeks before delivery and no later than 36 weeks. If labour occurs or delivery is indicated in a patient who is fully anticoagulated on warfarin, Caesarean section should be considered to protect the fetus from the risk of intracranial haemorrhage. If the INR is between 2.0 and 2.5 the risk of maternal bleeding during operation is low (Haemostasis and Thrombosis Task Force 1993).

CONCLUSIONS

Our first priority must be to bring proven prophylactic methods to obstetric patients who are at high risk of thromboembolic complications. No method is likely to be 100% effective, but present evidence indicates that low-dose heparin confers a high degree of protection against venous thrombosis and if necessary can be used throughout pregnancy by the woman herself.

The time of greatest danger is the immediate puerperium, especially in patients who have been delivered by Caesarean section. Prophylaxis with low-dose heparin should be given to all mothers who are in a high-risk category for thromboembolic complications. In addition to reducing the number of maternal deaths from pulmonary embolism, the judicious use of prophylactic methods should also decrease the incidence of the postphlebitic syndrome.

Clinicians must accept the fallibility of the clinical diagnosis of deep vein thrombosis. Treatment based solely on the history and clinical examination will be unnecessary in as many as 50% of patients. An accurate and objective diagnostic method should therefore be used whenever possible and the most reliable methods available at present are contrast phlebography, Doppler ultrasound and lung scanning.

REFERENCES

Aaro L A, Juergens J L 1974 Thrombophlebitis and pulmonary embolism as complications of pregnancy. Medical Clinics of North America 58: 829–834

Andrew M, Boneu B, Cade J et al 1985 Placental transport of low molecular weight heparin in the pregnant sheep. British Journal of Haematology 59: 103–108

Astedt B 1989 Prevention and treatment of deep vein thrombosis in pregnancy. In: Eklof B, Gjoies J E, Thulesius O et al (eds) Controversies in the management of venous disorders. Butterworths, London, pp 159–166

Aznar J, Gilabert J, Estelles A, Espana F 1986 Fibrinolytic activity and protein C in pre-eclampsia. Thrombosis and Haemostasis 55: 314–317

Bahnson R R, Wendel E F, Vogelzang R L 1985 Renal vein thrombosis following puerperal ovarian vein thrombophlebitis. American Journal of Obstetrics and Gynecology 152: 290–291

Barbier P, Janville A P, Autret E, Courean C 1992 fetal risks with Dextran during delivery. Drug Safety 7(1): 71–73

Bennett G G, Oakley C M 1968 Pregnancy in a patient with a mitral valve. Lancet i: 616–619

Berg E M, Fasting S, Sellevold O F 1991 Serious complications with Dextran 70 despite hapten prophylaxis. Is it best avoided prior to delivery? Anaesthesia 46(12): 1033–1035

Bonnar J 1975 Thromboembolism in obstetric and gynaecological patients. In: Nicolaides A N (ed) Thromboembolism. MTP, Lancaster, pp 311–340

Bonnar J 1976 Long-term self-administered heparin therapy for prevention and treatment of thromboembolic complications in pregnancy. In: Kakkar V V, Thomas D P (eds) Heparin—chemistry and clinical usage. Academic Press, London, pp 247–260

Bonnar J 1977 Acute and chronic coagulation disorders in pregnancy. In: Poller L (ed) Recent advances in blood coagulation, vol 2. Churchill Livingstone, Edinburgh, pp 363–379

Bonnar J 1981 Venous thromboembolism and pregnancy. Clinical Obstetrics and Gynecology 8: 455–473

Bonnar J, Ma P 1979 Prevention of venous thromboembolism in pregnancy with subcutaneous sodium and calcium heparin. IX World Congress of Gynecology and Obstetrics, Tokyo

Bonnar J, Walsh J J 1972 Prevention of thrombosis after pelvic surgery by British dextran 70. Lancet i: 614–616

Bousser M G, Chiras J, Bories J, Castaigne P 1985 Cerebral venous thrombosis—a review of 38 cases. Stroke 16: 199–213

Brandt P 1981 Observations during the treatment of antithrombin-III deficient women with heparin and antithrombin concentrate during pregnancy, parturition, and abortion. Thrombosis Research 22: 15–24

Brandt P, Stenbjerg S 1979 Subcutaneous heparin for thrombosis in pregnant women with hereditary antithrombin deficiency. Lancet i: 100–101

Browse N L 1977 The prevention of deep vein thrombosis and pulmonary embolism by pharmacological methods. Triangle 16: 29–32

Browse N L 1978 Diagnosis of deep vein thrombosis. British Medical Bulletin 34: 163–167

Coon W W 1977 Epidemiology of venous thromboembolism. Annals of Surgery 186: 149–164

Coon W W, Willis P W III, Keller J B 1973 Venous thromboembolism and other venous disease in the Tecumseh community health study. Circulation 48: 839–846

Dahlman T C 1993 Osteoporotic fractures and the recurrence of thromboembolism during pregnancy and the puerperium in 184 women undergoing thromboprophylaxis with heparin. American Journal of Obstetrics and Gynecology. 168: 1265–1270

Daniel D G, Campbell H, Turnbull A C 1967 Puerperal thromboembolism and suppression of lactation. Lancet ii: 287–289

Department of Health and Social Security 1991, 1994 Reports on Confidential Enquiries into Maternal Deaths in The United Kingdom 1985–87 and 1988–1990. HMSO, London

de Swiet M, Ward D, Fidler S et al 1983 Prolonged heparin therapy in pregnancy causes bone demineralisation. British Journal of Obstetrics and Gynaecology 90: 1129–1134

de Swiet M, Floyd E, Letsky E 1987 Low risk of recurrent thromboembolism in pregnancy (letter). British Journal of Hospital Medicine September, p 264

Ennis J T, Dowsett D J 1983 Radionuclide venography. In: Ennis J T, Dowsett D J (eds) Vascular radionuclide imaging. A clinical atlas. Wiley, Chichester, pp 5–11

Forestier F, Daffos F, Capella-Pavlovsky M 1984 Low molecular weight heparin (PK 10169) does not cross the placenta during the second trimester of pregnancy. Study by direct fetal blood sampling under ultrasound. Thrombosis Research 34: 557–560

Friend J R, Kakkar V V 1970 The diagnosis of deep vein thrombosis in the puerperium. Journal of Obstetrics and Gynaecology of the British Commonwealth 77: 820–825

Friend J R, Kakkar V V 1972 Deep vein thrombosis in obstetric and gynaecologic patients. In: Kakkar V V, Jouhan A J (eds) Thromboembolism. Churchill Livingstone, Edinburgh, pp 131–138

Ginsberg J S, Hirsh J, Rainbow A J, Coates G 1989 Risks to the fetus of radiologic procedures used in the diagnosis of maternal venous thromboembolic disease. Thrombosis and Haemostasis 61: 189–196

Greer I A, Barry J, Mackon N, Allan P L 1990 Diagnosis of deep vein thrombosis in pregnancy: a new role for diagnostic ultrasound. British Journal of Obstetrics and Gynaecology 97: 53–57

Greer I A, de Swiet M, 1993 Thrombosis prophylaxis in obstetrics and gynaecology. British Journal of Obstetrics and Gynaecology 100: 37–40

Hall J G, Pauli R M, Wilson K M 1980 Maternal and fetal sequelae of anticoagulation during pregnancy. American Journal of Medicine 68: 122–140

Haemostasis and Thrombosis Task Force 1993 Guidelines on the prevention, investigation and management of thrombosis associated with pregnancy. Maternal and Neonatal Haemostasis Working Party of the Haemostasis and Thrombosis Task. Journal of Clinical Pathology 46: 489–496

Halpern J P, Morris J G L, Driscoll G L 1984 Anticoagulants and cerebral venous thrombosis. Australian and New Zealand Journal of Medicine 14: 643–648

Hathaway W E, Bonnar J 1987 Thrombotic disorders in pregnancy and the newborn infant. In: Haemostatic disorders of the pregnant woman and the newborn infant. Elsevier, Amsterdam, pp 151–184

Hellgren M, Nygards E B 1982 Long-term therapy with subcutaneous heparin during pregnancy. Gynecologic and Obstetric Investigations 13: 76–89

Hellgren M, Tengborn L, Abildgaard U 1982 Pregnancy in women with congenital antithrombin III deficiency: experience of treatment with heparin and antithrombin. Gynecologic and Obstetric Investigations 14: 127–141

Hirsh J 1986 Mechanism of action and monitoring of anticoagulants. Seminars in Thrombosis and Haemostasis 12: 1–11

Hirsh J 1991 Heparin. New England Journal of Medicine 324: 1565–1574

Hirsh J, Cade J F, O'Sullivan E F 1970 Clinical experience with anticoagulant therapy during pregnancy. British Medical Journal 1: 270–273

Hull R, Delmore T, Carter C et al 1982 Adjusted subcutaneous heparin versus warfarin sodium in the long-term treatment of venous thrombosis. New England Journal of Medicine 306: 189–194

Johnson W C, Patten D H, Widrich W C, Nabseth D C 1974 Technetium 99 m isotope venography. American Journal of Surgery 127: 424–428

Kakkar V V 1987 Diagnosis of deep vein thrombosis. In: Bloom A L, Thomas D P (eds) Haemostasis and thrombosis, 2nd edn. Churchill Livingstone, Edinburgh, pp 779–792

Kakkar V V, Cohen A T, Edmonson R A et al 1993 Low molecular weight versus standard heparin for prevention of venous thromboembolism after major abdominal surgery. Lancet i: 259–265

Kline A, Hughes L E, Campbell H, Williams A, Zlosnick J, Leach K G 1975 Dextran 70 in prophylaxis of thromboembolic disease after surgery: a clinically orientated randomised double blind trial. British Medical Journal 2: 109–112

Lao T T, de Swiet M, Letsky E, Walters B N J 1985 Prophylaxis of

thromboembolism in pregnancy: an alternative. British Journal of Obstetrics and Gynaecology 92: 202–206

Lee P K, Wang R Y C, Chow J S F, Cheung K L, Wong V C W, Chan T K 1986 The combined use of warfarin and adjusted subcutaneous heparin during pregnancy in patients with artificial heart valves. American Journal of Cardiology 8(1): 221–224

Letsky E A 1985 Coagulation problems during pregnancy. In: Lind T (ed) Current review in obstetrics and gynaecology. Churchill Livingstone, Edinburgh, pp 29–55

Letsky E, de Swiet M 1984 Thromboembolism in pregnancy and its management. British Journal of Haematology 57: 543–552

Lisbona R, Rush C, Leparto L 1987 Technetium-99m red blood cell venography of the lower limb in symptomatic pulmonary embolization. Clinical Nuclear Medicine 12(2): 93–98

Malone L 1983 The fetus as the target organ: a special case. In: Ennis J T, Dowsett D J (eds) Vascular radionuclide imaging. A clinical atlas. Wiley, Chichester, pp 225–226

Melissari E, Parker C J, Wilson N V et al 1992 Use of low molecular weight heparin in pregnancy. Thrombosis and haemostasis 68: 652–656

O'Neill H, Blake S, Sugrue D, MacDonald D 1982 Problems in the management of patients with artificial valves during pregnancy. British Journal of Obstetrics and Gynaecology 89: 940–943

Paull J 1987 A prospective study of Dextran-induced anaphylactoid reactions in 5745 patients. Anaesthesia Intensive Care 15: 163–167

Royal College of Obstetricians and Gynaecologists 1995 Report of the RCOG Working Party on Prophylaxis against Thromboembolism in Gynaecology and Obstetrics. RCOG, London, p 19

Sasahara A A 1987 Diagnosis of pulmonary embolism. In: Bloom A L, Thomas D P (eds) Haemostasis and thrombosis, 2nd edn. Churchill Livingstone, Edinburgh, pp 792–801

Srinivasan K 1983 Cerebral venous and arterial thrombosis in pregnancy and puerperium. Angiology Journal of Vascular Disease 34: 731–746

Stevenson R E, Burton O M, Ferlauto G L, Taylor H A 1980 Hazards of oral anticoagulants during pregnancy. Journal of American Medical Association 243: 1549–1551

Tejani N 1973 Anticoagulant therapy with cardiac valve prosthesis during pregnancy. Obstetrics and Gynecology 42: 785–793

Thomas D P 1987 Pathogenesis of venous thrombosis. In: Bloom A L, Thomas D P (eds) Haemostasis and thrombosis, 2nd edn. Churchill Livingstone, Edinburgh, pp 767–778

Virchow R 1860 Cited in: Cellular pathology as based upon physiological and pathological histology. Churchill Livingstone, Edinburgh, pp 197–203

Wang R Y C, Lee P K, Chow J S F, Chen W W C 1983 Efficacy of low-dose, subcutaneously administered heparin in the treatment of women with artificial heart valves. Medical Journal of Australia 2: 126–128

Webber M M, Bennet L R, Cragin M D 1969 Thrombophlebitis demonstration by scintiscanning. Radiology 92: 620–623

Weiner C P, 1982 Anticoagulants and antiplatelet agents. In: Rayburn W F, Zuspan F P (eds) Drug therapy in obstetrics and gynecology. Appleton-Century-Crofts, Norwalk, Connecticut, pp 345–358

Weiner C P 1985 Diagnosis and management of thromboembolic disease during pregnancy. Clinical Obstetrics and Gynecology 28: 107–118

Whitfield L R, Lele A S, Levy G 1983 Effect of pregnancy on the relationship between concentration and anticoagulant action of heparin. Clinical Pharmacology and Therapy 34: 23–28

Wiebers D O, Whisnant J P 1985 The incidence of stroke among pregnant women in Rochester, Minnesota, 1955 through 1979. Journal of American Medical Association 254: 3055–3057

45. Psychological effects of perinatal death

Gillian Forrest

INTRODUCTION

The loss of a baby in the perinatal period is a traumatic event which has far-reaching consequences for the bereaved parents. Over the past few years, with dramatic improvements in perinatal and infant mortality rates, parents' expectations of the safe delivery of a healthy baby have become very high. When things do go wrong therefore, they are not only confronted with the loss of their baby, but also with the loss of their faith in modern medical care. In addition, as part of industrialized Western society which has lost its familiarity with death and bereavement, many parents do not even have the comfort of the mourning rituals which have traditionally helped the bereaved to cope. It is important, therefore, for professionals dealing with perinatal death to have an understanding of the bereavement process, and an awareness of the difficulties and dilemmas facing parents so that medical staff can offer the best possible care.

BEREAVEMENT

Our knowledge of bereavement is based partly on descriptive accounts of patients in psychiatric treatment, and partly on objective studies of groups of bereaved subjects. Parkes (1985) has recently reviewed the literature and classification of grief reactions. Normal grief reactions vary between individuals, but there are some common features. At first, there is usually a period of shock or numbness, which may last for hours or days and is more marked after an unexpected death. This is followed by acute episodes of intense emotional distress with weeping, protestation and anger, with accompanying somatic symptoms of anxiety such as palpitations or choking sensations in the throat. These pangs of grief are precipitated by any reminders of the loss and are set against a chronic background disturbance of depressed mood, disturbances of sleep, appetite and weight and social withdrawal (Worden 1982). Vivid dreams and hallucinations of the dead person or his* voice are quite common. There is an overwhelming need to rehearse the events around the death and this is one aspect of grief work, the process by which we accept the reality of the loss and withdraw psychologically from the relationship with the dead person, in order to continue our own life in a positive manner.

The chronic low mood and loss of purpose in life may continue for months or years, while the pangs of grief tend to decrease in intensity and frequency with time. There is an increase in psychosomatic and somatic illness in the year following bereavement, which may be a consequence of the disturbance of the immune system which has been reported (Bartrop et al 1977). Anniversary reactions are commonly experienced for some time.

Recovery from bereavement is marked by a return to psychological, social and physical well-being. Because of the enormous individual variations in response, it is not possible to provide a specific time scale. However, a successful outcome depends on the individual's personality and life experiences, the circumstances of the death, the relationship he had with the dead person and on the supportive network surrounding him (Raphael 1977). The style of an individual's grief reaction will be determined by his personality traits, for example, whether he grieves in private or openly expresses his emotions.

---

*Throughout this chapter the masculine pronoun 'he' has been used to avoid the awkward repetition of 'he or she'.

PERINATAL DEATH

Today, it is widely accepted that losing a baby late in pregnancy or soon after delivery is accompanied by the same sort of grief reaction described above. Since 1970 there has been a great deal of descriptive literature, with some objective studies on management and outcome and it is now clear that grief after perinatal death is no different, qualitatively, from that following the death of any loved person. See reviews by Zeanah (1989), Forrest (1990) and Bourne & Lewis (1992).

There are some special features. Anxiety and anger are frequently described, with blame being directed at the staff, other members of the family, or at one's self, in the form of guilt. This may be due in part to the suddenness of the death and is probably compounded when there is no scientific explanation available to help the parents understand exactly what went wrong (Newton et al 1986). Desperately seeking for a cause for the baby's death is also common. Clearly, it is easier for parents who do have an explanation such as malformations of the baby or extreme prematurity. *Empty arms* is another common and distressing symptom after the phase of numbness has passed and mothers are frequently tormented by hearing their dead baby crying, or feeling fetal movements. Some experience negative or aggressive feelings towards other babies and are fearful of losing control, while others long to hold a baby, any baby, however painful this might be. Many mothers do not expect to lactate once the baby has died, and find the fact that they do very upsetting. Most authors emphasize the great sense of loss of self-esteem experienced by bereaved mothers; they experience failure both as women and as wives.

Most young parents will not have been bereaved before and often experience difficulties coping with the complicated registration and funeral procedures (Forrest et al 1981). Many mothers are unprepared for the emotional turmoil of their grief reaction and of the exacerbation of symptoms which often accompanies the expected date of delivery or the return of menstruation. They may feel they should be over it after a few weeks. This view may be reinforced by well-meaning friends and relatives and even some medical practitioners, who may advise the couple to go ahead with another pregnancy long before they have sufficiently recovered from their loss to cope with this psychological stress. There is evidence that fathers recover from grief more quickly than mothers (Helmrath & Steinitz 1978, Clyman et al 1980, Forrest et al 1982) and this in itself may lead to relationship problems, particularly if the couple arc not used to sharing their feelings, or if one is blaming the other for the baby's death. Meyer & Lewis (1979) report that sexual and marital difficulties are common sequelae, although an increase in marital breakdown rate has not been reported.

Another difficult area is the reaction of other young children in the family to the loss of the baby. They may be very confused about what has happened to the baby and even feel responsible for his disappearance (Bowlby 1979). Behavioural changes are common and may take the form of over-activity, naughtiness, regression and school problems, as well as emotional problems (Van Eerdewegh et al 1985). These reactions are usually fairly short-lived—a few weeks or months is the time noted by most authors—unless the emotional state of the parents is such that there is an absence of normal warmth in family relationships for an extended period of many months (Black & Urbanowicz 1985) or if serious relationship difficulties develop between the mother and the surviving children (Halpern 1972, Lewis 1983).

There are particular problems associated with miscarriages and stillborn babies in which iatrogenic factors undoubtedly play a part. Miscarriages are frequently regarded by professionals and others as minor setbacks in successful childbearing. For some women, however, they represent a loss as painful as that of a full-term baby (Oakley et al 1984). This is particularly so if there have been difficulties conceiving, previous miscarriages, or if the pregnancy was terminated because of fetal abnormalities (Lloyd & Laurence 1985). Here there is the double loss of that baby and of the chance of childbearing. A previous termination of pregnancy has been reported by many clinicians as a complicating factor for normal grieving because of the associated guilt and sense of retribution that is experienced by the mothers. If the pregnancy was well advanced, beyond 20 weeks or so, some parents want to hold a funeral for their baby and this may present administrative difficulties.

Much has been written about unresolved grief after a stillborn baby, notably by Lewis (1976, 1983). He attributes this to the painful emptiness of the experience. There is no real object to mourn as the baby never lives outside the womb, and no memories to help either. It is similar to the situation in which someone is missing, believed dead. The problem is accentuated if the stillborn baby is rapidly removed from the delivery room before the parents have a chance to see or hold him, and if the hospital takes over the funeral arrangements without involving the parents. These babies are still often buried in unmarked graves.

The attitudes of friends and relations may also contribute to the difficulties. For example, one grieving mother was told: 'You can't have postnatal depression, you haven't got a baby'. For these reasons, successful mourning after stillbirth may be harder to achieve without the guidance of well-informed staff and greater understanding on the part of society in general.

Long-term effects of perinatal death

There have been few studies on the long-term effects of perinatal death.

In the largest study reported so far, Nicol et al (1986) followed up 110 women for 6–36 months after a perinatal death. They found 21% suffering from a pathological grief reaction, with continuing severe psychological symptoms (depression, anxiety, tiredness, etc.); social adjustment problems and marital difficulties, and a resolve to have no further children. Nicol et al also found that a poor outcome was associated with a crisis in the pregnancy, an unsupportive family network and seeing but not holding the baby.

There have been reports of serious relationship problems with babies conceived too quickly after a loss (Cain & Cain 1964, Poznanski 1972, Lewis & Page 1978, Bourne & Lewis 1984). It seems that if the dead child has been incompletely mourned before the start of a new pregnancy, mourning may be postponed until after the delivery of the baby, when it can reappear as postnatal depression (Lewis 1979). The new baby's identity can become confused with that of the idealized dead baby, causing great emotional problems. He may never be able to live up to his parents' expectations and may also become the focus of any unresolved anger which the parents feel as a result of their loss. The survivor of twins may also be involved in very similar problems if the dead twin is not properly mourned at the time. This has been called the replacement baby syndrome.

It seems therefore that about 1 in 5 bereaved families are likely to suffer adverse long-term effects after losing a baby. Good care should therefore aim to try and prevent these long-term sequelae.

CARE

In many countries now, the recommendations for care emphasize the important role of maternity unit staff as regards families facing the loss of their baby (Giles 1970, Klaus & Kennell 1976, National Stillbirth Study Group 1979, Kowalski 1980, Fetus and Newborn Committee, Canadian Paediatric Society 1983, Rousseau & Moreau 1984, Royal College of Obstetricians and Gynaecologists 1985).

This section brings together the recommendations for care made by individual clinicians and organizations concerned with helping parents cope with perinatal death. Their effectiveness was evaluated in our randomized study (Forrest et al 1982). It is generally agreed that the key task is to enable parents to overcome their fear of death and dying so that they can experience the painful reality of their loss and allow mourning to begin. This involves encouraging them to have as much contact as possible with their baby, both before and after death. There is widespread agreement by authors that it is particularly important for parents of stillborn babies to see, hold and name their baby.

Intrauterine death and stillbirth

When an intrauterine death is suspected, the fears for the baby's condition should be shared with the parents, together if at all possible, and not denied. If the mother is at the clinic, efforts should be made to contact her partner or a friend, so that she is not left to travel home alone and unsupported. The ultrasonographers in the scanning room have an important role to play when the confirmatory scan is done. They need to be sympathetic to the situation, relaxing any rules to allow the mother to be accompanied by anyone she chooses.

After intrauterine death has been confirmed, most women are very frightened at the prospect of delivering a dead baby, as well as being shocked by their loss. It helps if staff take time to explain carefully what will happen, that adequate pain relief will be available, and what the baby will look like at delivery. This is often successful in overcoming any reluctance the parents may have about seeing or holding their baby. If the baby is very malformed or macerated, it may help to show him first to the parents wrapped up. Even so, a few parents will not be able to cope with seeing and holding their baby at the time of delivery. A photograph should be taken and kept in the medical notes for possible use later and further opportunities for seeing the baby offered to parents over the next few days, as they often change their minds. Photographs, hand and footprints, and other mementos of the baby are in fact very important, as they provide tangible evidence of the reality of the baby's existence and of his loss. They should be available for parents as keepsakes, if they wish.

If a baby dies in labour, it is good practice to inform the consultant in charge immediately (or very soon if it is the middle of the night). The fact that a senior member of staff has come very promptly to try to help the parents from his own experience is nearly always deeply appreciated by parents, and can soften any resentful feelings the couple may have towards the hospital staff.

Neonatal death

When the baby lives long enough to be transferred to an intensive care unit, it is again very important for the staff to make time to keep parents as fully informed as possible about the baby's condition and encourage them to share in any possible part of the care. Photographs of the baby are very helpful, particularly for the fathers to keep at home, or if the mother is too unwell to visit the unit. In a randomized trial of the use of routine Polaroid photographs of sick babies in the first week of life (Pareira et al 1980), there was a significant increase in visiting by the parents of photographed babies compared with the non-photographed group. When the baby's condition is known to be terminal, it is important to try to involve the parents in the decision to cease life support and then to let them nurse their dying baby in their arms, free if possible from all the equipment that has been necessary until then. Guilt for removing the baby from the life support system has not been reported.

Many parents like to help with the laying-out of the baby's body and this should be encouraged. They often select special clothes or toys to be placed in the coffin with the baby.

Facilitating the parents' contact with the reality of the death of their baby in these ways facilitates their grief reactions. They also need privacy to express their grief and this should be provided, however busy the unit.

Aftercare

The choice of site of the aftercare of the mother is important as mothers differ in their requirements at this time. Some want to be on their own, far away from the sound of babies crying; others long to return to familiar faces on the ward. It is helpful if care can be as flexible as possible in this aspect; the mother will also need her partner to remain with her for the first night at least. Ideally, the hospital should provide a couch in the mother's room so that the couple can share their grief together. Help with the suppression of lactation has already been mentioned as an important issue for the mother whose baby has died. If the mother is physically fit to return home immediately and wishes to do so, it is essential to ensure that she has a good supportive network of family, friends and professionals before briskly discharging her.

The autopsy

Consent for autopsy should always be requested after a perinatal death, as it may provide invaluable information about the cause of death and help parents not only with their grief but also assist in the planning of future pregnancies. Most parents do consent although the decision is often painful. As one mother put it: 'She's been through enough; must she be cut up now as well?' There are, however, a small number of parents whose religion forbids autopsy and their dilemma needs to be acknowledged to avoid a situation in which they are subjected to intolerable pressure to obtain their consent.

Having consented, parents cherish great hopes that the findings will answer their questions about why their baby died. It is therefore very important for them to receive the results in a form which makes sense to them. The best person to do this is a senior member of staff who can interpret the pathologist's findings. This can be done as part of the follow-up interview.

Registration and funeral arrangements

Fundamental to good care is a knowledge not only of the bereavement process but also of the legal procedures required when a baby dies or is stillborn. (Stillbirth and Neonatal Death Society 1991). It is also necessary to be familiar with the registration and funeral arrangements in one's own unit or locality. Religious practices also vary greatly and an awareness of these and sensitivity to individual parents' wishes is crucial. A funeral may involve considerable expense and assisting parents in making difficult choices, helping those in financial straits and encouraging them to attend the funeral are therapeutic aspects of care. The unit should ensure that a suitable individual is available for this task.

Many units have prepared leaflets outlining their own procedures and providing helpful advice on various aspects of losing a baby; these can be very helpful for parents.

Communication

Good care hinges around good communication and parents often comment on communication failures in describing their experiences. Staff need to give bereaved parents opportunities for talking together about the loss of their baby and listen sympathetically to their expressions of grief. It is much harder to listen than talk oneself. In addition, staff need to try and help parents in their search for a cause of death and senior obstetric or paediatric staff need to discuss this with the parents. Seeing both parents together not only helps to strengthen their relationship as they share the experience of their baby's loss, but also helps prevent misunderstandings or inconsistencies in explanation. Arranging for the same members of staff to meet regularly with the parents also helps. Any information given in the first few days of the loss will probably have to be repeated later as the initial shock of bereavement passes. A follow-up interview a few weeks later seems to be the best way of overcoming this difficulty. Good communication between staff about the loss of the baby is also vital to prevent painful situations, such as an individual being unaware that a baby has died and breezily asking the mother when she is to be delivered. Communication between hospital and primary health care teams also needs to be good. The primary care team should be informed immediately about the baby's loss so that they can contact the family as soon as, or even before, the mother is discharged from hospital. Parents may want the support of their own religious adviser and the hospital needs to check on this and contact the person concerned.

The next pregnancy

The timing of the next pregnancy is important, as has already been discussed, to allow for the dead baby to be mourned first. From their members' experience, the Stillbirth and Neonatal Death Society (1984) recommends waiting 6–8 months. Our study (Forrest et al 1982) found that pregnancy occurring less than 6 months after the loss was strongly associated with high depression and anxiety scores at the 14-months' assessment. However, the enormous individual variation in bereavement response means that it is inappropriate to recommend a fixed time interval. The best advice appears to be to wait a while until the parents have had a chance to say goodbye to the dead baby and until the mother feels emotionally as well as physically strong enough to cope with another pregnancy. The next pregnancy will inevitably be an extremely anxious time and she will need extra support during it and in the first few months after delivery (Phipps 1985).

Follow-up

Most mothers will be discharged home within a few days of their baby's death, still too shocked to grasp properly what has happened or why. Careful follow-up is extremely important. Parents should be able to contact the staff who cared for them by telephone after they leave the hospital; and some units offer home visits by a social worker. An appointment should be made for both parents to see the consultant or a senior member of staff about 6 weeks later, as soon as the chromosomes and autopsy results are available and some form of perinatal mortality conference has taken place, to cover the following points:

1. To give the parents the opportunity of going over the events around the loss of their baby and releasing emotion.
2. To allow clarification of why the baby died, if at all possible. The autopsy results should be given to parents in an appropriate form.
3. To give obstetric counselling and in particular, advise about the timing of future pregnancies.
4. To make any necessary arrangements for genetic counselling.

Although returning to the maternity unit for these appointments is usually a harrowing prospect for parents, they almost always find it helpful. Perhaps this is because they have moved a step further in their grief work by once again facing the painful memories.

Checklists

Some units find it useful to have checklists to ensure that all practical aspects of care have been covered (White et al 1984). Although they can be helpful as *aides-mémoire*, checklists should not replace personal, compassionate contact with bereaved parents.

Care of the family at home

The general practitioner (GP), health visitor and the other primary health care workers form the professional supportive network for the family once the mother has been discharged home. These professionals can help by continuing to express concern, informing parents about the symptoms of bereavement and putting them in touch with any local support groups for parents who have lost a child (see Useful Addresses). The GP can watch for signs of a pathological grief reaction and refer for specialist help if necessary. These reactions are most likely to take the form of unremitting symptoms of depression, severe anxiety or the appearance of psychosomatic illness. There may also be drug or alcohol abuse.

Anger is another feature of grief reactions and the GP may need to deal with anger focused on the maternity unit. To do so, he needs to have good relationships with the obstetric and paediatric staff and to be fully informed about the course of events which led to the baby's loss. The parents may also blame the GP, of course. When this happens, it is essential for him to meet the family as soon as possible so that they can ventilate their feelings, and, hopefully, re-establish their relationship. Many parents remain angry simply because they were denied any compassionate response to their situation; no one on the staff said: 'I'm so sorry your baby has died'.

The GP or health visitor will probably be the people the family turn to for help with the reactions of their other children to the baby's death. Parents may need help in allowing their children to vent their feelings about such a painful subject and it must be remembered that young children will use play as a vehicle for expressing this emotion. Explaining death to the under-5-year-olds is also difficult, because developmentally, they are not yet able to grasp the concept (Lansdown & Benjamin 1985). Even very simple statements like: 'The baby's gone' will be interpreted literally and lead to questions about where, and when a visit can be made. The parents will need to provide more information as the child's capacity for understanding develops.

THE ROLE OF SPECIALIST COUNSELLORS

So far, this chapter has concentrated on the management of normal grief and the prevention of abnormal reactions through the care of the ordinary staff of maternity units and primary health care teams. However, about one in five families will show pathological reactions and all of these are likely to be accompanied by family relationship problems. In such cases, the help of specialist counsellors trained in grief work will be needed to advise staff on management or to take over the cases if necessary. The treatment required is often lengthy; antidepressant drugs and psychiatric surveillance may be necessary for severe depressive symptoms. Child and family psychiatrists may be particularly helpful in dealing with family relationship problems. Specialist counsellors can also help to promote normal grieving in parents who are most at risk of pathological reactions, and can also be useful in supporting the staff of the unit through regular staff meetings, case discussions, training sessions and offering advice to self-help groups (Lake et al 1983, Kellner et al 1981).

SELF-HELP GROUPS

Self-help can be very effective in providing appropriate support for parents facing many different problems and perinatal bereavement is no exception. In the UK, several national organizations exist—for example, the Stillbirth and Neonatal Death Society (SANDS) and the Compassionate Friends—and there are often locally based groups as well. SANDS have played a major part in changing attitudes and practices in hospitals and in the community and have campaigned for the reform of hospital funeral arrangements and registration anomalies. Their support groups are to be found in most parts of the UK. Parents can benefit from sharing their experiences together, discovering that they are not alone in their suffering and that time helps to heal their wounds. However, not everyone can cope with group support and it is not wise to rely entirely on local self-help groups to meet all the needs of bereaved families. While it is invaluable to give parents the telephone number or address of a local contact, this should not replace follow-up by the hospital and general practitioner.

TRAINING

The training of staff in the care of families who have lost their baby or who are faced with the birth of a malformed or handicapped baby deserves as much emphasis as the development of their technical expertise. Because we have lost our familiarity with death and bereavement at a personal level, staff need to be informed about the process of mourning as well as being trained in the basic skills of interviewing and counselling. They also need to explore their own feelings about death if they are to understand and help others. A good training programme should therefore combine formal with informal teaching, such as the use of group discussions, videotapes and role play. In addition, junior staff can learn a great deal from watching and listening while more experienced members of staff handle difficult and painful situations.

CONCLUSIONS

Good care does not end with a baby's death; much can be done to help the family cope with their loss and facilitate recovery from the bereavement. In this chapter, an attempt has been made to describe parental grief reactions and set out guidelines for care. But successful implementation depends on the attitudes of individual staff members and the importance attached to training in this area.

Effective care has implications for both maternity unit staff and professionals working in the community. Time needs to be spent with parents whose baby dies or is malformed, listening as well as talking. Attention also has to be paid to the details of follow-up in individual cases. The unit may have to review its procedures for postnatal care in order to be able to offer more flexibility; senior members of staff need to play a central role in caring for the parents, sharing their own experience and expertise with junior staff. Attention must be given to the practical aspects of the registration and funeral arrangements for babies and the primary health care team should monitor the bereavement process. Such changes in care improve rapport with grieving families; staff cope better with the painfulness of perinatal death because they feel able to help. Finally, families on the whole emerge from their grief able to continue functioning well, with positive attitudes towards the professionals who shared in the loss of their baby.

USEFUL ADDRESSES

Compassionate Friends, 53 North Street, Bristol BS3 1EN. Tel: 0117 9539639.

Stillbirth and Neonatal Death Society (SANDS), 28 Portland Place, London W1 3DE. Tel: 0171 436 5881.

REFERENCES

Bartrop R W, Lazarus L, Luckhurst E, Kiloh L G, Penny R 1977 Depressed lymphocyte function after bereavement. Lancet i: 834–836

Black D, Urbanowicz A 1985 Bereaved children—family intervention. In: Stevenson J E (ed) Recent research in developmental psychopathology. Pergamon, Oxford

Bourne S, Lewis E 1984 Pregnancy after stillbirth or neonatal death. Lancet ii: 31–33

Bourne S, Lewis E 1992 Psychological aspects of stillbirth and neonatal death—an annotated bibliography. Tavistock Clinic, London

Bowlby J 1979 Attachment and loss, vol 3. Hogarth, London

Cain H C, Cain B S 1964 On replacing a child. Journal of the American Academy of Child Psychiatry 3: 443–455

Clyman R, Green C, Rowe J, Mikkelsen C, Ataidc L 1980 Issues concerning parents after the death of their newborn. Critical Care Medicine 8: 215–218

Fetus and Newborn Committee, Canadian Paediatric Society 1983 Support for parents experiencing perinatal loss. Canadian Medical Association Journal 129: 335–339

Forrest G C 1990 Care of the bereaved. In: Chalmers I, Enkin M W, Keirse M J (eds) Effective care in pregnancy and childbirth. Oxford University Press, Oxford

Forrest G C, Claridge R S, Baum J D 1981 The practical management of perinatal death. British Medical Journal 282: 31–33

Forrest G C, Standish E, Baum J D 1982 Support after perinatal death: a study of support and counselling after perinatal bereavement. British Medical Journal 285: 1475–1479

Giles P 1970 Reactions of women to perinatal death. Australian and New Zealand Journal of Obstetrics and Gynaecology 10: 207–210

Halpern W 1972 Some psychiatric sequence to crib death. American Journal of Psychiatry 129: 398–402

Helmrath T A, Steinitz E M 1978 Parental grieving and the failure of social support. Journal of Family Practice 6: 785–790

Kellner K R, Kirkley-Best E, Chessborough S, Donnelly W 1981 Perinatal mortality counseling program for families experiencing stillbirth. Death Education 5: 29–40

Klaus M H, Kennell J H 1976 Maternal infant bonding. C V Mosby, St Louis

Kowalski K 1980 Managing perinatal loss. Clinics in Obstetrics and Gynaecology 23: 1113–1123

Lake M, Knuppel R A, Murphy J, Johnson T 1983 The role of a grief support team following stillbirth. American Journal of Obstetrics and Gynecology 146: 877–881

Lansdown R, Benjamin G 1985 The development of the concept of death in children aged 5–9 years. Child Care, Health and Development 11: 13–20

Lewis E 1976 Management of stillbirth—coping with an unreality. Lancet ii: 619–620

Lewis E 1979 Inhibition of mourning by pregnancy: psychopathology and management. British Medical Journal 11: 27–28

Lewis E 1983 Stillbirth: psychological consequences and strategies of management. In: Milunsky A (ed) Advances in perinatal medicine, vol 3. Plenum, New York

Lewis E, Page A 1978 Failure to mourn a stillbirth; an overlooked catastrophe. British Journal of Medical Psychology 51: 237–241

Lloyd J, Laurence K M 1985 Sequelae and support after termination of pregnancy for fetal malformation. British Medical Journal 290: 907–909

Meyer R, Lewis E 1979 Impact of stillbirth on a marriage. Journal of Family Therapy 1: 361

National Stillbirth Study Group 1979 The loss of your baby. Health Education Council/Mind, London

Newton R W, Bergin R, Knowles D 1986 Parents interviewed after their child's death. Archives of Disease in Childhood 61: 711–715

Nicol M T, Tompkins J R, Campbell N A, Syme G J 1986 Maternal grieving response after perinatal death. Medical Journal of Australia 144: 287–289

Oakley A, McPherson A, Roberts H 1984 Miscarriages. Fontana, London

Pareira G R, Talbot Y R, Boatwell W R, Parina P A, Musholt K S 1980 Photographs of sick neonates prior to transport; the effect on parental visiting pattern. Pediatric Research 14: 2662–2673

Parkes C M 1985 Bereavement. British Journal of Psychiatry 146: 11–17

Phipps S 1985 The subsequent pregnancy after stillbirth; anticipatory parenthood in the face of uncertainty. International Journal of Psychiatry in Medicine 15: 243–263

Poznanski E O 1972 The 'replacement child'; a saga of unresolved parental grief. Behavioral Pediatrics 81: 1190–1193

Raphael B 1977 Preventive intervention with the recently bereaved. Archives of General Psychiatry 34: 1450–1454

Rousseau P, Moreau K 1984 Le deuil perinatal. Extrait de la revue L'enfant de l'ONE no 5. Jolimont, Belgium

Royal College of Obstetricians and Gynaecologists 1985 Report of the RCOG working party on the management of perinatal deaths. RCOG, London

Stillbirth and Neonatal Death Society 1984 Preconceptual care of preparing for your next baby. SANDS, London

Stillbirth and Neonatal Death Society 1991 Miscarriage, stillbirth and neonatal death, guidelines for professionals. SANDS, London

Van Eerdewegh M M, Clayton P, Van Eerdewegh P 1985 The bereaved child; variables influencing early psychopathology. British Journal of Psychiatry 147: 188–194

White M P, Reynolds B, Evans T J 1984 Handling of death in special care nurseries and parental grief. British Medical Journal 289: 167–169

Worden W 1982 Grief counselling and grief therapy. Tavistock, London

Zeanah C H 1989 Adaptation following perinatal loss: a critical review. Journal of the American Academy of Child and Adolescent Psychiatry 28: 467–480

The newborn

46. Evaluation of the newborn

David Hull   Terence Stephenson

Material in this chapter contains contributions from the first edition and we are grateful to the previous authors for the work done.

ADJUSTMENTS AT BIRTH

Lung expansion and the onset of breathing

Once the infant emerges from the birth canal and the umbilical cord is occluded, clamped and cut, the infant's immediate priority is to establish an alternative oxygen supply. For this he or she needs to fill the lungs with air and to breathe regularly at an appropriate rate and depth.

At the time of birth the infant's sensory system is well in advance of the motor system, so the brain will record a kaleidoscope of new sensations as he or she is handled and squeezed and head, trunk and limbs drop into novel positions. In utero the hips are flexed so it is not surprising that dangling babies by their ankles at birth provokes a gasp and crying. The sensations are such that the majority of babies gasp at birth without noxious stimulus. If the gasp occurs whilst the airway is clear, then the gas–liquid interface moves down the respiratory tree as the lung fills with air. In healthy infants, the first inspiratory gasps can generate intrathoracic pressures of over $100\,\mathrm{cmH_2O}$ (Milner & Vyas 1982). The formation of the functional residual capacity depends on a number of factors, including diaphragmatic tone and the presence of surfactant, but the precise mechanisms are as yet ill understood (Milner 1993). Usually functional residual capacity is established to 70% of its final volume within a few gasps. Sometimes, despite gasps, little or no air is held. Only when the lungs are filled with air will tidal ventilation begin and only then will the infant have control of an

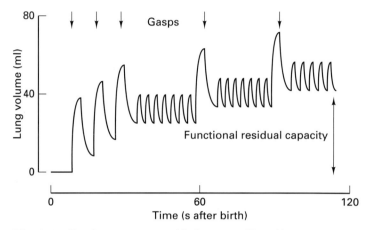

Fig. 46.1 Respiratory patterns with the onset of breathing.

independent oxygen supply. Most healthy infants achieve this by 1–2 minutes (Fig. 46.1; Chamberlain et al 1975, Palme-Kilander et al 1993). Asphyxiated, sedated and premature infants may have problems with the initial gasps and the establishment and maintenance of a functional residual capacity. Infants born by Caesarean section have lower gas exchange levels during the second minute after birth compared to infants born vaginally (Palme-Kilander et al 1993).

The closure of the fetal channels

Consequent upon clamping the umbilical cord, the venous return from the placenta stops abruptly, the ductus venosus collapses, the pressure in the right atrium falls and the foramen ovale closes. When the lungs expand and fill with air the pulmonary vascular resistance falls, the pulmonary blood flow increases, and the increased pulmonary venous return causes a rise in the left atrial pressure which further contributes to the closure of the foramen ovale (Dawes 1968; Fig. 46.2). The mechanical effect of lung inflation on the pulmonary vasculature is reinforced by the falling CO_2, rising pH and rising Po_2, all of which favour pulmonary vasodilatation. Hormonal

813

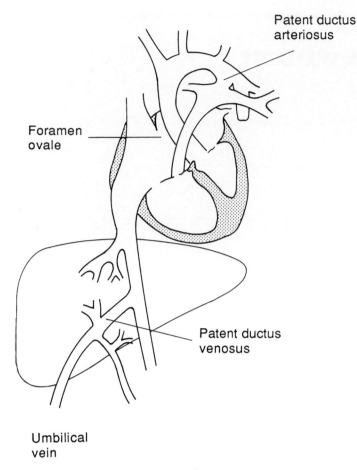

Patent ductus
arteriosus

Foramen
ovale

Patent ductus
venosus

Umbilical
vein

Fig. 46.2 The fetal channels.

changes may also influence pulmonary vascular resistance (Soifer et al 1985, Kuhl et al 1989, Davidson & Eldemerdash 1990, Hargrave et al 1990). In addition, there must be receptors responsive to recently described agents which have pulmonary vasodilator properties, such as magnesium sulphate and nitric oxide (Kinsella et al 1992).

With the fall in pulmonary pressure, the flow through the ductus arteriosus reverses so that oxygenated blood traverses the duct; the oxygen acts on the muscle in the duct wall causing it to contract (Heymann & Rudolph 1975), a mechanism which involves prostaglandins. Drugs inhibiting the synthesis of prostaglandins cause the duct to close (Heymann et al 1976), whereas an infusion of prostaglandin E_1 can keep the ductus open (Hallidie-Smith 1984). Prostaglandin-inhibitor drugs given to mothers, particularly during the second trimester, can cause intrauterine closure of the ductus, causing problems for the neonate, including persistent pulmonary hypertension (Friedman et al 1976). Indomethacin, a prostaglandin synthetase inhibitor, is used to close a persistent patent ductus in preterm infants (Rennie & Cooke 1992). Prostaglandin E_1 infusions are used to keep the ductus open in selected infants with congenital heart defects—those with duct-dependent pulmonary or systemic blood flow, such as severe pulmonary stenosis or coarctation of the aorta respectively; this can keep a child alive until corrective surgery can be performed (Silove 1986).

With muscle spasm, the ductus closes physiologically within a matter of minutes of birth but at this time, if an episode of hypoxia occurs, it may open again. However, over a matter of weeks the closed ductus slowly seals up and is replaced by a fibrous cord. With the closure of the fetal channels the chambers of the heart, previously working in parallel, begin to work in series. If one chamber is ill formed, for example hypoplasia of one ventricle, the other can no longer maintain both circulations and acute circulatory problems are precipitated.

Colour, tone and blood pressure

With birth, pulmonary arterial blood pressure falls and systemic pressure rises (Dawes 1968). Oxygenation after birth causes the infant to change from a pasty white or blue to a glowing pink. Birth is a stressful experience: fetal catecholamine levels are high and peripheral vasomotor control appears to be largely untried. Thus, during the first hours of life, the limbs and trunk of normal, healthy infants can appear to be mottled or even a striking harlequin pattern. Many infants have blue hands and feet for some time after birth. Birth also results in an increase in tone; within moments of this development the infant is usually wide awake and ready to suckle.

Temperature control

It is a cold world for the infant. In utero, the fetus is bathed in amniotic fluid at 37°C and because the fetal metabolic rate per kilogram is higher than the mother's, the fetal body temperature is higher by 0.3–0.6°C. At birth, the skin dries and the infant loses heat by evaporation. This has to be reduced to a minimum if a drop in body temperature is to be avoided. Drying down with a warm towel, followed by swaddling in a warm blanket and being cuddled by the parents is ideal. Even with precautions, an infant's rectal temperature often falls after birth and then rises slowly over the first hours of life. This subsequent rise may be in part associated with the rising minimal metabolic rate as the infant's systems begins to work to support independent existence (Smales & Kime 1978).

Even the term infant has a limited capacity to control body temperature (Hull & Chellappah 1983, Rutter 1986). Thus on exposure to cold he may reduce surface heat losses by vasoconstriction and double body heat production by thermogenesis in brown adipose tissue (Hull 1966). Even so, because of an infant's body weight : surface area ratio, if he is taken from a warm cot, undressed and prepared for a bath in a warm room at 25°C, he will not be able to maintain body temperature.

In a hot environment a baby can sweat a little (Rutter & Hull 1979) but this capacity is limited so he is even more vulnerable in hot environments. Infants have always been dependent on their parents for protection and this is particularly important with respect to body warmth in the first days of life. Cuddling and swaddling are not just comforting but also important for sensing and maintaining the baby's temperature.

Swallowing, digesting and evacuation

A total of 10% of an infant's body weight at birth is formed by adipose tissue of which half is fat, stored as tri-acylglycerol, which can provide sufficient calories to sustain the infant for some weeks after birth (Widdowson & Spray 1981). Thus, there is no great urgency for the bowel to become fully functional in the first hours of life. Indeed it has to develop and grow to accommodate its increasing workload (Weaver 1992).

In utero the fetus swallows amniotic fluid containing some protein (Friis-Hansen 1982). Although the fetus can swallow amniotic fluid, this is less of a physiological challenge than suckling in the newborn, when it is vital that milk is not aspirated into the air-filled lungs. Coordinated sucking and swallowing requires protective bulbar reflexes which are only achieved in the human infant by 35 weeks' gestation (Herbst 1989). Also at this gestational age, significant increases in circulating concentrations of intestinal regulatory polypeptides (gastrin, motilin, neurotensin) occur in response to milk feeds (Lucas et al 1978). Therefore, unlike other systems which mature earlier in gestation and can function adequately, although not perfectly, following extremely preterm delivery (e.g. the kidney and endocrine pancreas), the gastrointestinal system cannot support independent oral nutrition until well into the final trimester.

After birth, the bowel must not only accommodate a larger volume, digesting disaccharides and fats and many complex proteins, but it must also adjust to colonization with bacteria. These bacteria are usually introduced by parents or other attendants and are influenced by the intraluminal environment of the bowel, which in the main is determined by fed nutrients.

By the end of the first trimester, the neuromuscular development of the human gut is largely complete. Circular and longitudinal muscle are present in both small and large bowel and the autonomic neural plexi are identifiable. These structures, necessary for peristalsis, are morphologically mature long before enteral feeding is required or coordinated sucking and swallowing are possible. The preterm human infant passes an average of one stool per day from as early as 25 weeks' gestation, even if not enterally fed (Weaver & Lucas 1993). This suggests that there is an intrinsic pattern of large bowel motor activity which can function in a coordinated propulsive

fashion. This does not usually lead to defaecation in utero, though what prevents prenatal evacuation is not known; meconium-stained liquor is only rarely seen before term (Lucas et al 1979, Mathews & Warshaw 1979). At term, this is often not a normal event but, rather, occurs as a sympathetically mediated response to fetal distress.

The newborn infant has no voluntary control over evacuation and defaecation probably occurs as a reflex response to rectal load. Milk feeds entrain the intrinsic activity of the colon and induce regular defaecation at a frequency determined by the volume of the products of digestion which reach the rectum; the more feeds, the more stools (Weaver & Lucas 1993). Although the amount of stool varies, the water content remains within a narrow range (around 70%) consistent with the water reabsorptive function of the colon. After the first week of life, stool volume falls although milk intake continues to increase, partly due to a further maturation of the water-conserving capacity of the gut.

Babies often defaecate for the first time during delivery or, if not, within the first day of life; 95% of infants pass meconium by 24 hours and 98% by 48 hours; delayed passage of meconium raises the possibility of anal atresia, Hirschsprung's disease or meconium ileus due to cystic fibrosis. By contrast, they regularly micturate in utero, making a considerable contribution to the amniotic fluid (Hytten 1985). Thus infants with obstructive problems of the urinary tract usually declare themselves before delivery by oligohydramnios, and after birth by postural deformations and lung hypoplasia. However, babies who dribble urine may pass undetected, so the observation of a good stream of urine is also important.

Renal function

The kidneys receive a relatively small proportion of cardiac output in utero (2–3%) compared to postnatal life (Robillard & Nakamura 1988a). This low renal blood flow may be viewed as appropriate because the placenta performs many of the functions which the kidneys assume in postnatal life. After birth, the kidney takes up its key role in fluid and electrolyte balance and excretion of chemical waste. During labour and immediately after birth, there are large surges of antidiuretic hormone, renin, cortisol and angiotensin II, resulting in renal vasoconstriction and salt and water retention. In early postnatal life, renal vascular resistance falls and renal blood flow increases until the kidneys receive approximately 5–20% of cardiac output. Possible endocrine mediators of the fall in renal vascular resistance and increased renal blood flow include prostaglandins, the kallikrein–kinin system and atrial natriuretic peptide (Godard et al 1982, Robillard et al 1988, Robillard & Nakamura 1988b, Stephenson & Broughton-Pipkin 1990). The initial low renal blood flow may be beneficial in a term infant who usually has little fluid intake on the first days of postnatal life (Stephenson & Rutter 1992), particularly if breastfed. The glomerular filtration rate is also lower in the first 2 days of postnatal life than later in the first week. The subsequent increase in glomerular filtration rate postnatally may in part be caused by the hormonal changes mentioned above.

Postnatally, there is a rapid increase in the maximum urine osmolality attainable, from around 500–600 mOsm/kg H_2O in the first 2 weeks of postnatal life to greater than 1000 mOsm/kg H_2O after 6–8 weeks (Edelmann et al 1960). The increase in concentrating ability can be influenced by protein intake (Polacek et al 1965), which perhaps influences the tonicity of the renal medulla by increasing urea concentration. There is good evidence of an appropriate increase in antidiuretic hormone in response to stimuli such as haemorrhage, diuretics and hypertonic saline (Simpson & Stephenson 1993).

The newborn has the capacity to pass a dilute urine from a very early stage but the relatively low glomerular filtration rate, which is influenced both by postconceptional and postnatal age, means that there is a very limited ability to excrete a water load. In a similar manner to the rapid maturation of concentrating ability, there is a rapid postnatal increase in the ability to excrete a water load, primarily because of the increase in glomerular filtration rate.

RESUSCITATION

An infant will need active resuscitation if he or she fails to gasp, expand the lungs, maintain a functional residual volume or to begin breathing rhythmically.

Failure to gasp

The risk factors include maternal sedation and anaesthesia, prolonged labour, intrauterine asphyxia and immaturity (Chamberlain et al 1975). Perhaps the commonest factors are drugs crossing to the fetus prior to birth and suppressing brain activity, although it is amazing to see some infants bursting into life, whilst their mothers, heavily sedated or anaesthetized, are unaware of what is happening. Another cause for failure to gasp is fetal hypoxia, whatever the cause, but the fact that an infant cries immediately at birth does not mean that he has not been irreversibly damaged by intrauterine asphyxia. Fetal asphyxia may take any form between two extremes. At one end is the infant who suffers prolonged hypoxia which slowly drains the energy resources, particularly glycogen, causing acidosis and gradually developing widespread damage which may or may not be reversible. At the other extreme is the infant who suffers total acute asphyxia, as may occur with cord prolapse when the oxygen supply is suddenly completely cut off. Depending on the nature of the insult, infants differ both in their response to birth and in their recovery during resuscitation (Fig. 46.3). There are usually other complicating factors. Babies experiencing trauma during delivery, who may well have gasped frequently prior to delivery, may be suffering as much from shock (hypotension) and acidosis as from hypoxia, and this may be complicated further by aspiration of meconium into the respiratory tree.

Failure to open the lungs

An infant may gasp but fail to hold the gas in the lungs,

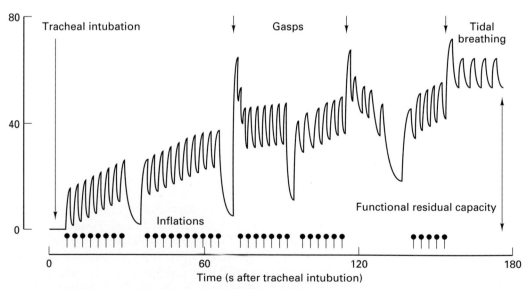

Fig. 46.3 Diagramatic representation of the establishment of the functional residual capacity (FRC) during artificial ventilation of an asphyxiated infant. Only when the FRC had formed, partly with inflations and partly after gasps did the infant begin spontaneous breathing.

Table 46.1   Reasons why gasps may not draw air into the lungs

Problem	Cause
Airway obstruction	Aspirated vernix, meconium or blood Large or floppy tongue Laryngeal spasm or stenosis Tracheal agenesis
Deformed thoracic cage	Thoracic dystrophy (many causes) Ill-formed or paralysed diaphragm
Thoracic cage filled with:	Pleural effusions (many causes) Bowel and liver (diaphragmatic hernia) Haematomas
Lung hypoplasia	Due to renal agenesis Due to chronic amniotic leak Associated with diaphragmatic hernia

perhaps because of the effect of drugs or hypoxia on the tone of the diaphragm and the muscles of the chest wall. The task is then to ventilate the infant, supplying oxygen and removing carbon dioxide until normal lung function returns.

However, it may be that with the gasp, no air enters the lungs because the airway is obstructed. With intra-uterine hypoxia or because of stimulation and handling, the fetus may gasp and draw amniotic fluid and birth canal debris, such as vernix, into the lungs. This can occur so that aspirating the airways is both an emergency and a priority (Gregory et al 1974). Until this is performed, attempts to push the oxygen into the lungs may be in-appropriate. Although aspiration of lung liquid from the upper airway is to some extent unavoidable, the baby's head should be held below the level of the lungs after birth, until the airways have been cleared.

There are many other reasons why gasps may prove ineffectual, but most are rare (Table 46.1).

Failure to begin tidal breathing and persisting cyanosis

Very occasionally it is possible to ventilate a child adequately but tidal breathing still does not occur. This can be due to severe asphyxia, very heavy sedation or gross brain abnormality. It may also be a consequence of the presence of the endotracheal tube or of inadvertent hyperventilation.

Occasionally, the lungs may ventilate but the infant remains pale or cyanosed. Pallor may be due to bleeding or shock. A tentorial tear or rupture of a viscera can cause either or both. Persisting cyanosis may be due to a persistent fetal circulation or to severe congenital heart disease.

Assessment

It is common practice to have scoring systems for the assessment and resuscitation of the newborn (Curnock 1986). Whilst there are advantages in such uniformity, it is a mistake to assume that all infants in need of resus-citation have similar problems and that all assessment criteria have the same meaning irrespective of these problems.

An internationally respected and understood method of assessment is the Apgar score. In essence it is a numerical interpretation of the infant's heart rate, respiratory efforts, colour, responsiveness and tone; the first three factors in the main reflect adequate oxygenation. It is customary to record the score at 1 and 5 minutes.

As a guide to what to do and when to do it, the infant's heart rate and respiratory efforts are the key features. Restoring the heart rate, expanding the chest and oxy-genating the baby are the objects of the exercise. Noting the changes in response to actions such as nasal stimu-lation are more important than adding up the score. In fact the score at 5 minutes may well reflect more of the activities of the resuscitator than the state of the infant.

Assessment based on more pertinent criteria, such as the time to first gasp or the time to establishing regular respirations, have their own merits (Chamberlain et al 1975) but have not been generally accepted. If the Apgar score is to remain the common language (Marlow 1992), it must be interpreted correctly (Table 46.2).

Minute 0   If an infant is asphyxiated prior to birth, and is born pale or blue and floppy with a heart rate below 100 beats/min, active resuscitation must begin at birth. There is no virtue in waiting.

Minute 1   The majority of infants are not asphyxiated at birth for asphyxia is not an inevitable consequence of the birth process. However, some do not gasp and open their lungs immediately; they have primary apnoea and may need to be encouraged to gasp. Again it is the falling

Table 46.2   The Apgar score

Factors	Score		
	0	1	2
Heart rate	Absent	Slow, < 100 beats/min,	> 100 beats/min
Respiratory effort	Absent	Slow, irregular	Good, crying
Muscle tone	Flaccid	Some limb flexion	Active motion
Reflex irritability	No response	Cry	Vigorous cry
Colour	Blue, pale	Body pink, limbs blue	Completely pink

heart rate and failure of the infant to make a respiratory effort which signal the need for appropriate resuscitation.

Minutes 2–5 Some babies start breathing and then give up; others do not respond to the simpler stages of resuscitation, so time becomes a premium and if the heart beat remains slow, or if blueness or pallor develop whatever the respiratory effort, informed action is required. Such a situation is a considerable challenge to the clinician.

Management

Handling

The clock is started as soon as the head (vertex presentation) or body (breech presentation) is delivered. At birth, the infant, whether asphyxiated or not, should be handled gently, the cord clamped and cut, and the baby dried in warm towels as expediently as possible. If a problem is anticipated the infant should be placed on a dry, warm surface under a radiant source in a good light and observed closely.

Clearing the airway

Gentle low-pressure suction is used to clear the mouth and pharynx, if necessary under direct vision using a laryngoscope. The current concern to prevent the possible transmission of HIV has precluded the use of mouth suction devices for clearing pharyngeal mucus or meconium and has created the need for readily available mechanical suction at all deliveries (Gamsu et al 1993). Injudicious prodding into the lower pharynx can cause laryngeal spasm or bradycardia from vagal stimulation and should be avoided.

Provoking a gasp

In a cold world and in an unaccustomed position, it may be assumed that the infant has been adequately stimulated. However, various powerful stimuli may provoke a response. If there is respiratory depression and the mother has received opiates within the last 6 hours, neonatal Narcan (naloxone 0.02 mg/ml solution) should be given (0.01 mg/kg intravenously or intramuscularly if venous access is not easy). This dose can be repeated six times at 3-minute intervals and naloxone 0.01 mg/kg can be given intramuscularly (maximum volume of 1 ml in each leg) to give an additional longer duration of action. The upper respiratory tract is the most appropriate site to stimulate. Cold oxygen blown on the nasal mucosa, for example, often works when handling has not and has the added advantage of ensuring that if the baby gasps, an oxygen-rich mixture is inhaled. The infant may also gasp during clearing of the airway. When all

this has failed and artificial ventilation is required, the first inflation often provokes an inspiratory effort, a reflex response which contributes considerably to the success of the procedure (Milner et al 1984).

Oxygenation

To deliver oxygen to the infant it is necessary to fill the lungs with gas. For the majority, it is probable that air is all that is necessary, though in practice pure oxygen is used. This has the disadvantage that if it is left in the lungs after resuscitation and the infant stops breathing again, all the oxygen may be absorbed, causing secondary atelectasis which may be more difficult to reverse. It is good practice to let the infant breathe air through an endotracheal tube before removing it, so that nitrogen remains in the lung and splints the air spaces open.

Gas can be pushed into the lungs either by a facemask and bag or by endotracheal intubation and inflation at a controlled pressure. Resuscitaires have a simple blow-off valve to prevent the inadvertent use of excessive pressures which may cause a pneumothorax.

Facemask and bag

This is perfectly adequate for most babies who fail to breathe. In Sweden it is the method of choice both in hospitals and in the community (Palme et al 1985). It has the advantage of being simple to apply, readily available and relatively safe. With pressure-limited systems, the stomach should not distend with gas (Vyas et al 1983). A variety of facemasks and bags are available (Palme et al 1985). In the resuscitation of infants it is often assumed that if the heart rate rises above 80–100 beats/minute the ventilation is satisfactory. In a recent study of mask ventilation, a transient increase in heart rate to 100 beats/minute in the absence of measurable gas exchange was recorded in 25% of infants. The effect of mask ventilation can be considered satisfactory if the heart rate rises to 130 beats/minute and the oxygen saturation measured in the right hand is 70% or more (Palme-Kilander & Tunell 1993). If an emergency arises away from a delivery room, mouth-to-mouth resuscitation can be effective. Use only the pressure that can be generated by the cheeks.

Tracheal intubation

The most certain way for experienced staff to resuscitate the baby is to intubate the trachea with a snug-fitting tube and expand the lung with intermittent inflations at a rate of 30–40/minute, holding each inflation for about 1 second and not exceeding a pressure of 30 cmH$_2$O. If meconium is seen around the vocal cords or in the trachea, a 10 gauge suction catheter should be inserted through the cords under direct vision, prior to intubation, and the meconium aspirated using an initial suction pressure of 70 mmHg, increasing as necessary. Avoid positive-pressure ventilation until as much meconium has been removed as possible. Repeated suctioning can be continued for up to 2 minutes provided the heart rate remains above 60 beats/minute, but if the baby is severely asphyxiated, positive pressure ventilation through an endotracheal tube should be commenced at 1 minute. Whatever method of lung inflation is used, it is essential to watch the chest cage for expansion and to avoid overinflation. This can occur with ball valve effects, for example from the endotracheal tube being pressed against the carina. Whilst observing the chest movement keep checking the pulse rate which is usually visible as pulsation at the root of the umbilicus.

If the infant fails to respond, the commonest errors are:

1. The endotracheal tube is in the oesophagus and not the trachea. Auscultating over the stomach is an unreliable method for assessing correct tube placement. If in doubt, take it out and revert to facemask and bag ventilation.
2. The chest is not moving. This is because either the airway is blocked with mucus or meconium or inadequate pressures are being used to inflate the lungs. The tubing may be disconnected or again the endotracheal tube is in the oesophagus. Tracheal stenosis or agenesis are rare possibilities.
3. The chest expands but the infant does not become pink. Check that the resuscitaire is connected to the wall oxygen supply or that the cylinders are not empty. Someone might be standing on the tubing or the oxygen tubing may have become disconnected from the endotracheal tube.

The following actions may be appropriate:

1. Cardiac massage (100 compressions/minute).
2. Correct any acidosis
   1 mmol/kg sodium bicarbonate intravenously = 2 ml/kg 4.2% $NaHCO_3$.

3. Tap pneumothorax or pleural effusion.
4. Consider shock or bleeding: give plasma 20 ml/kg intravenously.
5. If the heart rate remains below 100/minute after 2 minutes of effective positive-pressure ventilation, consider 0.25 ml/kg 1 : 10 000 adrenaline and 2 ml/kg 25% dextrose intravenously.
6. If intravenous access is difficult, adrenaline or naloxone can be given in double the above doses via the endotracheal tube followed by positive-pressure ventilation (O'Callaghan & Stephenson 1992). Absorption across the pulmonary circulation is good.

When not to resuscitate and when to stop

These are both difficult decisions, depending on clinical judgement. If an infant has a congenital abnormality incompatible with life, such as a severe meningomyelocele, renal agenesis or gross multiple anomalies, clearly no action should be taken. Antenatal diagnoses should not be assumed to be infallible and should always be confirmed by the attendance of a paediatrician at the time of delivery. With very immature infants, the decision is best left to those with experience of neonatal care. By far the majority of infants under 25 weeks' gestation die, and of those that survive under current management, 10–30% are severely handicapped. Increasingly, units are drawing up guidelines for the care of infants, born technically alive by virtue of a pulsating heart, but who, as a result of prenatal pathology or immaturity, would not survive even with intensive care (Tables 46.3, 46.4).

When there is doubt, or when time is required to make an informed choice, resuscitation should be performed. The additional information gained, of the infant's response to resuscitation, often helps in making decisions about whether and when to withdraw support. Such situations are often emotionally charged, due to staff concern as well as the parents' tragedy, so the timing is not solely dependent on biological factors (Stephenson & Barbor 1995). The following problems are not uncommon:

Table 46.3 Percentage of infants who survive to discharge home by gestation: 1992 data for a Nottingham hospital with approximately 5500 inborn deliveries. All infants born alive (i.e. with a beating heart) on the labour suite are included, irrespective of gestation, even if they did not survive to be admitted to the neonatal unit

	Gestational age (weeks)							
	< 26	26–27	28–29	30–31	32–33	34–35	36+	Total
Received neonatal care	13	23	43	57	89	56	179	460
Inborn (excluding in utero transfers)	9	18	35	42	77	51	176	408
In utero transfers	4	5	8	15	12	5	3	52
Outborn	1	7	12	10	11	9	28	78
Deaths (number of lethal congenital abnormalities in parentheses)	7 (0)	11 (0)	7 (0)	3 (0)	3 (0)	3 (2)	6 (5)	40 (9)
% Survival (excluding lethal congenital abnormalities)	46	52	84	95	99	98	99	

Table 46.4 Percentage of infants who survive to discharge home by birth weight: 1992 data for a Nottingham hospital with approximately 5500 inborn deliveries. All infants born alive (i.e. with a beating heart) on the labour suite are included even if they did not survive to be admitted to the neonatal unit

	Birthweight (g)						
	<750	750–999	1000–1499	1500–1999	2000–2499	2500+	Total
Received neonatal care							
Inborn (i.e. excluding in utero transfers)	18	17	53	97	70	153	408
In utero transfers	4	5	18	17	4	4	52
Outborn	2	5	20	16	11	24	78
Deaths (number of lethal congenital abnormalities in parentheses)	11 (0)	7 (0)	7 (0)	5 (0)	6 (2)	4 (0)	40 (2)
% Survival (excluding lethal congenital abnormalities)	50	68	90	96	95	97	

Severe asphyxia

In Britain, approximately one full-term baby per 1000 dies or is severely handicapped as the result of perinatal asphyxia. An infant experiencing severe asphyxia in the last stages of delivery may be born with no sign of life, but cardiac massage and artificial ventilation may restore the heart beat. Most paediatricians can recall a miraculous recovery from such a position.

Most infants who recover probably experienced acute total asphyxia immediately prior to birth but were previously in good shape. In these cases, recovery of a heart beat is usually followed quickly by gasping, and regular respirations are established within 20 minutes. Whereas early Apgar scores indicate the effectiveness of resuscitation and say little about ultimate outcome, a low Apgar score beyond 15 minutes is predictive of a poor neurological prognosis (Marlow 1992).

If an infant has experienced acute or chronic hypoxia then reversing a terminal situation at birth may be un-rewarding for the brain may well already be irreversibly damaged. Reports based on analyses of outcomes of infants with Apgar scores of 0–1 at birth (D'Souza 1983) are difficult to interpret because the investigators are unable to adjust for the degree of prenatal asphyxia. However, in general, it has been the view that if a structurally normal mature infant is not breathing spontaneously at 30 minutes, it is unlikely that he will survive; if he does, it will be with severe brain damage. It is important in making this decision to allow the infant full opportunity to breathe for himself. The endotracheal tube itself may inhibit the infant's spontaneous efforts and very occasionally, an infant may begin to breathe when the tube is removed. Some units treat cerebral oedema aggressively, guided by intracranial pressure monitoring, but it now seems unlikely that the outcome is altered (Svenningsen et al 1982, Levene 1988). The severity of hypoxic ischaemic encephalopathy is the most accurate clinical predictor of outcome after birth asphyxia in full-term infants (Levene 1993). Unfortunately, the degree of hypoxic ischaemic encephalopathy may deteriorate over the first few days and a decision on whether treatment

should be withdrawn may have to be deferred until this nadir is apparent (Table 46.5).

Congenital abnormality

Nothing is more challenging to the resuscitation than an apparently normally formed infant, born in good condition, who slowly dies because of failure to establish an alternative oxygen supply. While internal bleeding always has to be considered, the more likely explanation will be congenital abnormality. Always call a colleague. The possibilities include airway stenosis, bilateral lung hypoplasia, severe congenital heart abnormalities and cerebral anomalies. If the infant is pink but fails to breathe, transfer on a ventilator to the neonatal unit. If the infant remains blue or white and the heart beat slows, there is probably no point in continuing artificial ventilation after 30 minutes.

Immaturity

Lung maturity largely determines whether an infant survives the first 24 hours and lung maturity does not necessarily correspond to gestation. Lung performance can be compromised by asphyxia and aspiration. Some clinicians intubate and ventilate at birth most infants under 28 weeks' gestation to assist them to form a functional

Table 46.5 Severity and outcome of hypoxic-ischaemic encephalopathy (reproduced with permission from O'Callaghan & Stephenson 1992)

	Grade		
	I	II	III
Clinical	Hyperalert Staring Irritable Tone may be increased or decreased	Require tube feeding Asymmetric tonic neck reflex Difference in tone between upper and lower limbs	Hypertonia Seizures Coma Require ventilation
Outcome	>95% normal	75% normal	20% normal 50% die in newborn period

residual capacity but there have been no studies to show that such an aggressive policy is beneficial compared to an expectant approach. In some premature infants born in poor condition, lung inflation is virtually impossible. Such infants should be transferred immediately for neonatal intensive care, for they will need controlled ventilating for some days if they are to survive. Their colour can be a poor guide to Pa_{O_2}, for they can look pink with a low Pa_{O_2} (because of the predominance of fetal haemoglobin with high oxygen affinity) or blue with a normal Pa_{O_2} (because of the relative polycythaemia). If intensive care is not available, and if they appear lifeless despite lung inflation and being kept warm, it is wise to stop after 30 minutes.

IMMEDIATE SCRUTINY

The newborn is examined under three sets of circumstances:

1. Immediately at birth.
2. As a routine check within 48 hours, although there is some debate regarding the cost/benefit of an early repeat examination (Cartlidge 1992).
3. When necessary if a problem arises.

When a baby is born everybody wants to know what he or she looks like. The parents have first claim since they need to be reassured that everything is all right. The person conducting the delivery, usually a midwife, has to answer the question whether the baby is all right—occasionally this can be very difficult. The parents can reasonably expect their attendants to be as truthful as possible in as sympathetic a manner as possible.

To deal with the immediate question, it is important to check that all the external parts are present, that the head, eyes and ears appear normally formed, to count the number of digits, to examine the back, and decide, if possible, whether the child is a boy or girl. If there is doubt about the sex, do not guess: say that it is sometimes difficult to determine the sex from the external genitalia at the time of birth and that further examination and tests will be required. Reassure the parents that a definitive and lifelong gender will become clear within a week at most. The parents should be dissuaded from choosing a neutral name.

Assess the infant's adjustment to the birth and clamping the cord. Some infants cry at birth and then stop breathing. The baby can be handed on to the parents when the tone and colour are good.

The next question is whether or not the infant can go with the mother to the lying-in ward or whether special care is needed. About 15% of all infants used to go to special care, but with minimal neonatal nursing skill available in the lying-in wards, this can be reduced to below 8% (Chiswick 1986). The decision will depend on local policies, with particular regard to staffing levels and expertise on the postnatal wards. It will also involve birthweight and some estimate of gestation, an evaluation of risk based on antenatal and labour records, and the state of the infant at birth. Currently, in Nottingham, less than 5% of inborn deliveries are admitted to the neonatal unit.

A number of specific problems must be considered at this time.

Oesophageal atresia

In some units it is routine policy to pass a tube directly into the baby's stomach to exclude oesophageal atresia. Often the catheter which was used to aspirate the upper airways is used. The manoeuvre is certainly essential if there has been polyhydramnios. A firm tube which can be felt in the infant's abdomen is the most certain method of excluding atresia.

Rectal agenesis

This takes many forms. In some it is obvious at a glance; in others the anal dimple is present and the problem escapes detection. It is good practice to record the infant's rectal temperature before mother and baby are transferred from the labour suite. Some babies become cool despite warm towels, while others are chilled because of complications, changed priorities and breech delivery. Asphyxiated and preterm infants are at particular risk. Taking the rectal temperature is not without risk (Hull & Chellappah 1983), but properly performed it is safe and points to the need for keeping the infant warm. The need to insert the thermometer into the rectum ensures that rectal agenesis (except in the very rare cases of high membranes) is recognized early.

Infection

The most virulent neonatal infection is caused by group B streptococcus, an organism found in the vagina of up to 10% of pregnant women (Weindling et al 1981). For reasons which are unclear, a much smaller proportion of infants become infected but the mortality of those who are is approximately 50%. The infant may be born in very poor condition or the onset may be insidious and even of late onset. In either case, the signs are non-specific and may mimic hyaline membrane disease. Largely for these reasons, paediatricians have a low threshold for commencing intravenous benzyl penicillin in all babies at the onset of signs of respiratory distress, and broad-spectrum antibiotics in any infant seriously ill at birth (Baker 1990). There has been much recent debate over whether an antiseptic vaginal douche (Burman et al 1992) or maternal intrapartum antibiotics can reduce the transmission rate or the severity of the illness in the infant (Dashefsky 1990). Any type of perinatal preventive intervention requires the local availability of a rapid detection test for the organism to allow the at-risk group to be targetted (Editorial 1986). Otherwise, the programme cannot be cost effective and there is the risk of anaphylaxis to antibiotics in mothers who are not carrying the organism.

A baby may be born smelly or covered with turbid liquor, sometimes after prolonged rupture of membranes. The baby should be examined for signs of sepsis. If ill, or the baby has other problems such as prematurity, grunting respiration or birth asphyxia, he should be transferred to the neonatal unit for a full infection screen. This includes viral and bacterial swabs from ear, throat, umbilicus and any obvious septic site; additionally, suprapubic aspiration of urine (ideally under ultrasound guidance), full blood count, blood cultures, chest X-ray and lumbar puncture may be performed. Intravenous penicillin and gentamicin should be started immediately after the specimens have been obtained. The combination of a vague flu-like illness in the mother, green liquor, a neonatal rash and, rarely, abscesses on the placenta, suggests *Listeria monocytogenes* is the causative organism in which case ampicillin and gentamicin are a more powerful synergistic combination. Epidemiological studies have suggested that if the mother has eaten paté or shop-prepared salad, there is a greater risk of her acquiring listeria (SMAC Department of Health 1992).

If the baby is well, our policy is to admit the infant to the neonatal unit only if the three following conditions are met:

1. The mother has a pyrexia at the time of delivery or has been treated with antibiotics prior to delivery.
2. The liquor is offensive or there was a purulent or smelly vaginal discharge before birth.
3. The membranes have been ruptured for more than 24 hours.

For the well baby, the same swabs are taken as described and also a full blood count and blood culture, but antibiotics are not commenced unless his condition changes. If the baby is sent to the postnatal ward with his mother, he must be reviewed 4 hourly with regular temperature and respiratory rate observations. If staffing levels do not permit this, there should be a lower threshold for admission to the neonatal unit.

Often, however, these warning circumstances or signs are not present in infants who contract infection from the birth canal. If the mother is known to have genital herpes, streptococcal, gonococcal or listeria infections, it is essential that those responsible for the care of the newborn should be informed immediately (see Ch. 33). Primary herpes cervicitis is an indication for elective Caesarean section to protect the infant but this is not necessarily true for a recurrence. Recent studies have shown that only one-third of asymptomatic women who shed herpes simplex virus in early labour have recently acquired a primary infection. Infants of these mothers are ten times more likely to have neonatal herpes simplex infection than babies whose mothers have asymptomatic reactivation of herpes simplex (Prober et al 1987, Brown et al 1991). Whether fetal scalp electrodes are used depends on the significance of the information from fetal heart rate monitoring in each individual case.

Vitamin K

All infants should be given vitamin K as a prophylaxis against haemorrhagic disease of the newborn (VonKries 1991). Babies are more at risk if they are given oral vitamin K rather than parenteral vitamin K, if they are breastfed, or if they have liver disease (McNinch & Tripp 1991). A recent epidemiological study has shown a statistical association between neonatal vitamin K injection and subsequent risk of malignancy. However, the risk of haemorrhagic disease is certain; that of cancer is not (Ekelund et al 1993, Hull 1993).

Our present policy is to give intramuscular vitamin K only to infants on the neonatal unit (if > 1.5 kg birthweight, 1 mg; birthweight < 1.5 kg, 0.5 mg). This injection is never given on the labour suite because of the danger of inadvertent administration of ergometrine. All other infants receive 1 mg vitamin K orally. It is intended that further 1-mg doses will be given to breastfed infants at 1 week and 4–6 weeks after birth. However, implementation of this policy is hampered at present (early 1995) by the fact that there is no product licence for oral vitamin K (the parenteral preparation is given orally at present) and by the logistics of ensuring prescription and administration in the community. However an appropriate oral product may soon be available.

ROUTINE EXAMINATION

This is the service the infant receives before going out into the world. It is the first entry in a child's health records. Although it has developed casually, it is likely to become a more exacting and demanding examination. Doctors are now being sued for not doing it properly.

Ideally, it should be done at leisure, with the parents, and after appraising the essentials of the antenatal and labour records. Before approaching the parent and baby, the doctor should know the name and sex of the infant, the past obstetric history and whether any previous children have died. The only way to ensure thoroughness is to complete a checklist. Inevitably, it will not be possible to follow the same routine for each infant and occasionally full examination cannot be completed at one session. If the baby is asleep, complete as much of the examination as possible without waking him, especially the assessment of colour and respiratory rate which are more difficult if the infant is crying. Leave palpitation of femoral pulses, examination for dislocation of the hip, measurement of occipitofrontal circumference (the maximum of three measurements, not the mean) and assessment of neurological state until the end.

Minor problems

Parents often welcome reassurance about a variety of minor matters. Red marks over the eyes, bridge of nose and nape of neck (stork bites, salmon patches) usually disappear without trace within a year. White pimples in the glands on the butterfly area of the face (milia) can be prominent; these also disappear in time. Cysts on the gums (ranula) disperse spontaneously; primitive teeth need to be removed. Breast development with small amounts of milk secretion (witch's milk) occurs in 90% of term infants, boys and girls alike, and reflects the infant's rather than the mother's hormonal status (McKiernan & Hull 1980). In most infants, after initial swelling the breast tissue gradually disappears over a period of weeks. Girls may have a mucous plug in the vagina and a little withdrawal bleeding which has no significance.

Babies develop a surprisingly wide range of rashes. Neonatal urticaria (erythema toxicum) can be very florid, with a widespread fluctuating maculopapular rash most marked on the second day. It does not appear to distress the infant and requires no treatment. A different rash, characterized by red macular patches and superficial clear vesicles (miliaria), is called a heat rash and may be precipitated by a warm humid atmosphere, but this is not always evident.

Minor abnormalities

The significance of minor congenital structural abnormalities is more difficult to assess. They may provide clues to problems elsewhere.

Fontanelles

Large fontanelles and wide sutures are not uncommon and usually have no significance if the head circumference is normal. However, a third fontanelle is found in some chromosome abnormalities, e.g. Down's syndrome, and prominent Vermian bones are a feature of osteogenesis imperfecta.

Accessory auricles

These are usually isolated abnormalities but may also be associated with inner ear problems and deafness, and with syndromes involving hypoplasia of the mandible or maxilla. Abnormally formed ears are often associated with renal abnormalities and are a feature of many dysmorphic syndromes. All infants with accessory auricles, any malformation of the external ear, cleft lip or palate, a family history of deafness, and all preterm infants should ideally have their hearing screened prior to discharge from the hospital. This policy targets an at-risk subgroup in which deafness is much more common. Early (within the first 6 months of life) fitting of hearing aids is beneficial.

Palmar creases

Single creases (simian crease) occur in many normal individuals and are sometimes, though not invariably, a feature of Down's syndrome (trisomy 21).

Fused labia

Again these are often an isolated anomaly but may be a feature of masculinizing syndromes. Topical application of 0.01% orthodienoestrol each night for 1 month may avoid the need for surgical separation.

Two cord vessels

A single artery occurs in three per 1000 infants and raises the question of an underlying renal abnormality. Ultrasonography will reveal a renal anomaly in over 15% of these infants, almost half of whom will have a persisting and significant abnormality. There is more than a five-fold increase in the incidence of renal anomalies and vesicoureteric reflux for infants with a single umbilical artery over that found in the general population (Bourke et al 1993). An ultrasound scan to identify the presence and size of the kidneys is indicated in all infants with either a single umbilical artery or abnormal ears, for during embryogenesis the ears develop at a similar gestation as the kidneys.

Specific conditions

Examination of the newborn is primarily a surveillance procedure aimed at identifying problems that need further attention. In some it is secondary prevention—the early identification of a disorder to minimize its expression, e.g. dislocated hips. In others, it is concerned with tertiary prevention—recognizing a handicap so that care and support can be provided, thus reducing the accumulating problems which add to the child's and the family's disability, for example in Turner's syndrome.

Syndromes

If a child has dysmorphic features, it is important to document them precisely, and if their significance is not obvious expert advice should be sought. Occasionally the facial features of Down's syndrome are hard to recognize

Table 46.6 Percentage of Down's syndrome infants with the dysmorphic features indicated (reproduced with permission from Stephenson & Wallace 1991)

Flat facial profile	90%
Hypotonia	80%
Excess skin on back of neck	80%
Slanted palpebral fissures	80%
Anomalous auricles	60%
Clinodactyly (incurving) of fifth finger	50%
Single palmar crease	45%

in the first days of life (Table 46.6). Hypotonia and hyperextensibility are characteristic features and often help in the decision of whether to investigate further. Infants with Turner's syndrome (3/10 000) may pass undetected. Webbing of the neck, oedema of the feet or abnormal nails all indicate the need for further enquiry.

Deformations

The position in utero can deform the body shape. It is often helpful to try and fold the infant into his fetal position. Misshapen heads, asymmetrical faces, torticollis, chest wall depressions, unusual dimples or distorted hands and feet may all result from restricted intrauterine movement. They usually resolve when full movement is restored after birth. The parents may be shown stretching exercises for postural talipes but expert physiotherapy is required for a sternocleidomastoid tumour. Plagiocephaly is extremely common and may not resolve until the infant spends more time upright, allowing gravity to act symmetrically.

Club foot

There may be an element of deformation in all club feet. If the foot cannot be easily placed into its normal position orthopaedic opinion should be sought.

Dislocated hips

This condition may also be a consequence of intrauterine position. About 2% of infants have unstable hips at birth but in many of these cases the signs will resolve without treatment. However, in 10% of this group there will be signs of dislocation and another 10% show evidence of subluxation or dysplasia. Current policy recommends that all infants should be examined soon after birth as intervention, by splinting the hips in abduction, is more successful if started early. Anyone performing this examination must be well practised in the procedures; experience can be gained initially on models and then increased by examining infants under expert guidance. The more experienced the clinician, the higher the success rate; even

so the diagnosis can be missed. There is still controversy as to whether late dislocation can occur in the first year of life (Dunn 1986). It seems that it does occur very rarely. Ideally the hips of those at high risk of dislocation (family history, breech delivery, etc.) should be examined by ultrasound (Clarke et al 1985).

Cleft lip and palate

Cleft lip is easily identified. Cleft palate can be missed if the infant is reluctant to cry. Always ask how the infant copes with feeding. Sometimes a palatal defect can be felt when it cannot be seen easily, particularly a submucous cleft with an intact mucosal covering. The lip is usually repaired at 3 months, the palate at around 1 year. A Haberman teat often helps with bottlefeeding; breastfeeding is very difficult. Some parents choose a name without the consonants s and f.

Heart defects

Examination of the pulses may point to a patent ductus arteriosus (full and bounding) or coarctation of the aorta (absent femoral pulses). However, this is not reliable because in coarctation the femoral pulses are often palpable at the first neonatal check because the ductus arteriosus has not yet closed. Central cyanosis, peripheral collapse (extreme pallor) and signs of heart failure—tachycardia, tachypnoea, difficulty with feeding, excess sweating, an enlarged liver—all indicate the possibility of an underlying heart problem. The presence of a heart murmur in an otherwise healthy infant is far more difficult to interpret. Closing fetal channels lead to a variety of sounds which subsequently disappear. Conversely, in infants with severe defects no murmurs may be heard in the first days of life because the right-sided pressures are relatively high and there is little gradient for shunting between left and right.

If the heart is active and the murmur loud—3/6 and above—an ECG and chest X-ray are justified. The results of these may direct the echocardiographer as to the likely lesion. Expert cross-sectional echocardiography can delineate the anatomical diagnosis in most cases of congenital heart disease. Cardiologists reach a correct anatomical diagnosis on the basis of clinical features without echocardiography in only two-thirds of referred neonates; the score for neonatologists was one-third (Haworth & Bull 1993). However, an echocardiogram is not required on every child who has a murmur. If the infant is asymptomatic and the murmur is quiet—2/6 or less—then clinical review at discharge and 6 weeks is sufficient. The difficult task is to explain to the parents what you are doing without causing inappropriate anxiety. Nevertheless, the parents of all infants with a murmur should be told of the warning signs which would dictate earlier review—dusky or pale episodes, slow to feed or sweaty, breathlessness and poor weight gain.

BIOCHEMICAL SCREENING

Many inherited metabolic diseases, of which the great majority are recessive, present in the newborn period. It is pertinent to consider why this is so. For some it is because the placenta discharged the harmful metabolites; for others it is because milk feeds present a previously unfamiliar nutrient load, such as galactose in lactose and phenylalanine in milk proteins. Disorders such as galactosaemia and phenylketonuria only come to light as milk feeding is established.

For other babies, it is the accelerated metabolism of independent existence which reveals the disorder. Hypothyroidism is a good example. Such disorders may be detected in three ways: (i) by mass screening; (ii) by screening infants at risk by virtue of a family history, and (iii) by biochemical investigation of infants with a cluster of clinical features.

Mass screening

Mass screening is appropriate if the disease is an important problem, the natural history is known and there is a latent period before irreversible damage occurs. There must be an agreed approach with recognized treatment, a suitable test (few false positives and few false negatives) and adequate resources.

Mass screening has been practised for phenylketonuria, galactosaemia, syrup urine disease, tyrosinaemia, homocystinuria, histidinaemia, arginosuccinicaciduria and hypothyroidism, cystic fibrosis and muscular dystrophy. Screening programmes for phenylketonuria and hypothyroidism fulfil the desirable criteria and are in common use (Danks 1981). The dried spot of blood obtained at the time of the Guthrie test is also being used in some regions for measurement of immunoreactive trypsin, a significantly high concentration indicating that a sweat test is required after 6 weeks of age to exclude or confirm cystic fibrosis. Some centres also screen for galactosaemia.

Phenylketonuria

This rare condition (about one in 10 000) is detected by the Guthrie procedure on heelprick blood from an infant once feeding is established, on the fourth, fifth or sixth day. It is a screening test and all positive results require further investigation, since not all will have the classical disorder which inevitably results in brain damage unless a special demanding dietary regimen is adopted.

Hypothyroidism

Congenital hypothyroidism, due to agenesis or dyshormonogenesis, has an incidence of one in 4000. The same blood spot used to detect excess phenylalanine can also be used to assay thyroid-stimulating hormone, which is raised in hypothyroid states, before irreversible damage has occurred. Again a raised level is an indication for further investigations to define the problem (Barnes 1985).

Familial risk

If there is a known familial risk of an inborn error of metabolism, in particular a previously affected sibling or a history of unexplained infant deaths, it is mandatory to institute appropriate investigations as soon as possible. For example, galactosaemia can be diagnosed without exposing the child to galactose, or megavitamin therapy (coenzymes) can be given in an attempt to induce some enzyme systems and so avoid harm in certain inherited metabolic disorders.

Neonatal illness

A full description of the clinical situations in which investigations for metabolic disorders are indicated is found in Danks & Brown (1986). In general, appropriate investigations should be considered in infants who are lethargic and hypotonic; vomit in the absence of obstruction; convulse; have apnoeic spells or abnormal behaviour without obvious cause; suffer unexplained hypoglycaemic or acidaemia; have unexplained jaundice or a haemorrhagic tendency. Suspicion will be reinforced if the infant improves when feeds are stopped or if the infant or his urine smells unusual. Blood glucose, calcium, acid base status and amino acids, urinary sugars, ketones, ketoacids and amino acids would be initial estimations.

ILLNESS IN THE NEWBORN PERIOD

Parents or staff of the lying-in wards may become concerned about babies for a variety of reasons.

Grunting

It is not uncommon for infants who cry normally at birth and begin regular breathing to develop rapid or laboured respiration. The majority resolve spontaneously. The disorder has been labelled transient tachypnoea or mild respiratory distress, names which are at least descriptive and correct. If group B streptococcal infection is suspected (Weindling et al 1981, Editorial 1986), blood cultures should be taken and penicillin given immediately.

Enquiry about feeding performance is essential. If oesophageal atresia has not been excluded it should be. Babies with oesophageal atresia, unable to swallow their own saliva, sound very bubbly, so the diagnosis, once considered, usually becomes clear on careful clinical assessment alone. More commonly babies have some initial difficulty with effective swallowing, whether related to asphyxia or immaturity, although often it is unrelated. Gentle skilled feeding with small more frequent feeds is curative and only very occasionally is tube feeding required. There are many rare disorders resulting in oesophageal incoordination which also present at this time.

Going blue, apnoeic attacks and fits

Here again the challenge is to identify the infant with a serious problem. Cot deaths have been reported in lying-in wards, so one should not be overconfident about the survival of the apparently healthy. A clear history is very helpful. Did the episode or episodes occur with feeding or handling or whilst the baby was in the cot? Was the infant aware? Did he stop breathing? Did he cry before or after the episode? Was the baby floppy? If the body was jerking, what parts were affected?

Hypoglycaemia should be considered first and can be excluded by a quick heelprick blood test. It will have been anticipated in the dysmature type of infant described by Clifford—the child shows the features of intrauterine growth retardation with undernutrition, low body weight for gestational age—and also in infants of diabetic mothers, although hypoglycaemia can occasionally occur in infants without any of those predisposing clinical factors (Aynsley-Green & Soltesz 1986). Perinatal asphyxia, infections and cold exposure may contribute. Once the diagnosis is made the infant needs to be transferred to the neonatal unit for management. There are a number of rare metabolic disorders which present with hypoglycaemia in the newborn (Table 46.7).

Infections, in particular meningitis, can also present with fits or blue episodes, so if there is any doubt about what happened, culture of blood and cerebrospinal fluid, and antibiotic cover until the results are to hand, is the appropriate management (see Ch. 49).

Thorough clinical examination of the infant should exclude lung disorders and heart disease. If the infant has either a serious episode or recurrent minor episodes, observation in the neonatal unit with an apnoea alarm is indicated until these episodes have stopped.

A clear story of convulsions demands thorough neurological assessment. If the infant shows other neurological abnormalities further investigations are indicated. In hypoxic-ischaemic encephalopathy, the temptation to treat every abnormal movement with increasing doses of multiple anticonvulsants should be avoided. There is no evidence that this improves the outcome. Exaggerated startle responses and irritability, spasms and hypertonia on handling are common and are not true seizures.

Since the majority of blue attacks or apnoeic episodes or twitchings turn out to be of no lasting importance, it is a difficult judgement whether to reinforce parental and nursing anxiety by special observations and investigations which prove to be unnecessary, or to leave well alone and act only if new developments reinforce the initial concern. Whichever course is adopted, the parents must be kept fully informed and can make invaluable observations provided they know what is significant.

Jaundice

It is both normal and common for healthy newborn infants to become jaundiced (bilirubin above 85 μmol/l). In utero, unconjugated bilirubin is cleared by the placenta but after birth the load falls on the newborn liver so one

Table 46.7 Rare causes of neonatal hypoglycaemia (blood level below 2.2 mmol/l)

Insulin level	Cause
Transient	
Normal insulin levels	Small for gestational age (SGA)
	Asphyxia, starvation, cold, sepsis
High insulin levels	Maternal glucose infusions
	Infant of diabetic mother
	Erythroblastosis fetalis
	Idiopathic transient hyperinsulinism (often SGA)
	Beckwith–Wiedemann syndrome (macroglossia-exompthalmos)
Persistent	
Normal or low insulin levels	Congenital hypopituarism (small penis)
	Cortisol deficiency
	Glucagon deficiency
	Metabolic disorders (e.g. glycogen storage disorder)
High insulin levels	Tumours of islet cells (insulinomas)
	Immune-sensitive hypoglycaemia

factor is a delay in uptake by hepatocytes and the induction of glucuronyl transferase activity. Thus disorders of the liver or agents which interfere with glucuronyl transferase activity, such as drugs, will exaggerate the phenomenon. Another factor contributing to the raised level of unconjugated bilirubin is an increased bilirubin load due to red cell breakdown. Thus disorders which increase this burden, for example bruising or increased red cell fragility or breakdown, accentuate the bilirubin levels as in rhesus incompatibility. Bilirubin concentrations are also determined by the capacity of the serum binding proteins which may be reduced by raised free fatty acid levels, which compete for the binding sites following the initial establishment of feeding, and by various drugs. Bilirubin concentrations require monitoring to assess the underlying pathology and also because bilirubin is itself toxic. Further action is indicated in a healthy term infant if the unconjugated bilirubin level rises above 300 µmol/l, if clinical jaundice is present in the first 24 hours or lasts more than a week, if the conjugated level rises above 25 µmol/l or if bile is present in the urine (Mackinlay 1993).

The differential diagnosis of both unconjugated and conjugated bilirubin is considerable (Table 46.8), but it must again be emphasized that the majority of jaundiced infants are healthy and come to no harm and so the decision when to investigate further is not easy.

The management of hyperbilirubinaemia has become easier with the effective use of phototherapy. Each neonatal service has its own guidelines about when and how to use phototherapy (Dodd 1993). There is no reason why most term infants should not stay with their mothers on the lying-in wards. As a result partly of the fall in rhesus-affected infants and partly of more vigorous use of phototherapy, exchange transfusions are now rarely performed.

Temperature

The rectal temperature, measured by inserting a mercury thermometer 5 cm into the rectum and leaving it there for at least 2 minutes, is one of the observations routinely monitored by nursing staff. The interpretation of unusual variations, whether high or low, is not straightforward. In the newborn, the body temperature is far more under the influence of environmental conditions: if the buttocks are exposed because of a nappy rash it will be lower; if the infant is near a heat source and well swaddled so that opportunities for heat loss are limited, it will rise. Clinical assessment includes both an assessment of the infants's general well-being and of the environment immediately before the temperature was taken. If the infant is otherwise normal, adjusting the environment is all that is required, with the temperature being recorded 4 hourly until it returns to the normal range.

FEEDING

Once the infant has a firm grip on independent existence the next major step is to establish an alternative source of nutrition. While most infants root and suckle soon after birth, the volume they take is small for little is usually available and colostrum itself has relatively little energy content. Nevertheless, the experience is a first important step both in the infants' nutrition and in the induction of lactation, as well as an occasion for the emotional meeting of mother and child. In some cultures colostrum is avoided; since bottlefed babies do not receive it, colostrum per se is not essential.

The breastfed baby must then await the establishment of lactation until a point is reached when infant and mother together determine the supply and demand (see Ch. 42).

Breastfeeding

Breastfeeding does not appear to be instinctive; it has to be learnt. Breastfeeding is more likely to be established when the information programme before delivery has been thorough, when problems like inverted nipples have been dealt with, when mistaken notions about the effects of breastfeeding on breast shape have been discussed and when the mother knows who to turn to for advice and support.

The atmosphere in the postnatal ward and home is the key. It helps if both mother and baby are relaxed, if the baby suckles early, and if mother and infant have free and easy contact. Fixed schedules and unnecessary supplementary feeds can and often do interfere with the natural process. Babies and mothers are both individual in their feeding habits so there are many solutions, just

Table 46.8 Factors which may increase neonatal jaundice

Factors	Examples
Prebirth events	Maternal drugs, e.g. oxytocin Fetal disease, e.g. rubella Blood incompatibility, e.g. rhesus
Birth events	Asphyxia Delayed clamping of cord Bruising
Postbirth events	Delayed passage of meconium Dehydration and starvation Polycythaemia Infections, e.g. *Escherichia coli* and hepatitis Breast milk jaundice
Inherited disorders	In bile metabolism, e.g. Crigler–Najjar Which damage the liver, e.g. galactosaemia Hypothyroidism
Obstruction to bile secretion	Extrahepatic atresia Duodenal and low bile duct obstruction

as there are many problems. There are many excellent books and booklets on breastfeeding (Gunther 1970, Jelliffe & Jelliffe 1979, Royal College of Midwives 1993).

Obstetricians, paediatricians or family doctors are not particularly expert at counselling mothers on breast-feeding, and yet their advice is often sought if problems arise. The assessment of a nursing expert on the adequacy of the mother's supply of milk, the feeding position and technique and the suckling efforts of the baby is invaluable. Clearly if the mother is uncertain, tense, depressed, frightened or in pain the problem may lie in the supply. It is most unlikely that the breast is biologically unable to perform its task. Alternatively, a lethargic or irritable baby may not be sucking effectively. Some babies have to be encouraged whilst others are so lively they would test the patience of a saint. With support and encouragement, most mothers who wish to are able to breastfeed. A feeding problem may be a symptom of the mother's mood or a sign of a disorder in the infant.

There are very few absolute contraindications to breastfeeding. Severe illness in the mother or certain infectious diseases like tuberculosis or HIV (Ades et al 1993) are examples. Severe mental illness is a reason for the mother not to feed at all, either by breast or bottle. There are also rare contraindications to milk feeding, for example galactosaemia and phenylketonuria. Only rarely do drugs given to the mother pass to the infant in significant amounts (Current British National Formulary, Beeley 1987, MIMS 1988); some exceptions are given in Table 46.9.

In the UK it is recommended that breastfeeding should be continued for 3–4 months before a weaning diet is introduced (Department of Health and Social Security Report 1980, 1988). In practice, most mothers begin to wean before that period. The argument is that by 4 months the infant's ability to digest, metabolize and excrete a wider range of substances has increased and he is beginning to be able to chew. However, milk remains a good food for a growing infant and many mothers choose to breastfeed for much longer. In third-world countries continued breastfeeding brings with it many additional benefits and is a major factor in the survival and future well-being of infants and toddlers (Jelliffe & Jelliffe 1979).

It is an unhappy fact, however, that in the UK many mothers stop breastfeeding soon after they leave hospital. In 1980, a variety of reasons were given (Department of Health and Social Security 1980, 1988). These are probably at best only a crude index of underlying social attitudes—insufficient milk, painful breasts, the baby not sucking or rejecting the breast all suggest failure to establish feeding rather than secondary problems, and no doubt relate in part to the mother being unable to maintain at home what she had managed in hospital. Some mothers who are planning to return to full-time work choose to bottlefeed from birth on the basis that a short period of breastfeeding will not be worthwhile. However, a recent study has shown that breastfeeding for only 12 weeks confers significant protection against gastrointestinal illnesses and that this protective effect persists beyond the period of breastfeeding itself (Howie et al 1990). Although many studies suggesting an anti-infective role for breastfeeding have been flawed (Bauchner et al 1986), most have found a protective effect of breastfeeding against gastrointestinal infection and none have found an adverse effect.

Breast milk

Much has been written about the unique qualities of human milk. Certainly it is more than a quantitative mixture of protein, fat, carbohydrate, minerals and vitamins. The subject is dealt with fully in Chapter 42.

Bottlefeeding

Nurses are the experts at artificial feeding. A deliberate ritual is followed when preparing an artificial feed: filling the bottle, selecting the teat, choosing a time and a place to suit both baby and nurse and attending to the baby before feeding begins. Some babies will only willingly take a feed from one person—usually the mother—given in a certain way; others will feed from anyone in a variety of circumstances and conditions.

If there are problems with regurgitation, vomiting or failure to thrive, it is important to watch how the infant's mother prepares a feed and how the baby takes it. Better still, ask an expert nursing sister to advise. Sometimes there are obvious problems; the infant gobbles too fast, for example, or sucks hard with little reward, or swallows air. It is a particular skill to persuade a sick infant or an

Table 46.9 A guide to drugs in breast milk: unsuitable for administration to breastfeeding mothers

Gold salts
Indomethacin
Chloramphenicol
Tetracyclines
Clindamycin
Phenindione
Amiodarone
Doxepin
Lithium
Iodides
Oestrogens
Antineoplastics, immunosuppressants and radioactive pharmaceuticals
Atropine
Ergotamine
Vitamin A
Vitamin D

infant with a congenital anomaly (e.g. cleft palate) to feed. The availability of thin plastic nasogastric tubes which can be left in situ for days on end has taken much of the anxiety out of the management of the infant who is difficult to feed, for it is now technically easy to maintain adequate nutrition.

Artificial feeds

Modern food technology is now such that virtually any recipe can be formulated. However, we are by no means certain as to what is the best recipe. Worse, we do not know what is wanted of a feed: is it rapid growth, or is it optimal growth, increments of the body constituents which are the same as those which occur with human milk feeding? Is it a feed for health which protects against infection, avoids allergies or sets the scene for longevity? No doubt there will be feeds which favour some or all of these objectives, but they will not be the same, so choices are inevitable.

In the face of this, national and international advisory bodies have recommended that infant formulae, used as the sole feed, should resemble as far as possible the constituents of average human milk (Department of Health and Social Security 1980, 1988), and they do in quantity. It is ironic in the face of these recommendations that a soy-based feed, containing vegetable oil, vegetable protein and glucose syrup, should have been promoted so vigorously and is increasingly being offered to babies. Since there is little to choose between the other main products on the market, the price and convenience of the preparation become important factors in influencing the mother's selection.

For powdered milks the key to producing the correct mixture and the recommended calorie density is filling the scoop (Jeffs 1989, Lucas et al 1991). It should be neither heaped nor packed but carefully levelled. It is all too easy to give extra for good measure, but this produces a feed with an electrolyte load (especially sodium) which some infants cannot handle. The resulting hypernatraemia can be potentially dangerous if the infant becomes dehydrated by gastroenteritis. Since nursing staff are as likely to make errors as mothers, prepared liquid feeds are preferred in hospital.

PROGRESS

The neurological, psychological and behavioural responses of infants around the time of birth and particularly in the following few weeks have been the subject of many detailed observations in recent years (Volpe 1981). At the same time sophisticated imaging techniques (ultrasound (Trounce & Levene 1988), computerized tomography (Rorke & Zimmerman 1992), magnetic resonance imaging (Flodmark 1988) and spectroscopy (Wyatt et al 1989), near infrared spectroscopy (Edwards et al 1988) and sensitive analysis of evoked responses) have become available. So far, their impact on treatment has been relatively limited but ultrasonography now provides invaluable information about the infant's likely prognosis.

Initial neurological assessment might involve a review of the infant's posture, feeding and sucking patterns, spontaneous activity, muscle tone and strength and his response to being pulled to sit or being held in ventral suspension. The infant's response to some of these manoeuvres will vary with his state (Prechtl 1974). Primitive reflexes might be tested; the Moro is the favourite but others include the stepping reflex, Galant's reflex and the palmar grasp reflex. However, whilst these are of general interest, most of the essential information on tone and movement of the head, trunk and limbs can be assessed whilst handling the baby for other procedures during routine examination.

Abnormal neurological features

If the infant was damaged prior to or during birth, or the brain is ill formed, then a variety of features may occur which touch on most aspects of the infant's being.

Apnoea may occur at birth and hyperpnoea, hypopnoea, cyanotic episodes and irregular breathing and recurrent apnoeic attacks may follow. Rooting and sucking may be absent, weak or ineffectual, so that tube feeding is essential. The cry may vary in pitch and persistence but is rarely robust or easily soothed.

Extreme irritability with excessive startle response is usually accompanied by generalized hypertonia. Alternatively there may be hypotonia with little spontaneous movement. Depending on the tone, the posture varies from that of a rag doll to frightening opisthotonos. Finally, there may be convulsions, expressed as apnoeic attacks, focal fits, generalized twitching, myoclonic jerks and gross cycling movements.

The management, clinical course and prognosis will depend on the cause. If once the infant has adjusted to birth and independent existence, the features stay comparatively constant, an underlying abnormality should be considered. If they follow a sequence of hypotonia followed by hypertonia, irritability with fits followed by slow recovery, then ischaemic brain injury is more likely (Brown et al 1974). In drug withdrawal the infant is initially normal but then becomes irritable.

Everybody would wish to know whether the brain is irreversibly damaged or not. It is virtually impossible in the absence of specific syndromes with predictable clinical courses to give an informed answer at present. It may well be that with the newer imaging techniques, features will become evident in term babies (Rorke & Zimmerman

1992), as they appear to be in preterm infants (DeVries et al 1988, Edwards et al 1988, Flodmark 1988, Wyatt et al 1989), which point to a certain poor prognosis (Stewart et al 1987). Analysis of the EEG, evoked potentials or Doppler cerebral blood flow velocity may aid in predicting an adverse outcome (Levene 1993), but these techniques are not widely used at present.

Specific screening

There is no doubt that newborn infants can both hear and see. Already techniques are available and are being used in some centres to screen routinely at-risk infants for deafness. For diagnostic purposes both vision and hearing can be tested by evoked responses.

REFERENCES

Ades A, Davison C, Holland F et al 1993 Vertically transmitted HIV infection in the British Isles. British Medical Journal, 306: 1296–1299

Aynsley-Green A, Soltesz G 1986 Metabolic and endocrine disorders. In: Roberton N R C (ed) Textbook of neonatology. Churchill Livingstone, Edinburgh, pp 605–623

Baker C J 1990 Antibiotic therapy in neonates whose mothers have received intrapartum group B streptococcal chemoprophylaxis. Pediatric Infectious Disease Journal 9: 149–150

Barnes N D 1985 Screening for congenital hypothyroidism; the first decade. Archives of Disease in Childhood 60: 587–592

Bauchner H, Leventhal J, Shapiro E 1986 Studies of breast-feeding and infections. How good is the evidence? Journal of the American Medical Association 256: 887–892

Beeley L 1987 Safer prescribing. A guide to some problems in the use of drugs. Blackwell Scientific Publications, Oxford

Bourke W, Clarke T, Mathews T, O'Halpin D, Donoghue V 1993 Isolated single umbilical artery—the case for routine renal screening. Archives of Disease in Childhood 68: 600–601

Brown J K, Purvis R J, Fofar J O, Cockburn F 1974 Neurological aspects of perinatal asphyxia. Developmental Medicine and Child Neurology 16: 567–580

Brown Z, Benedetti J, Ashley R et al 1991 Neonatal herpes simplex virus infection in relation to asymptomatic maternal infection at the time of labor. New England Journal of Medicine 324: 1247–1252

Burman L, Christensen P, Christensen K et al 1992 Prevention of excess neonatal morbidity associated with group B streptococci by vaginal chlorhexidine disinfection during labour. Lancet 340: 65–69

Cartlidge P H T 1992 Routine discharge examination of babies: is it necessary? Archives of Disease in Childhood 67: 1421–1422

Chamberlain R, Chamberlain G, Howlett B, Claireaux A 1975 British births 1970, vol 1. The first week of life. Heinemann Medical, London

Chiswick M L 1986 Regional organisation of perinatal care. In: Roberton N R C (ed) Textbook of neonatology. Churchill Livingstone, Edinburgh, pp 803–813

Clarke N M P, Harcke H T, Mettugh P et al 1985 Real time ultrasound in the diagnosis of congenital dislocation and dysplasia of the hip. Journal of Bone and Joint Surgery 67B: 406–412

Curnock D A 1986 Neonatal resuscitation. Hospital Update 12: 679–692

D'Souza S W 1983 Neurodevelopment outcome after birth asphyxia. In: Chiswick M L (ed) Recent advances in perinatal medicine, vol 1. Churchill Livingstone, Edinburgh, pp 137–153

Danks D M 1981 Diagnosis of metabolic diseases after birth; neonatal screening and the investigation of symptomatic patients or babies at risk. In: Hull D (ed) Recent advances in paediatrics, vol 6. Churchill Livingstone, Edinburgh, pp 51–71

Danks D M, Brown G K 1986 Inborn errors of metabolism in the neonate. In: Roberton N R C (ed) Textbook of neonatology. Churchill Livingstone, Edinburgh, pp 644–658

Dashefsky B 1990 Prophylaxis against neonatal group B streptococcal disease. Pediatric Infectious Disease Journal 9: 147–149

Davidson D, Eldemerdash A 1990 Endothelium-derived relaxing factor: presence in pulmonary and systemic arteries of the newborn guinea pig. Pediatric Research 17: 128–132

Dawes G S 1968 Fetal and neonatal physiology. Year Book Medical Publishers, Chicago

Department of Health 1992 Standing Medical Advisory Committee. The diagnosis and treatment of suspected Listeriosis in pregnancy. Department of Health, London

Department of Health and Social Security 1980, 1988 Present day practice in infant feeding. Report on Health and Social Subjects 20 (1980) and 32 (1988). DHSS, London

DeVries L, Larroche J-C, Levene M 1988 Germinal matrix haemorrhage and intraventricular haemorrhage. In: Levene M, Bennett M, Punt J (eds) Fetal and neonatal neurology and neurosurgery. Churchill Livingstone, Edinburgh, pp 312–325

Dodd K 1993 Neonatal jaundice—a lighter touch. Archives of Disease in Childhood 68: 529–533

Dunn P M 1986 Screening for congenital dislocation of the hip. In: MacFarlane A (ed) Progress in child health, vol 3. Churchill Livingstone, Edinburgh, pp 1–12

Edelmann C, Barnett H, Troupkou V 1960 Renal concentrating mechanisms in newborn infants. Effect of dietary protein and water content, role of urea and responsiveness to anti-diuretic hormone. Journal of Clinical Investigation 39: 1062–1069

Ekelund H, Finnström O, Gunnarskog J, Källén B, Larsson Y 1993 Administration of vitamin K to newborn infants and childhood cancer. British Medical Journal 307: 89–91

Editorial 1986 Rapid detection of B haemolytic streptococci. Lancet i: 247–248

Edwards A D, Wyatt J S, Richardson C et al 1988 Cotside measurement of cerebral blood flow by near infra-red spectroscopy. Lancet ii: 770–771

Flodmark O 1988 Computed tomography and magnetic resonance imaging of the neonatal central nervous system. In: Levene M, Bennett M, Punt J (eds) Fetal and neonatal neurology and neurosurgery. Churchill Livingstone, Edinburgh, pp 122–138

Friedman W F, Hirschklau M J, Printz M P et al 1976 Pharmacologic closure of patent ductus arteriosus in the premature infant. New England Journal of Medicine 295: 526–529

Friis-Hansen B 1982 Body water metabolism in early infancy. Acta Paediatrics Scandinavia 296(suppl): 44–48

Gamsu H, Heggie M, Lissauer T, Milner A, Rosen M, Weaver J 1993 Resuscitation of the newborn. Working Party of the British Paediatric Association, College of Anaesthetists, Royal College of Midwives, Royal College of Obstericians and Gynaecologists, London

Godard C, Valloton M, Faure L 1982 Urinary prostaglandins, vasopressin and kallikrein excretion in healthy children from birth to adolescence. Journal of Pediatrics 100: 898–902

Gregory G A, Gooding C A, Phibbs R H, Tookey W H 1974 Meconium aspiration in infants—a prospective study. Journal of Paediatrics 85: 848–852

Gunther M 1970 Infant feeding. Methuen, London

Hallidie-Smith K A 1984 Prostaglandin E1 in suspected ductus dependent cardiac malformation. Archives of Disease in Childhood 59: 1020–1026

Hargrave B, Roman C, Morville P, Heymann M 1990 Pulmonary vascular effects of exogenous atrial natriuretic peptide in sheep fetuses. Pediatric Research 27: 140–143

Haworth S, Bull C 1993 Physiology of congenital heart disease. Archives of Disease in Childhood 68: 707–711

Herbst J 1989 Development of suck and swallow. In: Lebenthal E (eds) Human gastrointestinal development. Raven, New York, pp 229–239

Heymann M A, Rudolph A M 1975 Control of the ductus arteriosus. Physiological Reviews 55: 62–77

Heymann M A, Rudolph A M, Silverman 1976 Closure of the ductus

arteriosus by inhibition of prostaglandin synthesis. New England
Journal of Medicine 295: 530–533

Howie P, Forsyth J, Ogston S, Clark A, Florey C d V 1990 Protective
effect of breast feeding against infection. British Medical Journal
300: 11–16

Hull D 1966 The structure and function of brown adipose tissue.
British Medical Bulletin 22: 92–96

Hull D 1993 Vitamin K and childhood cancer. The risk of
haemorrhagic disease is certain; that of cancer is not. British Medical
Journal 305: 326–327

Hull D, Chellappah G 1983 On keeping babies warm. Recent
Advances in Perinatal Medicine 153–168

Hytten F E 1985 The physiology and pathology of amniotic fluid.
In: Fox H (ed) Haines and Taylor's textbook of gynaecological and
obstetrical pathology, 3rd edn. Churchill Livingstone, Edinburgh

Jeffs S 1989 Hazards of scoop measurements in infant feeding. Journal of
the Royal College of General Practitioners 39: 113

Jelliffe D B, Jelliffe P G F 1979 Human milk in the modern world.
Oxford University Press, Oxford

Kinsella J P, Neish S R, Shaffer E, Abman S H 1992 Low dose
inhalational nitric oxide in persistent pulmonary hypertension of the
newborn. Lancet 340: 919–820

Kühl P G, Cotton R B, Schweer H, Seyberth H W 1989 Endogenous
formation of prostanoids in neonates with pulmonary hypertension.
Archives of Disease in Childhood 64: 949–952

Levene M 1988 Management and outcome of birth asphyxia.
In: Levene M, Bennett M, Punt J (eds) Fetal and neonatal neurology
and neurosurgery. Churchill Livingstone, Edinburgh, pp 383–392

Levene M 1993 Management of the asphyxiated full term infant.
Archives of Disease in Childhood 68: 612–616

Lucas A, Bloom S, Aynsley-Green A 1978 Metabolic and endocrine
events at the time of first feed of human milk in preterm and term
infants. Archives of Disease in Childhood 53: 731–736

Lucas A, Christofides N, Adrian T, Bloom S, Aynsley-Green A 1979
Fetal distress, meconium and motilin. Lancet i: 718

Lucas A, Lockton S, Davies P S W 1991 Milk for babies and children.
British Medical Journal 302: 350–351

Mackinlay G 1993 Jaundice persisting beyond 14 days after birth.
British Medical Journal 306: 1426–1427

Marlow N 1992 Do we need an Apgar score? Archives of Disease in
Childhood 67: 765–767

Mathews T, Warshaw J 1979 Relevance of the gestational age
distribution of meconium passage in utero. Pediatrics 64: 30–31

McKiernan J, Hull D 1981 Breast development in the newborn.
Archives of Disease in Childhood 56: 525–529

McNinch A W, Tripp J H 1991 Haemorrhagic disease of the newborn
in the British Isles: two year prospective study. British Medical
Journal 303: 1105–1109

Milner A 1993 How does exogenous surfactant work? Archives of
Disease in Childhood 68: 253–254

Milner A D, Vyas H 1982 Lung expansion at birth. Journal of
Paediatrics 101: 879–886

Milner A D, Vyas H, Hopkin I E 1984 Efficacy of face mask
resuscitation at birth. British Medical Journal 289: 1563–1565

MIMS 1988 A guide to drugs in breast milk. MIMS 1 May, p 124

O'Callaghan C, Stephenson T 1992 Pocket paediatrics. Churchill
Livingstone, Edinburgh

Palme C, Nystrom B, Tunell R 1985 An evaluation of the efficiency of
face mask in the resuscitation of newborn infants. Lancet i: 207–210

Palme-Kilander C, Tunell R 1993 Pulmonary gas exchange during
facemask ventilation immediately after birth. Archives of Disease in
Childhood 68: 11–16

Palme-Kilander C, Tunell R, Chiwei C 1993 Pulmonary gas exchange
immediately after birth in spontaneously breathing infants. Archives
of Disease in Childhood 68: 6–10

Polacek E, Vocel J, Neugebaverova L 1965 The osmotic concentrating
ability in healthy infants and children. Archives of Disease in
Childhood 40: 291–295

Prechtl H F 1974 The behavioural state of the newborn infant. Brain
Research 76: 185–212

Prober C, Shullender W, Yasakawa L, Aru D, Yeager A, Arvin A 1987
Low risk of herpes simplex virus infections in neonates exposed to
the virus at the time of vaginal delivery to mothers with recurrent

genital herpes simplex virus infection. New England Journal of
Medicine 316: 240–244

Rennie J, Cooke R 1992 Prolonged low dose indomethacin for the
persistent ductus arteriosus of prematurity. Archives of Disease in
Childhood 66: 55–58

Robillard J E, Nakamura K T 1988a Hormonal regulation of renal
function during development. Biology of the Neonate 53: 201–211

Robillard J, Nakamura K 1988b Neurohormonal regulation of renal
function during development. American Journal of Physiology
254: F771–779

Robillard J, Nakamura K, Matherne G, Jose P 1988 Renal
haemodynamics and functional adjustment to postnatal life.
Seminars in Perinatology 12: 143–150

Rorke L, Zimmerman R 1992 Prematurity, postmaturity, and destructive
lesions in utero. American Journal of Neuroradiology 13: 517–536

Royal College of Midwives 1993 Successful breastfeeding. Churchill
Livingstone, Edinburgh

Rutter N 1986 Temperature control and its disorders. In: Roberton
N R C (ed) Textbook of neonatology. Churchill Livingstone,
Edinburgh, pp 148–162

Rutter N, Hull D 1979 Response of term babies to a warm
environment. Archives of Disease in Childhood 54: 178–183

Silove E D 1986 Pharmacological manipulation of the ductus
arteriosus. Archives of Disease in Childhood 61: 827–829

Simpson J, Stephenson T 1993 Regulation of extracellular fluid volume
in neonates. Early Human Development 34: 179–190

Smales O R C, Kime R 1978 Thermoregulation in babies immediately
after birth. Archives of Disease in Childhood 53: 58–61

Soifer S J, Loitz R D, Roman C, Heymann M A 1985 Leukotriene end
organ antagonists increase pulmonary blood flow in fetal lambs.
American Journal of Physiology 249: H570–H576

Stephenson T, Barbor P 1995 Ethical dilemmas of diagnosis and
intervention. In: Levene M, Lilford R, Bennett M, Punt J (eds) Fetal
and neonatal neurology and neurosurgery, 2nd edn. Churchill
Livingstone, London, pp 709–718

Stephenson T J, Broughton-Pipkin F 1990 Atrial natriuretic factor: the
heart as an endocrine organ. Archives of Disease in Childhood
65: 1293–1294

Stephenson T, Rutter N 1992 Thermoregulation and fluid balance in
the newborn. In: McIntosh N, Campbell A (eds) Forfar and Arneil's
textbook of paediatrics. Churchill Livingstone, Edinburgh, pp 158–165

Stephenson T, Wallace H 1991 Clinical paediatrics for postgraduate
examinations. Churchill Livingstone, Edinburgh

Stewart A L, Reynolds E O R, Hope E L et al 1987 Probability of
neurodevelopmental disorders estimated from ultrasound
appearances of brains of very preterm infants. Developmental
Medicine and Child Neurology 29: 3–11

Svenningsen N W, Blennow G, Lindroth M, Gaddlin P O, Ahstrom H
1982 Brain-orientated intensive care treatment in severe neonatal
asphyxia. Archives of Disease in Childhood 57: 176–183

Trounce J, Levene M 1988 Ultrasound imaging of the neonatal brain.
In: Levene M, Bennett M, Punt J (eds) Fetal and neonatal neurology
and neurosurgery. Churchill Livingstone, Edinburgh, pp 139–148

Volpe J J 1981 Neurology of the newborn. W B Saunders, London

VonKries R 1991 Neonatal vitamin K—prophylaxis for all. British
Medical Journal 303: 1083–1084

Vyas H, Hopkin I E, Milner A D 1983 Face mask resuscitation: does it
lead to gastric dilatation? Archives of Disease in Childhood
58: 373–375

Weaver L 1992 Breast and gut: the relationship between lactating
mammary function and neonatal gastrointestinal function.
Proceedings of the Nutrition Society 51: 155–163

Weaver L, Lucas A 1993 Development of bowel habit in preterm
infants. Archives of Disease in Childhood 68: 317–320

Weindling A M, Hawkins J M, Coombes M A, Stringer J 1981
Colonisation of babies and their families by Group B streptococci.
British Medical Journal 283: 1503–1505

Widdowson E M, Spray C M 1981 Chemical composition in utero.
Archives of Disease in Childhood 26: 205–214

Wyatt J S, Edwards A D, Azzopardi D I, Reynolds E C R 1989
Magnetic resonance and near infra-red spectroscopy of perinatal
hypoxic-ischaemic brain injury. Archives of Disease in Childhood
64: 953–963

47. Obstetrical responsibility for abnormal fetal outcome

Fiona J. Stanley

Material in this chapter contains contributions from the first edition and we are grateful to the previous author for the work done.

The extent to which improvements in obstetric care over the past three decades have resulted in improved population measures of fetal outcome such as perinatal mortality and cerebral palsy should be of great interest to obstetricians, paediatricians and those organizing perinatal services. Other changes may also have played a role in falling mortality rates—both stillbirth and neonatal death rates—such as increased proportions of better mothers (taller, of more optimal ages and parities and possibly other factors), fewer unwanted pregnancies resulting from wider availability of better contraceptives, and the general improvement of health of mothers in most developed countries (Grant 1993). Interestingly, rates of preterm birth and low birthweight, which seem to be strongly related to social and environmental factors such as poverty and smoking levels in communities, have changed very little over time (F. Stanley, 1994, unpublished data, Levin et al 1990, US Department of Health and Human Services 1993, Power 1994). Perinatal mortality has fallen coincident with changes in obstetric care but low birthweight has not, which suggests that medical care has influenced the death rates, but that neither social nor maternal improvements have been sufficient to influence the low birthweight rates. In this chapter, the abnormal fetal outcomes which will be considered include mortality, concentrate mainly on cerebral palsy but exclude low birthweight and preterm birth because the causes and prevention of these are much less well understood and thus far less amenable to current obstetric interventions.

Obstetricians believe that most of the fall in stillbirths and part of the fall in neonatal mortality in recent years have been due to better antenatal and perinatal care being made available to a larger proportion of pregnant women and those in labour. Until the last 5–10 years, there was an expectation that the wider availability of perinatal technologies aimed at reducing birth asphyxia, such as electronic fetal monitoring and Caesarean section, would also result in large falls in rates of cerebral palsy (Quilligan & Paul 1975, Amiel-Tison et al 1988). This expectation has, disappointingly, not been realized.

ANIMAL MODELS OF BRAIN DAMAGE

Since events during labour and delivery, notably trauma and asphyxia, have long been thought to be possible causes of cerebral palsy, it is not surprising that attempts to develop brain pathology in the animal fetus similar to that seen in the human with cerebral palsy first utilized the production of elements of asphyxia—decreased blood oxygen levels and increased carbon dioxide levels leading to lactic acidosis and a lowering of blood pH. It soon became evident that anoxia of at least 10–12 minutes duration in the animal model can result in damage to the brain stem, a pathology quite unlike the pathology usually seen in the human child with cerebral palsy and therefore of little interest in this chapter (Myers 1972). Prolonged partial asphyxia of the monkey fetus, however, produced a different pathology with involvement of the cerebral hemispheres, paracentral cortical regions etc.—a pathological picture more closely akin to that seen in the human with cerebral palsy (Myers 1972).

Thus, at least in the animal model, it appeared that severe fetal asphyxia might cause a pathological picture consistent with cerebral palsy. Of striking importance, however, was the rarity of this pathological outcome following partial asphyxia. The brain is not the only organ affected by hypoxia or asphyxia, and indeed it is probably not the first organ affected. Those animal fetuses which were severely asphyxiated usually died from the effects of the asphyxia on the heart, or they survived with an intact brain. Only a very few animals survived with the characteristic brain pathology.

At a later date and with further experiments, Myers et al (1981) concluded that the critical factors in the development of the brain damage were a very high level of lactic acid in the brain (reflected as metabolic acidosis in the blood) and poor perfusion of the brain caused by a shock-like state in the animal, probably due to the effect of asphyxia on the fetal heart. These authors also reported that a high serum glucose level seemed a critical element in the experimental production of asphyxial brain damage.

Other strategies for the induction of brain damage have also been successful in the experimental animal: these are techniques that do not depend on the presence of severe fetal asphyxia or acidosis. Clapp et al (1985) using a fetal sheep model, caused histological damage in the cortical white matter by firstly, partial intermittent cord occlusion late in pregnancy and secondly, by the induction of mild hyperglycaemia in a fetus which was growth retarded from a technique previously shown not to induce brain damage in itself. Neither of these experimental conditions was accompanied by significant fetal hypoxia or acidosis.

Gilles et al (1976) consistently produced perinatal telencephalic leukóencephalopathy (PTL), a pathology thought to be present in many humans with cerebral palsy, in the brains of newborn kittens up to 10 days of age by exposing them to the endotoxin of *Escherichia coli*. This finding seems to have clinical relevance when one considers that human infants with terminal bacteraemia were five times more likely to have had PTL than were infants who did not have bacteraemia (Leviton & Gilles 1973). The same authors found that 85% of infants with PTL and terminal bacteraemia had Gram-negative organisms. Thus, the possibility that an endotoxin, even without clinical evidence of infection, might cause brain pathology consistent with the presence of cerebral palsy must be considered. Broman (1978) has noted an increased risk of neurological dysfunction in children of mothers who had urinary tract infections during pregnancy.

Since factors other than asphyxia in the experimental animal can produce brain damage, it is apparent that we should not theorize that asphyxia is the only mechanism, or even necessarily the primary one, for the production of brain damage in the human fetus or newborn. This is particularly true in view of the well documented fact that even very severe acidosis in the human fetus at birth is only uncommonly followed by permanent brain damage (Brown et al 1974, Scott 1976). Similarly, only a minority of children subsequently shown to have cerebral palsy were asphyxiated or acidotic at the time of birth (Nelson & Ellenberg 1981). These issues will be discussed below.

Gilles (1985) has discussed what is known and what is not known about the pathology of cerebral palsy, with special emphasis on conclusions the pathologist may draw about the cause or causes of that pathology. On the question of asphyxia Gilles wrote: 'in current textbooks of neuropathology some 28 distinct morphologic abnormalities of the neonatal brain are attributed to asphyxia, hypoxia, or anoxia.' He further points out that the 'multiple risk factors of the perinatal leucoencephalopathy characterized by focal necroses do not include markers of hypoxia, anoxia, or systemic hypotension.' Thus he concludes that the many types of pathology attributed to hypoxia or asphyxia, coupled with the lack of prominence of hypoxia or asphyxia as a possible cause of perinatal leukoencephalopathy, mean that it cannot be concluded with certainty that there is a cause and effect relationship between the presence of neonatal asphyxia and brain pathology.

In spite of this strong evidence to the contrary, fetal asphyxia, especially intrapartum fetal asphyxia, continues to be the major theoretical cause of cerebral palsy. Most of the remainder of this chapter will discuss what is known and what is not known about the asphyxia–cerebral palsy relationship.

Gluckman and colleagues from New Zealand have developed models of perinatal asphyxia in the fetal sheep and rat (Gluckman & Williams 1991, Gluckman et al 1992, Williams et al 1993). They have clearly demonstrated that following an asphyxial insult neuronal death occurs in two phases—one associated with the event (primary neuronal death) and one which initiates over some 6–12 hours after the event and may last for several days (delayed neuronal death). Unless the initial insult is catastrophic or irreversible, this delayed death is a most important cause of neuronal loss. Much of Gluckman's work is investigating the role of cytokines and is aimed at possible new therapies to reduce the impact of this delayed neuronal death. Their studies support earlier animal work of Clapp et al (1985) and studies in humans which suggest that the preterm brain is less vulnerable to asphyxial events as it appears more able to recover (Kuban & Leviton 1994), and damage is more likely to result in white matter injury (Mallard et al 1994). Asphyxial damage to the heart and other organs resulting in fetal compromise has also been observed and is in accordance with the global mechanisms thought to be operating in the human fetus. Gluckman's group is now extending its work to look at models of global fetal asphyxia, which result in both hippocampal and cortical brain injury, more detailed studies of preterm lambs and to investigate perinatal asphyxia in the human fetus.

The continuum of reproductive wastage hypothesis (Lilienfield & Parkhurst 1951) is still believed by many to be logical—that very severe insult (e.g. from asphyxia) to the fetus causes death, a lesser insult causes cerebral palsy and less still might cause other milder problems such as attention deficit disorder. However there are now many data to refute this hypothesis and it seems that the major causes of perinatal death are not major causes of cerebral palsy. Animal and human data are now more supportive of an all or nothing theory, in which it is postulated that if asphyxia does not kill the fetus, usually from hypoxic cardiac rather than neurological effects, then the fetus survives intact, without brain damage (Williams et al 1993). Put simply, if there is enough asphyxia to cause brain damage, it usually causes irreversible damage to other vital organs as well. The unknown factors in all these studies, which are not usually well mimicked in animal models (because we are not yet sure what they are), are the contributions of prior vulnerabilities which exist in the fetus from a variety of causes. The focus of cerebral palsy research now is on the relative contributions of antenatal and intrapartum events to causation. From such research the relative contribution of poor care received in labour (and thus obstetric responsibility) to the occurrence of this disabling condition is likely to be ascertained.

For obstetric care to influence the level of abnormal fetal outcomes, it must either prevent the events that cause them or reduce their impact. This implies two things, first that we know the causes of abnormal fetal outcomes and secondly that obstetric care can prevent them or reduce their morbidity.

The worldwide expansion of scientific overviews into the Cochrane Collaboration had its origins in the perinatal arena (The UK Cochrane Centre, Oxford). The Oxford database of perinatal trials, which is regularly updated with new trial information, can now be accessed to provide unbiased and accurate data on best practice in obstetric care (Chalmers et al 1989, Cochrane Pregnancy and Childbirth Database 1993). The major drawbacks are that few trials are large enough, even when pooled, to have death or cerebral palsy as outcomes, nor have many of them been funded to follow up to a diagnosis of cerebral palsy, which may not be made accurately for 3–5 years after birth (Stanley 1994b). Thus since most randomized controlled trials of perinatal interventions such as electronic fetal monitoring, Caesarean section, antenatal steroids and surfactant have not usually been designed to ascertain cerebral palsy as an outcome, we need to use other data to elucidate whether these activities are of benefit in terms of neurological morbidity. It would of course be extremely useful if all such trials could be funded to follow up the cohorts until the age when most cerebral palsy is diagnosed so that meta-analyses could be done to give the best estimate of the impact of the interventions on cerebral palsy occurrence.

HOW MUCH PERINATAL MORTALITY IS NOW PREVENTABLE BY OBSTETRIC CARE?

The most recently published data on perinatal death, traditionally used as our universal measure of obstetric care in labour and shown for Western Australia in Figure 47.1, suggests that:

1. The rates are now very low in most developed countries (Stanley & Watson 1992).
2. Most causes could not have been prevented by any currently known obstetric practice (Tables 47.1, 47.2).
3. Other factors in the community such as the proportion of low birthweight or non-white births are more strongly associated with perinatal death than is obstetric care.

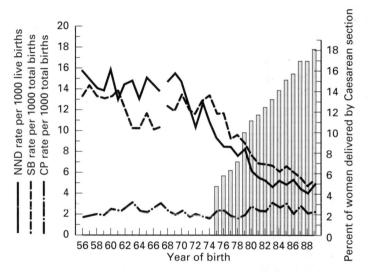

Fig. 47.1 Stillbirth (SB), neonatal death (NND) and cerebral palsy (CP) rates per thousand, 1956–89, shown against the percentage of women having Caesarean sections, 1975–89, in Western Australia (Gee 1990).

Table 47.1 Causes of stillbirth (20 weeks onwards) in Western Australia 1980–89 (Stanley et al 1994)

Cause	No.	%
Hypertension	152	8
Antepartum haemorrhage	254	14
Obstetric/labour/del	12	1
Unexplained < 2000 g	589	32
Unexplained ≥ 2000 g	325	17
Intrauterine infections	66	4
Cord conditions	92	5
Other	83	4
Lethal malformations	285	15
Total	1858	100

Table 47.2 Causes of neonatal deaths (0–27 days) in Western Australia, 1980–89 (Stanley et al 1994)

Cause	No.	%
Asphyxia	55	4
Antepartum haemorrhage	113	9
Postnatal infections	10	1
Low birthweight	451	35
Sudden infant death syndrome	46	4
Intrauterine infections	59	5
Other	19	1
Obstetric problems	69	5
Lethal malformations	466	36
Total	1288	100

Thus while the fall in perinatal mortality in recent decades may well have been attributable to obstetricians with some help from improved maternal characteristics, any further fall in abnormal outcomes awaits more research which would result in the primary prevention of birth defects, preterm birth or unexplained stillbirths, such as the exciting finding relating neural tube defects to periconceptional folate (Wald 1993). In societies with higher death rates and with a different set of causes, current obstetric practice still has the potential to make significant improvements in outcome; this brings in the issue of equitable use of resources. In Australia, for example, whilst much of the poor perinatal mortality amongst Australian Aboriginal infants is due to their poverty and other social problems, there is undoubtedly also an equity issue of poor care as well, reflected in their much higher rates of preventable perinatal and maternal mortality compared with Caucasian Australians (Gee 1992, Health Care Committee of National Health and Medical Research Council 1993).

Thus it is important to think carefully today before using unadjusted perinatal mortality rates as an index of obstetric care; even rates of intrapartum death amongst normally formed and full-term normal birthweight infants do not seem to vary much between areas and occur so rarely as to no longer be an adequate index. If they are higher and they do vary, as may occur between different regions (Levin et al 1990), then of course it is worth pursuing the reasons for those variations, recognizing that poor obstetric care may be but one factor responsible.

The suggestion that neonatal seizures might be a better index (Dennis & Chalmers 1982) has not received support from most researchers in this area because, like cerebral palsy and perinatal death, most infants with seizures have many causal pathways for their fits, most of which start well before the intrapartum period (Nelson & Leviton 1991).

WHAT IS CEREBRAL PALSY?

Cerebral palsy is defined as a group of non-progressive disorders of movement or posture due to a defect or lesion of the developing brain (Bax 1964, Nelson & Ellenberg 1978). Many syndromes, a great number of which are very rare, have as part of their clinical parameters a chronic non-progressive motor handicap. Interference with the developing brain includes the period from conception to well into childhood. Thus causes can be genetic or related to early antepartum, perinatal or postnatal problems. Whilst this broad grouping of children with similar handicaps due to such a variety of causes has been useful for management, considerable epidemiological challenges arise from the resulting heterogeneity. This has also caused confusion for parents who may well believe that a perinatal event must be the main reason for all cerebral palsy (Stanley & Blair 1991).

HOW MUCH CEREBRAL PALSY IS PREVENTABLE BY OBSTETRIC CARE?

There has been more interest in the area of cerebral palsy in relation to obstetric care in the last decade than in the many preceding it. Much of this has arisen out of the explosion in the number and costs of law suits related to the role of the obstetrician who is increasingly being accused of having been negligent in not preventing the cerebral palsy by some actions during labour and delivery (Freeman & Freeman 1992). This trend to sue arose in part, paradoxically, from the obstetricians themselves, who promised parents the perfect baby with the arrival of the New Obstetrics (Editorial 1989). The parents become angry and blame the obstetrician when the perfect baby does not arrive, which is unlikely to occur in 100% of births; our society has steady rates of birth defects—5% of all births (Bower et al 1993), cerebral palsy—2.5 per 1000 births (Stanley & Watson 1992) and intellectual disability—7–8 per 1000 births (Baird & Sadovnick 1985). Table 47.3 gives realistic expectations for abnormal pregnancy outcomes for parents based on the best available data from developed countries where women have access to modern obstetric and neonatal care.

What is the evidence that the introduction of new obstetrics technologies such as electronic fetal monitoring and Caesarean section has reduced cerebral palsy rates?

Table 47.3 Realistic expectations for abnormal pregnancy outcomes in Australia, based on 1992 birth numbers and applying Western Australian rates (data from WA Maternal and Child Health Research Data Base (Stanley et al 1994))

Of all conceptions:
   >15% (45 000) will miscarry   ✓
Of all births:
   5% (14 450) will have a birth defect   ✓
   6% (17 340) will deliver preterm   ✓
   0.2% (580) will have cerebral palsy by age 5   ✓
   0.8% (2312) will have intellectual disability by age 6   ✓

There are only a small number of population-based registries of cerebral palsy in the world which can be used to answer this question and none of them, unfortunately, are in America where the use of these interventions has tended to be more widespread. Swedish (Hagberg et al 1993), Mersey, UK (Pharoah et al 1990) and our own registry data here in Western Australia (Stanley & Watson 1992) are available as the best from which to extrapolate to the rest of the developed world. Overall cerebral palsy rates for Western Australia in relation to increasing Caesarean section rates are illustrated in Figure 47.1. Whilst there are differences in the levels of low birthweight, perinatal mortality and other social and demographic conditions between Australia, Sweden, the UK and other countries like the USA, these are the only data we have. When we want to extrapolate these data, the differences must be remembered (Bhusan et al 1993). However the similarities in the levels and trends of cerebral palsy in these different population registries is suggestive that they may be representative of other similar countries without such data. The epidemiological challenges and problems in using cerebral palsy birth prevalence rates has been more fully and critically discussed elsewhere (Stanley & Blair 1994).

TRENDS IN CEREBRAL PALSY RATES

Figure 47.2 shows the birth prevalence of cerebral palsy per 1000 total births for Sweden and Western Australia over the last 20 years and for the last 10 years for Mersey, UK (Stanley 1994b, Stanley & Blair 1994). Thus the best estimate we have for the developed world with increasing exposure to new obstetric technologies for diagnosing and preventing birth asphyxia is that the

prevalence of 2–2.5 per 1000 has not changed, and if anything is increasing. Closer analysis of these trends shows that the occurrence of cerebral palsy in children of normal birthweight has either remained unchanged (in Western Australia) or risen (in Sweden) and that in low birthweight infants has risen (in all places).

The hope that these interventions would reduce cerebral palsy was based on the assumptions that birth asphyxia was the major cause of cerebral palsy and that birth asphyxia could be diagnosed and prevented by these interventions. The evidence presented below refutes the widespread belief that intrapartum care commonly influences the risk of cerebral palsy and shows that there is insufficient evidence for a strong causal relationship between cerebral palsy and putative indicators of birth asphyxia, whether it was preventable or not.

PERINATAL FACTORS AND CEREBRAL PALSY

The various sequences that could result in cerebral palsy are illustrated in Figure 47.3. It is impossible to identify with any accuracy the causes or timing of irreversible brain damage as shown in the diagram. Determining the relationship between a pregnancy event and the later diagnosis of cerebral palsy has been attempted using both cohort (Ellenberg & Nelson 1988) and case-control methods (Blair & Stanley 1988).

The best-known method is the US Collaborative Perinatal Project which whilst now 30 years out of date, still provides the best data on the relationship between perinatal factors, particularly birth asphyxia and cerebral palsy. Table 47.4 shows data from the 50 000 US births in this study born between 1959 and 1963 (Ellenberg & Nelson 1988). The relationship between low Apgar score (<5 at 5 minutes), neonatal signs (decreased activity after the first day of life, need for incubator care >3 days, feeding problems, poor suck or respiratory difficulties), newborn seizures, and later cerebral palsy is well demonstrated. Most of the cerebral palsy cases (62.7%) occurred amongst the group of children without any perinatal signs. The highest risk of cerebral palsy (545.5 per 1000) was in the very small proportion of children (0.06%) with all

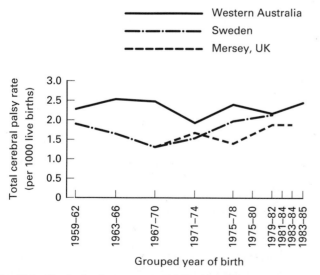

Fig. 47.2   Cerebral palsy rates per 100 live births from registries in Western Australia, Sweden, Mersey, UK, between 1959 and 1985 in grouped years (Hagberg et al 1989, Pharoah et al 1990).

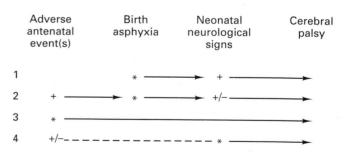

Fig. 47.3   Some possible sequences and timing of irreversible brain damage (*).

Table 47.4 Predicted risk of cerebral palsy (CP), percentage of population in each risk group, and percentage of CP contributed by perinatal characteristics, 1959–63 births, USA (reproduced with permission from Ellenberg & Nelson 1988)

| Early characteristics | | | | | |
Low Apgar score	Neonatal signs	Newborn seizures	Predicted risk* (CP/1000)*	Children in risk group (%)	Cases of CP in risk group (%)
–	–	–	1.3	90.1	62.7
+	–	–	2.9	0.9	1.3
–	–	+	1.3	0.06	0.0
+	–	+	2.9	0.01	0.0
–	+	–	3.2	8.1	13.3
+	+	–	7.0	0.7	2.7
–	+	+	96.8	0.08	4.0
+	+	+	545.5	0.06	16.0

* Predicted risk based on multiple logistic model with Apgar score, presence or absence of neonatal signs, or newborn seizures and their interactions as predictor variables. An Apgar score was considered low if < 5 at 5 minutes. Neonatal signs were decreased activity after the first day of life, need for incubator care > 3 days, feeding problems, poor suck or respiratory difficulties.

three early characteristics. Neonatal neurological signs, particularly seizures, were good predictors of cerebral palsy, but even these occurred in only 36% (13.3 + 2.7 + 4.0 + 16.0) of all cases. The most likely explanation for the strong associations is that these neonatal signs are the early manifestations of cerebral palsy, rather than being indicative of intrapartum asphyxial damage. The majority of these infants with newborn encephalopathy (abnormal neurological signs in the first week of life) were not born after complicated deliveries in which intrapartum asphyxia had been thought to have been present, and many had antenatal factors that could have been implicated in their brain damage. Nelson suggests that less than 10% of these cases of cerebral palsy were due to birth asphyxia, and the asphyxia in these cases tended to be severe and prolonged (Nelson & Ellenberg 1986, Nelson 1988).

Most researchers believe that it is important to separate term and preterm infants in the study of the relationship between birth asphyxia and cerebral palsy (Pharoah et al 1990, Hagberg et al 1993, Kuban & Leviton 1994). Many more preterm infants have markers of perinatal asphyxia than term infants but the association of these markers with cerebral palsy is weaker among preterm than term infants (Blair & Stanley 1988).

THE ASSOCIATION OF BIRTH ASPHYXIA WITH CEREBRAL PALSY

The relationship between intrapartum asphyxia and cerebral palsy has received more attention than any other relationship because of the hopes of obstetricians that cerebral palsy is related to intrapartum asphyxia.

Evidence is now available from several types of studies (Nelson & Ellenberg 1981, 1984, 1986, Ounsted & Radcliff 1987, Blair & Stanley 1988, Ellenberg & Nelson 1988, Freeman & Nelson 1988, Kuban & Leviton 1994) that suggests that:

1. Birth asphyxia may not be as important a cause of cerebral palsy as was previously thought.
2. Neonatal signs of birth asphyxia, such as difficulty in initiating and maintaining respiration, and abnormal neonatal neurological signs including seizures may be early manifestations of cerebral palsy from a variety of causes, of which birth asphyxia is only one.
3. Infants with birth asphyxia and neurological damage may not, even with alternative obstetric care, have fared better.
4. The majority of children with cerebral palsy probably had some antenatal insult or condition which either was the cause of their impairment or made them particularly vulnerable to birth events.

The scientific study of birth asphyxia in the human fetus is enormously challenging for several reasons. It poses problems for epidemiologists because possible confounding factors (gestational age, other morbidity) and the low incidence of the outcome (cerebral palsy 2.5/1000) demand populations from which to identify cases and because there is often selection bias in the groups studied. It challenges all researchers and obstetricians in their clinical practice as there is no direct measure of cerebral oxygenation to enable us to link it to fetal outcomes. Researchers and obstetricians have therefore used a variety of secondary measures of questionable validity to identify fetuses and neonates who may have had birth asphyxia which resulted in irreversible neuronal damage. Positron emission tomography measures metabolic changes and neuronal death, but can only be used on very small numbers of children (J Wyatt 1992, personal communication) and the same applies to near infrared spectrometry which measures cerebral impedance (a measure of cytotoxic oedema), electrocortical activity and cerebral haemodynamics. The first step with these new tools would be to use them in infants who are exhibiting signs of newborn encephalopathy and see how helpful they were in identifying stages of neuronal death and predicting long-term outcome.

A list of those markers used most commonly for birth asphyxia is shown in Table 47.5 (Low 1990). Their inadequacies in relation to low buffer base levels in the umbilical artery, which is perhaps the best available measure of fetal cerebral oxygenation, are clearly demonstrated. To interpret this table further, of those infants with acidosis as identified by low umbilical artery buffer base, only 50% had late decelerations on fetal heart rate tracing and more than 50% of those infants with late decelerations on fetal heart rate tracing did not have low umbilical artery buffer base levels. This exposé of the fetal heart rate trace as being of such low sensitivity and high false-positive rate is very important for obstetricians

Table 47.5 Adequacy of markers of fetal/birth asphyxia compared with umbilical artery buffer base < 34 mmol/l (from Low 1990)

	Sensitivity (%)	False positive (%)
Late decelerations fetal heart rate	50	> 50
Moderate/severe meconium	32	95
Apgar score 0–3 at 1 minute	46	84
Apgar score 0–3 at 5 minutes	8	73
NE* severe	23	79

* Defined as seizures and recurrent apnoea.

in training and medical students reading this textbook. There has been far too much trust placed on abnormalities of the fetal heart rate trace to diagnose later cerebral palsy from birth asphyxia, when it is obvious from these and many other data sets (Freeman 1990, Thacker 1991, Deans & Steer 1994) that there are a plethora of reasons for abnormal fetal heart rate traces, in addition to birth asphyxia, and that most children with cerebral palsy had normal heart rate traces in labour (or there was no indication even to perform a trace).

Most of these markers for birth asphyxia are poor predictors of later cerebral palsy (Dijxhoorn et al 1985, Freeman & Nelson 1988, Lumley 1988, Ruth & Raivio 1988), and the majority of children with cerebral palsy did not have any of these signs in the neonatal period (Nelson & Ellenberg 1986, Blair & Stanley 1988). Although neonatal seizures are strongly related to cerebral palsy (Table 47.4), it is obvious from Table 47.5 that many infants with seizures (79%) did not have low buffer base levels and that many infants with low buffer base levels did not have seizures or other signs of newborn encephalopathy (only 23% in the table).

Table 47.6 comes from the Western Australian case-control study of all spastic cerebral palsy occurring in the population in a 6-year period, in which two independent observers categorized their estimates as to whether the child had had birth asphyxia as a cause (Blair & Stanley 1988). Of the 183 cases, 124 (92 + 32; 68%) had no neonatal problems. Of the remainder (59), 30 had abnormal neurological signs at birth but no clinical evidence of birth asphyxia (fetal distress, low Apgar scores, prolonged

Table 47.6 Estimation of birth asphyxia or trauma having caused the brain damage in children with spastic cerebral palsy (from Blair & Stanley 1988)

Birth status	Estimation*				
	1	2	3	4	All
No birth asphyxia or newborn encephalopathy	92	0	0	0	92
Birth asphyxia but no newborn encephalopathy	32	0	0	0	32
Newborn encephalopathy but no birth asphyxia	22	5	3	0	30
Both birth asphyxia and newborn encephalopathy	10	7	3	9	29
Total	156	12	6	9	183

* 1 = definitely not, 2 = most likely, 3 = possible, 4 = very likely.

time to breath) and thus may well have had neurological signs as their first clinically observed indication of earlier brain damage. Among the 29 with signs of birth asphyxia and abnormal neonatal signs, in only 12 (8.2%) did the two observers agree that there was a definite or possible chance that in these children the cause may have been asphyxia. It was interesting that one of these 12 cases was later found to belong to a pedigree with cerebral palsy as a dominant genetic disorder (Blair et al 1992).

In this study we were unable to determine the proportion of the children with cerebral palsy that had had these markers of birth asphyxia because of existing problems. Nor could it be determined how many may have been preventable by better obstetric care. Studies investigating the relationship between obstetric care and cerebral palsy directly are reviewed later in this chapter.

Obstetricians should accept that they can only promise perfection at the end of labour, and it is even impossible to do so then. Few of the trials of interventions to reduce birth asphyxia, specifically those involving electronic fetal monitoring (Lumley 1988), have included follow-up to the age when cerebral palsy can be diagnosed confidently. One that has (Grant et al 1989), although showing significant reductions in neonatal seizures, did not demonstrate any difference in cerebral palsy occurrence. The implication is that monitoring may reduce birth asphyxia as measured by seizures, but not cerebral palsy, and thus few cases of cerebral palsy seem to be related to birth asphyxia.

Nigel Paneth wrote (1986), 'Determining the precise role of a specific asphyxia-related variable in the causal sequence leading to cerebral palsy will require more extensive analysis of its relation to antecedent factors.'

Attempts to investigate causal sequences using case-control data and the difficulties of doing so are illustrated in two recent papers (Blair & Stanley 1993a, b). Nearly 50% of cases and only 14% of controls had identified maternal, antenatal, intrapartum, immediate postpartum or neonatal risk factors. Most cases (35%) experienced their first risk factor before the intrapartum period and only 13% thereafter (both term and preterm together). When separated by birthweight and gestation, factors were identified more often in both antenatal and neonatal periods for low birthweight and low gestational age infants than in those heavier infants born at term. We concluded that there were many routes to spastic cerebral palsy, each contributing only a small proportion and many routes may be multifactorial, with most commencing before delivery. It was felt 'therefore unlikely that any single preventive activity will significantly reduce cerebral palsy rates.'

ANTENATAL FACTORS ASSOCIATED WITH CEREBRAL PALSY

Whilst the emphasis in this chapter is on obstetric care

and fetal outcomes, the strong associations of cerebral palsy with some maternal factors and antenatal conditions and problems should be mentioned. They may well be shown to be part of causal sequences which could include obstetric care. They include advanced maternal age, poor previous obstetric history including spontaneous fetal loss and need for infertility treatment, family history of epilepsy and/or intellectual disability, long birth intervals, maternal thyroxine dependence, maternal iodine deficiency, exposure to methyl mercury, abnormalities of amniotic fluid volume, premature prolonged rupture of membranes, presence of major or minor congenital malformation (other than CNS), antenatal death of co-twin or co-triplet, unhealthy placenta, severe antepartum haemorrhage at 21–30 weeks, maternal viral infection (cytomegalovirus, rubella) and being small for gestational age (Blair & Stanley 1990, Paneth 1993, Kuban & Leviton 1994, Stanley 1994a).

Many authors agree that most full-term cerebral palsy children without obvious intrapartum or postpartum events (the majority) probably experienced their brain-damaging event antenatally (Paneth 1993, Gaffney et al 1994). There are excellent reviews of abnormalities of neuronal migration that would fit the pattern seen in cerebral palsy (Barth 1987, Sarnat 1987), but the challenge is to be able to study them in human populations. Several papers are now appearing using new and sophisticated forms of cerebral scanning (Krägeloh-Mann et al 1992) and other methods to determine cerebral oxygenation (Wyatt 1986); it will be most interesting to see how these contribute to the determination of timing and aetiology of cerebral palsy in the future. The problems of inter- and intraobserver variation in the interpretation of scans is significant, but once they are addressed, clinicopathological correlations may be described. It is also possible that the study of cytokines such as interleukin-1, interleukin-6 and tumour necrosis factor alpha may give some clues as to the timing and sequence of neurological damage in the fetus (Adinolphi 1993, Leviton 1993). We still know too little about the role of many of these cytokines in normal pregnancy (Rutanen 1993), but they seem to reflect inflammation and infection which may play more of a role in preterm birth and cerebral palsy than is currently realized.

CEREBRAL PALSY, PERINATAL DEATH AND QUALITY OF OBSTETRIC CARE

The relationship between abnormal fetal outcome (cerebral palsy and perinatal death) and the quality of care during labour and delivery has been examined directly in only two studies, both case control and from Oxford, UK (Niswander et al 1984, Gaffney et al 1994). They attempt to answer the question mentioned earlier in this chapter—whilst only a small proportion of children with cerebral palsy or perinatal deaths are likely to have had intra-

partum problems (3–13%), could any of these could have been prevented by better management?

Niswander et al (1984) reported on 34 children with cerebral palsy and 92 infants who had died perinatally with what was described as terminal apnoea. The care these two groups had received compared with a group of normal livebirths (n = 377 for the cerebral palsy cases and n = 375 for the comparison with the deaths) was classified (without knowledge of case or control status) by a group of obstetricians as suboptimal or not, based on specific prior defined criteria. The criteria emphasized the recognition and management of fetal asphyxia as this was thought to be the most important cause of cerebral palsy.

The proportion of normal control children experiencing suboptimal care in labour was 14.6%, 16.3% for those who died and only 2.9% for the children who were diagnosed as having cerebral palsy. Thus this study did not support the hypothesis that suboptimal care was an important cause of cerebral palsy nor of terminal apnoea. However this study lacked power and the group with cerebral palsy included those who were preterm as well as term.

Using similar methodology, the more recent and much larger study from Oxford investigated the adverse antenatal factors and suboptimal intrapartum care (using predefined criteria) of 141 cases of cerebral palsy and 62 babies who died intrapartum or neonatally (Gaffney et al 1994). Only term infants who had cerebral palsy or who died were chosen, and any child with a congenital malformation was excluded. Term controls, also without malformations and born at term, were chosen from the births in the same regions in which the cases were born. Criteria for suboptimal obstetric care were decided upon beforehand by a consensus of all obstetricians in the Oxford region. Information about each criteria was obtained from the hospital records and blinded before being given to two independent assessors, including a consultant obstetrician. Antenatal data and postnatal information was collected as well.

Failure to respond to signs of severe fetal distress was 4.5 times more common in the cases of cerebral palsy (odds ratio 4.5 with 95% confidence interval 2.4–8.4) and 26 times more common in cases of death (26.1; 6.2–109.7) than among controls. This association persisted after controlling for increased incidence of complicated obstetric histories in the cases of cerebral palsy. Neonatal encephalopathy, regarded as the best clinical indicator of birth asphyxia, was present in only two-thirds (23/33) of the children with cerebral palsy in whom there had been a suboptimal response to fetal distress; these 23 formed 6.8% of all children with cerebral palsy born to residents of the region during the study period.

The authors concluded that there was an association between quality of intrapartum care and death. They also suggested that there was an association between some cases of cerebral palsy and suboptimal care, but this seems to have a role in only a small proportion of all cases of cerebral palsy. The contribution of adverse antenatal factors was much more important than suboptimal care or other intrapartum events in this group of term children.

The study of Gaffney et al (1994) is virtually the only well-conducted one which has directly investigated the relationship between suboptimal obstetric care and abnormal fetal outcome. The relationship was much stronger for death than for cerebral palsy and only a small proportion of cases of cerebral palsy (similar to previous studies' estimates of less than 10%) was classified as possibly preventable if care had been better. This study suggests that substandard obstetric care is not a common cause of cerebral palsy. Also it supports the earlier comments that birth asphyxia is not a common cause of cerebral palsy.

The difficulty is that even with this well-conducted study, the real cause of the brain abnormality is not known and whether it could have been prevented if the care had been optimal is still a moot point. This paper will undoubtedly be used to prove cases of negligence in obstetric care in relation to cerebral palsy cases, when in reality it proves the urgency to separate negligence from compensation and support for parents of children with cerebral palsy.

THE PRETERM INFANT AND ABNORMAL FETAL OUTCOME

Although the proportions are changing, most cerebral palsy still occurs in term infants; about 70% of all cerebral palsy in 1985–88 in the Western Australian Cerebral Palsy Register weighed more than 2500 g at birth. The emphasis in this chapter has been on the relationship between birth asphyxia and cerebral palsy in the term infant. However one of the strongest correlates in all studies of cerebral palsy is that between preterm birth, low birthweight and cerebral palsy (Stanley & Alberman 1984, Cooke 1990). Trends for total cerebral palsy shown earlier in this chapter mask the rather dramatic changes occurring amongst low birthweight and preterm infants.

The birth prevalence of cerebral palsy in very low birthweight (<1500 g) infants from the Mersey region, UK and Western Australian databases are shown in Figure 47.4. They show significant rises in the rates from the early 1970s to the late 1980s. These patterns coincide with the increases in survival in very low birthweight infants over the same time period: in Western Australia survival of babies under 1500 g rose from 20% in 1975 to 85% in 1988 (Stanley & Watson 1992). Similar survival patterns are reported from most developed countries (Department of Health 1990, Kleinman et al 1991, Bhushan et al 1993).

In spite of a variety of improvements in society generally and in the provision of maternal and child health services,

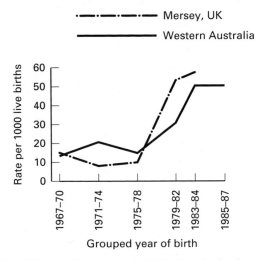

Fig. 47.4 Very low birthweight (< 1500 g) cerebral palsy rates per 1000 live births from registries in Western Australia and Mersey region (UK) between 1967 and 1987 in grouped years (Pharoah et al 1990) (reproduced with permission from Stanley 1994b).

the proportions of all live births born preterm or of low birthweight is actually increasing in some developed countries and none are showing a fall (Stanley 1994 unpublished data, Power 1994, US Department of Health 1994). Adding to the number of high-risk low birthweight infants are the increasing numbers of multiple births occurring as a consequence of the increasing use of infertility treatments such as drugs which stimulate the ovaries and the implanting of multiple embryos in IVF/GIFT procedures (Kiely et al 1992, Levene et al 1992, AIHW National Perinatal Statistics Unit 1993). The association of higher-order births and cerebral palsy occurrence has recently been investigated using the Western Australian Cerebral Palsy Register (Petterson et al 1993). The rates of cerebral palsy for singletons, twins and triplets are shown in Table 47.7. The risk of cerebral palsy is significantly higher in twins and triplets than in singletons. Although twins and triplets were more likely to be of low birthweight than singletons, their risks of cerebral palsy if low birthweight were similar. In contrast, in normal birthweight categories, twins had a higher rate of cerebral palsy than singletons. Rates of cerebral palsy were much higher in multiple births in which one co-twin or co-triplet had died before birth than in those in which all survived. This suggests that the obstetric practice of selective fetocide in multiple pregnancies (Lipitz et al 1994) should be questioned as it may not benefit the surviving fetuses.

The increased sophistication and use of neuroimaging has resulted in a much better understanding of aetiology of cerebral palsy in low birthweight infants. Ultrasound imaging of the brains of very preterm infants has demonstrated that images in the first few weeks of life correspond to the ischaemic or infarctive cerebral white matter lesions which are closely linked to cerebral palsy (de Vries et al 1985, Leviton & Paneth 1990, Krägeloh-Mann et al

Table 47.7 Prevalences (95% confidence intervals) of cerebral palsy in Western Australia, 1980–89. Plurality as recorded on midwives' notifications (Petterson et al 1993)

Category*	Singleton	Twin	Triplet
Per 1000 live births	1.60 (1.44, 1.77)	7.40 (5.25, 10.15)	26.67 (9.85, 57.14)
Per 1000 1-year survivors	1.60 (1.43, 1.77)	7.32 (5.14, 10.13)	27.91 (10.31, 59.75)
Per 1000 confinements	1.59 (1.43, 1.76)	13.24 (9.24, 18.36)	75.95 (28.38, 158.01)

* Four singletons and two twins with severe cerebral palsy who died before age of 1 year are counted in cerebral palsy among live births, but are not counted in cerebral palsy in survivors.

1992); the finding of echodense areas in the brain parenchyma is associated with a 50% risk of cerebral palsy and if the regions show cavitation and cyst formation the risk of cerebral palsy is nearly 100% (de Vries et al 1993). Paneth reports that in populations scanned regularly, at least one-half of all cases of cerebral palsy arising in the very low birthweight population are identified by these abnormal ultrasound findings in the neonatal period (Paneth 1993).

What if anything is the impact of obstetric care on the outcome of these babies or is care all in the province of the neonatal paediatrician? There are two schools of thought about the aetiology of cerebral palsy in these low birthweight infants. One is that most cases are due to the postnatal complications of preterm birth, with good evidence of developing white matter necrosis on ultrasound after birth, and without much interest in what might have gone on before birth or during it. The other is that many of these infants had been damaged before birth and are now surviving to be diagnosed as having cerebral palsy, whereas in the past they would have died. Not all preterm infants with cerebral palsy show ultrasound changes of postnatal white matter necrosis and thus it is likely that both antenatal and postnatal causes are involved in the preterm cerebral palsy story.

Leviton has put forward the hypothesis that an important sequence for preterm birth and white matter necrosis may well be initiated by ascending genital tract infection resulting in the release of cytokines (such as tumour necrosis factor) which could stimulate the release of prostaglandins initiating preterm labour, and cause irreversible neuronal cell damage as well (Leviton 1993). Until we have better markers of antenatal brain damage whether from infections or other causes, epidemiological studies cannot contribute much more useful information to this important question.

There is little evidence that obstetric care in labour has much influence on the occurrence of intraventricular haemorrhage and white matter necrosis in preterm infants as few randomized trials have been successful in this area. With the lack of randomized trials, evidence has to be sought from elsewhere. Kitchen and colleagues (1992) compared the outcomes at age 2 years of two cohorts of extremely low birthweight infants born in two different eras of obstetric care, 1977–82 and 1985–87. Caesarean delivery, electronic fetal monitoring, antenatal steroid

therapy and tocolytic therapy were analysed with attempts to control for possible confounders (a major problem with non-randomized studies). The only obstetric antenatal variable associated with an improved outcome was antenatal steroid therapy. The authors suggest: 'The obstetrician may aid the fetus of birth weight 500–999 grams by giving the mother steroids to accelerate lung maturity, but caesarean section cannot be recommended as the routine mode of delivery unless there are recognised maternal or fetal indications.' (Kitchen et al 1992)

Obviously any obstetric activity which results in a reduced rate of preterm delivery is to be actively sought. However, until the relationships between causes of preterm birth and cerebral palsy are better understood, it would be premature to promise that cerebral palsy rates will fall if preterm birth rates fall. The antenatal mechanisms of preterm birth and cerebral palsy may be different and not all cerebral palsy in preterm infants occurs postnatally.

CONCLUSION

The extent to which obstetric care can be claimed as responsible for abnormal fetal outcomes has been markedly overestimated over the past 20 years and has resulted in the justification of possibly unnecessary obstetric interventions and a most detrimental rise in litigation.

Research into cerebral palsy shows that birth prevalence has not fallen as anticipated with the widespread introduction of new technologies aimed at reducing birth asphyxia. It has also shown that there are many causes and causal sequences which result in cerebral palsy and that intrapartum asphyxia in a normal full-term infant without prior vulnerability is a rare event. Whether obstetric care could have prevented such cases is still unknown and it is very difficult to prove the specific cause of cerebral palsy in any one case.

Acknowledgements

I would like to acknowledge my hard-working colleagues in the Western Australian Cerebral Palsy Register (Linda Watson, Dr Eve Blair), Dr Jennifer Kurinczuk, ICHR, for critically reading the manuscript and Mrs Colleen Moylan for typing it.

The Western Australian Cerebral Palsy Register has been funded by the Child Health Research Foundation (formerly Telethon), the Charles and Sylvia Viertel Foundation and the National Health and Medical Research Council of Australia.

REFERENCES

Adinolfi M 1993 Infectious diseases in pregnancy, cytokines and neurological impairment: an hypothesis. Developmental Medicine and Child Neurology 35: 549

AIHW National Perinatal Statistics Unit, Fertility Society of Australia 1993 Assisted Conception, Australia and New Zealand, 1991. AIHW National Perinatal Statistics Unit, Sydney

Amiel-Tison C, Sureau C, Shnider S M 1988 Cerebral handicap in full term neonates related to the mechanical forces of labour. In: Patel N (ed) Baillière's Clinical Obstetrics and Gynecology 2: 145

Baird P A, Sadovnick A D 1985 Mental retardation in over half-a-million consecutive livebirths: an epidemiological study. American Journal of Mental Deficiency 89: 323

Barth P G 1987 Disorders of neuronal migration. Canadian Journal of Neurological Sciences 14: 1

Bax M C O 1964 Terminology and classification of cerebral palsy. Developmental Medicine and Child Neurology 6: 295

Bhushan V, Paneth N, Kiely J L 1993 Impact of improved survival of very low birth weight infants on recent secular trends in the prevalence of cerebral palsy. Pediatrics 91: 1094

Blair E, Stanley F J 1988 Intrapartum asphyxia: A rare cause of cerebral palsy. Journal of Pediatrics 112: 155

Blair E, Stanley F J 1990 Intrauterine growth and spastic cerebral palsy. I. The association with birthweight for gestational age. American Journal of Obstetrics and Gynecology 162: 229

Blair E, Stanley F J 1993a Aetiological pathways to spastic cerebral palsy. Paediatric and Perinatal Epidemiology 7: 302

Blair E, Stanley F J 1993b When can cerebral palsy be prevented? The generation of causal hypotheses by multivariate analysis of a case-control study. Paediatric and Perinatal Epidemiology 7: 272

Blair E, Stanley F J, Hockey A 1992 Intrapartum asphyxia and cerebral palsy (letter). Journal of Pediatrics 121: 170

Bower C, Rudy E, Ryan A, Forbes R, Grace L 1993 Report of the Birth Defects Registry of Western Australia. Health Department of Western Australia Statistical Series/36

Broman S 1978 Perinatal antecedents of severe mental retardation in school age children. Presented at the 86th Annual Convention of the American Psychological Association, Toronto

Brown J, Purvis R, Forfar J, Cockburn F 1974 Neurological aspects of perinatal asphyxia. Developmental Medicine and Child Neurology 16: 567

Chalmers I, Enkin M, Keirse M J N C (eds) 1989 Effective care in pregnancy and childbirth. Oxford University Press, Oxford

Clapp J, Peress N, Mann L 1985 Effect of intermittent partial cord occlusion or hyperglycaemia on neuropathologic outcome in the fetal lamb. Phoenix, AZ Society for Gynaecologic Investigation 32nd Annual Meeting (abstract)

Cochrane Pregnancy and Childbirth Database 1994 Derived from The Cochrane Database of Systematic Reviews. Cochrane Updates on Disk. Update Software, Oxford

Cooke R W I 1990 Cerebral palsy in very low birthweight infants. Archives of Disease in Childhood 65: 201

de Vries L S, Dubowitz L M S, Dubowitz V et al 1985 Predictive value of cranial ultrasound in the newborn baby: a reappraisal. Lancet ii: 137

de Vries L S, Eken P, Groenendaal F, van Haastert I C, Meiners L C 1993 Correlation between degree of periventricular leukomalacia diagnosed using cranial ultrasound and MRI later in infancy in children with cerebral palsy. Neuropediatrics 24: 263

Deans A C, Steer P J 1994 The use of fetal electrocardiogram in labour. British Journal of Obstetrics and Gynaecology 101: 9

Dennis J, Chalmers I 1982 Very early neonatal seizure rate: a possible epidemiological indicator of the quality of perinatal care. British Journal of Obstetrics and Gynaecology 89: 418

Department of Health 1990 Confidential Enquiry into Stillbirths and Deaths in Infancy. HMSO, London

Dijxhoorn M J, Visser G H A, Huisjes H J, Fidler V, Touwen B C L 1985 The relation between umbilical pH values and neonatal neurological morbidity in full term appropriate-for-date infants. Early Human Development 11: 33

Editorial 1989 Cerebral palsy, intrapartum care, and a shot in the foot. Lancet ii: 1251

Ellenberg J H, Nelson K B 1988 Cluster of perinatal events identifying infants at high risk for death or disability. Journal of Pediatrics 113: 546

Freeman R 1990 Intrapartum fetal monitoring—a disappointing story. New England Journal of Medicine 322: 624

Freeman J M, Freeman A D 1992 Cerebral palsy and the 'bad baby' malpractice crisis: New York State shines light toward the end of the tunnel. American Journal of Diseases of Children 146: 725

Freeman J M, Nelson K B 1988 Intrapartum asphyxia and cerebral palsy. Pediatrics 82: 240

Gaffney G, Sellers S, Flavell V, Squier M, Johnson A 1994 Case-control study of intrapartum care, cerebral palsy, and perinatal death. British Medical Journal 308: 743

Gee V 1990 Perinatal Statistics in Western Australia. Seventh Annual Report of the Western Australian Midwives' Notification System 1989. Health Department of Western Australia, Perth

Gee V 1992 The 1990 Western Australia Birth Cohort. Perinatal and infant mortality identified by maternal race. Health Department of Western Australia, Perth, Statistical Series/34

Gilles F 1985 Neuropathologic indicators of abnormal development. In: Freeman J (ed) Prenatal and perinatal factors associated with brain disorders. US Department of Health and Human Services NIH Publication (no 85–1149). Bethesda, Maryland, p 53

Gilles F, Leviton A, Kerr C 1976 Endotoxin leucoencephalopathy in the telencephalon of the newborn kitten. Journal of the Neurological Sciences 27: 183

Gluckman P D, Williams C E 1991 Cerebral function in the fetus—its assessment and the impact of asphyxia. In: Hansen M (eds) Fetal brainstem. Cambridge University Press, Cambridge

Gluckman P D, Williams C E 1992 When and why do brain cells die? Developmental Medicine and Child Neurology 34: 1010

Grant A, O'Brien N, Joy M-T, Hennessy E, MacDonald D 1989 Cerebral palsy among children born during the Dublin randomized trial of intrapartum monitoring. Lancet ii: 1233

Grant J 1993 The state of the world's children. Oxford University Press, Oxford

Hagberg B, Hagberg G, Olow I, von Wendt L 1989 The changing panorama of cerebral palsy in Sweden. V. The birth year period 1979–82. Acta Paediatrica Scandinavica 78: 293

Hagberg B, Hagberg G, Olow I 1993 The changing panorama of cerebral palsy in Sweden VI. Prevalence and origin during the birth year period 1983–1986. Acta Paediatrica 82: 387

Health Care Committee of National Health and Medical Research Council 1993 Report on Maternal Deaths in Australia 1988–90. Australian Government Publishing Service, Canberra

Kiely J L, Kleinman J C, Kiely M 1992 Triplets and higher-order multiple births. American Journal of Disease of Children 146: 862

Kitchen W H, Permezel M J, Doyle L W, Ford G W, Rickards A L, Kelly M A 1992 Changing obstetric practice and 2-year outcome of the fetus of birth weight under 1000 g. Obstetrics and Gynecology 79: 268

Kleinman J C, Fowler M G, Kessel S S 1991 Comparison of infant mortality among twins and singletons: United States 1960 and 1983. American Journal of Epidemiology 133: 133

Krägeloh-Mann I, Hagberg B, Petersen D, Riethmuller J, Gut E, Michaelis R 1992 Bilateral spastic cerebral palsy—pathogenetic aspects from MRI. Neuroepidemiology 23: 46

Kuban K C K, Leviton A 1994 Cerebral palsy. Review article. New England Journal of Medicine 330: 188

Levene M I, Wild J, Steer P 1992 Higher multiple births and the modern management of infertility in Britain. British Journal of Obstetrics and Gynaecology 99: 607

Levin J B, Macfarlane A, Bennett S 1990 The comparison of trends in perinatal mortality in small areas. International Journal of Epidemiology 19: 78

Leviton A 1993 Preterm birth and cerebral palsy: is tumor necrosis factor the missing link? Developmental Medicine and Child Neurology 35: 553

Leviton A, Gilles F 1973 An epidemiologic study of perinatal telencephalic leucoencephalopathy in an autopsy population. Journal of Neurological Sciences 18: 53

Leviton A, Paneth N 1990 White matter damage in preterm

newborns—an epidemiologic perspective. Early Human Development 24: 1

Lilienfeld A M, Parkhurst E 1951 Study of the association of factors of pregnancy and parturition with the development of cerebral palsy. American Journal of Hygiene 53: 262

Lipitz S, Reichman B, Uval J et al 1994 A prospective comparison of the outcome of triplet pregnancies managed expectantly or by multifetal reduction to twins. American Journal of Obstetrics and Gynecology 170: 874

Low J A 1990 The significance of fetal asphyxia in regard to motor and cognitive defects in infancy and childhood. In: Tejani N (ed) Obstetric events and developmental sequelae. CRC Press, Boca Raton, p 43

Lumley J 1988 Does continuous intrapartum fetal monitoring predict long term neurological disorders? Paediatric and Perinatal Epidemiology 2: 299

Mallard E C, Williams C E, Johnston B M, Gluckman P D 1994 Increased vulnerability to neuronal damage following umbilical cord occlusion in the fetal sheep with advancing gestation. American Journal of Obstetrics and Gynecology 170: 206

Myers R 1972 Two patterns of perinatal brain damage and their conditions of occurrence. American Journal of Obstetrics and Gynecology 112: 431

Myers R, Wagner K, de Courten G 1981 Lactic acid accumulation in tissue as cause of brain injury and death and cardiogenic shock from asphyxia. In: Lauersen N, Hochberg H (eds) Perinatal biochemical monitoring. Williams & Wilkins, Baltimore, p 11

Nelson K B 1988 What proportion of cerebral palsy is related to birth asphyxia? Journal of Pediatrics 112: 572

Nelson K B, Ellenberg J H 1978 Epidemiology of cerebral palsy. Advances in Neurology 19: 421

Nelson K B, Ellenberg J H 1981 Apgar scores as predictors of chronic neurologic disability. Pediatrics 68: 36

Nelson K B, Ellenberg J H 1984 Obstetric complications as risk factors for cerebral palsy or seizure disorders. Journal of the American Medical Association 251: 1843

Nelson K B, Ellenberg J H 1986 Antecedents of cerebral palsy. Multivariate analysis of risk. New England Journal of Medicine 315: 81

Nelson K B, Leviton A 1991 How much of neonatal encephalopathy is due to birth asphyxia? American Journal of Diseases of Children 145: 1325

Niswander K, Elbourne D, Redman C et al 1984 Adverse outcome of pregnancy and the quality of obstetric care. Lancet ii: 827

Ounsted M, Radcliff J 1987 Causes continua and other concepts II. Risks are not causes. Paediatric and Perinatal Epidemiology 1: 130

Paneth N 1986 Birth and the origins of cerebral palsy. (Editorial) New England Journal of Medicine 315: 124

Paneth N 1993 The causes of cerebral palsy. Recent evidence. Clinical and Investigative Medicine 16: 95

Petterson B, Nelson K B, Watson L, Stanley F 1993 Twins, triplets, and cerebral palsy in births in Western Australia in the 1980s. British Medical Journal 307: 1239

Pharoah P O D, Cooke T, Cooke R W I, Rosenbloom L 1990 Birthweight specific trends in cerebral palsy. Archives of Disease in Childhood 65: 602

Power C 1994 National trends in birth weight: implications for future adult disease. British Medical Journal 308: 1270

Quilligan E J, Paul R H 1975 Fetal monitoring: is it worth it? Obstetrics and Gynecology 45: 96

Rutanen E-M 1993 Cytokines in reproduction. Annals of Medicine 25: 343

Ruth V J, Raivio K O 1988 Perinatal brain damage: predictive value of metabolic acidosis and the Apgar score. British Medical Journal 297: 24

Sarnat H B 1987 Disturbances of late neuronal migrations in the perinatal period. American Journal of Diseases of Children 141: 969

Scott H 1976 Outcome of very severe brain asphyxia. Archives of Disease in Childhood 51: 712

Stanley F J 1994a Aetiology of cerebral palsy (Review). Early Human Development 36: 81

Stanley F J 1994b Cerebral palsy trends: implications for perinatal care. Acta Obstetrica et Gynecologica Scandinavica 73: 5

Stanley F J, Alberman E D 1984 Birthweight, gestational age and the cerebral palsies. Clinics in Developmental Medicine 87: 57

Stanley F J, Blair E 1991 Why have we failed to reduce the frequency of cerebral palsy. Medical Journal of Australia 154: 623

Stanley F J, Blair E 1994 Cerebral palsy. In: Pless I B (ed) The epidemiology of childhood disorders. Oxford University Press, New York, p 473

Stanley F J, Watson L 1992 Trends in perinatal mortality and cerebral palsy in Western Australia, 1967 to 1985. British Medical Journal 304: 1658

Stanley F J, Croft M, Gibbins J, Read A 1994 A population data base for maternal and child health research in Western Australia using record linkage. Paediatric and Perinatal Epidemiology (in press).

Thacker S B 1991 Effectiveness of safety of intrapartum fetal monitoring. In: Spencer J A D (eds) Fetal monitoring—physiology and techniques of antenatal and intrapartum assessment. Oxford Medical Publications, Oxford, p 211

US Department of Health and Human Services 1993 Health United States 1993 and Healthy People Review. No PHS 93–1232

US Department of Health and Human Services 1994 Health United States 1993. US Government Printing Office, Washington DC

Wald N J 1993 Folic acid and neural tube defects: the current evidence and implications for prevention. In: Neural Tube Defects Ciba Foundation Symposium 181. John Wiley, Chichester, p 192

Williams C E, Mallard C, Tan W, Gluckman P D 1993 Pathophysiology of perinatal asphyxia. Clinics in Perinatology 20: 305

Wyatt J S 1986 Quantification of cerebral oxygenation and haemodynamics in sick newborn infants by near infrared spectroscopy. Lancet ii: 1063

Vital statistics

48. Birth rates

Geoffrey Chamberlain

INTRODUCTION

Most countries in the developed world collect data on the numbers of births that take place; they also do regular population censuses. With these data, they can publish birth rates. In July 1837, the registration of live births started in England and Wales; from 1927 data on stillbirths were also collected. The Population (Statistics) Act 1938 was the beginning of the analysis of these data for statistical purposes and it was from this time that multiple births could first be distinguished in this country. The Population (Statistics) Act of 1960 required further questions about the father. Data from England and Wales are published regularly by the Registrar General through the Office of Population, Censuses and Surveys (OPCS), while those from Scotland and Northern Ireland came from their respective General Registry Offices.

Births have to be registered by law under the Births and Deaths Registration Act of 1836. The General Registrar Office and the Local Superintendent Registrars and Registrars were established by that Act, which requires a Registrar to inform him- or herself within 42 days of any birth occurring inside the district; it obliged the parents, or failing them the occupier of the tenement in which the birth took place, to provide such information to the local Registrar.

The amount of data collected has increased so that now details are obtained about:

1. The child
   a. date and place of birth
   b. sex
   c. legitimacy
2. The father
   a. place of birth
   b. occupation
   c. date of birth
3. The mother
   a. place of birth
   b. date of birth.

For legitimate births only, further data are collected about the parents' marriage and the number of children born to the mother. These data are checked locally.

As well as the system of registration, the midwife or doctor who attended the birth must notify the District Medical Officer (England and Wales) or the Chief Administrative Medical Officer (Scotland and Northern Ireland) within 36 hours. With this and the civil registration system quite separate, they act as a check of each other. The District Health Authority informs the local Registrar of Births of babies notified. In return, the Registrar returns the list of registered babies with their National Health Service number, a service the Registrars must initiate.

DEFINITIONS

The data about births can be expressed in various ways.

The absolute numbers of births is well known and can be expressed by various years (Fig. 48.1). This is helpful in knowing the numbers which may present in the population in coming years; these figures are refined in demograms. The crude birth rate is the number of viable births (live and dead) per thousand of the total population (Fig. 48.2). This is a simple mathematical fraction that can be derived from the birth data and the Census returns.

$$\text{Birth rate} = \frac{\text{Births per year} \times 1000}{\text{Mid-year population}}$$

In the above ratio, the denominator is the total population, including men and women below and above the reproductive age group. A denominator would be more

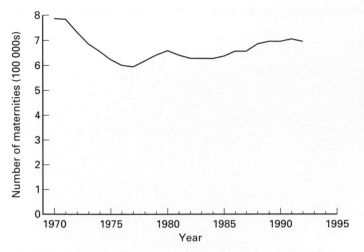

Fig. 48.1 Absolute numbers of women giving birth in England and Wales (1970–92).

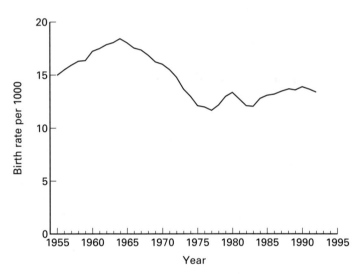

Fig. 48.2 Crude birth rates for England and Wales (1955–92).

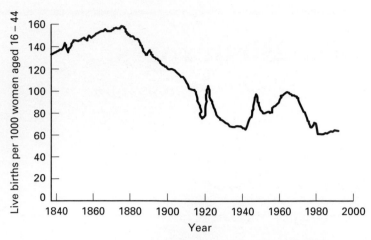

Fig. 48.3 General fertility rate for England and Wales (1838–1992).

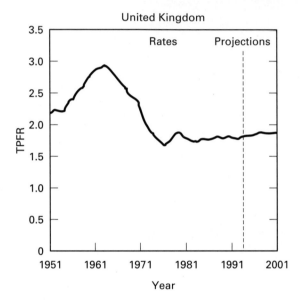

Fig. 48.4 Total period fertility rate (TPFR). Average number of children which would be born per woman if woman experienced the age-specific fertility rates of the period in question throughout their child-bearing lifespan. Data from Office of Population Censuses and Surveys 1994 Social Trends 24. HMSO, London.

appropriate if it consisted of all those, and only those, who might appear in the numerator. Hence a more appropriate measure of birth rates can be obtained by only looking at the births in comparison to the number of women in the reproductive age group. This is taken nominally from age 15 to 44 years (Fig. 48.3). Thus the general fertility rate is derived:

$$\text{General fertility rate} = \frac{\text{Births per year} \times 1000}{\text{Women 15–44 years in mid-year population}}$$

Another measure of this is the total period fertility rate, which is the summation of the fertility rates in any given year by the years the mother has left to an age when it is considered that reproduction will probably stop (arguably taken as 50 years). This measures the average number of children that might be expected to be born to a woman if she experienced the age-specific fertility rates of the calendar year in question throughout the rest of her childbearing life (Fig. 48.4).

This is a more precise measure than is that of completed family size, which can only be calculated in retrospect when a woman has completed her family. However, mean family size is an attractive index and often used in the popular press giving the coarse differences between countries. When the completed family size drops below two, replacement of the population has stopped and therefore that society is below zero population growth.

WORLD POPULATION CHANGES

Population dynamics examine how populations change

in countries and between countries. The relation of this to births and deaths can be shown simply as follows:

$$\text{Births} \longrightarrow \text{Population size} \longrightarrow \text{Deaths}$$
$$\Updownarrow$$
$$\text{Migration}$$

At times of economic stability, migration is not a major feature in many countries, although it obviously has a great part to play at times of rapid economic growth, such as immigration did in the USA at the beginning of the century, or emigration in times of economic hardship, such as in Ireland at the time of the potato famines.

Leaving migration aside, one can then calculate how a country is likely to expand. A good example would be the flourishing country of Kenya which has a large agricultural and tourist industry and virtually no migration either in or out. The birth rate is 48 per 1000; the death rate is 15 per 1000. Thus there will be a natural increase of 33 per 1000 in the year. From this, one can extrapolate approximately that in about 20 years' time, the population will have approximately doubled. In most countries of the Western world, the birth rate and death rate are roughly equal; if migration is not a major factor, they have reached zero population growth.

The classical factors which stabilized populations in the 19th century were:

1. Effects on death rate
   a. disease
   b. famine
   c. war
2. effects on birth rate
   a. celibacy of the population
   b. restraint.

While we do not live in a perfect world, the three influences which affect death rates are considerably curtailed. At the end of the 20th century, falling disease rates have been seen in the Western world although many diseases, particularly the infectious ones, still need to be overcome in the developing world. The effects of famine are mostly being overcome. Agricultural policies like those in the Punjab in India are leading the world away from starvation. Despite the campaigns of Korea, Vietnam and the Gulf War, there have been no world wars for 50 years and so deaths from this cause are greatly reduced in both the warrior class and civilians. Hence, reduction in birth rates has now become the major instrument in altering populations. In the latter part of the 20th century, in many countries celibacy has been overtaken as an influence on birth rates by contraception and wider family spacing.

The effects of changes in the birth rate can be seen by examining the information from age-specific rates in 5-year samples of the populations. From this, population

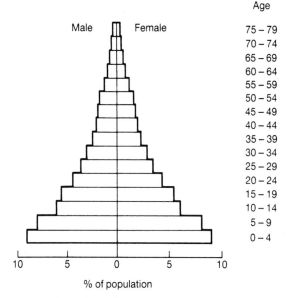

Fig. 48.5 Smoothed-off demogram for a rapidly developing country recording male and female populations in 5-year cohorts.

projections can be derived. Figure 48.5 depicts a typical developing country. Population data in 5-year age groups show that the numbers of the young are expanding whilst mean life expectancy is not very high. Figure 48.6 shows the same data in a more developed country where the 5-year cohorts are of approximately the same size until degenerative diseases start becoming a factor at about 55 years of age.

Figure 48.6 shows demograms from the same country (Hong Kong) over a 20-year period. Fifteen years after the war, the birth rate had been going up steadily and so in the mid 1960s, the Government began an intensive

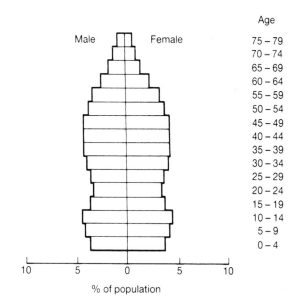

Fig. 48.6 Smoothed-off demogram for a developed country recording male and female populations in 5-year cohorts.

campaign to promote the use of contraception. The middle demogram shows that 10 years later this had worked, for the effect of contraception was a great reduction in the birth rate. In 1981, this reduced birth rate structure was sustained. The bulge of children born in the late 1950s had worked its way through and was represented by figures showing those aged in their 20s. The implication of this in the provision of facilities for schooling, universities and job opportunities is obvious and demograms are often used to make such social planning. If the population was to continue in this pattern, it would be expected that Hong Kong would require an enlargement in geriatric services in 30 years' time.

The demogram for the UK (Fig. 48.7) for recent years has shown a slight diminution in births from 1964 to the late 1970s. Generally, however, the demogram is reasonably straight-sided, as in other developed countries. With improvements in health and better nutrition, an ageing population will soon weigh down the upper end of this demogram. They require geriatric and social services now and over the next 30–40 years; this will be a constant strain on the social security system.

BIRTH RATES IN ENGLAND AND WALES

The birth rate in England and Wales is shown in Figure 48.3 for the last century. In the Victorian days, it was about 35 per 1000. This was just after the Industrial Revolution when Britain was a rich nation economically. Birth rates declined from then until the 1920s, when there was the Depression. The birth rate of the 1930s was slightly boosted by the threat of war and a recovery in

the activity of heavy industry. This caused a mild increase in birth rates; however, the birth rate has stayed at a generally lower level since the Second World War.

Examination of the more recent birth rate data shows that the postwar boom rose to an apex in 1964 when it was about 17 per 1000 and since then it has declined steadily (Fig. 48.2). There was a minor resurgence in 1980, when the birth rate was about 14 per 1000 and the total period fertility rate 1.89—a figure still below replacement rates for a population.

In mid 1986, the estimated population of England was 47 254 000. This was an increase of 143 000 from the previous year. Whilst half of this increase was the excess of immigrants over emigrants, the other half was due to the excess of the birth rate over the death rate. Increased birth rates are also reflected in the age structure, for while the 5–15-year group has fallen by 11% since 1981, the 1–4-year group is 4% up on 1985 and 6.8% increased on 1981 data. The implications for planning educational needs in a few years' time are not lost on politicians or teachers.

FACTORS THAT MODIFY THE BIRTH RATE

Family spacing

Obviously the earlier in life couples start reproducing, the more likely they are to have a larger family. In the Pacific Islands, girls often marry at 12 or 13 years of age and so have a greater exposure to intercourse and are more likely to have more babies. Conversely, in Sri Lanka the mean age of marriage is 28 years; birth rates are

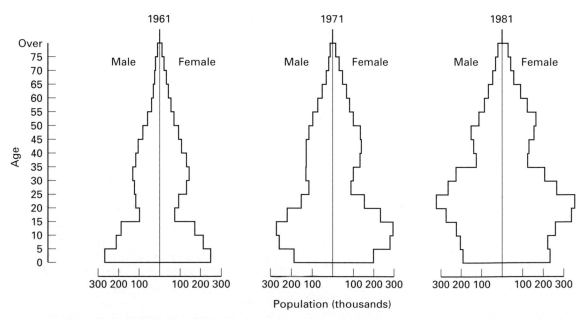

Fig. 48.7 Smoothed-off demogram of Hong Kong in 1961, 1971 and 1981 recording male and female populations in 5-year cohorts.

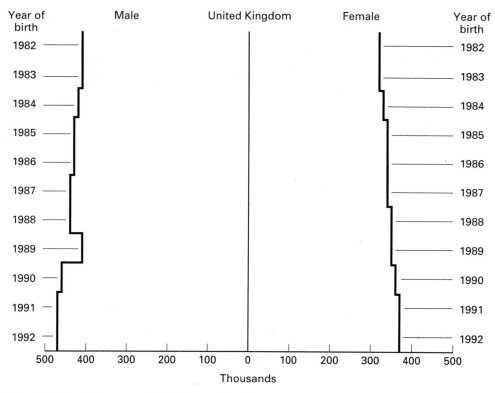

Fig. 48.8 Basal demogram of the UK population in 1991 in annual cohorts, i.e. data not smoothed-off. This shows changes in finer detail (redrawn from Social Trends 1994; HMSO, London).

dropping fast in that country. The frequency of intercourse itself influences the number of children, but more important is the spacing of families. In many parts of the world, breastfeeding is the most commonly used method of contraception and so pregnancy occurs every 2 or 3 years during reproductive life. Other methods of pharmaceutical and mechanical contraception are more common in the Western world and their use leads to a later start in reproduction and a wider spacing of families and so a lower birth rate.

Table 48.1 represents the average number of children born per woman at the current fertility rates in the major regions of the world. It is sharply divided into those areas where contraception is more widely used and those

where it is not. Apart from conventional contraception, in many parts of Eastern Europe induced abortion is considered a method of contraception. This is frowned upon in the Western world, partly because it has an unacceptable rate of medical sequelae.

Seasonal variations

There are inbuilt variations in birth rate. In the UK the seasonal pattern of birth rate changes has remained the same for over a century with only minor variations occurring during the years of World Wars I and II. The birth rate in England and Wales is highest in January to March and generally lowest from October to December. Several explanations have been put forward, ranging from the hypothesis that intercourse may be more frequent in the spring, for the tax year finishes in early April, to the idea that trace elements are entering the diet in different rates at different times of the year. All these are hard to substantiate for there have been changes shown in other parts of the world, such as Australia, where the peak of birth rate is from the spring to the autumn. Further, limited work based on 16th century baptismal data, which bears a strong relation to birth rate data, implies that these trends were in existence long before income tax was invented—though obviously not before intercourse was invented.

Table 48.1 Total fertility rates for some major regions of the world (1990–95)

Region	Total fertility rate
Western Europe	1.7
North America	2.0
USSR (former)	2.3
China	3.2
India	4.8
Central America	3.1
Africa	6.0

Total fertility rate = average number of children born per woman at current fertility rates.

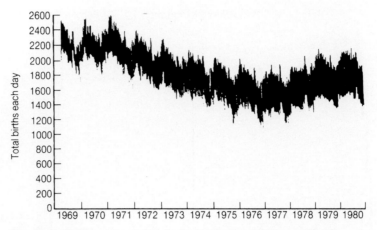

Fig. 48.9 Daily numbers of births for England and Wales (1969–80).

Figure 48.9 shows the variation in daily births for England and Wales from 1969 to 1980. It is remarkable for its consistency. A secondary peak in birth rates can be seen in September of each year. This is commonly associated with the fact that nine months before September was Christmas and New Year with their usual festivities.

Daily variation

A short-term cycle is seen in birth rates when one examines the day of the week on which people are born. Figure 48.10 explores this in a simplified way. The birth ratio is derived by dividing by 7 the total number of births in England and Wales in 1980. Thus, if the distribution were random, the expected number of births on any day would be one-seventh of all. This is designated at 1: any figures above 1 indicate an increase in the number of

births, while below 1 indicates a deficit in births on that day.

It can be seen that at the weekend there is a deficiency in the number of births; the lowest ratio is on Sunday and the next lowest on Saturday. It is not the purpose of this chapter to pursue the reasons for this in detail but it may be that some women have a lower threshold of the uterus going into spontaneous contractions. It might be that stimulation of the cervix could cause an unusual release of prostaglandins which, whilst not enough to cause labour to start in most women, could start the process in a woman who is very close to labour with a lower-onset threshold. It is as probable that in the UK sexual intercourse is more frequent on Friday and Saturday; this might be the stimulus to the release of prostaglandins. This hypothesis is being explored at the moment.

CONCLUSIONS

Examination of birth rates is not a dull, statistical process but one that gives information in a wide range of social and medical fields. A country that keeps proper data about its births and deaths is one that usually has a good health service. If the information is not counted then the people do not count.

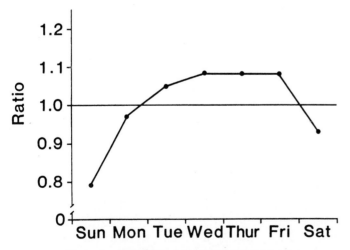

Fig. 48.10 Birth rates in 1980 by day of the week (see text).

Acknowledgements

There are no formal references in this chapter since all the data are easily available and are constantly being updated from Government sources. The author would like to acknowledge the great help he has had from two major sources:

McFarland A, Mugford M 1984 Birth counts, the statistics of pregnancy and childbirth. HMSO London
Office of Population Censuses and Surveys Birth statistics 1837–1991. Series FM1 nos 13,21. HMSO, London

49. Perinatal mortality

Jean Chapple

Material in this chapter contains contributions from the first edition and we are grateful to the previous author for the work done.

INTRODUCTION

Modern technology gives us countless methods of investigating and treating both health and disease. However, many of the procedures carried out by health professionals are ineffective and do not produce a better state of health for those individuals who have sought clinical help (Enkin et al 1989). In a tax-funded health-care system such as the National Health Service (NHS), it is inevitable that interest is focusing on funding good results, or outcomes, of health care rather than emphasizing the processes (such as numbers of operations or other procedures). One of the earliest outcome measures used in the NHS was perinatal mortality. This measure was first proposed in an article published in 1948 (Peller 1948) which suggested combining stillbirth and first week death rates, as the time trends for early neonatal deaths were more like those for stillbirths than other death rates in infancy. This chapter will look at how often and why perinatal deaths occur and discuss whether the perinatal death rate is a good measure of the effectiveness of maternity and neonatal services.

DEFINITIONS

The perinatal mortality rate (PNMR) per thousand births is calculated from:

$$\frac{(\text{Stillbirths} + \text{deaths at 0–6 days after live birth}) \times 1000}{\text{Live births} + \text{stillbirths}}$$

Definitions of live births and stillbirths and hence perinatal mortality vary with national policy and with time. A stillborn baby in the UK must be registered with the local Registrar of Births and Deaths and is currently defined (under section 41 of the Births and Deaths Registration Act 1953) as a child issuing forth from its mother after the 24th completed week of pregnancy which did not at any time after being completely expelled from its mother breathe or show any other signs of life. This definition came into force on 1 October 1992; prior to this, the cut-off gestational age was 28 weeks. This change in definition will increase the PNMR, as babies dying between 25 and 28 weeks will now be included in the figures, although the Office of Population Censuses and Surveys (OPCS) will continue to supply figures based on both definitions for some time. Stillborn babies are defined by the time after which they were born, rather than the gestation at which they died, so a papyraceous twin who has died months before its sibling is born should be registered as a stillbirth. In practice, this would rarely be implemented.

All liveborn babies must also be registered. A liveborn baby is a child who breathes or shows signs of life after complete expulsion from its mother, regardless of length of gestation. This categorization varies greatly from one country to another, as there are different legal definitions excluding live births below defined lower limits of gestational age or birthweight. Laws relating to the timing of registration may also affect whether the child is certified as live or stillborn (Macfarlane & Mugford 1984).

Individual judgement also plays a part in certification

of perinatal deaths (Keirse 1984) and judgements about viability (Fenton et al 1990). Some fetuses are born so early that they are not viable but may still show visible signs of life for a few minutes. The current abortion law in England, Wales and Scotland allows termination of pregnancy for severe fetal malformation at any gestational age. If the termination is carried out after 24 weeks' gestation and the fetus is dead at birth, it should officially be registered as a stillbirth, and the legal forms relating to termination of pregnancy must also be completed. If feticide is not carried out prior to delivery, such a fetus may be live born and die after delivery, and this should again be registered as a live birth and subsequent death, with official disposal of the body, and with completed termination documentation. However, it is not unknown for clinicians to be influenced by perceptions of how the parents will feel about official form filling and financial considerations for the parents with regard to maternity benefit and the cost of burial. This is understandable but technically illegal—the legal cut-off points are artificial and parental grief pays no regard as to what stage in pregnancy a baby is lost.

THE COLLECTION OF DATA ABOUT PERINATAL MORTALITY

Countries have different methods of collecting data about perinatal deaths as well as different definitions. This section deals with the situation in England and Wales. Greater detail can be found in volume 1 of *Birth Counts* (Macfarlane & Mugford 1984).

Civil registration of births

The industrialization of society with the population moving from villages to large cities led to major changes in the way data on births, deaths and marriages were collected. Authorities could no longer rely on information from parish baptismal and burial records. In 1837, a law was passed to make it a statutory requirement to register all births with the Registrar of Births and Deaths in the locality in England and Wales where the birth had taken place. Registration was required in Scotland in 1855 (Nissel 1987).

Parents are required to give details of the baby and demographic data, such as their own date and place of birth, to the Registrar within 42 days of the birth. Certain details, such as parity of the mother and the occupation of the father (to determine social class) are requested only for legitimate babies. As nearly one-third of babies are now born to parents who are not married, this information does not apply to an increasingly large proportion of births. Important information, such as birthweight, gestational age and ethnic group of parents, is completely omitted from initial collection of registration data.

Medical notification of births

An increasing interest in improving maternal and child health at the beginning of the 20th century led to the introduction of another system of collecting data about births in order to ensure that midwives, health visitors and doctors were aware that a baby had been born and could offer clinical support and advice. The attendant at the birth has to notify the designated medical officer (usually the Director of Public Health) of the local health authority of any birth occurring in that authority, in writing, within 36 hours of birth. This system gives the opportunity to collect information on birthweight, which since 1978 has been statutorily transferred from the notification system to the birth registration system to provide national statistics on birthweight. Birth attendants are also asked to notify OPCS about congenital malformations noted within 10 days of birth to give a national picture of the birth prevalence of malformations. This requirement started in 1964 in response to the thalidomide tragedy.

Death certification

Stillbirths and neonatal deaths must all be registered. The certificates made out by the Registrar of Births and Deaths include the medical cause of death, certified by the doctor in attendance. Stillbirth certificates act as both a birth and death certificate and the child's name can now be included, as well as the birthweight, gestational age and cause of death, which may be certified by a midwife. Since 1986, a new neonatal certificate has been issued, which, like a stillbirth certificate, collects data on maternal causes contributing to the death.

Linkage of birth and death certificates

Butler (1967) stated that a prerequisite to the reduction of perinatal mortality is to identify the obstetric and sociological associates of perinatal deaths. Heady & Heasman (1959) first demonstrated that linkage of the information on birth certificates with that on death certificates of infants who subsequently died would allow calculation of death rates by demographic factors collected for babies at birth, such as mother's country of birth and social class.

Some data collected by statute is for legitimate births only. As the proportion of illegitimate births has increased rapidly recently (Fig. 49.1), such data have less value. Other data, such as place of birth of mother, can no longer be used as an approximation of ethnic group because of the rising number of second- and third-generation children born to immigrant groups. There have also been problems in collecting timely and compatible data within rapidly changing NHS and OPCS organizations. This puts limits on the use of routinely collected national data and has led to increasing interest in more intensive surveys and enquiries.

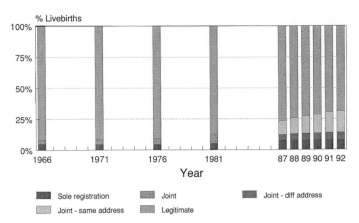

% Livebirths

Legend:
- Sole registration
- Joint - same address
- Joint
- Legitimate
- Joint - diff address

Fig. 49.1 Registration of live births by legitimacy, England and Wales 1966–91. Source: OPCS 1993.

SURVEYS OF PERINATAL DEATHS

The first of these national studies was done in 1946 (Joint Committee of the RCOG and the Population Investigation Committee 1948) but this was more concerned with examining maternity services in Britain at the time when the NHS was being planned than with looking at causes of death. In 1958 the British Perinatal Mortality study (Butler & Bonham 1963) evaluated nationally how and when British babies were born or died, how often they died and what clinicopathological features led to their death. The study used a cohort of births between 3 and 9 March 1958 plus deaths in the next three consecutive months. This cohort has been studied long term to look at the effects of prenatal factors in parents on the next generation (Emanuel et al 1992). The detailed first report contained statistical data on factors such as maternal age, parity, place of booking, gestation and birthweight, while the second report (Butler & Alberman 1969) used multivariate analysis of high risk influences on the outcome of pregnancy, such as smoking and sociobiological factors.

A third study was done in 1970 to look at all babies born alive or dead after the 24th week of gestation (Chamberlain et al 1975). This provided basic data in Britain for factors such as low birthweight and placental abnormalities and quantified them. These studies did not look at deaths individually but epidemiologically. A proposed fourth study in 1982 did not occur in England and Wales (Chalmers 1979). By this time, deaths had fallen to a level where it was possible to do a confidential enquiry on each case. A more unified routine data collection system for the far fewer births taking place in Scotland made a Scottish study feasible at this time (McIlwaine et al 1979).

PERINATAL ENQUIRIES

Staff working in maternity services have a long history of investigating deaths through confidential enquiries, a form of external clinical audit (Shaw 1980). In such studies, each death is reviewed individually by a group of clinicians from different disciplines concerned in maternity care, and *avoidable*, *adverse* or *notable* factors which may have contributed to the death are identified. Identification of less than optimal resources and practice can be fed back anonymously to all clinicians to make them rethink how they provide maternity care.

From 1928 onwards, the main concern of obstetricians was for maternal rather than perinatal deaths, as the maternal mortality rate was 4.4 deaths per 1000 total births, or 3000 mothers dying each year. This led to a national confidential enquiry into maternal deaths. The persisting differences in PNMRs between countries and between regions in England and Wales in the 1970s led to interest in applying the methodology of confidential enquiries to perinatal deaths—although, as there were then ten perinatal deaths for each maternal death, the task was much larger (Chalmers 1979, Chalmers & McIlwaine 1980). Several regions (Northern, South East Thames and Wessex) started enquiries at this time which have collected data to the present time.

Many of these enquiries were conducted on a regional basis. Some involved interviews with the bereaved parents and the primary care professionals involved (Paediatric Research Unit 1973, Mersey Region Working Party on Perinatal Mortality 1982, Mutch et al 1981, Wood et al 1984). A considerable amount of relevant data are available from statutory returns on births and deaths (Black & Macfarlane 1982, Clarke 1982). However, without good denominator data from detailed information on all births or a proper case-control study, it is impossible to put perinatal deaths in an enquiry into perspective and calculate a relative risk for factors leading to perinatal death (Coggon et al 1993). This is a major problem of current confidential enquiries. Adverse factors occur in the care of mothers and babies who survive as well as those who die. Lack of denominator data to put the risks in perspective makes it impossible to assess the sensitivity and specificity of screening for adverse risk factors. Most screening tests in pregnancy produce a high proportion of false positives, leading to unnecessary clinical intervention, and there is a danger that confidential enquiries may contribute to this.

A full national Confidential Enquiry into Stillbirths and Deaths in Infancy (CESDI) was instituted in England, Wales and Northern Ireland from 1 January 1993. Slightly contrary to its name, CESDI covers all deaths from the 20th week of pregnancy to the end of the first year of life. For the first year, confidential assessment by local regional multidisciplinary panels of obstetricians, paediatricians, midwives, general practitioners, pathologists and others was undertaken for all babies over 2500 g birthweight with no severe congenital malformations who died from a perinatal cause during labour or the first week of life. Annual reports will be produced by the National Advisory Body (NAB) for CESDI to highlight factors contributing to deaths. It is hoped that timely feedback will make clinicians aware of possible problems. Studies of sudden infant deaths with controls have been undertaken in three regions as a pilot study to look at the use of case controls in assessing adverse factors.

TRENDS IN PERINATAL DEATHS

Comparisons of the perinatal mortality rates between Western countries in the 1970s led the Committee on Child Health Services (1976) to refer to the infant mortality rate in the UK as a 'holocaust'. This led to a renewed interest in perinatal mortality and to the regionally based confidential enquiries into such deaths mentioned above. In 1976, the PNMR for England and Wales was 17.7 per 1000 births. By 1992, it had fallen to 7.6. This is similar to trends in other Western countries, which are all beginning to converge at rates of less than 10. There are now equal proportions of stillbirths to early neonatal deaths, but Figure 49.2 shows that this was not always the case. Stillbirth and early neonatal death rates began to converge in the mid 1950s, reaching the same levels by the mid 1970s.

CAUSES OF PERINATAL DEATHS

Classification of immediate causes

OPCS uses the International Classification of Diseases (ICD) codes to classify disease and injuries for national statistics. Since 1 January 1986, the certifier has been able to record separate main fetal and maternal conditions leading to the stillbirth or neonatal death without giving precedence to one particular condition. However, classifi-

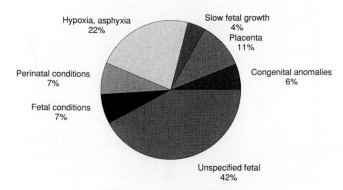

Fig. 49.3 Causes of stillbirths, main fetal cause (%), England and Wales 1991 ($n = 3254$). Source: OPCS Series DH6 No 5.

cation using International Classification of Disease (ICD) codes is not easy, and clinicians do not always complete death certificates as fully as they might. Figure 49.3 shows that in 1991 42% of stillbirths had no fetal or maternal condition recorded on the medical certificate. Allowing for this underreporting, nearly one-quarter of stillbirths were certified as due to intrauterine hypoxia and birth asphyxia and 7% as congenital anomalies (OPCS 1991). In the neonatal period, the main causes of death were congenital anomalies (24%) and prematurity (25%) (Fig. 49.4).

Pathological causes of death such as anoxia or prematurity give little precise information on the aetiology of deaths. Baird and his colleagues (1954) in Aberdeen therefore devised a clinical classification with an hierarchical structure—for example, if a baby weighing 1500 g dies shortly after an operative delivery done because of a placenta praevia and is found at postmortem to have a tentorial tear, it seems more logical to attribute the death primarily to placenta praevia than to prematurity or birth trauma. This classification was used as the basis of the British Perinatal Mortality Survey in 1958 (Butler & Bonham 1963) and a modified version of this clinicopathological approach (Cole et al 1986) is also used for the current national Confidential Enquiry into Stillbirths

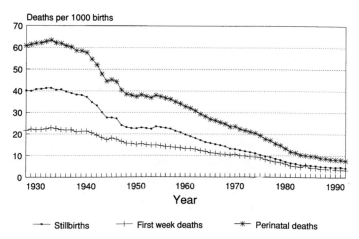

Fig. 49.2 Stillbirths, first week and perinatal deaths, England and Wales 1928–92. Source: OPCS statistics series DH3.

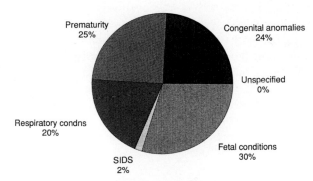

Fig. 49.4 Causes of neonatal deaths, main infant conditions, England and Wales 1991 ($n = 3052$). Source: OPCS Series DH6 No 5.

and Deaths in Infancy (CESDI), as it gives a classification of obstetric factors.

Other recent classifications have tried to relate the classification to the time in pregnancy, delivery or post-natal period when the factor causing eventual death occurred. This then allows health services to focus on preventive action at the appropriate time. Wigglesworth (1980) proposed a classification using a pathophysiological approach which did not need detailed pathological investigation and shows fetal and neonatal factors. It arranges causes of death in a mutually exclusive hierarchy: congenital malformations, stillbirths occurring before the onset of labour (both pregnancy related), neonatal deaths due to immaturity (neonatal period), deaths due to asphyxial conditions (related to labour and delivery) and other specific causes. This classification of fetal causes of death is also used in CESDI assessments.

Both these types of classification need to be used with data on the maturity of the baby at birth. Gestational age is not routinely collected in national statistics. It is considered difficult to categorize accurately, as the dates for calculation of gestational age given by the mother may differ from those calculated from ultrasound readings or may not be available at all. Birthweight is therefore often used as a proxy for gestational age, although this too has its drawbacks if the baby is at the extremes of the birthweight distribution for its gestation.

Figure 49.5 shows trends in perinatal rates and causes of death in the Northern region between 1981 and 1990 and Figure 49.6 shows comparable figures for three regions running long-term enquiries. These show that although the perinatal rates are different and interpretations of the classification may vary with different groups of assessors, the proportions of perinatal deaths for each cause are broadly similar.

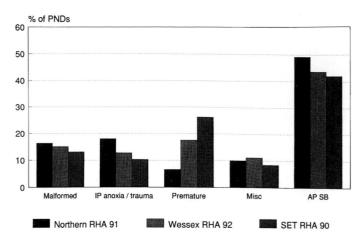

Fig. 49.6 Causes of perinatal death (PND), Northern, Wessex and South East Thames (SET) Regional Health Authorities. Source: Northern, Wessex and SE Thames RHAs.

Immediate cause of perinatal death

The three major determinants of perinatal mortality found in all studies (Chamberlain 1980) are:

1. Congenital anomalies.
2. Low birthweight (LBW) and very low birthweight (VLBW) (taken as less than 2500 g and less than 1500 g respectively).
3. Hypoxia.

It is difficult to analyse trends in causes of perinatal mortality as there have been changes in the international classification of causes of death (World Health Organization 1977) and the way in which deaths are coded.

Predisposing causes

It seems likely from what data are available that all causes of perinatal mortality are falling in incidence, mainly because predisposing factors are altering in prevalence. These can act at several different stages of pregnancy.

Prepregnancy risk factors

Deaths due to lethal congenital malformations are falling because of prenatal diagnosis with termination of affected pregnancies. Some families are aware that they carry genes for severe genetic disease and seek advice pre-pregnancy. In others, fetal anomaly scanning may reveal structural abnormalities such as spina bifida and allow a fall in perinatal mortality because of their detection (Saari-Kemppainen et al 1990). However, routine scanning has not been shown to reduce mortality and improve outcome from any other cause (Bucher & Schmidt 1993, Ewigman et al 1993).

Some maternal infections such as rubella and

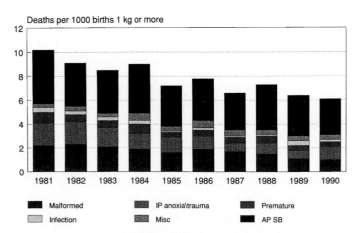

Fig. 49.5 Causes of perinatal morbidity, Northern Region collaborative survey. IP = intrapartum; AP = antepartum; SB = stillbirth. Source: Northern RHA.

toxoplasmosis may be transmitted vertically from mother to child and cause severe malformation. Although the birth prevalence of severe malformations and deaths due to these infections may be falling, it remains to be seen if public health programmes to immunize children against rubella, prevent the spread of toxoplasmosis through personal and food hygiene (RCOG Multidisciplinary Working Group 1992) and to prevent neural tube defects by periconceptional increase in maternal folic acid intake (MRC Vitamin Study Research Group 1991, Czeizel & Dudas 1992, Czeizel 1993) will actually result in primary prevention of malformations.

Maternal ill health or stunted growth may conspire against a normal fetal growth rate or even, as in the case of diabetes, accelerate fetal growth to a dangerous degree. Defects such as abnormal uterine shape may prevent normal placentation and anomalies of the cervix predispose to incompetence of the internal os and premature delivery.

Advanced maternal age is associated with antepartum haemorrhage (Butler & Alberman 1969), possibly as fibroids are commoner and may distort the uterus, leading to abnormalities of placentation.

Conceptional risk factors

Random errors of meiotic or early mitotic divisions can lead to fetal chromosomal abnormalities or multiple pregnancy, both of which are commoner in older mothers. Some trisomies, such as trisomy 18 (Edward's syndrome) and trisomy 13 (Patau's syndrome) are rapidly lethal, often in the middle or third trimester, but others such as trisomy 21 (Down's syndrome) may produce viable fetuses if there is no major structural abnormality such as a congenital heart defect.

Multiple births are exposed to many hazards and are becoming commoner with increasing use of infertility treatment. Multiple placentation and increased nutritional demands made by two or more fetuses can result in fetal growth retardation. In monozygous twins, cords can become entangled in a single amniotic sac, competition for placental tissues may occur or one twin may transfuse blood into the other, resulting in a marked size difference between them, or the death of one twin. Premature delivery is also very high, especially in higher-order births.

Environmental factors acting in pregnancy

External environment

There are many well-recognized teratogens and other fetal toxins which may play a small part in perinatal mortality in developed countries. These include viral infections such as fetal rubella, cytomegalovirus and toxoplasmosis which may cause minimal symptoms in a pregnant woman if caught during pregnancy, but can seriously damage a fetus, especially in the first trimester. Other organisms, such as listeriosis, salmonella and parvovirus (fifth disease) can cause death through prematurity with or without intrauterine or neonatal infection.

Altitude plays a part in producing low birthweight— about 30% of babies born in Colorado above 10 000 metres were low birthweight in Lubchencho's classic study (Lubchencho et al 1963) on birthweight distribution for gestational age, compared with 7% in the UK today. This may play a part in perinatal mortality in some countries.

Exposure to occupational or environmental hazards such as radiation or lead can contribute to perinatal mortality, but the literature is not clear on the risks, mainly because the numbers of births considered were generally too small to achieve sufficient statistical power to assess risk (Rosenberg et al 1987, Savitz et al 1989). A retrospective case control study of over 1000 perinatal deaths in Leicester between 1976 and 1982 showed that leather workers were at increased risk of perinatal deaths, particularly from congenital malformations and macerated stillbirths, compared to other manual workers in the same class (Clarke & Mason 1985). The effect of occupational hazards on perinatal mortality may also be mediated through an increased risk of prematurity or low birthweight, both of which have a major influence on the risk of a baby dying. One study has shown a dose-related association between blood lead and risk of preterm delivery (McMichael et al 1986). The risk of preterm delivery and low birthweight was shown to be over 50% higher in the children of women who worked with electrical, metal or leather goods than in other female manual workers and was more frequent in the children of mothers and fathers employed in manual rather than non-manual jobs in a large study in Scotland between 1981 and 1984 (Sanjose et al 1991).

In utero environment

The effects on the fetus of maternal smoking have been intensively studied and include deviations from normal placentation (Christianson 1979) and fetal growth retardation (Naeye 1978). The actual contribution made by maternal smoking to the risk of perinatal death is not direct but appears to depend on the presence of other adverse factors, as smoking reduces fetal growth rate and therefore adds to other detrimental influences. However, its importance even in a low-risk population is shown by the estimate that in England and Wales in 1984, 18% of babies of low birthweight were attributable to maternal smoking (Simpson & Armand Smith 1986).

The role of undernutrition and specific dietary constituents is still uncertain (Naismith 1981) but will also vary with the underlying health of the mother.

Complications specific to pregnancy

Hypertension in pregnancy is not only potentially dangerous for the mother (Report on Confidential Enquiries into Maternal Deaths in the UK 1988–90) but is associated with changes to placental blood vessels with a consequent reduction in blood flow and fetal growth retardation. It may also lead to prematurity, either by elective or spontaneous preterm delivery. Urinary tract infections can also predispose to preterm labour, as may infections of the amniotic sac (Peckham & Marshall 1983).

FETAL GROWTH AND MATURITY

Birthweight is the best predictor of perinatal mortality. In England and Wales in 1990, 59% of perinatal deaths occurred in the 6.5% of babies who weighed less than 2500 g at birth. Thirty-six per cent of perinatal deaths occurred in the 0.9% of babies who weighed less than 1500 g at birth.

Most of the factors which contribute to perinatal death do so by influencing fetal growth rate, gestational age or both. The size of any baby is influenced by genetic factors (including the presence of congenital malformations and parental height and weight), birth order, and ethnic group (Thomson 1983). These are all closely associated with socioeconomic status, as is risk of exposure to environmental health hazards, such as those at work, and personal health behaviour, such as smoking. All these factors produce very robust birthweight distributions which change only slowly with time. Table 49.1 shows that there has been virtually no change in the birthweight distribution in England and Wales between 1983 and 1990. The fall in mortality over these years is not due to a decrease in the proportion of LBW babies, but in improved survival rates, especially in LBW and VLBW babies. However, there is much debate as to whether there are limits to the gestational age and birthweight below which aggressive resuscitation and active treatment should not be instituted, as there is considerable short- and long-term morbidity in survivors (Walker & Patel 1987, Allen et al 1993). The cut off in improved survival appears to be at 25 weeks' gestation and 750 g birthweight (Hack & Fanaroff 1989).

Growth-retarded babies are at higher risk of perinatal mortality. A study in Sweden showed that growth-retarded babies had four times the PNMR of the general population, even after deaths due to congenital malformations were excluded (Wennergren et al 1988). In Ontario, preterm growth-retarded babies had a PNMR of 180 per 1000 (Fitzhardinge & Inwood 1989) and in Baltimore, 86% of perinatal deaths occurred in growth-retarded babies (Callan & Witter 1990).

Intrauterine growth retardation is also associated with an increased risk of perinatal death not only through its link with low birthweight, but through an increased association with major congenital abnormalities. Studies report a birth prevalence of 4.6% to 11% (Butler 1974, Wennergren et al 1988) in small for gestational age (SGA) infants and 31.6% in SGA infants under 1500 g birthweight (Drillien 1974).

DEMOGRAPHIC FACTORS

Some demographic factors will affect overall birthweight distribution, mainly by subtly influencing the birthweight distribution. This includes the proportion of multiple births, as the birthweight distribution for multiple births is considerably to the left of that for singletons (Fig. 49.7). Even small increases in multiple birth rates, such as have been occurring with increasing use of modern infertility treatments, will increase overall low birthweight. Even though birthweight-specific mortality rates for multiple births are lower than those for singletons (Table 49.2), this does not compensate for their disadvantageous weight distribution.

The distribution of birthweight is also shifted to the left in primiparity and in disadvantaged socioeconomic conditions. There is still great disparity between PNMR in different social classes in Britain (Fig. 49.8), although the increasing proportion of babies born to unmarried women has meant that illegitimate babies are now less disadvantaged at birth than they were. Hellier (1977) showed that almost a quarter of the reduction in PNMR that occurred in England and Wales between 1953 and 1978 was explained by the demographic changes in maternal age, parity and social class that had occurred.

Women from ethnic minority groups appear to have a higher risk of perinatal death than indigenous mothers. A minor part may be due to a difference in birthweight distributions, but the incidence of malformations may be very different. The increased incidence of lethal congenital malformations in British Pakistanis made a large contribution to a perinatal mortality rate of 18 per 1000 in 1984 for this group, compared to 12 per 1000 in other ethnic groups, a 50% excess (Balarajan & Botting 1989, Chitty & Winter 1989). Access to and use of maternity services may also affect outcome (Clarke et al 1988).

Cross-sectional and longitudinal birth data

Most PNMRs are calculated from cross-sectional information on the occurrence and rate of perinatal deaths in a given period, usually over a year, so that data do not follow a cohort of women through their reproductive careers. This is misleading; analysis of data on births and deaths within sibships to the same mother presents different demographic patterns associated with low birthweight and perinatal death, particularly in regard to parity (Roman et al 1978, Bakketeig & Hoffman 1979, 1981).

Table 49.1 Birthweight distribution (%) of births and birthweight-specific perinatal mortality rates per 1000 total births in England and Wales 1983–90 (Source: OPCS DH3 monitors)

Birthweight group (g)	1983		1984		1985		1986		1987		1988		1989		1990	
	%	PNMR/1000	%	PNMR/1000	%	PNMR/1000	%	PNMR/1000	%	PNMR/1000	%	PNMR/1000	%	PNMR/1000	%	PNMR/1000
<1500	0.8	384.0	0.9	365.9	0.9	350.1	0.9	345.5	1.1	322.8	1.1	319.2	1.1	275.6	1.0	279.6
1500–1999	1.3	106.9	1.3	94.7	1.3	93.7	1.4	85.0	1.4	86.5	1.4	82.7	1.3	75.6	1.3	75.7
2000–2499	4.6	29.7	4.5	30.4	4.6	28.3	4.7	27.3	4.6	22.4	4.4	24.1	4.4	22.3	4.4	19.5
2500–2999	18.6	7.5	18.4	7.3	18.4	7.2	18.1	6.6	17.7	6.5	17.1	6.6	16.7	6.1	16.5	5.4
3000–3499	38.6	2.8	38.5	2.8	38.3	2.9	38.1	3.0	37.8	2.6	37.5	2.7	36.2	2.4	36.0	2.5
3500–3999	27.3	2.2	27.6	2.1	27.5	1.8	27.7	2.0								
>3500									37.3	2.1	38.4	2.1	37.3	2.0	37.1	1.8
>4000	8.6	2.9	8.7	2.8	8.9	3.1	9.0	2.7								
Not known	0.1	228.2	0.1	242.0	0.1	195.0	0.1	187.1	0.1	246.7	0.1	119.9	3.1	21.9	3.9	20.8
Total	100	10.4	100	10.1	100	9.5	100	9.5	100	8.9	100	8.7	100	8.3	100	8.1

PNMR = Perinatal mortality rate.

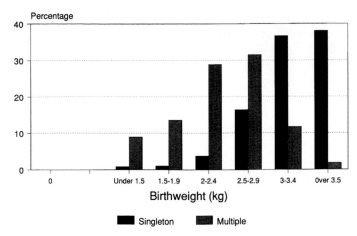

Fig. 49.7 Birthweight distribution, England and Wales, singleton and multiple births 1989. Source: OPCS 1990.

Table 49.2 Birthweight distribution (%) of births and birthweight-specific perinatal mortality rates per 1000 total births for single and multiple births in England and Wales 1989 (source: OPCS 1990)

Birthweight group (g)	Singleton		Multiple	
	%	PNMR/1000	%	PNMR/1000
<1500	0.9	275.3	9.0	279.7
1500–1999	1.1	88.7	13.6	33.5
2000–2499	3.8	24.5	28.9	10.3
2500–2999	16.4	6.2	31.5	6.0
3000–3499	36.7	2.4	11.7	(2.7)
<3500	38.1	2.0	1.9	(13.3)
Not known	3.1	19.6	3.2	129.4
Total	100	7.6	100	39.5

Figures in parentheses are rates based on less than 20 deaths.

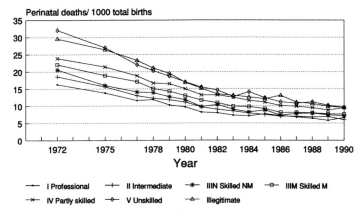

Fig. 49.8 Perinatal mortality by father's social class 1972–90. Source: OPCS Mortality Statistics, DH3 series.

Cross-sectional data suggest a U- or J-shaped pattern of risk with parity, with risk being high in primiparous women, falling in the second pregnancy and then rising with each subsequent pregnancy. Longitudinal studies show that within sibships, average risk seems to fall

steadily with increasing parity, with highest risks at all parities in the largest sibships. This may be caused by overrepresentation of highly parous mothers whose previous pregnancies had ended in a miscarriage, fetal or infant death.

Longitudinal studies can also examine the effects of birth interval—close spacing of pregnancy may contribute to an increased risk of perinatal death and there is also a tendency for repeated perinatal death in the same mothers.

ARE PERINATAL MORTALITY RATES A MEASURE OF MATERNITY AND NEONATAL CARE?

There are several factors which make the continued use of perinatal mortality rates as a measure of the effectiveness of maternity and neonatal care increasingly unsafe.

Perinatal rates include only deaths in the first week of life. Many babies who would previously have died within this period are now surviving into the late neonatal period, thanks to improved paediatric care, but they still die. There is a strong case for including late neonatal deaths in analyses of deaths occurring around the time of delivery to prevent the postponement of death from artificially lowering perinatal rates.

Place of delivery of premature babies of less than 28 weeks' gestation (on the delivery suite or on a gynaecology ward) may affect classification and hence figures for perinatal mortality (Fenton et al 1990). The onus of judgement regarding viability and classification is often placed on relatively junior staff. There is a theoretical possibility that there may be pressure on clinical staff to regard a fetus as non-registrable if the clinical performance of their unit is judged on its crude PNMR alone.

Crude comparisons of perinatal mortality, either by hospital or by district of residence, can be highly misleading because of the problems caused by statistics involving very small numbers in numerator data and large denominators—are the figures due to random variation? Increasingly small numbers and rates of deaths have led OPCS to publish rates for combined 3-year periods with 95% and 99% confidence limits to give some idea of the reliability of the crude figure.

Low and very low birthweight are such strong determinants of perinatal survival that any maternity hospital with a neonatal unit, especially one which takes tertiary referrals, will have a high crude perinatal rate simply because of the types of cases it cares for. Evaluating its services on this basis is akin to castigating a geriatric hospital because of its high numbers of deaths—units looking after high-risk patients have high death rates. Some effort should be made to adjust PNMRs for case mix and referral patterns to get a meaningful result (Clarke et al 1993). Calculating birthweight-specific perinatal rates may help (see Table 49.1), although numbers at individual hospitals will again be very small. Even when this is done, it is difficult to compare the effectiveness of hospital units using PNMRs because of the increasingly small subset of perinatal deaths that are amenable to medical intervention (Field et al 1988).

Other outcome or risk assessment scores may be much more useful. Reliable assessment of neonatal care is impossible without correcting for major risk factors, particularly initial disease severity (Tarnow-Modi et al 1990). One robust method of assessing initial neonatal risk which is more predictive of outcome than birthweight alone is the clinical risk index for babies (CRIB) score (International Neonatal Network 1993). This includes birthweight, gestational age, congenital malformations, maximum base excess in the first 12 hours, and minimum and maximum appropriate fraction of inspired oxygen in the first 12 hours. On the obstetric side, Buekens (1990) describes six outcome measures influenced by process of care and its quality: maternal and perinatal mortalities, postpartum haemorrhage, the sequelae of obstructed labour, Apgar scores and very early neonatal seizures.

While all perinatal deaths are tragic and should not be dismissed lightly, there is concern that death may be preferable to severe long-term impairment and anxiety about the quality of life for some very small babies who would have become part of the perinatal mortality statistics if modern technology had not been used to save them. It is important that in the future as much attention is paid to morbidity arising in the antenatal and perinatal period as has been paid to perinatal mortality in the past.

REFERENCES

Allen M C, Donohoe P K, Dusman A E 1993 The limit of viability—neonatal outcome of infants born at 22 to 25 weeks' gestation. New England Journal of Medicine 329: 1597–1601

Baird D, Walker J, Thomson A M 1954 The causes and prevention of stillbirths and first week deaths. Journal of Obstetrics and Gynaecology of the British Empire 61: 433–448

Bakketeig L S, Hoffman H J 1979 Perinatal mortality by birth order within cohorts based on sibship size. British Medical Journal 2: 693–696

Bakketeig L S, Hoffman H J 1981 Epidemiology of preterm birth. In: Elder M G, Hendricks C H (eds) Results from a longitudinal study of births in Norway in preterm labour. Butterworths International Medical Reviews, London

Balarajan R, Botting B 1989 Perinatal mortality in England and Wales: variations by mother's country of birth (1982–1985). Health Trends 21: 79–84

Black N, Macfarlane A 1982 Methodological kit: monitoring mortality statistics in a health district. Community Medicine 4: 25–33

Bucher H C, Schmidt J G 1993 Does routine ultrasound scanning improve outcome in pregnancy? Meta-analysis of various outcome measures. British Medical Journal 307: 13–17

Buekens P 1990 Outcome measures of obstetrical and perinatal care. Quality Assurance in Health Care 2: 253–262

Butler N R 1967 Causes and prevention of perinatal mortality. WHO Chronicle 21: 43–61

Butler N 1974 Late postnatal consequences of fetal malnutrition. Current Concepts in Nutrition 2: 173–178

Butler N R, Alberman E D (eds) 1969 Perinatal Problems: The Second Report of the 1958 British Perinatal Mortality Survey. E&S Livingstone Ltd, Edinburgh

Butler N R, Bonham D G 1963 Perinatal Mortality. The First Report of the 1958 British Perinatal Mortality Survey. E&S Livingstone, Edinburgh

Callan N A, Witter F R 1990 Intrauterine growth retardation: characteristics, risk factors and gestational age. International Journal of Gynecology and Obstetrics 33: 215–220

Chalmers I 1979 Desirability and Feasibility of a 4th National Perinatal Survey: report submitted to the Children's and Reproductive Research Liaison Group's Research Division of the DHSS. National Perinatal Epidemiology Unit.

Chalmers I, McIlwaine G (eds) 1980 Perinatal audit and surveillance. Proceedings of the 8th study group. RCOG, London

Chamberlain G 1980 Background to better perinatal health. Lancet i: 1–7

Chamberlain R, Chamberlain G, Howlett B, Claireaux A 1975 The first week of life. British births 1970, vol 1. Heinemann Medical, London

Chitty L S, Winter R M 1989 Perinatal mortality in different ethnic groups. Archives of Disease in Childhood 64: 1036–1041

Christianson R E 1979 Gross difference observed in the placentas of smokers and non-smokers. American Journal of Epidemiology 110: 178–187

Clarke M 1982 Perinatal audit: a tried and tested epidemiological method. Community Medicine 4: 104–107

Clarke M, Mason E S 1985 Leatherwork: a possible hazard to reproduction. British Medical Journal 290: 1235–1237

Clarke M, Clayton D G, Mason E S, MacVicar J 1988 Asian mothers' risk factors for perinatal death—the same or different? A ten year review of Leicestershire perinatal deaths. British Medical Journal 297: 384–387

Clarke M, Mason E S, MacVicar J, Clayton D G 1993 Evaluating perinatal mortality rates: effects of referral and case mix. British Medical Journal 306: 824–827

Coggon D, Rose R, Barker D J P 1993 Epidemiology for the uninitiated. BMJ Publishing Group, London

Cole S K, Hey E N, Thomson A M 1986 Classifying perinatal death: an obstetric approach. British Journal of Obstetrics and Gynaecology 93: 1204–1212

Committee on Child Health Services 1976 Fit for the future. Cmnd 6684 (Court report). HMSO, London

Czeizel A E 1993 Prevention of congenital abnormalities by periconceptional multivitamin supplementation. British Medical Journal 306: 1645–1648

Czeizel A E, Dudas I 1992 Prevention of the first occurrence of neural tube defects by periconceptional vitamin supplementation. New England Journal of Medicine 327: 1832–1835

Drillien C M 1974 Prenatal and perinatal factors in etiology and outcome of low birthweight. Clinics in Perinatalogy 1: 197–211

Emanuel I, Filakati H, Alberman E, Evans S J W 1992 Intergenerational studies of human birthweight from the 1958 birth cohort.1. Evidence for a multigenerational effect. British Journal of Obstetrics and Gynaecology 99: 67–74

Enkin M, Keirse J N C, Chalmers I 1989 A guide to effective care in pregnancy and childbirth. Oxford University Press, Oxford

Ewigman B G, Crane J P, Frigoletto F D, Lefevre M L, Bain R P, McNellis D 1993 Effect of ultrasound screening on perinatal outcome. New England Journal of Medicine 329: 821–827

Fenton A C, Field D J, Mason E, Clarke M 1990 Attitudes to viability of preterm infants and their effect on figures for perinatal mortality. British Medical Journal 300: 434–436

Field D J, Smith H, Mason E, Milner A D 1988 Is perinatal mortality a good indicator of perinatal care? Paediatric and Perinatal Epidemiology 2: 213–219

Fitzhardinge P M, Inwood S 1989 Long term growth in small for date children. Acta Paediatrica Scandinavica Supplement 349: 27–33

Hack M H, Fanaroff A A 1989 Outcomes of extremely low birth weight infants between 1982 and 1988. New England Journal of Medicine 321: 1642–1647

Heady J A, Heasman M A 1959 Social and biological factors in infant mortality. Studies on medical and population subjects No 15. HMSO, London

Hellier J 1977 Perinatal mortality 1950 and 1973. Population Trends 10: 13–15

International Neonatal Network 1993 The CRIB (clinical risk index for babies) score: a tool for assessing initial neonatal risk and comparing performance for neonatal intensive care units. Lancet 342: 193–198

Joint Committee of the RCOG and the Population Investigation Committee 1948 Maternity in Great Britain. Oxford University Press, London

Keirse M J N C 1984 Perinatal mortality rates do not contain what they purport to contain. Lancet i: 1166–1169

Lubchenco L O, Hansman C, Dressler M, Boyd E 1963 Intrauterine growth as estimated from liveborn birthweight data at 24 to 42 weeks of gestation. Pediatrics 32: 793–800

Macfarlane A, Mugford M 1984 Birth counts: statistics of pregnancy and childbirth. National Perinatal Epidemiology Unit, OPCS/HMSO, London

McMichael A J, Vimpani G V, Robertson E F, Baghurst P A, Clark P D 1986 The Port Pirie cohort study: maternal blood lead and pregnancy outcome. Journal of Epidemiology and Community Health 40: 18–25

McIlwaine G M, Howat R C L, Dunn F, MacNaughton M C 1979 The Scottish Perinatal Mortality Survey. British Medical Journal 2: 1103–1106

Mersey Region Working Party on Perinatal Mortality 1982 Confidential inquiry into perinatal deaths in the Mersey region. Lancet i: 491–494

MRC Vitamin Study Research Group 1991 Prevention of neural tube defects: results of the Medical Research Council Vitamin Study. Lancet 338: 131–137

Mutch L M M, Brown N J, Spiedel B D, Dunn P M 1981 Perinatal mortality and neonatal survival in Avon: 1976–79. British Medical Journal 282: 119–122

Naeye R 1978 Effects of maternal cigarette smoking on the fetus and placentae. British Journal of Obstetrics and Gynaecology 83: 732–737

Naismith D J 1981 Diet during pregnancy—a rationale for prescription. In: Dobbing J (ed) Maternal nutrition in pregnancy. Eating for two? Academic Press, London, pp 21–40

Nissel M 1987 People count; a history of the General Register Office. HMSO, London

OPCS 1990 Mortality statistics. Perinatal and infant: social and biological factors. Review of the Registrar General on Deaths in England Wales, 1990. Series DH3 No 3. HMSO, London

OPCS 1991 Annual reference volume Series DH6 No 5. Mortality statistics in childhood. HMSO, London

OPCS 1993 Population trends no 74. HMSO, London

Paediatric Research Unit, Royal Devon and Exeter Hospital 1973 A suggested model for inquiries into perinatal and early childhood deaths in a health care district. Children's Research Fund Report

Peckham C S, Marshall W C 1983 Infections in pregnancy. In: Barron S L, Thomson A M (eds) Obstetrical epidemiology. Academic Press, London, pp 209–262

Peller S 1948 Mortality past and future. Population Studies 1: 405–456

RCOG Multidisciplinary Working Group 1992 Prenatal screening for toxoplasmosis in the United Kingdom. RCOG, London

Report on Confidential Enquiries into Maternal Deaths in the UK 1988–90 1994. HMSO, London

Roman E, Doyle P, Beral V, Alberman E, Pharoah P 1978 Fetal loss, gravidity and pregnancy order. Early Human Development 2: 131–138

Rosenberg M J, Feldblum P J, Marshall E G 1987 Occupational influences on reproduction: a review of the recent literature. Journal of Occupational Medicine 29: 584–591

Saari-Kemppainen A, Karjalainen O, Ylostalo P, Heinonen O P 1990 Ultrasound screening and perinatal mortality: controlled trial of systematic one-stage screening in pregnancy. Lancet 336: 387–391

Sanjose S, Roman E, Beral V 1991 Low birthweight and preterm delivery, Scotland, 1981–1984: effect of parents' occupation. Lancet 338: 428–431

Savitz D A, Whelan E A, Kleckner R C 1989 Effect of parents' occupational exposures on risk of stillbirths, preterm delivery, and small for gestational age infants. American Journal of Epidemiology 129: 1201–1218

Shaw C D 1980 Aspects of audit. British Medical Journal 1: 1256

Simpson R J, Armand Smith N G 1986 Maternal smoking and low birthweight: implications for antenatal care. Journal of Epidemiology and Community Health 40: 223–227

Tarnow-Modi W, Ogston S, Wilkinson A R et al 1990 Predicting death from initial disease severity in very low birthweight infants: a method for comparing the performance of neonatal units. British Medical Journal 300: 1611–1614

Thomson A M 1983 Fetal growth and size at birth. In: Barron S L, Thomson A M (eds) Obstetrical epidemiology. Academic Press, London, pp 89–142

Walker E M, Patel N B 1987 Mortality and morbidity in infants born between 20 and 28 weeks gestation. British Journal of Obstetrics and Gynaecology 94: 670–674

Wennergren M, Wennergren G, Vilbergsson G 1988 Obstetric characteristics and neonatal performance in a four-year small for gestational age population. Obstetrics and Gynaecology 72: 615–620

Wigglesworth J S 1980 Monitoring perinatal mortality—a pathological approach. Lancet ii: 684–686

Wood B, Catford J C, Cogswell J J 1984 Confidential paediatric enquiry into neonatal deaths in Wessex, 1981 and 1982. British Medical Journal 288: 1206–1208

World Health Organization 1977 Manual of the international statistical classification of diseases, injuries and causes of death, vol 1. WHO, Geneva

50. Maternal mortality

Geoffrey Chamberlain

INTRODUCTION

Today, both maternal and perinatal deaths are so rare in the developed world that standards of obstetric care cannot be assessed in terms of mortality rates. Up to the 1930s, however, the maternal mortality rate (MMR) was the dominant statistic. The downward trend in overall death rates in Britain between the second half of the 19th century and the mid 1930s is well known. Figure 50.1 shows the death rate from all causes in women aged 15–44 in England and Wales between 1838 and 1993. It illustrates the steady reduction in death rate, interrupted only by the influenza epidemic of 1920. It is now generally agreed that this decline was largely due to improvements in social and economic conditions, primarily in hygiene and nutrition, as well as in medical care (Loudon 1987).

If social and economic improvements were responsible for the fall in the general death rate, the same factors should have produced a fall in MMR. In fact, as Loudon (1987) points out, the fall in maternal deaths should have been even steeper because of advances in obstetric care;

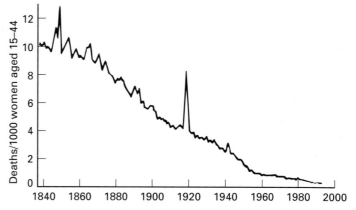

Fig. 50.1   Death rates from all causes in women aged 15–44 in England and Wales from 1838 to 1993. Modified from Loudon (1986a) with permission.

measures were introduced between the late 19th century and the 1930s which were capable of reducing MMR. These included antisepsis and asepsis in the 1870s and 1880s; Caesarean section as a safe technique for some obstetric emergencies, after 1900; the Midwives' Act of 1902; improvements in the teaching of obstetrics and the growing recognition of the importance of antenatal care in the 1920s and 1930s; improved organization of the specialty of obstetrics and gynaecology and higher standards of specialist care associated with the founding of the Royal College of Obstetricians and Gynaecologists in 1929.

Maternal deaths were defined as occurring in pregnancy, labour or the lying-in period. The latter was not clearly defined before the mid 19th century, and some very late deaths were included in early reports. It became the convention that the lying-in period lasted 1 month from birth: nowadays, for registration purposes, it is 6 weeks. Maternal deaths used to be classified as puerperal or associated deaths. Puerperal deaths were due either to puerperal fever (puerperal sepsis) or accidents of childbirth, the latter representing all other deaths and dominated by haemorrhage and toxaemia.

Despite the downward trend in deaths from all causes,

865

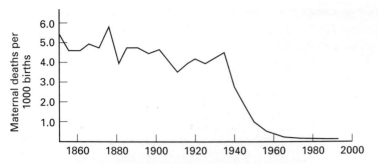

Fig. 50.2 Maternal mortality in England and Wales. Quinquennial rates per 1000 births from 1850 to 1970. Modified from Loudon (1986a) with permission.

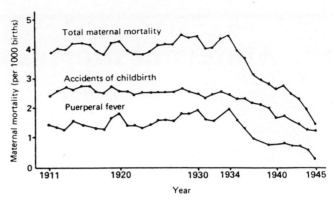

Fig. 50.3 Total maternal morbidity and mortality from puerperal fever and accidents of childbirth in England and Wales from 1911 to 1945. From Loudon (1987) with permission.

shown in Figure 50.1, and the seeming improvements in maternity care, maternal mortality paradoxically refused to fall. Instead, it remained on a plateau from the 1850s to the mid 1930s. Figure 50.2 shows the quinquennial MMR in England and Wales between 1850 and 1993.

The persisting high MMR became a public and political scandal by the 1920s. It was not confined to England and Wales, for the same trends were seen in Scotland, and the rates were even higher in the USA. Even in the Netherlands and Scandinavia, where maternal mortality was lower than in Britain or the USA, the rates stayed level rather than falling. The trends in maternal mortality over these years and the factors which predisposed to the lack of improvement have been reviewed by Loudon (1992).

In England and Wales, maternal mortality finally began to drop in the thirties and when it did, the fall was sudden, profound and sustained, continuing to the present time. There have been few more remarkable statistical changes during the 20th century. At about the same time the fall occurred in all the developed countries, in Europe, Scandinavia and the USA. There is little doubt that this change was first initiated by the introduction of sulphonamides, but after the first few years, they cannot have been the only explanation.

Figure 50.3 shows the importance of the reduction in deaths from puerperal fever in the overall fall in MMR after 1934. There was little reduction in deaths from accidents of childbirth between 1911 and 1934, after which a gradual fall began. By contrast, deaths from puerperal fever showed more variation, with peaks of high mortality in 1920, 1930 and 1934, and low rates in 1913 and 1918. After 1934, the reduction in deaths from puerperal fever was rapid; it accounted for 78% of the total reduction in maternal deaths in England and Wales between 1934 and 1940. Loudon (1987) argues convincingly that sulphonamides were generally available, widely used and known to be effective by late 1937. The possibility of a simultaneous decline in streptococcal virulence was suggested by several experienced observers, notably Colebrooke (1936), but the most likely hypothesis is nevertheless

that the improvement was due mainly to the introduction of sulphonamides. They probably brought about the sustained fall in MMR between 1937 and the early 1940s. As Loudon (1987) stresses, the first year with a notable fall in maternal mortality was 1937.

The death rates from puerperal fever were actually lower in 1913 and 1918 than they were in 1935 or 1936. Only in 1937, when deaths from puerperal fever reached a new low level, could it be said with confidence that a new factor had come into operation. After 1940, penicillin, blood transfusion and better obstetric care played increasingly important roles in lowering maternal mortality and tended to eclipse the early but vital contribution of the sulphonamides.

CAUSES OF UNDIMINISHED MATERNAL MORTALITY BEFORE 1937

The high MMR in England and Wales between 1850 and 1937 was not simply the result of lack of sulphonamides or other antibiotics. In general, the persistently high maternal mortality was probably due to either poor obstetric care, resulting from poor training or poor clinical application, or to social and economic deprivation, adversely influencing the health of the mother and her ability to withstand the stresses of pregnancy and birth.

After reviewing all the evidence, Loudon (1986a) concluded that poor obstetric care was much the more important. 'Maternal mortality appears to be remarkably resistant to the ill effects of social and economic deprivation, but remarkably sensitive to the good and bad effects of medical intervention.'

Between the mid 19th century and the 1930s, maternal mortality tended to be higher in the middle and upper social classes than in the working classes (Loudon 1986b). Most births took place at home under the care of midwives or general practitioners; there was a strong association between social class and attendance by doctors.

For first pregnancies, 82% of the wives of professional or salaried workers were delivered by doctors, compared with only 35% of the wives of manual workers. That study was conducted in 1946; the difference was probably even greater in the 1920s and 1930s. Because the vast majority of births were domiciliary the outcome of home delivery was largely responsible for the national level of maternal mortality.

Excessive obstetric intervention

In the second half of the 19th century there was a profound change in obstetric practice. During the preceding 80 or 90 years, practice had been extremely conservative. From the 1870s, however, obstetricians, especially those in general practice, began to intervene in normal labour to an astonishing extent. They took their lead from those who advocated the active use of forceps delivery, usually under general anaesthesia. From the end of the 19th century (Loudon 1986a), forceps delivery under chloroform or anaesthesia was used in 50 or even 70% of domiciliary deliveries. This was justified on the grounds that modern women should not be expected to bear the pains of normal labour. There was also widespread disregard of antiseptic practice and little interest in antenatal care.

By contrast, extremely good results were often reported in home confinements conducted by midwives trained by charities. The poor of the great cities were delivered by midwives. The Liverpool Ladies' Charity, for example, reported an MMR of 1.3 per 1000 in over 6000 deliveries, undertaken in the poorest homes in the city (Bickerton 1936). Such good results would have been unlikely if socioeconomic deprivation was a major cause of high maternal mortality.

THE ROCHDALE EXPERIMENT

Important evidence for the importance of good obstetric care came from the famous Rochdale experiment of the early 1930s. When Dr Andrew Topping was appointed Medical Officer of Health to Rochdale in 1930, the city had the highest maternal mortality in the country, just under nine per 1000 births. By vigorous reformation of the maternity services, but with no alteration to the diet or living conditions of the poor, the MMR was reduced to 1.7 per 1000 births by 1935, showing that obstetric care was the decisive factor. The measures introduced were simple. Publicity, with the help of the press, led to a high attendance rate at specially established antenatal clinics; general practitioners were alerted to the serious hazards of interference in labour; good cooperation was established between midwives, general practitioners and a consultant, recruited from Manchester; a puerperal fever ward was opened. When the Rochdale experiment

was reviewed (Oxley et al 1935), the previously high MMR could not be attributed to economic disabilities; it had been due much more to obstetrical factors which in many instances had proved preventable.

It would be a mistake, however, to conclude that poverty and malnutrition do not influence maternal mortality. The lesson of the period between 1850 and 1930 is that the persistence of a high MMR resulted from poor obstetric care, with excessive intervention by poorly trained general practitioner obstetricians at home confinements. In this situation, the better-off who could afford a general practitioner fared worse than the poor, who were looked after by a midwife whose care was likely to be less interventionist. Obstetric care has improved a great deal over the past 50 years and analysis nowadays demonstrates the expected trend, with MMR being lower in social classes 1 and 2 and higher in 4 and 5 (Confidential Enquiries into Maternal Deaths 1979–81).

CONFIDENTIAL AND MEDICAL ENQUIRY INTO INDIVIDUAL MATERNAL DEATHS

Although the MMR did not begin to fall significantly until 1937, an organization for recording and publicizing the causation of maternal deaths in England and Wales was originally set up in 1928 by the Minister of Health, Neville Chamberlain, when he established a Departmental Committee on Maternal Mortality and Morbidity. In that year alone there were 2920 maternal deaths in relation to 660 267 live births, an MMR of 4.42 per 1000 births or 442 per 100 000. In 1930, the departmental committee introduced the concept of a primary avoidable factor in maternal deaths in its interim report and published its final report in 1932. The investigation covered 5800 cases and proved so valuable that Medical Officers of Health were asked to continue the enquiries, submitting their confidential reports to the Chief Medical Officer of the Ministry of Health. This continued up to the end of 1951; summaries of the enquiries appeared in successive annual reports on the state of the public health. A primary avoidable factor was considered to be present in 46% of the cases investigated in the first report, but the proportion with avoidable factors altered very little in subsequent years, although the number of deaths diminished markedly from 1937. The diminishing urgency of maternal mortality, combined with other problems during the war years, led to enquiries being conducted in a decreasing proportion of registered maternal deaths. By 1951, reports were received for only about 60% of known deaths. New methods were clearly needed to study preventability in the smaller number of deaths then occurring.

In 1949, maternal mortality was the subject of a discussion at the 12th British Congress on Obstetrics and

Gynaecology and reference was made to a method of enquiry sometimes use in the USA—investigation by a local committee of experts, publication of case reports and comments in medical journals. The president of the congress, Sir Eardley Holland, suggested to the Minister of Health the possibility of adopting a similar method in this country. Consultations followed with the Royal College of Obstetricians and Gynaecologists and the Society of Medical Officers of Health, resulting in the adoption of a new system of enquiry involving the family doctor, the Medical Officer of Health, the midwife and the consultant obstetrician. These Confidential Enquiries into Maternal Deaths (CEMD) commenced in 1952 and the findings of the first triennial report, 1952–54, were published in 1957 by Her Majesty's Stationery Office. Triennial reports on these confidential enquiries have been published for the 11 triennia since then. That for 1982–84 was the last for England and Wales, because reports from 1985 have been published on a UK basis. Previously, Scotland had produced a quinquennial report and Northern Ireland a decennial report.

CEMD in England and Wales from 1952 to 1990

These 13 confidential enquiries have provided an unique monitoring system for maternal mortality during the past 38 years in England and Wales with the latest report incorporating data from the whole of the UK (England, Wales, Scotland and Northern Ireland). While studies of maternal mortality have been published in many countries, for example by Högberg (1985) on maternal mortality in Sweden, there is no national surveillance organization

for the detailed investigation of every maternal death in any country outside the UK.

Constant rate of fall in maternal mortality

Figure 50.4 is similar to the graph of maternal mortality shown in Figure 50.1, but based on annual rather than quinquennial rates between 1847 and 1982. Figure 50.4 appears to indicate that the main fall in maternal mortality began in 1937 and was at first extremely rapid, particularly during the was years and immediately afterwards. When the CEMD commenced in 1952, the death rate was only a fraction of what it had been in 1937 and the fall between 1952 and 1984 looks relatively insignificant. However, such a graph is unduly influenced by the very large number of deaths in the earlier years, which must have been potentially avoidable by relatively minor improvements in care. As triennia pass and the MMR falls even lower, the number of potentially avoidable deaths inevitably becomes smaller so that in the latest enquiry covering the years 1988–90 there were only 173 maternal deaths in the UK to be compared with 2 360 309 births—a rate of 7 per 100 000 deliveries (Fig. 50.5).

To avoid the bias resulting from the larger number of deaths in earlier years, the changing MMR may be expressed on a logarithmic scale. Figure 50.6 shows MMR between 1850 and 1970 expressed in this way and reveals that the rate of reduction in MMR has been maintained between 1937 and 1970. In other words, since the MMR first began to fall in England and Wales, the rate of improvement has been constant, approximately halving every 10 years. From over 4000 per million in

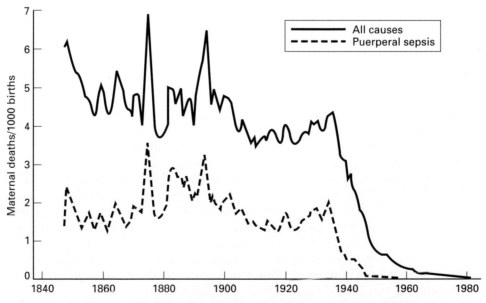

Fig. 50.4 Maternal mortality in England and Wales from 1847 to 1982. From Confidential Enquiries into Maternal Deaths in England and Wales 1982–84.

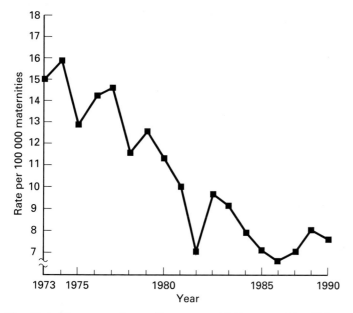

Fig. 50.5 The maternal mortality rate per 100 000 maternities, UK 1973–90. Source: Confidential Enquiry into Maternal Deaths in England and Wales 1988–90.

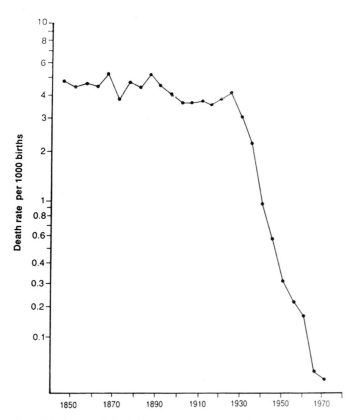

Fig. 50.6 Maternal mortality in England and Wales from 1850 to 1970. Quinquennial rates per 1000 births; semilogarithmic graph. From Loudon (1986a) with permission.

1937, the rate has fallen to 86 per million by 1982–84, so that after almost 50 years MMR has fallen to one-fiftieth of its original level. Since the rate of reduction between 1952 and 1984 has been just as fast as it was between 1937 and 1951, the findings of the CEMD between 1952 and 1984 are clearly of the greatest relevance for achieving continued improvement in the obstetric services.

The method for conducting the CEMD

At the start, enquiry into known or suspected maternal deaths was initiated by the Medical Officer of Health of the town or district. With re-organization of the National Health Service, this post became that of Area Medical Officer and, in turn, subsequently, District Medical Officer then Director of Public Health Services. The enquiry form (MCW97), which has been modified, developed and expanded over the years, is sent to all health staff concerned in the care of the woman, including the midwife, general practitioner, health visitor, community physician, consultant obstetrician and any other individual involved in the death. Every possible attempt is also made to obtain details of autopsy, including histology.

When all available local information has been collected, the Consultant in Public Health forwards the partially completed form to the Regional Obstetric Assessor, a senior consultant obstetrician in the region appointed by the Chief Medical Officer. The Regional Anaesthetic Assessor also reviews the enquiry forms of women who have had an anaesthetic. While there have been Regional Assessors in Obstetrics and Anaesthetics since the earliest years of the CEMD, it was only in 1981 that Regional Pathology Assessors were appointed. They also review the MCW97 forms and add their comments and opinions about the autopsy findings.

The MCW97 form is then sent to the Chief Medical Officer at the Department of Health and Social Security. The Department's Central Assessors in Obstetrics and Gynaecology, Anaesthetics and Histopathology review all facts recorded in each case and act as final arbiters in assessing the main cause of death, any contributing factors and whether or not care was of the accepted standard. Strict confidentiality is observed at all stages of the CEMD. The identity of the patient is erased from all forms so that the opinion of assessors cannot be related to a named individual. After the completion of each triennial report, all MCW97 forms are destroyed.

For each death a single main cause is allotted and classified according to the WHO *International Classification of Diseases, Injuries and Causes of Death*, 9th revision (ICD 9) (1975). Although deaths are assigned to one main cause, they may be referred to in other chapters. Thus, a death assigned to hypertensive diseases of pregnancy, in which haemorrhage and anaesthesia also played a part, might be mentioned in all three chapter, but would only be counted as a death from hypertensive diseases.

CLASSIFICATION OF MATERNAL DEATHS

Until the 1973–75 triennial report, deaths were coded under the *International Classification of Deaths*, 8th revision (WHO 1967). Up to that time, deaths classified under the heading of complications of pregnancy, childbirth and the puerperium were classified as true maternal deaths, while deaths with main causes coded elsewhere in the International Classification, in women known to have been pregnant at the time of death or to have been pregnant within 1 year of death, were classified as associated maternal deaths.

ICD 9, introduced in 1979, defined maternal deaths as:

1. *Direct*, resulting from obstetrical complications of the pregnant state (pregnancy, labour and the puerperium), from interventions, omissions, incorrect treatment or from a chain of events resulting from any of the above.
2. *Indirect*, resulting from previous existing disease, or diseases which developed during pregnancy and were not due to direct obstetric causes but aggravated by physiological effects of the pregnancy.
3. *Fortuitous*—deaths from other causes, which fortuitously occur in pregnancy or the puerperium, are excluded from maternal mortality as internationally defined. These have been defined as fortuitous deaths in the triennial reports on CEMD from 1976 to 1978.

This new classification has helped to overcome the type of difficulty noted in previous reports, when a death could be classified as associated, even if the pregnancy had brought it to light or caused exacerbation of a pre-existing condition, making it indirect.

A further recommendation of ICD 9 is that maternal death should be defined as the death of a woman while pregnant or within 42 days of termination of pregnancy, irrespective of the duration and the site of the pregnancy, from any cause related to or aggravated by the pregnancy or its management, but not from an accidental or incidental cause. This is in line with the definition adopted by the International Federation of Gynaecology and Obstetrics (FIGO) and is included in previous reports. In the CEMD, maternal death had always been defined as one occurring during pregnancy or labour, or as a consequence of pregnancy, within 1 year of delivery or abortion. This wider definition has the advantage of including deaths in which the period of the survival is longer than 42 days but in which pregnancy played an important role. Late deaths (after 42 days) have been included in all the triennial reports but their presence has been specifically indicated since they were not included within the FIGO definition. From the 1979–81 report onwards, late deaths have been documented separately in an additional chapter.

Denominators for calculation of incidence and rates

Historically, MMR was defined as the number of maternal deaths per 1000 total births. Strictly this is not a rate but a ratio for the denominator is not included in the numerator as it must in a rate. Deaths include those associated with ectopic pregnancy and abortions while the denominator refers to maternities, i.e. women giving birth to viable babies not all those pregnant. Thus the term ratio is mathematically correct but rate has been used for many years. The CEMD has based mortality rates on the number of maternitics. This is the number of mothers delivered as distinct from the number of babies born, which is larger because it includes infants from multiple births. As MMR has fallen, it has proved necessary to express the rate per 10^4, 10^5 and in the most recent reports, per 10^6 maternities. The change in the reports after 1985 when the total population of the UK was examined did not have a major effect on the resulting statistics. Table 50.1 shows that although the maternal mortality rate per 100 000 ranges from 2.4 to 7.4 in the four Kingdoms, the number of births in the three Celtic Kingdoms is too few to alter the total rate of 6.1 much from that of England at 6.2 per 100 000.

To provide realistic denominators for deaths occurring in early pregnancy, such as ectopic pregnancy or abortion, Office of Population Censuses and Surveys (OPCS) data have been used to calculate total pregnancies, a figure including legal and spontaneous abortions, ectopic pregnancies and total maternities (Table 50.2). Many rates have been calculated from this denominator since 1979–81.

Table 50.1 Direct maternal deaths in CEMD by area of residence: 1985–87 and 1988–90

Area	Total births (no.)	Direct deaths (no.)	Direct MMR (per 100 000)
UK	4 666 120	284	6.1
England	3 876 169	240	6.2
Wales	228 495	17	7.4
Scotland	396 509	23	5.8
N. Ireland	164 947	4	42.4

Table 50.2 Total maternities and total pregnancies in England and Wales from 1970 to 1984 (from Confidential Enquiries into Maternal Deaths 1982–84)

Triennium	Total maternities	Total pregnancies
1970–72	2 222 500	2 732 600
1973–75	1 851 900	2 366 800
1976–78	1 781 300	2 275 800
1979–81	1 910 900	2 437 800
1982–84	1 905 800	2 427 000

AVOIDABLE FACTORS OR SUBSTANDARD CARE

From 1930, when the Departmental Committee on Maternal Mortality identified a *primary avoidable factor* in some maternal deaths, the annual reports of the Chief Medical Officer up to 1950, and subsequently the triennial reports on the CEMD from 1952 to 1978, have included data on the incidence of avoidable factors. An avoidable factor was considered present if there was a departure from generally accepted standards of satisfactory care, or if the care provided was considered inappropriate in the circumstances. In the 1979–81 report, the term *substandard care* was substituted for avoidable factors to take into account not only failures in clinical care but also some of the underlying factors which may have produced a low standard of care for the patient. These included shortage of resources for staffing facilities, administrative failure in the maternity services or in back-up facilities such as anaesthetic, radiological or pathology services. It was considered that the term *avoidable factors* had often been misinterpreted as meaning that avoiding these factors would have prevented the death.

In 1952–54, the incidence of avoidable factors was approximately 45%. By 1976–78, the incidence had increased to approximately 58%. This apparent increase resulted more from increasingly high standards of assessment than from deterioration in management.

It has proved more difficult quantitatively to assess the incidence of substandard care since 1979. Apart from those due to pulmonary or amniotic fluid embolism, a high proportion of deaths due to other causes are still associated with substandard care. For example substandard care was evident in 88% of deaths due to hypertension, 63% of those due to haemorrhage and 37% of deaths following abortion. Considerable further improvement must therefore be possible, although maternal mortality has now fallen to such a low level.

TRENDS IN CAUSES OF MATERNAL MORTALITY FROM 1952 TO 1984

The numbers of deaths from individual causes from 1952 to 1969 are shown in Table 50.3, from 1970 to 1984 in Table 50.4 and 1988–90 (for UK) in Table 50.5. The direct maternal death rate by cause as a rate per million

Table 50.3 Numbers of direct deaths by cause from 1952 to 1969 in England and Wales (from Confidential Enquiries into Maternal Deaths 1982–84)

Causes	1952–54	1955–57	1958–60	1961–63	1964–66	1967–69
Hypertensive diseases of pregnancy	246	171	118	104	67	53
Pulmonary embolism	138	157	132	129	91	75
Abortion	153	141	135	139	133	117
Haemorrhage	188	138	130	92	68	41
Anaesthesia	Not classified separately				50*	50†
Ectopic pregnancy	No separate chapter			42	42	32
Amniotic fluid embolism	Not recognized			27	30	27
Sepsis (excluding abortion)	Included in abortion			33	57	26
Ruptured uterus	No separate chapter			38	30	18
Other direct causes	All other direct deaths					
	369	254	227	88	61	66
Total	1094	861	742	692	579	455

* Calculated later; † not in total.

Table 50.4 Numbers of direct deaths by cause* from 1970 to 1984 in England and Wales (from Confidential Enquiries into Maternal Deaths 1982–84)

Causes	1970–72	1973–75	1976–78	1979–81	1982–84
Hypertensive diseases of pregnancy	47	39	29	36	25
Pulmonary embolism	52	33	43	23	25
Abortion	71	27	14	14	11
Haemorrhage	27	21	24	14	9
Anaesthesia	37	22	27	22	18
Ectopic pregnancy	34	19	21	20	10
Amniotic fluid embolism†	16	14	11	18	14
Sepsis (excluding abortion)	30	19	15	8	2
Ruptured uterus	13	11	14	4	3
Other direct causes	13	22	19	17	21
Total	340	227	217	176	138

* Late deaths were excluded; †confirmed histologically.

Table 50.5   Number of direct deaths by cause from 1985 to 1990 in the UK (from Confidential Enquiries into Maternal Deaths 1988–90)

	1985–87	1988–90
Hypertensive diseases of pregnancy	27	27
Pulmonary embolism	32	33
Haemorrhage	10	22
Anaesthesia	6	4
Ectopic pregnancy and abortion	22	24
Amniotic fluid embolism	9	11
Genital tract sepsis	6	7
Genital tract trauma	6	3
Other direct deaths	21	14
Total	139	145

maternities from 1973 to 1990 is shown in Table 50.6. The first six triennia were dominated by deaths from hypertensive diseases of pregnancy, pulmonary embolism, haemorrhage and abortion. Bearing in mind the fluctuation in the number of maternities during the triennia between 1952 and 1990, the rates shown in Table 50.6 are more reliable indicators of trends than the numbers of deaths in Tables 50.3–50.5.

There was a dramatic reduction in the MMR from hypertensive diseases of pregnancy and from haemorrhage between 1952–54 and 1958–60, and perhaps because of this it may have been easy to improve on previously very poor standards of care. By comparison, the MMR from pulmonary embolism fell relatively little over these years. Since deaths from abortion showed no improvement, this became the main cause of death between 1958–60 and 1970–72. In these years, the reports comment repeatedly on the dangers of home confinement in women with a previous history of haemorrhage, of inadequate anticipation or treatment of the complications of hypertensive disease, on the need for better booking arrangements and for effective flying squad facilities.

With haemorrhage deaths, the introduction in 1962 of a combined preparation of oxytocin and ergometrine for intramuscular use must have helped to maintain the reduction in deaths from this cause over the first six triennia. Table 50.6 shows that between 1970 and 1984 deaths from haemorrhage continued to fall, perhaps because of better management, the avoidance of unwanted

high-risk pregnancy in women of high parity and possibly because of better prophylaxis in second- and third-stage labour.

Perhaps the most dramatic change in the CEMD has been the effect of the Abortion Act (1967) which came into force in 1968. Abortion remained the main cause of death in 1967–69 and although there was a marked reduction in deaths from criminal and spontaneous abortion in 1970–72, abortion was still the main cause of death in that triennium because there was an increase in therapeutic abortion deaths associated with many relatively late abortions and the continuing use of techniques such as hysterotomy, often combined with sterilization, or hysterectomy. By 1973–75, legal abortions were more often being performed earlier in pregnancy and more often by simple, vaginal techniques and the abortion MMR fell. By 1982–84, the death rate from abortion was very low indeed and for the first time there were no deaths from criminal abortion. This reflection of the changes since the Abortion Act continues in the reports of 1985–87 and 1988–90 when no deaths occurred from illegal abortions in any of the four kingdoms, thus continuing for nine consecutive years a nil return of deaths, while in the world data about a fifth of maternal deaths are from this cause.

Table 50.6 shows that in the six triennia between 1973 and 1990, there was little improvement in MMR from pulmonary embolism. A slight reduction was seen from hypertensive cause but this left this and pulmonary embolism as the equal main causes of death in 1990. Although the MMR from hypertensive diseases of pregnancy is lower in the 1980s than in the 1950s, the slow improvement in the last 15 years has been disappointing. The recent CEMD has highlighted the serious hazards of hypertensive diseases, which can develop insidiously and progress rapidly to a dangerous stage with little warning. Death is still mainly due to cerebral haemorrhage, probably the result of failure to control severe hypertension, but can also result from disseminated intravascular coagulation, renal failure or liver necrosis. These complications can all be anticipated by appropriate investigations (repeated platelet counts, blood urea, urate, creatinine and AST). Establishment of expert teams in each region has been suggested, either to advise about management or to

Table 50.6   Direct maternal death by cause, rates per million estimated pregnancies, England and Wales 1973–90*

	Pulmonary embolism	Hypertensive disorders of pregnancy	Anaesthesia	Amniotic fluid embolism	Abortion	Ectopic pregnancy	Haemorrhage	Sepsis, excluding abortion	Ruptured uterus	Other direct causes	All deaths
1973–75	12.8	13.2	10.5	5.4	10.5	7.4	8.1	7.4	4.3	8.5	88.0
1976–78	18.5	12.5	11.6	4.7	6.0	9.0	10.3	6.5	6.0	8.2	93.4
1979–81	9.0	14.2	8.7	7.1	5.5	7.9	5.5	3.1	1.6	7.5	70.0
1982–84	10.0	10.0	7.2	5.6	4.4	4.0	3.6	1.0	1.2	8.4	55.0
1985–87	9.1	9.4	1.9	3.4	2.3	4.1	3.8	2.3	1.9	7.5	45.6
1988–90	8.0	8.6	1.0	3.5	2.4	5.2	7.3	2.1	0.7	8.3	47.0

* Rates for the UK were not available as there was no information on pregnancies for Scotland and Northern Ireland.

take over cases if requested. In the 1988–90 survey, the authors report surveying UK obstetric units and finding that 9% still have not eclampsia prolocol and 24% no intensive care unit on the same site.

Pulmonary embolism remains a major problem largely because no effective method has been developed for preventing it or for detecting deep vein thrombosis early. The triennial reports have repeatedly stressed the importance of an awareness of factors predisposing to pulmonary embolism. The 1982–84 report draws attention to the hazard of pulmonary embolism in women delivered by elective Caesarean section for severe hypertensive diseases of pregnancy. This was re-emphasized in the 1988–90 report and additional warnings were given about older and plumper mothers. Further, much greater surveillance of antenatal potential thrombotic factors should be stressed and the value of prophylactic anticoagulation in pregnancy re-stressed.

While the period between 1952 and 1959 was dominated by four main causes of death, the period between 1970 and 1984 has seen the emergence of new major causes of death. Thus, in 1979–81, complications of anaesthesia were the third main cause of death, followed by ectopic pregnancy and amniotic fluid embolism. In 1982–84, anaesthesia was again the third commonest cause of death followed by amniotic fluid embolism, abortion, ectopic pregnancy and haemorrhage. By 1990 anaesthesia had dropped considerably in ranking order leaving ectopic pregnancy third in frequency.

There has been a reduction in deaths associated with anaesthesia sustained on the last two triennial reports of the UK. However numbers are small and perhaps they should be set against the general anaesthetics given. There is probably a reduction since 1953 for regional, epidural, and spinal blocks are much more frequently used for elective Caesarean sections and pudendal blocks for vaginal operative deliveries than in the middle years of the century. Intubation errors are not so commonly reported and the use of H_2 receptor blocking drugs is advised to prevent acid reflux. Pulsed oxymetry and CO_2 analysis of expired air is strongly recommended. The large number of women who died with adult respiratory distress syndrome is noted even though their cause of death is recorded elsewhere.

That deaths from amniotic fluid embolism are of relatively increasing importance is hardly surprising because no advance has been made in its prevention, detection or treatment. The MMR has remained practically unchanged.

Deaths from sepsis after abortion are mentioned in the CEMD chapter on genital sepsis, but are actually counted in the abortion chapter. Deaths from genital sepsis include deaths from puerperal sepsis, from sepsis after surgical procedures and from sepsis before or during labour. While the huge reduction in deaths from sepsis between 1952–54 and 1967–69 was impressive, the reduction in

the MMR from sepsis between 1970 and 1990 has in fact been equally rapid.

The incidence of ectopic pregnancy has not increased as much in England and Wales as in some European countries, the figures in the CEMD show that deaths following ectopic pregnancy have decreased in absolute numbers but the rank remains about the same because of reductions in the other indices. Since many of the deaths occur very early in pregnancy, improvements may be associated with increasingly sophisticated diagnostic tests, including rapid sensitive assays of beta-human chorionic gonadotrophin in urine or blood, improved ultrasound diagnosis including transvaginal scanning (Urquhart & Fisk 1988) and a more rapid recourse to laparoscopic investigation in women with pelvic pain of uncertain origin. Alternatively, it may transpire that the improvements since 1982–84 were simply due to chance.

Ruptured uterus deaths have fallen considerably, perhaps because of increasing awareness of the dangers of excessive uterine stimulation with oxytocic drugs, especially in women previously delivered by Caesarean section, or with possible cephalopelvic disproportion in labour.

Other direct deaths, also classified as miscellaneous, show a varying incidence over the triennia, reflecting the difficulty of reliably attributing to this category direct deaths not readily attributed to other causes.

CAESAREAN SECTION

If there was as little information about the total number of Caesarean sections as about anaesthetics, the MMR, expressed per million maternities, would show the same unsatisfactory trend. However, the increasing number of Caesarean sections in each triennium is clear; the rate has risen from 5.2% in 1970–72 to 10.9% in 1985–90. From these data, the fatality rate per 1000 Caesarean sections can be calculated and shows a steady rate of improvement (Table 50.7). In 1979–81 there was concern that despite a falling fatality rate, the number of Caesarean sections had increased so much that the number of deaths was actually increasing. However, the fall in the number of Caesarean section deaths since is reassuring, although the future trend must be watched. Figure 50.7 illustrates how the fatality rate has continued to fall steadily despite the rising Caesarean section rate.

Table 50.8 shows that when only direct deaths are considered, the Caesarean fatality rate over the past five triennia has fallen even more than the MMR from all causes until the last two reports when it rose. The percentage of direct deaths associated with Caesarean section has increased from 24% to 42%; this may mean that an increasing proportion of women with severe problems in late pregnancy are delivered by Caesarean section.

Further analysis of the 1982–84 figures showed that the incidence of direct deaths from elective Caesarean

Table 50.7 Estimated number of Caesarean sections performed and estimated mortality rate per 1000 Caesarean sections within 42 days in NHS hospitals in England and Wales for each triennium (from Confidential Enquiries into Maternal Deaths 1982–84)

	1970–72	1973–75	1976–78	1979–81	1982–84	1985–90
Total maternities in NHS hospitals	2 000 612	1 799 980	1 689 670	1 876 570	1 840 970	2 087 442
Estimated number of Caesarean sections	103 310	101 410	120 570	167 020	185 820	228 413
Percentage of maternities by Caesarean sections in NHS hospitals	5.2	5.6	7.1	8.9	10.1	10.9
Deaths after Caesarean sections (direct maternal and associated deaths from enquiry series)	102	77	80	87	69	85
Estimated fatality rate per 1000 Caesarean sections	0.99	0.76	0.66	0.52	0.37	0.37

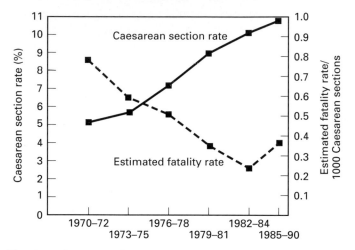

Fig. 50.7 Percentage Caesarean section rate and estimated fatality rate per 1000 Caesarean sections in England and Wales from 1970 to 1990. From Confidential Enquiries into Maternal Deaths with permission.

sections was only 0.09 per 1000 operations, compared with 0.37 per 1000 emergency operations. A similar difference was found in the previous triennium, but the 1982–84 report does not show the reason for the high mortality rate amongst the emergency group. Undoubtedly the conditions for which the operation is performed carry greater risks among women undergoing emergency procedures. Since it is rarely possible to predict the need for delivery by emergency Caesarean section, attempting to reduce the number by performing more elective operations would be likely merely to increase the overall Caesarean section rate. However, the comments about obstetric anaesthetic services are also relevant to the performance of Caesarean section.

DEATH ASSOCIATED WITH CARDIAC DISEASE

Maternal death rates associated with cardiac disease are dropping sharply. Table 50.9 shows this reduction over 30 years. Most of the improvement has come in the acquired heart disease category in the mid 1970s, while deaths from congenital abnormalities have reduced but not so dramatically. Among the acquired disease deaths, ischaemic heart disease now accounts for as many cases as rheumatic disease. It is a sad reflection that, in the latest Confidential Enquiry into Maternal Deaths, eight of the nine cases of acquired heart disease were judged to have had substandard care; four of these were women who had refused medical advice while the rest were professional shortcomings. Possibly, the women who disregarded professional advice had not been advised strongly enough; when faced with a life-threatening condition, a doctor should not hesitate to say so, for women now wish to be better informed and they should be. Prepregnancy counselling would be wise here to warn of forthcoming risks and possible intrusive management to care (e.g. hospital admission). If the woman then entered into pregnancy with known cardiac hazards, she should be seen at a special antenatal clinic with an obstetrician and a cardiologist attending also so they may see the woman together and consult on her condition.

Amongst the congenital lesions, a full spectrum of the conditions expected in this age group was found. The numbers have stayed fairly constant in the past 20 years but since the acquired disease cases are reducing, the proportion of congenital heart disease contributing to the total has now increased and is now about half the total.

Again, substandard care occurred in the majority of

Table 50.8 Number of direct maternal deaths within 42 days of Caesarean section (from Confidential Enquiries into Maternal Deaths 1982–84)

	1970–72	1973–75	1976–78	1979–81	1982–84	1985–87	1988–90
All direct deaths	340	227	217	175	138	139	145
Direct deaths from Caesarean section	81	60	61	59	44	42	58
Percentage of all direct deaths	24	26	28	34	32	35	42
Caesarean section rate (%)	5.16	5.63	7.14	8.90	10.09	NK	10.9
Estimated fatality rate/1000 Caesarean section	0.78	0.59	0.51	0.35	0.24	NK	0.25

NK = not known.

Table 50.9 Number of maternal deaths in England and Wales 1961–90 (Source: Confidential Enquiry into Maternal Deaths)

	All cases	Acquired			Congenital
		Ischaemic	Other	All	
1961–63	71	NA	NA	68	13
1964–66	50	NA	NA	43	7
1967–69	49	NA	NA	34	15
1970–72	42	NA	NA	33	9
1973–75	18	NA	NA	14	4
1976–78	17	NA	NA	14	3
1079–81	16	6	6	12	4
1082–84	17	8	3	11	6
1985–87	19	6	3	9	10
1988–90	14	4	4	8	6

cases of deaths from acquired heart disease. Much of this involved the professionals who had not recognized the heart condition or had underestimated its effects. It is important that when a woman presents for the first time in a pregnancy, a careful history and clinical examination are performed to exclude congenital heart disease. Further, comparatively minor symptoms in another woman should be treated with graver respect than one with heart disease, e.g. small pains in the chest in a woman with Marfan's syndrome.

MATERNAL MORTALITY IN DEVELOPING COUNTRIES

While the MMR in the developed countries ranges between 6 and 50 per 100 000 live births, the MMR in developing countries still remains between 100 and 3500 deaths per 100 000 live births (Högberg 1985).

For these countries, the experience of Europe and the USA should be helpful. In general, the present problems of the developing countries have similarities to those in the developed countries before 1850. As Walker (1986) pointed out, maternal mortality must rank with some infectious diseases as among the few instances where medical care has achieved a dramatic reduction in mortality rates. In support of the proposal that effective medical care has been more important than improved socio-economic status in reducing maternal mortality, he quoted the study of Kaunitz et al (1984) who reported that in a religious group avoiding obstetric care in the USA, MMR between 1975 and 1982 was 87 per 10 000 live births—a level over 90 times higher than in the remainder of the state of Indiana and comparable with that in many developing countries. Walker (1986) also noted that many maternal deaths in developing countries could be prevented if the number of births to older, high parity women could be reduced by appropriate family planning.

The position of women in society in many countries of the developing world is considerably inferior to that of men. They are less educated and have less say in the affairs of their family, society and country. This needs redressing but must be done from inside the country according to the wishes of the people and not imposed from the West as a catch-all cure. The birth rates are high in many developing countries and one of the major associations with maternal mortality is high parity. If a reduction of family size could be achieved, there would be a drop in maternal mortality; this comes not just with the wider use of family planning but with improved total health, for then less children would die in infancy and so the mother will be reassured that more of her babies would survive childhood. Reduced parity will also be followed by not just an improvement of the woman's health but a reduction in the risk of death in childbirth in future generations.

Further, the attitudes to the place of women in society leads to an underrating of care in childbirth. Changes in education and recognition of women in the governance of countries will improve and with it maternal mortality will decline.

While improving living conditions is a praiseworthy aim in every country, reducing excessive MMR in developing countries in not likely to be achieved without the provision of effective obstetric care for all pregnant women.

CONCLUSIONS

This has been a brief account of the successful efforts made by the maternity services in England and Wales and in developed countries in general to overcome the once huge problem of maternal mortality. The great improvements brought about in the past 50 years have been illustrated and the factors responsible for the improvement discussed.

Inevitably, review of the 13 triennial reports of the CEMD between 1952–54 and 1988–90 has been extremely limited. During the period of the enquiries more than 32 million births were registered in England and Wales, and between the introduction of the 1967 Abortion Act in 1968 and the end of 1990, nearly 2.3 million legal terminations of pregnancy were performed.

Although the rate of improvement in mortality in England and Wales has been linear between 1937 and 1984, reaching its lowest level of 7.4 per 10 000 total births in 1988–90, the high rate of substandard care shows that further improvement can and should be achieved. In Sweden, maternal mortality was only 6.6 per 100 000 total births between 1971 and 1980 (Högberg 1985).

Acknowledgements

I am grateful to the Controller of Her Majesty's Stationery Office for permission to use tables and figures from the Reports of the Confidential Enquiries into Maternal Deaths.

REFERENCES

Al-Meshari A 1993 Maternal mortality in Saudi Arabia (1989–1992). Ministry of Health, Saudi Arabia

Association of Anaesthetists 1987 Anaesthetic services for obstetrics—a plan for the future. Association of Anaesthetists of Great Britain and Ireland/Obstetric Anaesthetists' Association, London

Bickerton T H 1936 A medical history of Liverpool from the earliest days to the year 1920. John Murray, London

Colebrooke L, Kenny M (1936) Treatment with prontosil of puerperal infections due to haemolytic streptococci. Lancet ii: 1319–1322

Confidential Enquiries into Maternal Deaths in England and Wales. Thirteen triennial reports from 1952–1954 to 1988–1990, inclusive. HMSO, London

Högberg U 1985 Maternal mortality in Sweden. Umea University Medical Dissertation (new series) 156

Kaunitz A M, Spence C, Davidson T S, Rochat R W, Grieves D A 1984 Perinatal and maternal mortality in a religious group avoiding obstetric care. American Journal of Obstetrics and Gynecology 150: 826–831

Loudon I 1986a Deaths in child bed from the 18th century to 1935. Medical History 30: 1–41

Loudon I 1986b Obstetric care, social class, and maternal mortality. British Medical Journal 293: 606–608

Loudon I 1987 Puerperal fever, the streptococcus and the sulphonamides. British Journal of Medicine 295: 485–490

Loudon I 1992 Maternal mortality. Clarendon Press, Oxford

Oxley W H F, Philips M H, Young J 1935 Maternal mortality in Rochdale. An achievement in a black area. British Medical Journal 1: 304–307

Urquhart D R, Fisk N M 1988 Transvaginal ultrasound in suspected ectopic pregnancy. British Medical Journal 296: 465–466

Walker G 1986 Family planning, maternal mortality and literacy. Lancet ii: 162

WHO 1967 Manual of the international classification of diseases, injuries and causes of death. 8th revision, vol 1. WHO, Geneva

WHO 1975 Manual of the international classification of diseases, injuries and causes of death. 9th revision, vol 1. WHO, Geneva

Medicolegal aspects

51. Medicolegal problems in obstetrics

J. Brian Capstick

Material in this chapter contains contributions from the first edition and we are grateful to the previous author for the work done.

The need for a chapter on law in an obstetrics textbook is the result of a steady increase over the years in the number of major malpractice claims. In the UK, most large claims are brought on behalf of people afflicted with cerebral palsy which they attribute to shortcomings in the obstetric care. The number of such claims made nationally is thought to have risen from about 70 in 1984 to about 200 in 1989 (Acheson 1990) and perhaps as many as 600 in 1990 (Capstick & Edwards 1990).

More recent figures are difficult to obtain in the absence of a national database of claims but, in 1994, a typical NHS Acute Unit with an annual turnover of about £100 000 000 may expect to have 16 current brain-damaged baby claims, of which half will not be successfully defended at a cost of about £8 000 000, spread over 5 years. New claims of this type are likely to arise at the rate of three every 2 years, falling to one a year after 1996.

The upward trend in the number of claims has continued and health authorities and National Health Service (NHS) Trusts now face up to five times as many obstetric litigation cases as they did in 1988. The incidence of cerebral palsy itself has remained stubbornly constant, despite improvements in other obstetric outcomes, at about one in 400 live births, or 1500 cases a year.

A number of factors are responsible for this increase in claims. A change in the Civil Legal Aid Regulations in 1990 extended state funding to the majority of obstetric claims brought by or on behalf of the child. Until then, any application for legal aid on behalf of a child was subject to a means test based on the parents' income, but the means test is now carried out on the income of the child. In practice, this means that eligibility for legal aid is no longer an obstacle to pursuing the major claims.

Another factor in the rising number of claims is the widespread use of electronic fetal heart monitoring, which not only creates an opportunity to argue about the significance of alleged abnormalities but also fuels the argument in years to come by leaving behind a permanent record, in the form of the trace.

Advances in fetal and neonatal medicine have also added to the number of claims by ensuring that many more damaged babies now survive than in previous years. A severely growth-retarded baby with neurological impairments is nowadays more likely to live to be the subject of a litigation claim than in the not too distant past.

Finally, the efforts of patient support groups and the increasing expertise of solicitors in bringing claims on behalf of patients have ensured that compensation is pursued for many more patients and their families who may have suffered loss and damage as a result of obstetric malpractice.

The growing volume of litigation has given rise to concerns other than the cost of claims. The burgeoning Caesarean section rate is to some extent attributed to medicolegal pressures (Ennis et al 1991). In the USA it has risen from 5.5% in 1970 to 24% in 1987 and, in the UK, from 5.3% in 1970 to 13% in 1990/91 (Written Parliamentary Answers at V3/93), although many factors other than medicolegal pressures have contributed to this phenomenon. They include the reduction in family size, which has led to an increase in the proportion of primigravid births and a reduction in the penalty to future pregnancies (Boylan 1991), the trend towards repeat sections (Quam et al 1988), developments in anaesthetics that have changed the perceived risk–benefit ratio and, especially in America, the practice in private medicine of payment by item of service (Black 1990).

In the UK, as in other jurisdictions, there is also concern about the effect of litigation in reducing the number of men and women willing to practise obstetrics. This problem is aggravated by the perception that there is little that the individual practitioner can do to prevent litigation and that he or she will be engulfed by the rising tide of claims regardless of how assiduously they practise their craft. However, there is an emerging body of knowledge about claims from which it is possible to identify areas where practice might be improved in order to reduce the risk of accidents and there is also much that can be done to avoid or defend claims more reliably when outcomes are poor.

This chapter is therefore written in the hope that greater understanding of the causes of claims and the process for resolving them may reduce the apprehension that they cause to the practitioner.

THE BASIS OF LIABILITY

Legal liability to pay compensation to a patient who has suffered some injury as a result of a medical act or omission usually only arises when some fault is established. As Lord Denning said in *Hatcher* v. *Black* 'Every surgical operation involves risks. It would be wrong and, indeed, bad law to say that simply because a misadventure or mishap occurred, the hospital and the doctors are thereby liable.' In most cases, fault will have to be established by the patient proving negligence.

The law of negligence is made up of three elements, namely:

1. The existence of a duty to take care owed by the defendant to the plaintiff.
2. A breach of that duty occasioned by a failure to attain the standard of care prescribed by law.
3. Damage caused to the plaintiff by the breach.

Each of these elements will be considered in turn.

The duty of care

In the case of a private hospital, which merely provides a mix of hotel and medical facilities for use by physicians selected by the patient, the hospital's duty is confined to the proper working of those facilities and the doctors chosen by the patient are alone responsible for any shortcomings in the treatment they provide. It is axiomatic that a doctor owes his/her patients a duty to exercise reasonable care and skill in relation to their medical treatment, so the existence of a duty of care between doctor and patient is rarely in dispute.

On the other hand, in the case of a public hospital operated by the NHS, the patient goes to the hospital expecting treatment and the hospital owes him/her a duty to provide it to a reasonable standard. The duty of a hospital managed by the NHS to take reasonable care in the provision of medical treatment may arise in two ways. First, the hospital will be vicariously responsible for the

errors of the clinical staff, whom the hospital normally selects. The nature of vicarious liability is such that the hospital is responsible in addition to (and not instead of) the clinician for any breach of duty owed by the clinician to the patient.

In addition to their vicarious responsibility for the errors of their staff, health service and other public hospitals also owe a direct duty to their patients (see Kennedy & Grubb 1989). The distinction is important because more and more cases of error are linked in one way or another to the inadequacy of resources, particularly the the lack of senior cover for junior doctors, midwives and nurses, and the duty of care owed directly by hospital to the patient includes a duty to provide adequate resources. *Wilsher* v. *Essex Area Health Authority* [1987] QB 730, [1986] 3 All ER 801 is a case in point, in which the doctrine of direct liability was discussed by the Court of Appeal.

The plaintiff was an infant child who was born prematurely suffering from various illnesses, including oxygen deficiency. He was placed in the special care baby unit where, in order to monitor the level of oxygen in his bloodstream, an inexperienced junior doctor inserted a catheter into a vein rather than an artery. A registrar failed to notice the error and repeated it himself some hours later, with the result that the plaintiff was given excess oxygen that could have caused the child's retrolental fibroplasia, for which the trial judge awarded £116 199.

The judges in the Court of Appeal commented thus on the health authority's primary duty of care:

MUSTILL L J: . . it might have been said that the defendants owed a (direct) duty to ensure that the special care baby unit functioned according to the standard reasonably to be expected of such a unit. This approach would not require any consideration of the extent to which individual doctors measured up to the standards required of them as individuals, but would focus attention on the performance of the unit as whole.

SIR NICOLAS BROWNE-WILKINSON VC: In my judgement, a health authority which so conducts its hospital that it fails to provide doctors of sufficient skill and experience to give the treatment offered at the hospital may be directly liable in negligence to the patient.

..... Claims against a health authority that it has itself been directly negligent, as opposed to vicariously liable for the negligence of its doctors, will, of course, raise awkward questions. To what extent should the authority be held liable if (e.g. in the use of junior housemen) it is only adopting a practice hallowed by tradition? Should the authority be liable if it demonstrates that, due to the financial stringency under which it operates, it cannot afford to fill the posts with those possessing the necessary experience? But, in my judgement, the law should not be distorted by making findings of personal fault against individual doctors who are, in truth, not at fault in order to answer such questions. To do so would be to cloud the real issues which arise.

At present, cases are decided by reference to the duty owed vicariously for the fault of individual doctors rather than directly by the hospital to the patient, but an increasing proportion of claims would be more accurately and incisively adjudicated by reference to the direct duty and it is likely to become a more common feature of claims. Such an approach would be fairer to doctors, who should not be the scapegoats for resource issues, and would force hospital managers and the courts to confront the resource problem direct.

The doctor's duty begins at the moment he undertakes to care for the patient, which usually has to be inferred from the circumstances, as the undertaking is seldom given expressly. The leading case is *Barnett* v. *Chelsea and Kensington Hospital Management Committee* [1969] 1 QB 428, [1968] 1 All ER 1068, in which three nightwatchmen drank some tea which, unknown to them, had been laced with arsenic. They went to the casualty department of the defendant's hospital and complained to a nurse that they had been vomiting. She telephoned the casualty officer, who was himself unwell. He did not see the men, but said that they should go home and call their own doctors. One of the men died some hours later. On these facts the court decided that the hospital had undertaken a duty to care for the men although, in this instance, the plaintiff would have died in any event, so his widow could not recover damages.

The unborn child

Special arrangements have been necessary to define the duty owed to the unborn child, which are of particular relevance in the context of obstetrics. The starting point is that the unborn child is not endowed with a legal personality and therefore has no rights which others have a duty to respect other than those which have been created piecemeal, usually by statute. For example, a child, when born, had no right to sue in respect of injury inflicted prenatally until the thalidomide tragedy impelled Parliament to enact the Congenital Disabilities (Civil Liability) Act in 1976.

The Act confers a right of action on a child who was born alive but disabled on or after 22 July 1976, if the disability was caused by an occurrence which affected either parent's ability to have a normal healthy child, or affected the mother during pregnancy, or affected the mother or child in the course of its birth. The Act only confers rights on children who are born alive, and does not apply in cases where the defendant's negligence causes the death of the fetus in utero, although in such circumstances either or both parents may have an action that is independent of the Act.

It is important to bear in mind that the child's rights under the Act derive from a duty owed to the mother and that the Act does not go so far as to create duties owed independently to the unborn child. If such a legislative enterprise were ever attempted, it would have to define the stage of pregnancy at which fetal rights would accrue and reconcile them with termination of pregnancy, which is perhaps the ultimate compromise of any rights the unborn child might have. As it is, the possibility of a claim by the child against the mother is expressly excluded unless the mother is driving, in which case she owes her unborn child the same duty of care as she owes to any other person. This exception is permitted on policy grounds, because in most cases the true defendant in such a claim will not be the mother but the company which insures her while she is driving.

Refusal of treatment

The rules governing the rights of the unborn child have important practical consequences for the increasingly common situation where the woman refuses care which may be medically advisable. They confer on the woman the right to refuse treatment on the basis of a religious or purely idiosyncratic objection, even though the treatment might be necessary to save her own life or that of the unborn child. She may insist on a home confinement when a hospital delivery is more appropriate, or she may reject treatment, such as induction, electronic fetal monitoring or Caesarean section, which is medically advised. If, as a consequence, the child suffers brain damage, or any lesser injury, the Act bars any claim it may have against the mother and it has no claim against the obstetrician or midwife, who will have committed no wrong to the mother whose wishes they respected.

As a result, mothers will often deny or seek to minimize the extent to which they refused treatment which was offered and which might have benefited the child. Obstetricians and midwives therefore need to be scrupulous about maintaining records of any offers of treatment made and any warnings given when it is refused. An unreported case illustrates the point:

Mrs W was a primigravida whose birth plan stated that she wanted a natural delivery with minimum interference. Following admission to hospital at the start of labour, matters did not progress normally. In the opinion of the doctors, abnormalities on the CTG trace indicated that artificial rupture of membranes and application of fetal scalp electrode were required. Despite the best efforts of the midwife, sister, SHO and registrar, the patient refused that intervention.

The situation continued to deteriorate and the clinical decision was that the reassurance of a normal fetal blood sample was needed if labour was to continue normally. The same team of midwives and doctors again failed to persuade the patient of the need to intervene. At her insistence, the labour continued with only external monitoring.

The clinical picture continued to get worse to the point where the doctors felt they had no option but to perform a Caesarean section in the absence of reassurance that closer monitoring might have been given. Yet again, the patient initially refused, although she eventually agreed.

The baby was born in an asphyxiated condition, and died a few days later. The staff were devastated by what had happened, because they had tried so hard to avoid it.

Sometime later, a letter was received from Mrs W's solicitors blaming the hospital for the neonatal death. Mrs W claimed it was the fault of the doctors and midwives for not advising her properly on the need for intervention at the various stages. Had they done so, she would have followed their advice.

Eventually the claim was abandoned, partly because there were good midwifery notes that recorded the true history. However, without them the patient might have succeeded in her claim or at least put the staff involved through an unpleasant trial.

In extreme cases, a patient may jeopardize her own life or that of the fetus. In such a case, no one has a legal duty to seek a court order compelling a competent adult to submit to treatment and, theoretically, the court has no power to grant one. However, judges will usually strive to save life and, in Re S ([1992] 4 All ER 671) the court ordered an emergency Caesarean section against the patient's wishes to protect 'the vital interests of the patient and the unborn child'. As the unborn child had no right to the court's protection and the mother did not want it, the decision has been condemned by many lawyers as legally flawed, but perhaps bad law has a place in the occasional hard case. A recent paper (RCOG 1994) on the legal and clinical position of enforced surgery is helpful.

Wrongful life

A further twist in the story of the unborn child's rights, or lack of them, is provided by the *wrongful life* cases. These are instances in which a failed sterilization has led to the birth of an unplanned baby who turns out to be handicapped or in which there has been a failure to diagnose that the fetus is likely to be born handicapped in time for the woman to opt for a termination of pregnancy.

If such cases are due to negligence, the mother is normally entitled to the costs of bringing up the child (*Emeh* v. *Kensington and Chelsea and Westminster Area Health Authority* [1985] QB 1012 [1984] 3 All ER 1044), but the question also arises whether the child is entitled in its own right to additional compensation for the pain and suffering and loss of earnings following its handicap, on the basis that it should not have been born at all. In *McKay V. Essex Area Health Authority* [1982] QB 1166, [1982] 2 All ER 771, the plaintiff had been infected with rubella in utero and had been born with various handicaps as a consequence. She alleged negligence on the part of the doctor who treated her mother antenatally in that he knew, or should have known, of the infection and should therefore have advised the mother to terminate the pregnancy and thus prevent the birth of a handicapped child.

There were various other claims in the action which resulted in the payment of some compensation, but the Court of Appeal rejected a claim on this basis. Not only could the judges not accept that anyone can have a duty towards a person, whether or not in utero, to terminate

his life but, if there was any such right, it was impossible to say what should be the basis for the assessment of damages for a breach of it. The handicap was the result of the rubella, not the doctor's failure to advise the mother to terminate the pregnancy, so compensation could not be paid for the pain and suffering of handicap compared to a healthy person. The difference which followed the omission to terminate was between not existing at all and existing in a disabled state, a distinction which defied quantification in money terms.

The standard of care

Level of skill required

The standard of care expected of professional people in this country was authoritatively defined in *Bolam* v. *Friern Hospital Management Committee* [1957]: It is 'the standard of the ordinary skilled man exercising and professing to have that special skill... it is sufficient if (the practitioner) exercises the ordinary skill of an ordinary, competent man exercising that particular art'.

A general practitioner is not expected to possess specialist skills, but a specialist is expected to exercise the ordinary skill of his speciality. If the threshold of skill is raised for the specialist, the question arises whether it is lowered for the junior doctor. Some light is shed on the issue by the cases involving learner drivers. In *Nettleship* v. *Weston* [1971], a learner driver mounted the kerb, injuring the instructor and damaging a lamp-post. The defence that one could expect no more from a learner received short shrift from LORD DENNING M R:

It is no answer for him to say: "I was a learner driver under instruction. I was doing my best and could not help it." The civil law permits no such excuse. It requires of him the same standard of care as any other driver. 'It eliminates the personal equation and is independent of the idiosyncrasies of the particular person whose conduct is in question.'

Similarly, there is an irreducible minimum level of competence required of the trainee doctor. In *Wilsher* (above) MUSTILL L J put the matter thus:

To my mind, this notion of a duty tailored to the actor rather than to the act which he elects to perform, has no place in the law of tort. . . . It was suggested that the medical profession is a special case. Public hospital medicine has always been organised so that young doctors and nurses learn on the job. If the hospitals abstained from using inexperienced people, they could not staff their wards and theatres, and the junior staff could never learn. . . . . Nevertheless I cannot accept that there should be a special rule for doctors in public hospitals . . . To my mind it would be a false step to subordinate the legitimate expectation of the patient that he will receive from each person concerned with his care a degree of skill appropriate to the task which he undertakes.

He went on to say that trainee doctors must exercise the level of skill appropriate to their post, so a junior houseman will be expected to perform to the standards of a reasonably competent junior houseman. This cannot be the whole of the story, because it preserves the variable duty of care to the patient that the learned judge was anxious to avoid, but merely allows it to vary from post to post rather than from individual to individual.

Perhaps the position is that junior doctors and non-specialists are expected to know their limitations and to summon help when they get out of their depth. It is the consultant's responsibility to decide what he can reasonably delegate, according to post, qualifications and experience of his juniors. It is also the consultant's responsibility to ensure that junior doctors are aware of when they should seek help and to make him- or herself available to give it. If, as so often happens in the claims, help is sought but there is not enough consultant cover or other resources to provide the level of skill and care required in the circumstances, either at all or in time prevent a tragedy, the matter is then a resource issue for which the hospital is directly responsible.

Adequacy of resources

In obstetric practice, a lack of resources may be reflected in a number of ways—whether, for example, there is sufficient consultant cover to support junior staff with difficult traces, whether fetal scalp blood sampling is available to give a more accurate diagnosis than electronic fetal heart monitoring, whether, if the decision is made to intervene surgically, there is an unreasonable delay in doing so because facilities or anaesthetic cover are inadequate. All these are resource issues and consultants and hospital managers need to identify the point at which lack of resources exposes the hospital or the doctor to unacceptable risks.

Once a hospital has undertaken to provide treatment, lack of resources will not be accepted as an excuse for an inadequate standard of care. In the leading case (*Bull* v. *Devon Area Health Authority* 1989), the allocation of resources had led to a split site for the hospital's obstetric and gynaecological activities. In these circumstances, there was an inherent risk that an experienced obstetrician would not be able to attend within a reasonable time whenever required to do so. Despite the fact that the administrative arrangements were determined by the availability of resources, the court held that the delay in arrival of a qualified obstetrician was unreasonable and the cover arrangements negligent.

If resources are not available to provide a service to the required standard, hospital managers and clinicians have to choose whether to risk the claims or opt not to provide the service at all. If they choose the latter course, the courts will not usually intervene in such a way as to require a hospital to provide any particular service. For example, when patients on a lengthy waiting list for orthopaedic treatment sought judicial review of a decision not to approve funds for a new unit, the court indicated that funding decisions should be left to the Secretary of State and, through him, regional and district health authorities (*R. v. Secretary of State for Social Services ex parte Hincks* 1979).

The implications of these decisions are that a hospital may decline to provide a service but, if the service is provided, it must be to a reasonable standard. Lack of funds is not an excuse for insufficient experienced cover to meet the needs of all patients on the labour ward, although the law does permit the number of beds to be limited so as to reflect the availability of resources. Similarly, the provision of emergency theatres needs to be reviewed since it may not be sufficient, for litigation purposes, for a hospital to contend that delay in carrying out a Caesarean section was as a result of all theatres already being in use. It would be open to the court to find that the administrative arrangements which had led to this situation were negligent and award damages accordingly.

Differences of opinion

It frequently happens that ordinary, skilled professional men do not agree with each other about appropriate methods. Some means must therefore be found for a court to deal with the situation where the experts for one party aver that a particular practice was acceptable, whereas experts for the opposing party prefer another practice and may even condemn the suggested alternative as unacceptable. The approach adopted by English law was phrased in a manner familiar to every student of medical law in the *Bolam* case (above) by MCNAIR J:

A doctor is not guilty of negligence if he has acted in accordance with a practice accepted as proper by a responsible body of medical men skilled in that particular art. . . . Putting it the other way round, a doctor is not negligent, if he is acting on accordance with such a practice, merely because there is a body of opinion that takes a contrary view.

This formula, known as the *Bolam* test, was developed further in *Maynard* v. *West Midlands Regional Health Authority* [1985] 1 All ER 635. In cases in which there are differences of medical opinion and practice, doctors will not be found negligent if a body of competent professional opinion supports their judgement and practice, even if another equally competent body of opinion considers that what they did was wrong. As Lord Scarman said, quoting an earlier case, 'The true test for establishing negligence in diagnosis or treatment on the part of a doctor is whether he has been proved to be guilty of such failure as no doctor of ordinary skill would be guilty if acting with ordinary care . . .'

A further matter which has been considered by the courts in dealing with standards of care is the time at which the prevailing standard should be assessed. In many medical negligence cases, the incident which is the subject of the claim will have taken place many years before the case comes to trial. In the interval, medical practice in the area may have moved on considerably, but the medical treatment will be judged by the prevailing standards at the date of treatment. Whilst this may impose practical problems in identifying whether a practice accorded with a responsible body of opinion at the time in question, any other approach would be inequitable.

CAUSATION

If the patient can prove that her treatment fell below the required standard of care, she then has to prove that the lapse caused, or materially contributed to, her loss or injury. Proving causation is often the most difficult task facing a plaintiff in a medical negligence action and, as a result, there have been several attempts to challenge the traditional legal requirement that the plaintiff must prove, on the balance of probabilities, that treatment falling below the requisite standard has caused or materially contributed to the damage.

However, the orthodox approach was restated when the case of *Wilsher* (above) reached the House of Lords. The retrolental fibroplasia from which the infant plaintiff in that case suffered could have been caused by the negligent administration of excess oxygen, but could also have occurred as a result of a number of other conditions common in premature babies, all of which had afflicted the plaintiff. At the trial, the medical evidence was inconclusive as to whether the excess oxygen had caused the condition.

The House of Lords decided that, in cases where a plaintiff's injury was attributable to a number of possible causes and only one of these was the defendant's negligence, the combination of a breach of duty and the plaintiff's injury did not give rise to a presumption that the defendant had caused or materially contributed to the injury. The burden of proof remained on the plaintiff to prove a causative link between the defendant's negligence and his injury. In the case of baby Wilsher, as the retinal condition could have been caused by any one of a number of different agents and it had not been proved that it was caused by the failure to prevent excess oxygen being given, the burden of proof as to causation had not been discharged and the claim therefore failed.

This approach to causation imposes a heavy burden on plaintiffs in many obstetric malpractice cases, particularly so in claims relating to children who allegedly suffered neurological damage as a result of perinatal asphyxia.

CONSENT

Cases where the patient refuses altogether treatment which is advised medically have been dealt with above in the context of the duty of care owed to the unborn child.

Other questions of consent generally arise where consent was given at the time but the patient subsequently argues that it was given on the basis of an inadequate warning of risks, or where the patient is under 16 years of age, or is otherwise legally or practically unable to consent to medical treatment.

Inadequate warning of risks

The most common situation in the consent cases concerns not the total absence of consent but rather the contention that consent was given on the basis of an inadequate warning of risks. The lack of full disclosure is not regarded as vitiating consent (if it did, the doctor's subsequent treatment of the patient would constitute a battery) but rather as a negligent omission to properly inform the patient (*Sidaway* v. *Board of Governors Bethlehem Royal Hospital* [1985] 1 All ER 643 (HL)). Most consent cases are therefore decided by reference to the same principles as apply to cases which involve a challenge to other areas of clinical competence.

We have already commented on the Bolam test in relation to the standard of care—'a doctor is not negligent if he is acting in accordance with a practice accepted as proper by a responsible body of medical men skilled in that particular art, merely because there is a body of such opinion which takes a contrary view'. This criterion applies equally to consent cases but subject, in such cases, to a power for a court to override a medical consensus if it seems to the court manifestly wrong (*Sidaway* 1985).

The extent to which a doctor must warn a patient of the risks inherent in a proposed course of treatment has been the subject of much recent litigation. It is important to bear in mind that most cases concern how much information about risks a doctor must volunteer to his patient unasked. If a patient asks specific questions, the doctor must answer them truthfully. In one typical case (*Blyth* v. *Bloomsbury Health Authority* (1985) Times 24 May, on appeal (1987) Times 11 February) the court held that a health authority was negligent in administering the contraceptive drug Depo-Provera without warning of possible side-effects, despite a reasonable request by the plaintiff for detailed information, where the plaintiff would not have agreed to the administration of the drug had she been in receipt of all available material.

Generally, a doctor must volunteer a warning where there is a substantial risk of grave adverse consequences, unless there is a cogent clinical reason for not doing so. Verbal warnings are ephemeral and disputes concerning exactly what a patient was told are common. A patient's recollection may be unreliable, but the doctor's will be even less so when a claim is made months or years later. A doctor's best protection, therefore, is to make a contemporaneous written record of warnings given. Similarly, if there was a clinical reason for not giving a patient the warnings appropriate in routine cases, then that reason must also be noted.

Minors

The ability to give consent to treatment comes into being on the patient's 16th birthday (Family Law Reform Act 1969, s.8). Younger patients have limited powers to give consent. In *Gillick* v. *West Norfolk and Wisbech Area Health Authority* [1986] AC 112, [1985] 3 All ER 402 the House of Lords set out the circumstances in which a doctor may rely on the consent of a girl under 16. That case concerned the lawfulness of prescribing the contra-ceptive pill to an under-age girl, although the House of Lords also made it clear that similar principles applied to terminations of pregnancy.

The requirements are that the girl can understand the doctor's advice, that she cannot be persuaded to inform her parents or allow the doctor to do so, and that her physical or psychological health is likely to suffer without advice or treatment. In the case of contraceptive advice, there is the further requirement that the girl is very likely to begin or continue having sex with or without contra-ceptive treatment.

A person aged 16 or more certainly has the power to consent to treatment, but he or she may not always have an untrammelled right to refuse it. An additional mechanism for treating patients under 18 is to use the court's power of wardship or, alternatively, the provisions of the Children Act 1990 to obtain a court order allowing treatment. In a recent example, the court ordered the feeding of a 16-year-old anorexic as being in her best interests (Re W (a minor) [1992] 4 All ER 627), and in Re S (above) a woman was ordered to undergo a Caesarean section in her own interests and that of her baby.

Incapacity

Patients may sometimes be incapable of giving informed consent either permanently (e.g. because of mental inca-pacity) or temporarily (e.g. when unconscious). In these circumstances a doctor is under a duty to do what is necessary to prevent a deterioration in the patient's con-dition or to improve her health. Irreversible elective procedures, in particular termination or sterilization, must not be carried out other than as an emergency life-saving procedure without an express consent. In the case of a person permanently incapacitated, a doctor contem-plating either procedure must obtain court approval as in Re F (1990) 2 AC 1, where the court ruled that the sterilization of a girl with a severe learning disability was in her best interests.

A patient who cannot consent because she is under anaesthetic or otherwise temporarily unconscious must be allowed to recover and consent must then be sought in the usual way. Even in emergencies, treatment may not legally be given if a patient has previously refused it and that refusal was intended to continue in times of incapacity. For example, if an adult patient states that she does not want a blood transfusion during an operation in any circumstances, then those wishes should be respected. Even so, many of the lawyers who advise doctors point out that it is not clear what penalty, if any, a court would impose on a doctor who disregarded these instructions in order to save the life of a patient or her baby. As we have seen, when judges are themselves confronted with the dilemma, they have (in the reported cases at least) invariably chosen the life-saving option.

DAMAGES

Once a patient has shown that negligence led to loss, the remaining issue is the quantum, or amount, of dam-ages. Damages are intended to restore the patient to the position she would have been in but for the negligence. In personal injury cases, this is often a somewhat artificial exercise, but the principle of English law that damages are compensatory and not punitive has avoided the exces-sive awards which are sometimes said to exist in other jurisdictions.

An example of damages in a cerebral palsy claim comes from *Cassel* v. *Riverside Health Authority* (1992), one of the most recent cases to have been reported fully. The Court of Appeal awarded the infant plaintiff £1191 900 broken down as follows:

1. Pain, suffering and loss of amenity—8%.
2. Past medical treatment and nursing care by parent and professionals—8%.
3. Future nursing care—38%.
4. Housing—3.5%.
5. Equipment—5%.
6. Plaintiff's future loss of earnings—26%.
7. Fees for court management of the award—7%.
8. Interest—4.5%.

The various categories by reference to which damages are assessed are called heads of damage. Damages which attempt to compensate in money for pain, suffering and loss of amenity are also called general damages and are calculated by reference to a judge-made tariff. At the time of writing, the maximum awards under this head are in the region of £125 000.

The other heads of damage are known collectively as special damages and are particular to the circumstances of each case, with the result that each side in a case which cannot be successfully defended will expend substantial effort in order to strike as good a bargain on the quantum of damages as circumstances permit. There is an element of horse trading but, in large claims at least, it is not uncommon nowadays for the plaintiff's case on quantum to run to several hundred pages of close argument, often prepared by accountants with the help of experts in the various regimens of therapy that are available. Bargaining down the quantum of claims is an equally complex activity, where skill counts as much as in many disputes about liability and where a competent defence team can save large amounts of money. Some comment is appropriate about certain heads of special damage.

Nursing care

A plaintiff is entitled to medical treatment and nursing care to such extent as the court finds reasonable. Inevitably, the court will look sympathetically at the needs of a brain-damaged child who may need continuous nursing care for the rest of his life. Increasingly sophisticated medical and nursing care not only adds directly to these costs, but has led to increased life expectancy for even the most severely handicapped, which in turn leads to increasing awards to cover the cost of future care.

The cost of future care to defendants is exacerbated by the fact that it is open to a plaintiff to claim for the cost of private medical care, notwithstanding that care could be provided free to him by the NHS (Law Reform (Personal Injuries Act) Act 1948 s.2 (4)). To remove the abuse whereby successful plaintiffs receive awards based on the cost of private care and then obtain free care from the NHS, it should be presumed that health service care will be provided to the extent that it is available.

Housing costs

This head covers the cost of purchasing and/or converting a property to fit the needs of the brain-damaged child, and his later needs as an adult. The accommodation must also be large enough to accommodate parents and/or other carers. The damages awarded do not reflect the full cost of accommodation needs, because the courts apply a substantial discount to the capital costs of purchasing a house to account for the fact that there will be a windfall to the next of kin when the patient dies.

Loss of earnings

This covers the loss of future earning capacity of the brain-damaged child. The courts try to speculate as to the career path that the plaintiff might have had but for his disability. This exercise involves looking at the rest of the family before deciding such issues as whether the child would have gone to Eton and a career at the Bar (as in one case), or else would have enjoyed a less prosperous life. A sum is awarded after a substantial discount to allow for the acceleration of earnings that the plaintiff would not normally have received until many years after the trial.

Structured settlements

The traditional award of damages comprises a one-off lump sum. An alternative that is becoming more common in large cases is for the patient to accept a structured settlement (Hay & Capstick 1993), in which some of the damages awarded are used to purchase an annuity guaranteeing the patient an income for life. Arrangements made with the Inland Revenue encourage this approach with a tax concession.

A variation on the theme which is becoming more common within the NHS is for the defendant hospital to self-fund the structured settlement by retaining some of the damages and making the periodic payments itself, without an insurer as intermediary.

No-fault compensation?

In the last few years calls have increased for a reappraisal of the way in which the victims of medical accidents should be compensated. Many people feel that the current tort-based system is too complicated, slow and expensive and imposes too great a burden on victims of medical accidents. In 1987, a BMA working party recommended a scheme for medical accident compensation without apportionment of blame—so-called no-fault compensation. The proposals came before Parliament in the form of a private member's bill, only to be resoundingly rejected. Established no-fault compensation schemes in New Zealand and Sweden have been running into financial and other difficulties and for the time being the issue of no-fault compensation has dropped from the health policy agenda.

Any revival of proposals for a no-fault scheme will have to overcome some intractable problems (Capstick et al 1991). If compensation levels remain the same but the need to establish fault is removed, the cost may well undermine the overall provision of health care. On the other hand, if levels of compensation were reduced to cover more successful claims, the victims of medical accidents would then be worse off than, say, the victims of road accidents.

If, in order to overcome this anomaly, the tort system were retained alongside the no-fault scheme (which would have been the position had the private member's bill succeeded), the benefits of better use of resources and greater equity that are said to follow from no-fault schemes would not be achieved. The tort system would cost as much as ever, and the existing inequity between victims of medical accidents where there is fault and victims where there is no fault would simply be replaced with another inequity between a privileged class of victims of medical accidents generally and the victims, for example, of hereditary diseases or any other of life's numerous misfortunes.

Furthermore, even if the burden of proving negligence was removed from claimants, there would still be the difficulty of proving causation, which is most acute in the brain-damaged baby cases which are the very cases that proponents would most want dealt with under a no-fault scheme.

BE PREPARED FOR CLAIMS

Limitation periods

The time within which patients' claims can be brought (the limitation period) is governed by the Limitation Act 1980. The usual time limit for bringing a claim for personal injury caused by negligence is 3 years from the date upon which the incident giving rise to complaint occurred, subject to various exceptions. One of these is that, in cases involving children, the 3-year time period does not begin to run until the child's eighteenth birthday. Moreover, if the individual suffers mental impairment at birth to an extent that permanently prevents capacity to manage his or her own affairs, (s)he never attains legal majority and a claim in negligence can be brought on their behalf at any time.

In addition to the specific exceptions, the court has a general discretion to extend the limitation period and allow cases to proceed where this is considered to be equitable. In practice, this discretion is freely exercised in the patient's favour. One recent case involved a claim in respect of surgery carried out on a 17-year-old boy in 1967. A writ was issued on his behalf in 1989 and a defence raised on the basis of limitation. The judge held that the claim had been brought within the limitation period and, even if it had not, he would exercise his discretion in the plaintiff's favour despite the fact that the surgeon who had carried out the initial operation had died in the interim.

The effect of these rules is that the defendant in many obstetric cases is not given the protection against stale claims which the law gives defendants in most other personal injury actions. It is one of the ironies of the legal system that it usually takes several years in obstetric cases to adjudicate on a delay by a doctor of hours or minutes. Hospitals often have to face claims which relate to births which occurred many years ago. One study (Capstick & Edwards 1990) of 49 brain-damaged baby claims found that the average interval between the date of birth and the hospital being notified of a claim was over 5 years, with 25% taking more than 7 years.

Delays of this kind are particularly prejudicial to the defence of obstetric claims because of the memory gap. For the woman giving birth, the experience is one that she will not repeat very often and is likely to be vivid. She will remember what happened and what was said to her at the time and subsequently. She will also have the opportunity to present the case to her lawyers while her memory is still fresh and they will be able to prepare her case at leisure before notifying the hospital that there is to be a claim.

The position of the defending doctor, midwife or hospital is quite different. They assist at many deliveries and the experience for them is a normal part of a working day. Individual cases are soon forgotten and the chances of remembering why one decision was made and not another, or what was said to a patient in the way of warnings or advice that went unrecorded, soon become very remote. The longer the delay in investigating a claim, the greater is the likelihood that the defence will be handicapped by being unable to locate key witnesses or having to rely on a skimpy written record or witnesses who have no direct recollection of the events at issue.

Nor do problems end when the claim is made. The plaintiff will have had an opportunity to prepare her case down to the last detail over a period of years, but will press the court to allow the defence only a matter of months to prepare its case, which is usually the more complex, and the courts will often comply with such requests.

The hospital that does not inquire into a bad outcome until the claim arrives is therefore well on the way to coming second in the ensuing litigation. The solution to this problem is to set up a system for reporting and reviewing bad obstetric outcomes, so that potential litigation claims may be identified as soon as possible after the birth and the appropriate inquiries made.

Outcome reporting

A procedure for identifying and following up bad obstetric outcomes is the single most time- and resource-saving step that it is open to most hospitals to take in order to reduce the cost of claims.

Identifying potential claims

The likelihood that a person will become a plaintiff in an obstetric claim is determined mainly by the size of the potential damages award. The potential award of damages for a child born with cerebral palsy is over a million pounds, while the potential award in respect of a stillbirth is between £10 000 and £15 000 (Edwards et al 1993), thus greatly reducing the prospects of a claim, even if the parent has a strongly arguable case on liability. The prospects of a claim recede further for a minor maternal injury, because the likely damages will be low and entitlement to legal aid more limited than for claims brought on behalf of children.

Serious injury to the baby is therefore likely to give rise to a claim. However, in the neonatal period, it is difficult to identify all of the babies who may suffer lasting physical or mental impairment, as it may take up to a year before brain damage is diagnosed. The result is that some other marker has to be used as the indicator for a potential claim:

Paediatricians now recognise the presence of hypoxic ischaemic encephalopathy (HIE), also called neonatal encephalopathy, in the first 72 hours of life as being the most accurate marker of clinically significant asphyxia at birth (Hall 1989). By no means all infants who show signs of fitting will turn out to be brain damaged, but the number who suffer from HIE is not so great as to make a review of the obstetric management of all of them impracticable. Every case of moderate to severe HIE should be reported and investigated as a potential claim, particularly where it appears that the baby was born in poor condition, perhaps with low Apgar scores requiring resuscitation and admission to a special care baby unit.

The objective of an outcome reporting system is to ensure that, if there is a bad outcome, a thorough review of the obstetric management is carried out and the evidence which may subsequently be necessary to account for a particular course of obstetric care is not lost. This requires proper documentation of the intrapartum and neonatal care, including statements from the midwives and doctors involved. An accurate diagnosis should also be sought which, apart from its clinical value, may also help to establish whether the infant's condition was caused by any shortcomings in the obstetric management. Details of the infant's condition at birth may be of considerable evidential value, so it is important to ensure where possible that such evidence is preserved during the neonatal period. The body of evidence thus gathered should be used for the purpose of obtaining legal advice and case planning against the possibility of a claim. (Capstick 1994)

Outcome reporting and its ensuing investigations should be a standard practice in cases of moderate to severe neonatal ecephalopathy. The procedure should be documented and should identify clearly who has responsibility for making and receiving reports, for following them up and securing appropriate legal advice.

Privilege and disclosure

An important consideration for doctors and hospital managers that frequently arises in the context of access to medical records is the question whether documents that are generated in the course of any inquiry following the birth may be the subject of a court order for compulsory disclosure to a potential plaintiff. The answer depends entirely on the circumstances in which the inquiry was carried out.

The law is that documents which are created for the dominant purpose of seeking legal advice or to assist with the conduct of litigation are protected (privileged) from disclosure (*Waugh* v. *British Railways Board* 1980). The purpose of an outcome reporting process is to permit the hospital to investigate the obstetric management in cases which have had a poor outcome while memories are still fresh. The information thus collected will be used to obtain legal advice whether a claim is in prospect and,

if so, to prepare a case plan to ensure that the hospital is ready for the claim when it arrives.

Moreover, it is not necessary that the proceedings which are intended to be the subject the legal advice sought should necessarily have been begun. If litigation is 'reasonably in prospect', documents brought into existence for the purpose of enabling solicitors to advise whether a claim shall be made or resisted are protected by privilege, whether or not a decision to instruct solicitors has been made at the time the documents are brought into being (*Guinness Peat Properties Ltd* v. *Fitzroy Robinson Partnership* [1987]). From the statistical analysis that introduced this chapter, it appears that there are about 1500 cases of cerebral palsy in a year and, nowadays, at least 600 claims. The implication is that there is a 40–50% chance that a child afflicted with cerebral palsy will at some time pursue a claim for damages, which must constitute a reasonable prospect that there will be a claim.

The final consideration is that, if a document is brought into being by direction or under the authority of an employer or insurer, it is their intentions that determine the dominant purpose, not those of the author. As a result of these considerations, documents prepared as a result of inquiries into the obstetric management of babies that develop neonatal encephalopathy should normally attract privilege if they are carried out under the authority of a properly drafted procedure for investigating potential claims.

Disclosure of casenotes

Medical records which are not privileged are usually disclosable to the patient. Traditionally, medical malpractice claims were initiated by a letter before action from the plaintiff's solicitors, indicating a likely claim against the hospital/health authority and requesting access to medical records. The Supreme Court Act 1981 at section 33 provides for prospective litigants in claims for personal injuries and death to apply for access to relevant case notes. Provided the potential litigant is able to indicate the grounds upon which it is considered likely that (s)he and the hospital in question will be parties to an action for personal injury, and there is no medical reason why the records should not be disclosed, access can be secured in this way with comparative ease.

Since November 1991, an additional route has been available to potential litigants who wish to see their medical records. Following the implementation of the Access to Health Records Act, all patients now have a right to obtain copies of all medical records prepared in respect of them since November 1991. Although this right is subject to one or two procedural safeguards, in practice the Act means that any patient can obtain copies of their notes without even intimating that a medical malpractice claim is likely. Thus, in many cases, the early warning system of letters before action will be removed and this in turn makes it all the more imperative that obstetricians and hospital managers take full account of the need for an outcome reporting procedure.

COMMON ISSUES IN CLAIMS

By analysing a number of claims, it is possible to build up a profile of common risks. Studies conducted in England (Capstick & Edwards 1990, Ennis & Vincent 1990, Vincent et al 1991) and in America (Julian et al 1985) show that a small number of risks arise in obstetric malpractice litigation with unerring regularity. If obstetricians wish to reduce their exposure to claims, it is necessary for them to reduce risks in these areas.

The major risk in obstetrics relates to those cases where the child is subsequently diagnosed as having cerebral palsy allegedly caused by some defect in the obstetric care. The allegation is usually that signs of fetal distress were not acted upon in time to prevent the damage. Sometimes the delay is said to have arisen because the early warning signs went unnoticed or unheeded, sometimes because of a decision not to intervene and sometimes because, once a decision was made to intervene, too much time was allowed to elapse between the decision and the action.

The assessment of fetal well-being on the labour ward, and the response to any abnormalities which are revealed, therefore constitute the most common major litigation risk within obstetrics. These activities are usually delegated to midwives for whom guidance on the subject of claims exists in the form of a booklet published by the Royal College of Midwives (Edwards et al 1993).

Supervision

A common feature of the claims is that avoidable delays occur in reacting to signs of fetal distress because insufficient supervision is available from senior obstetric staff. Any shortcomings on the part of the midwifery staff in appreciating fetal distress may be compounded by the failure of the junior doctor to take appropriate action. In some cases, a midwife's line of communication to more senior medical staff may be impeded by a junior doctor who has less experience of labour ward practice than she does.

Clinical directors should review the lines of communication within their units to ensure that, in appropriate circumstances, midwives will be able to make contact through the sister in charge of the labour ward with the duty registrar or consultant. Clear guidelines should be introduced for those circumstances in which personal involvement by a consultant is essential.

A related issue is the amount of time that consultants spend on the labour ward. A study group convened by the Royal College of Obstetricians and Gynaecologists to consider the problems of litigation concluded that consultants do not spend sufficient time in the labour ward (Chamberlain et al 1985) and health authorities have been instructed under HC(90)16 to review the work programmes of their consultants.

Staff levels and turnover

A high turnover of staff is destructive of quality in any service organization and its reduction is a priority in many obstetric departments in the NHS. Locum doctors, agency staff and trainees on short-term appointments are not subject to the same standard of selection as permanent staff and, if they are only on short-term appointments, will inevitably be an unknown quantity for much of the time, thereby increasing the risk of accidents.

Record keeping

Inadequate record keeping continues to expose doctors to claims unnecessarily and, while generations of them have resisted exhortations to do the job more thoroughly, this author is not yet entirely ready to abandon the attempt. The areas which need most attention relate to meconium staining of the amniotic liquor and decisions to wait and see in the presence of unfavourable cardiotocography (CTG) traces.

The significance of meconium staining of the amniotic liquor is often debated in the context of claims. Clinically, both the volume and colour of the amniotic liquor released on rupture of the membranes are significant. It is desirable from a legal point of view that the volume of liquor is recorded and that the record specifies that the liquor is clear or whether meconium is thick, fresh or stale. Staff should at the same time record their response, even if it is only to maintain or initiate careful monitoring of fetal well-being. The absence of any record of these distinctions is a common feature of records that makes claims more difficult to defend.

The correct interpretation of and response to abnormalites revealed by CTG is at the heart of most claims. Partly because of the proportion of false positives associated with CTG, clinicians often prefer to wait and see how a labour progresses in the face of possible alarm signals before coming to any decision to intervene. The majority of claims, on the other hand, comprise allegations that the medical team did not respond quickly enough to abnormal traces. There is therefore a conflict between the medical and legal interests and, in such circumstances, clinicians have to be prepared to support decisions to wait and see in the face of abnormal or equivocal traces.

In particular, if the signs of possible distress are recorded at the time, perhaps automatically by a machine, but the decision to wait and see is not documented, the image of events that will appear in the rear-view mirror of legal proceedings is that the warning signs were there, but that nothing was done about them. A sequence of warning signs, even if they are trivial or inconsequential, coupled with the absence of a record that progress was assessed in the light of them, may easily create an impression of neglect or indifference, even if what happened in fact was that a proper degree of care was provided but not recorded.

The solution is to maintain a clear record of any indications of potential fetal distress, and to record decisions that were made in the light of them, even if the decision was only to maintain an appropriate level of monitoring.

Training

The analysis of claims will not reduce accidents unless practice is improved by training in the areas which are vulnerable to claims. It is the clinical director's responsibility to ensure that junior staff are adequately trained.

A particular objective should be to improve the use and interpretation of CTG, where gross errors still occur. Staff should be made familiar with the main abnormalities which can be revealed, and how these should be interpreted within the overall clinical picture. If such training encourages good quality notes, including observations of the CTG trace and the appropriate response, a number of legal claims might be avoided.

Limitation of losses

Once an accident has happened, there are various means open to a hospital to limit the amount that it will cost. The first is to operate an outcome reporting procedure of the type described above in order to reduce the length of time that elapses between the occurrence and the date the hospital finds out.

Once a hospital has found out about a claim, the principal factor within its control that will affect how much it costs is the calibre of the legal and medical team engaged to defend it. The defence team has two jobs to do. One is to form a view on liability, preferably at a relatively early stage in the action so that money is not thrown away defending the indefensible. Liability issues are mainly the responsibility of the medical experts, although they have to be properly instructed. The other task for the defence team is to negotiate the quantum of damages in those cases that cannot be successfully defended, which requires skill and experience.

Dealing with potential litigants

It is often said on behalf of plaintiffs that the main motivation for commencing a legal claim is to obtain an explanation of the treatment provided or the outcome (Clements 1992). It is unlikely that the quality of any explanation given to the parents of a child suffering from cerebral palsy will prevent litigation, but claims may be prevented in many cases of stillbirth or neonatal death by dealing candidly with the parents. Quite apart from reducing the likelihood of claims, such an approach may help the parents to cope and, in any event, parents should not be left in a situation where they feel that litigation is the only way to obtain an accurate explanation of their tragedy.

Clinicians often fear that expressions of regret at the outcome may be confused with an admission of liability. Sometimes they are, but the risk may be reduced by training with reference to case studies and simulated interviews. In cases where the hospital is thought to be at fault, liability should never be admitted until the hospital has:

1. completed a thorough investigation
2. satisfied itself that the injury complained of has been caused by the negligence to be admitted
3. taken competent legal advice about the consequences.

CONCLUSION

It is easy to become despondent about the prevailing level of litigation in the practice of obstetrics. However, the hope is that this chapter may illustrate that claims are not merely the product of chance and that there is a growing body of knowledge that will help to reduce the number of accidents that give rise to claims and to confine the number of claims that cannot be successfully defended to those where there has been some fault on the hospital's part in treating the patient and not just poor preparation for the possibility of a claim. The competent and conscientious practitioner has much less to fear from litigation than is often supposed, and practising and aspiring obstetricians should not allow the possibility of claims to blight what should be an enjoyable and rewarding specialty.

REFERENCES

Acheson D 1990 William Power Memorial Lecture to the royal College of Midwives, 5 December 1990 (reprinted in Hospital Doctor 10 and 17 January 1991)

Barnett v. *Chelsea and Kensington Hospital Management Committee* [1969] 1 QB 428, [1968] 1 All ER 1068

Black N 1990 Medical litigation and the quality of care. Lancet 335: 35–37

Blyth v. *Bloomsbury Health Authority* (1985) Times 24 May, on appeal (1987) Times 11 February

Bolam v. *Friern Hospital Management Committee* [1957] 1 All ER 118, [1957] 1 WLR 582

Boylan P C 1991 Current problems in obstetrics, gynaecology and fertility. Mosby Yearbook, London

Bull v. *Devon Area Health Authority* (1989) Medico Legal Journal 57: (2); AVMA Medical and Legal Journal 1990, (January) 11

Capstick B 1994 Risk management in obstetrics. In: Clements R V (ed) Safe practice in obstetrics and gynaecology. Churchill Livingstone, Edinburgh

Capstick B, Edwards P 1990 Trends in obstetric malpractice claims. Lancet 336: 931–932

Capstick B, Edwards P, Mason D 1991 Compensation for medical accidents. British Medical Journal 302: 230–232

Cassel v. *Riverside Health Authority* [1992] PIQR Q168

Chamberlain G V P, Orr C J B, Sharp F 1985 Litigation in obstetrics and gynaecology. In: Proceedings of the 14th Study Group of the RCOG.

Clements R V 1992 Defensive medicine—is this where risk management leads? Health Service Journal 102: 5298 (Supplement Managing Risk) 16th April 1992

Edwards P, Mason D, Capstick B (ed) 1993 Risk management for midwives. Joint publication by Royal College of Midwives and Capsticks, Solicitors

Emeh v. *Kensington and Chelsea and Westminster Area Health Authority* [1985] QB 1012, [1984] 3 All ER 1044, CA

Ennis M, Vincent C A 1990 Obstetric accidents: a review of 64 cases. British Medical Journal 300: 1365–1367

Ennis M, Clark A, Grudziniskas J G 1991 Change in obstetric practice in response to fear of litigation in the British Isles. Lancet 338: 616–618

Gillick v. *West Norfolk and Wisbech Area Health Authority* [1986] AC 112, [1985] 3 All ER 402

Guiness Peat Properties Ltd v. *Fitzroy Robinson Partnership* [1987] 2 All ER 716, CA

Hatcher v. *Black* (1954) Times 2 July

Hall D M B 1989 Birth asphyxia and cerebral palsy. British Medical Journal 299: 279–282

Hay K, Capstick B 1993 Future gains and future losses. International Insurance Law Review 1: (8)

Julian T M, Brocker D C, Butler J C et al 1985 Investigation of obstetric malpractice closed claims: profile of event. American Journal of Paediatrics 2: 320–324

Kennedy I, Grubb A 1989 Medical law: text and materials. Butterworths, London

Maynard v. *West Midlands Regional Health Authority* [1985] 1 All ER 635

McKay v. *Essex Area Health Authority* [1982] QB 1166 [1982] 2 All ER 771

Nettleship v. *Weston* [1971] 2 QB 691, [1971] 3 All ER 591, CA

Quam L, Dingwall R, Fenn P 1988 Medical malpractice claims in obstetrics and gynaecology: comparisons between the United States and Britain. British Journal of Obstetrics and Gynaecology 95: 454–461

R. v. *Secretary of State for Social Services ex parte Hincks* (1979) Solicitor's Journal 123: 436; Butterworths Medico Legal Reports 1: 93–97

RCOG 1994 Legally enforced surgery. RCOG, London

Re F (1990) 2 AC 1 [1989] 2 WLR 1025, [1990] 2 AC 1

Re S ([1992] 4 All ER 671)

Re W (a minor) [1992] 4 All ER 627

Sidaway v. *Board of Governors of the Bethlem Royal Hospital and the Maudsley Hospital* (1985) 1 All ER 643 (HL)

Vincent C A et al 1991 Obstetric accidents: the patient's perspective. British Journal of Obstetrics and Gynaecology [1980] 98: 390–395

Waugh v. *British Railways Board* AC521; [1979] JWLR 150; [1979] 2 All ER 1169, HL

Wilsher v. *Essex Area Health Authority* [1987] QB 730, [1986] 3 All ER 801

Turnbull's Obstetrics

Index